7th EDITION

MASSAGE THERAPY
Principles and Practice

Susan G. Salvo, EdD, BCTMB, LMT

Program Coordinator and Lead Instructor
Louisiana Institute of Massage Therapy
Lake Charles, Louisiana
New Mexico School of Massage
Program Coordinator and Instructor
Albuquerque, New Mexico

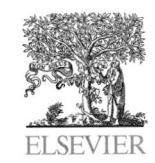

ELSEVIER

Elsevier
3251 Riverport Lane
St. Louis, Missouri 63043

MASSAGE THERAPY: PRINCIPLES AND PRACTICE, SEVENTH EDITION   ISBN: 978-0-323-87815-9
Copyright © 2023 by Elsevier Inc. All rights reserved.

Previous editions copyrighted 1999, 2003, 2007, 2012, 2016 and 2020.

Director, Content Development: Laurie Gower
Publishing Director: Kristin Wilhelm
Content Strategist: Melissa Rawe
Content Development Specialist: Brooke Kannady
Publishing Services Manager: Deepthi Unni
Project Manager: Thoufiq Mohammed
Designer: Margaret Reid

Printed in India

Last digit is the print number: 9 8 7 6 5 4 3 2

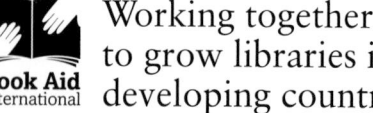

This book is, once again, dedicated to a special person in my life.

To Michael Breaux—my childhood friend, domestic partner, business partner, study partner, proofreader, collaborator, father of my children, travel companion, chef extraordinaire, and real-life superhero.

We've laughed, cried, and dreamed together. We've shared the highs and lows of marriage, business, and parenting, as well as supported each other through the joys and sorrows of life. With you by my side, good times are twice as good and hard times are half as bad.

Honorable mention goes to our dog Duke, a Corgi-Dachshund mix rescue dog who has been my constant companion during most of my book revisions. He curls up in my office keeping me company while the others are off at work and school, ready to alert me to visitors at the door and coaxing me to take breaks from my desk to let him outside several times a day. There is probably no other dog on the planet who is as loyal, or as spoiled (we pour gumbo over his dog food).

My writing career would have been less fulfilling without their love and support.

SUSAN SALVO

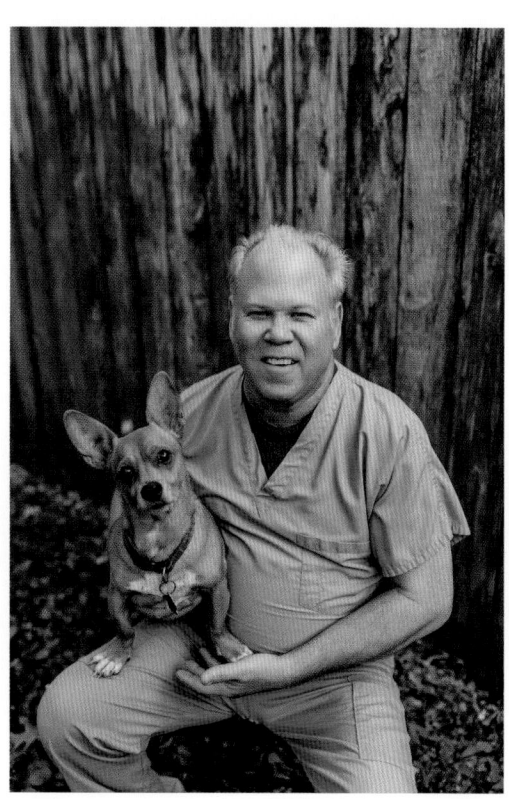

ACKNOWLEDGMENTS

I have gathered together a wonderful group of contributors. They are my "dream team," and I could not have done this book without them. A big warm THANK YOU to contributors and co-contributors Michele Renee, JoEllen Sefton, Ana Bott, and Jennifer Breaux. Also, special thanks to Chris Salvo and Suzanne Salvo for their wonderful photography for this and previous editions.

I relied heavily on the advice of brilliant and trusted colleagues while revising this particular edition and would like to acknowledge them: Nancy Triplett, Sandra K. Anderson, James Robert Black, Michelle Cordero, and James L. Murrin II.

The editorial team can make or break a project. I was blessed with a great group of individuals such as Brooke Kannady, Melissa Rawe, Thoufiq Mohammed, and Maggie Reid.

I also want to thank my Facebook friends, massage students, massage instructors, massage clients, university professors, and massage practitioners who have provided continual support and inspiration. I love the massage profession, and it is my wish to use education and research to move it forward into a bright future.

Dr Susan Salvo

CONTRIBUTORS AND REVIEWERS

CONTRIBUTORS

Ana Bott, ACMT
LGBTQ Specialist Massage Therapist
The Real Massage
Brighton, United Kingdom

Jennifer Breaux, Esq
Counselor
District of Columbia Bar
Washington, DC

Michele J. Renee, DC, Mac
Director of Integrative Care
Massage Therapy Program Director
Northwestern Health Sciences University
Bloomington, Minnesota

JoEllen M. Sefton, PhD, ATC, CMT
Director, Warrior Research Center
School of Kinesiology, Auburn University
Auburn, Alabama

REVIEWERS

Sandra K. Anderson, BA, LMT, ABT
Certification in Massage Therapy, Zen Shiatsu, and Thai
    Massage
Instruction, Continuing Education Provider
Costa Rica School of Massage Therapy
Samara, Costa Rica

James Robert Black, LMT, RM
Education Manager
Cortiva Institute & Hollywood Institute
Maitland, Florida

Michelle Cordero, BA, LMT, CIMT
Director of Education
ASIS Massage Education
Mesa, Arizona

James L. Murrin II, BA, AAS, Diploma LMT, MLT
Academic Program Director
Medical Massage Therapy
Daymar College
Columbus, Ohio

PREVIOUS EDITION CONTRIBUTORS

Laura Allen, BA, LMBT, NCTMB
Approved Provider of Continuing Education under the
    NCBTMB
Rutherfordton, North Carolina

Sandra K. Anderson, BA, LMT, NCTMB
Co-Owner, Tucson Touch Therapies
Tucson, Arizona

Celia Bucci, MA, LMT
Chicago, Illinois

Kim Corpus, LMT, CBE, CPMS, Doula
Massage Therapist and Educator
Crouse Hospital
Syracuse, New York

Judith Delany, LMT
Director and Certified NMT Instructor
NMT Center
St. Petersburg, Florida

Richard Gold, PhD, LAc
President and Executive Producer of Metta Mindfulness
    Music
Pacific College of Oriental Medicine
San Diego, California

Allissa Haines, BS, LMT
Owner, Haines Massage
Guest Faculty, Bancroft School of Massage Therapy
Plainville, Massachusetts

Megan E. Lavery, LAPC, LMT, BCTMB
Faculty, Zero Balancing Health Association
Former Faculty, Natural Health Institute of Bowling Green
Fernandina Beach, Florida

Rita S. Lebleu, LMT, MA
Rhetorical and Interpersonal Communication
DeQuincy, Louisiana

Til Luchau, BA NCTMB, CMP
Director and Lead Instructor, Advanced-Trainings.com
Faculty, Rolf Institute of Structural Integration®
Boulder, Colorado

Sandy Grover Mason, BA, LMBT 4403, CMT, AMTA, NCTMB
Clinical Education Coordinator and Instructor, Therapeutic Massage
Forsyth Technical Community College
Owner, Body Therapeutic
Winston-Salem, North Carolina

Monica J. Reno, LMT
Continuing Education Provider
Touch Education, LLC
Lady Lake, Florida

Hayley A. Salvo
Bachelors in Journalism, Magna Cum Laude
The English Centre
Málaga, Spain

Alice Sanvito, LMT
Licensed Massage Therapist
St. Louis, Missouri

Ralph R. Stephens, BSEd, LMT, NCTMB
President, Ralph Stephens Seminars, LLC
Coralville, Iowa

H. Micheal Tarver, PhD
Professor of History, Arkansas Tech University
Russellville, Arkansas

Kenneth G. Zysk, PhD, DPhil
Associate Professor
Institute for Cross-Cultural and Regional Studies
Department of Asian Studies
University of Copenhagen
Copenhagen, Denmark

As the practice of massage evolves, so must this textbook. *Massage Therapy Principles and Practice*, the seventh edition, continues with its focus on evidence-informed practice and citations of scholarly sources, while maintaining the textbook's characteristic intuitive organization, readability, and respect for tradition. This textbook simplifies difficult concepts, is packed with meaningful and vibrant images, detailed illustrations, and has a commonsense approach, all of which enhance learning.

With the widening range of massage practices across the globe, massage practitioners are in high demand, particularly those cross-trained to work in a variety of settings, including spas, health clubs, hospitals, oncology wards, physical therapy, and chiropractic clinics. As author, my goal is to focus on key concepts required to achieve massage licensure, which forms the foundation of a massage practice in all these settings.

ORGANIZATION

The book covers important subjects of massage practice required in curricula and programs approved by the Commission on Massage Therapy Accreditation (COMTA) and content areas outlined in professional standards-setting documents such as the Core: Entry Level Analysis Project (ELAP) and the Massage Therapy Body of Knowledge (MTBOK). This prepares students for successful passing of the Massage and Bodywork Licensing Exam or MBLEx. Each chapter begins with learning objectives that correspond with its chapter headings. Key concepts are bolded, helping students identify and learn vocabulary terms and their definitions. Concepts are presented from simple-to-complex to help students build or scaffold knowledge, which promotes academic success. Even though the information used by massage practitioners is rapidly expanding, we are committed to keeping the content manageable, relevant, and well organized.

The textbook has two units and 30 chapters.

- Unit One contains 17 chapters and focuses on foundational subjects such as history, ethics, boundaries, research, evidence-based practice standards and treatment planning, body mechanics, draping, self-care, infection control, and massage techniques, as well as essential skills of clinical hydrotherapy and spa methods, complementary and integrative methods such as reflexology, seated massage, Asian bodywork, clinical applications, and business practices. Also included in Unit One is how to adapt massage for special populations such as pregnant and frail elderly clients, and clients in hospice care.
- Unit Two contains 13 chapters and provides the essentials of anatomy, physiology, kinesiology, and pathology with an emphasis on treatment planning for these conditions and safe practice procedures. Also included are massage modifications for medical treatments such as dialysis and conditions such as musculoskeletal injuries.

New for Seventh Edition

New Assessments in every chapter—Along with the tried-and-true activities designed for application of knowledge in real-world scenarios, each chapter now has a multiple-choice question section to help vocabulary building and critical thinking.

More Emphasis on Evidence-Informed Practice—This is a central focus of massage education and enhances the safety and efficacy of the profession. Two chapters are devoted to this. Chapter 5 teaches students how to develop a clinical question and how to search for, evaluate, and apply evidence when formulating treatment plans. Chapter 6 features a review of massage research by body system and populations, and includes over 80 new studies, which adds to our body of knowledge. Chapter 6 also has the new educational directives for massage schools from the Massage Therapy Foundation.

Evidence-based Approaches to Body Mechanics and Endangerment Sites—Chapters 7 and 8 discuss these topics and integrate evidence from research studies to enhance the safety and practice of massage therapy.

Updated Protocols for Infection Control and Disinfection—Chapter 9 includes the most up-to-date procedures from the CDC for safe practice including disinfecting of office surfaces, massage tools, and laundry.

Empathy-based Ethics—This edition features an expanded discussion of cultural competency, how to develop and express empathy when communicating with clients and colleagues in cross-cultural work settings, recommendations for a LGBTQ+ inclusive practice, and decision-making approach that can be used to manage mild, moderate, and severe ethical dilemmas.

New Kinesiology Images—This edition features new action-oriented illustrations of body movements, origins, and insertions to help students accurately identify, locate, palpate, and treat muscles.

Expanded Clinical Massage, Sports Massage, and Hospital-Based Massage Sections—This chapter expounds on the current pain and biopsychosocial models with special emphasis on pain management. Michele Renee and I collaborated to create a user-friendly list of orthopedic assessments (complete with statistics) and guidance on how to use muscle energy techniques, proprioceptive neuromuscular facilitation, positional release, strain/counterstrain, manual lymphatic drainage, myofascial release, instrument-assisted soft tissue mobilization, cupping, and taping. Also included in this chapter is how to modify the massage for soft tissue injury during the acute phase and post-surgery considerations. The chapter is jam-packed with knowledge and skills massage practitioners need when working in rehabilitation or sports clinics, physician-referred practices, or multidisciplinary clinics.

Spa Procedures—As requested, spa procedures are back in Chapter 12 and include protocols for body wraps, body scrubs, floatation tanks, hot stone massage, and more.

Special Populations—Chapter 11 now includes expanded sections regarding quality-of-life assessments, working with clients who have disabilities or impairments, and mandatory reporting requirements. This chapter also includes the most updated information for use of essential oils, hydrotherapy, and CBD products during pregnancy.

Distinctive Features

Terms and Their Meanings—These tables help students learn word origins used in science and medicine. This knowledge improves comprehension as well as test scores.

Biographies—Biographical profiles and candid interviews provide a real-world perspective from the most-respected authorities and pioneers in massage and pain management. This edition adds the biography of researcher Niki Munk.

Activities and Assessments—Robust activities and assessments such as matching questions, multiple choice questions mentioned previously, case studies, and discussion questions are provided to promote critical thinking, encourage dialogue, foster open-mindedness, and enhance cultural competencies.

Evolve Online Resources—The text includes an extensive collection of online resources, available at http://evolve. elsevier.com/Salvo/MassageTherapy. Students have access to educational activities, flash cards, videos to demonstrate massage techniques, routines, procedures, and client intake interviews, as well as photo galleries, audio glossaries, downloadable forms, and a practice test with over 600 questions.

CONTENTS

CHAPTER 1

The farther backward you can look, the farther forward you can see.
—Winston Churchill

History of Massage: Prehistoric Times to the Modern Era and Professional Societies, Organizations, and Associations

---

LEARNING OBJECTIVES

After completing this chapter, the student should be able to:

1. Define massage, and discuss massage during the prehistoric times, the ancient world, the Middle Ages, and the European Renaissance.
2. Describe the impact the modern era and professional societies, organizations, associations, and human trafficking has had on the massage profession.

INTRODUCTION

Massage therapy is the manipulation of soft tissue using compression and decompression/traction for clinical, therapeutic, and palliative purposes or for wellness and self-care purposes (DeDomenico, 2007; Ernst et al., 2006). The history of massage is long and multifaceted. Archeologic and historical evidence indicates massage, in various forms, has been practiced for thousands of years across the globe (Field, 2002). Over the centuries, massage has been referred to in history and literature as well as by physicians and philosophers. This chapter provides an overview of massage history, spotlighting key figures and important events chronologically (Fig. 1.1).

Most literature about massage prior to the 1800s is devoid of the word "massage." In fact, the origin of the word "massage" is unclear but can be traced to numerous sources: the Hebrew *mashesh*, the Greek *masso* and *massin*, the Latin *massa*, the Arabic *mass'h*, the Sanskrit *makeh*, and the French *masser*. By the early 1800s, the term *massage* was used by most European-based cultures (DeDomenico & Wood, 1997). The terms *masseur* and *masseuse* are French terms that came into the English language to denote males and females who practiced massage; these terms have since been replaced by the current nongendered term *massage therapist* or *massage practitioner* (Wood, 1974). In addition, there is a lack of detailed or comprehensive definitions of massage in historical documents. For example, *Thomas Medical Dictionary* (1886) defined massage as "from the Greek, meaning to knead." Massage was often referred to by its techniques such as friction or rubbing. The next sections include the history of massage from prehistoric times to the modern era.

PREHISTORIC TIMES

Prehistoric times refer to the period between the appearance of humans and the invention of writing systems. Historians and archeologists have uncovered artifacts depicting the use of massage during this time. For example, European cave paintings (c. 15,000 BCE) portray what appears to be the use of massage after battle. Massage-like grooming behaviors are also observed in animals such as primates, which may play a role in social structures (DeDomenico & Wood, 1997).

ANCIENT WORLD

The ancient world is the period from the invention of writing systems to the end of the Roman Empire in 476. The use of massage during this period is well recorded, and there are extensive written and pictorial records. Countries where evidence exists on the use of massage include China, India, Egypt, Persia, Japan, Greece, Italy (Rome), and the Americas. Most ancient cultures described massage combined with other traditional treatments, particularly herbal remedies and various types of baths.

China

Written records regarding the practice of massage go back to 3000 BCE in China. At the time of Hwang Ti, various ideas and beliefs were compiled under the name of the Yellow Emperor (died in 2599 BCE) which later became the classic scripture of traditional Chinese medicine known as the *Nei Chang*. The Nei Chang was written about 2760 BCE, and this work contains detailed descriptions of massage procedures as well as herbal medicines (DeDomenico & Wood, 1997).

During the Tang dynasty, four primary types of medical practitioners were recognized: physicians, acupuncturists, masseurs, and exorcists. The term used to describe massage was *amma, amna,* or *anmo*. In fact, amma is now regarded as the original massage technique and precursor to all other Chinese therapies, manual and energetic. Amma later became tuina (written as 推拿 and pronounced twee-nah). Tuina translates in English to "push/pick up". This translation correlates with compression/decompression, which is our current definition of massage. Acupuncture was not mentioned in Chinese medical writing until 90 BCE.

India

Knowledge of amma massage traveled to the subcontinent of India from China, and massage became part of Hindu tradition. Massage is described in India's first great medical texts, the Ayurveda books of wisdom (approximately 1800 BCE), which recommend massage as an indispensable healing procedure (Hentschel & Schneider, 2004). Later Ayurvedic texts, such as the Samhitas (c.1700 to 1100 BCE) and the Manav Dharma Shastra (c.300 BCE), also mention massage.

Egypt and Japan

Massage traveled from China to Egypt and Japan by the sixth century BCE, and these ancient cultures used massage in conjunction with plant essences such as essential oils (Calvert, 2002; DeDomenico & Wood, 1997). The temple of the ancient Egyptian pharaoh Nyuserre Ini (Fifth Dynasty during the Old Kingdom period) depicts the king enjoying what appears to be a foot massage. The tomb of Ankhmahor (Sixth Dynasty during the Old Kingdom) is a drawing that depicts two people massaging the hands and feet of two other people (Fig. 1.2). There is much debate whether this image is of massage or another type of procedure such as manicures, pedicures, or surgery. In addition, the ancient Egyptians were the first to study essential oils and codify their effects.

In Japan, amma was practiced for many years and evolved into shiatsu, which means finger pressure. Shiatsu is a Japanese method based on the same traditional Chinese medicine concepts as Chinese acupuncture—energy flows in the body through streams called *channels* or *meridians*. Pain, discomfort, and illness may occur when these channels are blocked or depleted. Acupuncturists use needles at specific points to balance the flow of energy, whereas shiatsu practitioners use their fingers, thumbs, forearms, elbows, and even their knees and feet to press into points called *tsubos*. Tsubos are openings into the channels.

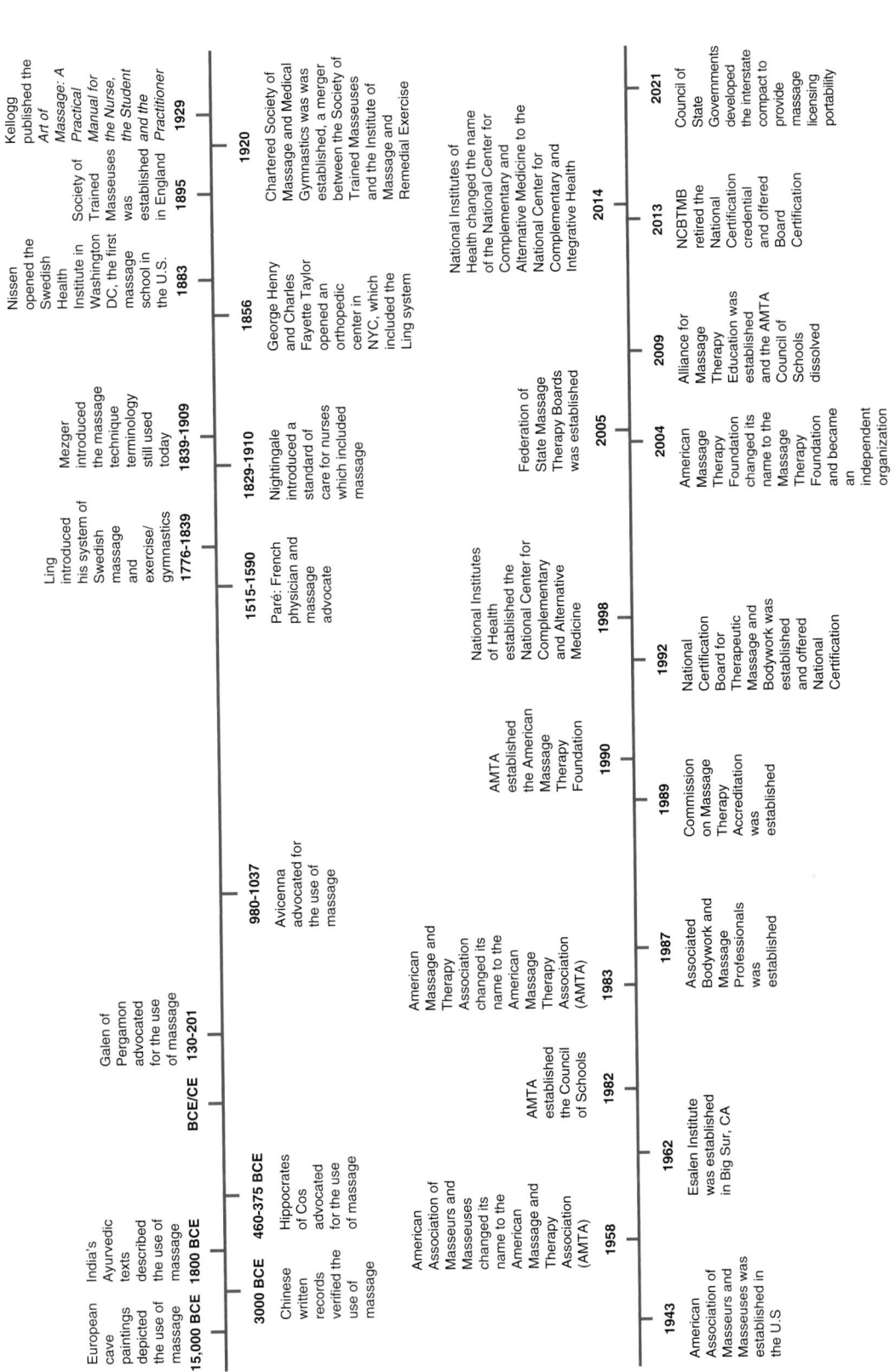

FIG. 1.1 Massage timeline.

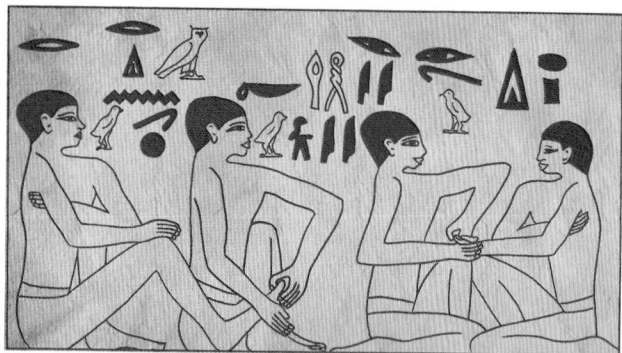

FIG. 1.2 Drawings found in the tomb of Ankhmahor of two people massaging the hands and feet of two other people.

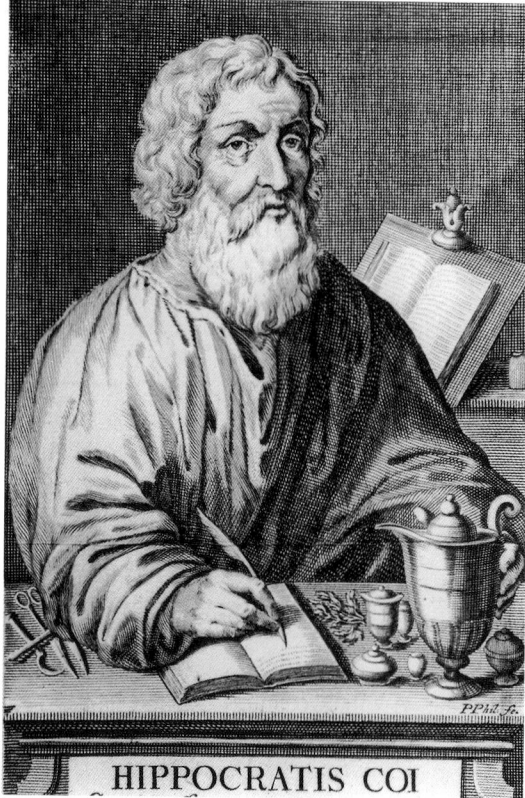

FIG. 1.3 Hippocrates of Cos (460 to 375 BCE), the father of Western medicine, advocated for the use of massage. (Courtesy U.S. National Library of Medicine, Bethesda, MD.)

Greece and Rome

The ancient Greeks used massage widely to maintain health and promote beauty. Various ideas of healing treatments in Greece merged into a *techne iatriche,* or healing science. Among the followers of this new science was **Hippocrates of Cos** (460 to 375 BCE) (Fig. 1.3). Hippocrates is believed to have been a fine physician, founder of a medical school, author of numerous books, and advocated for the use of massage or "rubbing." These works are collectively known as the *Corpus Hippocraticum* and summarized much of what was known about disease and medicine in the ancient world. Hippocrates is generally recognized as the father of

modern Western medicine, and he believed physicians should avoid causing harm to patients. In an essay titled *On Joints,* Hippocrates discussed treatment of a shoulder dislocation after reduction and wrote, "And it is necessary to rub the shoulder gently and smoothly. The physician must be experienced in many things, but assuredly also in rubbing; for things that have the same name have not the same effect. For rubbing can bind a joint, which is too loose and loosen a joint which is too tight. However, a shoulder in the condition described, should be rubbed with soft hands and above all things, gently; but the joint should be moved about, not violently, but as so far as it can be done without producing pain" (Coulter, 1932; Johnson, 1866). In Homer's book *The Odyssey* (800 to 701 BCE), he described how "war torn" soldiers were massaged back to health.

The ancient Greeks, perhaps more than any other culture, are responsible for giving massage a high degree of social acceptance. The Greeks built elaborate bathhouses where massage and exercise were available, but bathhouse patrons were seeking luxury instead of health, and Grecian bathhouses became the playgrounds of the rich and powerful (Wood, 1974).

The Romans inherited much of their massage tradition from the Greeks, and it was widely used, especially in combination with hot baths. Roman politician Julius Caesar (100 to 44 BCE) is said to have had himself pinched all over as a remedy for a condition similar to epilepsy. **Aulus Cornelius Celsus** (25 BCE to CE 50) compiled numerous volumes collectively called *De Medicina.* This is the primary source of medical knowledge in ancient Rome, and it included pathology, pharmacology, surgery, and orthopedics; the latter discussed the use of friction or massage.

A later follower of Hippocratic medicine was **Galen of Pergamon** (130 to 201). Galen was the most famous physician in the Roman Empire and wrote extensively on the topic of massage (DeDomenico & Wood, 1997). In at least 100 treatises, Galen combined the Greek knowledge of anatomy and medicine and included the use of exercise, baths, and massage. Galen strongly recommended gladiators be rubbed or pinched all over until their skin was red in preparation for combat. Galen's influence on all aspects of medical thinking cannot be overstated, and it is probably because of him, massage survived long after the fall of Rome.

Do not seek to follow in the footsteps of the wise. Seek what they sought.

Matsuo Basho

MIDDLE AGES

The Middle Ages began after the collapse of the Roman Empire in CE 476 and ended in the 15th century with the fall of Constantinople in 1453. The use of massage continued but fell into decline in Europe and Asia during the early part of the Middle Ages. This era was "the Dark Ages," when many aspects of ancient culture and practice were abandoned. However, many of Galen's medical texts had been translated into Arabic; Muslims incorporated the Greco-Roman *medical* knowledge into the Islamic medical framework. One example of the integration of medical knowledge was a text titled *Kitabu'l Hawi Fi't-Tibb,* or *Comprehensive Book of Medicine,* which included the use of massage. This text was written by the Persian physician **Rhazes** (854 to 924), also known as Abu Bakr Muhammad ibn Zakariya al-Razi.

Another example of Greco-Roman and Islamic medical knowledge integration was a text titled *al-Qānūn fī aṭ-Ṭibb,* or *Canon of Medicine.* This text was written by one of the greatest Persian physicians of this era, **Avicenna** (980 to 1037), also known as *Ibn Sina.* The *Canon of Medicine* is the most famous book in the history of medicine in both the East and the West. Avicenna excelled in the assessment of conditions and comparison of signs and symptoms. He also advocated for the use of analgesics, or pain-relieving agents, which included massage. The *Canon of Medicine* became the standard medical text at many medieval universities and remained in use until 1650 (Calvert, 2002).

Much of ancient culture and traditions, including massage, were abandoned during the Middle Ages (or Dark Ages), with the exception of a few of the aforementioned Persian physicians. Massage did remain an important procedure for folk healers and midwives, but no compilations of techniques and procedures were undertaken during this time period. However, the revival of the Galenic tradition centuries later played an important part in the rise of scientific thought during the Renaissance (DeDomenico & Wood, 1997).

EUROPEAN RENAISSANCE

The European Renaissance began in the 14th century and ended in the 16th century. The word *renaissance* means rebirth, and it was an exciting period in the history of medicine and medical treatments. Classical Greek learning resurfaced and Western medicine was revitalized by new translations of old Greek and Latin texts. Among the newly revived texts was Celsus's *De Medicina,* which came into circulation again, thanks to German Johannes Gutenberg's (c.1400 to 1468) printing press.

Ambroise Paré (1515 to 1590), the famous French surgeon, was among the earliest individuals in this era to discuss the effects of massage, and he used friction to treat dislocated joints and other orthopedic conditions. Paré also invented several surgical instruments and established new surgical procedures.

In England, **William Harvey** (1578 to 1657) discovered the circulation of blood in 1628, and his writings did much to promote the acceptance of massage as a treatment measure. Harvey observed the hearts of living animals and determined the active phase of the heart muscular contraction (systole) was the mechanism that pumps blood through arteries and veins. He was also able to show valves in veins support blood to flow only in one direction, or toward the heart. Harvey stated "we are able to influence the circulation both by voluntary exertion and by passive massage in muscles and we should expect both of these measures would influence the constituents of blood generally" (Brunton, 1894). Although Harvey's work was important, massage did not gain popularity in Europe until the 18th century.

> *Knowledge is the true organ of sight, not the eyes.*
> **Panchatantra, fifth century**

MODERN ERA

The modern era began in the 17th century and is the current era; it is also referred to as the *Information Age.* The modern era has seen the creation of new medical systems that incorporated the anatomic, physiologic, and chemical discoveries of the previous 200 years. During this time, a wide variety of physicians and authors advocated for the use of massage and some developed their own systems.

The most famous and enduring influence on massage is the contribution made by Swede **Pehr Henrik Ling** (1776 to 1839). Ling accepted a post as gymnastic and fencing master at the University of Lund in Sweden in 1804. He developed his own system of massage and exercises or gymnastics, the latter of which consisted of four types—educational, military, medical, and esthetic (Fig. 1.4). This system was called the *Swedish Remedial Massage and Exercise,* the *Swedish Movement Cure,* or simply the *Ling system.* Ling quickly gained international recognition, and modifications of his basic concepts have been used throughout the globe. The term *Swedish massage* was used to describe the massage component of Ling's system. For this reason, Ling is regarded as the father of Swedish massage.

In 1813, Ling founded the Central Institute of Gymnastics in Stockholm and began teaching his system to others.

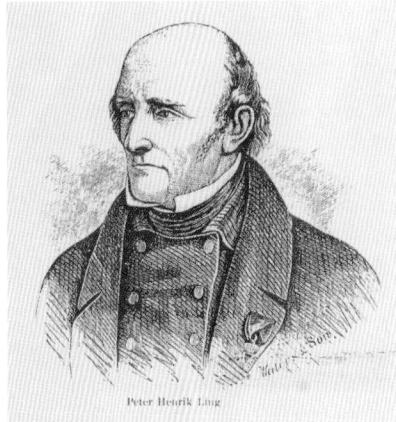

FIG. 1.4 Pehr Henrik Ling (1776 to 1839), the father of Swedish massage, developed his own system of massage and exercises/gymnastics called the Swedish Remedial Massage and Exercise, the Swedish Movement Cure, or simply the Ling system. (Courtesy Calvert, R. N. [2002]. *The history of massage: An illustrated survey from around the world.* Rochester: Healing Arts Press.)

Physicians could complete the program in 1 year, compared with 2 or 3 years for nonphysicians. By 1839, the year of Ling's death, 38 schools throughout Europe were teaching his system, including in London, Berlin, Dresden, Leipzig, Vienna, Paris, and St. Petersburg in Russia. Many of Ling's original ideas have faded from popularity, but his work remains an important influence in the early development of the physical therapy and massage professions (Kellgren, 1890).

Dutch physician **Johann Mezger** (1839 to 1909) also developed his own style of massage and made massage a fundamental component of physical rehabilitation. French was the international language in the 19th century, and Mezger is credited with introducing the terminology to describe massage techniques (e.g., effleurage, pétrissage, tapotement), which is still used in massage legislation, medical insurance billing codes, and massage curricula.

Florence Nightingale (1829 to 1910) of England, founder of modern nursing, took care of wounded soldiers during the Crimean War (1853 to 1856). She developed a standard of care for patients, and massage was an integral part of care (Fig. 1.5). When nurse training was developed, massage was included in the curriculum and massage was provided to patients as part of their comfort measures (Ruffin, 2011). The use of massage declined as analgesics become more popular, and massage was removed from the nursing curriculum in the 1970s (Lewis et al., 2010).

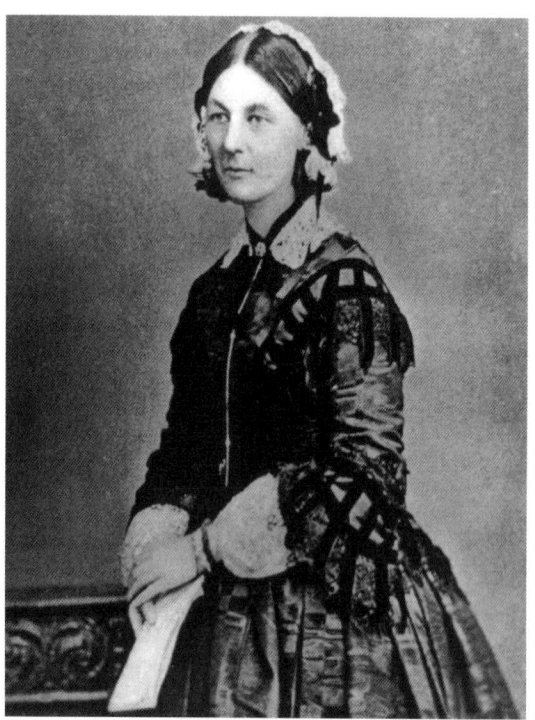

FIG. 1.5 Florence Nightingale (1829 to 1910), the founder of modern nursing. Massage was an integral part of the nursing standard of care for soldiers during war times. (From Yoost, B. L., & Crawford, L. R. [2016]. *Fundamentals of nursing* [1st ed.]. St. Louis, MO: Elsevier.)

World War I provided countless opportunities for the use of massage and exercise to rehabilitate injured soldiers. French physician **Just Lucas-Championniere** (1843 to 1913) advocated for the use of massage and passive movements to treat soft tissue injuries and fractures. British physicians **James B. Mennell** (1880 to 1957) and **Sir William Bennett** (1852 to 1931) were impressed with Lucas-Championniere's work and began using massage at the St. Thomas Hospital and the St. George's Hospital, respectively; both hospitals are in London (Wood, 1974).

In the United States Drs. **George Henry Taylor** (1829 to 1899) and **Charles Fayette Taylor** (1827 to 1899) sailed to Sweden to study the Ling system and returned to the United States to open the Remedial Hygienic Institute of New York City in 1856. The institute was an orthopedic clinic specializing in Ling's system of massage and exercise. "Water cures" and nutrition were incorporated into their treatment regimen. The two physicians published many important works on Ling's system, and George Taylor wrote the first American textbook on the subject, titled *An Exposition of the Swedish Movement Cure* (1860).

It should be noted massage and exercise were referred to simultaneously and little distinction was made between the two. For example, massage and exercise or gymnastics were combined in Ling's system. It was not until 1886 that massage was separated from exercise. Credit for this distinction is given to two individuals, namely Drs. **Emil A. G. Kleen** (1847 to 1923) of Sweden and **William Murrell** (1853 to 1912) of England. In fact, Murrell provided one of the earliest definitions of massage in his book titled *Massage as a Mode of Treatment* (1886) and stated massage is the "scientific mode of treating certain forms of a disease by systematic manipulations" (Wood, 1974).

American physician **Douglas Graham** (1848 to 1928) authored several texts on massage, including *A Practical Treatise of Massage* (1884), which focused on massage for specific conditions. Graham described massage as "a term now generally accepted by European and American physicians to signify a group of procedures usually done with the hands, such as friction, kneading, manipulations, rolling, and percussion to the external tissues of the body in a variety of ways, either with a curative, palliative, or hygienic object." Graham defined massage more comprehensively than Murrell and stated the *what* (usually done with the hands), the *where* (external tissues of the body), the *how* (friction, kneading, manipulations, rolling, and percussion), and the *why* (curative, palliative, or hygienic) (Wood, 1974).

Norwegian gymnast **Hartvig Nissen** (1857 to 1924) opened the Swedish Health Institute of Washington, D.C., in 1883. This is considered the first massage school in the United States. Nissen wrote an article titled *Swedish Movement and Massage* (1888), which was subsequently published in several medical journals. The result of the publication was numerous letters from physicians who wanted to know more about Ling's system, and this inquiry led Nissen to publish a book of the same title later the same year. Taken together, Nissen's and Graham's works are generally

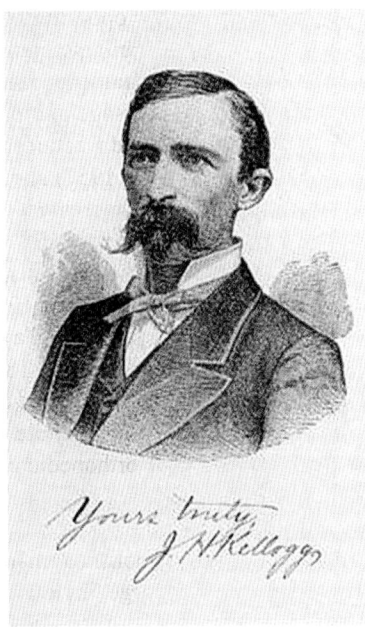

FIG. 1.6 John Harvey Kellogg (1852 to 1943) promoted massage to the general public by writing articles and books, publishing a magazine, and directing the Battle Creek Sanitarium, which provided massage as part of the health regimen for its patrons. (© Judi Calvert.)

credited with promoting the use of massage within the United States medical profession.

While the Taylor brothers, Graham, and Nissen, were advocating for massage within the medical community, Dr. **John Harvey Kellogg** (1852 to 1943) of Battle Creek, Michigan, promoted massage to the general public. Kellogg wrote numerous articles and books on massage and published a magazine called *Good Health* (Fig. 1.6). Kellogg also published the *Art of Massage: A Practical Manual for the Nurse, the Student and the Practitioner* (1929). Kellogg was the director of the Battle Creek Sanitarium founded by members of the Seventh-day Adventist Church. Under his directorship, massage and hydrotherapy were a central aspect of the health regimen for patrons.

When you steal from one author, it's plagiarism; if you steal from many, it's research.

Wilson Mizner

PROFESSIONAL SOCIETIES, ORGANIZATIONS, AND ASSOCIATIONS

The massage profession began to take shape during the beginning of the 20th century. As massage gained popularity, unscrupulous schools began to offer massage training in which schools provided students lodging while they were enrolled in the program and work after their graduation. However, the work establishments were often brothels (Beck, 2016). In 1894 the Commissioners of the British Medical Journal published a report titled "The Scandals of Massage" to expose these practices. This prompted nine British nurses and midwives to form a council of trained masseuses. The following year (1895), the council established the **Society of Trained Masseuses**. The founders of the Society acted to legitimize massage, which had become tarnished by its association with prostitution. The Society established a massage practice model, which regulated massage through a published massage curriculum and accreditation of massage schools, which included regular inspections and use of only qualified massage instructors. The Society quickly embraced wider methods of treatment, including medical gymnastics and water cures (which would later be called therapeutic exercise and hydrotherapy, respectively). Members of the Society were required to pass examinations and were subject to routine surveillance (Nicholls & Cheek, 2006). In 1900, the Society was incorporated and became the **Incorporated Society of Trained Masseuses**. By the end of World War I (1918), the Society had nearly 5000 members. In 1920 the Society merged with the **Institute of Massage and Remedial Exercises**. These two bodies were then granted a Royal Charter by King George and became the **Chartered Society of Massage and Medical Gymnastics**. By 1939, the Society has approximately 12,000 members (Callaway & Burgess, 2009).

World War II saw the emergence of physical therapy as large numbers of soldiers returned from the war. Massage as a specific and exclusive manual modality played a smaller role in physical rehabilitations as other methods were developed. Hence massage became one procedure in the arsenal of rehabilitation and part of an overall treatment plan for patients. For this reason, the Chartered Society of Massage and Medical Gymnastics decided to change its name in 1943 and become the **Chartered Society of Physiotherapy**, which remains today. By 1947 the field of physical therapy and rehabilitation was established as a separate medical specialty. Massage remained part of the physical therapy curriculum and is often referred to as *manual therapy*. An important distinction is massage techniques used in physical therapy to address specific conditions applied on specific areas rather than applied in a whole-body session (Federation of State Boards of Physical Therapy [FSBPT], 2012).

In 1943, postgraduates from the College of Swedish Massage in Chicago created the **American Association of Masseurs and Masseuses**, the first massage association in the United States. In 1958 the American Association of Masseurs and Masseuses changed its name to the **American Massage and Therapy Association** and, in 1983, dropped the "and" to become the **American Massage Therapy Association** (AMTA). Currently, AMTA is the largest massage organization, with state chapters in all 50 states and Washington, D.C. In 1987 the **Associated Bodywork and Massage Professionals** (ABMP) was founded and is currently the second organization serving the massage profession.

In 1962, Michael Murphy and Richard Pierce founded the Esalen Institute in Big Sur California, a retreat center and think tank for the human potential movement. After World Wars I and II, many European scholars immigrated to the United States. Several scholars ended up at Esalen, where they debated and exchanged ideas. Scholars include psychologist Wilhelm Reich (Reichian therapy), Moshe Feldenkrais (Feldenkrais method), Ida Rolf (structural integration or Rolfing) (Fig. 1.7), Alexander Lowen (bioenergetics), Fritz Smith (Zero Balancing), Andrew Weil, Deepak Chopra, Dub Leigh (Zen Bodywork), Betty Fuller (Trager), Judith Aston (Aston Kinetics), John Upledger (Craniosacral Therapy), Til Luchau (Advanced Myofascial Techniques), and Dean Juhan (author of *Job's Body*). For many people, Esalen was their first exposure to massage and where many came to learn massage. Massage practitioners at Esalen developed a distinct style, called *Esalen Massage.* In the 1980s, the **Esalen Massage and Bodywork Association** was founded. Many styles of massage have been developed since the 1960s, and a large majority have their roots at Esalen.

Founded in 1982, **AMTA Council of Schools** was created to support and innovate massage education. The Council was dissolved in 2009. The same year, the **Alliance for Massage Therapy Education** (AFMTE) formed to strengthen and elevate educational practices and standards. AFMTE published a set of massage instructor competencies in 2013 and launched a program certifying massage instructors in 2018.

Commission on Massage Therapy Accreditation (COMTA) was founded in 1989 to establish and maintain quality and integrity in massage education. The United States Department of Education (USDE) granted COMTA recognition in 2002, and COMTA remains the only specialized accrediting agency approved by the USDE to accredit massage programs and schools.

In 1990, the **American Massage Therapy Foundation** was established by the AMTA to advance the massage profession through supporting scientific research and evidence-informed practice. In 2004 the foundation became an independent organization and changed its name to the **Massage Therapy Foundation** (MTF).

In 1992, the **National Certification Board for Therapeutic Massage and Bodywork** (NCBTMB) was founded after significant encouragement from the AMTA and other industry leaders. The objective was to create a national certification to facilitate massage licensing reciprocity throughout the United States. A national certification examination was launched, and many states adopted the examination as part of their licensing requirements. In 2013, NCBTMB began providing board certification, which is currently the highest voluntary credential in the massage profession. NCBTMB is actively involved in the massage continuing-education approval process. The practice of offering the examination as part of state licensure was retired in 2014. Licensing and certification are discussed in Chapter 17.

The **Touch Research Institute** (TRI) at the University of Miami's School of Medicine was also established in 1992 under the directorship of Dr. Tiffany Field. This institute is the first in the world to focus on the effects of massage and touch and its applications in the treatment of diseases. Their research efforts continue today and have shown massage and touch have numerous beneficial effects on health and wellbeing. Another important event in 1998 was the formation of the *National Center for Complementary and Alternative Medicine* (NCCAM) within the **National Institutes of Health** (NIH) by the United States Congress. NCCAM's mission was to investigate and evaluate unconventional health practices.

In 2005, the **Federation of State Massage Therapy Boards** (FSMTB) was formed after the ABMP convened a meeting of massage regulators and educators. One of the initial goals of the Federation was to create a valid and reliable licensing examination, and this came to fruition in 2008 with the publication of the Massage and Bodywork Licensing Examination (MBLEx). In 2014 the MBLEx became the only licensing examination in the United States.

In 2014, Congress changed the name *National Center for Complementary and Alternative Medicine* (NCCAM) to *National Center for Complementary and Integrative Health* (NCCIH), stating the use of "alternative medicine" was rare. The new center within the NIH blends medical and healthcare practices and products with mainstream medicine. NCCIH has two subgroups—products such as herbal supplements and probiotics; and practices such as massage, acupuncture, chiropractic, and yoga (NIH, 2018). Massage has been shown to be beneficial for many people and has become a respected and popular modality.

Human Trafficking

Human trafficking is a form of modern-day slavery in which traffickers use force, fraud, or coercion to obtain some type of labor or commercial sex acts (Homeland Security, n.d.). Human trafficking is the third largest

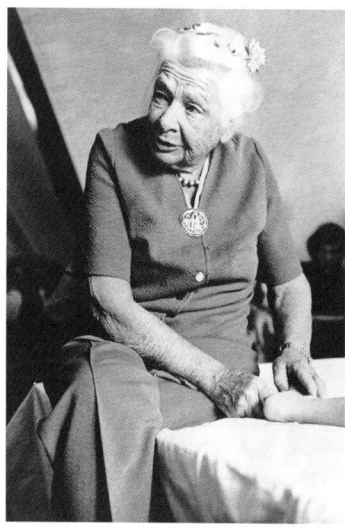

FIG. 1.7 Ida Rolf (1896 to 1972), founder of structural integration or Rolfing, was one of the many scholars who taught at the Esalen Institute. (Courtesy the Rolf Institute—David Kirk-Campbell.)

source of revenue for organized crime, just behind drugs and guns/firearms trafficking. In human trafficking, the trafficker uses humans as slaves for a profit, usually forcing them into prostitution and sexual slavery. Poor socioeconomic conditions and promises of a good job, an education, and a better life are often part of the first encounter between traffickers and victims. They arrive in the United States to find they are indebted, have no job, no legal status, and no choices. To hold up their end of the bargain, victims are forced to provide services; these services range from commercialized sexual exploitation (the most common form of human trafficking) to work in farms, factories, or hotels. It can also involve organ removal and surrogacy. Slaves are moved frequently from state to state and are not able to create a support network. There are also an increasing number of victims who are American minors, recruited or forced into prostitution as young as 12 years old.

Although great strides have been made in the massage industry toward professionalism, the use of massage as a cover for human trafficking is still prevalent today. According to a report published by the Federation of State Massage Therapy Boards (2017), an estimated 9000 illicit massage businesses are currently active, and this type of commercial-front massage business is one of the top venues for sex trafficking.

According to data provided by the Polaris Project (n.d.), forerunners of human trafficking research, outreach, and victim identification, victims of trafficking who work under the cover of massage are often young females from Asia, South America, and the former Soviet Union. Underage Americans are also trafficked across state borders to work in massage parlors as prostitutes.

Several diploma-mill "massage schools" have arisen that fabricate training and sell massage diplomas and transcripts to traffickers who distribute the documents to their sex trade workers. This is an attempt to impart a cover of legitimacy to an illegal practice of massage. There is also much fraud committed involving targeting testing centers and licensing boards, as reported by the FSMTB. To combat problems associated with human trafficking, the Federal Bureau of Investigation is working to help free people. Congress passed the Trafficking Victims Protection Act (TVPA) in 2000, which created public awareness programs in countries from which females are usually trafficked. At the state level within the United States, Congress also established a visa program for victims who want to return to their families. There are also severe penalties for traffickers. The TVPA created the Office to Monitor and Combat Trafficking in Persons in 2001 and launched the Innocence Lost National Initiative, which helped rescue nearly 900 children and convict more than 500 pimps and other individuals involved with human trafficking.

Several issues can arise for legal massage practitioners from human sex trafficking. Practitioners can be threatened, harassed, intimidated, and even assaulted. This may result in additional operational costs for practitioners to increase security. Personal and business establishment reputations may be compromised. It also erodes public trust as the integrity of massage educational institutions, testing authorities, and state licensing boards is questioned, especially if they have allowed unqualified individuals to enter the massage profession (FSMTB, 2017). Many states require licensed massage practitioners to display antitrafficking awareness posters and report when human trafficking situations are suspected.

The FSMTB recommends all massage state boards report to a national accrediting agency and all massage schools become regulated by a common accreditation agency. These measures might make it difficult for traffickers to move their victims and their illegal business from state to state. Another recommendation is to require licensing of massage establishments. This measure would allow law enforcement to investigate the business owners and arrest traffickers. The implementation and enforcement of these recommendations may reduce human trafficking and the negative impact it has on the massage profession.

THE FUTURE OF MASSAGE

Today, massage practitioners play an important role in the management of a variety of medical conditions. Research continues to be conducted, and this new knowledge elevates the overall standing of the massage profession in the healthcare, wellness, medical, and rehabilitation communities. Of clients who discussed massage with their healthcare providers, 9% were referred to a massage practitioner, 24% were strongly recommended to get a massage, and 29% were encouraged to get a massage (AMTA, 2020). Massage is one of the complementary therapies with the highest physician referral rates (Wahner-Roedler et al., 2006), and massage is rated among physicians as the complementary therapy most likely to be beneficial and least likely to be harmful (Ernst, 1999). Hospitals across the United States and Canada are using massage for their patients and staff (Healey, 2010; Kania-Richmond et al., 2015).

In addition, the occupational outlook for massage practitioners is bright, with employment opportunities projected to grow 26% from 2016 to 2026, which is much faster than the average for all occupations (U.S. Department of Labor, 2020). Employment opportunities are found not only in medical centers but also in spas, cruise ships, hotels, resorts, and wellness centers. Private practice is another career option for massage practitioners. In fact, in 2021, the Council of State Governments began working on an interstate compact which provides massage licensing portability between states.

E-RESOURCES

http://evolve.elsevier.com/Salvo/MassageTherapy

- Chapter challenge
- Flash cards
- Additional information

PEHR HENRIK LING

Did you ever wonder what is so Swedish about Swedish massage, when the language often used to talk about it is French and the movements are used throughout the world? The answer lies in the life of Pehr Henrik Ling, known everywhere as the father of Swedish massage.

Ling was born in Småland (the traditional province in southern Sweden) in 1776. Far from showing promise in his studies, he was expelled from school for bad behavior, then traveled Europe for a while before finally returning to Sweden. Upon his return he took up fencing, the classical sport of sword fighting. Eventually, he accepted a position at the University of Lund, where he taught fencing and gymnastics and studied anatomy, physiology, and kinesiology.

Naturally, Ling's growing understanding of the human body started to affect his teaching. He noticed the movements his students made were far from ideal from a physiologic perspective but were so habitually ingrained it was difficult for students to learn more efficient movements. Ling decided to dedicate himself to teaching better movement, feeling that this would be good not only for students and athletes but also the Swedish military, which had recently lost Finland in a war with Russia.

Ling's new system of movement education for physical rehabilitation and retraining (called Swedish gymnastics) required very little equipment and focused on the use of simple stretches. Some were active movements done by the student alone. Some were passive movements, during which the student relaxed and another student guided the body's movement. Others were cooperative movements, in which the student provided the impetus for the movement and another student would either assist or resist.

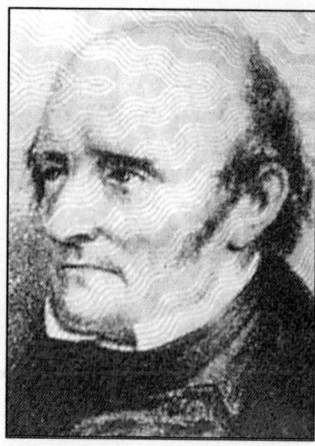

From Calver, R. N. (2002). *The history of massage: An illustrated survey from around the world.* Rochester: Inner Traditions/Bear & Company. All rights reserved. http://www.Innertraditions.com. Reprinted with permission of publisher.

Ling's work took on a new dimension in 1813, when he opened the Swedish Royal Central Institute of Gymnastics. It was here he expanded on his system of rehabilitative gymnastics and exercise, which was known variously as the Ling system, Swedish movements, and the Swedish Movement Cure. Although Ling's main focus was on the medical use of movement training (which laid the foundations of the modern field of physical therapy), massage was also a part of the Swedish Movement Cure, giving rise to the term Swedish massage.

Ling died in 1839, after years of failing health, but his impact on the medical world has only spread further with time. The fields of physical therapy, massage therapy, kinesiology, and gymnastics all owe a huge debt to Pehr Henrik Ling, the renegade remedial gymnastics teacher and father of Swedish massage.

Although the use of movement and massage for health promotion and rehabilitation is now well established, the medical profession did not always take kindly to Ling's new system during his lifetime. This is not surprising given his background; imagine what would happen if a high school dropout and football coach decided to open up a physical therapy clinic today.

Although Ling's lack of formal education in medicine aggravated many in the medical establishment, quite a few of his students were physicians, and these students spread rave reviews of Ling's system all across the country, even publishing success stories in reputable medical journals. By 1851, Ling's system was so popular that 38 schools were teaching his signature combination of gymnastics and massage all across Europe, which goes to show what one can do with solid observations when faced with prejudices rooted in tradition.

REFERENCES

American Massage Therapy Association (AMTA). (2020). *Massage therapy industry fact sheet.* Retrieved from https://www.amtamassage.org/publications/massage-industry-fact-sheet/.

Beck, M. (2016). *Theory and practice of therapeutic massage* (6th ed.). Boston, MA: Cengage Learning.

Brunton, T. L. (1894). The Harveian oration on modern developments of Harvey's work: Delivered at the Royal College of Physicians. *British Medical Journal,* 2(1764), 894–899.

Callaway, L., & Burgess, S. (2009). History of massage. In: L. Casanelia & D. Stelfox (Eds.), *Foundations of massage* (3rd ed., chapter 2). Australia: Churchill Livingstone.

Calvert, R. N. (2002). *The history of massage: An illustrated survey from around the world.* Rochester, VT: Healing Arts Press.

Coulter, J. S. (1932). *Clio medica VII, Physical therapy* (pp. 39–40). New York: Paul B. Hoeber.

DeDomenico, G. (2007). *Beard's massage: Principles and practice of soft tissue manipulation* (5th ed.). Philadelphia: Elsevier Saunders.

DeDomenico, G., & Wood, E. C. (1997). *Beard's massage* (4th ed.). Philadelphia: WB Saunders.

Ernst, E. (1999). Massage therapy for low back pain: A systematic review. *Journal of Pain and Symptom Management,* 17(1), 65–69.

Ernst, E., Pittler, M. H., Wider, B., & Boddy, K. (2006). *The desktop guide to complementary and alternative medicine* (2nd ed.). Edinburgh: Elsevier Mosby.

Federation of State Boards of Physical Therapy. (2012). *The birth of our federation.* Retrieved from http://history.fsbpt.org/.

Federation of State Massage Therapy Boards. (2017). *Human trafficking task force report.* Retrieved from https://www.fsmtb.org/consumer-information/human-trafficking/.

Field, T. (2002). Massage therapy. *Medical Clinics of North America,* 86(1), 163–71.

Healey, D. (2010). *The hospital environment.* Retrieved from https://www.amtamassage.org/publications/massage-therapy-journal/the-hospital-enviornment/.

Hentschel, H. D., & Schneider, J. (2004). The history of massage in the ways of life and healing in India. *Wurzburger Medizinhistorische Mitteilungen,* 23, 179–203.

Homeland Secuirty. (n.d.). *What is human trafficking?* Retrieved from https://www.dhs.gov/blue-campaign/what-human-trafficking.

Johnson, W. (1866). *The anatriptic art.* London: Simkin Marshall and Co.

Kania-Richmond, A., Reece, B. F., Suter, E., & Verhoef, M. J. (2015). The professional role of massage therapists in patient care in Canadian urban hospitals—A mixed methods study. *BMC Complementary and Alternative Medicine,* 7, 15–20.

Kellgren, A. (1890). *The technic of Ling's system of manual treatment.* Edinburgh and London: Young J. Pentland.

Lewis, S. L., Dirksen, S. R., Heitkemper, M. M., Bucher, L., & Lewis, I. (2010). *Medical-surgical nursing: Assessment and management of clinical problems* (8th ed., pp. 94–95). St. Louis: Elsevier.

National Institutes of Health. (2018). *Complementary, alternative, or integrative health: What's in a name?* Retrieved from https://nccih.nih.gov/health/integrative-health.

Nicholls, D. A., & Cheek, J. (2006). Physiotherapy and the shadow of prostitution: The society of trained masseuses and the massage scandals of 1894. *Social Science & Medicine,* 62(9), 2336–2348.

Polaris. (n.d.). *Human trafficking.* Retrieved from https://humantraffickinghotline.org/type-trafficking/human-trafficking.

Ruffin, P. T. (2011). A history of massage in nurse training school curricula (1860–1945). *Journal of Holistic Nursing: Official Journal of the American Holistic Nurses' Association,* 29(1), 61–67.

Thomas Medical Dictionary. (1886). Philadelphia: J. B. Lippincott Co.

United States Department of Labor: Bureau of Labor Statistics. (2020). *Summary report for massage therapists.* Retrieved from https://www.onetonline.org/link/summary/31-9011.00.

Wahner-Roedler, D. L., Vincent, A., Elkin, P. L., Loehrer, L. L., Cha, S. S., & Bauer, B. A. (2006). Physicians' attitudes toward complementary and alternative medicine and their knowledge of specific therapies: A survey at an academic medical center. *Evidence-based Complementary and Alternative Medicine: eCAM,* 3(4), 495–501.

Wood, E. C. (1974). *Beard's massage: Principles and techniques* (2nd ed.). Philadelphia: WB Saunders.

BIBLIOGRAPHY

Basham, A. L. (1976). The practice of medicine in ancient and medieval India. In C. Leslie (Ed.), *Asian medical systems.* Berkeley, CA: University of California Press.

Buikstra, J. E. (1993). Diseases of the pre-Columbian Americas. In K. F. Kiple (Eds.), *The Cambridge world history of human disease.* New York: Cambridge University Press.

Castiglioni, A. (1947). *A history of medicine* (Translated by E. B. Krumbhaar). New York: Alfred A Knopf.

Graham, D. (1884). *A practical treatise on massage.* New York: William Wood.

Hippocrates. (1928). *Hippocrates, Vol III. On wounds in the head. In the surgery. On fractures. On joints. Mochlicon* (Translated by E. T. Withington). Cambridge, MA: Harvard University Press.

Kleen, E. A. G. (1921). *Massage and medical gymnastics* (2nd ed.). New York: Wm. Wood and Co.

Liddel, L. (1984). *The book of massage: The complete step-by-step guide to eastern and western techniques.* New York: Simon & Schuster.

McMillan, M. (1921). *Massage and therapeutic exercise.* Philadelphia: WB Saunders.

Means, P. A. (1931). *Ancient civilizations of the Andes.* New York: C Scribner and Sons.

Meintz, S. L. (1995). Alternatives and complementary therapies: Whatever became of the back rub? *RN,* 58(4), 49–501.

Murrell, W. (1886). *Massage as a mode of treatment* (pp. 38–40). Philadelphia: P. Blakinston Son.

Nissen, H. (1905). *Practical massage in twenty lessons.* Philadelphia: FA Davis.

Pettman, E. (2007). A history of manipulative therapy. *Journal of Manual and Manipulative Therapy,* 15(3), 165–74.

Rahman, F. (1987). *Health and medicine in the Islamic tradition: Change and identity.* New York: Crossroad Press.

Veith, I., & Huang, T. (1949). *Nei ching su wen.* Baltimore: Williams & Wilkins.

Wanning, T. (1993). Healing and the mind/body arts: Massage, acupuncture, yoga, t'ai chi, and feldenkrais. *AAOHN Journal: Official Journal of the American Association of Occupational Health Nurses,* 41(7), 349–351.

Wide, A. G. (1905). *Handbook of medical and orthopedic gymnastics.* New York: Funk and Wagnall.

Zysk, K. G. (1985). *Religious healing in the Veda, with translations and annotations of medical hymns in the Rgveda and the Atharvaveda and renderings from the corresponding ritual texts.* Philadelphia: American Philosophical Society.

REVIEW AND APPLY YOUR KNOWLEDGE

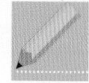 **MATCHING ONE: CONCEPT REVIEW**

Place the letter of the answer next to the number of the term or phrase that best describes it.

A. 3000 BCE
B. Amma
C. *Canon of Medicine*
D. Ayurveda books of wisdom
E. China
F. Hippocrates of Cos
G. Pehr Henrik Ling
H. Massage therapy
I. Johann Mezger
J. American Association of Masseurs and Masseuses
K. Nei Chang
L. Swedish Movement Cure

_____ 1. A method of manually manipulating soft tissues using compression and traction for therapeutic, palliative, and self-care or wellness purposes.
_____ 2. Written records of massage go back as early as _____.
_____ 3. The original Chinese massage technique.
_____ 4. The country in which the first written accounts of massage originated.
_____ 5. The father of modern Western medicine.
_____ 6. The classic scripture of traditional Chinese medicine.
_____ 7. The father of Swedish massage.
_____ 8. The first massage organization in the United States founded in 1943 by postgraduates of the College of Swedish Massage in Chicago.
_____ 9. India's first great medical works.
_____ 10. Credited with introducing French terminology to describe massage techniques.
_____ 11. The most famous book in the history of medicine in both the East and the West.
_____ 12. The name given to Ling's system of massage and exercises or gymnastics.

MATCHING TWO: CONCEPT REVIEW

Place the letter of the answer next to the number of the term or phrase that best describes it.

A. Human trafficking
B. Federation of State Massage Therapy Boards
C. Touch Research Institute
D. National Certification Board for Therapeutic Massage and Bodywork
E. Esalen Institute
F. John Harvey Kellogg
G. Galen of Pergamon
H. Middle Ages
I. Florence Nightingale
J. Hartvig Nissen
K. Shiatsu
L. Essential oils

_____ 1. Japanese method based on the same traditional Chinese medicine concepts as acupuncture.
_____ 2. Facility that opened in 1962 and, for many people, was their first exposure to massage.
_____ 3. The person who opened the Swedish Health Institute of Washington, D.C. in 1883, which is considered the first massage school in the United States.
_____ 4. The first institute in the world which focused its research efforts on the effects of massage and touch and its applications in the treatment of diseases.
_____ 5. Use of massage continued but fell into decline in Europe and Asia during this era.
_____ 6. The most famous physician in the Roman Empire and who wrote extensively about massage.
_____ 7. Form of modern-day slavery in which traffickers use force, fraud, or coercion to obtain some type of labor or commercial sex acts.
_____ 8. Founder of modern nursing who developed a standard of care for patients which included massage.
_____ 9. The Egyptians were the first to study and codify the therapeutic effects of _____.
_____ 10. Director of the Battle Creek Sanitarium who made massage and hydrotherapy a central part of their health regimen.
_____ 11. Organization providing licensure examination for the massage profession.
_____ 12. Organization providing board certification for the massage profession.

MULTIPLE CHOICE: TEST YOUR KNOWLEDGE

Place the letter of the answer next to the number of the term or phrase that best describes it.

_____ 1. The Sanskrit term for massage is:
A. *mashesh.*
B. *massin.*
C. *mass'h.*
D. *makeh.*

_____ 2. The earliest recorded portrayal of massage are:
A. Renaissance medical treatments.
B. prehistoric cave paintings.
C. Chinese written records.
D. Indian medical texts.

_____ 3. The early Greek physician who advocated for the use of "rubbing" was:
A. Hippocrates of Cos.
B. Galen of Pergamon.
C. Rhazes.
D. Avicenna.

_____ 4. The printing press was created by:
A. Ambroise Paré.
B. William Harvey.
C. Johannes Gutenberg.
D. Matsuo Basho.

_____ 5. Who founded the Central Institute of Gymnastics in Stockholm?
A. James Mennell
B. Johann Mezger
C. Just Lucas-Championniere
D. Pehr Henrik Ling

_____ 6. Who is considered the founder of modern nursing?
A. Sir William Bennett
B. George Henry Taylor
C. Florence Nightingale
D. William Murrell

_____ 7. Who authored *A Practical Treatise of Massage*?
A. Johann Mezger
B. Douglas Graham
C. Florence Nightingale
D. Emil A.G. Kleen

_____ 8. The emergence of physical therapy occurred after large numbers of soldiers returned from which armed conflict?
A. Crimean War
B. World War II
C. Korean War
D. Vietnam War

_____ 9. The original name of the first massage association in the United States was the:
A. American Massage and Therapy Association.
B. American Massage Therapy Association.
C. Associated Bodywork and Massage Professionals.
D. American Association of Masseurs and Masseuses.

_____ 10. The current massage licensing examination, the MBLEx, was created by the:
A. Touch Research Institute.
B. National Certification Board for Therapeutic Massage and Bodywork.
C. Federation of State Massage Therapy Boards.
D. National Institute of Health.

_____ 11. Human trafficking is the _____ largest source of revenue for organized crime.
A. second
B. third
C. fourth
D. fifth

_____ 12. The United States Department of Labor projects opportunities for massage practitioners to grow ___ than the average for all occupations.
A. much faster
B. slightly faster
C. slightly slower
D. much slower

CRITICAL THINKING

What Does This Have to Do With Me?

How do you think the issue of human trafficking can affect you as an individual massage practitioner? Do you think you should be concerned about it when you become a practicing professional? Why do you answer the way you do? What do you think you can do to address human trafficking?

Answers can include but are not limited to:

Several issues can arise for legal massage practitioners because of human trafficking. Practitioners can be threatened, harassed, intimidated, and even assaulted. This may result in additional operational costs for massage practitioners to address the need for security. Personal and business establishment reputations may be compromised. It also erodes public trust as the integrity of massage educational institutions, testing authorities, and state licensing boards is questioned, especially if they have allowed unqualified individuals to enter the massage profession (FSMTB, 2017).

Individual massage practitioners can become involved in professional massage organizations that advocate for high educational and licensure standards, can become aware of illicit massage offices in their municipalities that may be covers for human trafficking, and can report suspicions to law enforcement. Massage practitioners should not "look the other way" and hope someone else will take care of the problem. In addition, massage practitioners need to have the utmost integrity and ethics and conduct themselves professionally at all times. This modeling of professional behavior informs the public of the difference between legitimate massage practitioners and those who are not.

PROFESSIONAL PRACTICE

Those Who Cannot Remember the Past...

Bodhi and Joanna are classmates in their massage program. While they are studying the history of massage and bodywork, Bodhi confides to Joanna he does not understand why they are bothering to learn about the origins of massage. After all, it is just ancient history; it does not have anything to do with today, and it sure will not help them get a job massaging after they graduate. He asks Joanna, "Why are we wasting time learning this when we could be spending more time learning techniques?" If you were Joanna, how would you respond to Bodhi? What historical information would you include to support your answer? How would you relate this information to becoming a professional massage practitioner?

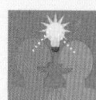

DISCUSSION

The Many Faces of Massage

This chapter mentions many methods and styles of massage, and there are many not mentioned. Choose a method and write a 50- to 75-word summary. You can use the Internet or call a local practitioner who has received training in the method you have selected as a resource. If you used a website, include the link at the end of your summary. Post your summary on an Internet-based discussion board monitored by your instructor (if available).

I would like to thank H. Michael Tarver and Til Luchau for their prior contributions on this chapter.

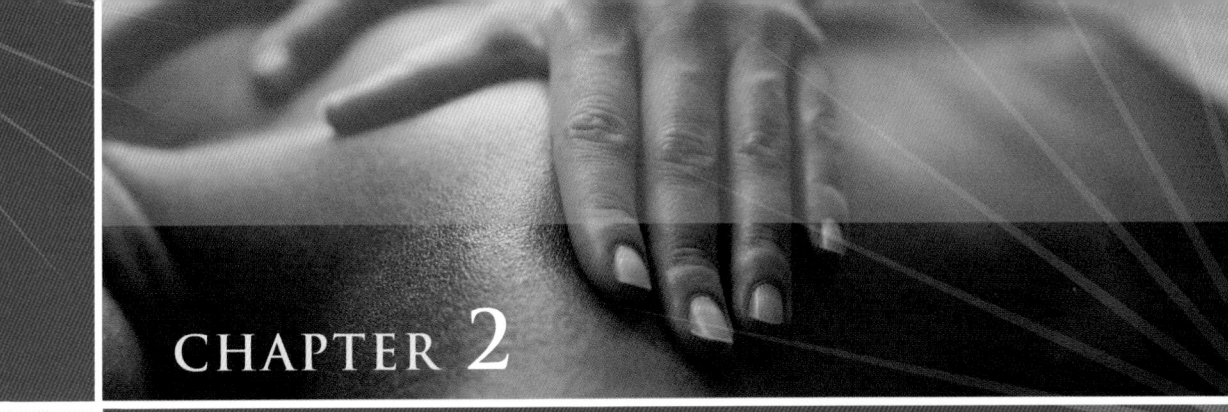

CHAPTER 2

The Therapeutic Relationship: Ethics, Cultural Competencies, and Boundaries

Today I shall behave, as if this is the day I will be remembered.

—Dr. Seuss

LEARNING OBJECTIVES

After completing this chapter, the student should be able to:

1. Define ethics, professionalism, and discuss their key principles.
2. Discuss cultural competencies.
3. Define professional boundaries and types of boundaries.
4. Compare and contrast professional relationships with dual relationships, and discuss types of dual relationships.
5. Identify steps of making professional decisions using the turbulence theory.
6. Outline sexual misconduct, sexual harassment, risk management, and how to terminate a session.

http://evolve.elsevier.com/Salvo/MassageTherapy

INTRODUCTION

Ethical principles and interpersonal skills form and inform the relationship between massage practitioners and their clients. This relationship, called the *therapeutic* or *professional relationship,* is the basis of all treatment approaches, regardless of their specific aim. So why do clients receive and continue to receive massage? Several themes emerged from an investigation by Smith et al. (2009a). The most commonly reported reason was a positive outcome, such as pain relief, which was often immediate. Another reason for continued use by clients was that expectations and treatment goals would be met based on previous positive massage outcomes which they scheduled at regular intervals. Another reason was the client-practitioner relationship, which contributed to the positive outcomes received. Smith et al. (2009b) later investigated specific elements of the massage valued most by repeat clients. Findings included: a pleasant unhurried atmosphere; firm, confident, and appropriate touch; good rapport with a friendly practitioner who was caring, knowledgeable, skilled, competent, and genuinely interested in their wellbeing. Walach et al. (2003) found massage as effective as standard medical care in chronic pain syndromes, and the positive outcomes in the massage group lasted longer, possibly because of psychologic influences. Furthermore, a strong relationship between the client and the practitioner is one of the best predictors of positive outcomes (Horvath & Symonds, 1991).

As we shall see, supportive relationships themselves act as nervous system regulators in which behavioral, physiologic, and biochemical rhythms of individuals in close relationships become synchronized (Field, 2012). Although the relationship serves the best interest of clients, practitioners bring their own uniqueness and creativity to the table. However, practitioners are the professionals and, therefore, are responsible for most of the session.

ETHICS AND PROFESSIONALISM

Ethics are moral principles governing behavior. Ethics involve judgments about what is right and wrong. Moreover, ethical issues are not always legal issues. In this chapter, we will focus on **professional ethics**, principles, values, and ideals a profession creates for itself, which are disclosed in a document called a **code of ethics**. This code represents a set of standards of ethical conduct for members of a profession. If a professional is unethical, they may be suspended or evicted from the professional organizations in which they hold membership, and may lose their license to practice. **Standards of practice** is a broader document which includes guidance for business practices, prevention of sexual misconduct, and ethical principles such as confidentiality.

The concept of ethics has had several meanings over time. Initially ethics, derived from the Greek word *ethos* for customs, referred to a group to which a person belonged and the characteristics of the group that distinguishes it from other groups. Ethics later came to mean a person's disposition, character, and conduct or behaviors. Ethics include the acquisition of knowledge to improve conduct, reflection upon core values, and putting clients'/patients' best interest and welfare first. Begley (1999) argued that ethics involves decision-making where "preferred alternatives are selected and others are rejected."

Professionalism is the adherence to a set of values and obligations; formally agreed-upon codes of conduct; and reasonable expectations of clients, colleagues, and co-workers. The overarching principle of professionalism is **fiduciary responsibility**, acting in a client's best interest and putting that interest before your own. Other key values of professionalism include maintaining standards expected of other members of the profession, and staying current with changes and discoveries in the field. Knowing and abiding by the laws and standards governing the profession are also part of our professional responsibilities or *duties.* Professionalism must be understood, practiced, refined, and adhered to with the same intensity and focus as knowledge of massage techniques. Both professionalism and ethics share the same principles of confidentiality, integrity, decency, accountability, responsibility, and honor. Massage professionals should possess psychosocial and humanistic qualities, such as caring, empathy, humility, compassion, social responsibility, and sensitivity to the culture, beliefs, and values of others.

Following this further, professionals must understand the principles beneath the codes, as no code of ethics can address every situation that massage practitioners will encounter. Next, let's examine other key principles of ethics, which include *autonomy, veracity, beneficence, nonmalfeasance, fidelity, justice,* and *confidentiality* (Burch, 2010).

Autonomy

Professionals have an obligation to uphold **autonomy**, which is respecting the rights of competent individuals to make their own decisions. Informed consent is largely based on principles of autonomy (informed consent is discussed in Chapter 10). Respecting autonomy requires professionals to honor the treatment decisions of clients. Professionals should not hinder these decisions unless acting on them is detrimental to the client or to society. An example is refusing to work in an endangerment site or when a contraindication is present (endangerment sites and contraindications are discussed in Chapter 8). Professionals who have clients with diminished autonomy (e.g., minors or people declared incompetent by a judge) require prior consent from parents or legal guardians/representatives.

Veracity

Veracity is the obligation to tell the truth. Veracity is rooted in autonomy because competent individuals base decisions largely on what professionals tell them, and to what degree. Veracity is concerned with the client's right to know the truth about the professional's credentials and about techniques, products, and procedures, including their risks and benefits. Veracity is violated by lying, exaggerating, deliberately withholding all or part of the truth, or deliberately cloaking information in language that would be easily misunderstood by or intentionally misleading to the client. Veracity includes the obligation of honesty in advertising.

Beneficence and Nonmalfeasance

Beneficence obligates professionals to act in ways that benefit the wellbeing of others. **Nonmalfeasance** requires professionals to "do no harm" and to act in ways that avoid harm. Both beneficence and nonmalfeasance mean professionals weigh the benefits of treatment against their potential risks before treatment is administered. Professionals may encounter situations where providing safe beneficial treatment may conflict with the client's autonomy. For example, being beneficent and nonmalfeasant requires that a practitioner discontinue treatment when it is determined that the client's skin is being damaged from hot stone massage, even if the client states the treatment should continue.

Fidelity

The principle of **fidelity** requires that professionals remain loyal and dedicated to clients, keep their promises, and honor their commitments. Fidelity includes promises and commitments made to individual clients and also to the public by practicing within the standards of care (standards of care is discussed in Chapter 10). Fidelity demands professionals continually update their knowledge and skills and avoid techniques that can injure clients.

Justice

Justice is the obligation to act on the basis of fairness, equality, and nondiscrimination. Justice seeks not to **discriminate**, which is unjust or prejudicial treatment of others based on a perceived difference (e.g., race, nationality, age, marital status, gender, gender identity, sexual orientation, religion, disability, cognitive reasoning, level of physical fitness, political affiliations, socioeconomic factors, pregnancy status, employment status, veteran status, immigration status, or history). Justice includes equitable access to care. Antidiscrimination laws vary by jurisdiction. Professionals should be familiar with the laws where they practice.

Confidentiality

Confidentiality refers to the obligation of professionals or professional organizations to safeguard entrusted information. This includes protecting information from unauthorized access, release, loss, theft, or modification. Fulfilling the duty of confidentiality is essential to building trust among professionals and between professionals and the public.

Client interviews should be conducted in private, never public, areas. Confidentiality also needs to be ensured within massage rooms; they should be soundproof, so people nearby cannot hear conversations in the room with the door shut.

Disclosing a client's identity is a violation of confidentiality. When receiving referrals from clients, avoid sharing client information about the common acquaintance with either client. This includes not disclosing when the other has an appointment, even when asked directly. Following this further, if a massage practitioner has two clients in a domestic partnership, the practitioner should refrain from answering questions from one about the other. Avoid answering even caring questions such as, "Was my spouse's neck range of motion better when you saw them yesterday?" Your reply might be, "Because of confidentiality I cannot share this information. I hope you understand," or "I can't answer, but they might."

In social settings where both practitioners and their clients are present, confidentiality is compromised when a practitioner initiates conversation with the client. The professional may make eye contact, smile, and give a nod of politeness. If the client initiates conversation, the practitioner should refrain from discussing treatment information. Because social settings exist in which both practitioners and their clients may be present, practitioners may wish to discuss these situations with clients in advance.

If clients instruct their massage practitioners to share information, practitioners may be obligated to do so. Clients have a right to have their records released to other service providers so complementary treatment plans can be developed. Clients may instruct practitioners to release their records to lawyers or insurance companies, or even translators to reduce language barriers. In these cases, obtain the client's dated signature on a release form before releasing their records (release forms are on Evolve under Chapter 10 resources). Know your state law regarding charging for copies of medical records.

The increasing use of computerized medical records, and the ease with which information can be accessed, is also an ethical concern, and is discussed in Chapter 10.

Limits to Confidentiality

There are some exceptions or limits to confidentiality. The code of ethics published by the National Certification Board for Therapeutic Massage and Bodywork (2017) states certificants will safeguard the confidentiality of all client information, unless disclosure is requested by the client in writing, is medically necessary, is required by law, or is necessary for the protection of the public. Confidentiality exceptions should be discussed with clients, perhaps during the initial visit when discussing informed consent and office policies. Ethical conflicts regarding confidentiality limits can be minimized by disclosing the type of information shared and with whom. Exceptions to confidentiality include *consultations, medical emergencies, court proceedings, insurance filing and billing, collections, responding to complaints,* and *child or elder abuse/neglect* (Fisher, 2018).

Consultations – Massage practitioners can consult with colleagues about their cases. Information shared should not include any identifying information about the client, and be done in a manner that preserves client anonymity from the consultant. Consultants are required to keep shared client information confidential.

Medical Emergencies – If a client is experiencing health problems making it difficult or impossible to obtain consent before releasing information to first responders, the practitioner may share client relevant information during medical emergencies.

Court Proceedings – If clients are involved in court proceedings and requests are made for client records, the practitioner may be legally required to release those records, and the client/practitioner relationship may not be privileged under state law. The ability to disclose the receipt of a subpoena, and the fact that there is an investigation, can vary. Read all of the paperwork attached to the subpoena and contact the issuer or your attorney before disclosing any information to anyone other than the issuer of the subpoena.

Insurance Filing and Billing – The practitioner may release client records if the practitioner is billing an insurance or workers' compensation company for services provided. Records usually include information regarding treatment, dates of service, and progress reports.

Collections – If collection action becomes necessary, practitioners can legally disclose client information to collection agencies or attorneys to help settle outstanding account balances. The practitioner must make reasonable attempts to collect outstanding balances before soliciting legal assistance. In these cases, information disclosed is limited to demographic information and dates of service, but not treatment notes or progress reports.

Responding to Complaints – Massage practitioners may disclose relevant information regarding client treatment to support professional judgments and actions when clients file complaints or lawsuits against practitioners. Little data is available regarding types of complaints made against massage practitioners. Lavery (2018, personal communication) noted most complaints involve one of the following issues: (1) fraudulent transcripts used to apply for licensure; (2) practicing without a license or with an expired license; (3) working outside scope of practice or standards of care; (4) fraudulent financial documentation, including bartering; (5) drug or alcohol use; (6) sexual misconduct, including draping and inappropriate touch; and (7) prostitution.

Child or Elder Abuse/Neglect – If practitioners suspect abuse or neglect of children, elderly, or incapacitated adults, they may be legally required to file a report and provide information to appropriate agencies. **Abuse** is any action by a person in a position of trust or power that causes harm to another person. **Neglect** is failure by a caregiver to provide necessary food, shelter, healthcare, or supervision to the person for whom they are caring. The legal requirement is called *mandatory reporting*. Mandatory reporting is discussed in Chapter 11.

THERAPEUTIC RELATIONSHIPS

The **therapeutic relationship** is the relationship between a practitioner and a client that allows practitioners to apply their professional knowledge and expertise to help clients achieve their treatment goals. This relationship protects a

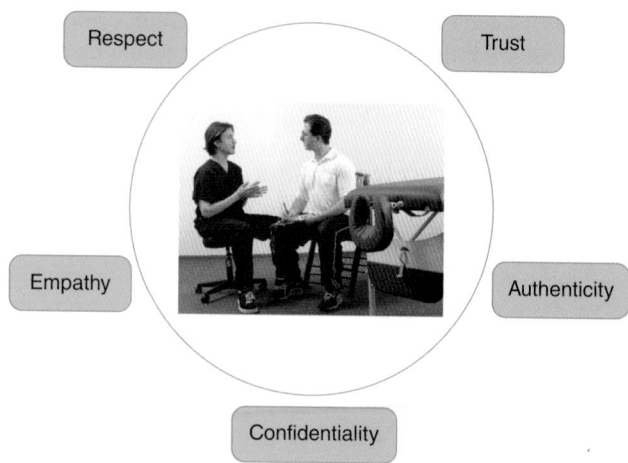

FIG. 2.1 Professional relationships: key principles of respect, authenticity, empathy, trust, and confidentiality.

client's dignity and provides a framework for ethical principles to be applied. Underlying principles of the relationship are respect, authenticity, empathy, trust, and confidentiality—the latter was previously discussed in the "Ethics" section (Sheldon & Foust, 2014). These principles are essential to the relationship, regardless of its length, which may range from a single session to a lifetime (Fig. 2.1). The therapeutic relationship is also called the *therapeutic alliance, helping alliance, working alliance,* or *therapeutic use of self.*

Respect

Respect is the ability to accept another person's beliefs despite your own personal feelings, and the choice to treat them with value and consideration. Respect can be given to yourself, to others, and to situations regardless of conflicting beliefs. Respect is exhibited through words and actions. It is important to remember clients bring their own way of responding to stress, pain, and injury, as well as to massage. Massage practitioners will encounter many clients, some with values and behaviors difficult for the practitioner to understand. For example, some clients may have personal hygiene standards different from the massage practitioner's standards, or political beliefs conflicting with the massage practitioner's beliefs.

In addition, practitioners may not understand why clients become sad or angry, but these feelings need to be acknowledged. In these situations, it is important the practitioner withhold judgment. When practitioners respect their clients, they accept them unconditionally as unique human beings, validating their humanity with their actions. Respect in the relationship is an acceptance of the client as a whole person—as the client is in that moment, and not how you want the client to be. Acceptance does not necessarily mean agreement; it means valuing and validating all thoughts, feelings, and beliefs without judgment. This validation has the potential to be deeply healing for clients. Psychologist Carl Rogers (1902–1987) called this *unconditional positive regard*, the acceptance of another person regardless of what they say or do. When we accept the whole person unconditionally, we validate and respect their humanity and accept them physically, mentally, spiritually, and emotionally.

We show respect when we take care of ourselves by making healthy choices, eating the right foods in the right amounts, exercising regularly, getting enough rest, expressing our emotions appropriately, and using proper body mechanics. We show respect for emotions when we acknowledge our feelings and the feelings of others. We show respect for privacy when we deliberately refrain from disclosing personal information. We show respect when we explain the who, how, why, and when of treatment. We show respect when we listen to clients and respond to their questions. We show respect when we modify pressure during the massage when requested by the client. We show respect by having and implementing professional boundaries. We show respect when we refer clients to appropriate healthcare providers as needed to help clients fulfill treatment goals. We show respect to our colleagues and to other healthcare providers by not denigrating them or their methods. We show respect to our profession and other professions by not performing services for which we are not licensed (such as joint manipulations, prescriptive exercise, or counseling, all of which are under the practice of chiropractic, physical or occupational therapy, and psychotherapy, respectively). We show respect by following our code of ethics and dutifully following laws that apply to the society in which we live. We show respect for people from other cultures by our willingness to learn about them and their customs, beliefs, and way they view the world.

Massage practitioners who are respectful take into account the client's preferences, expectations, predispositions, social and cultural values, and religious or spiritual beliefs when developing the plan of care, without inserting their own agenda. For example, when clients request a relaxation massage, avoid turning the session into a clinical massage, as this action would be disrespectful and invalidate the client's preference. Respect and unconditional positive regard also mean the practitioner accepts the client's progress or lack of progress.

Authenticity

Authenticity is the ability to be oneself while in a professional role. Rogers (1961) described this quality of the professional relationship as being open and congruent. Congruency occurs when the external presentation of your words and actions harmonize with your internal world of thoughts and feelings. When we are not exhibiting authenticity, others usually detect it and may feel we aren't being truthful, which can hurt the relationship. Being authentic means maintaining a conscious awareness of where our thoughts and attention are during the session. This heightened self-awareness and focused attention is called *mindfulness* (mindfulness is discussed in Chapter 7). We hold all feelings as normal, be it fear, anxiety, joy, peace, or boredom. We notice our own body, visceral sensations, breath patterns, and heart rate, and can modulate them when we are feeling

anxious. Mindfulness helps us develop qualities such as empathy, openness, acceptance, and compassion (Bruce et al., 2010). Authenticity is a part of professional behavior because it allows the integration of shared humanity into the relationship (Sheldon & Foust, 2014).

Empathy

Empathy is the desire to understand what another person is experiencing without mistaking it for your own experience. Empathy involves the ability to sense, accurately perceive, and appropriately respond to one's personal, interpersonal, and social environment. Empathy is educated compassion or intellectual understanding of another person's perspective and emotions (Sheldon & Foust, 2014). Cozolino (2006) added that professionals should keep their "own perspective in mind while simultaneously imagining what it is like to be the other. In order to have empathy, we need to maintain an awareness of our inner world as we imagine the inner world of others."

The term empathy comes from the German *Einfühlung*, which means "feeling into." The term described a deep and transformative feeling from looking at art, watching a theater production, or listening to music. The term was later used in psychosocial science to describe perspective-taking within relationships. Riess (2012) stated empathy can be taught and learned. Empathy also helps us live together in a multicultural society by reducing the emotional fight, flight, or freeze reaction that may occur when our viewpoints are challenged.

In contrast, **sympathy** is the commingling of your own feelings and the feelings of others without differentiation. Sympathy comes from the Latin *sympatheia*, which means "suffering together." Massage and bodywork professionals should avoid sympathy when providing client care, as emotional involvement may impair professional judgment.

One effective way to be culturally competent is to express empathy nonverbally. The nonverbal aspect of the techniques is important, as it transcends language and cultural barriers. Being mindful or aware of our own mental/emotional state and what we might be projecting is valuable and we should occasionally observe ourselves interacting with clients as if in the audience instead of as actors on the stage; this reflective activity is called the "witnessing self," "observing self," or the "balcony perspective."

Rogers (1961) thought it was important for professionals to express empathy nonverbally when interacting with clients.

So how can massage practitioners express empathy? Riess and Kraft-Todd (2014) identified seven essential nonverbal empathetic behaviors, and created the acronym **E-M-P-A-T-H-Y**. to help professionals remember them (E - Eye contact; M - muscles of facial expression; P - posture; A - affect; T - tone of voice; H - hearing the whole person; and Y - your response). These are briefly discussed next.

E: Eye Contact

Make meaningful eye contact right away with the client. Consider making a mental note of the client's eye color.

Once eye contact is established, hold it for 4 to 5 seconds, slowly glance to the side, and reestablish eye contact. Consider using the 50/70 rule. Maintain eye contact for 50% of the time while *speaking* and 70% of the time while *listening*. This action conveys interest and will keep eye contact from being perceived as staring. Be sure to blink normally. In addition, limit the amount of time looking at electronic devices such as computers, mobile phones, and smartwatches. If you must look at your device, explain to the client why you are doing it, then put it away after its use and give the client your undivided attention. Be aware that in some Eastern and Caribbean cultures, eye contact may be perceived as aggression or disrespect. In other cultures and some religions, long eye contact between two people may be perceived as flirtatious. In contrast, some cultures avoid eye contact with persons in an authoritative role as a sign of respect. However, in the United States, Canada, and most of Europe, professional eye contact is appropriate and necessary in professional relationships. Finally, keep in mind that eye contact may be difficult or uncomfortable for some people, such as those who are neurodiverse (i.e., persons with autism or neurologic atypical behaviors), or who have experienced trauma. Always respect the client's choice to look elsewhere while you focus your attention on them.

M: Muscles of Facial Expression

Look at the clients' facial expression and mimic this expression to some degree. Ask yourself "What is my client feeling?" Empathy is largely based on the ability to decode facial expressions. There is extensive literature on the seven basic facial expressions of universal emotions: surprise, fear, disgust, anger, happiness, sadness, and contempt/hate. By studying faces, we cannot tell what people are thinking, only what they are feeling about what they are thinking.

P: Posture

Postures send powerful signals of approach or avoidance. When conversing with clients, mimic their posture. If they are seated, sit down. If they are standing, stand up. Avoid standing while clients are seated, as this demonstrates dominance. Express respect and social/emotional openness by using an open posture, which includes facing clients at eye level, head erect or slightly side-tilted, shoulders back, and hands apart. While sitting, hands on the arms of the chair conveys interest in and time for clients. In contrast, closed posture may involve arms folded, legs crossed, and the body positioned at a slight angle. Closed postures convey disinterest or even discomfort.

A: Affect

Affect is expressed emotion. While listening, try to determine clients' affect or what they are feeling, such as happiness, fear, apprehension, or sadness. Making a mental note of the person's emotional state deepens empathy. Remember, empathy is the *desire to understand* another person's experience.

T: Tone of Voice

Note the client's tone of voice. Mimic their voice tone initially, and then modulate yours to convey warmth, concern, and curiosity. The voice is a window into emotions, because the area of the brain that receives and interprets sounds and facial expressions is the same area that generates fight or flight reactions (Chapter 23). This means when we are stressed out, our voice and facial expression mirrors the experience—other people can literally hear and see our emotions.

H: Hearing the Whole Person

Listen intently and curiously while suspending judgment until you understand the other person's perspective. When you hear the whole person, you are putting all information gathered into context. Ask, what is the client asking for or trying to convey? Are they frustrated and need to vent? Do they just need to be heard? Is there a deeper concern ("I need home care suggestions on how to reduce stress"), beyond their chief complaint ("I need a relaxing massage")?

Y: Your Response

Note how you are responding. We often mirror each other's feelings so if you are feeling calm, it will help your client to feel calm. If you are feeling anxious, take a few slow deep breaths to calm yourself. Field (2012) noted that nervous systems synchronize when we empathize. Expressing empathy will be easier if you are calm and can manage emotions such as anger. Responding calmly when communicating with clients will ultimately improve rapport.

Empathy is increasingly important as our society becomes more culturally diverse and multilingual. We may also find, through nonverbal empathic behaviors, practitioners experience beneficial effects such as reduced risk of burnout and increased career longevity.

Trust

Trust is confidence in and reliance upon others, whether individuals or organizations, to act in accordance with accepted social, ethical, or legal norms. Erikson (1963) described trust as the reliance on consistency, sameness, and continuity of experiences that are familiar and predictable. Trust is established by verbal communication and by nonverbal empathic behaviors mentioned previously. Trust is the foundation of all relationships and is essential when individuals are placed in vulnerable situations. Clients need to view their practitioner as someone who is trustworthy as well as knowledgeable, honest, dependable, open to the client's concerns, and accepting of who they are as people.

In addition, clients will be more forthcoming and honest in their disclosures if they feel disclosures are held in confidence. Client disclosures lead to clearer communication and better identification of treatment goals, which may result in improved outcomes. Trust is increased and reinforced by favorable outcomes and when the client's expectations are fulfilled or exceeded.

Trust can be easily upset by important issues as well as by seemingly insignificant things. For example, it is best not to tell clients they can call you anytime. Although you may be sincere in wanting to help, you may be uncomfortable receiving a call at 3:00 AM. A careless statement may mislead the client and weaken trust.

When we work from a place of compassion, it is a place of non-judgment, non-comparison, without the need to understand. With compassion we are not entrained in the drama of the client's story, we are just with them.
~ **Fritz Frederick Smith**

CULTURAL COMPETENCY

To build empathy and trust, practitioners must be aware of their own culture as well as the cultures of their clients and coworkers, and display competency, inclusion, and respect diversity during intercultural interactions. **Culture** is an accumulated pattern of values, beliefs, and behaviors shared by an identifiable group of people with a common history and verbal and nonverbal symbol systems. **Cultural competency** is a set of behaviors, attitudes, and policies enabling professionals to interact effectively with others in cross-cultural situations (Denboba et al., 1998). **Intercultural communication** is communication between people of different cultures and ethnicities. **Intercultural communication competency** is the degree to which you can effectively adapt verbal and nonverbal messages to the appropriate cultural context. These processes require you to have some awareness and knowledge about the person's culture with whom you are communicating, with whom you are motivated to communicate, and that you have the appropriate verbal and nonverbal skills to understand messages during the encounter. Cultural competency and intercultural communication competence acknowledge that individuals are unique; this allows clients to hold their own beliefs, characteristics, and cultural practices. This process involves adopting behaviors that honor a client's right to the highest quality of care apart from religious, cultural, or personal beliefs or other characteristics listed in the previous section titled "Justice." Statements reflecting cultural incompetency include:

- "If they want to come to America, then they need to live by our culture."
- "If she had not gained all this weight, none of this would have happened. I do not feel sorry for her."
- "It's just a sprain; I have known people with worse pain."
- "She should have used common sense. She brought it on herself and now has HIV infection."
- "If you do not want a male practitioner giving you a massage, then go to another clinic."
- "It is against my religion to massage a transgender person. I just think it is wrong. God wouldn't want it."

Professionals cannot simply be tolerant of cultural differences, as tolerance has both positive and negative aspects. *Positive tolerance* is open acceptance of differences and the

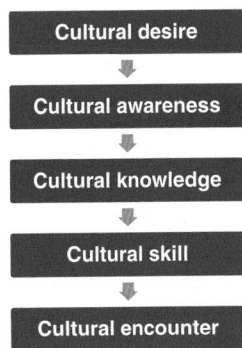

FIG. 2.2   Model of cultural competency. This diagram outlines five milestones toward cultural competency based on the work of Campinha-Bacote (2002).

ability to empathize and value another person's differences; this demonstrates cultural competence. However, *negative tolerance* is tolerance that grudgingly accepts differences because there is no choice in the matter (Boatwright, 2014). Thoughts or statements such as, "The clinic has a policy to ensure I care for you. I will follow it, but I will not like it," demonstrates negative tolerance. This suggests your thoughts and beliefs are the only correct ones, or **ethnocentrism**, and demonstrates a lack of acceptance, acknowledgment, or respect for cultural and ethnic differences. At the other end of cultural competency is intolerance. *Intolerance* is the unwillingness to accept the views, beliefs, or behaviors that differ from one's own. Culturally competent practitioners know that culture matters, and they are good at relating to people from other cultures.

Many microcultures exist in the United States. The formation of microculture groups is often because of immigration, occupation, or colonization. These include Hispanic/Latinx; Black Americans; Asian Americans; Native Americans/American Indians/Indigenous Peoples; Arab Americans; and Lesbian, Gay, Transgender, and Queer/Questioning Americans. Hispanics/Latinx is the largest microculture.

Campinha-Bacote (2002) developed a model of five milestones that views cultural competence as an ongoing process in which healthcare practitioners continuously strive toward working effectively in cross-cultural environments by valuing and responding appropriately to cultural differences. The milestones are: (1) cultural desire; (2) cultural awareness; (3) cultural knowledge; (4) cultural skill; and (5) cultural encounters (Fig. 2.2). Although not in order, the acronym A-S-K-E-D will help remember the milestones of cultural competence. **A-S-K-E-D** stands for **A**wareness, **S**kill, **K**nowledge, **E**ncounter, and **D**esire. Next is a brief discussion of each milestone.

Cultural Desire

Practitioners must be motivated to become culturally competent—it should not be forced or coerced.

Cultural Awareness

Cultural awareness is conducting a self-exploration and examination of one's own cultural and professional background and biases toward other cultures, including the existence of xenophobia (prejudice of people from other countries), racism (prejudice of people from different races), and other forms of cultural phobias and "-isms." Prejudiced individuals may not act on their biased attitude. This means someone can be prejudiced towards a certain group but not discriminate against them. Discrimination involves unjust or prejudicial treatment.

Cultural Knowledge

This is acquiring information about culturally diverse groups and, since this model applies to healthcare settings, cultural knowledge includes gathering information about cultural beliefs and values regarding health and health-related practices as well as medical statistics such as incidence and prevalence rates related to a client's condition.

Cultural Skill

This is the ability to collect culturally relevant information about the client's presenting concern, as well as performing culturally-sensitive assessments and integrating this information into the treatment plan.

Cultural Encounter

Practitioners are encouraged to engage in face-to-face interactions with people from culturally diverse backgrounds to potentially modify existing beliefs about cultural groups and prevent possible stereotyping. Cultural encounters provide the impetus to continue the journey toward cultural competence.

Cultural competency does not happen overnight; it is a carefully thought-out learning process. We each have prejudices and beliefs that may impede cultural competency. We must empathize and respond compassionately and empathetically when interacting with clients from other cultures. Professionals must be vigilant in curbing tone or body gestures demonstrating cultural incompetency. Examples of common issues that may arise include the appropriateness of eye contact and handshakes, or the need to include spouses and/or family members in decision-making. Massage practitioners do not need to know everything or be perfect, but do need to demonstrate cultural competence when interacting with individuals from diverse cultural backgrounds within our communities.

LGBTQ+ Communities and Cultural Competency

Cultural competency, diversity, and inclusion extend to the lesbian, gay, bisexual, transgender, and queer or questioning (LGBTQ+) community. The plus sign (+) is a symbol of recognition for current and emerging subgroups such as asexual, gender variants, or allies within the LGBTQ+ community.

The plus sign can also include those who are intersex, but it is important to recognize that being intersex, transgender, or other LGBTQ+ identities are not mutually exclusive. LGBTQ+ persons can be of any age, sex, race, ethnicity, nationality, religion, occupation, socioeconomic status, or other demographic group. The distinguishing cultural trait among LGBTQ+ community members is sexual orientation and/or gender identity.

What does LGBTQ+ mean? Here are a few terms and definitions to facilitate mutual understanding (Human Rights Campaign, n.d.; Stonewall, 2017a). These terms will be used throughout this section. Their correct use shows respect, and enables the practitioner to provide the best possible care for the client. These terms will change over time as our understanding of them evolves, and individuals may identify themselves in different ways during different stages of their journey.

- **Ally (Straight Ally).** Someone who is cisgender or heterosexual and supports equal rights, gender equality, and LGBTQ+ social movements, challenging homophobia, biphobia, and transphobia.
- **Bisexual (Bi).** Someone who has a romantic and/or physical attraction to more than one sex, gender, or gender identity, though not necessarily simultaneously, in the same way, or to the same degree.
- **Cisgender (Cis).** Someone whose gender identity is the same as the sex they were assigned at birth. Some individuals also use the term "non-trans."
- **Gay.** A male who has a romantic and/or physical attraction toward males. This term is also used by lesbians and non-binary people to describe same-sex attraction and further to identify with the LGBTQ+ community.
- **Intersex.** A person who is born with both or neither biologic attributes, reproductive organs, or sexual anatomy of males and females. Intersex people may identify as any of the terms within the LGBTQ+ community, or may choose not to identify with the community.
- **Lesbian.** A female who has romantic and/or physical attraction toward females. Non-binary people may also use this term to describe themselves.
- **Nonbinary.** People who do not identify with the binary genders of male or female. Non-binary people may identify as being both a man and a woman, somewhere in between, or as falling completely outside these categories. Although many also identify as transgender, not all nonbinary people do. Nonbinary people may also at times feel gender-fluid with shifts in their identity at various points in their life.
- **Queer.** Umbrella term for people within the LGBTQ+ community who fall under any of the identities and orientations counter to the mainstream. While the word was previously used as a homophobic slur, it has been reclaimed by LGBTQ+ people who now embrace it and use it to reject previous stigmas. This can also include the term "genderqueer."
- **Trans Female.** Someone whose assigned gender at birth was male but identifies and lives as a female. This can also include the terms male to female (MtF), assigned male at birth (AMAB), trans woman, or trans feminine.
- **Trans Male.** Someone whose assigned gender at birth was female but identifies and lives as a male. This can also include the terms female to male (FtM), assigned female at birth (AFAB), trans man, or trans masculine.

- **Transgender (Trans)**. Someone whose gender is not the same as the sex they were assigned at birth. Being transgender does not imply any specific sexual orientation. Therefore, transgender people may identify as straight, gay, lesbian, bisexual, etc. Transgender is also used to signify a range of identities, including but not limited to nonbinary and gender-fluid.

As with any demographic, LGBTQ+ people have specific and prevalent pathologies. They are more likely to experience mental health issues, with nearly 50% of transgender people having experienced suicidal ideations. In physical health, LGBTQ+ people are more likely to develop physical issues such as obesity, cancers, and cardiovascular diseases compared with the general population (Hafeez et al., 2017).

Although many strides have been made, there still remains a large stigma attached to "coming out." Transgender and nonbinary individuals have only recently become a gender marker in some countries, but not all. Numbers we do have do not account for those unable to express their sexuality and gender for fear of retribution or discrimination. Indeed, studies on experiences of homophobic and transphobic hate crimes indicate they are rising in the US and the UK, which may be reasons why LGBTQ+ individuals may feel unsafe in disclosing information (Bradley, 2020; Ronan, 2020; Stonewall, 2017b).

Gender dysphoria is experienced by many, but not all, transgender and nonbinary people. *Gender dysphoria* is a series of symptoms experienced by someone whose biologic sex and gender identity do not match. It is characterized by high levels of uneasiness and anxiety around physical presentation of the body. Gender dysphoria can lead to anxiety, depression, isolation, and issues of bodily dissociation and rejection of the physical body. Massage can positively impact gender dysphoria through empathetic nonjudgmental touch. Guidelines when working with clients who have or may have gender dysphoria are:

- If your client opens up to you about their identity, ask about how they experience gender dysphoria in terms of massage. This will help to identify where the client feels dysphoria the most, and its severity. For example, a trans male client may feel dysphoric about their chest, but not their back. Use this as a starting point for discussing where they would and wouldn't feel comfortable receiving a massage.
- Being mindful of hand placement during the massage. For example, areas associated with dysphoria are not only sensitive and a source of anxiety, but the areas surrounding them may be also. Recognize this and verbalize the boundary by statements such as "I'm just coming around into your waist, but going no higher there. Does that feel okay?"

Secondly, clients may be experiencing physical pain in response to attempts to reduce dysphoria. For example, clients who are trans men may be using binders to compress the chest muscles. This can create significant tension in the upper torso, the neck, and jaw. Another example is trans female clients who may alter their body posture to accentuate their femininity. This may lead to pain in the quadratus lumborum. Discussing this with clients allows them to feel safe and able to say where their tension is located.

There are studies which document LGBTQ+ youth growing up and facing discrimination as a form of childhood trauma. This may lead to posttraumatic stress disorder in this population. See Chapter 15 in *Mosby's Pathology for Massage Professionals* to learn more about PTSD and how to modify the massage for these clients.

How to Create a LGBTQ+ Inclusive Practice

It is important to reduce barriers for LGBTQ+ individuals so everyone has equal access to high-quality care (Box 2.1). Indeed, clients who are LGBTQ+ may not feel comfortable disclosing information relating to their health and body. To reduce this barrier, practitioners must create an environment which understands the specific health needs of LGBTQ+ people and empowers them to feel safe enough to come into our practices and share their health information. There are a number of ways in which this can be achieved.

LGBTQ+ individuals report they often search for subtle cues to determine acceptance. For example, display LGBTQ+-friendly symbols such as rainbows or pink triangles, and post a nondiscrimination statement that includes gender identity and sexual orientation. If you decide to use symbols in your office, be sure to have the cultural knowledge to follow it up, as that could potentially lead to a traumatic experience for LGBTQ+ clients. Add information in your profiles, websites, and social media platforms that you are LGBTQ+ inclusive and welcoming (American Medical Association [AMA], n.d.; Ard & Makadon, n.d.; Eliason & Schope 2001). It is important these clients see you as someone with whom it is safe to share information. Other recommendations include:

- **Gender-neutral bathrooms**. Mark single-occupancy bathrooms as gender-neutral, or post a sign stating all are welcome to use the bathroom stall of their choice if your business has only female and male bathrooms.
- **Revise client intake forms**. Include a space for preferred pronouns, which range from she/her/hers, he/him/his, to genderless pronouns such as they/them. Include a space for clients to indicate their preferred names, as those may be different from their legal names or the names on insurance policies. Use their preferred names and pronouns during conversations. A LGBTQ+ intake form is on Evolve under Chapter 10 resources. Include boxes for information around hormone treatments or gender reassignment surgeries. This option allows people to share or not share information that is often deeply personal.
- **Use gender-neutral draping, language, and scents**. Drape all clients the same way (see Chapter 7). Consider your language in the massage room. Chest, not breast. Sides, not hips. Have neutral or unscented options in massage products, and allow clients to make scent-related choices.
- **Learn about gender reassignment procedures**. If the client is taking feminizing or masculinizing hormone

---

BOX 2.1

In the Service of Life

In recent years the question "How can I help?" has become meaningful to many people. But perhaps there is a deeper question we might consider. Perhaps the real question is not how can I help, but how can I serve?

Serving is different from helping. Helping is based on inequality; it is not a relationship between equals. When you help, you use your own strength to help those of lesser strength. If I am attentive to what is going on inside of me when I am helping, I find I am always helping someone who is not as strong as I am, who is needier than I am. People feel this inequality. When we help, we may inadvertently take away from people more than we could ever give them; we may diminish their self-esteem, their sense of worth, integrity, and wholeness. When I help, I am very aware of my own strength. But we do not serve with our strength; we serve with ourselves. We draw from all of our experiences. Our limitations serve, our wounds serve, even our darkness can serve. The wholeness in us serves the wholeness in others and the wholeness in life. The wholeness in you is the same as the wholeness in me.

Helping incurs debt. When you help someone, they owe you one. But serving, like healing, is mutual. There is no debt. I am as served as the person I am serving. When I help, I have a feeling of satisfaction. When I serve, I have a feeling of gratitude. These are very different things.

Serving is also different from fixing. When I fix a person, I perceive them as broken, and their brokenness requires me to act. When I fix, I do not see the wholeness in the other person or trust the integrity of the life in them. When I serve, I see and trust that wholeness. It is what I am responding to and collaborating with.

There is distance between ourselves and whatever or whomever we are fixing. Fixing is a form of judgment. All judgment creates distance, a disconnection, an experience of difference. In fixing, there is an inequality of expertise that can easily become a moral distance. We cannot serve at a distance. We can only serve to which we are profoundly connected, which we are willing to touch. This is Mother Teresa's basic message. We serve life not because it is broken but because it is holy.

If helping is an experience of strength, fixing is an experience of mastery and expertise. Service, on the other hand, is an experience of mystery, surrender, and awe. A fixer has the illusion of being causal. A server knows he or she is being used and has a willingness to be used in the service of something greater, something essentially unknown. Fixing and helping are very personal; they are very particular, concrete, and specific. We fix and help many different things in our lifetimes. But when we serve, we are always serving the same thing. Everyone who has ever served through the history of time serves the same thing. We are servers of the wholeness and mystery in life.

The bottom line, of course, is we can fix without serving. And we can help without serving. And we can serve without fixing or helping. I think I would go so far as to say fixing and helping may often be the work of the ego, and service the work of the soul. They may look similar if you are watching from the outside, but the inner experience is different. The outcome is often different, too.

Our service serves us as well as others. That which uses us strengthens us. Over time, fixing and helping are draining and depleting. Over time we burn out. Service is renewing. When we serve, our work itself will sustain us.

Service rests on the basic premise: the nature of life is sacred, life is a holy mystery which has an unknown purpose. When we serve, we know we belong to life and to that purpose.

Fundamentally, helping, fixing, and service are ways of seeing life. When you help, you see life as weak. When you fix, you see life as broken. When you serve, you see life as whole. From the perspective of service, we are all connected: All suffering is like my suffering and all joy is like my joy. The impulse to serve emerges naturally and inevitably from this way of seeing.

Lastly, fixing and helping are the basis of curing but not of healing. In 40 years of chronic illness I have been helped by many and fixed by a great many others who did not recognize my wholeness. All fixing and helping left me wounded in some important and fundamental ways. Only service heals.

By Rachel Naomi Remen, M. D. "In the Service of Life," adapted from a talk given by Rachel Naomi Remen at IONS fourth annual conference, first appeared in the Noetic Sciences Review (Spring 1996, issue number 37), published by the Institute of Noetic Sciences (IONS), and is reprinted with permission of IONS (www.noetic.org), all rights reserved. Copyright 1996.

---

therapy, ask about routes of administration and side effects. Chapter 3 in *Mosby's Pathology for Massage Professionals* discusses gonadal hormones. If the client is having or has had gender reassignment surgeries, the usual contraindications apply (see Chapter 14). Be aware that some surgical scars are previous sites of gender dysphoria. Show compassion and consideration when working in these areas, and always obtain consent.

PROFESSIONAL BOUNDARIES

The therapeutic relationship exists to meet the needs of clients while providing them with safe, effective, and competent care. **Professional boundaries** are the spaces between the practitioner's power and the client's vulnerability. Power comes from the practitioner's position, knowledge, and access to client information. In contrast, clients know (or should know) little about their practitioners. This imbalance of power is called the **power differential**, the inherently greater power and influence that helping professionals (i.e., practitioners) have compared to the people they help (i.e., clients). Massage clients arrive at their appointments looking for help, often seeking reduction of pain or stress, and hoping for improved function. Massage practitioners use their knowledge, skills, and abilities to address client needs. Vulnerability may be accentuated when clients lie down, often undressed and draped, while their practitioners stand fully clothed over them.

Massage practitioners should make every effort to respect the power imbalance and use their position of greater power to serve clients. This is accomplished through setting and respecting healthy boundaries. Boundaries also protect a client's integrity and foster predictability with repeat sessions—boundaries promote trust.

Problems can arise when practitioners do not acknowledge or are uncomfortable with this power. New practitioners may not view themselves as powerful. There may be a belief that practitioners and clients are equals because of the collaboration that occurs during treatment planning, but even during collaboration, practitioners are still in the position of power. Not accepting and respecting this power can make it difficult for practitioners to maintain boundaries.

Boundaries are important, both legally and ethically. The law holds professionals to a higher standard of behavior because of the power imbalance. Strategies for maintaining professional boundaries are: (1) have clearly defined roles and responsibilities, including who can participate in the relationship; (2) establish clear boundaries between yourself and others; (3) develop and follow a treatment plan; (4) recognize that different cultures and ethnic groups may have varying rules for interactions and that these rules must be factored into professional decisions and actions; (5) meet personal needs outside of the practitioner/client relationship; (6) develop self-awareness; and (7) create and follow a self-care plan. Self-care is discussed in Chapter 4.

Self-awareness allows practitioners to identify their thoughts and feelings and to discern which are their own and which belong to their clients. Self-awareness allows practitioners to recognize signs and symptoms of emotional exhaustion, compassion fatigue, burnout, and over-involvement with a client. Self-awareness fosters balanced use and alignment of our professional and personal lives, allowing practitioners to be genuine—an essential characteristic of the relationship discussed previously.

Professional relationships are not places to have personal needs met. Doing so opens the door to dual relationships (where more than one role exists), transference (when a client transfers feelings and behaviors from the past into the present relationship), and countertransference (same principle as transference, except the direction is reversed—from practitioner to client), which can occur when practitioners lack self-awareness. Dual relationships, transference, and countertransference are discussed later in this chapter.

Clients often want to know who their practitioners are as people. Clients may be disclosing personal information to their practitioners, and may feel more comfortable knowing something about the person with whom they are engaging in a professional relationship. This curiosity may lead clients to ask personal questions. Revealing thoughts, feelings, and personal history to clients is called **self-disclosure**. There is a fine line between disclosing too much and too little. This topic is much debated among professionals. Many scholars in the fields of psychotherapy, medicine, ethics, and massage recommend we disclose little about our personal selves; we are a blank slate so the relationship can center on the client. Others argue that giving clients some personal information helps them relax and feel comfortable, knowing we are human. Personal information that might be appropriate to share is how long we have lived in the area and why we moved there. Clients often want to know about our family. A small degree of information sharing is generally considered appropriate.

However, too much self-disclosure or inappropriate self-disclosure can be confusing for clients, especially if practitioners disclose their own current needs or problems without a clear connection to the client's goals. Especially important is not disclosing personal experiences related to a similar problem your client is having. This type of self-disclosure may lead clients to minimize their own experience and perceive your experience as more significant because of the power differential. For example, if your client is grieving after the death of a parent and you share your own experience of a parent who died the previous year, the client may feel overly concerned about your feelings and discontinue talking about their grief. This may prevent a client from having needs met because they are more concerned with taking care of you. Too much self-disclosure can also lead to transference (see "Emotional Boundaries").

When disclosing personal information, consider your reason for doing so. Does it serve the relationship, the client, or you? Does it create boundary issues? One clear sign it is not in your client's best interest is when you self-disclose to satisfy your own social needs. Finally, ask yourself if you are disclosing personal information without realizing it. Social media makes our personal lives more accessible to clients. Are you disclosing more than intended? What would clients find if they did a Google search on you? How will you respond to a client's friend request on Facebook, Snapchat, Instagram, Twitter, or some other social media account? How will a client respond to seeing you at a party? Or on vacation skiing? Or wearing revealing clothing? Could transference be inflamed? What might happen if clients see you doing something that does not fit with their views of you as a practitioner? How will they feel or react if they see you support a group or viewpoint they disagree with? All of the information about you online is available for your clients to see.

There is a difference between crossing a boundary and violating a boundary. *Crossing a boundary* involves actions supporting the client's treatment plan or health and wellbeing, culturally welcomed by the client, motivated by the client's best interests, and considered professionally appropriate and acceptable. For example, offering to hug a grieving client to express empathy is considered acceptable. *Violating a boundary* involves actions unwelcomed by the client, motivated by the practitioner's personal needs or desires, and that may be harmful to the client. The practitioner must also consider the client's history when determining appropriate professional behaviors; hugging a client who has a history of sexual abuse is inappropriate professional behavior (Shallcross, 2011).

Physical Boundaries

Physical boundaries represent circumstances under which practitioners physically touch and massage their clients; this includes the who, what, when, where, why, and how of physical contact. It should be noted that physical boundaries and physical contact are the most controversial boundaries of all, as they can cross into emotional boundaries. When obtaining consent for treatment, practitioners should inform their clients about the areas massaged or avoided, and about techniques likely used to address treatment goals. Other aspects of physical boundaries include:

- Letting clients choose the level of disrobing.
- Employing best practices with regard to how clients are draped and how the drape is moved.
- Refraining from working under a drape.
- Exercising professional judgment with regard to how deep or how long areas are massaged.
- Using only hands or forearms to massage the client. Massage practitioners should not allow other parts of their body to come into contact with the client during the massage; they should be mindful when leaning over the client. Exceptions are massage methods using other areas of the practitioner's body such as feet and knees (e.g., barefoot shiatsu, ashiatsu, Thai massage).
- Empowering clients to speak up if they feel uncomfortable with anything or want to make a change.

Physical Boundaries: Hugs Between Clients and Practitioners

There is plenty of debate regarding hugs between practitioners and clients. Massage practitioners are expected to be empathetic with their clients in ways to support the client's health and wellness. Most nursing and mental healthcare guidelines regarding hugs suggest not initiating a hug. If the client requests a hug, the practitioner should evaluate its appropriateness from the standpoint of what is in the best interest of the client, and balance this assessment with the potential risk to the practitioner.

In some cases, a client-initiated hug is safe and appropriate—the hug is given without harm. But what if the hug was perceived by the client as sexual, longer than the client wanted or expected, or if the practitioner's hands or body were not where the client expected them to be, or if the hug was too tight and experienced as painful or even frightening? The practitioner takes a risk when touching a client in a way that isn't required or part of the treatment plan. Laws protect individuals who receive unwanted touch even with prior consent. If practitioners want to be safe legally, they should consider not hugging their clients. If the practitioner wants to respond empathetically to a client-initiated hug, give the hug but realize the associated risks (Buppert, 2014). Suggestions include ensuring that the client is completely dressed, that no hugs are given while the client is on the massage table, that the door is open, and that the hug is delivered briefly as a side hug with no frontal body contact.

In addition, practitioners are not required to hug their clients. Massage practitioners who decide not to hug their clients can nonverbally discourage hugs from clients by several methods, such as holding a clipboard when greeting clients, or standing or sitting behind a desk or counter when clients exit the massage room.

Emotional Boundaries

Emotional boundaries involve the capacity to be aware of, to control, and to express one's emotions. They also involve identifying which emotions are yours, which ones are not yours, and keeping these feelings separate. Feelings of trust can grow in the relationship when clients feel they can express their feelings in a safe, supportive, and nonjudgmental environment, and when their practitioners understand them and accept them for who they are and how they feel. Keep in mind that emotions and touch are often interconnected as mentioned previously; clients may have an emotional reaction to touch. Client emotional reactions to touch include crying and transference. Countertransference, a practitioner's unconscious emotional reaction toward clients, is also discussed in this section.

Emotional Boundaries: Emotional Reactions and Crying

Crying is a universal human experience and a tool to communicate emotions. Clients may cry to express current or suppressed emotions—some clients may not know why they are crying. Changes in hormones, stress, and sleep deprivation have been linked to increased crying episodes. Clients in counseling or psychotherapy are more likely to cry. In these events, it is appropriate to discuss how these situations will be addressed if and when they occur. Keep in mind how crying is perceived, and that the degree to which it is accepted varies across genders and cultures. For example, females report crying more often compared with males (Vingerhoets & Scheirs, 2000). Crying is more accepted in Western cultures and less accepted in Eastern cultures.

The safety of the relationship and the relaxation experienced during massage may facilitate emotional reactions. For example, a client may suppress feelings of grief over the death of a loved one too painful to bear at the time, but which are expressed as crying during the massage. A guiding principle regarding emotional reactions and crying in professional relationships is an attitude of compassion and to "seek not, forbid not." When the client becomes tearful or begins to cry, it is within our scope of practice to make empathetic statements and gestures to reassure the client you accept them unconditionally. Here are a few suggestions.

- When the client begins to cry, pause the massage and do not break physical contact.
- Use compassionate statements such as, "Crying is normal," "You are in a safe place," "I am comfortable with your tears." While the client is crying, it may be appropriate to rest a hand on the client's shoulder as a gesture of empathy (Fig. 2.3).

When clients stop crying, help them acclimate to their surroundings with statements such as, "Take a few deep

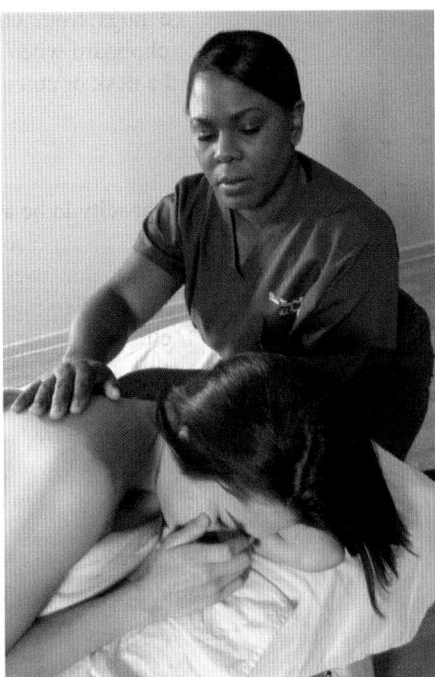

FIG. 2.3   If you take a break from the massage and remain in the room while the client is crying, it may be appropriate to rest a hand on the client's shoulder as a gesture of empathy.

breaths," and "Feel the massage table beneath you." Use statements that feel comfortable to you. Ask if they want to continue with the massage, take a break from the massage, or stop the massage before the scheduled time. Regardless of which option is chosen, be calm and accepting, and avoid encouraging or discouraging a particular response. The client may feel confused. If the client asks for an explanation of what happened, state only what you observed without your own interpretations or conclusions.

Note that clients may feel embarrassed or ashamed after crying and may choose not to return to your office for a massage. Their decision must be respected.

When a client has an emotional release such as crying, massage practitioners need to have a solid understanding and impeccable boundaries regarding the types of help they offer a client. Legal statutes do a good job of outlining scope of practice. Be absolutely sure that treatments, advice, and focus are on the soft tissues of the body. We can recognize the imprint that thoughts, feelings, and emotions make on the structures of the body, but we should refrain from engaging in conversations or exercises that address the human psyche directly. It is not within our scope of practice to do the following:

- Encourage clients to share emotional content.
- Process the emotions.
- Delve for deeper-held emotions.
- Offer unsolicited "insights."
- Intentionally evoke emotional responses in the client.

Whenever the focus of massage becomes more about the client's emotions than about the client's body, a boundary has been crossed. Another reason we do not cross emotional boundaries is that massage practitioners are not trained to differentiate between emotional experiences that are helpful to clients and those that are harmful. There is mounting evidence that cathartic therapies may feel good in the moment, but have no lasting benefits for the mental health and well-being of the client and may be harmful to the healing process by causing additional trauma. Unless the practitioner has obtained the appropriate education and licensure in professions such as psychotherapy and counseling, massage practitioners are not trained to differentiate between which emotional experiences may be helpful or harmful. A massage practitioner's scope of practice does not allow for the intentional eliciting or processing of emotions. When clients share their emotional concerns with their massage practitioners, the practitioner should act to bring the focus back to the body by using questions such as, "Where do you feel that in your body?" or "Can you tell me what you notice in your body as you say that?"

Clients may feel self-conscious and embarrassed during or after crying, even while feeling safe within the relationship. Recall a time you have cried unexpectedly in front of someone. How did you feel? Were you concerned the person would judge you or think less of you? Because of these feelings, clients may choose not to reschedule or return to your office for a massage. Their decision must be respected.

Refrain from mentioning a crying incident to a client during subsequent sessions, unless the client brings it up. However, do obtain verbal consent before working on areas that led to the expressed emotions. For example, if a client began to cry during a foot massage, obtain consent before working on the feet during the next session. In addition, avoid mentioning the emotional reactions when obtaining consent, as this action demonstrates respect for emotional boundaries.

Emotional Boundaries: Transference

Transference occurs when a client *transfers* or projects feelings and behaviors they have for someone onto an entirely different person. In the professional relationship, transference occurs when the practitioner assumes a different role in the client's life, more than just someone providing massage services. The assigned feelings and behaviors can be positive (love, affection, adoration, worship) or negative (hatred, hostility, aggression, jealousy). They can also grow as your feelings toward the person grow.

Transference may occur when needs that are not being met in the client's personal life are now being met in the professional relationship. These needs include the need for physical contact, focused attention, being listened to, and validation. Vulnerability may facilitate transference, as can unresolved events in a client's life.

Transference, in essence, is the "casting of roles." For example, if the practitioner reminds the client of their father and they act on these feelings, the client may start behaving inappropriately. The behaviors depend on the type of relationship clients have/had with the father. Was the relationship loving and nurturing, or was it filled with violence and abandonment? During positive transference, the client may bring the practitioner cookies their father liked, and want to be treated as a special child/client, such as spending extra time on them or scheduling appointments outside normal office hours. A client experiencing positive transference is not likely to question the practitioner's actions (even ones that deserve questioning), and the client may invite the practitioner to lunch or ask questions encouraging a personal relationship. When the practitioner does not reciprocate by providing preferential treatment, the client's feelings may be hurt, or they could feel angry. And if the practitioner displays favoritism, client transference may continue and even intensify. After all, who would not be willing to bend the rules for a client who brings gifts and provides favors? Deliberate reinforcement of transference by the practitioner serves to perpetuate the problem, distorts the true nature of the professional relationship, and removes the focus from the client's treatment goals.

Keep in mind that practitioners cannot control how clients feel or behave. When practitioners know or suspect their clients are experiencing transference, it is important to maintain professional boundaries and not encourage transference or lead clients to feel their affection is reciprocated. For example, have set hours to which you adhere, and apply it to all clients. Successful navigation requires maturity, integrity, professionalism, and ethical behaviors. Massage practitioners are encouraged to seek professional supervision when needed.

Emotional Boundaries: Countertransference

Countertransference is similar to transference, except the direction is reversed—transferring from practitioner to client. Countertransference may occur from the practitioner's unmet personal needs, unresolved emotions, or internal conflicts brought into the relationship unknowingly. Countertransference can also occur when practitioners view clients as people from their past.

Countertransference can also occur when practitioners see aspects of themselves in their clients. For example, clients may be of the same age, recently married or divorced, or have children with ages similar to the practitioner's children. Because of these similarities, practitioners may believe clients will be best served by the same type of work or by solutions that helped the practitioner. Remember, both transference and countertransference involves seeing another as someone else—not as they truly are. Countertransference may prevent practitioners from determining a client's unique history and treatment goals, or from acting in their best interests. Signs of countertransference are:

- Having intense feelings, positive or negative, toward a client.
- Becoming angry or depressed when a client cancels an appointment.
- Becoming impatient, angry, or depressed when a client is not progressing with treatment.
- Being argumentative with a client.
- Seeking to or becoming involved in a client's personal life.

- Thinking excessively about the client between appointments.
- Making excuses for a client's inappropriate behavior.
- Giving a particular client additional time during appointments.
- Fantasizing about the client romantically or sexually.
- Ignoring or relaxing professional boundaries.

If practitioners discover they are experiencing countertransference, they should self-reflect and identify what might be causing it. Are personal needs getting met? If not, develop a self-care plan so personal needs can be met outside the relationship. If the practitioner cannot identify reasons behind the countertransference, it may continue or repeat itself with other clients. In these cases, help should be sought from a trusted colleague or mental health counselor.

If countertransference cannot be managed or becomes a problem, it might be best to terminate the professional relationship and refer the client to a different practitioner. Use caution during termination and referral, because the client may feel rejected. Again, consider seeking guidance from a trusted colleague or mental health counselor before talking with the client.

Keep in mind that feelings are just feelings; they are not permanent. If the practitioner has an emotional or even physical attraction to a client, this does not mean that something is wrong with the practitioner or that the practitioner is being unprofessional. Feelings are normal—just do not act on those feelings. Feelings, including infatuation, typically have a short lifespan of a few hours or a few days. Again, supervision can be helpful in some situations.

Personalization can occur in all professional relationships and, under certain conditions, may be helpful to the client. Massage practitioners will remind clients of other people in their lives, past, and present. Clients will remind practitioners of people in their own lives. Transference and countertransference, however, are more serious, complex, and interrelated. It is important to recognize transference and countertransference and reduce their negative impact to best serve the client's highest good. These topics become even more complicated in dual relationships, which are discussed in some depth later in this chapter.

Intellectual Boundaries

Intellectual boundaries encompass beliefs, thoughts, and ideas, as well as safeguarding self-esteem. When others agree with us, we tend to feel safe, validated, and close to the like-minded person. Conversely, when someone disagrees with us, we may feel uncomfortable, especially if the disagreeing person is in a more powerful or authoritative position. Massage practitioners should respect a client's own unique way of knowing and understanding. For example, clients may believe their shoulder pain is inherited, karmic, or resulting from stored emotions or nutritional deficiencies.

To maintain intellectual boundaries, practitioners should avoid discussing their political, religious, or spiritual views with clients, especially when clients have differing views on the same topic. This may extend to objects in the office conveying personal beliefs, such as artwork, posters, and even screensavers. Exceptions to this principle are if the service institution is supported by political or religious organizations. In this case it may be appropriate to display alignment with the organization's philosophy.

In addition, practitioners should avoid recommending self-care activities to their clients unless these are requested. Massage practitioners should base their professional advice on evidence and phrase it accordingly. For example, when discussing treatment plans with clients, disclose how the plan was devised, such as the research supporting the use of the proposed intervention (e.g., massage, essential oils, hydrotherapy). See Chapter 5 for discussions on evidence-informed practice. Furthermore, practitioners should avoid criticizing the client's self-care plan which they have personally constructed or the self-care plans provided by other practitioners unless there is actual potential for harm.

Time Boundaries

Time boundaries are concerned with professional communication, including when appointments are scheduled, and the duration of time spent on professional activities (e.g., intake, massage). Unlike personal relationships in which time is somewhat flexible, a professional's time is structured, limited, purposeful, and monetized. As mentioned previously, boundaries create a sense of predictability.

Massage clients essentially hire practitioners for a session, which is time-bound. Time boundaries include: (1) being ready when clients arrive, having clean linens on the table; (2) beginning and ending the session on time; and (3) focusing on the client during the session while avoiding distracting activities such as talking or texting on mobile devices or conversing with other people in the waiting room.

Some practitioners begin charging for the session at the onset of the massage. Other practitioners begin charging when the health assessment and client interview begins. Convey this information when clients schedule their initial appointment, as they may be confused when they think they are paying for a 60-minute massage and the hour actually consists of a 15-minute intake and a 45-minute massage. Poor time boundary management exists when a 1-hour massage requested by the client lasts 60 minutes one session, 75 minutes the next, and 50 minutes during another session.

Time boundaries also include the days of the week and times of the day when appointments are scheduled. Under what circumstance are appointments scheduled if clients request a different day or different time, if at all? Determine how situations will be handled when clients are running late, or if you are running late. Would you allow sessions to run over time? Under what circumstances? Would you ask permission if you wish to extend the session time? Although you may have an extra 5 or 10 minutes to spend on a given massage, your client may not. Even if the client did have time, it may create an unrealistic expectation that you will exceed the time in future sessions.

Other aspects of time boundaries are how cancellations and no-shows are handled. These situations may cross time and financial boundaries. Determine the cancellation policy, how far in advance you expect clients to cancel, and if a full amount or partial session charge will be expected. Determine a no-show policy and whether a full amount or partial session charge will be expected. In addition, determine a policy if clients cancel or do not keep appointments because of emergencies. It is also recommended to have a policy for when you, the practitioner, must cancel an appointment. These should be clearly articulated for clients as a part of your initial intake when you review policies, protocols, and procedures. Suggestions include scheduling a half-hour break between clients to allow time to work over if a client arrives late, or if the practitioner is running behind schedule because of unforeseen interruptions.

Time boundaries have become complicated in the digital age; practitioners should consider having a policy regarding how quickly they respond to client communications (e.g., voice, text, email).

Location Boundaries

Location boundaries provide guidelines about where professional activities are conducted, and include an office, clinic, spa or wellness center, client residence, or institutional care facility. Many practitioners work in their homes. Ideally, the client entrance and work areas are separate from the living areas. If this is not possible, work areas should be clutter-free and contain few or no personal items. Compliance with local zoning ordinances is required for most home offices. See Chapter 17 for more information about zoning.

When doing an outcall or mobile massage, know in advance about the space where massage equipment such as a massage table or chair will be set up. Inquire about parking and distances between the parking area and the location where the massage will be given, as mobile massage usually requires practitioners to transport equipment and supplies. Develop a policy for outcalls with new clients, such as contacting a third party as to the location, time, and duration of the session in order to maintain practitioner safety. Because this involves disclosing client information, the client must give consent before such disclosure. When providing services at the client's residence, there is an increased risk of becoming involved in the client's private life, and more vigilance may be needed to maintain professional boundaries.

Public spaces and/or social events are inappropriate locations for impromptu massage. This standard applies to practitioners and to students. If a practitioner or student has a friend who requests a neck massage in a shopping center, a reply may be, "I am shopping now and can do a better job at my office. Here is my business card. Please contact me for an appointment." This action demonstrates respect for both location and time boundaries—in this case, the practitioner's time off. Avoid giving professional opinions or advice during social events. Massage practitioners are held accountable for professional activities, regardless of where they are conducted; this includes social events. The practitioner may not have access to all resources needed to formulate professional opinions and may ill-advise current or potential clients. Instead, offer clients a business card and suggest they contact you for an appointment.

Financial Boundaries

Financial boundaries involve issues of money and include fee schedules, payment arrangements and procedures, and policies of nonpayment. Professional relationships are also business relationships, and practitioners offer time and expertise to clients in exchange for money. If practitioners are uncomfortable with money or have issues about money, it may be more difficult to establish and maintain financial boundaries.

Determine a fee schedule and inform clients about it when they schedule appointments. Some practitioners have sliding-scale fees, allowing clients to pay differing amounts depending on the client's ability to pay. Sliding-scale fees can become a boundary issue when money gets in the way of practitioners being fully present in their professional capacities. For example, it may be problematic if clients receive a reduced rate and then arrive at their appointments discussing their upcoming Caribbean vacation or expensive new car. What if the practitioner had not been on vacation in years or drives an older car because of a lack of financial resources? Also, determine how payments will be received, including cash, check, credit or debit card, or digital payment methods. Communicate policies for when payment agreements are not fulfilled and collection procedures apply. Inform clients in advance when fee schedules and payment policies change, perhaps by posting them in the office and on a website. Remind clients of financial policies when obtaining consent.

Financial boundaries include how payment arrangements are handled when receiving massages from colleagues. Will you offer and/or expect a professional discount? Will you trade for services? What if you charge more for an hour than your fellow practitioner? How will you address a difference in fees for the same time spent, if at all? If trading services, when will trades be scheduled? What happens if the practitioner you are trading with has scheduled the third session with you and you have only received one session from them? Will you stop trading until the number of trades is equal? Or will payment be expected for the next session? Ideally, these types of situations should be discussed beforehand and mutually agreed upon.

Financial Boundaries and Conflicts of Interest

A **conflict of interest** is "any financial or other interest which conflicts with the service of the individual because it (1) could significantly impair the individual's objectivity or (2) could create an unfair competitive advantage for any person or organization" (Institute of Medicine, 2009). This definition uses the phrases "could impair" and "could create," and even if competing interests do not impair objectivity or professional judgment or create an unfair competitive advantage, it is still a conflict of interest. Although financial conflicts of interest are the most common type,

other conflicts can occur that might impair objectivity, such as hiring a less qualified friend or family member for a position. Another example of a nonfinancial conflict of interest is performing techniques the practitioner believes in strongly but which do not address or fulfill the client's goals, or recommending products or procedures preferred by the practitioner, but which the client does not need or does not want. Cosgrove et al. (2013) stated conflicts of interest affect decisions in complex and unintended ways. Professionals have a duty to be honest and disclose financial and nonfinancial conflicts of interest that may impair professional judgment.

One of the most common conflicts of interest is selling products to clients. In these situations, practitioners may be faced with choosing between the client's best interests and the practitioner's financial interests when profits are received from the sale. The practitioner also assumes a salesperson role and, because of the power differential, disempowers the client to decline the sale. The client may purchase the product just to please the practitioner or because the sales pitch felt uncomfortable. These feelings may lead clients to schedule their next massage with practitioners who do not sell products. What if clients do not believe they received benefits from the product claimed by the practitioner? How will these and similar situations be addressed?

In some work situations, practitioners are expected to sell products. Discuss product sales with supervisors to determine their expectations before accepting a position which involves financial conflicts of interest. Under some circumstances, it may be possible to have another individual, such as a receptionist, handle product sales.

Digital Boundaries

Digital boundaries limit how much of personal information other people can access. Indeed, digital media, including social media and electronic communications, introduce a new boundary for practitioners, and this may create dual relationships and issues with confidentiality and privacy. For example, email does not safeguard confidentiality unless encrypted with a Health Insurance Portability and Accountability Act (HIPAA)–compliant service (Reamer, 2013). Sabin and Harland (2017, p. 55) recommend emails end with an electronic signature that discusses security and privacy, such as:

> *Notice of Confidentiality: This email, and any attachments, are intended only for use by the addressee(s) and may contain privileged or confidential information. Any distribution, reading, copying, or use of this communication and any attachments by anyone other than the addressee is strictly prohibited and may be unlawful. If you have received this email in error, please immediately notify me by email (by replying to this message) or telephone (xxx-xxx-xxxx), and permanently destroy or delete the original and any copies or printouts of this email and any attachments.*

Texting also does not safeguard confidentiality. However, Reamer (2013) states texting is acceptable for booking and confirming appointments, but not solicitation. Be mindful of the Telephone Consumer Protection Act (TCPA), which was modified to include SMS/text messaging. TCPA requires businesses and/or organizations to receive written consent from individuals before sending SMS/text messages. Obtaining an individual's phone number, whether it is a potential client, existing client, or former client, is not receiving consent or permission to contact them.

Social media such as Facebook and Instagram introduce another challenge. Soliciting or accepting friend requests from clients creates dual relationships. Clients may have access to private information from the practitioner's personal page, which may lead to confusion, transference, or countertransference (Barnett, 2010; Reamer, 2013). Best practices are to not friend clients, or to have separate personal and professional social media pages. Even with separate pages, personal pages are not private, and may be viewed by clients.

Finally, digitally transmitted information via text, email, or social media sites should be documented in client files if transmissions are related to client care. Policies regarding use of social networking sites, emails, text messages, and other electronic tools should be included in informed consent, which includes guidelines on what kinds of information are and are not appropriate for transmission via text and email (Sabin & Harland, 2017).

> *Compassion is what makes our lives meaningful. It is the source of all lasting happiness and joy. And it is the foundation of a good heart, the heart of one who acts out of a desire to help others. Through kindness, through affection, through honesty, through truth and justice toward all others we ensure our own benefits. This is not a matter for complicated theorizing. It is a matter of common sense. ...we cannot escape the necessity of love and compassion.*
>
> **~ Dalai Lama**

DUAL RELATIONSHIPS

Dual relationships are any situation where multiple roles exist between practitioners and clients. Examples of dual relationships are when clients are also friends, family members, or business associates. Nonsexual dual relationships are not always unethical, as some do not lead to exploitation or harm.

A power imbalance exists in professional relationships—it is not a relationship of equals. Clients expect practitioners to perform professional duties and responsibilities. Massage practitioners expect clients to comply with treatment plans, keep appointments, follow office policies, and pay for treatments. Massage practitioners cannot promise clients entering into a dual relationship that doing so will not affect their professional relationship.

It can be challenging to maintain professional boundaries when more than one role exists. Treating all clients equally can be difficult when some are friends and others are not. Professional boundaries can become blurred and interactions can become complicated. When additional roles exist, for instance if your client is also your accountant, a different set of expectations may exist. Maintaining professional boundaries and preserving ethics is the practitioner's responsibility, not the client's. Professionals are held accountable for negative consequences arising from dual relationships.

This section focuses only on nonsexual dual relationships.

Social Relationships

Social dual relationships include friendships and clients who are "friends" on social media (e.g., Facebook, Instagram). Social, or communal, dual relationships also include relationships with clients who live in the same community and participate in the same activities at the same time with their massage practitioners. A practitioner who shops where their client works, or belongs to the same church, synagogue, or mosque is in a communal dual relationship. Social relationships are easier to avoid in larger cities. However, in smaller communities, there are fewer places to worship, conduct business, and shop. Social dual relationships may be unavoidable in some cases.

Friendships

The most common social dual relationship is friendship. Being in a professional role is challenging when clients are also friends. Imagine how hard it would be not to chat with friends during the massage. Massage practitioners and clients/friends may treat appointments as opportunities to develop the friendship; sessions may become social events, which may lead to reduced focus on the needs of the client/friend.

How do professional relationships differ from friendships? Friendships usually involve choice, mutuality (both parties voluntarily enter the relationship), trust, delight or pleasure (both parties enjoy the relationship), and reciprocity. In friendships, the relationship is ideally a 50/50 exchange where a certain amount of give-and-take exists. You know as much about your friends as they know about you. You also support each other. In professional relationships, you know much more about your clients than they know about you. Mutual familiarity is uncommon in professional relationships. A power differential exists, not an equal partnership. You support them through professional services. Professional relationships involve choice, mutuality, trust, and pleasure, but not reciprocity (Fig. 2.4). Some professional relationships feel close, but they are not as intimate as friendships. Each party is receiving something of worth from the relationship, but it is not equal or reciprocal.

Besides, can we call what develops between clients and practitioners a friendship? McIntosh (2010) examines this question. Do we go to our client's office, remove our clothing, lie on their desk, get a massage, and pay for their time? And we typically do not show clients our lower selves, the part of us reserved only for those closest to us. These include our pettiness, neediness, jealousies, idiosyncrasies, and quirks. Ideally, we project our higher selves in professional settings. Positive aspects of our higher selves include respect, authenticity, empathy, and trust.

Friendships

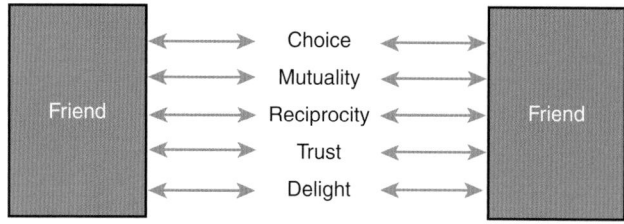

Professional Relationships

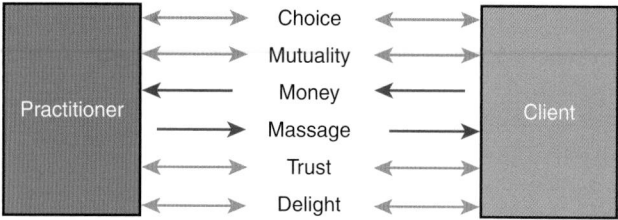

FIG. 2.4 Friendships versus professional relationships. Note reciprocity is part of friendships, but not part of professional relationships.

Turning clients into friends may also interfere with our relationships with other clients. How would you feel if your practitioner, Michael, was friends with his client, Mary, and not with you? If not hurt, you might question Michael's professional boundaries.

Friends and Massage School

Massage students will practice on fellow students while in school. These sessions need to be treated with the same respect and acknowledgment of professional boundaries as with future clients. This means staying focused on the client/student, not talking with students at the next massage table, and recognizing the power differential exists for the time they are on the table.

Massage students also often practice on their friends while in school. Let friends know that, after licensure, a fee may be attached to the massage. If you know what the fee will be, let them know early so they will be prepared to pay the requested fee at the appropriate time. This is also an opportunity to practice your role of practitioner with professional boundaries intact and to treat practice sessions as you would in professional settings.

Dating Clients

What if practitioners and clients want to date each other? The decision to date an ex-client should be considered carefully. The National Certification Board for Therapeutic Massage and Bodywork's (NCBTMB) Standards of Practice (Standard VI. A) recommends discontinuing the client–practitioner relationship for a minimum of 6 months before initiating dating relationships and possible sexual contact (unless a relationship existed prior to the date the professional relationship began). This time period is a minimum

and, in some cases, 6 months is not enough. Issues to consider include the length of time both parties were in the professional relationship, the level of client disclosure while in the professional relationship, whether transference occurred, and if the client still sees you in an authoritative role. When the latter occurs, it may be difficult for clients to see themselves as equal partners in the new relationship.

There are some cases where no amount of time between discontinuing the client–practitioner relationship and initiating a romantic relationship is adequate. Compare the level of disclosure with a client who you have been seeing for 2 weeks for a hamstring tear and a client you have been seeing weekly for 3 years, during which time he went through a divorce and lost a parent. It is easy to imagine the second client may have leaned on you more for emotional support. In fact, you may be a major part of their support network. There may be significant transference, and no amount of time will put the two of you on equal footing because of the deep bond your client experienced. This client may always see you as their savior, even as you attempt to establish a different role. The client may enter into a romantic relationship with you willingly but later feel taken advantage of because of previous disclosure. No matter who initiated the change in the relationship, if the client later feels harmed by it, licensing and certification boards will often rule in favor of the client and discipline the practitioner. Such situations can easily damage relationships with other clients and damage your professional reputation. The best and safest decision is to not become romantically or sexually involved with clients.

Familial Relationships

Maintaining professional boundaries is more challenging with family members. It can be a source of great joy to work with family, particularly when they are in pain. However, there is a tendency to carry over family dynamics into the professional relationship. If there is a strain in the familial relationship, there will likely be a strain in the professional relationship. For example, if you have always wanted your sibling's approval, you may use massage as a way to gain it. This places unrealistic expectations on the professional relationship, removing the focus from your sibling/client to your needs.

Other considerations are how appointments and fees are handled. When will you work on family? During normal office hours or only during your time off? How will you handle missed appointments? Will you charge family members? If so, is this fee different from what you charge other clients? And if you work with one family member and not another, will this negatively affect family dynamics? If so, how?

Yet another aspect of treating family members is the possibility of abuse in the family history. Greene and Boodrich-Dunn (2013) suggest if the practitioner has been abused sexually, physically, or otherwise by a family member, they should not massage that person or anyone associated with the abuse. People who have been abused may deny or minimize the abuse and not fully understand the implications and impact of touching people directly or indirectly associated with these events.

Business Relationships

Business dual relationships exist when the practitioner and client are also professional colleagues. You may know these people in a variety of ways, including working in the same office or training institution, co-presenting at professional conferences, coauthoring books, or as business partners, coworkers, or employer–employees. Business dual relationships include having clients who are also business partners or persons who provide business support, such as legal or accounting services. As with social and familial dual relationships, practitioners should keep the focus on the client and limit non-massage-related conversations during the session.

MAKING PROFESSIONAL DECISIONS

Practitioners make numerous decisions to address problems that arise during the day over the course of their professional careers. It is helpful to determine how serious the problem is so appropriate action can be taken. Some problems require no action, while others demand reasoned or considerable action.

Turbulence Theory

The turbulence theory is the categorization of situations into different levels so that appropriate decisions can be made. Gross (2019) classifies turbulence into four levels, ranging from light to extreme. Practitioners should ask themselves, "How serious is the situation? Can I handle this myself or do I need the aid of others inside or outside of my organization?" The turbulence theory was originally used by pilots to help them make decisions based on the amount of disturbance or "turbulence" they experienced while operating an aircraft.

- **Light Turbulence**. These are normal ongoing business problems and cause little to no disruption. An example of light turbulence is a client who arrives 15 minutes late and you either shorten the session or give them the full session time and finish later than originally expected. Most business problems are light turbulence.
- **Moderate Turbulence**. These are noticeable disturbances and require considerable action to solve. An example of moderate turbulence is a client who removes the drape during the massage, causing the practitioner to replace the drape, and tell the client that this behavior is not allowed, and that there will be consequences if the same or similar behaviors are repeated. Another example is when a fellow practitioner calls in sick and either a replacement practitioner must be found, or a day of clients rescheduled.
- **Severe Turbulence**. These involve administrative action and may affect the entire organization. To solve the problem, assistance from outside the organization may be required. An example of severe turbulence is being served a lawsuit for malpractice because of alleged substandard care given to a client that may have led to an adverse event and an attorney must be consulted.
- **Extreme Turbulence**. Extreme turbulence involves possible business closure. Forces are so great that control is lost. No one in the organization knows what to do, and a new approach is needed to solve the problem. An example

is a global pandemic, wherein you must cease operations until permission is granted by local authorities to resume operations.

Solving Light to Moderate Problems

Most business problems are light to moderate turbulence. Clients have differing values and priorities, opinions will vary, and miscommunication and misunderstandings occur. The following is an effective and empathetic approach using 6 steps to manage and resolve problems (Steinbrecher, 2013).

1. **Be Respectful**. If a client has been late for an appointment twice in 1 month, use polite language such as, "I noticed you've been arriving late this month, which seems out of character for you—you always arrive on time," rather than, "You are late for the second time this month." Notice the use of "I" messages in the respectful example.

2. **Be Specific**. If a client is late for an appointment twice in 1 month, say, "I noticed on Tuesday the 8th, as well as Friday the 18th, you were late." Being specific lets the client know that you are aware of the situation and that it will be addressed. This also creates an opportunity for the client to explain and for you to listen.

3. **State How You and Others Were Affected**. Again, use "I" messages. For example, say, "I am not sure you are aware of the problems created by clients showing up late. It decreases the time I can spend with the client who arrives late, and affects the next client and clients scheduled the rest of that day." The client gets a glimpse of how the problem affects other people, not just in their session, but all sessions for the rest of the day.

4. **Seek Perspective**. Actively solicit their perspective by asking, "From your perspective, what is happening?" While you are listening, display empathy nonverbally. Avoid the word "but," as this negates everything positive you have said.

5. **Solicit Solutions**. Actively solicit solutions. For example, "What do you think would help solve the problem? What are you willing to do?" This last question brings in accountability. You can also ask, "I can imagine this is challenging—and we need to come up with a solution. What ideas do you have?"

6. **Take Action**. Once you have respectfully discussed the issue and how it affected you, asked why it happened, and come up with possible solutions by soliciting the other person's opinions and ideas, recap the steps and settle on a win-win resolution. For example, "It appears you are overcommitted on certain days. Would it be better to shorten your appointment time from 60 to 30 minutes or consider a weekend appointment?" Or, "Would it help if I gave you a reminder call or text the morning of your appointment?" and "What do you think?"

Massage practitioners can benefit by learning empathetic and respectful approaches to problem-solving involving authentic communication. It can make the difference between positive and negative outcomes. It takes courage to confront difficult issues, and many people would rather avoid conflict. However, the benefits of a positive resolution outweigh the anxiety that some individuals have about addressing problems.

Solving Severe to Extreme Problems

When solving severe or extreme problems, consider a problem-solving approach that examines problems from numerous perspectives, and consider several courses of action before settling on an appropriate response. The following process contains several steps, considers ethical guidelines and legal ramifications, and puts empathy into the forefront. Corey et al. (2011) recommend an 8-step process for making decisions.

1. **Identify the Problem**. Reflect on the issue and consider all aspects of the problem. Is it an ethical, moral, or legal issue? Other? Frame and Williams (2005) suggest reflective questions such as "What is the central theme?" and "Are cultural or historical factors involved?"

2. **Identify Issues Around the Problem**. List and describe critical issues and stakeholders. Realize stakeholders include the client, family/friends of the client(s), other clients, business owners, co-workers, the community, and the profession. What are their preferences, values, and vulnerabilities? Where are power imbalances?

3. **Review Ethical Guidelines**. Look at codes of ethics, including those associated with state licensing boards and professional organizations, such as the American Massage Therapy Association, Associated Bodywork and Massage Professionals, Federation of State Massage Therapy Boards, and NCBTMB. If codes conflict, follow the strictest guideline. Apply ethical principles of autonomy, veracity, beneficence, nonmalfeasance, fidelity, justice, and confidentiality to the situation, and note if conflicts exist among principles.

4. **Review Laws and Regulations**. Apply state laws and regulations, including reporting mandates for vulnerable populations (e.g., children, elderly), scope of practice and professional activity restrictions (i.e., no diagnosing), and standards of care. Consider the rights and responsibilities of various stakeholders. Be aware that some ethical issues may also be legal issues. For example, not renewing a state license yet continuing to practice massage is illegal. In contrast, offering hot stone massage after watching a video may be unethical but not illegal. The primary purpose of massage laws is to protect the public from injury or fraud. This protection is partially provided by laws regarding rules for obtaining and maintaining licensure. If laws are broken, civil or criminal charges may occur. Convicted individuals may be fined, imprisoned, have their licenses revoked, or receive other penalties determined by the courts. If laws specify all licensed massage practitioners must adhere to the state board's code of ethics, an action that violates the code of ethics would not only be unethical (i.e., dating a client or providing services without adequate training), but would also be illegal. Penalties for these illegal activities might include fines or suspension of license.

5. **Obtain Consultation**. Seek counsel from mentors, teachers, peers, or other trusted professionals—they can help identify any blind spots. Prejudices, biases, privilege, and personal unmet needs or emotions can impair objectivity. If there are legal questions, seek legal counsel. Many ethical dilemmas are in "gray" areas, and ethical codes cannot foresee every ethical situation.

6. **Consider Several Actions**. Synthesize the results of all consultations and create a list of possible actions.

7. **Think about Possible Consequences of Various Actions**. Examine the list and reflect on possible consequences each action might have on stakeholders. Consider risks and benefits. Consider ethical and legal implications. Also consider short-term and long-term consequences. Frame and Williams (2005) suggest asking, "How do these actions fit with the ethical codes? How were the client's preferences, values, and vulnerabilities taken into consideration? How were my own values affirmed or challenged? How is power used in each action? How would others appraise each action?" Discuss these options with your client, if possible.

8. **Decide on the Best Course of Action**. Make a decision, and carry it out. Document each step of the process, even steps not acted on. If the problem is investigated by an ethics or legal committee, documentation of the steps followed demonstrates thoughtful and thorough exploration of the issue. Documentation displays professionalism, even in situations where the final action is called into question.

SEXUAL MISCONDUCT AND SEXUAL HARASSMENT

Ethical guidelines, such as codes of ethics and standards of practice, often state that dual relationships should be avoided for the protection of clients. Sex with current clients is unethical, but not always illegal. For example, a practitioner may be fired from a job and have their license revoked because of sexual misconduct, but they might not go to jail. In addition, the person in the subordinate position may allege sexual harassment, which may be illegal.

Sexual misconduct and harassment is of particular concern to the massage profession because physical touch is our primary mode of treatment, often on a client's bare skin. This, combined with the private setting, low lighting, and soft music where massage takes place, could be perceived as a context for pursuing sexual contact. Touch may be misinterpreted. Massage practitioners are touching clients sometimes with the gentleness and attentiveness commonly shared with an intimate partner. Clients may be survivors of sexual abuse and subject to touch misinterpretation. In addition, clients with an abusive (physical or sexual) past may dissociate, reducing the ability to detect or stop a practitioner's inappropriate behavior because the client felt they were previously unable to stop this event from happening. Massage practitioners who are survivors themselves may not realize they are being sexually inappropriate with clients.

Because practitioners are likely to deal with issues of sexuality and sexual harassment, it is important that these discussions take place during one's training. Talking about them early is best done while in school. Through talking about these issues, we learn how to make sound judgments and good decisions. Classroom discussions are extremely important, as we learn from instructors' and classmates' experiences. The sensual pleasure inherent in massage is one of its greatest assets, but also one of its liabilities, and can lead to situations of seduction and exploitation.

Sexual misconduct is a range of sexual behaviors, consensual and nonconsensual, between someone in an authoritative role and someone in a subordinate role—these are relationships with power differentials. This includes practitioners and their clients, physicians and their patients, teachers and their students, mentors and their mentees, clergy and their congregants, and employers and their employees. Sexual misconduct is a broad, blanket term and includes sexual harassment.

Sexual harassment is sexual or sexually suggestive unwanted behaviors perceived as offensive, threatening, or embarrassing (Viglianti et al., 2018). Sexual harassment can substantially interfere with someone's work, educational, or social setting by creating an intimidating or hostile environment. Sexual harassment denies an individual dignity and respect; its behaviors range from unwelcome verbal, written, or physical conduct that denigrates an individual or an individual's relatives, friends, or associates; derogatory comments, innuendos, insults, slurs, nicknames, negative stereotyping, and other similar conduct; and placement, dissemination, or circulation of written or graphic material (hard copy or electronic forms). Specific examples of sexual harassment include:

1. Flirtatious behavior and comments made about a client's body or clothing.
2. Seductive or sexual gestures or expressions.
3. Sexual innuendos or sexually provocative remarks.
4. Telling sexually explicit jokes.
5. Discussing sexual problems, sexual performance, sexual preferences, or fantasies.
6. Kissing a client.
7. Unnecessary examination or treatment of breasts or pelvic area.
8. Filming a client without permission.
9. Entering the room before clients are completely draped or dressed.
10. Failure to ensure proper draping.
11. Offering sexual services to clients.
12. Asking a current client on a date.
13. Sexual self-arousal or stimulation in the presence of clients, including rubbing part of your body against the client's body or the table.
14. Any sex act.

Sexual Harassment by Massage Clients

Sexual harassment is prevalent in the workplace, with both males and females subjected to sexual harassment. Prevalence rates are higher toward females, with between 25% and 85% experiencing some form of sexual harassment at work (Vuleta, 2021). Massage practitioners are no different, with 75% reporting sexual harassment by their clients (Richard et al., 2020); most practitioners were young when the reported incident(s) occurred. The majority of practitioners stated these experiences did have an effect on their

practice going forward, and they became more cautious. Furthermore, the feelings practitioners had about the incident were largely anger, discomfort, and shock rather than fear. Here are a few more findings from the investigation:

• Verbal forms of sexual harassment were more common than physical forms. Verbal forms included commenting on the practitioner's appearance or requesting sexual favors. Physical forms included a client exposing their genitals, grabbing the practitioner without consent, or trying to force the practitioner to touch various parts of the body. There were no reports of forced sexual activity. Other forms of harassment were clients sending sexually suggestive or explicit messages on social media or in text messages.

• Most perpetrating clients were male. Richard et al. (2020) noted sexual harassment centers on males exerting power over females, and the power differential inherent in professional relationships did not outweigh this cultural power distance.

• Over half of offending clients booked their appointments several days in advance. Others were same-day bookings, the day prior, or walk-ins. First-time clients and repeat clients were both perpetrators, with more incidents occurring with repeat clients—most episodes occurred during the session.

• Incidences occurred most often in multi-practitioner offices and multidisciplinary clinics. It occurred least often in home offices, physiotherapy and sports clinics, and outcalls.

Sexual Risk Management

There are several actions practitioners can take that may reduce the risk of sexual harassment. Even with proactive measures, closeness felt by a client may lead to misunderstandings. Every practitioner should take proactive measures. Ways to reduce the risk of sexual misconduct and sexual harassment are:

• Display a zero-tolerance policy for sexual harassment by clients at the front desk. This warning may prevent clients who plan to sexually harass their practitioners.

• Avoid terms of endearment (e.g., honey, sweetie) because clients may misread them.

• Avoid terms such as "release," "available anytime," "open 24 hours," "my place or yours," "total relaxation," "complete relaxation," "full service," "full body massage," and "happy endings."

• Avoid using the term *bed* when referring to a massage table.

• Note the demeanor, tone of voice, and language used when booking new clients. Note any discomfort you are feeling. Be leery of clients who ask about the age, race of the practitioner, or distinct physical features such as hair color.

• Avoid sexual signals you may be sending inadvertently, such as wearing tight or revealing clothing. Although how you dress never justifies unwanted sexual advances, in the case of a client who mistakenly believes massage is a sexual service, dressing in revealing clothing can reinforce this impression.

- Avoid working on a client if you are in danger of *acting* on your feelings of physical attraction.
- Recognize the lack of safety associated with a home office. Leading clients through your home to the bedroom (now massage room) can make clients feel uneasy and may give mixed messages.
- Be aware of body contact during the massage. Pay attention to the way you lean into your client's body. Be conscious of what part of your body touches the client during massage techniques, including joint mobilizations and stretches.

Massage and Erections

Sexuality is a biologic fact, rooted in our brains, neural pathways, and hormones (Fox, 2007). Sexual activity has no place in the professional relationship. However, your client may experience a sexual response to touch. Sexual responses such as erections can occur naturally from massage or be triggered by sights, sounds, and/or smells, without sexual motivation. Erections are not necessarily sexual harassment. Acting on an erection is sexual harassment. Your response to these situations will depend on several factors.

If you believe the erection is a reflex response (which may not be easy to determine), simply ignore it. You can ask questions to distract the client from thoughts or feelings or sensations leading up to the erection. Or you can alter the speed and/or depth of the massage techniques or ask them to roll over into the prone position and continue the massage. Avoid any areas that might restimulate the erection, such as the lower abdomen, inner thighs, and lumbosacral region. If the erection occurs repeatedly, consider having a neutral but forthright conversation with your client. The client may be unaware of the erection or embarrassed and unsure about how to address it. Be mindful of what occurred prior to the erection, and make appropriate modifications. For example, if an erection happens every time you massage the feet, do not massage the feet in subsequent sessions, or only massage the feet when the client is prone.

However, if the client has an erection followed by inappropriate behavior, the client is likely sexualizing the massage. Behaviors range from subtle to overt, and may include: noises such as moaning; repetitive movements of the pelvis; touching their pelvis or penis; or removing part of, or the entire drape. The client may also touch you, even in a seemingly casual or accidental way. If you have discussed how these situations will be handled when obtaining consent, proceed with those actions, such as terminating the session (see the section titled Terminating a Session). If actions taken for these situations were not discussed with the client previously, consider removing your hands from the client, stepping back and toward the door, and saying something like, "I do not like the way in which you are behaving. If you do not stop immediately, I will end this session." If the client agrees to stop, you may continue with the massage if you feel comfortable. However, if you feel uncomfortable or if the client makes excuses about their behavior or tries to minimize your reactions, it is best to terminate the session. You have the right to refuse massage to a client who makes you feel uncomfortable, or unsafe, or who sexualizes the massage. Some state licensing boards require the licensee to immediately discontinue the session when a client behaves in any way meant to arouse or sexually gratify either the practitioner or the client (Texas Department of Licensing and Regulation [TDLR], 2021).

Terminating a Session

Practitioners need to be prepared to implement session termination protocols when circumstances require them (mentioned previously). This decision should not be taken lightly. Once the decision has been made, consider these guidelines:

- Remove your hands from the client; step back and toward the door.
- Tell the client the massage is over.
- Inform the client you will wait outside the massage room while they get dressed, and exit the room.
- Avoid answering questions until the client is dressed and has stepped out of the massage room.
- If the circumstances leading to the session termination are extreme, or if you are alone and become frightened, lock yourself in a room until the client has left, or call 911 and stay on the telephone until the client leaves.
- Document the entire incident, including the events leading to the decision of session termination, the actions taken, and client responses. Document statements verbatim and describe the situation in detail.
- If you feel fearful as a result of the session termination, some form of intervention should be taken, such as filing a police report. You may also choose to file a police report if you are stalked or further harassed by the client.

Sexual Misconduct by Colleagues

When practitioners engage in sexual misconduct or sexually harass their clients, they abuse their position of power and authority and take advantage of a client's vulnerability. In many states, there is a "duty to report" sexual misconduct and harassment by practitioners. If there is firsthand knowledge (i.e., we witnessed it ourselves or it was disclosed by the offending practitioner), practitioners may be required to file a report with the state licensing boards. If allegations are secondhand or obtained by hearsay (i.e., learned from other persons, such as the client), practitioners should encourage the client/victim to file a report. Agencies such as licensing boards and professional organizations are most able to respond to a complaint when filed by the victim. Some boards and organizations allow anonymous complaints, but these are not as strong as ones filed by victims, and are more difficult to address, resolve, or prosecute.

E-RESOURCES

http://evolve.elsevier.com/Salvo/MassageTherapy

- Chapter challenge
- Flash cards
- Additional information
- Downloadable forms

NINA MCINTOSH

Everybody studies ethics, right?

Today, ethics training is mandatory for massage students all across the country, and it feels impossible it could ever have been otherwise. All sorts of texts are available covering issues such as professional boundaries, dual relationships, and projection. But as hard as it is to believe, in 1999 there was only one: *The Educated Heart* by Nina McIntosh.

McIntosh was born and raised in Memphis, Tennessee, in 1943 and lived there until heading to study psychology at the Newcomb College of Tulane University. After a few years of employment in New Orleans, she then continued her education, earning her Master of Social Work (also from Tulane).

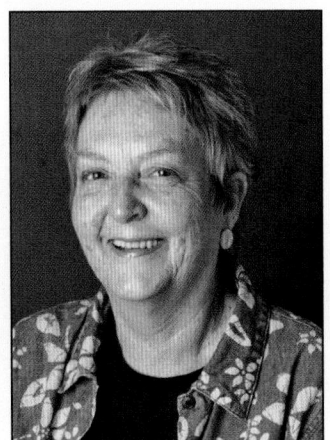

From Associate Body Work and Massage Professionals, A Tribute to Nina McIntosh, http://www.abmp.com/news/a-tribute-to-nin-mcintosh/.

Armed with her freshly minted MSW, McIntosh moved to Denver and began working as a psychiatric social worker. The experience was educational, but also distressing. She watched as the staff in the psychiatric hospital where she worked set up extremely rigid personal boundaries between themselves and their patients. They were discouraged from having physical contact with the patients, who were there because of their mental health issues, not body-related illnesses. McIntosh became convinced both the body and the mind needed careful and compassionate attention, and neglecting the body could only be detrimental to mental health, even when ostensibly done in the name of professionalism. This experience began McIntosh's lifelong fascination with appropriate boundaries in professional settings, as well as the importance of the health-promoting role of touch.

Determined to explore this idea further, in 1978 McIntosh enrolled in the Boulder College of Massage Therapy and then went on to study at the Rolf Institute in Boulder, becoming a Certified Rolfer. During her career as a Rolfer, she traveled widely and settled for a while in California before returning to her hometown of Memphis to care for her aging parents.

McIntosh's parents died in 1995, leaving her with the free time to write down her understandings about professional boundaries in the massage field, inspired by her experiences in psychology, social work, and massage.

This became *The Educated Heart*, which is still used in massage schools today.

McIntosh moved to Asheville, North Carolina, in 2005. Although she retired from Rolfing, McIntosh never stopped thinking or writing about massage ethics and remained an active member of the massage community for the rest of her life. Her popular ethics column in *Massage and Bodywork,* "The Heart of Bodywork," ran for nearly 10 years, and *The Educated Heart* finally found a publisher in Lippincott Williams & Wilkins, who published not only the second edition of the book in 2005 but also a third edition in 2010. The book, which is still one of the best-selling ethics textbooks in the massage community, is immediately useful, easy to read, and occasionally hilarious, with its real-life stories about professional boundaries gone wrong, and those done right. If your brain is exhausted from too many anatomy exams, reading *The Educated Heart* is the perfect way to fit some more studying into your life without it actually feeling like work. There is a reason it is such a classic.

In 2009, McIntosh was diagnosed with amyotrophic lateral sclerosis, better known as Lou Gehrig disease. As her physical health began a rapid decline, she maintained her sense of compassion and justice, volunteering with her church, advocating for wheelchair accessibility, and befriending a man who had been unjustly imprisoned for 15 years. She also kept up her wry sense of humor as her body failed her in an increasing number of ways, eventually losing even the ability to speak.

In 2010, she was awarded the Aunty Margaret Humanitarian Award at the World Massage Festival in Berea, Kentucky. She was too weak to attend the ceremony, and with typical humility said, "I don't think I'm much of a humanitarian." McIntosh died 1 month later, with joy and dignity. Her work lives on in her writings, and her ethics classes are still taught by Laura Allen, fellow massage practitioner, educator, and McIntosh's personal friend.

What started out as a self-published book by one woman with a devotion to ethical bodywork has since blossomed into a nationwide conversation about the ethics of professional touch.

REFERENCES

American Medical Association (AMA). (n.d.). *Creating an LGBTQ-friendly practice.* Retrieved from https://www.ama-assn.org/delivering-care/creating-lgbtq-friendly-practice.

Ard, K. L., & Makadon, H. J. (n.d.). *Improving the health care of lesbian, gay, bisexual and transgender people: Understanding and eliminating health disparities.* Boston, MA: The Fenway Institute. Retrieved from https://www.lgbthealtheducation.org/wp-content/uploads/Improving-the-Health-of-LGBT-People.pdf.

Barnett, J. (2010). Psychology's brave new world: Psychotherapy in the digital age. *Independent Practitioner, 30,* 149–152.

Begley, P. T. (1999). Value preferences, ethics and conflicts in school administration. Values and educational leadership (pp. 237–252). New York, NY: State University of New York Press.

Boatwright, W. M. (2014). *Champions for culturally competent care.* Retrieved from http://www.hpoe.org/resources/chair-files/1689.

Bradley, C. (2020). *Transphobic hate crime report.* Retrieved from https://www.galop.org.uk/transphobic-hate-crime-report-2020/.

Bruce, N., Shapio, S. L., Constantino, M. J., & Manber, R. (2010). Psychotherapist mindfulness and the psychotherapy process. *Psychotherapy, 47*(1), 83–97.

Buppert, C. (2014). *Is it ok for a nurse to hug a patient?* Retrieved from https://www.medscape.com/viewarticle/835233.

Burch, S. (2010). *Ethics: Medical settings.* New York: Natural Wellness.

Campinha-Bacote, J. (2002). The process of cultural competence in the delivery of healthcare services: A model of care. *Journal of Transcultural Nursing, 13*(3), 181–184.

Corey, G., Corey, M. S., & Callanan, P. (2011). *Issues and ethics in the helping professions* (8th ed.). Belmont, CA: Brooks/Cole.

Cosgrove, L., Bursztajn, H. J., Erlich, D. R., Wheeler, E. E., & Shaughnessay, V. B. (2013). Conflicts of interest and the quality of recommendations in clinical guidelines. *Journal of Evaluation in Clinical Practice, 19*(4), 674–681.

Cozolino, L. (2006). *The neuroscience of human relationships.* New York, NY: Norton.

Denboba, D. L., Bragdon, J. L., Epstein, L. G., Garthright, K., & Goldman, T. M. (1998). Reducing health disparities through cultural competence. *Journal of Health Education, 29*(Suppl. 5), S47–S53.

Eliason, M. J., & Schope, R. (2001). Does "don't ask don't tell" apply to health care? Lesbian, gay, and bisexual people's disclosure to health care providers. *Journal of the Gay and Lesbian Medical Association, 5*(4), 125–134.

Erikson, E. (1963). *Childhood and society.* New York: Norton.

Field, T. (2012). Relationships as regulators. *Psychology (Savannah, GA), 3*(6), 467–479.

Fisher, M. A. (2018). *Confidentiality and its limits in my practice.* Retrieved from http://www.centerforethicalpractice.org/ethical-legal-resources/ethical-information/ethical-obligations-confidentiality/confidentiality-limits-practice/.

Fox, S. (2007). *Relating to clients.* Philadelphia: Kingsley, Jessica Publishers.

Frame, M. W., & Williams, C. B. (2005). A model of ethical decision making from a multicultural perspective. *Couns Values, 49*(3), 165–179.

Greene, E., & Boodrich-Dunn, B. (2013). *The psychology of the body* (2nd ed.). Philadelphia: Lippincott Williams & Wilkins.

Gross, S. J. (2019). *Applying turbulence theory to educational leadership in challenging times.* Philadelphia: Routledge.

Hafeez, H., Zeshan, M., Tahir, M. A., Jahan, N., & Naveed, S. (2017). Health care disparities among lesbian, gay, bisexual, and transgender youth: A literature review. *Cureus, 9*(4), e1184.

Horvath, A. O., & Symonds, B. D. (1991). Relation between a working alliance and outcome in psychotherapy: A meta-analysis. *Journal of Counseling Psychology, 38*(2), 139–149.

Human Rights Campaign. (n.d.). *Glossary of terms.* Retrieved from https://www.hrc.org/resources/glossary-of-terms.

Institute of Medicine. (2009). Committee on conflict of interest in medical research, education, and practice. In B. Lo & M. J. Field (Eds.), Conflict of interest in medical research, education, and practice. Washington, DC: National Academies Press (US).

McIntosh, N. (2010). The educated heart: Professional guidelines for massage therapists, bodyworkers, and movement therapists (3rd ed.). Baltimore, MD: Lippincott Williams & Wilkins.

National Certification Board for Therapeutic Massage and Bodywork. (2017). *Standards of practice.* Retrieved from https://www.ncbtmb.org/standards-of-practice/.

Reamer, F. G. (2013). Social work in a digital age: Ethical and risk management challenges. *Social Work, 58*(2), 163–172.

Richard, M. E., O'Sullivan, L. F., & Peppard, T. (2020). Sexual harassment of massage therapists by their clients. *Canadian Journal of Human Sexuality, 29*(2), 205–211.

Riess, H., Kelley, J. M., Bailey, R. W., Dunn, E. J., & Phillips, M. (2012). Empathy training for resident physicians: A randomized controlled trial of a neuroscience-informed curriculum. *Journal of General Internal Medicine, 27*(10), 1280–1286.

Riess, H., & Kraft-Todd, G. (2014). E.M.P.A.T.H.Y.: A tool to enhance nonverbal communication between clinicians and their patients. *Journal. Association of American Medical Colleges, 89*(8), 1108–1112.

Rogers, C. (1961). *On becoming a person.* New York: Houghton Mifflin Harcourt.

Ronan, W. (2020). *New FBI hate crimes report show increases in anti-LGBTQ attacks.* Retrieved from https://www.hrc.org/press-releases/new-fbi-hate-crimes-report-shows-increases-in-anti-lgbtq-attacks.

Sabin, J. E., & Harland, J. C. (2017). Professional ethics for digital age psychiatry: Boundaries, privacy, and communication. *Current Psychiatry Reports, 19*(9), 55.

Shallcross, L. (2011). *Do the right thing.* Retrieved from http://ct.counseling.org/2011/04/do-the-right-thing/.

Sheldon, L. K., & Foust, J. (2014). *Communication for nurses.* Burlington, MA: Jones & Bartlett Learning.

Smith, J. M., Sullivan, S. J., & Baxter, G. D. (2009a). Massage therapy services for healthcare: A telephone focus group study of drivers for clients' continued use of services. *Complementary Therapies in Medicine, 17,* 281–291.

Smith, J. M., Sullivan, S. J., & Baxter, G. D. (2009b). The culture of massage therapy: Valued elements and the role of comfort, contact, connection and caring. *Complementary Therapies in Medicine, 17,* 181–189.

Steinbrecher, S. (2013). *Resolving conflict: Six simple steps to keeping the peace.* Retrieved from https://www.huffingtonpost.com/susan-steinbrecher/resolving-conflict-six-si_b_4171635.html.

Stonewall. (2017a). *Glossary of terms.* Retrieved from https://www.stonewall.org.uk/help-advice/faqs-and-glossary/glossary-terms.

Stonewall. (2017b). *LGBT in Britain: Hate crime and discrimination.* Retrieved from https://www.stonewall.org.uk/lgbt-britain-hate-crime-and-discrimination.

Texas Department of Licensing and regulation. (2021). Massage Therapy Program Administrative Rules: 117.92(e). *Sexual misconduct.* Retrieved from https://www.tdlr.texas.gov/mas/masrules.htm#11792.

Viglianti, E. M., Oliverio, A. L., & Meeks, L. M. (2018). Sexual harassment and abuse: When the patient is the perpetrator. *Lancet, 392*(10145), 368–370.

Vingerhoets, A., & Scheirs, J. (2000). Sex differences in crying: Empirical findings and possible explanations. In A. H. Fischer (Ed.), Studies in emotion and social interaction. Second series. Gender and emotion: Social psychological perspectives (pp. 143–165). Cambridge University Press.

Vuleta, R. (2021). *Sexual harassment in the workplace statistics.* Retrieved from https://whattobecome.com/blog/sexual-harassment-in-the-workplace-statistics/.

Walach, H., Güthlin, C., & König, M. (2003). Efficacy of massage therapy in chronic pain: A pragmatic randomized trial. *Journal of Alternative and Complementary Medicine (New York, N.Y.), 9*(6), 837–846.

REVIEW AND APPLY YOUR KNOWLEDGE

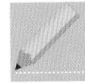

MATCHING ONE: CONCEPT REVIEW

Place the letter of the answer next to the number of the term or phrase that best describes it.

A. Abuse
B. Sympathy
C. Professional boundaries
D. Confidentiality
E. Discrimination
F. Self-disclosure
G. Dual relationships
H. Empathy
I. Neglect
J. Respect
K. Sexual misconduct
L. Transference

_____ 1. Unjust or prejudicial treatment of others based on perceiving them as different, such as a person's race, nationality, age, marital status, gender, gender identity, sexual orientation, religion, disability, cognitive reasoning, level of physical fitness, political affiliations, socioeconomic factors, pregnancy status, employment status, veteran status, immigration status, or history.

_____ 2. Commingling of feelings without differentiation between which feelings are the practitioner's and which are the client's.

_____ 3. A range of sexual behaviors, consensual and nonconsensual, between someone in an authoritative role and someone in a subordinate role.

_____ 4. Spaces between the practitioner's power and the client's vulnerability.

_____ 5. When a person projects feelings and behaviors they have for someone onto an entirely different person.

_____ 6. Obligation of professionals or professional organizations to safeguard entrusted information.

_____ 7. Situations where multiple roles exist between clients and practitioners.

_____ 8. Ability to accept another person's beliefs despite your own personal feelings.

_____ 9. Any action by a person in a position of trust or power that causes harm to another person.

_____ 10. Massage practitioner revealing thoughts, feelings, and personal history to clients.

_____ 11. Desire to understand what another person is experiencing without mistaking it for one's own experience.

_____ 12. Failure by a caregiver to provide necessary food, shelter, healthcare, or supervision to the person for whom they are caring.

MATCHING TWO: CONCEPT REVIEW

Place the letter of the answer next to the number of the term or phrase that best describes it.

A. Autonomy
B. Cultural competency
C. Emotional boundaries
D. Nonmalfeasance
E. Financial boundaries
F. Intellectual boundaries
G. Professionalism
H. Fidelity
I. Confidentiality
J. Sexual harassment
K. Therapeutic relationship
L. Unconditional positive regard

_____ 1. Affiliation between a practitioner and a client which allows practitioners to apply their professional knowledge and expertise to help clients achieve their treatment goals.

_____ 2. Boundaries encompassing our beliefs, thoughts, and ideas, as well as safeguarding self-esteem.

_____ 3. Boundaries separating personal feelings from the feelings of others.

_____ 4. Principle that requires professionals to remain loyal and dedicated to clients, to keep their promises, and to honor their commitments.

_____ 5. The obligation of professionals or professional organizations to safeguard entrusted information.

_____ 6. A set of behaviors, attitudes, and policies enabling professionals to interact effectively with others in cross-cultural situations.

_____ 7. Acceptance of another person regardless of what they say or do, validating and respecting their humanity.

_____ 8. Respecting the rights of competent individuals to make their own decisions.

_____ 9. Sexual or sexually suggestive unwanted behavior perceived as offensive, threatening, or embarrassing which can substantially interfere with someone's work, educational, or social setting by creating an intimidating or hostile environment.

_____ 10. Boundaries involving issues of money, including fee schedules, payment arrangements and procedures, and policies of nonpayment.

_____ 11. Adherence to a set of values and obligations, formally agreed-upon codes of conduct, and reasonable expectations of clients, colleagues, and co-workers.

_____ 12. Requires professionals to do no harm and to act in ways that avoid harm.

MULTIPLE CHOICE: TEST YOUR KNOWLEDGE

Place the letter of the answer next to the number of the term or phrase that best describes it.

_____ 1. Moral principles that govern behavior are:
   A. laws.
   B. codes.
   C. ethics.
   D. rules.

_____ 2. What principle of ethics obligates professionals to act in a way that benefits the wellbeing of others?
   A. Autonomy
   B. Beneficence
   C. Confidentiality
   D. Fidelity

_____ 3. The ability to be oneself while in a professional role describes:
   A. respect
   B. trust
   C. autonomy
   D. authenticity

_____ 4. Meaningful eye contact can be demonstrated by the _____ rule while speaking/listening.
   A. 30/30
   B. 50/70
   C. 20/10
   D. 100/100

_____ 5. The perspective that only your thoughts and beliefs are correct is called:
   A. cultural competency.
   B. positive tolerance.
   C. ethnocentrism.
   D. intolerance.

_____ 6. What is the Campinha-Bacote cultural competence milestone that describes acquiring information about culturally diverse groups?
   A. Cultural desire
   B. Cultural awareness
   C. Cultural knowledge
   D. Cultural skill

_____ 7. Revealing thoughts, feelings, and personal history to clients is called:
   A. self-disclosure.
   B. dual relationship.
   C. transference.
   D. countertransference.

_____ 8. Avoiding giving professional opinions or advice during social events is an example of:
   A. physical boundaries.
   B. emotional boundaries
   C. intellectual boundaries.
   D. location boundaries.

_____ 9. What is the most common social dual relationship?
   A. Friendship
   B. Familial
   C. Communal
   D. Business

_____ 10. Under what level of turbulence theory do most problems faced by practitioners fall?
   A. Light
   B. Moderate
   C. Severe
   D. Extreme

_____ 11. At what stage of training should practitioners begin to discuss the topic of sexual harassment?
   A. During school
   B. During examination
   C. After graduation
   D. After licensure

_____ 12. The most common form of sexual harassment reported by massage practitioners according to the Richard et al. study was:
   A. physical.
   B. verbal.
   C. forced activity.
   D. text message.

CRITICAL THINKING

What Did You Just Ask For?!

You have been working on a regular client every week for the last 6 months. The client is appreciative of the work you have done to resolve a stubborn shoulder issue, and you need the income from this steady client. At the end of your last session with the client, before you exit the massage room, the client asks for sexual favors. How do you handle this?

Answers can include but are not limited to:

It can be very upsetting when trust is broken by the client. When the massage practitioner has behaved professionally and ethically, and the client has decided to cross boundaries by asking for something that destroys the relationship, the practitioner has several options. One is to explain very clearly that massage does not include sexual activity of any kind, and that the client must agree to this before receiving another treatment. Another option is to explain very clearly that massage does not include sexual activity of any kind, and tell the client to never come back. It may be difficult to do this if the practitioner depends on the income. However, if the practitioner does not feel safe with this client, then no amount of money is worth continuing to have this client come to the practitioner's treatment space. A third option is to call the police. This depends on whether the practitioner feels safe setting a firm boundary, or if the practitioner feels unsafe with this client in the office. What the practitioner should NEVER do is laugh off the request and hope that the client does not ask for sexual favors again. The chances are good that the client will ask again, and could even escalate the situation from that point. The practitioner needs to remain calm, act professionally, and leave no doubt in the client's mind that there are very firm boundaries that the practitioner will NOT cross.

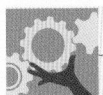

PROFESSIONAL PRACTICE

A Taxing Situation

Alice has been your accountant for 7 years. Two years ago, she needed help with a stiff shoulder. Alice was so pleased with the other benefits of massage that she now receives weekly massages by you. Her standing appointment is Thursday at 4 pm. On Monday, you receive a letter from the IRS stating a mistake was made on your last year's tax returns and you have underpaid by $800. How do you handle this situation?

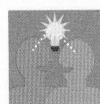

DISCUSSION

NCBTMB's Code of Ethics

Given the complexity of professional relationships, how can they be managed ethically? NCBTMB's Code of Ethics provides guidelines and supports professional judgment (http://www.ncbtmb.org/code-ethics). Visit the webpage that lists the Code of Ethics and Standards of Practice. After reading them, select the one you feel is most important, and explain why you feel this way.

I would like to thank Megan Lavery for her past contributions on this chapter.

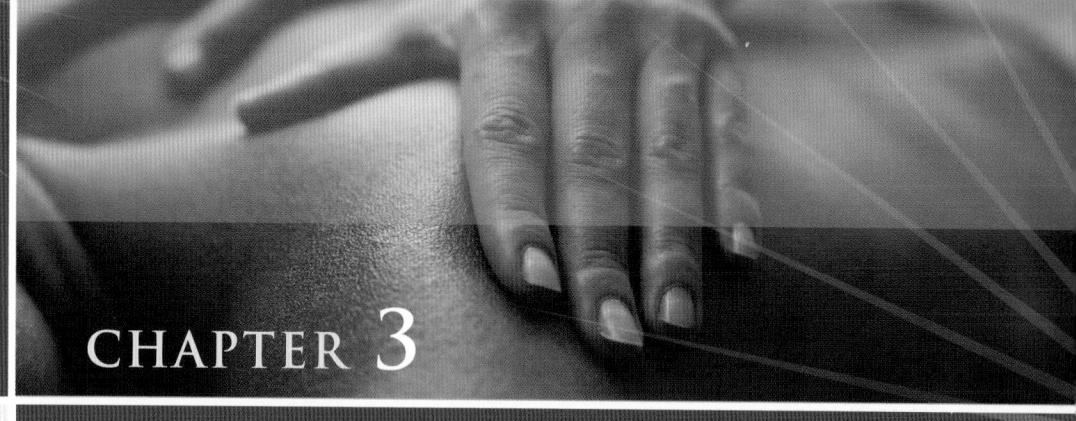

CHAPTER 3

Tools of the Trade: Tables, Accessories, Linens, Lubricants, Aromatherapy, Essential Oils, and the Massage Environment

I'm going to pretend that everybody is my brother or my sister. And if they are temporarily behaving like they're not, I'm going to pretend that they're just confused. I'm going to insist, through my mannerisms and my tone of voice, that I see them at their highest.
—George Saunders

LEARNING OBJECTIVES

After completing this chapter, the student should be able to:

1. Define massage table features, and state how to care for table fabrics.
2. Discuss massage table accessories, such as face rests and bolsters, and massage linens.
3. Discuss massage lubricants, including how to choose, dispense, apply, and store them.
4. State the use of aromatherapy and essential oils in a massage practice.
5. Describe the massage room environment and safety guidelines.

INTRODUCTION

A successful and fulfilling massage career depends on the quality of education the individual receives and the ability to use the tools of the trade wisely. Although "hands" are important, massage practitioners usually need additional equipment such as a massage table and related supplies, including linens and lubricants.

The atmosphere and environment of the massage room are also important aspects of a treatment because certain colors, aromas, and sounds promote relaxation. This chapter will examine tools of the massage trade and offer practical suggestions to assist in decision-making. Also included are safety considerations for your massage equipment and your massage room to reduce the risk of injury from slips, trips, and falls for you and your client. Disinfection procedures are in Chapter 9.

MASSAGE TABLES

Massage tables are used to position clients in various ways to facilitate receiving the massage and adjunct techniques (e.g., stretching, joint mobilizations). The most frequently purchased massage table type is a portable table, which accounts for approximately 95% of massage table sales. Portable massage tables are hinged in the middle and can be folded in half and transported (Fig. 3.1). When the two folded sides are latched together, the portable table resembles an oversized suitcase. An advantage of portable massage tables is they can be moved with relative ease, increasing the locations massage practitioners work. Electric lift tables are becoming more popular and offer the practitioner quick and easy change of table height. Due to the weight of the table, electric tables are usually stationary rather than portable and require clients to come to the practitioner.

Selecting a Table Manufacturer

When choosing a massage table or chair, look for a manufacturer with an excellent reputation. This is important for

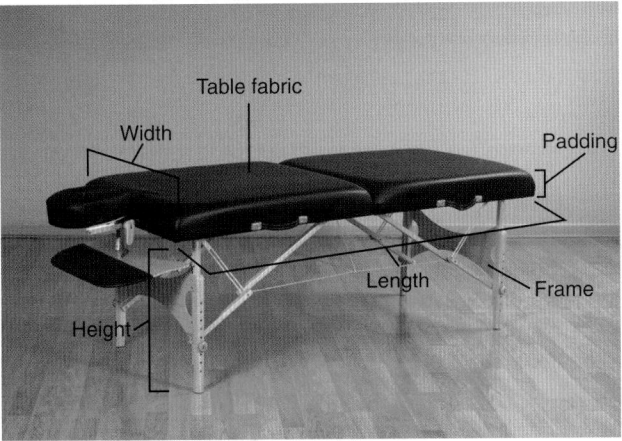

FIG. 3.1 Portable massage table with features of height, length, frame, width, padding, and fabric labeled.

several reasons. Respected, well-established companies usually have quality, well-made products that have withstood the test of time. These companies often provide excellent customer service before and after the purchase and may offer a trial period with all or part of the purchase price refunded once the product is returned if the customer is not satisfied. In addition, massage tables and chairs sold by reputable companies often hold their value and bring a higher resale price.

Currently, there is no national standard for determining weight ratings for massage tables and chairs. Consumers must rely on weight ratings supplied by the company. The more reputable the company, the more trustworthy their published weight ratings are. Most tables and chairs will be used for extended periods, commonly 10 or more years. If a face rest needs to be replaced or if a new accessory is needed, single accessory purchases are available. This may not be the case for tables sold by department stores, membership clubs, or massage warehouses, and these businesses may be unable to assist you in contacting the manufacturer if problems arise. As with most things in life, you get what you pay for, and:

The bitterness of poor quality remains long after the sweetness of low price is forgotten.
~ Benjamin Franklin

MASSAGE TABLE FEATURES

Most manufacturers offer several table feature options, including width, frame material, padding, and fabric. These and other features need to be factored into your decision about which table to buy and are presented next. Suggestions for selecting a massage chair are discussed in Chapter 15.

Width

Most massage tables have a width between 28 and 33 inches, with most tables being 30 to 31 inches wide. Massage table width preference depends on the size of the massage room; the type of client position most frequently used, such as side-lying versus prone (face down) position; and the type of clientele such as frail, disabled, or large-framed—who may all prefer a wider more spacious table.

Height

Massage table height range is usually between 22 and 34 inches. Adjustment is achieved by lengthening or shortening the table legs, usually in 1-inch increments. Aluminum table legs are typically nested tubes, with adjustments made quickly by pushing a spring-loaded button and changing the leg length longer or shorter. Wooden table legs are generally two sections held together by a tongue and groove system and one or two bolts. Height adjustments are made by unscrewing the knob(s), repositioning the lower section, and rescrewing the knob(s) to secure the two sections of the table leg.

Some practitioners may rarely change table height. However, client girth may vary enough to make ease of height adjustability a major consideration. This is especially true when working on the fourth, fifth, or sixth client of the day, when energy conservation and need for proper body mechanics become more of a consideration. Quick height adjustments are also important when a table is used by multiple practitioners. See Chapter 7 for table height suggestions.

Length

Most massage table lengths are 72 to 73 inches. Face rests and bolsters are frequently used—a face rest adds 10 to 12 inches to table length, and a 6- or 8-inch bolster reduces the client's length when placed behind the knees or in front of the ankles. Therefore a 6-foot or taller client will have ample room lying on a massage table.

Frame

Massage table frames, as well as its undercarriage, provide support and are made of wood, aluminum, or a combination of the two materials. Wood-frame portable massage tables usually weigh a few pounds more compared with aluminum-framed portable massage tables.

Padding

Massage table padding should be comfortable to the client while adapting to and supporting the client's body. In addition, some table pads have recesses for female breasts and for pregnant clients to lie prone (see Fig. 11.4). When selecting table padding, consider its density, loft, and durability. Let us examine each of these features.

Density

Most top-of-the-line massage tables use several grades of foam density, or degree of table padding mass, volume, and compactness. The foam pads are divided into grades of density, including light, medium, and high grade. High-grade density generally has better *memory,* or ability of the foam pad to return to its original height after being compressed.

Loft

Loft refers to the thickness of the table padding, and it can range from 1.5 (firm) to 4 inches (ultraplush). Practitioners who often use deep-pressure techniques tend to prefer firm loft, as clients will less likely sink into the table padding as downward pressure is applied. Loftier or fluffier padding increases client comfort while lying on the table and is preferred for practitioners who frequently apply techniques under the client's body.

Durability

The cellular structure of massage table padding breaks down over time. This rate depends on several factors such as foam density and how often the table is used. Certain table foam pads, such as AeroCel and UltraCell, are manufactured to be more durable and last longer compared with others. Some

practitioners reduce unequal padding wear and tear by switching the end of the "head" of the table (where the face rest frame is inserted) with the "foot" of the table. Rotate the table position within the massage room horizontally 180 degrees if you use this method.

TABLE FABRIC

Fabric covers the massage table, table accessories, and massage chairs. Most good-quality massage tables and products use polyurethane fabrics and do not contain polyvinyl chlorides (PVCs), which makes them environmentally friendly. Keep in mind that, although table fabrics are not easily damaged by blunt force, they can be perforated by sharp objects such as keys, hairpins, jewelry, and pet (cat) claws.

Keep It Covered

Keeping your table covered while not in use and during transport (e.g., in a case) helps keep the table fabric blemish-free. Table fabrics are smooth, which means massage linens may slip on their slick surfaces during use. This can be alleviated by placing a fitted table pad, a fitted sheet, or a flat sheet stretched snug across the table and tied at the corners in knots before adding massage sheets.

Keep It Clean

Clean massage table fabric and accessory fabric when needed. Most cleansers and detergents are too strong when used at full strength and, if used undiluted, will damage the fabric. Contact the manufacturers and request their approved cleaning product list. Many massage table manufacturers recommend a 4:1 diluted solution of green Windex, 409, Fantastik, or other nonabrasive, nonalcohol cleaning products. Vinegar may also be used. Avoid citrus oil–based cleaners because they can damage the fabric. Chlorine bleach is used for disinfecting but not routine cleaning of table and accessory fabric. Information regarding disinfecting contaminated surfaces such as table fabric is in Chapter 9.

Keep It Cool

Massage table fabrics are similar to fine wine; they do not like wide temperature ranges. Extreme hot or cold (>95°F/35°C or <32°F/0°C) can damage table and accessory fabrics. Examples of fabric damage by extreme temperatures are brittleness, cracking, and stretch marks. For this reason, do not place a massage table for long periods in a car, near a heat source, in direct sunlight, or in spaces not climatically controlled. If a massage table has been exposed to extreme temperatures, allow the fabric to return to room temperature (range of 68°F/20°C to 75°F/23°C) before allowing a client to sit or lie on it. Otherwise, the fabric may sustain a permanent stretch mark or crack if pressure is applied while the fabric is warm and stretchy or cool and stiff.

The pessimist sees difficulty in every opportunity. The optimist sees the opportunity in every difficulty.
—**Winston Churchill**

MASSAGE TABLE ACCESSORIES

Massage table accessories help position clients for the massage, provide client comfort and safety, and support effective body mechanics. Examples of accessories are face rest, arm shelf, bolsters, and stools (Fig. 3.2). Some table accessories help with table transport. Also included in this section are carry cases and table carts. Cover face rest cushions, arm shelves, and bolsters with a clean cloth before use. This cloth must be laundered or discarded (if disposable) after each use.

Face Rest

A face rest, or face cradle, allows clients to keep their heads and necks aligned while lying prone (see Fig. 3.2B). A face rest consists of two parts: a crescent-shaped cushion and a frame. The cushion is usually covered with the same fabric as the massage table and is generally attached to the frame by Velcro. The fasteners allow the cushion to be widened or narrowed and accommodate a wide range of facial structures. Face rest cushions are usually filled with foam padding similar to the table padding, but newer face rest cushions may contain water spheres. Because the cushion will migrate laterally over time with continued use, remove it

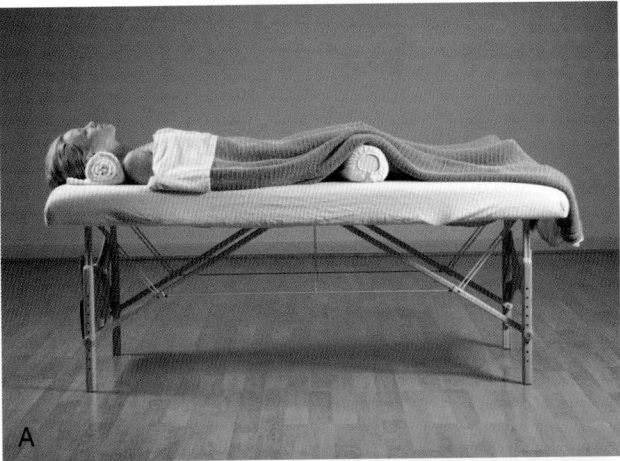

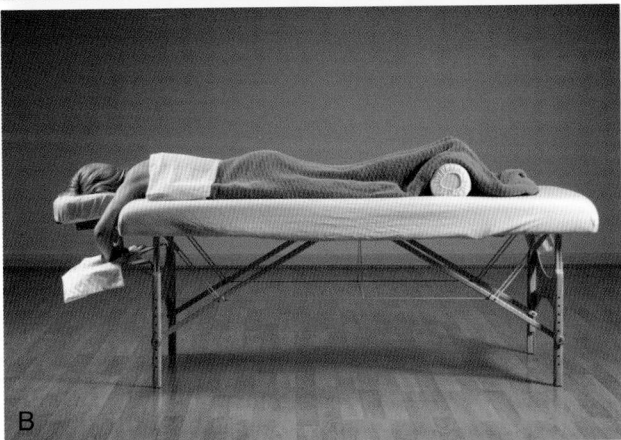

FIG. 3.2 Bolsters placed on a supine-lying client (A) and prone-lying client (B). Note the use of a face rest and arm shelf in B and that the table and all table accessories are draped

from the frame periodically to reshape it using a few firm squeezes.

The face rest frame is attached to the end of the table by support rods which insert into grommets. Face rest frames are not universal and usually only fit tables made by the same company. *Standard frames* allow the head and neck to be in one position—parallel to the tabletop. *Adjustable frames* can be raised, lowered, and tilted, allowing the neck to be flexed or extended for client comfort and for functionality such as practitioner access to the base of the skull. Adjustable frames can be folded down to lie against the table when not in use. Adjustable frames run the risk of breaking under increased pressure such as if the client pushes down against the frame. This situation can occur while the client is repositioning and leans on the face rest frame for support instead of the table. To prevent this from happening, instruct the client to scoot down on the table before repositioning.

Arm Shelf

The arm shelf provides a resting place for forearms while the client is lying prone (see Fig. 3.2B). The shelf is either a small platform suspended below the face rest or a hammock-style sling suspended by straps from the face rest frame. If the arm shelf is attached to the table frame by screws, the shelf is usable only at one end of the massage table.

If using arm shelves attached to the sides of the table, insert them after the client transfers onto the table and remove them before the client transfers off the table. Side arm shelves left in place while the client transfers are potentially hazardous if the client mistakes the removable arm shelf for the sturdy massage table.

Bolsters and Cushions

Bolsters and cushions, including pillows, provide additional support for the client's posterior neck, knees, and ankles. The most popular bolster height is 6 inches, but 3- and 8-inch heights are available. Covered bolsters are often placed behind the knees and behind the neck on a supine-lying client or when lying face up (see Fig. 3.2A). The knee bolster placement may also decrease excessive lordosis. Covered bolsters are placed in front of the ankles on a prone-lying client (see Fig. 3.2B). Other cushions for client positioning include cervical pillows and standard- and king-size pillows; the latter may be needed for side-lying massage. Some practitioners use positioning cushion systems designed to have pieces used singly or arranged in ways to fit a wide range of body types.

Stool

Stools allow the practitioner to sit while performing massage. Areas of the body easily massaged while the practitioner is seated include the face, neck, hands, and feet (Fig. 3.3). A covered stool can also be used as an arm shelf or as a small table for items such as massage lubricant or a box of tissue. Stool seats are shaped round, like a chair

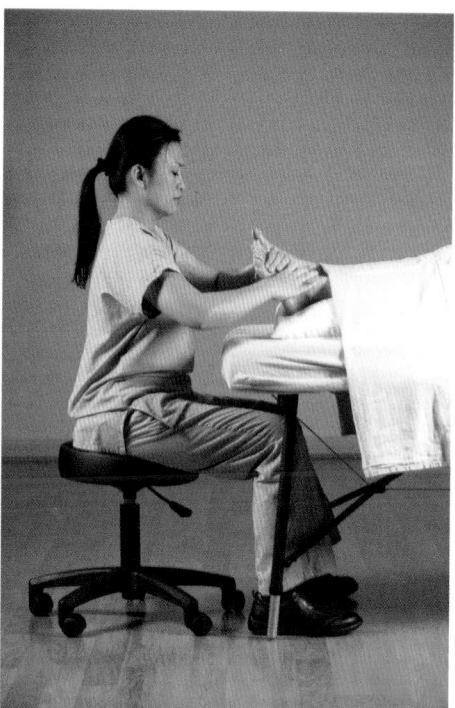

FIG. 3.3 Practitioner sitting in a stool to massage a supine-lying client's foot.

seat, or like a saddle. Stool height is usually adjustable, and many stool feet are on casters so the stool can easily roll across the floor when needed. An adjustable rolling stool offers practitioners height options and more mobility while seated. However, some practitioners prefer a non-rolling adjustable stool, as they are less likely to roll backward while applying pressure laterally. A large inflatable physioball can also be used as a stool.

Electric Table Warmer

Electric table warmers are used to keep the client warm during the massage. Ensure electric cords are in a safe location and do not create a fall risk. Turn on the table warmer before the client arrives, and set the temperature according to the client's preference.

Carrying Case

A carrying case helps the practitioner transport a portable massage table by providing padded handles and straps, making it easier to lift and carry the table. Most carry cases have several wide and deep zippered pockets for storing supplies. The carry case also protects table fabric from damage. Some carrying cases have wheels built in to make transport easier.

Table Cart

Table carts allow portable tables to be pushed or pulled rather than lifted and carried. Most table carts are attached to the table by an adjustable quick-clip strap. The table cart may require the massage table be within a carry case before it is loaded onto the cart.

MASSAGE LINENS

Massage linens are used to drape the clothed, partially clothed, or unclothed client, as well as drape over massage equipment such as the massage table and related accessories. Examples of massage linens are sheets, bolster covers, face rest covers, pillowcases, towels, and blankets. Popular linen colors are white, ivory, or soft pastels. Light solid colors do not overemphasize lubricant stains compared with dark solid colors. Chapter 7 contains draping techniques, and Chapter 11 contains draping modifications for special populations such as pregnant and elderly clients.

Popular sheet fabrics are cotton, cotton blends, and flannel. Avoid thin, clingy, or see-through fabrics such as jersey knit because these types of fabrics reveal details of the client's body. If revealing fabrics cannot be avoided, use an additional drape such as a blanket over the sheet. Sheets can be purchased singly or in prepackaged twin-sized sheet sets and include a fitted sheet, a flat sheet, and a standard-sized pillowcase; the pillowcase can be used to drape the bolster, face rest, or arm shelf.

Towels are made with terrycloth and are designed to absorb water easily, making them ideal for spa treatments. Towels are also used to drape the client during the massage, used over a sheet to provide additional warmth, or used to apply massage techniques such as friction. Do not place a towel on the massage table and then position the client over it, as the pressure of the client's body will cause the towel to leave compression marks on the skin.

Blankets help warm a chilled client and help the client relax (see Fig. 3.2). Heavier blankets are preferred over lighter blankets. In two studies, weighted blankets were effective in reducing anxiety among adults in mental health settings (Champagne et al., 2015; Mullen et al., 2008), with the majority of users preferring weighted blankets for their calming effect (Mullen et al., 2008). Moreover, there were no significant differences in vital signs between the control group and treatment group, indicating weighted blankets are safe (Champagne et al., 2015).

Sheets and accessory covers are used once for each client and then need to be laundered. Linens should be replaced as needed, including when they become odorous and smell rancid. Information regarding disinfecting contaminated linens is in Chapter 9.

MASSAGE LUBRICANTS

The primary purpose of a massage lubricant is to reduce friction between the practitioner's hands and the client's skin. Friction is a force that holds back the movement of a sliding object. Massage lubricants reduce friction so hands or massage tools used to provide massage can slide over by pushing or pulling while changing the shape of the tissue beneath. Too much lubricant = too much slide. Not enough lubricant = too much friction. If the right amount of lubricant is used, tissues can be moved but the friction is not uncomfortable or irritating to the skin.

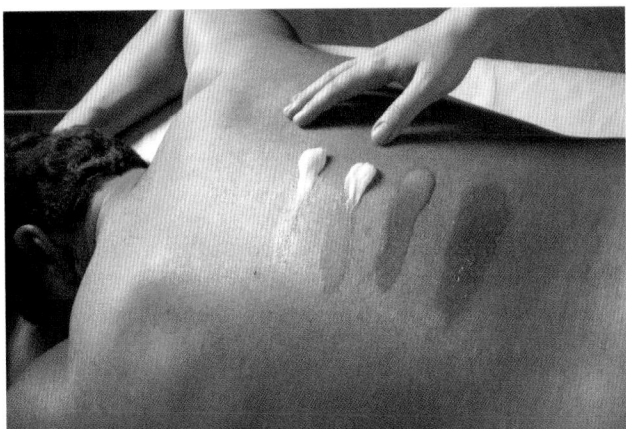

FIG. 3.4 Some massage lubricant choices. From left to right, they are butter, crème, gel, and oil.

Types of massage lubricant are crèmes, lotions, butters, waxes, oils, and gels (Fig. 3.4). Powders such as cornstarch are used when friction reduction should be minimal; an example is when applying lymphatic massage techniques. Some professional situations will require the practitioner to apply massage techniques through clothing or through a drape. Therefore the practitioner should know how to give a massage without the use of lubricants.

Lubricants used in hospital or medical settings must be preapproved by the infection control manager or appropriate staff member. In these situations, submit a product ingredient list, and, once approved, the product's safety data sheet or material safety data sheet remains on the premises and is available during inspections.

Oil-based and Water-based Lubricants

Massage lubricants can be oil-based or water-based. Oil-based lubricants provide more glide; less product is needed because it remains on the skin for longer periods, and these lubricants are less likely to cause chilling, as oil creates a layer of insulation to reduce loss of body heat. Conversely, water-based lubricants are less effective at reducing friction and are appropriate for techniques requiring more friction. These are marketed as "deep tissue" products because they contain more water and less oil.

Deep tissue massage products absorb more quickly compared with oil-based lubricants and are applied more frequently. In addition, water-based lubricants are more likely to cause the client to feel cold because of evaporative cooling. Consider using a blanket or table warmer as a proactive measure to keep the client warm.

Lubricant Types: Crèmes, Lotions, Oils, Gels, Butters and Waxes

Massage crèmes and lotions are the top-selling massage lubricants. Crèmes and lotions are moisturizing, hydrating, and more emollient, which means possessing skin softening or soothing qualities. Crèmes and lotions are also less likely to stain clothing and massage linens. The thickness of crème makes it less likely to spill out of its container.

Oils and gels are derived from nuts, seeds, and vegetables. Sesame, grape, coconut, and hemp seed oils tend to be well tolerated. One disadvantage of oils and gels is staining of linens and clothing and of odors remaining on massage sheets and bolster covers frequently in contact with these products. Some massage oil manufacturers sell washing machine additives that state they remove oils, stains and smells, but these additives have mixed reviews.

Butters are derived from fruit, nuts, or seeds. The most common butters used in massage lubricants are cocoa butter and shea butter. Cocoa butter, also known as Theobroma oil, is obtained from cacao seed, and shea butter is extracted from the tree's fruit (called tree nut). Butters will melt and liquefy when in contact with body heat, so use sparingly. **NOTE**: If clients are allergic to latex, they may also have an allergic reaction to shea butter because of cross-reactivity (Grier, 2012). Avoid shea butter as a massage lubricant or lubricant ingredient in these cases.

Massage waxes are a combination of wax blended with oils such as sweet almond oil or grapeseed oil. These offer reduced glide and are suitable for myofascial and scar tissue massage. Commonly used waxes in massage are beeswax, tribehenin, or candelilla.

Massage and Topical Cannabinoid Products

In some states, massage practitioners can use topical agents containing cannabinoids (CBDs). Research suggests transdermal delivery of CBD is safe, effective, and non–habit forming, partially because drug levels rise slowly when applied topically (Paudel et al., 2010). Hammell et al. (2016) found transdermal CBD reduced inflammation and decreased pain in rats with arthritis. Hunter et al. (2018) found transdermal CBD did not produce any statistically relevant results regarding knee pain from arthritis in humans. Schultz (2020) stated there is little scientific evidence CBD-infused products are more effective compared with other topical pain-relieving agents such as Tiger Balm, BenGay, Icy Hot, or Biofreeze. More will be learned about the effects of topically applied CBD, and there appears to be no evident side effects (Hammell et al., 2016). However, using CBD products in any form during pregnancy or while breastfeeding is not recommended (U.S. Food and Drug Administration [FDA], 2019). This caution includes topical applications.

Choosing Massage Lubricants

When choosing a massage lubricant, several factors are considered. Lubricants containing high-quality ingredients are more expensive. In general, crèmes and butters are more expensive compared with oils and gels. However, practitioners who use oils and gels more frequently need to replace their linens, requiring the cost of linen replacement to be considered. Some practitioners avoid products containing mineral oil and parabens. Mineral oil is thought to clog pores and may be a carcinogen (cancer-causing agent). Parabens are thought to mimic the hormone estrogen when they are absorbed into the skin; estrogens may play a role in breast cancer development. In response to these concerns, many massage lubricant manufacturers are removing mineral oils and parabens from all or part of their product lines.

No matter what lubricants and other massage products you use, it is essential you disclose the ingredients during the consent process with clients so they have a complete understanding of the substances you are applying to their skin.

Scented and Unscented Lubricants

Massage lubricants and similar products are available as scented and unscented or fragrance free. Scented products are selected according to client preference; the practitioner should obtain consent before their use on individual clients. Some scents are initially pleasant but become unpleasant as scented products are applied over larger areas of the client's body, especially in an enclosed space.

Hypoallergenic products are less likely to cause allergic reactions. They are used when the client has allergies to ingredients in nonhypoallergenic lubricants, has sensitive or hyperreactive skin, or skin conditions such as eczema (atopic dermatitis) or psoriasis. If you are unsure what product to use, choose an unscented, hypoallergenic lubricant.

Dispensing Massage Lubricants

Take proactive measures to reduce the risk of cross-contamination. Cross-contamination occurs when microorganisms such as bacteria are transferred from one source to another. Sanitize the outside of the container with soap and water before dispensing lubricant from it. Use the same hand washing procedure listed in Chapter 9 for the outside of the lubricant container. Do not place sanitized containers on unclean surfaces such as countertops and flooring.

When dispensing *thick lubricants* such as crèmes or butters, use a clean spatula to remove a sufficient amount of product for single-client use from the jar and place it in a sanitary disposable or reusable dish. Discard unused product after treatment. Discard the disposal dish, or sanitize the reusable dish. When dispensing *thin lubricants* such as lotions, gels, or oils, either use a container with a pump mechanism or a squeezable bottle or tube.

In hospital or medical settings, use only single-use lubricant containers. Once the lubricant container has been opened in a patient's room, the container and unused contents must be disposed of in the same room. This prevents contaminated lubricant from being used by anyone, including the patient's visitors.

Applying Massage Lubricants

When applying lubricant, determine which area will be treated and the amount of product required for the treatment area. Place the predetermined amount of product into the palm of your hand and rub it with the opposite hand to warm the product before applying it to the client's skin. If too much lubricant is dispensed, remove the excess product with a clean cloth. Apply more product as needed during the massage. As mentioned previously, too little lubricant can cause excess friction and can be uncomfortable and irritate the skin. Dry skin and body hair may require additional lubricant. Techniques applied in an up-and-down direction (i.e., vertically, horizontally, or diagonally) are less likely to mat and tangle body hair compared with techniques applied in a circular direction.

In hospital or medical settings, application of massage lubricants or touching a patient's skin usually involves the use of disposable gloves. Massage practitioners who do not glove may be in violation of infection control guidelines and hospital policies.

Storing Massage Lubricants

Store your massage lubricants in a cool, dark location away from direct sunlight. Under these conditions, most lubricants remain blended and unrancid for approximately 18 months. The product's shelf life can be extended for an additional year with refrigeration or freezing; allow the product to return to room temperature before use.

AROMATHERPY AND ESSENTIAL OILS

Aromatherapy is the use of fragrant essential oils by inhalation or by applying a diluted form to the skin. René-Maurice Gattefossé was the first to coin the phrase aromatherapie, from which aromatherapy is derived. Aromatherapy is also called *essential oil therapy*. **Essential oils** are concentrated essences of plants and possess characteristic fragrances of the plants from which they are extracted. Essential oils are so concentrated only small amounts, or drops, are used. Essential oils are extracted from many parts of plants using several methods, most often by steam distillation. Here are a few essential oils and parts of the plant they are derived.

- Flowers (e.g., lavender, jasmine)
- Fruits (e.g., bergamot, lemon)
- Grasses (e.g., citronella)
- Leaves (e.g., eucalyptus, peppermint)
- Roots (e.g., ginger, vetiver)
- Seeds (e.g., black pepper, fennel)
- Tree blossoms (e.g., ylang-ylang, clary sage)
- Woods and resins (e.g., sandalwood, frankincense)

Choosing Essential Oils

In general, essential oils can have calming or stimulatory effects. Ask the client before dispensing a particular essential oil(s) as they may not like the scent. **NOTE**: Essential oils used in massage products have been linked to contact dermatitis (Lakshmi, 2014); these include laurel (Adişen & Onder, 2007) and turmeric (Lopez-Villafuerte & Clores, 2016), as well as ayurvedic oils, particularly Dhanwantharam tailam and Eladi tailam (Eladi coconut oil), so caution is warranted. In addition, practitioners who use essential oils in their practice are at increased risk for occupational contact dermatitis (Crawford et al., 2004; Trattner et al., 2008). Crawford et al. (2004) found 15% to 23% of massage practitioners had contact dermatitis on their hands, and risks were greater among practitioners with a history of eczema.

Next are 10 popular essentials with some associated anecdotal effects.

1. **Lavender**. The most widely used essential oil, it combats insomnia, calms and balances the mind and emotions, and helps ease irritability.

2. **Eucalyptus**. Widely used for respiratory congestion, eucalyptus may also bring comfort when experiencing loss and grief. This oil can be used during periods of physical and mental fatigue and exhaustion.

3. **Lemon**. Lemon is used for increased energy and a sense of mental clarity, which makes it useful during times of indecisiveness. Lemon essential oil may irritate the skin.

4. **Peppermint**. Peppermint adds a sense of excitement and enthusiasm, as well as raising attention levels, such as what is needed to take a test. It is great for a pick-me-up or after a period of depression. This oil is used for headaches, nausea, and motion sickness. If your client is taking homeopathic remedies, then avoid using peppermint because it can act as an antidote.

5. **Rose geranium**. Relaxing and soothing, rose geranium also can enhance sensuality and assist in confidence building.

6. **Rosemary**. Aiding in stimulating mental clarity, concentration, and memory, rosemary promotes cerebral activity (and is used by some students during examinations). Do not use on clients with seizure disorders.

7. **Sandalwood**. Sandalwood promotes deep relaxation, abates depression, and calms the mind and emotions. Sandalwood is one of the more costly essential oils, along with chamomile, rose, and frankincense.

8. **Tangerine**. Tangerine is said to clear away negativity and opens up the heart by inspiring sensitivity and empathy. It also helps calm an overactive nervous system.

9. **Tea tree**. Tea tree acts as an antiseptic, so it can be used to disinfect contaminated items, as well as being antifungal and antibacterial. It also helps strengthen the immune response.

10. **Ylang-ylang**. This oil can calm the nervous system, ease depression, and reduce frustration. Used topically, ylang-ylang can irritate the skin.

Dispensing Essential Oils

Essential oils enter the body through mucous membranes by inhalation or are absorbed through the skin. Use only three or four oils at a time until you gain considerable training and experience in aromatherapy, because blends can become overpowering and even nauseating.

- **Inhalation**. Place 5 to 10 drops of essential oil on the center flap of a face rest cover, on a corner of a pillowcase, or on a tissue placed on the arm shelf while the client is prone.
- **Diffuser**. Place 10 to 15 drops of essential oils to a diffuser. Add more drops as needed.
- **Room Mister**. Add 2 to 10 drops per 1 oz of water in a spray bottle. Shake before use.
- **Baths (Immersion or Steam)**. For immersion baths, add 5 to 10 drops of essential oil in a tub for a single user. Be sure the water is moving while the client is in the water. For a steam bath, add 5 to 10 drops in the water well.
- **Compress**. Add 2 to 5 drops of essential oil to a small dish of water. Drench washcloth in scented water. Wring out excess water and apply to the skin.
- **Massage Lubricant**. Add 15 to 20 drops of essential oil to 1 oz of oil-based lubricant for a full-body massage.

This gives a 2.5% to 3% dilution. For massaging a localized area (e.g., muscle spasm in the shoulder), a slightly stronger dilution can be used. Add 12 to 15 drops of essential oil to ½ oz of carrier oil or lubricant for this purpose.

- **Body Treatment Product (Masks or Scrubs)**. Mix the essential oil in an oil-based carrier (discussed next), then add it to the body treatment product.

Carrier or Base Oils

Most essential oils must be diluted in a carrier or base oil to "carry" them to skin because they are potent and can cause irritation. Carrier oils, such as vegetable and nut oils, contain fat. Other fatty products used as carriers are jojoba, whole milk, oil-based creams, lotions, shampoos, and conditioners. In general, the higher the fat content, the more stable the carrier oil will be. Stability refers to its shelf life and resistance to oxidation and resultant rancidity. Jojoba is very stable. Safflower oil is not very stable and will go rancid quickly. Vitamin E, which helps stabilize carrier oils, can be added to lengthen shelf life.

Even though essential oils are not soluble in water, they can be added to water if they are properly dispersed, as in shaking a mist bottle before spraying, in a steam bath, or an immersion bath with moving water through a pump. If not dispersed, the essential oil will then float, concentrated, on top of still water.

A few essential oils can be applied undiluted or "neat" and include lavender, tea tree, Roman chamomile, and rose.

Essential Oil Safety

The Epilepsy Society (2019) recommends avoiding rosemary, fennel, sage, eucalyptus, hyssop, camphor, and spike lavender when working with people who have seizure disorders. Use of essential oils appears to be safe during pregnancy as there have been no reports of abnormal fetuses or aborted fetuses from the use of essential oils, either by inhalation or by topical application (Buckle, 2014). Next are suggestions for safe use of essential oils.

- Use oils you are familiar with and you can use on yourself (you are inhaling and absorbing them, too).
- Avoid using them on infants.
- Cut a single dose in half for children.
- Avoid using essential oils near the eyes
- Be sure the massage room has adequate ventilation.
- Blend them with carrier or base oils. (Exceptions: lavender, tea tree, Roman chamomile, and rose, as stated previously.)
- Do not apply any of the following essential oils before direct exposure to sunlight because they are photosensitive and may cause a skin rash: angelica, lavender, lemon, orange, tangerine, mandarin, and bergamot.

Storing Essential Oils

Essential oils are sold in dark, airtight containers usually made from glass and not plastic. Store essential oils in a cool, dry place away from direct sunlight. Under these conditions, essential oils last up to 7 years. However, when mixed with carrier oils (discussed later), shelf life is reduced to the shelf life of the carrier oil. Although classified as oils, essential oils have a property similar to water. When exposed to air for extended periods of time, essential oils evaporate because they are volatile (French, "to fly"). Replace the bottle top after use, and keep them out of children's reach.

THE MASSAGE ENVIRONMENT

Massage facilities can be scented or fragrance free. If scents are used, lavender, vanilla, valerian, jasmine, or any scent clients enjoy may promote calmness and relaxation (National Sleep Foundation [NSF], n.d.). Steady, low sounds, including white noise, will facilitate relaxation by blocking out distracting noise. Adequate lighting is needed to conduct assessments and in areas where clients transfer from one location to another or to and from the massage table. During the massage, low lighting facilitates relaxation. If bulbs are used, the recommended wattage is between 45 and 60 watts (Better Sleep Council [BSC], n.d.). Several studies indicate music during massage reduced anxiety and decreased depression (Cooke et al., 2007; Jones & Field, 1999).

Consider using calming hues rather than vibrant hues on walls (BSC, n.d.). Neutral colors such as taupe, gray, beige, and white or muted tones and light pastels help individuals feel calmer. Rich shades of red, orange, and yellow can create a warm cozy feeling. Certain blues and blue-greens, or cool colors, can have a soothing effect and can make a room feel cooler.

Ideal room temperatures for massage practitioners are between 68° and 76°F (Occupational Safety and Health Administration [OSHA], 2003). The higher end of this temperature range is recommended for clients. If clients have cold intolerance (sensitivity to cold temperatures) or feel chilled during the massage, provide comfort measures such as a blanket, an electric table warmer, raising the room temperature, or a combination of these. **NOTE**: Appropriate practitioner attire is discussed in Chapter 7.

Safety Guidelines

Slips, trips, and falls are the most common cause of office-related injuries (Centers for Disease Control and Prevention [CDC], 2018; Einstein College of Medicine [ECM], n.d.). The leading causes of slips, trips, and falls are slippery floors, materials left in walkways, inadequate lighting, tripping over open desk drawers or file cabinets, falling over electrical cords or wires, and bending or reaching for something while seated in an unstable chair. The following is a list of safety guidelines to make your facility accessible and safe and keep yourself, coworkers, and clients free from injury.

- Provide safe and unobstructed human passage in the public areas. Safe passage includes level flooring.
- Secure carpet edges and remove throw rugs.
- Avoid waxy floors. Clean up spills immediately.
- Remove low furniture and objects on the floor.
- Remove cords and wires on the floor.
- Install a raised toilet seat if the seat is too low.
- Use bright lights in walkways and hallways.
- Place handrails on stairways and grab bars in bathrooms.
- Bathrooms should have toilets that are wheelchair-height and sinks with lever-style faucets.
- Use lever-style handles on passage doors.
- Slopes, not steps, are needed between the parking space and the building. Exterior ramps should be designed so they drain well and do not hold water.
- The street address should be outside the building in clear view, which will make locating your building easier for emergency assistance (see Chapter 9).
- Ensure your table is barrier free during the transfer of clients on and off the table. Safely tuck bolsters and pillows not in use beneath the table or in a cabinet.
- Maintain all equipment in safe working condition. This includes checking and tightening massage table hinges, knobs, and locks before each business day.

EVOLVE RESOURCES

http://evolve.elsevier.com/Salvo/MassageTherapy

- Chapter challenge
- Flash cards
- Downloadable forms

STEPHEN HALPERN

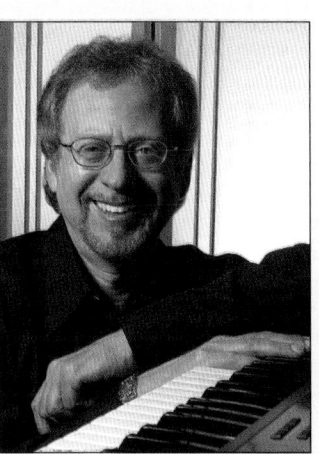

Music has been variously described as the "food of love," a "revelation," and "a ladder to the soul." Music provides the auditory landscape of a massage as much as the hands, lotions, and linens create a tactile one. We know this feeling of ease and relaxation that comes from certain kinds of music (and the stimulation and energy arising from other kinds) is not a figment of our imagination but a reaction of our nervous system. However, this was not always the case, and the pioneer who brought these facts to light was musician and researcher Steven Halpern.

Halpern has always been engaged in making music. As a musician, he has played everything from rock to jazz to rhythm-and-blues. His experiences as both a creator and consumer of music led him to wonder, as a curious college student in the late 1960s, about the effects of music on the human body.

At the time, there was little research on the subject. In fact, it was not even considered a respectable area of study, and few schools would allow Halpern to do the research he was drawn to. Eventually, he ended up at the University of California at Sonoma, where he had access to biofeedback equipment and permission to engage in his unusual research. He carefully studied the body's responses to music, using subtle rhythms, gentle tones, and nontraditional harmonics.

He soon discovered rhythms of the human body are affected by the rhythms in music, a phenomenon called entrainment. Faster music causes one's heart rate and breathing to speed up, whereas a slow, steady beat results in the opposite. Halpern notes, "Trying to relax to music with a fast beat is like drinking three cups of coffee and trying to relax. The 'audio caffeine' makes it virtually impossible."

Halpern combined his experience as a researcher and musician to compose music taking advantage of this same phenomenon. Naturally, it became very popular with massage practitioners. Halpern has even been hired by massage clients to play live music while they receive a massage. Massage practitioners who use his music in their practice sometimes state their clients start relaxing even before the massage begins, making their sessions easier and more effective.

Halpern notes that sound is always with us, whether we are deliberately listening or not: "Mother Nature gave us eyelids. She didn't give us ear-lids or body-lids." That being a given, he suggests paying attention to the sounds of our massage practices is just as important as keeping it visually appealing. The body is affected by the hum of an air conditioner, the ticking of a clock, or the creak of a floorboard, even though our brains may have developed a habit of ignoring these sounds as irrelevant.

Halpern's music, so appreciated by massage practitioners, has received praise from the wider community as well. His 2013 album, *Deep Alpha,* was nominated for a Grammy award for Best New Age Album. Just a few of his other popular albums include *Ocean Suite, Relaxation Suite,* and *Music for Sound Healing.* Although he composes music, Halpern's goal in doing so is far more than providing entertainment: "My mission statement has always been to create more peace, harmony, and healing on the planet. Every recording begins by setting the intention to bring through healing, relaxing, and beautiful music which nurtures body, mind, and spirit. I open my heart and tune in to a place of peace and love, and seek to share feelings with all who hear the recordings."

Although massage practitioners engage primarily with the tactile senses, the body is a whole, and the other senses cannot be ignored. Steven Halpern continues to serve the massage community by providing tools to help massage practitioners provide an environment of healing and serenity so lacking in the outside world of busyness, but it is up to every individual massage practitioner to take those tools and use them in ways to serve their clients best.

REFERENCES

Adişen, E., & Onder, M. (2007). Allergic contact dermatitis from Laurus nobilis oil induced by massage. *Contact Dermatitis*, 56(6), 360–361.

Better Sleep Council (BSC). (n.d.). *Extreme remake: Bedroom edition*. Retrieved from https://bettersleep.org/better-sleep/the-ideal-bedroom/.

Buckle, J. (2014). *Clinical aromatherapy: Essential oils in healthcare* (3rd ed.). Philadelphia: Elsevier Science.

Centers for Disease Control and Prevention (CDC). (2018). *Ergonomics and musculoskeletal disorders*. Retrieved from https://www.cdc.gov/niosh/topics/ergonomics/.

Champagne, T. T., Mullen, B., Dickson, D., & Krishnamurty, S. (2015). Evaluating the safety and effectiveness of the weighted blanket with adults during an inpatient mental health hospitalization. *Occupational Therapy in Mental Health*, 31(3), 211–233.

Cooke, M., Holzhauser, K., Jones, M., Davis, C., & Finucane, J. (2007). The effect of aromatherapy massage with music on the stress and anxiety levels of emergency nurses: Comparison between summer and winter. *Journal of Clinical Nursing*, 16(9), 1695–1703.

Crawford, G. H., Katz, K. A., Ellis, E., & James, W. D. (2004). Use of aromatherapy products and increased risk of hand dermatitis in massage therapists. *Archives of Dermatology*, 140(8), 991–996.

Einstein College of Medicine (ECM). (n.d.). *What are the top injuries in a typical office and how can you avoid them?* Retrieved from https://www.einsteinmed.edu/administration/environmental-health-safety/accident-injury-reduction-campagin/top-injuries.aspx.

Epilepsy Society. (2019). *Complementary therapies*. Retrieved from https://www.epilepsysociety.org.uk/complementary-therapies

Grier, T. (2012). *Is there cross-reactivity between shea butter and natural rubber latex?* American Latex Allergy Association, The Alert Newsletter, Dec issue. Retrieved from http://www.latexallergyresources.org/sites/default/files/newsletter-attachments/The%20ALERT%20Dec%202012.pdf.

Hammell, D. C., Zhang, L. P., Ma, F., Abshire, S. M., McIlwrath, S. L., Stinchcomb, A. L., & Westlund, K. N. (2016). Transdermal cannabidiol reduces inflammation and pain-related behaviours in a rat model of arthritis. *European Journal of Pain*, 20(6), 936–948.

Hunter, D., Oldfield, G., Tich, N., Messenheimer, J., & Sebree, T. (2018). Synthetic transdermal cannabidiol for the treatment of knee pain due to osteoarthritis. *Osteoarthritis and Cartilage*, 26(Suppl. 1), S26.

Jones, N. A., & Field, T. (1999). Massage and music therapies attenuate frontal EEG asymmetry in depressed adolescents. *Adolescence*, 34(135), 529–534.

Lakshmi, C. (2014). Allergic contact dermatitis (type IV hypersensitivity) and type I hypersensitivity following aromatherapy with ayurvedic oils (Dhanwantharam thailum, Eladi coconut oil) presenting as generalized erythema and pruritus with flexural eczema. *Indian Journal of Dermatology*, 59(3), 283–286.

Lopez-Villafuerte, L., & Clores, K. H. M. (2016). Contact dermatitis caused by turmeric in a massage oil. *Contact Dermatitis*, 75(1), 52–53.

Mullen, B., Champagne, T., Krishnamurty, S., Dickson, D., & Gao, X. R. (2008). Exploring the safety and therapeutic effects of deep pressure stimulation using a weighted blanket. *Occupational Therapy in Mental Health*, 24(1), 65–89.

National Sleep Foundation (NSF). (n.d.). *Five fragrant options to help transport you to dreamland*. Retrieved from https://www.sleep.org/articles/scents-for-relaxation/.

Occupational Safety and Health Administration (OSHA). (2003). *Office temperature and humidity*. Retrieved from https://www.osha.gov/pls/oshaweb/owadisp.show_document?p_table=interpretations&p_id=24602.

Paudel, K. S., Hammell, D. C., Agu, R. U., Valiveti, S., & Stinchcomb, A. L. (2010). Cannabidiol bioavailability after nasal and transdermal application: effect of permeation enhancers. *Drug Development and Industrial Pharmacy*, 36(9), 1088–1097.

Schultz, R. (2020). *Should you try CBD or Cannabis creams for pain relief?* Retrieved from https://www.shape.com/fitness/tips/should-you-try-cannabis-creams-pain-relief.

Trattner, A., David, M., & Lazarov, A. (2008). Occupational contact dermatitis due to essential oils. *Contact Dermatitis*, 58(5), 282–284.

U. S. Food and Drug Administration. (2019). What you should know about using cannabis, including cbd, when pregnant or breastfeeding. Retrieved from https://www.fda.gov/consumers/consumer-updates/what-you-should-know-about-using-cannabis-including-cbd-when-pregnant-or-breastfeeding

Ziegner, U. (n.d). Riviera Allergy Medical Center. *Allergic reactions trigger by shea butter for skin and hair*. Retrieved from https://www.rivieraallergy.com/blog/allergic-reactions-triggered-by-using-shea-butter-for-your-skin-and-hair

REVIEW AND APPLY YOUR KNOWLEDGE

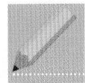 **MATCHING ONE: CONCEPT REVIEW**
Place the letter of the answer next to the number of the term or phrase that best describes it.

A. 18 months
B. Aromatherapy
C. Cross-contamination
D. Table width
E. Household bleach
F. Hypoallergenic
G. Terrycloth
H. Parabens
I. Memory
J. Cotton, cotton blends, and flannel
K. Reduce friction
L. Nonabrasive and nonalcohol

_____ 1. Product used for disinfecting table and accessory fabric but not for routine cleaning.

_____ 2. Ingredient thought to mimic the hormone estrogen when absorbed into the skin.

_____ 3. Popular sheet fabric material.

_____ 4. The shelf life of the majority of massage lubricants if stored in a cool, dark place.

_____ 5. Primary purpose of massage lubricant.

_____ 6. Massage product used on clients with sensitive or hyperreactive skin or who have skin conditions such as eczema (atopic dermatitis) or psoriasis.

_____ 7. Transfer of microorganisms from one source to another.

_____ 8. Ability of the massage table foam pad to return to its original height after being compressed.

_____ 9. Fabric ideal for spa use because it can absorb water easily.

_____ 10. Use of fragrant essential oils by inhalation or by applying a diluted form to the skin.

_____ 11. Type of products recommended by massage table manufacturers for cleaning table and accessory fabric in 4:1 diluted solution.

_____ 12. Should be 31 to 33 inches wide for large-framed clients.

 MATCHING TWO: CONCEPT REVIEW
Place the letter of the answer next to the number of the term or phrase that best describes it.

A. Behind the knees
B. 68° to 76°F
C. Slope
D. Face rest
E. Loft
F. Throw rugs
G. Polyurethane
H. Lavender, vanilla, jasmine
I. In front of the ankles
J. Spatula
K. Warm; cool
L. Butters

_____ 1. Scents recommended by the National Sleep Foundation to promote calmness and relaxation.

_____ 2. Derived from fruit, nuts, or seeds.

_____ 3. Where to place a bolster on a supine-lying client to reduce excessive lordosis.

_____ 4. Type of floor covering that should not be used in a massage office.

_____ 5. Red, yellow, and orange are _____ colors; blue and green are _____ colors.

_____ 6. Needed between parking spaces and buildings instead of steps to increase accessibility.

_____ 7. Tool that can be used to dispense thick lubricants such as crèmes or butters.

_____ 8. Used by the massage practitioner to help keep a prone-lying client's head and neck relatively aligned.

_____ 9. Where a bolster is placed on a prone-lying client.

_____ 10. Ideal room temperature range for workers, according to Occupational Safety and Health Administration (OSHA).

_____ 11. Fabric most often used by manufacturers to cover high-quality massage tables.

_____ 12. Term used to describe the thickness of foam padding.

MULTIPLE CHOICE: TEST YOUR KNOWLEDGE

Place the letter of the answer next to the number of the term or phrase that best describes it.

_____ 1. Most massage tables measure _____ inches wide.
A. 22 to 24
B. 28 to 30
C. 30 to 31
D. 31 to 33

_____ 2. Wood-frame portable massage tables usually weigh ____ than aluminum-framed portable massage tables.
A. substantially less
B. a few pounds less
C. a few pounds more
D. substantially more

_____ 3. The degree of table padding mass, volume, and compactness is called:
A. density.
B. memory.
C. durability.
D. loft.

_____ 4. Which bolster's placement may help decrease excessive lordosis?
A. Neck
B. Chest
C. Knee
D. Ankle

_____ 5. Which fabric should be avoided when selecting linens, due to its thin and clingy nature?
A. Flannel
B. Cotton
C. Cotton blends
D. Jersey knit

_____ 6. What size linens should be purchased for a massage table?
A. Twin
B. King
C. Full
D. Queen

_____ 7. Which lubricant would be best suited for scar tissue to minimize friction reduction?
A. Crème
B. Wax
C. Oil
D. Gel

_____ 8. Water-based lubricants are sometimes marketed as _____ products because they are appropriate for techniques requiring less friction.
A. Swedish massage
B. deep tissue
C. reflexology
D. hydrotherapy

_____ 9. Which lubricant is likely to stain linens?
A. Crème
B. Lotion
C. Oil
D. Butter

_____ 10. Which lubricant should not be used on clients with latex allergies due to the possibility of cross-reactivity?
A. Cocoa butter
B. Shea butter

C. Sesame seed oil
D. Grape seed oil

_____ 11. Which essential oil is derived from a root?
A. Black pepper
B. Clary sage
C. Bergamot
D. Ginger

_____ 12. Which essential oil is used for respiratory congestion and comforting grief?
A. Lavender
B. Sandalwood
C. Eucalyptus
D. Rosemary

CRITICAL THINKING

Most Value for Your Money

If a new graduate of massage school has limited funds to buy equipment and supplies to start a massage practice, what advice would you give them? What factors should the new graduate take into consideration?

Answers to this question can cover but are not limited to:

Select professional-grade equipment manufactured from a reputable, well-established company. This is important for several reasons. Reputable, well-established companies have quality, well-made products whose designs have stood the test of time. These companies usually provide superior customer service before and after the purchase and provide a trial period with all or part of the purchase price refunded once the product is returned if the customer is not satisfied with the product. In addition, previously owned massage tables and chairs manufactured from reputable companies often hold their value and bring a higher resale price.

Choose massage table accessories to help position the client for comfort and safety, such as a pillow and a bolster. Other accessories, such as additional bolsters and arm shelves, can be purchased later when the massage practitioner has more money.

Choose high-quality, white or light-colored linens, all in the same color. This way they will all match, and lubricant stains do not show easily on them. The high quality will make the linens last longer before they need to be replaced.

The best lubricant option is an unscented, hypoallergic crème or lotion. This can be used on all clients, and because crèmes and lotions do not stain sheets the way oils and gels do, laundry expenses will be minimized.

PROFESSIONAL PRACTICE

Almond Scented Oil Is the Best?

Tiffany has owned and operated a massage business, Southern Style Comfort, for 10 years in her hometown. She has two associate practitioners, Juanita and Suzanne, who have worked with her for 5 years each, and has recently hired a new massage school graduate, Rebecca.

Tiffany requires all the practitioners at Southern Style Comfort use the same lubricant, an almond-scented oil, to ensure clients receive a uniform experience. She also says almond is the signature scent of her business. Tiffany has bought the oil from the same distributor since she opened her business and gets a 10% discount for buying in bulk.

Within 2 weeks of using the oil, Rebecca notices a rash on her forearms. She mentions this to Juanita and Suzanne, who say they have each had a couple of clients through the years who have developed rashes after receiving a massage and Tiffany has had to refund them the price of their treatments.

What type of response is Rebecca most likely having to the oil? If you were Rebecca, how would you approach Tiffany about suggesting other lubricant options? What information could Rebecca give to Tiffany about lubricants? What would you recommend Rebecca do if Tiffany chooses to continue using only almond-scented oil?

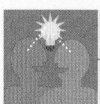

DISCUSSION

Past and Present Massage Experiences

Think about the massages you have received. Do not focus on the techniques you received or the practitioner's appearance but instead on the sounds, aromas, and sights. Can you describe the table, the accessories, linens, and lubricant used during the session? Were you given choices about scents and lubricants? What did you like about the session, and what did you not like?

If available, post your reflections on an Internet-based discussion board monitored by your instructor.

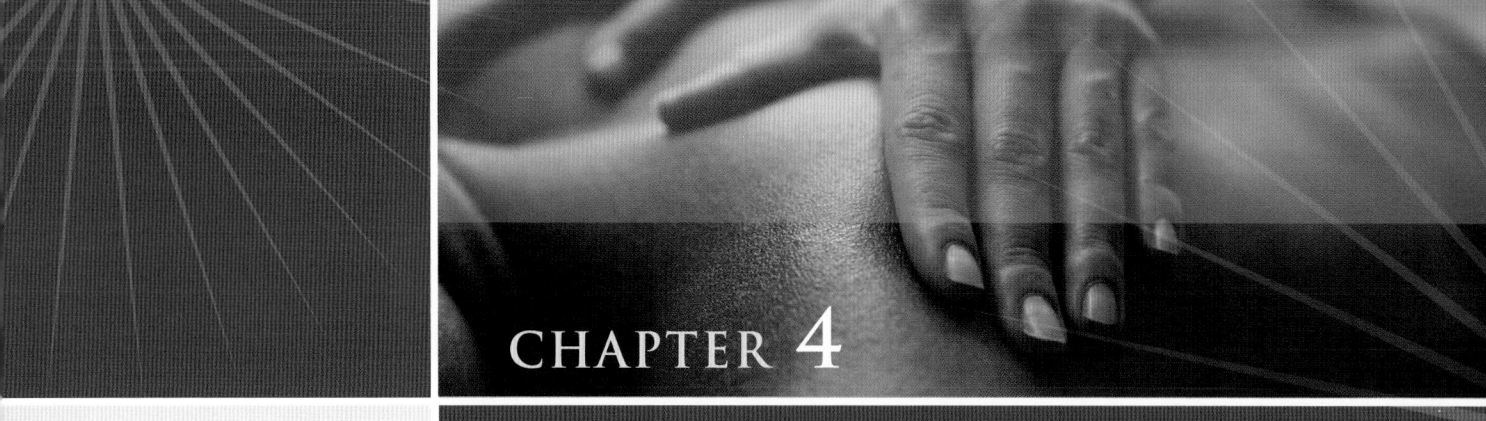

CHAPTER 4

Keep working on yourself, because the more you invest in yourself, the more you invest in your ability to serve others.

—Barry Green

Career Longevity: Wellness, Wellbeing, and Self-Care

Susan G. Salvo and Michele J. Renee

LEARNING OBJECTIVES

After completing this chapter, the student should be able to:

1. Define career longevity, wellness, wellbeing, self-care, and the wellness and biopsychosocial models.
2. Discuss the physical dimension of wellness.
3. Outline the occupational, intellectual, emotional, social, and spiritual dimensions of wellness.

INTRODUCTION

Career longevity is the length of time spent in service or employment within a field. There are several factors that promote career longevity such as a sense of pride and passion for the job, a supportive network and positive interactions with administration and team members, balance between work and family life, feelings of optimism, and education. Many professionals persisted in their careers and prevented burnout by utilizing self-care strategies such as exercising, talking with peers and supervisors, spending time with family, and practicing spirituality (Alexander et al., 2015; Killian, 2008; Mazerolle et al., 2016; Pustułka-Piwnik et al., 2014). Although investigations into factors contributing to career longevity in massage have not been conducted, the above data was extracted from studies in nursing, education, and athletic training. This information can be applied to the massage profession because of several commonalities—care of others and physicality in the performance of professional activities.

Wellness refers to activities, choices, and lifestyles oriented toward optimal health and wellbeing to live more fully within a community. Wellness has several dimensions, which are discussed in a wellness model featured in the next section. **Wellbeing** is the experience of health and includes feelings of comfort, safety, contentment, happiness, high life satisfaction, sense of meaning or purpose, and ability to manage stress—wellness is the behavior, and wellbeing is the state or outcome of wellness. Wellbeing can be measured with some degree of accuracy. Results from research experiments find that wellbeing is associated with self-perceived health, life and career longevity, reduced mental and physical disorders, social connectedness, and productivity (Centers for Disease Control and Prevention [CDC], 2018).

Wellness encourages better **self-care**, care of oneself that is learned, proactive, deliberate, purposeful, and continuous to improve or preserve health and wellbeing. Self-care can reduce stress, avoid occupational burnout, prevent illness and injury, and help individuals live a more balanced lifestyle. In medical models, self-care is at one end of the wellness spectrum and healthcare is at the other end. It is vital that massage practitioners actively practice self-care to perform quality massage sessions throughout the day, day after day, year after year, for the span of their career (Segall & Goldstein, 1989; Taylor & Renpenning, 2011).

WELLNESS AND BIOPSYCHOSOCIAL MODELS

In 1976, Hettler published a **wellness model** using the holistic integration of the six dimensions of wellness, including physical wellness, occupational wellness, intellectual wellness, social wellness, emotional wellness, and spiritual wellness (Fig. 4.1). Some wellness models include an environmental dimension, but Hettler states that environmental wellness is an aspect of occupational and social wellness. For example, work environments are part of occupational

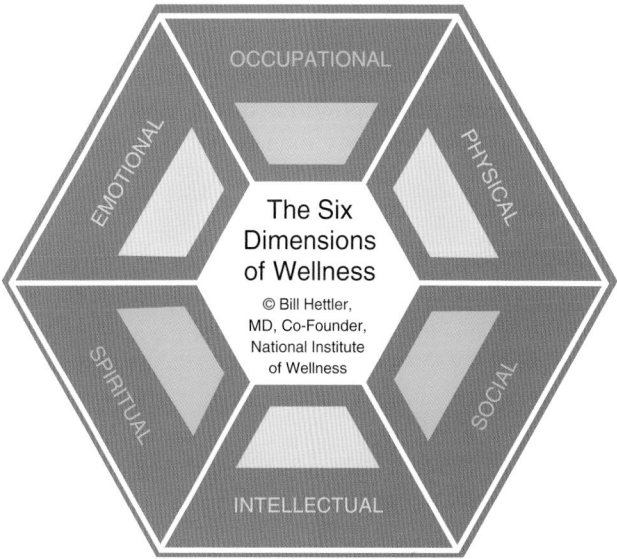

FIG. 4.1 Six dimensions of wellness. (Dimensions of Wellness Model ©1976 Bill Hettler, MD. Reprinted with permission from the National Wellness Institute, Inc., NationalWellness.org.)

wellness, and living environments (which include communities) are part of social wellness.

About the same time that wellness and self-care models were published, the medical community began revising its healthcare models. In 1977, Engel published a **biopsychosocial (BPS) model**, which views health, disease, and pain as products of complex interactions between biologic factors (i.e., genetics, biochemical), psychologic factors (i.e., moods, behaviors, personality, beliefs), and social conditions (i.e., culture, family relationships, socioeconomic status, community/social support). Engel created the BPS model partially because the biomedical model did not adequately address psychiatric, psychosomatic, and psychologic conditions.

The wellness model is a foundation for an evidence-informed approach of career longevity, self-care, and burnout prevention, and includes exercising (physical wellness), having a balance between personal life and work life, spending time with family, friends, and coworkers (social and occupational wellness), taking educational courses (intellectual wellness), reducing stress (emotional wellness), and practicing spirituality (spiritual wellness). Massage practitioners identified areas important for success and longevity, including building professional relationships, knowledge of running a successful business, learning from others in the field, and cultivating and maintaining relationships with mentors, colleagues, and friends (Kennedy & Munk, 2017). These topics are discussed in this chapter and in Chapters 2 and 17.

PHYSICAL WELLNESS

Physical wellness promotes proper care of our body for optimal health and functioning, and includes regular physical activity or exercise, balanced nutrition, rest and good sleep habits, hygienic practices such as routine bathing, and regular medical and dental examinations. These safeguard health and improve the quality of life. Physical wellness prepares the body for tasks of daily living and emphasizes core strength, balance, and endurance so that individuals can meet personal, familial, and professional goals. Prudden (1980) classifies massage as a strenuous occupation (Table 4.1). Participation in a wide range of exercises, proper nutrition, rest, and sleep help keep the body fit and able to meet the demands of the massage profession.

Physical Activity

Physical activity is movement produced by skeletal muscles and requires energy expenditure (World Health Organization [WHO], 2018). Types of exercise are cardiorespiratory, resistance, flexibility, and neuromotor. Recommendations for adults are listed next within their appropriate categories (American College of Sports Medicine [ACSM], (2011). Begin exercise with warm-up activities such as easy walking or low-intensity, sport-specific routines for a few minutes to increase temperature and blood flow to muscles, which lead to improved binding of contractile proteins (actin, myosin) in muscle fibers.

Static stretching of greater than 60 seconds has negative effects on subsequent strength and power, which could impact performance. Short-duration static stretching (of less than 60 seconds) as part of a warm-up can have a positive effect on flexibility and prevention of musculotendinous injury, and is still one of the most debated topics in sport science literature (Chaabene et al., 2019). Consult a physician or other qualified healthcare provider before beginning any exercise program. Gradual progression of exercise time, frequency, and intensity is recommended for best adherence and least risk of injury.

TABLE 4.1 Occupations, Activity Levels, and Related Areas of Pain

SITTING	STANDING	WALKING	ACTIVE	STRENUOUS
Accountant	Bank teller	Detective	Carpenter	Athlete
Administrator	Barber and beautician	Flight attendant	Carpet layer	Construction worker
Anesthetist	Bartender	Librarian	Electrician	Dancer
Architect	Butcher	Nurse	Farmer	Diver
Artist	Cafeteria server	Orderly	Fireman	Heavy equipment operator
Author	Clerk	Postal carrier	Forester	Linesman
Bookkeeper	Cook	Real estate agent	Maintenance person	Longshoreman
Bus, truck, and cab driver	Dental hygienist	Restaurant wait staff	Mason	Martial arts instructor
Chauffeur	Dentist	Security guard	Mechanic	Massage practitioner
Computer programmer	Electrologist		Painter	Miner
Crane operator	File clerk		Photographer	Steel worker
Dispatcher	Machinist		Plumber	
Draftsman	Physician		Police officer	
Editor	Sales clerk		Ski instructor	
Engineer	Surgeon		Soldier	
Executive	Teacher		Sports coach	
Jeweler	Veterinarian			
Lawyer				
Pilot				
Psychiatrist				
Secretary				
Student				

- **Sitting.** Sitting occupations often put trigger points in the chest, posterior neck, shoulders, and upper and lower back. Because the body is constantly bent, the groin may be involved. If excessive weight impairs circulation, then legs and buttocks, which are constantly compressed against chairs, become involved.
- **Standing.** Occupations requiring long hours of standing in one place contribute to the risk of lower back pain. The upper back is also in danger, as are arms, shoulders, and posterior neck. Swelling may also occur in feet and ankles.
- **Walking.** Occupations requiring ordinary walking are not at risk. However, when walking includes carrying (i.e., postal carrier, restaurant wait staff), the back is in danger.
- **Active.** Active occupations all entail danger. For example, carpenters damage their elbows and experience tennis elbow, the plumber working with pipe threaders and large wrenches puts trigger points in chest muscles, the mason strains the back, and the ski instructor damages the legs and lower back.
- **Strenuous.** Strenuous occupations often result in back pain, and injuries often involve torque, such as the ladder that gets away, the barrel that rolls the wrong way, or anything that pulls the torso with a twisting motion.

Modified from Prudden, B. (1980). *Pain erasure: The Bonnie Prudden way.* Lanham, MD: M. Evans & Co.

Cardiorespiratory Exercise

Cardiorespiratory exercises are activities involving prolonged body movements that increase heart and respiration rates. Benefits of cardiorespiratory exercise include improved stamina, weight loss or weight maintenance, and reduced risk of heart disease, lung cancer, type 2 diabetes, and stroke. Cardiorespiratory exercise is also called aerobic or cardio exercise.

Activity levels range from low to moderate to high intensity, or vigorous, depending on the amount of movement, and each level creates corresponding increases in heart and respiration rates.

- **Low Intensity**. This includes casual walking, bike riding at an easy pace, a stretch session, or beginner's yoga or tai chi classes.
- **Moderate Intensity**. Many low intensity activities become moderate intensity by increasing the pace—brisk walking of at least 4 miles an hour (mph), biking with light effort or 10 to 12 mph, walking or biking uphill, strenuous yoga classes, or playing tennis doubles. Lap swimming or water aerobics is also moderate intensity if it increases heart rate.
- **High Intensity**. Examples of high intensity activities include jogging at least 6 mph, biking 14 to 16 mph, swimming laps, playing tennis singles, circuit training, vigorous forms of weight training, or anything that causes you to pause in delivering a sentence to take a breath.

Recommendations for cardiorespiratory exercise are 150 minutes (2 hours and 30 minutes) to 300 minutes (5 hours) a week of moderate-intensity, or 75 minutes (1 hour and 15 minutes) to 150 minutes (2 hours and 30 minutes) a week of vigorous-intensity physical activity, or an equivalent combination of moderate- and vigorous-intensity activity. Preferably, activities should be spread throughout the week. Individuals unable to meet a minimum recommendations still benefit from some activity and may need a slower progression rate.

Resistance Exercise

Resistance exercises involve contracting muscles against resistance with effort. The resistance can be weighted bars, dumbbells, rubber tubing, your own body weight, gravity, bricks, bottles of water, or any other object that causes the muscles to contract. Benefits of resistance exercise are improved muscle tone, strength, stamina, and bone density. Resistance exercise is also called strength training or weight-lifting.

Recommendations for resistance exercises are two or three nonconsecutive days a week on all major muscle groups. Major muscle groups include the biceps, triceps, shoulders (trapezius or *traps,* deltoids or *delts*), chest (pectorals or *pecs*), back (latissimus dorsi or *lats*), abdomen or *abs,* quadriceps or *quads,* and hamstrings. For each exercise, perform one set of 8 to 12 repetitions or *reps.* Two to four sets of each exercise are recommended. Very light or light intensity is best for older or frail adults and for previously sedentary adults starting exercise.

Flexibility Exercise

Flexibility exercises are movements or positions designed to stretch or lengthen specific muscles or muscle groups. Benefits from flexibility exercises include improved mobility and range-of-motion. Stretching can be passive (produced by external forces without voluntary contraction) or active (produced by voluntary contraction without external forces). Passive stretching is discussed in Chapter 8. Muscle energy techniques and proprioceptive neuromuscular facilitation (combines isometric contraction and stretching) are discussed in Chapter 14.

- **Static Stretching**. Slowly moving a muscle or muscle group to its end range-of-motion and holding the position for a period of time, usually 10 to 30 seconds, but it can be longer. The end of the stretch should create light-to-moderate discomfort, but not pain. Examples of static stretching are hamstring and quadriceps stretches. Static stretching should be performed after exercise or done on its own.
- **Dynamic Movements**. Gradual transition from one body position to the next with progressive increases in range of motion as movements are repeated. Examples of dynamic stretching are arm circles, leg swings, and torso twists.
- **Ballistic Stretching/Movements**. Static stretching or dynamic movements with a bouncing motion at the end of available range-of-motion. Ballistic stretching/movements should only be used by persons who know their limitations or are working under supervision of a trainer, as this flexibility exercise does not allow muscles to adjust to and relax into the stretch or movement. Ballistic moves may cause muscles to tighten by activating the stretch reflex. An example of a ballistic stretch is bending forward to touch your toes and bouncing at the end of the stretch.

Recommendations for flexibility exercises are 2 or 3 days a week. Each stretch should be held for 10 to 30 seconds to the point of tightness or slight discomfort. Repeat each stretch 2 to 4 times, accumulating to 60 seconds for each stretch. Muscle groups most often tight are the hamstrings, hip flexors, calves, and chest muscles, and these muscles can be stretched using different positions.

Neuromotor Exercise

Neuromotor exercises incorporate resistance and flexibility with slow, focused movements and/or sustained body postures. Examples of neuromotor exercises are yoga, tai chi, or Pilates. Neuromotor exercises can improve agility, balance, coordination, gait, proprioception (self-awareness of movements and body positions), and reduce fall risk and fear of falling. Most exercises combine all or part of three elements to achieve these benefits.

- **Changing Your Base of Support**. This may involve standing with feet together, on 1 foot, and other forms of upright positions.
- **Move Away From Your Center of Gravity**. Lean forward, backward, or sideways.

- **Limit or Remove Visual Feedback**. Eyes can be partially or fully closed or done in a dimly-lit area.

Performing exercises while barefoot or wearing minimal footwear increases strength, improves balance, and may reduce fall risk (Curtis et al, 2021). Recommendations for neuromotor exercises are 20 to 30 minutes, two or three days a week.

> *You can't turn back the clock, but you can wind it up again.*
> ——**Bonnie Prudden**

Nutrition

Nutrition is derived from ingesting food and drink to help the body function properly, to support tissue growth and repair, and to supply the energy needed for daily activities. Nutritional needs vary throughout life, and factors such as age, activity levels, and disease should be considered when determining what and how much to eat. **Nutrients** are substances in food and drink that provide nutrition. Nutrients can be grouped into two categories—macronutrients and micronutrients.

- **Macronutrients**. These are proteins, carbohydrates, and fats, and are called macronutrients because they are needed in relatively large amounts. Macronutrients are also called the calorie group because they provide nutrients through **calories**, which are units of energy received from nutrients. Massage practitioners burn approximately 177 calories while performing a 60-minute classic massage (Więcek et al., 2018). This is about the same amount of calories spent walking or weightlifting.
- **Micronutrients**. These are vitamins and minerals and are called micronutrients because they are needed in smaller amounts, but play a central role in metabolism and tissue function. Because micronutrients lack caloric value, they are called the no-calorie group.

Proteins

Proteins are chains of amino acids. The body uses approximately 20 amino acids. Nine are essential and must be supplied by diet (histidine, isoleucine, leucine, lysine, methionine, phenylalanine, threonine, tryptophan, and valine)—the body can synthesize the others. Proteins assist the body's growth and energy needs, help build and repair tissues, and help form antibodies, which fight infection. Proteins can be classified as complete and incomplete.

- **Complete Proteins**. Foods containing all essential amino acids. Sources of complete proteins are meat, fish, poultry, eggs, milk, cheese, yogurt, quinoa, and soy products such as tofu, tempeh, edamame, and miso.
- **Incomplete Proteins**. Foods containing some, but not all, essential amino acids such as legumes (beans, peas, lentils), nuts and seeds, whole grains, and vegetables. Many plant-based foods are incomplete proteins, and must be eaten with other incomplete proteins to provide all essential amino acids. Combining beans and whole grains (hummus and pita bread; refried beans and tortillas), nuts or seeds with whole grains (peanut butter on whole wheat toast), or beans with nuts or seeds (salad with chickpeas and sunflower seeds) are examples of combining incomplete, plant-based proteins to meet the body's protein needs.

Carbohydrates

Carbohydrates are sugars that turn into glucose (blood sugar) after they are consumed. These are used by the body as energy. There are two main forms of carbohydrates—simple and complex. The main differences between the two are how quickly they are digested and absorbed, and their chemical structure.

- **Simple Carbohydrates**. Simple carbohydrates (carbs) are digested and absorbed quickly, causing a rapid rise in blood sugar. Simple carbs are monosaccharides or disaccharides. Monosaccharides are a single, simple sugar unit and include glucose, fructose, or galactose. Disaccharides are two monosaccharides bonded together and include sucrose (glucose bonded to fructose), lactose (glucose bonded to galactose), and maltose (glucose bonded to glucose). High fructose corn syrup is a manmade disaccharide and contains fructose bonded to fructose. Simple carbs provide little to no nutritional value aside from energy and are often referred to as empty calories. Sources of simple carbohydrates are honey, syrup, and table sugar.
- **Complex Carbohydrates**. Complex carbs contain more nutrients as well as dietary fiber and take longer to digest and absorb. Complex carbs containing three or more monosaccharides bonded together and are either oligosaccharides (3 to 10 monosaccharides) or polysaccharides (greater than 10 monosaccharides). There are numerous further subdivisions. Sources of complex carbohydrates are whole-grain breads, fiber-rich fruits (apples, blueberries, raspberries, oranges), and fiber-rich vegetables (corn, acorn squash, peas, beans).

Fats

Fats and oils are found in animal and plant foods, are sources of energy, and help the body absorb certain vitamins and minerals. Trans fats are a type of fat with no nutritional value and are harmful to health. They can be found in processed foods such as baked goods, snack foods, fried foods, shortening, margarine, and certain vegetable oils. The WHO is currently working to eliminate transfats from food by 2023. Fats can be classified as saturated and unsaturated.

- **Saturated Fats**. These are solid at room temperature and are mainly found in animal products such as butter, lard, full-fat milk and yogurt, full-fat cheese, and high-fat meat.
- **Unsaturated Fats**. These tend to be liquid at room temperature. Foods rich in omega-3s, a type of unsaturated fatty acid, should be included in the diet. Good sources of healthy fats are nuts, seeds, olive oil, avocados, eggs, and fatty fish, such as sardines, tuna, salmon, trout, mackerel, and herring.

Vitamins

Vitamins are essential for growth and metabolism. They can be soluble in water or fat and differ in how they are absorbed and stored in the body.

- **Water-Soluble Vitamins**. These dissolve in water, are easily absorbed into tissues, are not stored in the body, and are quickly excreted in urine. Water-soluble vitamins must be consumed regularly. Examples of water-soluble vitamins are B-complex group and vitamin C.
- **Fat-Soluble Vitamins**. These dissolve in fat, are absorbed slowly, and are stored in the liver and in fat cells for future use. Examples of fat-soluble vitamins are A, D, E, and K. Table 4.2 provides an overview of vitamins, including function, sources, and recommended daily intake.

Minerals

Minerals are chemical elements found in the earth's crust and vital in regulating many body functions. Plants take up minerals as they grow, and then we eat the plants. Minerals also leach into groundwater, which we drink. Minerals act as coenzymes (iron), support organs (potassium), build bone (calcium), relax muscles (magnesium), and aid healthy growth and development (zinc). Minerals often work with vitamins to perform bodily functions such as calcium and vitamin D. Minerals are divided into two categories: macro (bulk) minerals such as calcium and micro (trace) minerals such as iron. Table 4.3 provides a list of a few mineral examples.

TABLE 4.2 Vitamins: Functions, Sources, and Recommended Daily Intake

VITAMINS	FUNCTIONS	SOURCES	RDI[a]
Vitamin A (retinol)	Acts as an antioxidant, supports immune function, promotes healthy eyes, helps maintain skin smoothness and clarity, and helps bone growth.	Liver, spinach, sweet potatoes, pumpkin, collard greens, and milk	900 μg/700 μg
Vitamin B complex	There are more than 20 B vitamins such as B_1, B_2, B_3, B_5, B_6, B_7, B_9, and B_{12}.		
B_1 (thiamine)	Promotes heart function and helps convert carbohydrates and fats into energy.	Pork, whole grains, spinach, wheat germ, and fortified cereals	1.2 mg/1.1 mg
B_2 (riboflavin)	Promotes red blood cell formation and helps prevent cataracts.	Asparagus, organ meats, milk, yogurt, almonds, soybeans, and fortified cereals	1.3 mg/1.1 mg
B_3 (niacin)	Promotes adrenal function, assisting in expelling wastes, and helps maintain muscle tone.	Beets, chicken, turkey, veal, salmon, tuna, sunflower seeds, and peanuts	16 mg/14 mg
B_5 (pantothenic acid)	Promotes red blood cell production, aids in the breakdown of fats and carbohydrates for energy, and helps maintain a healthy digestive tract.	Brewer's yeast, corn, tomatoes, egg yolks, beef, duck, sweet potatoes, whole grains, and lobster	5 mg/5 mg
B_6 (pyridoxine)	Promotes nerve and brain function, aids DNA and RNA production, and helps with absorption of vitamin B_{12}.	Brown rice, whole-grain flour, bran, shrimp, lentils, fish, and nuts	1.3 mg/1.3 mg
B_7 (biotin, vitamin H)	Aids in metabolism of carbohydrates, fats, and amino acids.	Brewer's yeast, organ meats, nut butters, soybeans, legumes, and cooked eggs (raw egg white can interfere with biotin absorption)	30 μg/30 μg
B_9 (folic acid)	Aids in DNA and RNA production and crucial for brain development and function.	Spinach, whole grains, orange juice, wheat germ, asparagus, salmon, avocado, root vegetables (carrots, potatoes), and milk	400 μg/400 μg (600 μg during pregnancy)
B_{12} (cobalamin)	Promotes iron function and regulates red blood cell formation.	Fish, dairy, organ meats (liver, kidney) eggs, beef, and pork	2.4 μg/2.4 μg
Vitamin C (ascorbic acid)	Acts as an antioxidant, helps the body resist infection, promotes adrenal function, aids in collagen production, and can reduce high blood pressure and cholesterol.	Citrus fruits (oranges, limes), strawberries, broccoli, and sweet red peppers	90 mg/75 mg
Vitamin D (cholecalciferol)	Promotes bone development, helps absorb and metabolize calcium, and aids immune function.	Fortified milk, fish liver oils, and sun exposure (sunlight helps skin to synthesize vitamin D)	5 μg/5 μg
Vitamin E (tocopherol)	Powerful antioxidant, repairs tissue, reduces blood pressure, promotes sperm development, helps prevent cataracts, and increases maternal circulation during pregnancy.	Almonds, peanuts, sunflower seeds, spinach, avocado, oils (wheat germ, safflower), and carrot juice	15 mg/15 mg
Vitamin K	Aids in blood clotting and maintains bone health. Bacteria found in the intestines produce this vitamin.	Beef liver, green tea, spinach, dark green lettuce, asparagus, broccoli, and kale	120 μg/90 μg

[a]*RDI*, Recommended daily intake and includes both adult male and female values (e.g., 10 mg/6 mg).
mg, Milligram; μ*g*, microgram.

TABLE 4.3	**Minerals: Functions, Sources, and Recommended Daily Intake**		
MINERALS	**FUNCTIONS**	**SOURCES**	**RDI[a]**
Calcium (Ca)	Supports the development and maintenance of strong bones and teeth and promotes heart, nerve, and muscle function. Calcium requires other nutrients to function, such as vitamin D.	Cheese, ice cream, yogurt, broccoli, almonds, Swiss chard, and milk	1000 mg/1000 mg
Potassium (K)	Essential for kidney function; supports heart function and aids digestion.	Unprocessed foods, including meat, fish, vegetables (especially potatoes), fruit (especially avocados, bananas, and orange juice), dairy, and whole grains	2000 mg/2000 mg
Iron (Fe)	Attaches to hemoglobin in red blood cells, thereby supporting delivery of oxygen to tissues.	Liver, lean red meat, fish, poultry, oysters, whole grains, dried beans, legumes, and fortified breads and cereals	18 mg/18 mg (27 mg during pregnancy)
Zinc (Zn)	Acts as an antioxidant; promotes immune function; and helps regulate appetite, taste, and smell. Essential for growth and development and supports reproduction.	Oysters, red meats, poultry, cheese, shellfish, legumes, whole grains, and mushrooms	11 mg/8 mg

[a]*RDI,* Recommended daily intake and includes both adult male and female values (e.g., 10 mg/6 mg).
mg, Milligram.

Water

Drinking water helps regulate body temperature; lessens the burden on the kidneys and liver by flushing out waste products; helps dissolve minerals and other nutrients, making them more accessible to the body; helps prevent or reduce constipation; and moistens mucosal membranes such as those found in the mouth. Drinking water can help weight loss or weight management by reducing caloric intake when substituted for drinks containing calories such as soda and juice. Drinking water can also prevent dehydration, a condition that can lead to fatigue, headaches, decreased performance, mood changes, mild cognitive impairment, constipation, and kidney stones. Massage practitioners should be well hydrated when taking care of clients to reduce the risk of dehydration and to meet the demands of professional activities.

Currently there are no recommendations for how much water adults should drink daily. How much water you need depends on a lot of things and varies from person to person. Most healthy individuals adequately meet their daily needs by letting thirst be their guide. On the average, females drink 11.5 cups (91 ounces or 2.7 L) of water a day and males drink 15.5 cups (125 ounces or 3.7 L) of water a day from all beverages and foods (CDC, 2020).

Nutritional Guidelines: Food Labels and the Healthy Eating Plate

The Food and Drug Administration (FDA) and Harvard School of Public Health have created tools to help Americans make food choices. **Food labels** are found on packaged foods made in the United States and imported from other countries. They contain nutritional facts such as serving size, calories per serving, macro- and micronutrients, and a list of ingredients. The label also includes the daily values based on a 2000-calorie diet. Some health conditions warrant specialized diets; consultation with your healthcare provider is recommended to ensure optimal nutritional health.

In 2016, food labels were updated to reflect new scientific information. Research found that previous food labels were confusing and did not provide usable information. The new design has calories and serving sizes in a larger and bolder font. It includes the amount and percentage of total sugars, and added sugars. Types of fat eaten are more important than amount of fat, so new labels show percentages of calories from unhealthy saturated and transfats rather than a percentage of calories from all fats. Some labels contain two columns—one column of calories and nutritional information in a single serving and the other column of information when consuming the entire package. The recommended limit on sodium levels decreased from 2400 mg to 2300 mg a day. Vitamins A and C are no longer required to be identified on labels, as deficiencies are rare.

The **Healthy Eating Plate** is an infographic that helps people make food choices and plan portion sizes at mealtimes. It was developed by Harvard Health Publishing and nutrition experts at the Harvard School of Public Health. It offers more specific and more accurate recommendations compared with MyPlate, created by the U.S. Department of Agriculture. In addition, Healthy Eating Plate is based on research, and is not influenced by food industries or agriculture policies.

The Healthy Eating Plate divides a meal plate into food portions of fruits and vegetables, whole grains, and healthy proteins. It also contains use of healthy oils such as olive oil, drinking water, an icon for physical activity, and guidance to help individuals make healthy eating choices such as avoiding sugary drinks and limiting intake of milk/dairy and juice (Fig. 4.2).

Rest and Sleep

Rest includes behaviors used to promote health and wellbeing by temporarily discontinuing a previous stressful or a

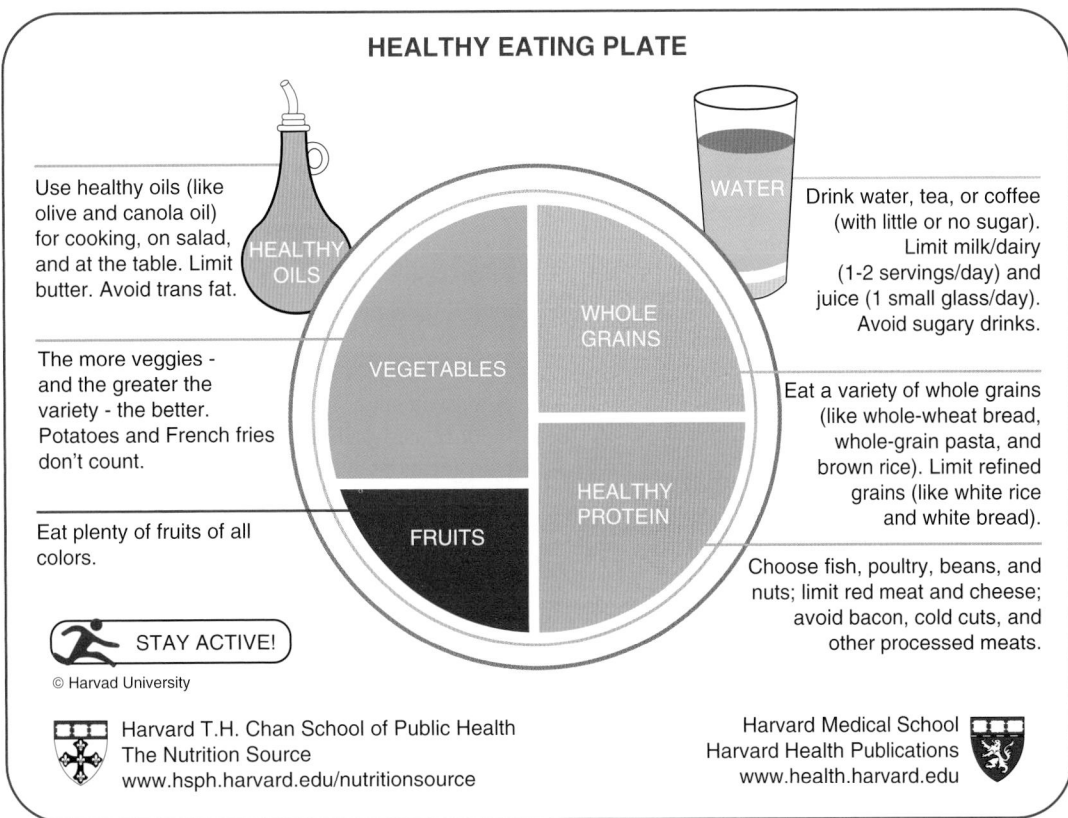

FIG. 4.2 Healthy Eating Plate developed by Harvard School of Public Health. This helps individuals make healthy eating choices and includes an icon for physical activity. (Copyright © 2011 Harvard University. For more information about The Healthy Eating Plate, please see The Nutrition Source, Department of Nutrition, Harvard T.H. Chan School of Public Health, http://www.thenutritionsource.org and Harvard Health Publications, health.harvard.edu. Harvard Health Publishing, 2017.)

demanding activity. Rest is both a process (to rest) and a condition (being in rest). There are several elements associated with rest.

- Freedom from stress.
- Freedom to do what is liked and enjoyed.
- State of calmness, open-mindedness, lack of demands, peace, and/or tranquilly.
- Relaxation and restoration.

Rest can be active or passive. Active rest includes walking in nature, stretching, and many forms of yoga and massage. It also includes engaging in the world outside of work and home life such as taking a vacation to see and experience something new. Active rest may also be enjoying and appreciating the arts. Passive rest is sitting or lying down, napping, praying, and/or meditating (Asp, 2015).

Sleep is a recurrent state of relaxation characterized by an altered state of consciousness, inhibited sensory activity, muscular inhibition, and reduced interactions. Adults need between 7 and 9 hours of sleep per night. Sleep allows the body to rest, recharge, and heal from the day's wear and tear. The amount and quality of sleep achieved daily affects many aspects of life. Adequate sleep is important for learning and memory, weight control, mood, health, and safety. Sleep deprivation contributes to slips/falls and errors in

judgments, including medical mistakes and road accidents. Sufficient sleep is a key to the body's ability to recuperate from the mental, emotional, and physical work of massage (CDC, 2017; Harvard Medical School, Division of Sleep Medicine, n.d.).

The best way to achieve sufficient sleep is to go to bed at the same time each night and wake up at the same time the next morning. Most individuals follow a familiar sleep pattern. Morning people generally go to bed between 9 and 11 p.m. and wake between 5 and 7 a.m. Night people go to bed between 11 p.m. and 3 a.m. and wake between 9 and 11 a.m. Knowing your individual preferred sleep pattern will help create the optimal client schedule. For example, massage practitioners who are "morning people" might avoid scheduling clients late in the day.

OCCUPATIONAL WELLNESS

Occupational wellness is the ability to balance work and leisure time, manage workplace stress, and build good relationships with co-workers and colleagues. Occupational wellness includes searching for and finding a career that provides a feeling of purpose and productivity. This means acknowledging talents and skills, and the opportunity to achieve personal satisfaction through work. Occupations include paid and unpaid roles because being paid to work, working as an unpaid caregiver, or working as a volunteer all possess similar work-related characteristics. Periodic reflection on the reasons that led to a career choice helps identify when changes are needed. This section examines ways to promote occupational wellness by reducing or preventing burnout and massage-related injury.

Burnout

Burnout is a syndrome resulting from chronic workplace stress not successfully managed. It is characterized by several dimensions.

- **Emotional Exhaustion**. Fatigue from continuous stress from excessive job and personal demands.
- **Depersonalization**. Cynicism, lack of empathy for others, and detachment from one's emotions.
- **Diminished Sense of Personal Accomplishment**. Decline in feelings of competence and achievement, believe their work is not important, or they are failing in their mission.

Maslach (2015) places burnout in both a personal and social context—the burned-out individual has feelings of incompetence and low self-confidence, and negative feelings toward the people they serve. Burnout is different from clinical depression in that depression is more pervasive and affects all aspects of life, whereas burnout focuses on work and people at work. Furthermore, the experience of fatigue, and fatigue recovery, is different in someone who is burned out. Someone who is not burned out recovers relatively quickly from work-related fatigue, but recovering from work-related fatigue takes longer if you are burned out. This includes both physical and emotional fatigue. In addition, people who are burned out describe work-related fatigue differently compared with people who are not burned out. For example, non-work-related fatigue is described by those who are not burned out as positive, with feelings of accomplishment and achievement. Work-related fatigue is described by someone who is burned out as negative, with feelings of failure, being weighed down, or burdened. People who are burned out are more likely to leave their chosen profession or current employer in search of another job.

Numerous studies have been conducted on risk factors affecting burnout (Adriaenssens et al., 2015; Pustułka-Piwnik et al., 2014; Shoji et al., 2015). These include feelings of dissatisfaction with work–life balance, lack of accomplishment, and low self-efficacy. Other contributing factors were:

- High job demands.
- Lack of job control.
- Lack of social support.
- Working in hospitals.
- Seniority or years of employment.
- Less formal education.

Burnout can manifest itself in several ways, including disinterest in work, dreading the next client, boredom, restlessness, inability to focus, depression, lack of productivity, tardiness and absenteeism, decline of social skills, workaholism, and deterioration of professional boundaries.

Burnout is associated with **compassion fatigue** and **empathy-based stress**, which are essentially emotional strain from working with individuals who are suffering from consequences related to traumatic events (Rauvola et al., 2019). These can reduce empathy toward those who are suffering. Self-care strategies listed in this chapter help reduce or prevent burnout and related conditions such as compassion fatigue and empathy-based stress.

Massage-Related Injuries

Approximately 70% of massage practitioners experience work-related pain and musculoskeletal symptoms. Common pain locations were fingers and thumbs, wrists, elbows, and shoulders, followed by the neck and lower back (Albert et al., 2008; Greene & Goggins, 2006; Jang et al., 2006). Practitioners who worked at least 6 hours a day or had more than 6 clients per day are more likely to experience lower back pain (Sathya et al., 2016). Being female was also a risk factor for injury-related work loss, perhaps because they generally have less upper body strength compared with males (Blau et al., 2013; Miller et al., 1993). Pain, fatigue, and injuries can have a major impact on a massage practitioner's income and may ultimately cause practitioners to leave the profession and seek less physically demanding employment (Mohr, 2010).

Preventing Burnout and Massage-Related Injuries

Using evidence as a foundation, featured next are methods used to prevent burnout and injury. Each practitioner should weigh all the pros and cons of each work situation to see what a good fit is for them while respecting the decisions of others who may choose to work in a different situation.

Prepare Physically

Blau and colleagues (2013) concluded that physical exhaustion had the strongest relationship to work loss from massage-related injuries. This section includes suggestions to prepare physically for work and ways to reduce or prevent fatigue and injury while using applied pressure that maximizes benefit to the client (Mohr, 2010; Turkeltaub et al., 2014). Prudden (1980) classifies massage as a strenuous occupation (see Table 4.1). To meet the physical demands of the profession, practitioners should follow these commonsense measures, which are discussed previously in this chapter and can be found in Chapter 7.

- Participate in regular physical activity.
- Eat a healthy balanced diet.
- Get enough rest and sleep.
- Warm-up before you begin your massage workday.

Increasing strength may reduce physical exhaustion, especially for females. Blau et al. (2013) suggested female practitioners strengthen their upper muscular limbs (e.g., shoulder, arms, neck) and all massage and manual practitioners continue strength exercises throughout their careers.

Prepare Mentally

Blau et al. (2013) also found a correlation between mental fatigue (feeling overwhelmed and emotionally drained) and injury-forced work loss. Riess and Kraft-Todd (2014) developed techniques that use nonverbal empathetic behaviors to help professionals express empathy. These techniques may reduce the risk of mental fatigue, compassion fatigue, and burnout. These techniques are in Chapter 2. Massage practitioners should use mindfulness to help them give their full attention to their clients. Mindfulness is needed so practitioners can make adjustments during the massage when they notice physical discomfort in their body.

Evaluate and Modify Environmental Factors

To improve occupational wellness, massage practitioners should evaluate and possibly modify the following. These and other factors are discussed in Chapter 7.

- An area of 3 feet (1 meter) of open space around all sides of the table to allow practitioners to stand or sit comfortably in relaxed, efficient, and aligned postures while administering techniques.
- Stow bolsters in easy-to-access locations between knee and waist height, so they can be lifted without bending or reaching.
- Perform massage on traditional wood, carpet with cushioned backing, or foam-backed vinyl flooring, if possible. Antifatigue mats can be placed around the table.
- Use a correct table height to allow practitioners to generate sufficient downward force.

Follow these Application Principles

Once you have prepared physically and mentally, and evaluated and/or modified environmental factors, apply the following principles to deliver pressure that maximizes benefits to clients. These application principles are discussed in Chapter 7.

- Engage the core.
- Stack the joints.
- Use body weight and gravity when applying force.
- Use a variety of techniques.
- Perform some techniques while seated.
- Stay hydrated.
- Rest between clients.
- Keep a consistent, reasonable workload.

Be Part of a Positive Supportive Work Community

Blau et al. (2013) noted that the mental fatigue mentioned previously may be from feelings of isolation, as many massage practitioners work alone without supervisor or co-worker interactions. Isolation is also a risk factor for burnout. Positive interactions with co-workers and talking with peers and supervisors promote career longevity. Therefore, it is vital that massage practitioners build and maintain a positive and supportive work community and participate in team-building activities to reduce feelings of isolation. Find ways to experience recognition and offer support through professional fellowship (Adriaenssens et al., 2015; Fortune & Gillespie, 2010).

Have Work–Life Balance

Have a work–life balance, as this can significantly reduce burnout and promote career longevity. Find a work schedule that leaves plenty of time to enjoy leisure activities.

Keep Learning Through Educational Efforts

Keep learning, even after massage school graduation. Education, both the amount of education and reduced cost, has a protective effect on burnout and injury (Blau et al., 2013; Pustułka-Piwnik et al., 2014). Use newly acquired techniques in ways that replenish rather than deplete your energy.

INTELLECTUAL WELLNESS

Intellectual wellness is the continuous acquisition, development, and creative application of critical thinking in the quest for a more satisfying existence. It involves recognizing one's own creative abilities and finding ways to increase your knowledge and skills. Intellectual wellness allows you to expand your ability to analyze, critique, understand, evaluate, problem solve, predict, and comprehend. Pursuing intellectual wellness includes engaging in mentally stimulating activities as well as sharing what we learn with others. Intellectual wellness can also be developed through cultural involvement, community involvement, and personal hobbies. This may also involve keeping current with information on healthy living, visiting art galleries and museums, traveling, and learning about new places, and open to new experiences. Writing poetry or seeing a play or a foreign film also fall within this dimension. Intellectual wellness may also include respectful discussions about religion and politics with someone who has differing philosophies. This domain allows us to develop a love for learning and philosophy for "life-long learning."

EMOTIONAL WELLNESS

Emotional wellness involves the capacity to be aware of, to control, and to appropriately express a wide range of emotions such as humor, joy, fear, anger, sadness, and appreciation, and accepting rather than denying your feelings. It includes developing positive emotions about yourself though a healthy self-concept and self-esteem, and exploring and clarifying your own sexual or gender identity. Emotional wellness means developing assertiveness and confrontation skills as well as awareness and acceptance of the emotions of others. Establishing and maintaining intimate and loving relationships, and handling interpersonal relationships judiciously and empathetically, are part of emotional wellness, as is enjoying life despite its occasional disappointments, irritations, and frustrations. Indeed, emotional wellness involves developing the skills to cope with stress.

Stress

Stress is the response of the body to any demand placed on it by stressors. A **stressor** is something that triggers the stress response. Hungarian Hans Selye, a 29-year-old endocrinologist at McGill University, first wrote about stress in a short letter he sent to *Nature* magazine, which was subsequently published (Selye, 1936). He noted harmful agents (stressors) caused pathophysiologic changes with common characteristics (stress response). Stress can include the following factors.

- **Environmental Factors**. Crowding, deadlines, excessive noise, or destructive weather.
- **Societal Factors**. Verbal aggression or conflict from family, friends, supervisors, co-workers, or customers.
- **Situational Factors**. Starting or losing a job, relocating, marriage, or divorce.
- **Chemical Factors**. Stimulants such as caffeine, irritants such as inflammation, and hormone/neurotransmitter imbalances such as thyroid-stimulating hormones and serotonin.

Selye (1974) stated there are several types of stress, classified by how it is perceived by the individual as positive (eustress) or as negative (distress). **Eustress** is perceived as positive and within our ability to meet the demands of the situation—it keeps us focused on a goal, improves performance, and gives us personal satisfaction. **Distress** is perceived as negative and beyond our capacity to cope. How individuals respond to stress is determined by their emotional reactions, their unique perceptions, their feelings of self-efficacy, or their ability to complete required tasks or play specific roles within the stressful situation. Neurobiologically, stress involves activation of the sympathetic division of the autonomic nervous system, which prepares the body to confront the stressor, usually in a fight-or-flight response (see Chapter 23). Ways to manage stress are listed next.

Managing Stress

Stress can reduce wellness and negatively affect physical and mental health. Evidence-based approaches to manage stress include practicing diaphragmatic breathing, gratitude, progressive muscle relaxation, guided imagery, mindfulness-based stress reduction, expressive writing, self-affirmations, and physical activity as mentioned previously (Creswell et al., 2013; Kim & McKenzie, 2014; Niles et al., 2014; Varvogli & Darviri, 2011; Wong et al., 2018). Talking to a therapist or counselor about stress can also be a key part of addressing and reducing it in the long term. Several studies found massage reduced stress among various populations (Brennan & DeBate, 2006; Cady & Jones, 1997; Engen et al., 2012; Haraldsson et al., 2005; Smith et al., 1999). Field et al. (2005) conducted a literature review and found that massage had beneficial effects on a variety of medical conditions and stressful experiences. In studies analyzed, cortisol levels decreased an average of 31%, serotonin increased an average of 28%, and dopamine increased an average of 31%. Massage also reduces anxiety

in the person giving the massage (Jensen et al., 2012). The American Institute of Stress (n.d.) suggests the use of massage as self-care to relieve stress (Fig. 4.3). The next section includes a brief summary of various methods of stress reduction.

Diaphragmatic Breathing

Diaphragmatic breathing is voluntary, slow deep breathing with the abdomen expanding downward rather than the chest expanding upward during inhalation. Practice diaphragmatic breathing by placing one or both hands on your abdomen. Breathe in through your nose (as if smelling something) for about 2 seconds. Your belly should fill like a balloon and your hand(s) should rise with your abdomen. Breathe out slowly through pursed lips (as if blowing bubbles) for about 4 seconds. Your hand(s) should lower as you exhale. Repeat breathing cycles for several minutes. **NOTE**: Stop if you feel faint or dizzy. Diaphragmatic breathing is also called abdominal/belly breathing or deep breathing.

Gratitude

Gratitude is thankful appreciation for all the wonderful things in life. Engage in the practice of gratitude by keeping

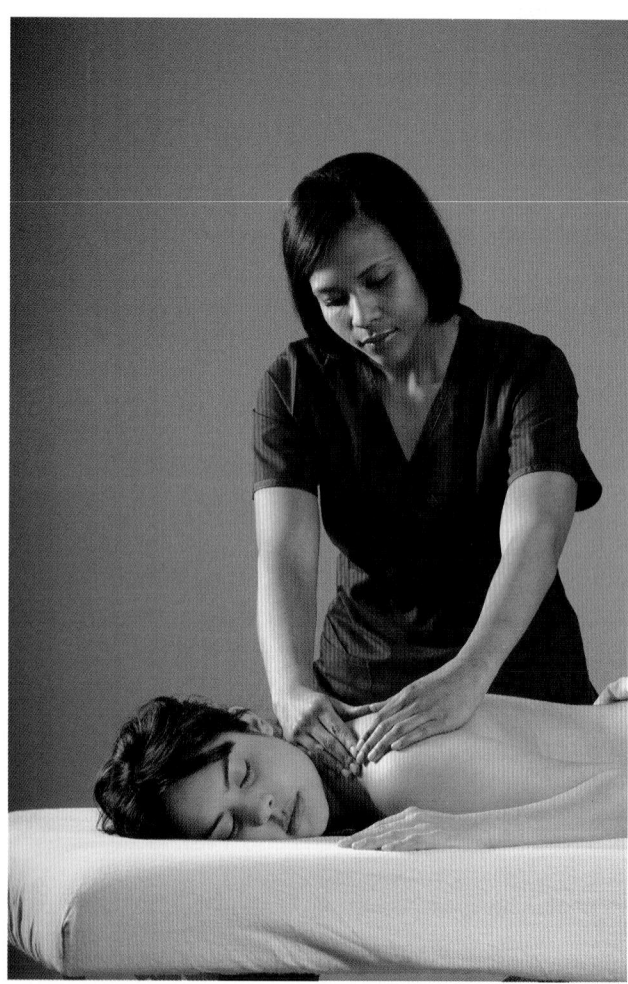

FIG. 4.3 Massage practitioner receiving massage as self-care to relieve stress.

a gratitude journal. Participate in a gratitude visit by writing a letter of gratitude to someone who is alive, delivering it in person, and reading it to them or ask them to read it. This activity can be a meaningful experience for both parties. You can also take pictures of things for which you are grateful. Be sure to take time to savor and enjoy the feelings of gratitude.

Progressive Muscle Relaxation

Progressive muscle relaxation is alternately squeezing and releasing muscles, focusing on distinctions between the feelings of muscle tension and relaxation. To practice progressive muscle relaxation, contract and relax muscles in different areas of the body in a sequential pattern, usually beginning in the legs, buttocks, back, abdomen, shoulders, then arms, and the face last. The squeeze or muscle tension phase is approximately 10 seconds and the release or muscle relaxation phase is approximately 20 seconds. Perform each squeeze/release sequence 2 to 3 times with eyes closed.

Guided Imagery

Guided imagery is a facilitated exploration of an imagined place. Guiding imagery involves recruitment of visual, auditory, olfactory, tactile, and kinesthetic sensory qualities, while linking the relaxation of the imagery with the relaxed state experienced by the individual. To practice guided imagery, sit or lie down and close your eyes. Take a few deep breaths and picture a calm and peaceful place. This could be a beach, a mountain setting, a meadow, or a library. Add some detail. For example, walk through your scene and notice what you touch and feel, see, smell, or hear. Take a few minutes to breathe slowly and feel calm and relaxed. When you are ready, slowly take yourself out of the scene and back to the present. Count to 3, and open your eyes. Notice your feelings. It may help to have an instructor or audio recording to follow.

Mindfulness-Based Stress Reduction

Mindfulness-Based Stress Reduction (MBSR) combines mindfulness mediation with an activity. To practice MBSR, focus your attention to present moments and observe the bodily sensations and the emotions felt while participating in the chosen activity. The activity can be breathing, walking, stretching, yoga, or eating a sandwich. The activity can be repeating a sound or phrase or thinking about a virtue such as compassion, gratitude, or love. Do the activity for 10 to 20 minutes. Mindfulness is also discussed in Chapters 2 and 7.

Expressive Writing

Expressive writing, as a stress reduction technique, is writing down words that symbolize your feelings about stressful and traumatic events. To practice expressive writing, write these events and how they made you feel—it can include your thoughts and your ideas. Writing can be structured or unstructured, but the most important thing is to let words flow freely. Do not be concerned about spelling errors or what others might think. Reduce barriers to writing by keeping a pen and paper handy, or a journal on your mobile phone. Keep your journal private or share some of your feelings with trusted friends and loved ones. Expressive writing can be done daily as a 15- to 20-minute session or only occasionally, with no feedback sought about what was written.

Self-Affirmations

Self-affirmations are positive statements spoken or read to affirm one's worthiness and value. They can be used to facilitate change, or to promote self-confidence and the belief in your own abilities. Examples of self-affirmations are "All I can do is my best," and "I know I can accomplish anything I set my mind to." Rev. Reinhold Niebuhr's serenity prayer is an example of a self-affirmation, which reads "God, grant me the serenity to accept the things I cannot change, the courage to change the things I can, and the wisdom to know the difference." To practice self-affirmations, say your statement when waking up and getting into bed, and perhaps throughout the day. Repeat the affirmation approximately 10 times. Listen to yourself and focus on the words as they leave your mouth. Believe the phrase is true. Perhaps ask a trusted friend or loved one to say it to you, as listening to someone else say your affirmation may reinforce your belief in it. Be patient as it may take several days to several weeks before changes are noted. Posting written self-affirmations that are seen on a daily basis can help solidify the message to yourself.

SOCIAL WELLNESS

Social wellness is the positive interaction with others and involves good use of communication skills, developing and maintaining meaningful relationships, valuing diversity and treating others with respect, and creating a social support system. The social support system includes family, friends, teachers, classmates, and others. Social wellness also involves participating in community events such as celebrations and festivals. Involvement in massage organization–sponsored continuing education within a learning community and attending conferences and conventions can be part of social wellness. Sharing experiences and challenges with colleagues can also fulfill a social need.

Social wellness includes interacting with people of other cultures, backgrounds, values, and beliefs. It means taking time for leisure and recreational activities. Following this further, social wellness emphasizes our interdependence with others and with nature. In fact, social wellness can be met by taking part in preserving the environment for others through recycling and conservation efforts.

SPIRITUAL WELLNESS

Spiritual wellness is searching for the meaning and purpose of human existence, with or without religious affiliation. According to Rickhi (2013), spirituality is the life we live inside ourselves, versus the life we live outside ourselves through our occupations and social networks. Although spiritual wellness can be obtained through religious practice, spiritual wellness is deeply personal and provides systems of faith, beliefs, values, ethics, principles and morals, things that involve harmony with oneself and others. Spiritual wellness may involve attending worship services as well as contemplative acts such as prayer and meditation.

E-RESOURCES

http://evolve.elsevier.com/Salvo/MassageTherapy

- Chapter challenge
- Flash cards
- Stress-busting tips for massage students
- Additional information
- Video

LORIMER MOSELEY

Like many of us, Lorimer Moseley had a wide variety of interesting jobs before finding his true passion. He worked as a truck driver, farmhand, musician, footballer, fence construction worker, and finally physiotherapist. It was at this point he noticed the gap between what he was doing clinically and the problems his patients were actually struggling with: chronic pain.

Have you noticed how differently pain affects one person compared with another? Or maybe why one injury can result in chronic pain lasting for years, whereas a similar injury in another person might resolve with no problem at all? Or even how some people don't experience any pain initially when they have severe injuries, like car accidents or wounds on a battlefield? Struggling with his own nagging injury from football, Moseley set out to better understand some of these questions as a doctor of neuroscience.

Moseley earned his doctorate at the University of Sydney Pain Management. In 2011 he was appointed Professor of Neuroscience and Foundation Chair in Physiotherapy at the University of South Australia. He leads the Body in Mind Research Group, a robust interdisciplinary team that researches pain in humans. Moseley is a prolific writer and speaker, having authored hundreds of research papers and several books, including *Painful Yarns,* which is the second best-selling pain book in the world. It is his attempt to bridge the gap and help clinical sciences begin to "listen" to what is known by pain scientists.

Pain occurs for one primary reason: to warn us of danger. It can be important for us to become aware of potential harm in our environment so we can assess the situation and make decisions to keep ourselves safe. Pain is contextual. Moseley demonstrated through research that when people feel something very hot or very cold, they look to cues in their environment to decide. For example, if people see red, they will likely perceive it as hot, and if they see blue, they will likely perceive it as cold. In other words, the brain is constantly collecting data to explain what it senses in the tissue. Why does this matter? Because the brain may gather information and apply it incorrectly, causing it to make incorrect decisions or

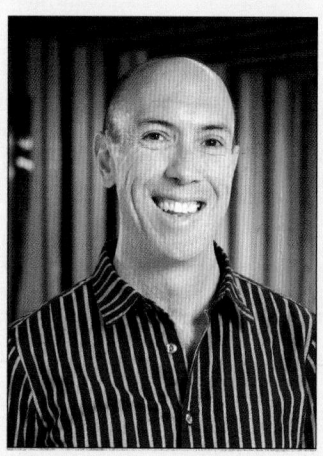

(Courtesy Lorimer Moseley.)

responses to experiences. That may be a factor in the development of chronic pain.

His passion for the topic of chronic pain stems from the huge problem we have in healthcare successfully treating it. In the West, it costs more to treat chronic pain (and not necessarily successfully) than cancer, cardiovascular disease, and diabetes combined. If the brain keeps identifying pain in the body, then it becomes more and more efficient about sounding the pain alert. Even more troubling, the brain becomes less and less specific in where the problem is!

Tissue damage is neither necessary nor sufficient for pain. The more we learn about pain, the more this becomes apparent, most significantly when we consider the 20% of people for whom quality of life is reduced by a chronic pain problem. I undertake studies that aim to increase our understanding of why things hurt, why things keep hurting and how we can better prevent and manage chronic pain in the community.

Moseley asks this important question: How do we convince people who are in pain that their pain is not entirely about what is happening in the tissues? If you begin to read Moseley's many articles and books or watch him speak, you will find he communicates in a way accessible to everyone. He helps nonscientists understand complex ideas. By using amusing, creative, and elegant metaphors and stories, he's helping people all over the world understand pain differently.

It can be extraordinarily challenging to explain complex concepts like neuroscience to nonscientists. Despite being a highly educated pain scientist, Lorimer Moseley has done just that. He is the embodiment of remaining in the learner's mind: curious, creative, and searching for new ways of understanding the world. He inspires us as practitioners to continue embracing and applying new ways of thinking about what we do.

Our body is not a machine. It is a garden. We're a single organism.

—**Lorimer Moseley**

REFERENCES

Adriaenssens, J., Gucht, V. D., & Maes, S. (2015). Determinants and prevalence of burnout in emergency nurses: A systematic review of 25 years of research. *International Journal of Nursing Studies*, 52(2), 649–661.

Albert, W. J., Currie-Jackson, N., & Duncan, C. A. (2008). A survey of musculoskeletal injuries amongst Canadian massage therapists. *Journal of Bodywork and Movement Therapies*, 12(1), 86–93.

Alexander, R. K., Diefenbeck, C. A., & Brown, C. G. (2015). Career choice and longevity in U.S. Psychiatric-mental health nurses. *Issues in Mental Health Nursing*, 36(6), 447–454.

American College of Sports Medicine (ACSM). (2011). Quantity and quality of exercise for developing and maintaining cardiorespiratory, musculoskeletal, and neuromotor fitness in apparently healthy adults: guidance for prescribing exercise. *Medicine and Science in Sports and Exercise*, 3(7), 1334–1359.

American Institute of Stress. (n.d.). *Management tips*. Retrieved from http://www.stress.org/management-tips/.

Asp, M. (2015). Rest: a health-related phenomenon and concept in caring science. *Global Qualitative Nursing Research*, 29(2), 2333393615583663.

Blau, G., Monos, C., Boyer, E., Davis, K., Flanagan, R., Lopez, A., & Tatum, D. S. (2013). Correlates of injury-forced work reduction for massage therapists and bodywork practitioners. *International Journal of Therapeutic Massage and Bodywork*, 6(3), 6–13.

Brennan, M. K., & DeBate, R. D. (2006). The effect of chair massage on stress perception of hospital bedside nurses. *Journal of Bodywork and Movement Therapies*, 10(4), 335–342.

Cady, S. H., & Jones, G. E. (1997). Massage therapy as a workplace intervention for reduction of stress. *Perceptual and Motor Skills*, 84(1), 157–158.

Centers for Disease Control and Prevention. (2017). *How much sleep do I need?* Retrieved from https://www.cdc.gov/sleep/about_sleep/how_much_sleep.html.

Centers for Disease Control and Prevention. (2018). *Wellbeing concepts*. Retrieved from https://www.cdc.gov/hrqol/wellbeing.htm.

Centers for Disease Control and Prevention. (2020). *Nutrition and healthy eating: water*. Retrieved from https://www.mayoclinic.org/healthy-lifestyle/nutrition-and-healthy-eating/basics/nutrition-basics/hlv-20049477.

Chaabene, H., Behm, D. G., Negra, Y., & Granacher, U. (2019). Acute effects of static stretching on muscle strength and power: An attempt to clarify previous caveats. *Frontiers in Physiology*, 10, 1468.

Creswell, J. D., Dutcher, J. M., Klein, W. M., Harris, P. R., & Levine, J. M. (2013). Self-affirmation improves problem-solving under stress. *PLoS One*, 8(5), e62593.

Curtis, R., Willems, C., Paoletti, P. & D'Aout, K. (2021). Daily activity in minimal footwear increases foot strength. *Scientific Reports*, 11(1), 18648. https://doi.org/10.1038/s41598-021-98070-0

Engel, G. L. (1977). The need for a new medical model: a challenge for biomedicine. *Science*, 196(4286), 129–136.

Engen, D. J., Wahner-Roedler, D. L., Vincent, A., Chon, T. Y., Cha, S.S., Luedtke, C. A., et al. (2012). Feasibility and effect of chair massage offered to nurses during work hours on stress-related symptoms: A pilot study. *Complementary Therapies in Clinical Practice*, 18(4), 212–215.

Field, T., Hernandez-Reif, M., Diego, M., Schanberg, S., & Kuhn, C. (2005). Cortisol decreases and serotonin and dopamine increase following massage therapy. *International Journal of Neuroscience*, 115(10), 397–413.

Fortune, L. D., & Gillespie, E. (2010). The influence of practice standards on massage therapists' work experience: A phenomenological pilot study. *International Journal of Therapeutic Massage and Bodywork*, 3(3), 5–11.

Greene, L., & Goggins, R. W. (2006). Musculoskeletal symptoms and injuries among experienced massage and bodywork professionals. *Massage and Bodywork*. Jan, 48–58.

Haraldsson, K., Fridlund, B., Baigi, A., & Marklund, B. (2005). The self-reported health condition of women after their participation in a stress management program: A pilot study. *Health and Social Care in the Community*, 13(3), 224–230.

Harvard Medical School: Division of Sleep Medicine. (n.d.). *Benefits of sleep*. Retrieved from http://healthysleep.med.harvard.edu/healthy/matters/benefits-of-sleep.

Jang, Y., Chi, C. F., Tsauo, J. Y., & Wang, J. D. (2006). Prevalence and risk factors of work-related musculoskeletal disorders in massage practitioners. *Journal of Occupational Rehabilitation*, 16(3), 425–438.

Jensen, A. M., Ramasamy, A., Hotek, J., Roel, B., & Riffe, D. (2012). The benefits of giving a massage on the mental state of massage therapists: A randomized, controlled trial. *J Altern Complement Med*, 18(12), 1142–1146.

Kennedy, A. B., & Munk, N. (2017). Experienced practitioners' beliefs utilized to create a successful massage therapist conceptual model: A qualitative investigation. *International Journal of Therapeutic Massage and Bodywork*, 10(2), 9–19.

Killian, K. D. (2008). Helping till it hurts? A multimethod study of compassion fatigue, burnout, and self-care in clinicians working with trauma survivors. *Traumatology*, 14(2), 32–44.

Kim, J. H., & McKenzie, L. A. (2014). The impacts of physical exercise on stress coping and wellbeing in university students in the context of leisure. *Health*, 6(19), 2570–2580.

Maslach, C. (2015). *Burnout: The cost of caring*. Los Altos, CA: Institute for Study of Human Knowledge.

Mazerolle, S. M., Eason, C. M., Lazar, R. A., & Mensch, J. M. (2016). Exploring career longevity in athletic training: factors influencing persistence in the NCAA division I setting. *Journal of Athletic Training*, 21(6), 48–57.

Miller, A. E., MacDougall, J. D., Tarnopolsky, M. A., & Sale, D. G. (1993). Gender differences in strength and muscle fiber characteristics. *European Journal of Applied Physiology*, 66(3), 254–262.

Mohr, E. G. (2010). Proper body mechanics from an engineering perspective. *Journal of Bodywork and Movement Therapies*, 14, 139–151.

Niles, A. N., Haltom, K. E., Mulvenna, C. M., Lieberman, M. D., & Stanton, A. L. (2014). Effects of expressive writing on psychological and physical health: the moderating role of emotional expressivity. *Anxiety Stress Coping*, 27(1), 1–17.

Prudden, B. (1980). *Pain erasure: The Bonnie Prudden way*. M. Evans & Company. New York, NY.

Pustułka-Piwnik, U., Ryn, Z. J., Krzywoszański, Ł., & Stożek, J. (2014). Burnout syndrome in physical therapists: demographic and organizational factors. *Medycyna Pracy*, 65(4), 453–462.

Rauvola, R. S., Vega, D. M., & Lavigne, K. N. (2019). Compassion fatigue, secondary traumatic stress, and vicarious traumatization: A qualitative review and research agenda. *Occupational Health Science*, 3(3), 297–336.

Rickhi, B. G. (2013). *The cosmic game*. Self-publication.

Riess, H., & Kraft-Todd, G. (2014). E.M.P.A.T.H.Y.: a tool to enhance nonverbal communication between clinicians and their patients. *Journal of the Association of American Medical Colleges*, 89(8), 1108–1112.

Sathya, P., Ramakrishnan, K. S., & Gowda, H. (2016). Prevalence of musculoskeletal problems in masseuse. *International Journal of Rehabilitation Research*, 5(5), 140–148.

Segall, A., & Goldstein, J. (1989). Exploring the correlates of self-provided healthcare behavior. *Social Science and Medicine*, 29(2), 153–161.

Selye, H. (1936). A syndrome produced by diverse nocuous agents. *Nature*, 138(3479), 32.

Selye, H. (1974). *Stress without distress*. Philadelphia: Lippincott Williams & Wilkins.

Shoji, K., Cieslak, R., Smoktunowicz, E., Rogala, A., Benight, C. C., & Luszczynska, A. (2015). Associations between job burnout and self-efficacy: A meta-analysis. *Anxiety Stress Coping*, 29(4), 367–386.

Smith, M. C., Stallings, M. A., Mariner, S., & Burrall, M. (1999). Benefits of massage therapy for hospitalized patients: a descriptive and qualitative evaluation. *Alternative Therapies in Health and Medicine*, 5(4), 64–71.

Taylor, S. G., & Renpenning, K. (2011). *Self-care science, nursing theory and evidence-based practice*. New York: Springer Publishing Company.

Turkeltaub, P. C., Yearwood, E. L., & Friedmann, E. (2014). Effect of a brief seated massage on nursing student attitudes toward touch for comfort care. *Journal of Alternative and Complementary Medicine*, 20(10), 792–799.

Varvogli, L., & Darviri, C. (2011). Stress management techniques: evidence-based procedures that reduce stress and promote health. *Health Science Journal*, 5(2), 74–89.

WHO: World Health Organization. (2018). *Physical activity*. Retrieved from https://www.who.int/health-topics/physical-activity#tab=tab_1

Więcek, M., Szymura, J., Maciejczyk, M., Szyguła, Z., Cempla, J., & Borkowski, M. (2018). Energy expenditure for massage therapists during performing selected classical massage techniques. *International Journal of Occupational Medicine and Environmental Health*, 31(5), 677–684.

Wong, Y. J., Owen, J., Gabana, N. T., Brown, J. W., McInnis, S., Toth, P., & Gilman, L. (2018). Does gratitude writing improve the mental health of psychotherapy clients? Evidence from a randomized controlled trial. *Psychotherapy Research*, 28(2), 192–202.

REVIEW AND APPLY YOUR KNOWLEDGE

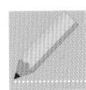 ## MATCHING ONE: CONCEPT REVIEW

Place the letter of the answer next to the number of the term or phrase that best describes it.

A. Self-care
B. Burnout
C. Calorie
D. Physical activity
E. Wellness model
F. Intellectual wellness
G. Macronutrients
H. Micronutrients
I. Nutrients
J. Strenuous
K. Stress
L. Occupational wellness

_____ 1. The occupational category Bonnie Prudden places massage practitioners in.

_____ 2. The holistic integration of the six dimensions of wellness, including physical wellness, occupational wellness, intellectual wellness, social wellness, emotional wellness, and spiritual wellness.

_____ 3. Care of oneself that is learned, proactive, deliberate, purposeful, and continuous to improve or preserve health and wellbeing.

_____ 4. Category of nutrients that include vitamins and minerals and are needed in small amounts.

_____ 5. The ability to balance work and leisure time, manage workplace stress, and build good relationships with co-workers and colleagues.

_____ 6. Unit of energy received from nutrients.

_____ 7. The continuous acquisition, development, and creative application of critical thinking in the quest for a more satisfying existence.

_____ 8. Substances in food and drink that provide nutrition.

_____ 9. Movement produced by skeletal muscles and requires energy expenditure.

_____ 10. The body's response to demands placed on it by stressors.

_____ 11. Syndrome resulting from chronic workplace stress not successfully managed and is characterized by a state of emotional exhaustion, depersonalization, and diminished sense of personal accomplishment.

_____ 12. Category of nutrients that include proteins, carbohydrates, and fats, and are needed in relatively large amounts.

MATCHING TWO: CONCEPT REVIEW

Place the letter of the answer next to the number of the term or phrase that best describes it.

A. Carbohydrates
B. Nutrition
C. Self-affirmations
D. Fats
E. Fat-soluble vitamins
F. Healthy Eating Plate
G. Incomplete
H. Food label
I. Protein
J. Sleep
K. Water-soluble vitamins
L. Neuromotor

_____ 1. These are absorbed slowly, are stored in the liver and in fat cells for future use, and include Vitamins A, D, E, and K.

_____ 2. Recurrent state of relaxation characterized by an altered state of consciousness, inhibited sensory activity, muscular inhibition, and reduced interactions.

_____ 3. Macronutrient containing chains of amino acids, and assists the body's growth and energy needs, while helping to build and repair tissues.

_____ 4. Type of physical activity that incorporates resistance and flexibility with slow, focused movement and/or sustained body postures.

_____ 5. Macronutrient naturally found in animal and plant foods, are sources of energy, help the body absorb certain vitamins and minerals, and include saturated and unsaturated classifications.

_____ 6. Positive statements (spoken or read) to affirm one's worthiness and value, and can be used to facilitate change in the individual who uses them.

_____ 7. Panels on packaged foods and contains nutritional facts such as serving size, calories per serving, macro- and micronutrients, and a list of ingredients.

_____ 8. These are readily absorbed into tissues, are not stored in the body, are quickly excreted in urine, and include Vitamins B and C.

_____ 9. Macronutrient that turns into glucose (blood sugar) and is used by the body as energy.

_____ 10. Ingesting food and drink to help the body function properly, to support tissue growth and repair, and to supply the energy needed for daily activities.

_____ 11. An infographic that helps people make food choices and plan portion sizes at mealtimes.

_____ 12. Term for foods containing some, but not all, essential amino acids in proteins.

MULTIPLE CHOICE: TEST YOUR KNOWLEDGE

Place the letter of the answer next to the number of the term or phrase that best describes it.

_____ 1. What is the experience of health and includes feelings of comfort, safety, contentment, happiness, high life satisfaction, and sense of meaning or purpose?
   A. Physical activity
   B. Wellbeing
   C. Self-care
   D. Healthcare

_____ 2. Which dimension of wellness promotes balanced nutrition, rest, and regular medical examinations?
   A. Physical
   B. Occupational
   C. Emotional
   D. Social

_____ 3. Which dimension of wellness promotes positive interaction with others, valuing diversity and treating others with respect, and creating a support system?
   A. Physical
   B. Occupational
   C. Environmental
   D. Social

_____ 4. Brisk walking of at least 4 miles an hour, biking with light effort or 10 to 12 mph, walking or biking uphill, strenuous yoga classes, or playing tennis doubles are examples of what type of activity level?
   A. Low intensity
   B. Moderate intensity
   C. High intensity
   D. Vigorous intensity

_____ 5. Yoga and tai chi are examples of what type of exercise?
   A. Cardiovascular
   B. Resistance
   C. Flexibility
   D. Neuromotor

_____ 6. Nuts and seeds are examples of:
   A. complete proteins.
   B. incomplete proteins.
   C. simple carbohydrates.
   D. complex carbohydrates.

_____ 7. Burnout is a condition that relates to which dimension of wellness?
   A. Physical
   B. Occupational
   C. Emotional
   D. Social

_____ 8. Approximately _____% of massage practitioners experience work-related pain and musculoskeletal symptoms.
   A. 50
   B. 60
   C. 70
   D. 80

_____ 9. An environmental modification that can help reduce practitioner injury is to stow bolsters between:
   A. foot and hip height.
   B. knee and waist height.
   C. foot and ankle height.
   D. knee and ankle height.

_____ 10. Which method of stress reduction involves recruitment of visual, auditory, olfactory, tactile, and kinesthetic sensory qualities?
   A. Diaphragmatic breathing
   B. Expressive writing
   C. Guided imagery
   D. Self-affirmation

_____ 11. Which dimension of wellness may include keeping current with information on healthy living, visiting art galleries and museums, and being open to new experiences?
   A. Physical
   B. Intellectual
   C. Emotional
   D. Spiritual

_____ 12. Which dimension of wellness involves searching for meaning and purpose, with or without religious affiliation?
   A. Social
   B. Intellectual
   C. Emotional
   D. Spiritual

CRITICAL THINKING

The Go-Getter

Sophia has just graduated from massage school and has been hired by a massage franchise. She is eager to start practicing and earning money, so she takes every shift her manager asks her to and agrees to substitute for several other massage practitioners who want to take some time off. What advice would you give to Sophia?

Answers can include but are not limited to:

Try to have some choice about the number of massage sessions done per day or per week. Blau et al. (2013) found physical exhaustion or being fatigued from energy expenditure had the strongest relationship to injury, and researchers recommended taking sufficient time between massages to reduce injury. Find ways to recuperate from the physical exertion of massage, which may include a brief rest, an easy walk, or refreshments to rehydrate and refuel before the next massage.

Positive interactions with co-workers and talking with peers and supervisors promoted career longevity. Build and maintain a positive work community, and participate in team-building activities. This helps us feel simultaneously as though we are a necessary part of the team and we are not alone.

Alexander et al. (2015) found that, oftentimes, members of helping professions enter because of past experiences, it was important on a personal level, or they had potential for success. Feelings of lack of accomplishment and low self-efficacy contributed to burnout (Shoji et al., 2015). Find ways to experience professional recognition and reward through contact and fellowship with a massage peer group. Your professional social network can include colleagues within your place of business as well as massage practitioners from your geographic region and beyond, met by attending state and national conferences.

PROFESSIONAL PRACTICE

More Than Just an Accident

Mark has been a massage practitioner for 7 years. He is in private practice and sees approximately 25 clients a week, most of whom come to him for the deep tissue treatments for which he is known. Recently he took a week off when his father died so he could travel to the funeral. His house is in the middle of being remodeled, so he has been adding new clients into his schedule to pay for the renovations. Lately, Mark's girlfriend, Samantha, has noticed Mark seems to be reluctant to leave for his office in the morning, and when he comes home at night, he talks very little and just parks himself in front of the TV. A few days ago, Samantha suggested they go hiking or out to brunch on Sunday, but Mark just stared at her and said he didn't feel like it. What could Mark be experiencing? What advice would you give Mark?

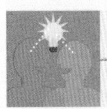

DISCUSSION

Physician, Heal Thyself

What is meant by the proverb, "Physician, heal thyself"? How can massage practitioners apply this principle to their practice? Look up the word salutogenesis, a term introduced by Antonovsky in 1979. Reflecting on the definition, write a self-care plan. Use these resources while developing a self-care plan.

https://www.heart.org/en/healthy-living/fitness/fitness-basics/aha-recs-for-physical-activity-in-adults

https://health.gov/sites/default/files/2019-09/Physical_Activity_Guidelines_2nd_edition.pdf

https://www.acsm.org/read-research/trending-topics-resource-pages/physical-activity-guidelines]

If available, post your reflections on an Internet-based discussion board monitored by your instructor.

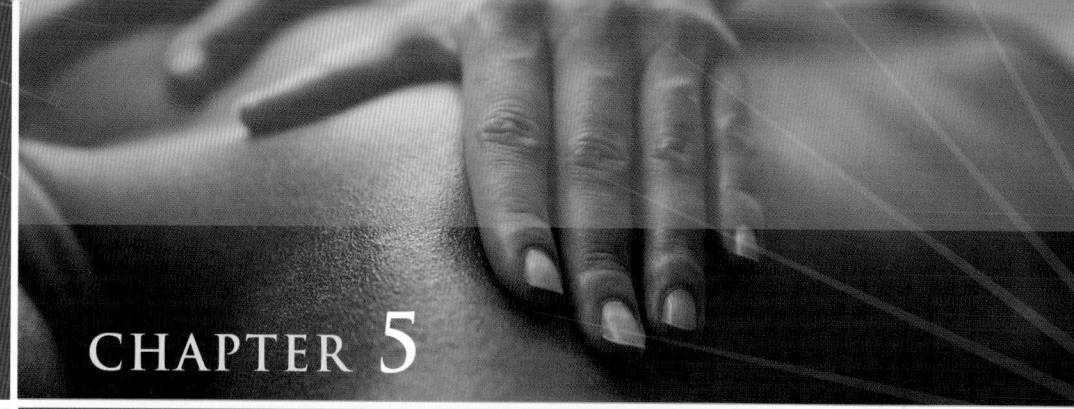

CHAPTER 5

Evidence-Informed Practice and Research Literacy

LEARNING OBJECTIVES

After completing this chapter, the student should be able to:

1. Define evidence-informed practice, research literacy, and approaches to research.
2. Explain evidence, the research process, the levels of practitioner expertise, and client preferences and how each plays a role in evidence-informed practice.

http://evolve.elsevier.com/Salvo/MassageTherapy

INTRODUCTION

Evidence-informed practice (EIP) has attained a position of importance and plays an integral part of healthcare practices and government health policies (Jack, 2006; National Institutes of Health [NIH], 2019; Webster, 2002). Massage, in various forms, has been used for thousands of years (Field, 2002). Early research studies focused on touch deprivation, with most led by psychologists examining relationships between lack of touch in early life and developmental delays (Spitz, 1965). Other types of studies investigating touch and massage were conducted over the next few decades. However, scientific investigation became more prevalent in the 1980s.

Field et al. (1986) studied the effects of massage and tactile stimulation on preterm infants. This and similar studies led to the establishment of the Touch Research Institute (TRI) at the University of Miami's School of Medicine in 1992 under the directorship of Field. The TRI was the first center in the world devoted solely to the study of touch and massage in its application in science and medicine (Touch Research Institute [TRI], n.d.). Research efforts continuing today have shown touch and massage have numerous beneficial effects on health and wellbeing. Other types of interventions studied at TRI include aromatherapy, tai chi, and yoga.

Another important research organization in the massage profession is the Massage Therapy Foundation (MTF). The MTF was started by the American Massage Therapy Association in 1990 with the mission of advancing the knowledge and practice of massage. Currently, the MTF is an independent organization and continues to support scientific research, education, and community service projects. Research and evidence are important so massage practitioners can select methods and techniques to help clients achieve optimal results.

Each year the quality and quantity of massage research studies increase. Many studies are funded by major organizations such as the National Institutes of Health (NIH). The NIH is made up of 27 institutes and centers, each with a specific research agenda. Examples include the National Institute on Aging, the National Library of Medicine, and the National Center for Complementary and Alternative Medicine (NCCAM), which was founded in 1998. In 2014, Congress changed the name of this center to National Center for Complementary and Integrative Health (NCCIH), stating that the use of massage and chiropractic and other practices as "alternative medicine" was rare. The new center blends complementary and integrative healthcare with mainstream medicine. NCCIH has two subgroups—products such as herbal supplements and probiotics; and practices such as massage, acupuncture, chiropractic, and yoga. Massage and chiropractic and osteopathic care are among the most common practices used by the general public (NIH, 2018).

EVIDENCE-INFORMED PRACTICE

Evidence-informed practice is a problem-solving approach used when making treatment decisions that integrates relevant

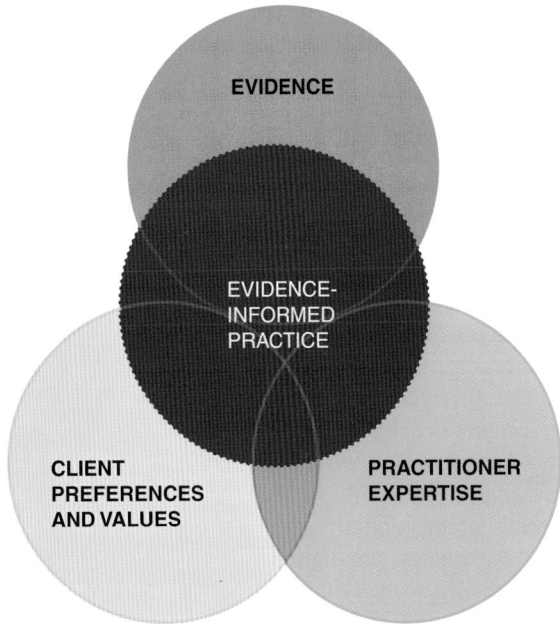

FIG. 5.1 Evidence-informed practice. All three elements are important and needed to support an evidence-informed massage practice.

evidence, the client's preferences and values, and the practitioner's professional expertise to achieve desired patient/client goals (Fineout-Overholt et al., 2005) (Fig. 5.1). Practitioners in the complementary and integrative health (CIH) sciences are required to be committed to an evidence-informed approach. *Patients* are recipients of services performed in medical settings, and *clients* are recipients in nonmedical settings. In this chapter, the terms patients and clients are used interchangeably.

There is a demand for research-literate massage practitioners who are willing and able to respond to a changing knowledge base and use evidence to inform and support their professional decisions (Evans et al., 2011). EIP is the response to the demand for cost-effective services and increased transparency in professional decision-making. The public and stakeholders need to know what service providers are doing, why they are doing it, and why they are choosing the selected intervention instead of a different one. EIP seeks to improve outcomes, protect the public from unsafe practices, protect service providers from litigation, and promote professional accountability and integrity. EIP also exposes gaps in knowledge and conflicts between evidence-based sources (Grainger, 2013). The essence of EIP is to *base treatment decisions on what was shown to be effective and not what was thought to be effective* (Sullivan, 1998).

EIP evolved from evidence-based medicine, which is "the conscientious, explicit, and judicious use of current best evidence in making decisions about the care of individual patients" (Sackett et al., 1996). The concept of evidence based was adopted by other professionals and became evidence-based practice (EBP). The primary focus of both approaches was evidence, usually high levels of evidence such as systematic reviews (SRs), meta-analyses, and randomized controlled trials (RCTs). However, some scholars suggest EBP is too restrictive and rigid, ignoring a professional's expertise, as well as the client values and preferences, and reduces the emphasis on client-centered care (Emanuel et al., 2011; Titler, 2008). Critics of EBP claim evidence exists to inform and guide, rather than to dictate practice, and professional decisions should draw on and integrate multiple sources, including emerging theories, expert opinion, and qualitative research. EIP includes the missing pieces of EBP previously mentioned and provides flexibility regarding the nature of evidence, how evidence is used, and different types of evidence are needed to support client-centered decisions.

In addition, advances in information technology had a radical impact on healthcare delivery. In fact, EIP is partly the result of the digital age with the arrival of wireless internet technology, the digitization of information, and the prevalence of personally owned web-enabled electronic devices (Webster, 2002). Assuredly, information literacy is the foundation for EIP, and further advances in information technology will likely affect the success of EIP (Webster, 2002).

Barriers to Evidence-Informed Practice

Barriers to EIP include (Bertulis, 2008; Grainger, 2013):
1. Lack of information literacy skills.
2. Lack of research skills.
3. Limited or poor access to quality information.
4. Lack of time (speed of access).
5. Negative staff attitudes and resistance.
6. Lack of administrative support.
7. Preference for colleagues as information sources over printed or computerized sources.
8. Reading barrier (health literacy).
9. Language barrier (English as a second language).
10. Lack of statistical knowledge.

Students and practitioners must overcome personal, professional, and institutional barriers to EIP. Take steps to acquire and utilize EIP skills in order to maintain progress with other service providers and with governmental standards. Actions may include discussing the value of evidence in professional practice with fellow colleagues and describing how you use evidence in your practice. Keep up-to-date with the latest research through publications provided by trade organizations.

RESEARCH LITERACY AND RESEARCH

Research literacy is cognitive and social understanding of the purpose, process, and value of research (Brody et al., 2012). To be research literate, massage practitioners must possess a set of skills, including the ability to locate, read, understand, and evaluate research literature.
- Locating research depends on the ability to use information technology, such as databases and search engines to retrieve studies.
- Reading and understanding research mean practitioners understand the research process itself, as well as the terminology used in the studies.
- Evaluating research depends on understanding of the hierarchies or levels of evidence to determine their strength or trustworthiness.

Research is systematic inquiry using prescribed methods to validate or refine existing knowledge or to develop new knowledge. Research is the backbone of the healthcare profession and can validate, provide efficacy, and innovate treatment protocols. The interrelationship between practitioners, clients/patients, and researchers is important to understand. Each group is involved as new knowledge is developed and old knowledge is tested and authenticated or invalidated (Fig. 5.2). Clients report results and experiences to their practitioners. Practitioners document results and tell researchers what they learn from their clients and infer from their experiences. Researchers develop research questions and design experiments to answer these questions. Practitioners read the published studies and use the information in their practices. Practitioners provide feedback to researchers, and the cycle continues.

Approaches to Research

There are three general approaches to research. They are *quantitative research, qualitative research,* and *literature reviews* (Creswell, 2013). All approaches collect and analyze **data** or recorded factual information used to validate research results.

Quantitative Research

Quantitative research is used to establish generalizable facts about a topic and focuses on testing theories and hypotheses. Quantitative methods are largely objective, and results can be replicated. Data are often collected in the form of questionnaires, surveys, or polls using closed-ended multiple-choice questions, depending on the type

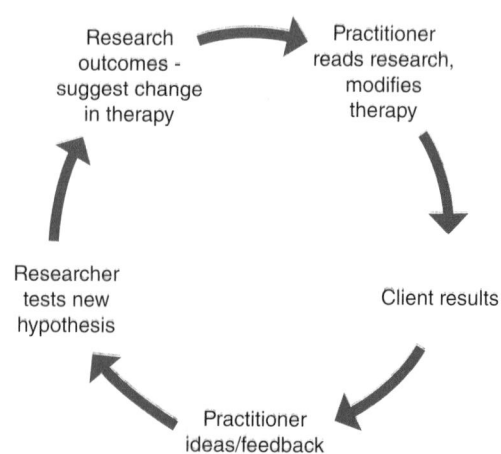

FIG. 5.2 The interrelationship between practitioners and clients/patients. Each group is involved as new knowledge is developed and old knowledge is tested and authenticated or invalidated.

of data needed. Data are analyzed mathematically, often using statistical analysis and findings are expressed in numbers.

Qualitative Research

Qualitative research is used to explore ideas and formulate theories or hypotheses. Qualitative methods are largely subjective and narrative based. Data are often collected by observations or interviews with open-ended questions to gather information about individual or collective experiences, or common themes. Data are analyzed by summarizing, interpreting, and categorizing commonalities to better understand concepts and their context and to gain insights on topics not well understood. Findings are expressed in words.

Although the scientific community prefers quantitative research (Emanuel et al., 2011; Sullivan, 1998), scholars are advocating for qualitative research as well as mixed methods because they provide insights into human behavior, including pain perception (Jack, 2006; Miller, 2010).

Literature Review

A **literature review** is a study, or survey, of existing scholarly work with the aim of discussing all published information about a specific topic or research question. It includes quantitative research, qualitative research, or both in the report. Literature reviews are also part of the research process mentioned later in this chapter.

Literature reviews are in great demand in most scientific fields because of the increasing output of scientific publications. Consumers of research find it both advantageous and necessary to rely on regular summaries of scientific literature rather than examine in detail every single new paper relevant to their interests. A literature review provides context, avoids duplicative research, and ensures professional standards are met.

> *It's time again. Tear up the violets and plant something more difficult to grow.*
>
> ~ **James Schuyler**

Types of Evidence

Evidence is information supporting an idea or conclusion (Higgs & Jones, 2000). Evidence is used to support or refute arguments and helps us to make professional decisions by knowing which methods are effective and what is not and how those methods should be applied to achieve documented results (e.g., length of session, frequency of sessions).

In the context of EIP, types of evidence are research, practitioner expertise, and client preferences. Once a good working knowledge of evidence is acquired, practitioners can apply these concepts in treatment planning by using PICO. PICO is a framework used to form a question about a specific client problem. Keywords contained in the question are used to search for relevant studies via the Internet or in databases. PICO stands for **P**atient/client or population;

Intervention; **C**omparison or control (not always used); and **O**utcome(s) of interest. For more information, see "Treatment Planning and Evidence-Informed Practice: PICO" in Chapter 10. But now, let's examine each type of evidence more closely.

Evaluating Evidence

Although all research evidence is valuable, some studies are given more "weight" when informing a treatment plan. Hence a ranking system is needed to evaluate their strength. The ranking system, called a **hierarchy of evidence**, is often denoted by a pyramid, with the strongest evidence near the peak and the weakest evidence near the wide base (Fig. 5.3). The system was first introduced by the Canadian Task Force to rank the effectiveness of healthcare interventions based on evidence quality (Canadian Task Force Report, 1979). In 1988 the United States created its own system based to some degree on the Canadian version (U.S. Preventive Services Task Force Edition, 1989).

Higher levels indicate stronger evidence and that bias was less likely to influence the results of the study. Lower levels indicate weaker evidence and that bias could have influenced the study's results. **Bias** is a researcher's preference for an outcome. In research, bias may occur when the investigator(s) select or encourage one outcome or answer over others. A researcher may unconsciously or consciously look only at data that support an opinion (called confirmation bias). Sponsor bias may occur if the researchers skewed data to support the interests of the organization funding the study. These are just two types of bias.

Most researchers use multiple methods to reduce bias, such as various people to code data, asking participants to review the results (member checks), asking peers to review the results (external audit), using more than one data source (triangulation), consciously suspending beliefs and judgments about the research topic (bracketing), withholding test information from participants (single-blinded) or from participants and data collectors (double-blinded), or randomly assigning groups (randomization).

A brief description of each level of the pyramid, starting at the top, is featured next.

Level 1

These are SRs and RCTs. A **systematic review** (SR) is a critical analysis of many studies. An example of an SR is Wilkinson et al. (2008), which found that massage had a short-term effect on pain reduction among cancer patients. Sometimes you will come across the term **meta-analysis**, which is a type of SR that uses statistics to determine the strength of the evidence. An example of a meta-analysis is Lee et al. (2015), which found massage had a beneficial effect for relief of cancer pain, especially for surgery-related pain, and foot reflexology appeared to be more effective than body massage or aroma massage.

A **randomized controlled trial** (RCT) is a study that randomly assigns participants to either a treatment group or

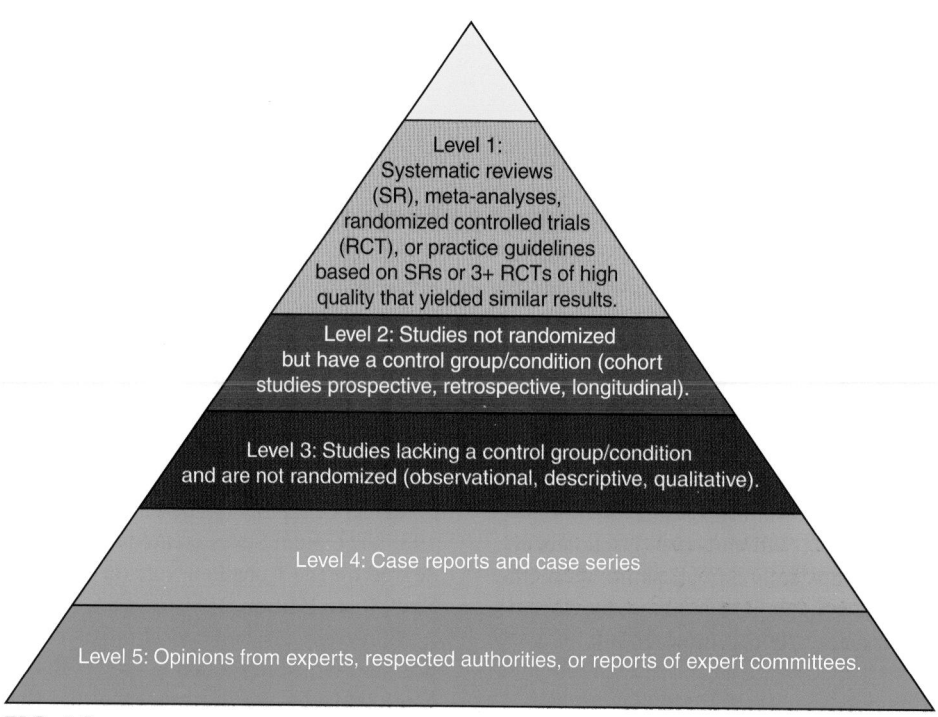

FIG. 5.3 Hierarchy of evidence. The strongest evidence is near the peak, and the weakest evidence near the wide base. Note the top is blank to indicate there is no perfect level of evidence.

a control group. The gold standard of research is random assignment into several groups. Many types of studies place participants into groups, not just RCTs.

- **Treatment (Experimental) Group**. Receives the intervention under investigation.
- **Control Group**. Does not receive the intervention under investigation or receives comparison or alternative treatment. The comparison treatment can be a sham treatment or an alternative treatment. A sham treatment, also called a placebo treatment, is a fake treatment. For example, participants may receive ultrasound from a machine that is unplugged. An alternative treatment is an intervention different from the one under investigation. For example, participants may receive local heat application. Alternative treatments are often used to compare results or costs of different interventions for the same condition (e.g., massage vs. warm foot bath for peripheral neuropathy).

An example of a single-blind randomized control trial is Momeni et al. (2020), in which massage on the legs and feet of intensive care unit patients administered daily for 6 days significantly reduced pain. The control group experienced more pain during the same timeframe. Level 1 also includes practice guidelines based on SRs of RCTs or three or more RCTs of high quality that yielded similar results.

Level 2

The second level contains cohort studies and includes longitudinal, retrospective, and prospective studies. **Longitudinal studies** look at the effect of a condition(s) over an extended period of time (e.g., low carb diets and weight loss).

Retrospective studies look back in time and examine exposures to suspected risk or protective factors in relation to an outcome (e.g., lung cancer). **Prospective studies** look at outcomes during the study period in relation to suspected risk or protective factors (e.g., vaccines). A **cohort** is a group of individuals who share a common characteristic such as birth, occupation, geographic area, or condition (e.g., they consumed tobacco products or received a certain vaccine). The comparison cohort does not share the characteristic studied, and the study looks for differences between groups. An example of a prospective cohort study is Hamre et al. (2007), who found patients with chronic disease who received massage over a 4-year time span experienced reduced chronic disease symptoms and improved quality of life. Level 2 is considered good evidence but not as strong as level 1 because the groups are not randomized.

Level 3

Level 3 studies lack a comparison group or condition and are not randomized. These include some observational, descriptive, and qualitative studies mentioned previously. **Observational studies** simply observe a phenomenon (e.g., how many people use massage). **Descriptive studies** describe the phenomenon or characteristics of a population (e.g., demographics, educational levels, socioeconomic factors). Surveys and questionnaires are to collect data for observational and descriptive studies. An example of a qualitative study is Garakyaraghi et al. (2014), which found that females who received a 10- to 15-minute Swedish massage 3 times a week for a total of 10 sessions reported they felt more relaxed, slept better, had less anxiety, tension, and fatigue, and felt more invigorated, less lonely, and more connected to their family and friends.

Level 4

Level 4 includes case reports and case series. A **case report** describes a single case, the intervention used, and the treatment outcome. A **case series** is a collection of case reports in which the same intervention was used or participants had the same condition. These represent **anecdotes**, or descriptions of personal experiences. Without controls and comparisons, we do not know to what extent the intervention contributed to the participants' outcomes, if at all.

Unlike the research process, which takes considerable planning and includes methods to reduce the influence of bias, anecdotal reports are based on hearsay. Hearsay is unsubstantiated, second-hand information and therefore is not considered as highly reliable evidence. Anecdotal accounts are common in nonscholarly professional journals. For instance, practitioners might write an article describing their experiences with a severely disabled client who achieved improved range of motion in his shoulder and neck while receiving massages, but as a contribution to science, anecdotes are seriously deficient. Without controls and comparisons, we do not know to what extent this practitioner contributed to the client's progress, if at all. Perhaps the client would have improved without the practitioner's efforts because of a newly installed home device that improved his quality of life or because of a drug prescribed by a physician without the practitioner's knowledge. However, case reports may suggest new areas of research. An example of a case report is Cunningham et al. (2011), who found massage applied to the extremities of a 45-year-old male diagnosed with chemotherapy-induced peripheral neuropathy greatly reduced his symptoms and improved his quality of life.

Level 5

Level 5 is the weakest level of evidence and includes expert opinions, the opinions of respected authorities, or reports of expert committees. **Expert opinions** are from people who have acquired vast amounts of information and offer experienced views on specified topics. Expert opinion is also a major source of ideas. On the downside, because experts draw heavily from their experiences, they may become biased about what works and what does not.

The Research Process

The research process is used to conduct investigations and pursue knowledge within a field. The terms *research process* and *scientific method* are often used interchangeably. In general, the process includes seven main steps which are (1) formulating a research question, (2) reviewing the literature, (3) selecting the best method to answer the research question, (4) conducting the experiment or investigation, (5) collecting the data, (6) analyzing the data, and (7) presenting the research results or findings (Fig. 5.4). Research is read and discussed in academic and professional communities,

which may lead to additional research—and the process repeats. The research process attempts to produce results that minimize bias and are reliable and valid.

- **Reliability**. Consistency of the study and indicates that, if the experiment or test was repeated by the same or different investigators, the results would be the same. For example, a reliable oral thermometer or weight scale would measure correctly each time it was used.
- **Validity**. The accuracy of the study and indicates that the experiment measured what it was supposed to measure. For example, if an experiment sought to measure knowledge of biology among freshman students and some students' primary language was Spanish, are we measuring their knowledge of biology or of English language? The experiment would need to control those variables for the experiment to be valid.

Ethics should be applied in all stages of research, including planning, conducting, and analyzing data. The researcher must consider all implications of how participation in a study might adversely affect, although unintentionally, its participants. This includes possible physical, mental, or even financial harm. Risks and benefits are disclosed to participants during the informed consent process (see Chapter 10). Specific rules or laws guiding research ethics did not exist until 1947, after World War II. Until this time, researchers were left to their own standards, with little or no consideration given to potential harm to participants. Now, rules and laws guide ethical standards when research involves humans. These include the Nuremburg Code, the Declaration of Helsinki, and the Belmont Report. Furthermore, researchers are required to complete courses offered by the Collaborative Institutional Training Initiative (CITI) and/or the NIH: Office of Extramural Research. In addition, Institutional Review Boards (IRBs) and research project advisory boards approve and oversee studies involving humans. More information on IRBs is found in the section titled "Describe the Methods and Conduct the Experiment."

Step 1: Formulate a Research Question

A research question is an answerable inquiry into a specific concern or issue and defines what the researcher wants to know. Choosing a research question is central to both quantitative and qualitative approaches. In quantitative approaches, the research question is usually followed by a hypothesis. A **hypothesis** is the presumed outcome of an experiment and what is expected to happen given a certain set of circumstances. Hypotheses are largely derived from the literature review, featured next. Furthermore, hypotheses define or describe relationships between variables in an attempt to answer the research question. The researcher may also include a *null hypothesis*, which states no statistically significant relationships exist between variables. Not all experiments include hypotheses and some have more than one. A **variable** is anything that can *vary* or change in an experiment and this change can be measured. Two main variables are independent and dependent.

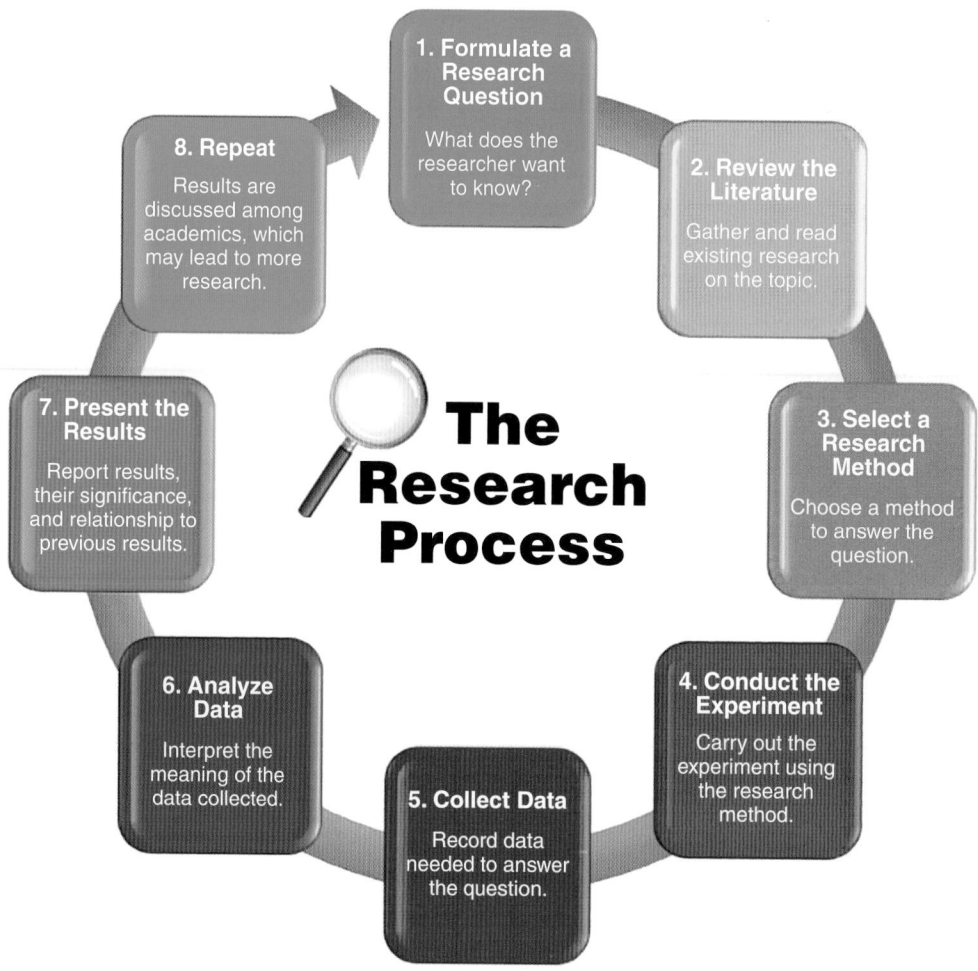

FIG. 5.4 The research process. This is used to conduct investigations and pursue knowledge within a field.

- **Independent Variable**. The focus of the experiment or intervention under investigation. It is the condition manipulated or controlled and is the presumed "cause" of the effect. The independent variable is stable, unaffected, and *independent* of other variables in the experiment. An example of an independent variable is massage.
- **Dependent Variable**. The condition expected to change because of the independent variable and is the presumed "effect." The dependent variable is *dependent* on other variables. Examples of dependent variables are heart rate, pain levels, and blood pressure.

Researchers are also being mindful of **extraneous variables** or variables not under investigation but may influence the outcome or relationship between dependent and independent variables. For example, the act of taking blood pressure may promote anxiety, causing their blood pressure to increase; or the act of lying on a massage table may promote relaxation, causing their blood pressure to decrease. In these two examples, the action caused the effect instead of the independent variable under investigation.

Confounding variables are extraneous variables related to the independent variable but may affect the dependent variable. For example, a study was conducted to determine whether massage (independent variable or "cause") reduces stress in self-report (dependent variable or effect) among emergency room personnel. The actual massage received (varying pressures and speed) and the years of experience of the practitioner are confounding variables because they could influence the results. A good research design controls the influence of confounding variables and ensures all participants received the same type and amount of massage from the same practitioner or from practitioners with similar backgrounds and expertise.

The researcher must also define terms and concepts used in the experiment. **Conceptual definitions** clarify what is measured and the population or condition/pathology under investigation. For example, a study among individuals with cancer must define massage (e.g., manipulation of soft tissues using compression and traction), the population studied (e.g., females), and type of cancer the population has (e.g., stage III breast cancer). **Operational definitions** describe how dependent variables were measured. For example, if blood pressure is a dependent variable, the study must describe how blood pressure was measured, including what instrument was used and where on the participant's body measurements were taken. Defining terms and concepts ensures clarity to anyone reading the study and allows future researchers to replicate the experiment.

Step 2: Review the Literature

As stated previously, *literature reviews* represent existing scholarly works with the aim of discussing all published information about a specific topic or research question. These are often found in professional literature and academic journals. Once researchers have formulated a question, they must become familiar with all existing knowledge on the topic by searching for and reading existing research literature. The literature is summarized, synthesized, and organized chronologically or into subcategories. A literature review might include tracing the intellectual progression within a field of study, placing previous work in context of how it has contributed to our current understanding of the research topic, identifying areas of prior research to prevent duplication of effort, revealing gaps existing in the literature, and validating the need for additional research.

Step 3: Select a Research Method

Next, the researchers must choose one or more methods to answer the research question. During the literature review process, methods used in previous studies are noted and often inform the current study. The researchers may choose to use questionnaires, surveys, polls, interviews, observations, archival records, or other instruments. Methods include details about the participant selection, if a control group was used, and if group selection was randomized.

Participants in the study must meet certain criteria; the methods section states the criteria used in the selection process. **Inclusion criteria** are characteristics participants must possess to be included in the experiment (e.g., age, gender, health status, or demographics). **Exclusion criteria** are characteristics disqualifying participants. Once participants have been selected, consent must be obtained. Informed consent indicates the person agrees to participate in the experiment and are thoroughly informed what involvement might entail, the potential risks and benefits of participation, what they will have to do during the study, how some information will be safeguarded and other information will be used, and they can withdraw participation from the study at any time. Informed consent is discussed more fully in Chapter 10. The final group of participants is called a **sample**, a subset of the population that is used to represent the entire population. Research makes inferences about the population studied from the sample from which it was drawn.

The methods section also discusses anticipated problems and steps researchers plan to take to prevent them from occurring. **Delimitations** are things the researchers can control (e.g., research question, choice of variables, population). **Limitations** are things the researchers cannot control (e.g., participant compliance, dropout rate).

The methods section includes where the investigation took place and how data will be collected and analyzed. This information allows readers to critically evaluate a study's overall validity and reliability. Methods are also called *protocols* or *procedures.*

After the methods are determined and before participant recruitment begins, the study must be approved by a committee such as an IRB. This process protects participants from undue harm caused by involvement in the study, monitors the study throughout data collection, investigates incidents occurring during the study, and evaluates the final report.

Step 4: Conduct the Experiment

Next, the researchers conduct the experiment using the selected method. If problems arise, the researcher describes ways in which they were minimized or why these problems did not have a meaningful impact on the data.

Step 5: Collect Data

Data are needed to answer the research question and are collected using the methods the researchers selected (i.e., questionnaires, surveys, polls, interviews). During this process, researchers assume the information disclosed by participants is true (e.g., self-reports of age and experiences of pain or stress reduction).

Step 6: Analyze the Data

Once data are collected, it is analyzed and aligned with the research question. Next the researchers begin to draw conclusions. There are several ways to analyze data; each perspective reveals something different. Data analysis of quantitative studies determines if the research hypotheses were supported or rejected. A supported hypothesis means results of data analysis were statistically significant. **Statistical significance** means there was a relationship between variables—something other than chance. A rejected hypothesis means results were statistically insignificant. **Statistical insignificance** means there was no relationship between variables or small differences can be accounted for by chance.

Keep in mind a rejected hypothesis is not a failed study. Researchers can learn as much from statistically insignificant results. For example, if a study shows no effect of massage on weight loss, practitioners can share this information with clients.

Next, it is important to determine whether results were *clinically significant.* **Clinical significance** is the practical importance of statistical significance to professional practice. An intervention could be "statistically" significant, but unless it is also "clinically" significant, it may not warrant a change in treatment protocols. For example, if instrument-assisted soft tissue mobilization (IASTM) increased shoulder range of motion by 3 degrees, how likely would practitioners use it? This 3-degree change could be statistically significant but would the increase improve your client's quality of life? If not, the study results would be statistically significant but *clinically insignificant.* This may be important, especially if the protocol is costly, is time consuming, had negative side effects, or led to adverse events. Any evidence-informed protocol change must be worth time and money and reduce negative effects on clients.

Step 7: Present the Results

Results are the study's outcome. Research results are also called *findings*. Results apply only to what was found after data analysis. For example, if a study found massage increased range of motion in the neck of healthy adults, the results could not state massage had the same effect in the shoulder or in children. When presenting the results, researchers reflect on its significance and its relationship to previous research. The investigator should suggest future research, which may include replicating the study with a different population or in a different area of the body. Research is an endless process, and research does not "prove" anything. Research is an effort to get as close to the "truth" as possible.

Presenting research is accomplished in several ways. The researcher(s) can write an article and submit for publication to a scholarly journal, which includes peer review. Peer review is evaluation of scientific, academic, or professional work by a group of experts in the same or similar field. The group decides collectively if the investigation was scientifically sound and contributes to the body of knowledge within a field. Peer review is a widely accepted indicator of quality scholarship; it is a red flag if a study is not published in a peer-reviewed journal. The **abstract** is at the beginning of a published paper and provides a brief overview of the entire study (typically 250 to 300 words). Most research papers have four main sections and follow the "IMRaD" format. IMRaD stands **I**ntroduction, **M**ethod, **R**esults, **a**nd **D**iscussion. Here is a brief summary.

- **Introduction**. Explains why this study is necessary or important. It begins by describing the problem that motivated the study and the current research in the field, revealing a gap of knowledge. Then it explains how the present study is a solution to the problem or the gap. If the study has hypotheses, this is stated at the end of the introduction.
- **Method**. This section states how the study was conducted and includes information about the participants, methods, and any instruments used to gather data.
- **Results**. The study findings are presented in this section and often include tables, figures, or graphs. Typically, this section contains only the findings and not any discussion or explanation of the findings.
- **Discussion**. In this section the researchers summarize the findings, connect them to other studies, and discuss their implications. Also found in this section are limitations of the study. This section makes use of these limitations as reasons to suggest future research studies.

Once published, each article becomes a permanent record of the field's body of knowledge and will be read and discussed in academic and professional communities. The investigation can also be presented in person at a professional conference. This may lead to additional investigations to learn more about specific topics.

PRACTITIONER EXPERTISE

A practitioner's professional **expertise** is a combination of formal education, knowledge accumulation, previous treatment decisions, and past outcomes. Development of expertise occurs when theoretical and practical knowledge are "tested" and "refined" in actual professional situations, which leads to improved judgment and quality of client care. Expertise also includes client assessments, information garnered from colleagues and client caregivers, presentations at professional development events, scientific theories, and nonresearch publications such as websites and blogs (Grainger, 2013). Sackett et al. (1996) stressed the importance of expertise, stating "external evidence can inform, but never replace, clinical expertise and it is this expertise that decides whether the external evidence applies to the individual patient at all and if so, how it should be integrated into a clinical decision; individual clinical expertise is needed to decide how the external evidence matches the patient's clinical state, predicament and preferences and whether it should be applied" (p. 72).

EIP skills develop over time through a sound education foundation and plethora of experiences. Benner (1982) wrote extensively about the acquisition of professional expertise in nursing and proposed five stages with accompanying capacities beginning at the novice stage and proceeding to the expert stage called the *novice to expert theory*. This model can be applied to the development of professional expertise. Benner stated the development of understanding in the applied health sciences is composed of practical knowledge and practitioner expertise (or the "know how"), research, and the client's reasons for seeking help and their preferences (or the "know why"). Benner's stages of professional expertise are listed next.

Stage 1: Novice

Novices, or beginners, are new students who have no experience in situations they are expected to perform. Novices usually lack confidence, and their professional behaviors are rule governed and relatively inflexible. Novices often require continual verbal and physical cues, are unable to use discretionary judgment, and have limited ability to predict what might happen in particular situations.

Stage 2: Advanced Beginner

Advanced beginners are newly employed graduates and demonstrate marginally acceptable performances because they have prior experiences in actual situations. Advanced beginners require occasional supportive cues. Knowledge is still developing; principles rather than rules begin to govern their actions.

Stage 3: Competent

Competence is demonstrated by practitioners who have been on the job in the same or similar situations for 2 or 3 years. They are confident and demonstrate conscious and deliberate planning, which helps them achieve efficiency. They complete tasks within a suitable time frame without supporting cues.

Stage 4: Proficient

Proficient practitioners perceive situations as wholes rather than chopped-up parts. Because of this perspective, they can better predict what might happen in given situations and what needs to change to alter outcomes. This holistic understanding improves decision-making.

Stage 5: Expert

Experts have an intuitive grasp of each situation, and they operate from a deep understanding. Their performance is fluid, flexible, and highly proficient without wasteful consideration of unfruitful alternative solutions. When experts encounter a situation for which they have no experience, they use analytic tools and external resources to attain goals.

CLIENT PREFERENCES

Client preferences are a collection of goals, expectations, predispositions, social and cultural values, and religious or spiritual beliefs creating partiality for certain decisions and their outcomes. Client preferences may include family involvement in decision-making; values surrounding quality-of-life issues; personal priorities; and personal beliefs about health, responsibility, and accountability. The beneficiary of EIP is the client; practitioners must construct a plan of care that benefits and is in the client's best interest as the client defines it (Guyatt et al., 2015). Inclusion of client preferences in EIP affects client adherence and compliance, client satisfaction, and treatment outcomes.

To elicit client preferences, use effective communication skills. Understanding the situations from the client's point of view and sociocultural perspective are important aspects of client engagement during the treatment planning process (Grainger, 2013). Professional communications should be

TIFFANY FIELD

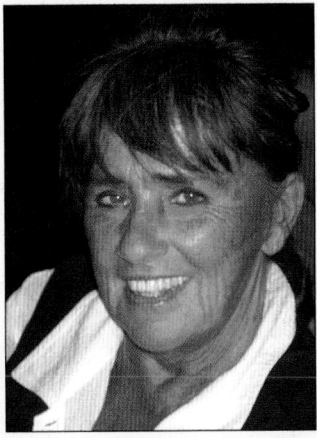

If you have ever used PubMed to find peer-reviewed research on massage, you will see a handful of names popping up over and over again. FIELD T is one of those names. Massage for rheumatoid arthritis: FIELD T. Yoga and massage for prenatal depression: FIELD T. Massage for preterm infants: FIELD T. Who is this Field person, and how did she come to be so involved in massage research?

Tiffany Field is not a massage practitioner, but she is passionate about massage. Inspired by the positive results when she massaged her own premature daughter, Field, a psychiatry professor, began formally researching the physiologic effects of touch. At the time (the early 1980s), there was virtually no research in this area. In 1992, she founded the Touch Research Institute at the University of Miami, School of Medicine. The Touch Research Institute is still the only center of its kind, devoted completely to the study of touch as it relates to science and medicine.

Field's research credits are too numerous to list but include many studies focused on infants and children. Her team's research found premature infants gained weight faster when they were massaged. Weight gain = shorter hospital stays = money saved. When hospitals discovered they could stand to save millions of dollars, they started to take serious notice of Field's work.

Field encourages massage practitioners to combine the practice of massage with further education. If massage research is going to truly take off, there need to be more massage practitioners who go on to earn advanced degrees. On the other hand, academics who want to research massage would do well to learn the hands-on side of things as well. In one of Field's studies on preterm infants, they found moderate pressure was more effective than the very light pressure others used in their studies. Why the move to try more pressure? The infants seemed to like it more. Sometimes there's no substitute for firsthand experience.

Tiffany Field is still enthusiastically engaged in touch research, collaborating with others and making surprising findings. Her published studies on massage for females with breast cancer showed improved immune response after massage, even though cancer used to be seen as a contraindication.

Massage research is a fascinating area of study. Whether your participation in massage research involves writing case reports as part of your massage practice, going on to earn a doctorate degree and become a researcher, or just looking up scholarly articles, we owe a great deal to those pioneers who got the ball rolling, and Tiffany Field is a pioneer.

free of unnecessary intellectual judgments and comparisons. Most importantly, the practitioner must be an empathetic and active listener. Active listening and nonjudgmental statements demonstrate empathy skills (Fowler & Tong, 2013). The client's circumstances and experiences are unique. A huge step in professional growth occurs when practitioners understand a client's rationale is not necessary and clients have the right to make treatment decisions. More information about client communication is in Chapter 10.

E-RESOURCES

http://evolve.elsevier.com/Salvo/MassageTherapy

- Chapter challenge
- Flash cards

REFERENCES

Benner, P. (1982). From novice to expert. *The American Journal of Nursing*, 82(3), 402–407.

Bertulis, R. (2008). Barriers to accessing evidence-based information. *Nursing Standard*, 22(36), 35–39.

Brody, J. L., Dalen, J., Annett, R. D., Scherer, D. G., & Turner, C. W. (2012). Conceptualizing the role of research literacy in advancing societal health. *Journal of Health Psychology*, 17(5), 724–730.

Canadian Task Force Report. (1979). *The periodic health examination*. Retrieved from https://www.ncbi.nlm.nih.gov/pmc/articles/PMC1704686/pdf/canmedaj01457-0037.pdf.

Creswell, J. W. (2013). *Educational research: Planning, conducting, and evaluating quantitative and qualitative research* (4th ed.). Upper Saddle River, NJ: Pearson.

Cunningham, J. E., Kelechi, T., Sterba, K., Barthelemy, N., Falkowksi, P., & Chin, S. H. (2011). Case report of a patient with chemotherapy-induced peripheral neuropathy treated with manual therapy (massage). *Supportive Care in Cancer*, 19(9), 1473–1476.

Emanuel, V., Day, K., Diegnan, L., & Pryce-Miller, M. (2011). Developing evidence-based practice among students. *Nursing Times*, 107(49/50), 21–23.

Evans, R., Delagran, L., Maiers, M., Kreitzer, M. J., & Sierpina, V. (2011). Advancing evidence informed practice through faculty development: The northwestern health sciences university model. *Explore (New York, N.Y.)*, 7(4), 265–268.

Field, T. (2002). Massage therapy. *The Medical Clinics of North America*, 86(1), 163–171.

Field, T. M., Schanberg, S. M., Scafidi, F., Bauer, C. R., Vega-Lahr, N., Garcia, R., Nystrom, J., & Kuhn, C. M. (1986). Tactile/kinesthetic stimulation effects on preform neonates. *Pediatrics*, 77, 654–658.

Fineout-Overholt, E., Melnyk, B. M., & Schultz, A. (2005). Transforming healthcare from the inside out: Advancing evidence-based practice in the 21st century. *Journal of Professional Nursing*, 21(6), 335–344.

Fowler, M. E., & Tong, V. (2013). *Religious cultural competency and improved patient care: Trends and best practices*. Retrieved

from http://www.hpoe.org/resources/hpoe-live-webinars/1365.

Garakyaraghi, M., Givi, M., Moeini, M., & Eshghinezhad, A. (2014). Qualitative study of women's experience after therapeutic massage. *Iranian Journal of Nursing and Midwifery Research*, 19(4), 390–395.

Grainger, P. (2013). *Evidence-informed practice: The basics for ensuring best practice [Video File]*. Retrieved from https://www.youtube.com/watch?v=gopBtDKDlRw.

Guyatt, G., Jaeschke, R., Wilson, M. C., Montori, V. M., & Richardson, W. S. (2015). What is evidence-based medicine? In G. Guyatt, D. Rennie, M. O. Meade, & D. J. Cook (Eds.), *Users' guides to the medical literature: A manual for evidence-based clinical practice* (3rd ed., pp. 7–14). New York, NY: McGraw Hill Education.

Hamre, H. J., Witt, C. M., Glockmann, A., Ziegler, R., Willich, S. N., & Kiene, H. (2007). Rhythmical massage therapy in chronic disease: A 4-year prospective cohort study. *Journal of Alternative and Complementary Medicine*, 13(6), 635–642.

Higgs, J., & Jones, M. (2000). Will evidence-based practice take the reasoning out of practice? In J. Higgs & M. Jones (Eds.), *Clinical reasoning in the health professions* (2nd ed., pp. 307–315). Oxford, UK: Butterworth Heineman.

Jack, S. M. (2006). Utility of qualitative research findings in evidence-based public health practice. *Public Health Nursing*, 23(3), 277–283.

Lee, S. H., Kim, J. Y., Yeo, S., Kim, S. H., & Lim, S. (2015). Meta-analysis of massage therapy on cancer pain. *Integrative Cancer Therapies*, 14(4), 297–304.

Miller, W. R. (2010). Qualitative research findings as evidence: Utility in nursing practice. *Clinical Nurse Specialist CNS*, 24(4), 191–203.

Momeni, M., Arab, M., Dehghan, M., & Ahmadinejad, M. (2020). The effect of foot massage on pain of the intensive care patients: A parallel randomized single-blind controlled trial. *Evidence-Based Complementary and Alternative Medicine: eCAM*, 13:3450853.

National Institutes of Health (NIH). (2018). *Complementary, alternative, or integrative health: What's in a name?* Retrieved from https://www.nccih.nih.gov/health/complementary-alternative-or-integrative-health-whats-in-a-name.

National Institutes of Health (NIH). (2019). *National center for complementary and integrative health: Mission*. Retrieved from https://www.nih.gov/about-nih/what-we-do/nih-almanac/national-center-complementary-integrative-health-nccih.

Sackett, D. L., Rosenberg, W. M., Gray, J. A., Haynes, R. B., & Richardson, W. S. (1996). Evidence-based medicine: What it is and what it isn't. *BMJ (Clinical Research Ed.)*, 312(7023), 71–72.

Spitz, R. A. (1965). *The first year of life. A psychoanalytic study of normal and deviant development of object relations*. New York, NY: International Universities Press.

Sullivan, P. (1998). Developing evidence-based care in mental health nursing. *Nursing Standard*, 12(31), 35–38.

Titler, M. G. (2008). The evidence for evidence-based practice implementation. In R. G. Hughes (Ed.), *Patient safety and quality: An evidence-based handbook for nurses* (Vol. 1, Chapter 7). Rockville, MD: Agency for Healthcare Research and Quality.

Touch Research Institute. (n.d.). *History of the Touch Research Institute*. Retrieved from http://pediatrics.med.miami.edu/touch-research/about-us.

U.S. Preventive Services Task Force Edition. (1989). *Guide to clinical preventive services*. Retrieved from https://catalog.hathitrust.org/Record/001530036.

Webster, P. (2002). Evidence based practice—what is it and how can it be encouraged in orthopaedic nursing? *Journal of Orthopedic Nursing*, 6(3), 140–143.

Wilkinson, S., Barnes, K., & Storey, L. (2008). Massage for symptom relief in patients with cancer: Systematic review. *Journal of Advanced Nursing*, 63(5), 430–439.

REVIEW AND APPLY YOUR KNOWLEDGE

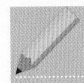

MATCHING ONE: CONCEPT REVIEW

Place the letter of the answer next to the number of the term or phrase that best describes it.

A. Evidence-informed practice
B. Control group
C. Evidence
D. Barriers to evidence-informed practice
E. Extraneous
F. Hierarchy of evidence
G. Delimitations
H. Sham
I. Quantitative
J. Randomized controlled trial
K. Qualitative
L. Variable

_____ 1. System used to rank the strength of various types of research studies.
_____ 2. Information supporting an idea or conclusion.
_____ 3. Type of research that is exploratory, more subjective, and narrative based.
_____ 4. Lack of information literacy skills and lack of research skills.
_____ 5. The gold standard of research.
_____ 6. Anything that can change in an experiment and this change can be measured.
_____ 7. Group that does not receive the intervention under investigation or receives a comparison treatment.
_____ 8. Fake treatment or placebo.
_____ 9. Problem-solving approach that integrates relevant evidence, client's preferences and values, and the practitioner's professional expertise to achieve desired patient/client goals.
_____ 10. Boundaries the research sets that are under their control.
_____ 11. Variable not under investigation but can influence the outcome.
_____ 12. Type of research emphasizing objective measurements and statistic, mathematic, or numeric data analysis.

MATCHING TWO: CONCEPT REVIEW

Place the letter of the answer next to the number of the term or phrase that best describes it.

A. Sample
B. Bias
C. Case report
D. Findings
E. Hypothesis
F. Independent variable
G. Methods
H. Reliability
I. Research
J. Research literacy
K. Systematic review
L. Treatment group

_____ 1. Ability of an experiment to yield the same results if repeated by the same or different investigator.
_____ 2. A subset of the population in a research study that represents the entire population.
_____ 3. Systematic inquiry using prescribed methods to validate or refine existing knowledge or to develop new knowledge.
_____ 4. Critical analysis of many studies.
_____ 5. Group that receives the intervention under investigation.
_____ 6. Results or outcome of an investigation.
_____ 7. Presumed outcome of an experiment.
_____ 8. Cognitive and social understanding of the purpose, process, and value of research and includes the ability to locate, read, understand, and evaluate research literature.
_____ 9. The focus of the experiment or intervention under investigation.
_____ 10. Preference for an outcome.
_____ 11. The protocols or procedures used in an experiment.
_____ 12. A single case describing a participant's health history, the intervention used, and the treatment outcome.

MULTIPLE CHOICE: TEST YOUR KNOWLEDGE

Place the letter of the answer next to the number of the term or phrase that best describes it.

_____ 1. Basing treatment decisions on what has been shown to be effective is the essence of:
A. evidence-informed practice.
B. hierarchy of evidence.
C. research literacy.
D. literature reviews.

_____ 2. Which approach to research is based on studying existing scholarly works with the aim of discussing all published information about a specific topic or research question?
A. Quantitative research
B. Qualitative research
C. Systematic review
D. Literature review

_____ 3. In what level in the hierarchy of evidence are randomized controlled trials?
A. Level 1
B. Level 2
C. Level 3
D. Level 4

_____ 4. What is a description of a personal experience?
A. Case report
B. Case series
C. Anecdote
D. Bias

_____ 5. Another name for the research process is the:
A. scientific method.
B. systematic review.
C. delimitations.
D. limitations.

_____ 6. Which factor of a study indicates its accuracy and indicates the experiment measured what it was supposed to measure?
A. Validity
B. Reliability
C. Variable
D. Hypothesis

_____ 7. Which is the variable that is expected to change and is the presume effect of an experiment?
A. Independent
B. Dependent
C. Extraneous
D. Confounding

_____ 8. Which describes how the dependent variable is measured?
A. Inclusion criteria
B. Exclusion criteria
C. Conceptual definitions
D. Operational definitions

_____ 9. Potential weaknesses or problems in an experiment that are beyond the researcher's control (e.g., participant compliance, dropout rate) are called:
A. limitations.
B. delimitations.
C. confounding variables.
D. extraneous variables.

_____ 10. The practical importance of results or findings of a study to professional practice is called:
A. statistical significance.
B. statistical insignificance.
C. clinical significance.
D. clinical insignificance.

_____ 11. The part of a research paper that presents the findings and often includes tables, figures, or graphs is the:
A. abstract.
B. introduction.
C. results.
D. discussion.

_____ 12. In which stage of Benner's "novice to expert theory" are professional behaviors relatively inflexible and rule governed?
A. Novice
B. Competent
C. Proficient
D. Expert

CRITICAL THINKING

What's Your Barrier?

Think about the 10 barriers to evidence-informed practice listed in the section "Barriers to EIP." What barriers do you have regarding research literacy? What are three steps you can take to overcome these barriers so you can enrich your massage practice?

Answers to this question can cover but are not limited to:

Taking a course on research literacy; contacting a mentor to help strengthen research literacy; looking through paper journals and online sites to become familiar with research; setting aside time to develop research literacy skills; discussing research with peers, covering topics such as relevant research topics and what determines whether information is quality or not; participating in the Massage Therapy Foundation's Student or Professional Case Report contest; attending research symposiums; attending conventions in which research is presented; contacting people who have conducted research for answers to questions about research; presenting research information to employers and discussing how it directly benefits clients.

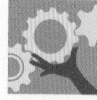

PROFESSIONAL PRACTICE

Form and Function

Dr. Theresa wanted to integrate less-invasive, nonpharmaceutical treatments for her patients with chronic pain. She contacted Sally, a massage practitioner, and Harold, an acupuncturist, and asked them to give her one research study explaining the benefit of their approach to lower back pain.

Sally submitted a peer-reviewed study titled "Reduction of anterior pelvic tilt using massage reduces low back pain." The study included five participants with lower back pain and no history of disk pathology, nerve pathology, broken bones, or pathology known to contribute to chronic pain. Each participant presented with hyperlordosis, noted specifically by an increased anterior pelvic tilt of 5 to 10 degrees. Each participant was treated by the same practitioner, using the same techniques. Participants were instructed to not use pharmaceuticals within 4 hours of each treatment and to note the use of pharmaceuticals during the duration of the study. They were also instructed not to receive other treatments for the condition. Each participant received five 40-minute treatments over the course of 1 month. Four of five participants had significant pain relief. One participant had moderate relief after the first two treatments but no significant improvement subsequently. The study concluded massage reduces lower back pain resulting from anterior pelvic tilt. It was funded by Healing Hands, Inc., a privately owned chain of massage studios, and conducted at one of their facilities.

Harold submitted a peer-reviewed study titled "Acupuncture significantly reduces lower back pain." The study was conducted over 24 months and included 121 participants. Nineteen of the original participants dropped out because their healthcare provider disapproved. Participants were evaluated for potential causes of lower back pain and were accepted if it was from one of three categories: herniated disk, lumbar sprain, or strength imbalance between the hip flexors and lumbar extensors. Acupuncture treatments differed depending on the cause of pain and followed the traditional model of Chinese medicine used for each condition. Each participant was consistently treated by 1 of 10 acupuncturists who received training from different institutions. Sixty percent of participants reported complete relief of symptoms; 20% reported moderate relief; 10% reported moderate relief but experienced new pain in a different area of the body; and 10% had no significant changes. The study was conducted at a respected university and funded by the National Institutes of Health.

What are the pros and cons of each study design? Are there elements in either affecting the reliability of outcomes? Are the study designs too narrow or too broad? Explain. Describe how you would improve each study. If you were to submit either of these studies for your client's consideration, would you explain the shortcomings even if you believe the outcome is reliable?

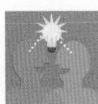

DISCUSSION

Massage Research

Locate a research study on massage published in a scientific journal. After reading the article, answer the following questions: (1) What did you learn from the study? (2) How will you apply what you have learned in your massage practice? If available, post your reflections on an Internet-based discussion board monitored by your instructor and include a link to the study (if possible).

I thank JoEllen Sefton for her past contributions on this chapter.

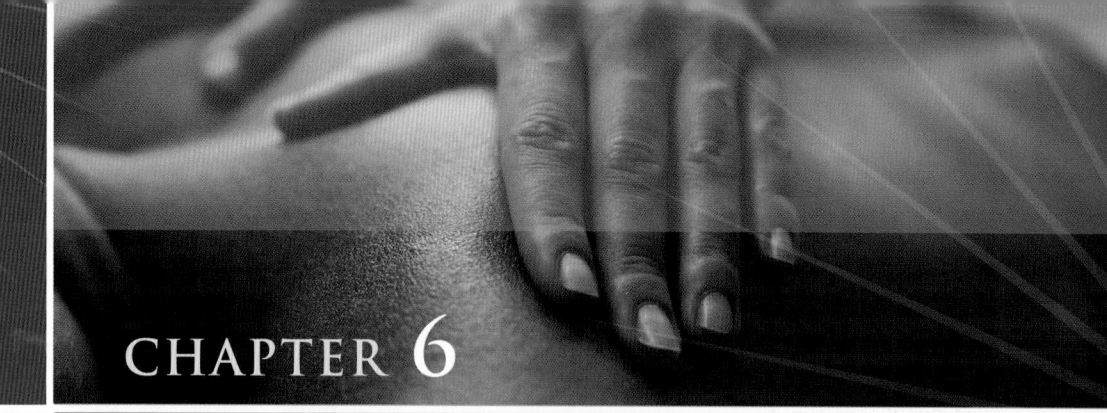

CHAPTER 6

Massage Therapy Research

JoEllen M. Sefton

LEARNING OBJECTIVES

After completing this chapter, the student should be able to:

1. State the value of a research agenda for the massage profession, general areas covered by the Massage Therapy Foundation (MTF) research agenda, and why this agenda is important for massage schools, instructors, students, practitioners, and their clients.
2. Explain the effects of massage on the musculoskeletal, cardiovascular, and lymphatic systems, and immunity.
3. Describe the effects of massage on connective tissues, skin, nervous and endocrine systems, other body systems, and internal organs, as well as its neuropsychological and whole-body effects.
4. Discuss the effects of massage for specific conditions/outcomes and state the value of massage education research.

http://evolve.elsevier.com/Salvo/MassageTherapy

INTRODUCTION

Massage and bodywork have evolved over thousands of years, from simple laying on of hands to the current evidence-informed practice. Throughout the years, massage has been shown to produce beneficial effects for clients. These effects can be specific, such as reduction of lower back pain, or general effects such as an overall feeling of wellbeing and improved quality of life. The continuing challenge for the profession is to improve our understanding of how massage produces its outcomes and how to use these to benefit our clients. We can meet our goal of providing the best client care possible through strong, evidence-informed practice.

If you are asked "How does massage work?" what would you say? Where would you even begin to answer this important question? If you love massage, you might immediately think about the relaxation massage can produce and answer with a description of the importance of self-care, wellness, and stress reduction. If you work with athletes, you might answer about how massage increases performance and postexercise recovery. If you work in a hospital, you might discuss how massage reduces anxiety associated with cancer treatments or those in hospice care. Massage is an expansive profession encompassing a variety of techniques and methods. This diversity makes answering the question challenging. We might answer the question successfully if we were to break this question down into particular outcomes or influence on specific body systems. Answering the question using a framework of body systems may help, but keep in mind everything is interrelated and the body is wonderfully complex; changes in one body system influence all others.

It is important to separate fact from myth. Much of what was once thought or known about the benefits and mechanisms of massage has been brought into question. Research is necessary to improve our understanding and is a constant process of discovery—we investigate, learn new things, replace old ideas, and investigate more. It is also important to keep in mind the placebo effect is an important component in healthcare. As discussed in Chapter 5, it is vital that massage practitioners stay current on new knowledge, use this knowledge during treatment planning, and share this knowledge with clients and colleagues. As we learn more about how massage works, we may change the techniques we use and how we use them to improve client outcomes.

Healthcare providers are including massage as part of an overall approach to address health concerns. More than 60% of clients seek out massage for improving health and wellness, while approximately 30% receive massage for pain management or relief. Fifty percent of clients who discussed massage with their physicians received a massage recommendation (American Massage Therapy Association [AMTA], 2021). Massage is one of the complementary therapies with the highest physician referral rates. Massage is also rated among physicians as the complementary therapy most likely to be beneficial (65% among rheumatologist and 39% of pediatricians) and least likely to be harmful (Ernst, 1999; Stussman et al., 2020). This positive outcome is the result of research elevating the overall standing of the massage profession in the healthcare, wellness, medical, and rehabilitation communities.

The good news is that a large amount of new research has been completed since the last edition of this book. In just 5 months, from January 2021 to June 1, 2021, 91 articles have been published in the research literature on massage. This constant update of our knowledge makes it vital that you become a good consumer of research (see Chapter 5). The goal of this chapter is to provide massage students and practitioners with a summary of some of what is currently known about the effects of massage on body systems, including the musculoskeletal, cardiovascular, lymphatic and immunity, connective tissues, integumentary or skin, nervous, and endocrine systems. It will look at psychological and whole-body effects. It will also discuss the massage research agenda and why research on massage education is important. This chapter is not intended to be an in-depth assessment of the actual research but rather a survey of what we know, what we do not know, and where our knowledge base currently stands. Hopefully this will lead you to a further and continued investigation of new research in these areas.

Keep in mind there are frequently conflicting results in research studies, which may be frustrating. However, this is common as research teams seek answers to difficult problems. Newer studies will correct or contradict previous studies as we continue to develop new knowledge. This is one reason you must stay up to date, read research studies, and keep an open mind as our knowledge base evolves.

This chapter primarily discusses research exploring how massage influences the body. There are also other areas of massage inquiry. Ongoing research is exploring how to best teach massage students (pedagogy and andragogy). Massage educational materials are based on curricula and materials from healthcare professions (e.g., nursing). This work looks at how to best train massage practitioners, organize massage curricula, and develop programs of continuing competence and education for the massage profession. Research is also exploring how to integrate massage into the Western healthcare system, how to improve awareness and acceptance of massage by healthcare providers, and best practices for providing massage access in different populations. This chapter will touch on some of this work, but space does not allow a full exploration of these topics. If you are excited about these research areas, it is an opportunity to learn more by using your research skills to explore them on your own.

THE MASSAGE RESEARCH AGENDA

A research agenda is an organizational statement identifying specific research priorities. The agenda will often include plans to address specific questions or fill specific needs. The research agenda helps individuals and organizations make decisions on research activities following a clear and well thought out framework. Research agendas are updated on a regular basis (e.g., annually, every 5 or 10 years) as the knowledge base grows and new directions and questions are identified.

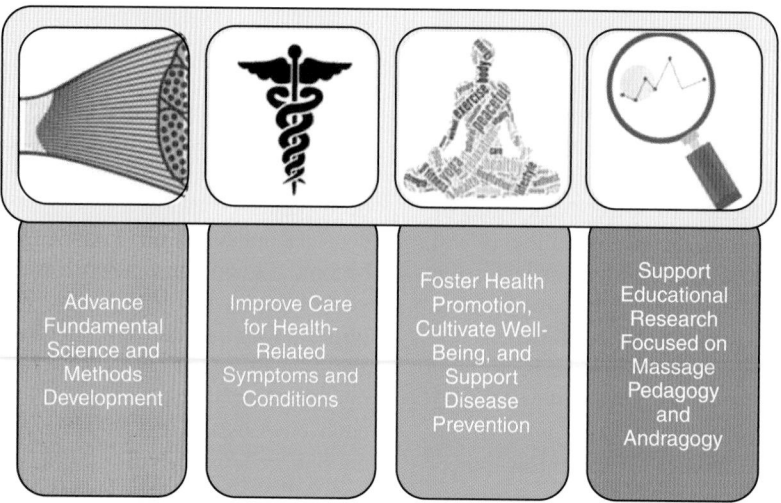

FIG. 6.1 Summary of the Massage Therapy Foundation's research agenda. (Modified from Summary of the MTF 2020 Massage Therapy Research Agenda. Sefton, J. M., Dexheimer, J., Munk, N., Miccio, R., Kennedy, A. B., Cambron, J., et al. [2020, December]. A Research Agenda for the Massage Therapy Profession: a Report from the Massage Therapy Foundation. *International Journal of Therapeutic Massage & Bodywork, 13*(4), 42–46. https://www.ncbi.nlm.nih.gov/pmc/articles/ PMC7704039.)

The massage research agenda was recently updated by the Massage Therapy Foundation (Sefton et al., 2020). The agenda identifies four research areas and specific goals within each area (Fig. 6.1).

1. Advance fundamental science and methods development.
2. Improve care for health-related symptoms and conditions.
3. Foster health promotion, cultivate wellbeing, and support disease prevention.
4. Support establishment of educational research focused on massage pedagogy and andragogy.

The research agenda includes specific ways organizations, researchers, practitioners, students, clients, and educators can become involved in helping to move the agenda forward. As you read through the research agenda (https://www.ncbi.nlm.nih.gov/pmc/articles/PMC7704039), you should be able to see how the topics in this chapter relate to the goals of the research agenda and ways you can help move the agenda forward.

MASSAGE EFFECTS ON THE MUSCULOSKELETAL SYSTEM

It makes sense to start with what is known about how massage influences muscles and nerves of the body. Massage students will likely think massage has significant effects on the musculoskeletal system because most massage is prescribed or sought out for muscular aches and pains. However, much of what we know about massage and muscles has been passed down with little supporting evidence. That does not mean massage is not beneficial to muscle function. It simply means the research will validate some theories and invalidate others. The skeletal system is discussed in Chapter 19, and the muscular system is discussed in Chapter 20.

As practitioners, we can see and feel changes. We often observe improved client outcomes even if mechanisms of action are unclear. It is up to researchers to discover ways to assess and quantify effects and enable us to move forward with the next generation of evidence-informed approaches. Next, let us look at how researchers have tried to do just that.

Beginning in 2012, a series of high-quality studies examined how the mechanical properties of skeletal muscle are modified when forces similar to massage are applied to the tissue (Haas et al., 2012). Researchers developed a model to apply consistent, massage-like force to muscle tissue. Removing the variables inherent in using human hands allowed researchers to focus on changes brought about by applied force, which provided a starting point for a series of studies progressing from tissues to animals, and eventually to massage treatment with humans (Best et al., 2014; Crawford et al., 2014; Haas et al., 2013a, 2013b; Wang et al., 2014). These studies suggest the importance of timing of the massage treatment, and a dose response for magnitude and frequency for recovery of muscle properties. Further studies show some influence of massage on muscle remodeling, and protein turnover during muscle disuse (Hunt et al., 2019; Lawrence et al., 2020). Research is continuing to better understand how massage treatment influences muscle repair and function.

Research suggests massage may reduce muscular tension, reduce hypertonicity, improve soft tissue function, decrease stiffness and fatigue after exercise, improve exercise performance, decrease delayed-onset muscle soreness (DOMS), and reduce serum creatine kinase post exercise. Although many of these studies are older and have small numbers of participants and significant limitations in their research methods, this work lays the foundation for additional research to further clarify how massage influences the musculoskeletal system. A clearer picture should appear as larger studies with more rigorous research designs are completed.

Several studies have indicated increased range of motion (ROM) after massage (Billhult et al., 2008; Sefton et al., 2010, 2011; Yarar-Fisher et al., 2010). This may be due to decreased pain or stiffness, decreased muscle tightness, or changes in the joint itself. Clinically, improved ROM is an important treatment goal that may result in overall improvements in activities of daily living and general wellbeing. One small study found calf massage had a positive impact on muscle strength and ankle proprioception after exercise-induced muscle damage (Shin & Sung, 2015). Flexibility is closely related to ROM. Although most studies do not indicate improvement in flexibility after massage (Badke & Boissonnault, 2006; Boissonnault & Badke, 2008; Hernandez-Reif et al., 2001; James et al., 2009; Perlman et al., 2006), there is evidence that massage reduces tension in muscle tendon units (Weerapong et al., 2005) which may influence how muscles lengthen.

Trigger points are a common area of interest. Massage to trigger points has been shown to relieve pain, increase ROM, and restore function (Arroyo-Morales et al., 2008; McNicol et al., 1981). Pressure over trigger points has been shown to affect parasympathetic nervous system activity and influence heart rate and other factors (Barlow et al., 2007; Takamoto et al., 2009). Massage to trigger points has been shown to reduce headaches (Lavelle et al., 2007) and back and neck pain (Arroyo-Morales et al., 2008; Bell, 2008; Delaney et al., 2002; Vernon et al., 2007; von Stülpnagel et al., 2009). Similarly, a 2016 study found Thai massage decreased overall pain in individuals with myofascial pain syndrome, increased cervical ROM, and improved overall quality of life (Boonruab et al., 2016). However, studies often include self-massage and other treatment measures, which make it difficult to control the intervention or compare results between studies. Although the positive results are encouraging, much remains to be learned.

Increases in blood flow and temperature may also optimize muscle function and decrease muscle spasm and tightness. Several studies (Billhult et al., 2008; Losito & O'Neil, 1997; Sefton et al., 2010; Wiktorsson-Möller et al., 1983) have assessed muscle electrical activity using electromyography (EMG) before and after massage. These studies indicated decreases in EMG activity (Fig. 6.2). However, EMG assesses multiple factors, which makes the interpretation of these findings difficult. A decreased EMG signal does not necessarily mean a decrease in muscle strength or function; it may suggest decreases in electrical activity only. For example, a fatigued muscle recruits additional motor units to complete a task; this causes an increased EMG signal. Thus lower EMG signals can represent a more efficient muscular contraction.

Massage after athletic events has been thought to "flush out toxins" and decrease postexercise soreness, called *delayed-onset muscle soreness* (DOMS). This has been taught for decades, possibly as an attempt to explain postmassage

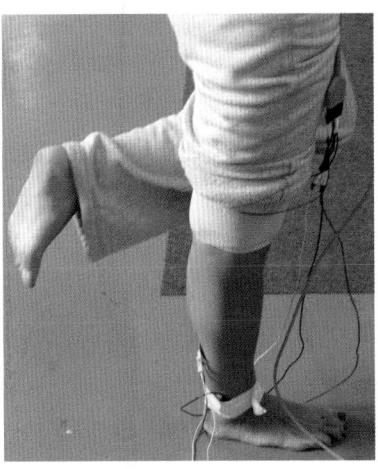

FIG. 6.2 Measuring massage-associated changes in muscle electrical activity during a research investigation using electromyography. (Auburn University Neuromechanics Research Laboratory).

soreness. Research investigating DOMS has yielded inconsistent results (Hong, 2002; Offenbacher & Stucki, 2000). One study demonstrated a decrease in DOMS, edema, and creatine kinase levels (an indicator of muscle function and damage) after massage (Trujillo, 1998). Another study found possible improvements in perceived soreness but not muscle swelling or ROM (Cheung et al., 2003). Other studies have failed to show any conclusive benefit (Ernst, 1998; Weerapong et al., 2005; Zainuddin et al., 2005). A literature review found massage had a slight effect on DOMS, but the effect was clinically insignificant. This same report found cryotherapy, stretching, and low-intensity exercise to have no effect on DOMS. Newer studies found massage decreased muscle soreness in rats, suggesting the effect might involve mitochondrial function (Urakawa et al., 2015), and decreased soreness and improved recovery in male bodybuilders (Kargarfard et al., 2016). Clearly, additional work is needed to understand whether there is any effect in this area and how to best treat or prevent DOMS.

Massage may improve muscle health and function, as discussed previously, especially when combined with active or passive movements. Massage has also been reported to influence balance and postural control (Cieslik et al., 2017; El Hage et al., 2013; Sefton et al., 2012a, 2012b; Wikstrom et al., 2017) (Fig. 6.3). Massage reduces spasms and assists in restoration of symmetric neuromuscular functioning, so it is possible massage may positively affect postural control. However, a large meta-analysis found little supporting evidence for improving neck pain or overall function (Cheng & Huang, 2014). This work strongly suggests randomized controlled studies are needed to further our knowledge in this area.

Finally, what effect does massage have on the skeletal system? Some research indicates massage of preterm infants improves weight gain and bone development, although recent reviews bring this into question (Bakowski et al., 2008; Connolly et al., 2003; Moraska, 2005). A small study suggests traditional Thai massage increased bone formation in

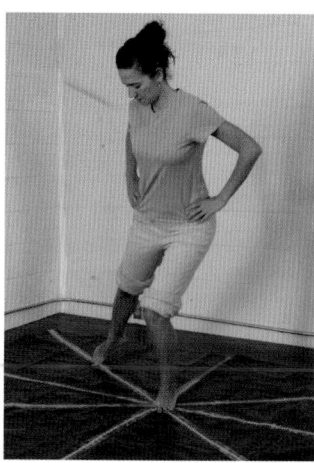

FIG. 6.3 Measuring massage-associated changes in balance and posture control during a research investigation. (Auburn University Neuromechanics Research Laboratory).

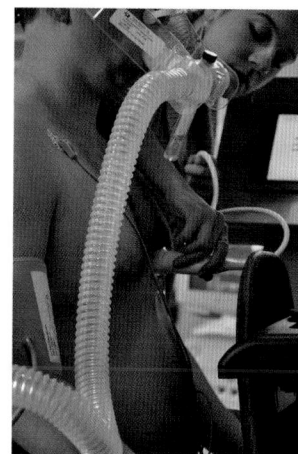

FIG. 6.4 Measuring massage-associated changes in blood pressure, respiration rate, and heart rate during a research investigation. (Auburn University Neuromechanics Research Laboratory).

some postmenopausal women (Saetung et al., 2013). Restoration of joint motion, increased circulation, decreased muscle spasm, and other massage benefits may influence bone health or healing.

To summarize, research suggests massage may:
- Directly affect muscular and skeletal systems through combined physiologic and psychological effects.
- Affect the viscoelastic response and muscle healing.
- Increase ROM.
- Decrease pain and may activate the parasympathetic nervous system, causing relaxation through massage of trigger points.
- Decrease EMG activity, suggesting increased muscle relaxation and decreased muscle fatigue.
- Reduce headaches, back pain, and neck pain.

MASSAGE EFFECTS ON THE CARDIOVASCULAR SYSTEM

Massage has been reported to decrease blood pressure, reduce heart rate, and cause variations in heart rate (Takamoto et al., 2009; Weerapong et al., 2005). These effects may promote cardiovascular health (Fig. 6.4). Decreases in systolic, diastolic, and arterial pressure and in heart rate were found after 45 to 60 minutes of massage in a study of 236 individuals (Kaye et al., 2008). Current theories suggest these changes result from reduced activity of the sympathetic nervous system by physiologic and psychological mechanisms, hypothalamus-pituitary-adrenocortical axis function, and increased blood flow, which affect endothelial function (Nelson, 2015). A randomized controlled trial found massage decreased blood pressure, reduced heart rate, and lowered inflammatory markers in hypertensive women (Supa'at et al., 2013). Massage may reduce the workload on the heart by reducing blood pressure. Research indicates massage is safe for individuals with cardiovascular disease who are undergoing treatment, surgery, or rehabilitation

(Kshettry et al., 2006; Okvat et al., 2002). Thus, under normal scenarios, there is no reason to believe massage would cause or contribute to a pathologic cardiac event. It is always a good idea for clients to inform their primary healthcare provider when they are receiving any type of complementary and integrative healthcare. The cardiovascular system is discussed in Chapter 26.

Physiologically based clinical studies support changes in peripheral blood flow and blood perfusion after massage treatment (Crane et al., 2012; Hinds et al., 2004; Mori et al., 2004; Rapaport et al., 2010; Sefton et al., 2010). This may be the mechanism through which massage influences leukocyte migration, weakening the inflammatory response to exercise. Research also indicates that massage mediates inflammation by reducing proinflammatory cytokines and tumor necrosis factor-α and decreases edema and muscle fiber damage after exercise (Crane et al., 2012; Haas et al., 2013b; Rapaport et al., 2010, 2012)—all which may reduce tissue damage and speed healing (Best & Crawford, 2017). Research assessing the influence of massage on myofascial trigger points suggests massage may break down adhesions and create changes in bradykinin, calcitonin gene–related peptide, serotonin, and substance P, which may decrease pain and movement restrictions (El-Hafez et al., 2020; Moraska et al., 2015, 2018; Morikawa et al., 2017; Simons & Mense, 2003). Most of these investigations are small, quality studies that need to be replicated in larger studies with diverse populations.

Blood platelets play a role in repair and regeneration of connective tissues, vascular tissues, and wound healing. Platelet counts are reactive to many factors such as exercise, mental stress, and several pathologies. Early studies (Aggeler et al., 1945; Lucia & Richard, 1933) demonstrated increases in blood platelet count after massage. Similar increases were found in immune responses when comparing massage with aromatherapy massage (Kuriyama et al., 2005). Increases in platelet count after massage suggest massage promotes tissue healing. Well-designed studies are needed to determine how big a role massage plays in this area.

One of the most commonly held beliefs in the profession is massage promotes healing and wellness through improved blood circulation. Improved circulation to tissues would theoretically enhance delivery of metabolic fuel, promote removal of metabolic by-products, and improve gas exchange. These effects would stimulate tissue healing and help to maintain tissue function. Improved lymph flow would promote immunity. Research has shown muscle contraction is an important component of blood and lymph circulation. This has led many to infer the force used during massage (squeezing, lifting, and shaking tissues) would have the same effect. Furthermore, we observe hyperemia (reddened skin associated with increased blood flow) during massage and we feel skin becoming warmer and softer.

However, it is challenging to assess changes in circulation from massage. Techniques used to measure changes in circulation also influence circulation or affect body tissues in other ways. An additional challenge comes from the fact there are several types of circulation. When discussing circulation, are we referring to arterial flow, venous flow, capillary exchange, or lymph drainage? If we decide to look at only arterial flow, do we examine changes in larger arteries or smaller arteries? For example, massage of the thigh may bring about minor blood flow changes in the femoral artery, which may go undetected. Examining changes in small arteries that supply the tibialis anterior muscle may reveal a significant change in blood flow. Finally, we feel the skin warm after a massage, but do changes in circulation occur in muscle below the skin, and do these changes improve healing of muscle injuries? As you can see, these are complex issues. Progress in the form of research is slowly being made, and a clearer picture is emerging.

Liu et al. (2004) measured the effects of mechanical pressure on capillary flow rate and blood viscosity after traditional Chinese medical massage (specifically called "swing," which included finger pushing, kneading, and rolling). This study revealed massage increased tissue pressure, which produced increases in capillary flow rate and decreased blood viscosity. Other attempts to measure blood flow directly during massage have been hampered by technical constraints. Nonetheless, findings from several studies using indirect blood flow assessment suggest massage may increase superficial flow to the treated area (Hovind & Nielsen, 1974; Weerapong et al., 2005). Drust et al. (2003) revealed increased intramuscular temperature within the quadricep muscle after massage, and Hinds et al. (2004) found increased skin temperature and blood flow with no corresponding increases in blood flow of the femoral artery. This study concluded massage may divert blood flow from muscles and questioned the efficacy of postexercise massage as a part of the recovery process. Other studies using Doppler ultrasound and laser Doppler also found no effect on blood flow within arteries after massage over both large and small muscle groups (forearm and thigh muscles) (Shoemaker

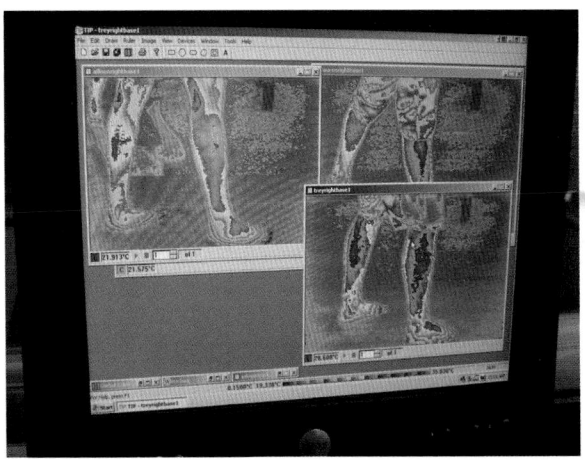

FIG. 6.5 Measuring massage-associated surface temperature and blood flow changes during a research investigation using infrared thermography. (Auburn University Neuromechanics Research Laboratory).

et al., 1997). Evaluation of noncontact surface temperature (via infrared thermography) has also been used to indirectly measure blood flow (Fig. 6.5). This technique allowed temperature assessment at specific points or changes across large areas. Studies using this technique indicated significant increases in surface temperature not only in areas of massage treatment (i.e., neck, shoulders) but also in the middle to lower back and down the arms in healthy adults (Sefton et al., 2010, 2011). The effect of skin friction during treatment was a possible source of temperature increase but only in the areas receiving treatment.

The next question is, do these findings represent changes in just skin temperature or does increased skin circulation indicate increased circulation? In a follow-up study, changes in blood oxidation levels in muscles were found in conjunction with changes in skin temperature after massage (Yarar-Fisher et al., 2010). A study on a pathologic population concluded connective tissue reflex massage on individuals with type 2 diabetes improved skin blood circulation (Castro-Sanchez, 2011b). Finally, a study examining the effect of massage techniques on blood flow found massage promoted blood flow but a device delivering vibration was more effective (Taspinar et al., 2013). There is still much to learn; however, we have evidence that massage does influence superficial blood circulation at some level.

To summarize, research suggests the effects of massage on cardiovascular functions and blood circulation are:

- Increases in capillary flow rate and decreases in blood viscosity.
- Increases in blood flow to the skin and possibly muscular tissue.
- Increases in blood oxidation levels.
- Increases in surface tissue temperatures of the treated and adjacent areas.
- Increases in platelet count.
- Decreases in heart rate, reduction of blood pressure, and decreases in heart rate variations.

MASSAGE EFFECTS ON THE LYMPHATIC SYSTEM AND IMMUNITY

There is evidence that massage promotes lymphatic flow and drainage. This is a well-researched area with studies showing the effectiveness of massage for decreasing edema and lymphedema (Bernas et al., 2005; Jeffs, 2006; Szuba, 2005). Massage, especially manual lymph drainage (MLD), either alone or combined with similar treatments, has become a commonly prescribed intervention after breast cancer surgery and plastic surgery.

Research examining the physiologic effects of massage on immunity is intriguing. Animal models help researchers get at the possible mechanisms of action. For example, Major et al. (2015) showed massage-like techniques improved immune system function measured in mice. A 2012 randomized controlled trial indicated massage was associated with higher immune responses, or natural killer cell cytotoxicity, and increased daily weight gain in stable preterm infants (Ang et al., 2012). Several small studies indicate massage increased killer T-cell levels and stimulated immune responses in individuals with human immunodeficiency virus (HIV) infection and cancer (Cohen et al., 2001; Hernandez-Reif et al., 2005; Shor-Posner et al., 2004). There are also studies suggesting massage combined with other treatments increased white blood cell counts in cancer patients (Diego et al., 2001; Hennenfent et al., 2006). However, one study did not draw the same conclusion (Hennenfent & Feliciano, 1998). The lymphatic system and immunity are discussed in Chapter 27.

Several studies have evaluated the effectiveness of massage as a nonsurgical treatment to prevent lymphedema after breast cancer treatments (Merchant & Chen, 2015). These studies often include multiple types of interventions, which makes it difficult to attribute findings to massage (Lacomba et al., 2010). One study found women had no significant increase in arm volume after surgery when using MLD compared with those who did not undergo treatment (Zimmermann et al., 2012), whereas another study found no benefit of MLD 12 months post intervention (Devoogdt et al., 2011). In a 2012 randomized controlled trial, Fernandez-Lao et al. (2012) found the attitudes of cancer patients influenced how massage affected pain sensitivity and immune response in breast cancer survivors. Collectively, research indicates cancer patients are likely to benefit from massage by increased lymph flow, decreased anxiety and stress, and reduced pain.

Studies on HIV/acquired immunodeficiency syndrome (AIDS) clients suggest similar results, such as decreased stress, improved quality of life, and improved immune response. Studies suggest massage improved the development in infants who were HIV positive (Perez et al., 2015), and massage was found to support immune function in HIV-positive children who did not have access to antiretroviral therapies (Shor-Posner et al., 2006).

Work assessing MLD, traditional massage, and a no-massage control group on persons with migraines found a significant decrease in migraine frequency and decreased intake of analgesics in the MLD group (Happe et al., 2016). Although this 8-week study was completed on mostly White, female participants, it was a sizable study (64 participants) and provided important input on choosing MLD as an intervention for migraine sufferers.

Clearly, much remains to be done in this area of study. We still need definitive results on the physiologic mechanisms of action of massage on the lymphatic system and immunity. However, research to date suggests a clear rationale for its use on individuals with compromised immune function, cancer, and related diseases for general promotion of immune response and overall health and wellbeing.

To summarize, research suggests the effects of massage on the lymphatic system and immune response are to:
- Improve lymphatic drainage.
- Reduce edema and lymphedema.
- Promote increases in lymphocyte levels.
- Promote immune health and function and overall wellbeing through combined physiologic effects.

MASSAGE EFFECTS ON CONNECTIVE TISSUES

Connective tissues become more fascinating as we learn more about how they function. Several connective tissues are included in other sections of this chapter (i.e., blood, lymph, bone). In this section, we will focus on loose and dense connective tissues. It was originally thought these tissues filled in space, held things together, and provided a framework for other structures. As we learn about fascia and techniques to work with this tissue, it is becoming more apparent that connective tissue is an integral and important part of massage. Newer studies suggest different types of connective tissue respond as excitable tissue—more like muscle or nerve tissue.

Massage techniques such as deep cross-fiber friction massage are frequently used to reduce scar tissue, decrease adhesion formation, and treat tendonitis. A few studies have examined effects of massage on connective tissue (Chaves et al., 2018; Miyaji et al., 2018), most completed in quality animal studies. A study investigating the effects of massage treatment on tendons in rats found a beneficial effect on the metabolic activity of tendon fibroblasts (Kassolik et al., 2013). Another study on rats revealed massage of the skin increased proliferation of epidermal cells, which can stimulate skin regeneration and tissue repair (Ratajczak-Wielgomas et al., 2018). Massage was also found to reduce inflammatory infiltration and mast cells in inflammatory skin lesions and reduce epidermal thickness in rats (Han et al., 2018); treatment also reduced anxiety before treatment for severe burns and reduced anxiety, redness, lichenification, scaling, excoriation, and pruritus associated with eczema in pediatric populations (Field, 2005).

To summarize, research suggests the effects of massage on connective tissues may:
- Reduce scar tissue formation.
- Increase scar tissue strength to aid in tendon healing.
- Assist in the treatment of tendonitis and ligament injuries.
- Reduce pain and itching in burn scars.

MASSAGE EFFECTS ON SKIN

As mentioned previously, massage increased skin temperature through changes in peripheral blood flow. Several studies assessed the effect of massage on the skin itself, but studies indicate improvements in eczema, including decreases in redness, lichenification (i.e., rough, thickened, dry skin), scaling, excoriation (i.e., crusting skin), and pruritus (i.e., itching) (Field, 2005). One study looked at the effects of 1 minute of mild massage on skin cells twice a day for 10 days. They found massage at some frequencies increased synthesis of some structural proteins compared with controls (Caberlotto et al., 2017). The same study found 8 weeks of facial massage combined with commercial anti-wrinkle cream improved skin texture and sagging compared with use of the cream alone. Massage also reduced scarring after burns (Cho et al., 2014; Field et al., 2000). The use of massage lubricant, the stimulation of blood flow, and the improvement of nutrient exchange may contribute synergistically to the health of the skin itself. Skin and the integumentary system are discussed in Chapter 22.

To summarize, research suggests the effects of massage on skin may:

- Reduce scarring after burns.
- Decrease symptoms of eczema and other skin conditions.
- Increase skin temperature.
- Contribute to the overall health of skin tissue.

MASSAGE EFFECTS ON THE NERVOUS SYSTEM

The nervous system is a vast and complex network involved in every aspect of how the body responds to its environment, including physical and psychological responses to massage. Several small studies have examined how massage influences neural tissue. Massage-like forces using a foam roller (sometimes called roller massage) were found to induce neural inhibition and decrease pain (Cavanaugh et al., 2017). Several studies assessing the Hoffmann reflex (H-reflex) found a decrease in neuromotor excitability after massage, suggesting massage reduces muscle tension through changes in neuromotor excitability (Morelli et al., 1990, 1991, 1998, 1999). Another group found occipital nerve massage reduced migraine attacks (Piovesan et al., 2007). The results in both studies were attributed to neural inhibition. It has been suggested that neural inhibition, reduction in substance P, and/or the gate control mechanism may contribute to the decrease in pain after massage across several populations (Boyd et al., 2016; Celebioglu et al., 2015; Chen et al., 2016; Field, 2016b; Field et al., 2011, 2014, 2015; Hernandez-Reif et al., 2001; Silva Gallo et al., 2013). Massage may also delay atrophy of denervated skeletal muscle through increasing or decreasing protein production (Wan et al., 2019). Changes in neural function may also contribute to changes seen in balance and posture after massage (Park et al., 2017; Sefton et al., 2012a, 2012b; Tütün Yümin et al., 2017). Several groups have found massage influenced neural processes and are working to discover the physiologic mechanisms involved (Kassolik et al., 2014; Shourabi et al., 2020; Tsai et al., 2016; Young et al., 2018). The nervous system is discussed in Chapter 23.

It is exciting to think massage is influencing the very core of the nervous system rather than just affecting surface tissues, but what do these changes mean to clients? The next step is connecting this response to improved treatment outcomes. One study found decreases in spinal reflexes, accompanied by decreases in EMG and increases in ROM after neck and shoulder massage (Sefton et al., 2011). This suggests decreased excitability may decrease tension and muscle firing, allowing for increased ROM in the cervical spine. More research is needed, but the potential connection between spinal cord function and improved treatment outcomes is promising.

Heart rate variability (HRV) is being assessed more and more as a measure of autonomic nervous system function. A randomized controlled study assessing the influence of a 10-minute Chinese head massage on HRV found those in the massage group had a significant shift from sympathetic to parasympathetic nervous system activity after treatment (Fazeli et al., 2016). Another small study using 24 female participants found head massage had a "relaxing and refreshing" effect, decreased anxiety, and may be used to provide comfort (Murota et al., 2016). Finally, Lee (2016) investigating head meridian acupoint massage and autonomic nervous system responses through HRV found a stress-relaxing effect.

Research on massage and the nervous system often focuses on how massage increases relaxation and reduces stress and anxiety (Listing et al., 2010; Lucini et al., 2009) and depression (Field et al., 2010; Hadfield, 2001; Hart et al., 2001; MacDonald, 1998). Many of these studies are small and used subjective measures. Some studies examine the effects of massage on neurotransmitters. Neurotransmitters are chemicals facilitating neurologic functions. Examples of neurotransmitters are endorphins, dopamine, and serotonin. Endorphins reduce pain. Serotonin regulates mood, appetite, sleep, memory, learning, and muscle contraction. Dopamine helps regulate heart rate and blood pressure and indirectly affects pituitary function and muscle movements. Massage studies using electroencephalography (EEG) of the brain have shown changes in pulse frequency (Diego et al., 2004; Wu et al., 2014) and cerebral blood flow in premature infants (Guzzetta et al., 2011; Rudnicki et al., 2012) and changes in brain activity in scapulocostal syndrome (Buttagat et al., 2012). Finally, beginning studies using magnetic resonance imaging (MRI) indicate both massage and reflexology produced changes in brain activity, although in different regions of the brain (Miura et al., 2013; Sliz et al., 2012).

Fibromyalgia is a disorder of widespread pain accompanied by disorders of sleep, mood, and memory. Once thought to be a muscular problem, fibromyalgia may be a nervous system disorder resulting from how the brain interprets and responds to pain signals. Clients with fibromyalgia often seek relief from massage. Some research indicates massage may relieve pain and symptoms (Baranowsky et al., 2009; Brattberg, 1999; Castro-Sanchez et al., 2011a; Çıtak-Karakaya et al., 2006; Field et al., 2003; Kalichman, 2010; Melillo et al., 2005; Morris et al., 2005; Tsao, 2007); however, evidence from randomized clinical trials is lacking. One systematic review suggested massage was not recommended for persons with fibromyalgia, whereas other systemic reviews found massage should be recommended (Kong et al., 2011; Tsao, 2007; Yuan et al., 2015). There may be a strong psychological component to massage, and much remains to be done, to understand the mechanisms of action, and to optimize treatment protocols.

If massage has an effect on neurotransmitters, it stands to reason massage would have direct effects on the parasympathetic nervous system, lowering heart rate and reducing blood pressure. Moreover, as noted previously, massage has been shown to directly affect brain wave activity and assist in those with sleep disorders, whether from decreases in pain, depression, or anxiety or from increased relaxation (Diego et al., 2004). Finally, a well-designed study indicated massage influenced brain development (Guzzetta et al., 2009). There is a great deal of work to be done in this area. Stay tuned.

To summarize, research suggests the effects of massage on the nervous system are to:

- Decrease nervous system excitability.
- Decrease stress, depression, and anxiety.
- Increase relaxation.
- Influence brain wave activity.
- Improve cognitive and memory functioning.
- Activate the parasympathetic response.

MASSAGE EFFECTS ON THE ENDOCRINE SYSTEM

Like the nervous system, the endocrine system influences almost every tissue in the body. This makes it difficult to measure the effects of massage on the endocrine system because its functions are interrelated with other body systems. Hormones are critical to physiologic functioning. The influence of massage on hormones, especially stress hormones (e.g., cortisol, catecholamine), has a long history of investigation in multiple settings and with varying populations with inconsistent results (Adib-Hajbaghery et al., 2015; Angelopoulou et al., 2020; Asadollahi et al., 2016; de Oliveira et al., 2018; Field, 2019; Hernandez-Reif et al., 2001; Pinar & Afsar, 2015; Van Dijk et al., 2020). Differences are often attributed to the massage type, timing, and methods used in data collection. Multiple studies show beneficial decreases in cortisol and blood pressure and other measures associated with stress and anxiety after massage compared with a control group (Field, 2016b; Kim et al., 2016; Lamas et al., 2016; Lindgren et al., 2010; Schaub et al., 2018; Sefton et al., 2012a, 2012b). Massage increases oxytocin and reduces adrenocorticotropic hormone (Morhenn et al., 2012; Rapaport et al., 2010, 2012). Work examining the influence of massage on plasma glucose,

insulin, gastrin, and somatostatin has found changes in gastrointestinal hormones (Ruan, 2019). Li et al. (2019) noted that foot massage increased oxytocin levels and activated regions in the brain associated with emotional touch. Moreover, the machine-administered massage was less effective in producing these results. The endocrine system is discussed in Chapter 24.

Type 2 diabetes can have detrimental effects on the cardiovascular system, nervous system, tissue healing, vision, and other sensory systems, as well as overall health and wellness. This and other problems associated with obesity are fast becoming a primary concern for the medical community, and federal research dollars are used to learn how to address these issues. An exciting area of research is the influence of massage on insulin production. Clinical evidence indicates improvement in diabetic symptoms with regular massage treatments. One animal study indicated improved insulin production after massage-like treatment in rats (Holst et al., 2005). Studies also indicate changes in insulin production and absorption after massage (Dillon, 1983; Field et al., 2008; Hildebrandt, 1991; Linde & Philip, 1989). Other studies suggest massage has positive effects on peripheral arterial disease by slowing disease progression through improved superficial circulation (Castro-Sanchez et al., 2011b); this cardiovascular disease is common in individuals with long-term diabetes mellitus. Research in this area is promising, and any positive effect massage can have on clients with diabetes would be a wonderful result.

To summarize, research suggests the effects of massage on the endocrine system may:

- Influence levels of hormones in multiple populations.
- Improve the production and absorption of insulin.
- Influence other massage-related outcomes and effects.

MASSAGE EFFECTS ON OTHER BODY SYSTEMS AND INTERNAL ORGANS

Changes in circulation, blood pressure, nutritional exchange, and other factors affect tissues throughout the body. Massage may influence individual internal organs and other body systems as part of the general effects of massage. It has been suggested massage specifically influences the urinary and digestive systems. Massage has been shown to decrease the severity of gastrointestinal symptoms, especially constipation and abdominal pain. Massage may also reduce nausea and vomiting under certain conditions and may promote a healthy gut microbiome (Chen et al., 2021).

Abdominal massage was shown to decrease stress in infants suffering from gastroesophageal reflux disease through a reduction in cortisol (Neu et al., 2014). Another study found abdominal massage reduced postoperative pain after a colectomy (LeBlanc-Louvry et al., 2002). These findings are likely a result of massage effects on systems other than directly on the internal organs involved. Several recent studies assessed the impact of massage on constipation. Canbulat Sahiner and Demirgoz Bal (2017) found no potential benefit for the use of reflexology to address constipation in children, whereas McClurg et al. (2016a) noted both abdominal massage and lifestyle advice beneficial in relieving symptoms of constipation in persons with Parkinson disease. Turan and Ast (2016) found abdominal massage applied to patients diagnosed with postoperative constipation reduced constipation symptoms, decreased time intervals between defecation, and increased quality of life. Moreover, McClurg and Lowe-Strong (2011) reviewed observational studies, case reports, and randomized controlled trials and determined abdominal massage is effective in relieving constipation by stimulating peristalsis, decreasing transit time, and increasing the frequency of bowel movements. They also noted abdominal massage reduced discomfort and pain, induced relaxation, and improved quality of life.

Massage has been suggested to be effective in chronic obstructive lung diseases, although a recent systematic review found evidence conflicting this. There are also multiple studies indicating massage as an effective treatment for asthma symptoms, especially in children (Field, 1995; Field et al., 1998; Pepino et al., 2013; Wu et al., 2017). A systematic review by Pepino et al. (2013) found evidence for the use of manual therapies for children with respiratory disease. It is important to note complementary and integrative health (CIH) therapies have been poorly researched in children although use in this population is growing. Wu et al. (2017) conducted a meta-analysis to determine the impact of treatments for children with asthma. Twelve of the 14 studies investigated included massage with or without other treatments. A significant effect of massage was observed compared with control groups. Moreover, four studies found significant improvements in forced expiratory volume and three found significant improvements in maximal expiratory flow. This is strong evidence supporting the use of massage for relief of asthma symptoms in children.

MASSAGE AND NEUROPSYCHOLOGICAL EFFECTS

The influence of massage on the neuropsychological aspects of our clients is a vast area, and an in-depth analysis of this work is well beyond the scope of this text. That being said, research is being developed to investigate how the mind influences the body, and new fields of science are being created. The mind-body connection results from the interrelationship between one's physical health and the state of one's mind. We have discussed the interplay of body systems and how difficult it is to separate individual systems in order to research the effects of massage. This holds true for the cognitive and emotional aspects of the body as well.

Stress, depression, and anxiety affect our health, whereas massage has been shown to decrease stress, depression, and anxiety. Massage has been shown to reduce anxiety and depression to a similar degree to improvements found with psychotherapy (Moyer et al., 2004). Reductions in neurotransmitters and hormones associated with anxiety have been found, along with positive effects on depression in

individuals with HIV and anxiety in cancer patients and military veterans. Multiple studies show massage decreases symptoms of stress. Physiologic measures of stress such as HRV, blood pressure, oxygen consumption, and cortisol show improvement after massage. Positive changes have been shown in healthy populations, healthcare providers, and patients.

A heightened sense of connection between the mind and body reported after massage may generate an overall feeling of health, wellness, and wellbeing. This is an exciting new area of research but an area difficult to quantify. A quick review of the literature using the terms *massage* and *wellness* results in more than 3000 peer-reviewed articles. For example, one study supports the use of mind-body therapies in pediatric oncology (Haun et al., 2009). Work has also been done in this area with female veterans with posttraumatic stress disorder (PTSD) (Price, 2007). Many studies that have been completed in differing populations show massage produces an improved state of mind and positive attitudes. This is one area thoroughly researched with solid conclusions.

One area of research is using massage in the treatment of hyperactivity disorders (attention-deficit/hyperactivity disorder, attention-deficit disorder, etc.). Several studies have found improved levels of focus, concentration, and overall functioning after massage (Arnold, 2001; Khilnani et al., 2003; Sawni, 2008). However, little new work has been completed in this area. Other studies indicate massage is useful for victims of trauma and abuse (Field, 2002; Price, 2005, 2007). Massage has also been successfully used with psychiatric patients for a variety of desired outcomes (Elkins et al., 2005). There are also studies suggesting massage influences communication, improves body image, improves mood, and helps us deal with strong emotions (Levine & Silver, 2007; Price, 2005, 2007). This is a vast field of study that will continue to evolve.

To summarize, research suggests the psychological effects of massage are to:
- Reduce anxiety, depression, and stress.
- Promote feelings of wellbeing.
- Promote a mind-body connection.
- Useful in treating hyperactivity disorders.
- Helpful in treating victims of violence and abuse (provided the practitioner has proper training).

MASSAGE AND WHOLE-BODY EFFECTS

As we indicated earlier, few changes brought about by massage are isolated to one tissue type or body system. Massage influences the nervous system, endocrine system, cardiovascular system, circulation of blood and lymph, connective tissues, and neuropsychological factors. The effects of massage on pain and fatigue are whole-body effects deserving special mention. It is important to remember that different types of tissue work in concert to produce health, wellness, disease, and healing. Massage likely influences multiple tissue types and processes simultaneously. However, researchers must break questions down into manageable pieces as they strive to learn how massage "works." They then will bring different parts of that new knowledge together to build an understanding of how massage influences the human body. Research to date suggests that some overall effects of massage on the body have been demonstrated and individual massage techniques act on physiologic processes in different ways (Waters-Banker et al., 2014). It will be important for future work to examine the physiologic effects of specific techniques, pressure, dose, and timing and examine how this new knowledge relates to the desired outcomes for health and wellness and for various pathologies and disease states.

Massage has long been used for pain resulting from multiple causes. Pain comes from muscle spasm and injury, tendonitis, bone fracture, skin conditions, trigger points, headaches, cancer treatments, osteoarthritis, orthopedic injury, fibromyalgia, labor and delivery, surgery, and other sources. How massage influences pain in each case may vary depending on the type and source of pain. Increased circulation, decreased spasms, changes in neurotransmitters and hormone levels, or even the simple act of touch and comfort all likely influence how the client perceives pain.

Fatigue is another area that responds to massage. Massage influences numerous factors that cause fatigue and interfere with sleep. Massage has been shown to improve sleep (Ejindu, 2007; Richards, 1998; Zhou et al., 2007); decrease chronic pain, which often results in overwhelming fatigue (Cardenas & Jensen, 2006; Cassileth et al., 2007; Suresh et al., 2008; Tsao, 2007; Walach et al., 2003); treat fibromyalgia, which often is associated with fatigue (Baranowsky et al., 2009; Berman & Swyers, 1999; Brattberg, 1999; Field et al., 2002); and generally improve overall wellbeing that would reduce symptoms of fatigue (Afari et al., 2000; Jones et al., 2007; Yao et al., 2007). Recent research has demonstrated the importance of sleep on factors such as immune system function, mental and physical recovery and performance, disease, obesity, mental health, wellness, and longevity. Studies suggest massage improves sleep in children, adolescents, adults, and the elderly; in patients who are hospitalized or institutionalized; those with different types of pain, including migraine; those recovering from heart surgery; and those with diseases/conditions such as cerebral palsy and cancer, as well as caregivers. If massage only improved sleep and had no other physiologic effect, we would find it has a positive effect on the overall health of individuals.

MASSAGE FOR SPECIFIC CONDITIONS AND OUTCOMES

This section discusses the effects of massage on specific conditions (Parkinson disease, cancer, arthritis, diabetes, aging) and for specific outcomes (decreasing pain and improving health and wellness). Further information can be found in their respective chapters through the textbook.

Parkinson Disease

Multiple studies have explored massage as a treatment for Parkinson disease (Casciaro, 2016; Craig et al., 2006; Donoyama & Ohkoshi, 2012; Donoyama et al., 2014; Duval et al., 2002; Ferry et al., 2002; Kim et al., 2009; King 2016; McClurg et al., 2016a, 2016b; Miyahara et al., 2018: Rajendran et al., 2001; Suoh et al., 2016; Törnhage et al., 2013). A 2020 systematic review of the use of massage as a clinical treatment of Parkinson symptoms found relaxation following massage contributed to a reduction in stress hormones and symptom improvement (Angelopoulou et al., 2020). Quality of life, motor skills, sleep, and fatigue improved, and decreases were found in anxiety, depression, and pain. Treatment methods included a wide range of massage types and styles, with no data supporting one over the other. Suspected underlying mechanisms mirror those mentioned earlier, especially influences on brain-derived neurotrophic factor (BDNF) levels and insulin-like growth factor (IGF)-1 pathways which are involved in neuroprotective effects for dopaminergic neurons (Mercado et al., 2017). The positive changes and the absence of negative side effects suggest further research on methods, doses, and timing are warranted. Parkinson disease is discussed in Chapter 23.

Cancer

The role of massage in cancer treatment has been more widely researched (Darabpour et al., 2016; Dilaveri et al., 2020; Dion 2016; Donoyama et al., 2018; Genik et al., 2020; Gentile et al., 2018; Ho et al., 2017; Izgu et al., 2019; Karagozoglu & Kahve, 2013; Kinkead et al., 2018; Massingill et al., 2018; Mazlum et al., 2013; Miladinia et al., 2017; Pan et al., 2014; Pinar & Afsar, 2015; Silverdale et al., 2019; Somani et al., 2013; Son et al., 2019; Toth et al., 2013; Uysal et al., 2017; Warpenburg, 2014). Work has also been completed on massage for healthcare providers and families of cancer patients (Cowen & Tafuto, 2018; Hand et al., 2019; Kozak et al., 2013; MacDonald, 2014). Several systematic reviews have been completed in the past 20 years. One review reports some evidence that massage reduces symptoms in children with cancer (Rodriguez-Mansilla et al., 2017), and another found weak evidence for the use of massage for the treatment of cancer-related pain (Boyd et al., 2016). All reviews reported weak evidence and the need for larger, well-designed studies for the use of massage for cancer patients. Cancer is discussed in Chapter 14 of *Mosby's Pathology for Massage Professionals*.

Arthritis

Massage as a treatment for arthritis is another area that has received a good deal of focus (Atkins & Eichler, 2013; Bahr et al., 2018; Cortes Godoy et al., 2014; Efe et al., 2019; Field et al., 2013; Ganji, 2019; Juberg et al., 2015; Nasiri & Mahmodi, 2018; Pehlivan & Karadakovan, 2019; Qingguang et al., 2015; Tosun et al., 2017; Zhu et al., 2016). One review found significant improvements in movement and pain with massage, yoga, or tai chi (Field, 2016a). Low to moderate evidence was found showing massage as a superior treatment to nonmovement therapies in reducing pain and improving functional outcomes (Nelson & Churilla, 2017). A 2017 study evaluating patient-reported quality of life after the use of massage for knee osteoarthritis found patients reported increased empowerment and quality of life after massage treatment (Ali et al., 2017). A small 2015 study found increased ROM, decreased pain, and improved sleep after massage (Field et al., 2015); similar results were found in a study of massage for osteoarthritis or the cervical spine (Field et al., 2014). One randomized controlled trial found massage to be a safe and effective short-term treatment for knee osteoarthritis, with longer biweekly treatments maintaining benefits (Perlman et al., 2019). However, a related commentary questioned the value of the results and noted a lack of available high-quality research data (Jackson et al., 2019). These discussions reinforce the need for larger, randomized studies to determine the effectiveness and methods for the use of massage for arthritis treatment. Arthritis is discussed in Chapter 19.

Diabetes

Several studies have explored the use of massage with persons with diabetes (Bayat et al., 2016; Lyu et al., 2019; Sajedi et al., 2011; Wändell et al., 2012). Several of these used massage or self-massage to improve blood flow in the feet, a common problem in this population (Chatchawan et al., 2015; Tütün Yümin et al., 2017). One study reported massage or self-massage improved foot skin blood flow and ROM in the feet and ankles in persons with diabetic peripheral neuropathy (Chatchawan et al., 2020). Another study found massage with hydrotherapy improved balance and glycemic markers in this same population (Shourabi et al., 2020), and a small study found improvements in adiponectin, adiponectin-leptin, adiponectin–hemoglobin A1c (HbA1c) levels (diabetes biomarkers) (Wändell et al., 2013). Results of the few studies in this area are promising and suggest the need for further research on effectiveness and how to optimize massage treatment for this population. Diabetes is discussed in Chapter 24.

Aging

The use of massage for health conditions associated with aging has also been explored (Bahrami et al., 2018; Davis & Srivastava, 2003; King, 2016; Liu et al., 2018; Mok & Woo, 2004; Pehlivan & Karadakovan, 2019; Rodriguez-Mansilla et al., 2013; Sansone & Schmitt, 2000; Satou et al., 2013; Thanakiatpinyo et al., 2014). There is some overlap between aging and the conditions noted earlier. Work has been done on the special considerations and conditions associated with older populations. Two studies found full body massage may improve balance and posture in active older adults (Sefton et al., 2012a, 2012b). One study found abdominal massage improved constipation symptoms in rest home residents (Çevik et al., 2018). A small study indicated massage may improve sleep, EEG,

and psychological factors (Nakano et al., 2019). Several studies included massage with other treatments (e.g., warm bath or herbal compresses) without a massage control group for comparison, making it impossible to determine the influence of massage on the outcomes (Kudo & Sasaki, 2020; Laosee et al., 2020). As with other populations and conditions, research shows areas of promise and suggests that there is more work to be done to determine massage benefits for the aging population. Aging and Massage for the Elderly is discussed in Chapter 16 of *Mosby's Pathology for Massage Professionals*.

Pain

Assessing the use of massage for the reduction of pain has overlap with some of the conditions and populations already discussed. Multiple studies of differing levels of evidence support the use of massage to reduce pain in a wide range of populations with varying causes of pain (Buttagat et al., 2020; Cyganska et al., 2020; Demir & Saritas, 2020a, 2020b; Gönenç & Terzioglu, 2020; Harrison et al., 2020; Horner et al., 2020; Kim et al., 2020; Laosee et al., 2020; Lasocki et al., 2020; Mizrak Sahin et al., 2021; Momeni et al., 2020; Roshanray et al., 2020; Rosmiarti et al., 2020; Skillgate et al., 2020; Sözen & Karabulut, 2020; Türkmen & Oran, 2021; Zerkle & Gates. 2020). A meta-analysis found massage was effective in reducing postoperative pain in cardiac patients (Boitor et al., 2017). Other meta-analyses and systematic reviews also suggest massage is effective in reducing shoulder pain (Yeun, 2017), primary dysmenorrhea (Sut et al., 2017), labor pain (Ranjbaran et al., 2017), general postoperative pain (Kukimoto et al., 2017), and cancer pain (Boyd et al., 2016). Evidence in many of these cases is still weak, and all suggest larger and more rigorous research is required to confirm these findings and suggest protocols for clinical implementation (Miake-Lye et al., 2019). Pain is discussed in Chapter 14.

Health and Wellness

Quality research on the influence of massage on the areas of overall health, wellness, resiliency, healing, and wellbeing is surprisingly lacking (Best et al., 2013; Hall et al., 2021; McFeeters et al., 2016; Musial & Weiss, 2014; Oumeish, 2005; Rosenbaum & Velde, 2016; Williams et al., 2019). The terms health, wellness, resiliency, healing, and wellbeing are broad and are often described in overlapping ways. When looking to progress in these areas, it will be important to specifically define terms and outcomes. One study found including massage as a part of an anatomy curriculum improves student wellness (Hoffmann et al., 2019). Several studies have shown positive effects of massage on mental health of different populations (Espí-López et al., 2020; Hall et al., 2021; Zhou et al., 2020), whereas others found no effects (Kanitz et al., 2015). Researchers have also found improved sleep (often using aromatherapy massage) and other indicators of health (Arbianingsih et al., 2020; Arslan et al., 2021; Ayik & Ozden, 2018; Cheraghbeigi et al., 2019; Efe Arslan & Kilic Akca, 2020; Hsu et al., 2019; Kanitz et al.,

2015; Kawabata et al., 2020; Kobayashi et al., 2020; Kudo & Sasaki, 2020; Mindell et al., 2018; Rafii et al., 2020). Investigators have also examined massage practitioners as educational providers in areas of health promotion and the barriers to this practice (Kennedy et al., 2018). Wellness and wellbeing are discussed in Chapter 4.

MASSAGE EDUCATION RESEARCH

Research into how to develop massage curricula, train massage practitioners, and provide continuing education is a growing field (Baskwill et al., 2020; Baskwill, 2011, 2018; Chunco, 2010; Finch, 2004, 2009; McQuillan, 2010; Menard, 2014; Munk, 2013; Munk et al., 2019; Weaver et al., 2018; Werner, 2010). It is especially important to improve evidence-informed educational materials and provide research continuing education for massage educators. Effective virtual education, researcher–massage school collaborations, and opportunities for students and educators to become involved in research are important goals needed to improve massage education and practice. There is also important work being done to determine optimal body mechanics to reduce practitioner injury and extend massage careers (Anderson, 2018). Finally, there is ongoing work on increasing insurance reimbursement, improving client satisfaction, and enhancing health and sanitation protocols in an effort to keep massage practitioners safe, practicing with fewer injuries, and supporting longer and more satisfying careers in the future.

E-RESOURCES

http://evolve.elsevier.com/Salvo/MassageTherapy

- Chapter challenge
- Flash cards
- Additional information

NIKI MUNK

Historically, massage research studies were conducted by people in the medical field who did not know trigger points from tapotement. Massage research has come a long way in 30 years and continues to evolve. Currently it includes a body of knowledge from massage practitioners and guidelines on how massage practitioners can be more involved in ongoing research by providing case reports. Niki Munk is a massage practitioner turned researcher.

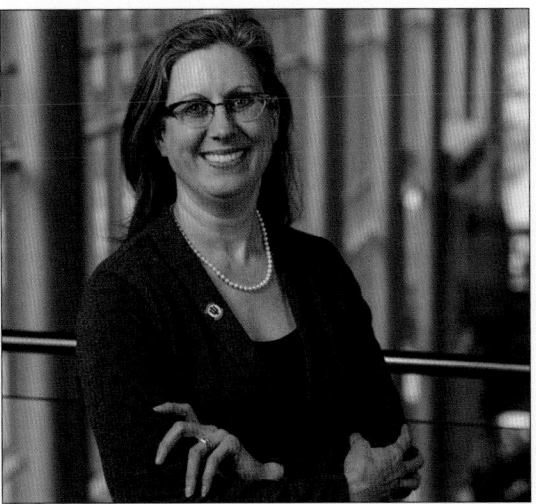

"More, better research," seems to be her mantra. Although she may not practice massage today, she has and she understands its benefits. "As evidence-informed practice improves, I believe there will be more potential for third-party payers, and research can help elevate the profession," she said. She wants to see massage as a field more "professionalized" and "systematically more robust," salaried positions with benefits, and fewer practitioners with burnout. She believes the right research—and agreement between stakeholders about the future of the industry—can help make that happen.

Munk is the chair at the Department of Health Sciences at Indiana University-Purdue University of Indianapolis who "stumbled not only into massage but also into research." Her undergraduate degree is in theater from the University of Alabama, where she graduated cum laude. After she received her massage license in 2005, Munk decided to accompany her parents on national bicycle tours and became interested in the impact of massage on the aging body. However, her massage training had not prepared her to feel confident in delivering geriatric massage, and she found little research to pull from. So, she pursued her Doctorate of Philosophy in gerontology, completing the program in 2011. "I only thought I knew what research was," she said.

She now oversees undergraduate and graduate students and teaches classes on the physically aging body, health sciences, health administration, and health policy. Her position allows her the opportunity to do research in areas that interest her most, including studies on pregnancy massage, and how massage impacts pain and mental health. Currently, Munk is the co-investigator in a Veteran's Administration and Department of Defense funded TOM-CATT study, which examines the care-ally–assisted and practitioner-provided massage for veterans with chronic neck pain. She sees her legacy as helping launch the research careers of future massage practitioners, nurses,

occupational therapists, and other healthcare professionals. While she acknowledges that scholarly research is not a trajectory for every practitioner, one need not be headed toward an advanced degree to complete a case report. According to Munk:

There are many resources to which massage practitioners can turn to for guidance in writing a case report including the Therapeutic Massage and Bodywork Adapted CARE Guidelines (which anyone can access in full in the open access International Journal of Therapeutic Massage and Bodywork—IJTMB).... If you have ever found yourself starting the relaying of a clinical case "story" with something like, "the most interesting thing happened today," or "I had a client who was able to [fill-in-the-blank] for the first time in ages," you likely have the beginnings of a really great case report.

Munk, N. (2019) All massage and myotherapy clinicians can contribute to research, Massage & Myotherapy Journal (Australia).

By her own admission, Munk is not popular with everyone in the massage industry, and that includes educators, practitioners, and even professional organizations. "The U.S. therapeutic massage and bodywork field seems to be at a professional precipice regarding the direction of its education and practice in regard to healthcare. Will the massage field work to professionally align itself to work with and in the medical healthcare setting and practice; remain as is with no definitive and recognized professional credential or qualification for work with and in the medical healthcare settings and practice; or shift completely away from alignment as complementary to medical healthcare settings and practice?"

"In my humble opinion," she said, "it's best if there is a clear divide—a split. If people want to work independently from a cosmetology or hair dresser standpoint, then that's what they do... The conversation in our field of a tiered system has not been well received."

"The impact of massage in most settings goes beyond helping manage pain," she said.

Whether it is the actual touch, the ongoing relationship between practitioner and client, the massage practitioner's ability to adapt to exactly what is needed during a session, or the pressure on skin that produces the outcome, she cannot say. But she continues to study its impact and encourages educators and students to do the same.

REFERENCES

Adib-Hajbaghery, M., Rajabi-Beheshtabad, R., & Ardjmand, A. (2015). Comparing the effect of whole body massage by a specialist nurse and patients' relatives on blood cortisol level in coronary patients. *ARYA Atherosclerosis*, 11(2), 126–132.

Afari, N., Eisenberg, D. M., Herrell, R., Goldberg, J., Kleyman, E., Ashton, S., et al. (2000). Use of alternative treatments by chronic fatigue syndrome discordant twins. *Journal of Integrative Medicine*, 2(2), 97–103.

Aggeler, P. M., Howard, J., Lucia, S. P., & Mills, E. (1945). Platelet counts and platelet function. *Proceedings of American Federation for Clinical Research, 2*, 110.

Ali, A., Rosenberger, L., Weiss, T. R., Milak, C., & Perlman, A. I. (2017). Massage therapy and quality of life in osteoarthritis of the knee: A qualitative study. *Pain Medicine*, 18(6), 1168–1175.

American Massage Therapy Association (AMTA). (2017). *Consumer views and use of massage therapy*. Retrieved from https://www.amtamassage.org/research/Consumer-Survey-Fact-Sheets.html.

American Massage Therapy Association (AMTA). (2021). *Industry fact sheet*. Retrieved from https://www.amtamassage.org/publications/massage-industry-fact-sheet/.

Anderson, R. B. (2018). Improving body mechanics using experiential learning and ergonomic tools in massage therapy education. *International Journal of Therapeutic Massage & Bodywork*, 11(4), 23–31.

Ang, J. Y., Lua, J. L., Mathur, A., Thomas, R., Asmar, B. I., Savasan, S., et al. (2012). A randomized placebo-controlled trial of massage therapy on the immune system of preterm infants. *Pediatrics*, 130(6), e1549–e1558.

Angelopoulou, E., Anagnostouli, M., Chrousos, G. P., & Bougea, A. (2020). Massage therapy as a complementary treatment for Parkinson disease: A systematic literature review. *Complementary Therapies in Medicine*, 49, 102340.

Arbianingsih, A., Amal, A. A., Hidayah, N., Azhari, N., & Tahir, T. (2020). Massage with lavender aromatherapy reduced sleep disturbances on infant. *Enfermería Clínica*, 30(Suppl. 3), 62–65.

Arnold, L. E. (2001). Alternative treatments for adults with attention-deficit hyperactivity disorder (ADHD). *Annals of the New York Academy of Sciences*, 931, 310–341.

Arroyo-Morales, M., Olea, N., Martínez, M. M., Hidalgo-Lozano, A., Ruiz-Rodríguez, C., & Díaz-Rodríguez, L. (2008). Psychophysiological effects of massage-myofascial release after exercise: A randomized sham-control study. *Journal of Alternative and Complementary Medicine*, 14(10), 1223–1229.

Arslan, G., Ceyhan, O., & Mollaoglu, M. (2021). The influence of foot and back massage on blood pressure and sleep quality in females with essential hypertension: A randomized controlled study. *Journal of Human Hypertension*, 35(7), 627–637.

Asadollahi, M., Jabraeili, M., Mahallei, M., Asgari Jafarabadi, M., & Ebrahimi, S. (2016). Effects of gentle human touch and field massage on urine cortisol level in premature infants: A randomized, controlled clinical trial. *Journal of Caring Sciences*, 5(3), 187–194.

Atkins, D. V., & Eichler, D. A. (2013). The effects of self-massage on osteoarthritis of the knee: A randomized, controlled trial. *International Journal of Therapeutic Massage & Bodywork*, 6(1), 4–14.

Ayik, C., & Ozden, D. (2018). The effects of preoperative aromatherapy massage on anxiety and sleep quality of colorectal surgery patients: A randomized controlled study. *Complementary Therapies in Medicine*, 36, 93–99.

Badke, M. B., & Boissonnault, W. G. (2006). Changes in disability following physical therapy intervention for patients with low back pain: Dependence on symptom duration. *Archives of Physical Medicine and Rehabilitation*, 87(6), 749–756.

Bahr, T., Allred, K., Martinez, D., Rodriguez, D., & Winterton, P. (2018). Effects of a massage-like essential oil application procedure using Copaiba and Deep Blue oils in individuals with hand arthritis. *Complementary Therapies in Clinical Practice*, 33, 170–176.

Bahrami, T., Rejeh, N., Heravi-Karimooi, M., Vaismoradi, M., Tadrisi, S. D., & Sieloff, C. L. (2018). Aromatherapy massage versus reflexology on female elderly with acute coronary syndrome. *Nursing in Critical Care*, 23(5), 229–236.

Bakowski, P., Musielak, B., Sip, P., & Biegański, G. (2008). Effects of massage on delayed-onset muscle soreness. *Chirurgia Narzadow Ruchu I Ortopedia Polska*, 73(4), 261–265.

Baranowsky, J., Klose, P., Musial, F., Haeuser, W., Dobos, G., & Langhorst, J. (2009). Qualitative systemic review of randomized controlled trials on complementary and alternative medicine treatments in fibromyalgia. *Rheumatology International*, 30(1), 1–21.

Barlow, A., Clarke, R., Johnson, N., Seabourne, B., Thomas, D., & Gal, J. (2007). Effect of massage of the hamstring muscles on selected electromyographic characteristics of biceps femoris during sub-maximal isometric contraction. *International Journal of Sports Medicine*, 28(3), 253–256.

Baskwill, A. (2011). Changing the culture of clinical education in massage therapy. *International Journal of Therapeutic Massage & Bodywork*, 4(4), 33–36.

Baskwill, A. (2018). Developing capability: Transforming massage therapy education through inquiry-based learning. *International Journal of Therapeutic Massage & Bodywork*, 11(3), 10–14.

Baskwill, A., Sumpton, B., Shipwright, S., Atack, L., & Maher, J. (2020). A Canadian massage therapy education environmental scan. *International Journal of Therapeutic Massage & Bodywork*, 13(4), 12–24.

Bayat, D., Vakilinia, S. R., & Asghari M. (2016). Non-drug therapy and prevention of diabetes mellitus by Dalk (massage). *Iranian Journal of Medical Sciences*, 41(Suppl. 3), S45.

Bell, J. (2008). Massage therapy helps increase range of motion, decrease pain and assist in healing a client with low back pain and sciatica. *Journal of Bodywork and Movement Therapies*, 12(3), 281–289.

Berman, B. M., & Swyers, J. P. (1999). Complementary medicine treatments for fibromyalgia syndrome. *Baillieres Best Practice & Research: Clinical Rheumatology*, 13(3), 487–492.

Bernas, M., Witte, M., Kriederman, B., Summers, P., & Witte, C. (2005). Massage therapy in the treatment of lymphedema. rationale, results, and applications. *IEEE Engineering in Medicine and Biology Magazine*, 24(2), 58–68.

Best, T. M., & Crawford, S. K. (2017). Massage and postexercise recovery: The science is emerging. *British Journal of Sports Medicine*, 51(19), 1386–1387.

Best, T. M., Crawford, S. K., Haas, C., Charles, L., & Zhao, Y. (2014). Transverse forces in skeletal muscle with massage-like loading in a rabbit model. *BMC Complementary and Alternative Medicine*, 14(1), 393.

Best, T. M., Gharaibeh, B., & Huard, J. (2013). Stem cells, angiogenesis and muscle healing: A potential role in massage therapies? *British Journal of Sports Medicine*, 47(9), 556–560.

Billhult, A., Lindholm, C., Gunnarsson, R., & Stener-Victorin, E. (2008). The effect of massage on cellular immunity, endocrine and psychological factors in women with breast cancer: A randomized controlled clinical trial. *Autonomic Neuroscience: Basic and Clinical*, 140(1–2), 88–95.

Boissonnault, W. G., & Badke, M. B. (2008). Influence of acuity on physical therapy outcomes for patients with cervical disorders. *Archives of Physical Medicine and Rehabilitation*, 89(1), 81–86.

Boitor, M., Gelinas, C., Richard-Lalonde, M., & Thombs, B. D. (2017). The effect of massage on acute postoperative pain in critically and acutely ill adults post-thoracic surgery: Systematic review and meta-analysis of randomized controlled trials. *Heart & Lung*, 46(5), 339–346.

Boonruab, J., Niempoog, S., Pattaraarchachai, J., Palanuvej, C., & Ruangrungsi, N. (2016). Effectiveness of the court-type traditional Thai massage versus topical diclofenac in treating patients with myofascial pain syndrome in the upper trapezius. *Indian Journal of Traditional Knowledge*, 15(1), 30–34.

Boyd, C., Crawford, C., Paat, C. F., Price, A., Xenakis, L., Zhang, W., et al. (2016). The impact of massage therapy on function in pain populations-a systematic review and meta-analysis of randomized controlled trials: Part II, cancer pain populations. *Pain Medicine*, 17(8), 1553–1568.

Brattberg, G. (1999). Connective tissue massage in the treatment of fibromyalgia. *European Journal of Pain*, 3(3), 235–244.

Buttagat, V., Eungpinichpong, W., Kaber, D., Chatchawan, U., & Arayawichanon, P. (2012). Acute effects of traditional Thai massage on electroencephalogram in patients with scapulocostal syndrome. *Complementary Therapies in Medicine*, 20(4), 167–174.

Buttagat, V., Techakhot, P., Wiriya, W., Mueller, M., & Areeudomwong, P. (2020). Effectiveness of traditional Thai self-massage combined with stretching exercises for the treatment of patients with chronic non-specific low back pain: A single-blinded randomized controlled trial. *Journal of Bodywork and Movement Therapies*, 24(1), 19–24.

Caberlotto, E., Ruiz, L., Miller, Z., Poletti, M., & Tadlock, L. (2017). Effects of a skin-massaging device on the ex-vivo expression of human dermis proteins and in-vivo facial wrinkles. *PLoS One*, 12(3), e0172624.

Canbulat Sahiner, N., & Demirgoz Bal, M. (2017). A randomized controlled trial examining the effects of reflexology on children with functional constipation. *Gastroenterology Nursing*, 40(5), 393–400.

Cardenas, D. D., & Jensen, M. P. (2006). Treatments for chronic pain in persons with spinal cord injury: A survey study. *Journal of Spinal Cord Medicine*, 29(2), 109–117.

Casciaro, Y. (2016). Massage therapy treatment and outcomes for a patient with Parkinson's disease: A case report. *International Journal of Therapeutic Massage & Bodywork*, 9(1), 11–18.

Cassileth, B. R., Deng, G. E., Gomez, J. E., Johnstone, P. A., Kumar, N., & Vickers, A. J. (2007). Complementary therapies and integrative oncology in lung cancer: ACCP evidence-based clinical practice guidelines (2nd edition). *Chest*, 132(Suppl. 3), 340S–354S.

Castro-Sanchez, A. M., Mataran-Penarrocha, G. A., Granero-Molina, J., Aguilera-Manrique, G., Quesada-Rubio, J. M., & Moreno-Lorenzo, C. (2011a). Benefits of massage-myofascial release therapy on pain, anxiety, quality of sleep, depression, and quality of life in patients with fibromyalgia. *Evidence-Based Complementary and Alternative Medicine*, 2011, 561753.

Castro-Sanchez, A. M., Moreno-Lorenzo, C., Mataran-Penarrocha, G. A., Feriche-Fernandez-Castanys, B., Granados-Gamez, G., & Quesada-Rubio, J. M. (2011b). Connective tissue reflex massage for type 2 diabetic

patients with peripheral arterial disease: Randomized controlled trial. *Evidence-Based Complementary and Alternative Medicine*, 2011, 804321.

Cavanaugh, M. T., Doweling, A., Young, J. D., Quigley, P. J., Hodgson, D. D., Whitten, J. H. D., et al. (2017). An acute session of roller massage prolongs voluntary torque development and diminishes evoked pain. *European Journal of Applied Physiology*, 117(1), 109–117.

Celebioglu, A., Gurol, A., Yildirim, Z. K., & Buyukavci, M. (2015). Effects of massage therapy on pain and anxiety arising from intrathecal therapy or bone marrow aspiration in children with cancer. *International Journal of Nursing Practice*, 21(6), 797–804.

Çevik, K., Cetinkaya, A., Yigit Gokbel, K., Menekse, B., Saza, S., & Tikiz, C. (2018). The effect of abdominal massage on constipation in the elderly residing in rest homes. *Gastroenterology Nursing*, 41(5), 396–402.

Chatchawan, U., Eungpinichpong, W., Plandee, P., & Yamauchi, J. (2015). Effects of Thai foot massage on balance performance in diabetic patients with peripheral neuropathy: A randomized parallel-controlled trial. *Medical Science Monitor Basic Research*, 21, 68–75.

Chatchawan, U., Jarasrungsichol, K., & Yamauchi, J. (2020). Immediate effects of self-Thai foot massage on skin blood flow, skin temperature, and range of motion of the foot and ankle in type 2 diabetic patients. *Journal of Alternative and Complementary Medicine*, 26(6), 491–500.

Chaves, P., Simoes, D., Paco, M., Pinho, F., Duarte, J. A., & Ribeiro, F. (2018). Deep friction massage and the minimum skin pressure required to promote a macroscopic deformation of the patellar tendon. *Journal of Chiropractic Medicine*, 17(4), 226–230.

Chen, H., Tan, P. S., Li, C. P., Chen, B. Z., Xu, Y. Q., He, Y. Q., & Ke, X. (2021). Acupoint massage therapy alters the composition of gut microbiome in functional constipation patients. *Evidence-Based Complementary and Alternative Medicine*, 2021, 1416236.

Chen, T. H., Tung, T. H., Chen, P. S., Wang, S. H., Chao, C. M., Hsiung, N. H., & Chi, C. C. (2016). The clinical effects of aromatherapy massage on reducing pain for the cancer patients: Meta-analysis of randomized controlled trials. *Evidence-Based Complementary and Alternative Medicine*, 2016, 9147974.

Cheng, Y. H., & Huang, G. C. (2014). Efficacy of massage therapy on pain and dysfunction in patients with neck pain: A systematic review and meta-analysis. *Evidence-Based Complementary and Alternative Medicine*, 2014, 204360.

Cheraghbeigi, N., Modarresi, M., Rezaei, M., & Khatony, A. (2019). Comparing the effects of massage and aromatherapy massage with lavender oil on sleep quality of cardiac patients: A randomized controlled trial. *Complementary Therapies in Clinical Practice*, 35, 253–258.

Cheung, K., Hume, P., & Maxwell, L. (2003). Delayed onset muscle soreness: Treatment strategies and performance factors. *Sports Medicine*, 33(2), 145–164.

Cho, Y. S., Jeon, J. H., Hong, A., Yang, H. T., Yim, H., Cho, Y. S., et al. (2014). The effect of burn rehabilitation massage therapy on hypertrophic scar after burn: A randomized controlled trial. *Burns*, 40(8), 1513–1520.

Chunco, R. (2010). The ethical implications of research and education in the massage therapy profession. *International Journal of Therapeutic Massage & Bodywork*, 3(3), 17–19.

Cieslik, B., Podsiadly, I., Kuczynski, M., & Ostrowska, B. (2017). The effect of a single massage based on the tensegrity principle on postural stability in young women. *Journal of Back and Musculoskeletal Rehabilitation*, 30(6), 1197–1202.

Çıtak-Karakaya, İ., Akbayrak, T., Demirtürk, F., Ekici, G., & Bakar, Y. (2006). Short and long-term results of connective tissue manipulation and combined ultrasound therapy in patients with fibromyalgia. *Journal of Manipulative and Physiological Therapeutics*, 29(7), 524–528.

Cohen, S. R., Payne, D. K., & Tunkel, R. S. (2001). Lymphedema: Strategies for management. *Cancer*, 92(Suppl. 4), 980–987.

Connolly, D. A., Sayers, S. P., & McHugh, M. P. (2003). Treatment and prevention of delayed onset muscle soreness. *The Journal of Strength and Conditioning Research*, 17(1), 197–208.

Cortes Godoy, V., Gallego Izquierdo, T., Lazaro Navas, I., & Pecos Martin, D. (2014). Effectiveness of massage therapy as co-adjuvant treatment to exercise in osteoarthritis of the knee: A randomized control trial. *Journal of Back and Musculoskeletal Rehabilitation*, 27(4), 521–529.

Cowen, V. S., & Tafuto, B. (2018). Integration of massage therapy in outpatient cancer care. *International Journal of Therapeutic Massage & Bodywork*, 11(1), 4–10.

Craig, L. H., Svircev, A., Haber, M., & Juncos, J. L. (2006). Controlled pilot study of the effects of neuromuscular therapy in patients with Parkinson disease. *Movement Disorders*, 21(12), 2127–2133.

Crane, J. D., Ogborn, D. I., Cupido, C, Melov, S., Hubbard, A., Bourgeois, J. M., & Tarnopolsky, M. A. (2012). Massage therapy attenuates inflammatory signaling after exercise-induced muscle damage. *Science Translational Medicine*, 4(119), 119ra113.

Crawford, S. K., Haas, C., Butterfield, T. A., Wang, Q., Zhang, X., Zhao, Y., & Best, T. M. (2014). Effects of immediate vs. delayed massage-like loading on skeletal muscle viscoelastic properties following eccentric exercise. *Clinical Biomechanics*, 29(6), 671–678.

Cyganska, A., Truszczynska-Baszak, A., & Tomaszewski, P. (2020). Impact of Exercises and Chair Massage on Musculoskeletal Pain of Young Musicians. *International Journal of Environmental Research and Public Health,* 17(14), 5128.

Darabpour, S., Kheirkhah, M., & Ghasemi, E. (2016). Effects of Swedish massage on the improvement of mood disorders in women with breast cancer undergoing radiotherapy. *Iranian Red Crescent Medical Journal,* 18(11), e25461.

Davis, M. P., & Srivastava, M. (2003). Demographics, assessment and management of pain in the elderly. *Drugs Aging,* 20(1), 23–57.

Delaney, J. P., Leong, K. S., Watkins, A., & Brodie, D. (2002). The short-term effects of myofascial trigger point massage therapy on cardiac autonomic tone in healthy subjects. *Journal of Advanced Nursing,* 37(4), 364–371.

Demir, B., & Saritas, S. (2020a). Effect of hand massage on pain and anxiety in patients after liver transplantation: A randomised controlled trial. *Complementary Therapies in Clinical Practice,* 39, 101152.

Demir, B., & Saritas, S. (2020b). Effects of massage on vital signs, pain and comfort levels in liver transplant patients. *Explore (NY),* 16(3), 178–184.

de Oliveira, F. R., Visnardi Goncalves, L. C., Borghi, F., da Silva, L. G. R. V., Gomes, A. E., Trevisan, G., et al. (2018). Massage therapy in cortisol circadian rhythm, pain intensity, perceived stress index and quality of life of fibromyalgia syndrome patients. *Complementary Therapies in Clinical Practice,* 30, 85–90.

Devoogdt, N., Christiaens, M. R., Geraerts, I., Truijen, S., Smeets, A., Leunen, K., et al. (2011). Effect of manual lymph drainage in addition to guidelines and exercise therapy on arm lymphoedema related to breast cancer: Randomised controlled trial. *British Medical Journal,* 343, d5326.

Diego, M. A., Field, T., Hernandez-Reif, M., Shaw, K., Friedman, L., & Ironson, G. (2001). HIV adolescents show improved immune function following massage therapy. *International Journal of Neuroscience,* 106(1–2), 35–45.

Diego, M. A., Field, T., Sanders, C., & Hernandez-Reif, M. (2004). Massage therapy of moderate and light pressure and vibrator effects on EEG and heart rate. *International Journal of Neuroscience,* 114(1), 31–44.

Dilaveri, C. A., Croghan, I. T., Mallory, M. J., Dion, L. J., Fischer, K. M., Schroeder, D. R., et al. (2020). Massage compared with massage plus acupuncture for breast cancer patients undergoing reconstructive surgery. *Journal of Alternative and Complementary Medicine,* 26(7), 602–609.

Dillon, R. S. (1983). Improved serum insulin profiles in diabetic individuals who massaged their insulin injection sites. *Diabetes Care,* 6(4), 399–401.

Dion, L. J., Engen, D. J., Lemaine, V., Lawson, D. K., Brock, C. G., Thomley, B. S., et al. (2016). Massage therapy alone and in combination with meditation for breast cancer patients undergoing autologous tissue reconstruction: A randomized pilot study. *Complementary Therapies in Clinical Practice,* 23, 82–87.

Donoyama, N., & Ohkoshi, N. (2012). Effects of traditional Japanese massage therapy on various symptoms in patients with Parkinson disease: A case-series study. *Journal of Alternative and Complementary Medicine,* 18(3), 294–299.

Donoyama, N., Satoh, T., Hamano, T., Ohkoshi, N., & Onuki, M. (2018). Effects of Anma therapy (Japanese massage) on health-related quality of life in gynecologic cancer survivors: A randomized controlled trial. *PLoS One,* 13(5), e0196638.

Donoyama, N., Suoh, S., & Ohkoshi, N. (2014). Effectiveness of Anma massage therapy in alleviating physical symptoms in outpatients with Parkinson's disease: A before-after study. *Complementary Therapies in Clinical Practice,* 20(4), 251–261.

Drust, B., Atkinson, G., Gregson, W., French, D., & Binningsley, D. (2003). The effects of massage on intra muscular temperature in the vastus lateralis in humans. *International Journal of Sports Medicine,* 24(6), 395–399.

Duval C, Lafontaine, D., Hebert, J., Leroux, A., Panisset, M., & Boucher, J. P. (2002). The effect of Trager therapy on the level of evoked stretch responses in patients with Parkinson's disease and rigidity. *Journal of Manipulative and Physiological Therapeutics,* 25(7), 455–464.

Efe Arslan, D., & Kilic Akca, N. (2020). The effect of aromatherapy hand massage on distress and sleep quality in hemodialysis patients: A randomized controlled trial. *Complementary Therapies in Clinical Practice,* 39, 101136.

Efe Arslan, D., Kutluturkan, S., & Korkmaz, M. (2019). The effect of aromatherapy massage on knee pain and functional status in participants with osteoarthritis. *Pain Management Nursing,* 20(1), 62–69.

Ejindu, A. (2007). The effects of foot and facial massage on sleep induction, blood pressure, pulse and respiratory rate: Crossover pilot study. *Complementary Therapies in Clinical Practice,* 13(4), 266–275.

El Hage, Y., Politti, F., Herpich, C. M., de Souza, D. F. M., de Paula Gomes, C. A. F., Amorim, C. F., et al. (2013). Effect of facial massage on static balance in individuals with temporomandibular disorder—a pilot study. *International Journal of Therapeutic Massage & Bodywork,* 6(4), 6–11.

El-Hafez, H. M., Hamdy, H. A., Takla, M. K., Ahmed, S. E. B., Genedy, A. F., & Abd El-Azeim, A. S. S. (2020). Instrument-assisted soft tissue mobilisation versus stripping massage for upper trapezius myofascial trigger points. *Journal of Taibah University Medical Sciences,* 15(2), 87–93.

Elkins, G., Rajab, M. H., & Marcus, J. (2005). Complementary and alternative medicine use by psychiatric inpatients. *Psychological Reports,* 96(1), 163–166.

Ernst, E. (1998). Does post-exercise massage treatment reduce delayed onset muscle soreness? A systematic review. *British Journal of Sports Medicine,* 32(3), 212–214.

Ernst, E. (1999). Massage therapy for low back pain: A systematic review. *Journal of Pain and Symptom Management,* 17(1), 65–69.

Espí-López, G. V., Monzani, L., Gabaldon-Garcia, E., & Zurriaga, R. (2020). The beneficial effects of therapeutic craniofacial massage on quality of life, mental health and menopausal symptoms and body image: A randomized controlled clinical trial. *Complementary Therapies in Medicine,* 51, 102415.

Fazeli, M. S., Pourrahmat, M., Liu, M., Guan, L., & Collet, J. (2016). The effect of head massage on the regulation of the cardiac autonomic nervous system: A pilot randomized crossover trial. *Journal of Alternative and Complementary Medicine,* 22(1), 75–80.

Fernandez-Lao, C., Cantarero-Villanueva, I., Diaz-Rodriguez, L., Fernandez-de-las-Penas, C., Sanchez-Salado, C., & Arroyo-Morales, M. (2012). The influence of patient attitude toward massage on pressure pain sensitivity and immune system after application of myofascial release in breast cancer survivors: A randomized, controlled crossover study. *Journal of Manipulative and Physiological Therapeutics,* 35(2), 94–100.

Ferry, P., Johnson, M., & Wallis, P. (2002). Use of complementary therapies and non-prescribed medication in patients with Parkinson disease. *Postgraduate Medical Journal,* 78(924), 612–614.

Field, T. (1995). Massage therapy for infants and children. *Journal of Developmental and Behavioral Pediatrics,* 16(2), 105–111.

Field, T. (2002). Violence and touch deprivation in adolescents. *Adolescence,* 37(148), 735–749.

Field, T. (2005). Massage therapy for skin conditions in young children. *Dermatologic Clinics,* 23(4), 717–721.

Field, T. (2016a). Knee osteoarthritis pain in the elderly can be reduced by massage therapy, yoga and tai chi: A review. *Complementary Therapies in Clinical Practice,* 22, 87–92.

Field, T. (2016b). Massage therapy research review. *Complementary Therapies in Clinical Practice,* 24, 19–31.

Field, T. (2019). Pediatric massage therapy research: A narrative review. *Children (Basel),* 6(6), 78.

Field, T., Delage, J., & Hernandez-Reif, M. (2003). Movement and massage therapy reduce fibromyalgia pain. *Journal of Bodywork and Movement Therapies,* 7(1), 49–52.

Field, T., Diego, M., Cullen, C., Hernandez-Reif, M., Sunshine, W., & Douglas, S. (2002). Fibromyalgia pain and substance P decrease and sleep improves after massage therapy. *Journal of Clinical Rheumatology,* 8(2), 72–76.

Field, T., Diego, M., Delgado, J., Garcia, D., & Funk, C. G. (2011). Hand pain is reduced by massage therapy. *Complementary Therapies in Clinical Practice,* 17(4), 226–229.

Field, T., Diego, M., Delgado, J., Garcia, D., & Funk, C. G. (2013). Rheumatoid arthritis in upper limbs benefits from moderate pressure massage therapy. *Complementary Therapies in Clinical Practice*, 19(2), 101–103.

Field, T., Diego, M., Gonzalez, G., & Funk, C. G. (2014). Neck arthritis pain is reduced and range of motion is increased by massage therapy. *Complementary Therapies in Clinical Practice*, 20(4), 219–223.

Field, T., Diego, M., Gonzalez, G., & Funk, C. G. (2015). Knee arthritis pain is reduced and range of motion is increased following moderate pressure massage therapy. *Complementary Therapies in Clinical Practice*, 21(4), 233–237.

Field, T., Diego, M., & Hernandez-Reif, M. (2010). Prenatal depression effects and interventions: A review. *Infant Behavior and Development*, 33(4), 409–418.

Field, T., Diego, M., Hernandez-Reif, M., Dieter, J. N. I., Kumar, A. M., Schanberg, S., & Kuhn, C. (2008). Insulin and insulin-like growth factor-1 increased in preterm neonates following massage therapy. *Journal of Developmental and Behavioral Pediatrics*, 29(6), 463–466.

Field, T., Henteleff, T., Hernandez-Reif, M., Martinez, E., Mavunda, K., Kuhn, C., & Schanberg, S. (1998). Children with asthma have improved pulmonary functions after massage therapy. *The Journal of Pediatrics*, 132(5), 854–858.

Field, T., Peck, M., Hernandez-Reif, M., Krugman, S., Burman, I., & Ozment-Schenck, L. (2000). Postburn itching, pain, and psychological symptoms are reduced with massage therapy. *Journal of Burn Care & Rehabilitation*, 21(3), 189–193.

Finch, P. (2004). The motivation of massage therapy students to enter professional education. *Medical Teacher*, 26(8), 729–731.

Finch, P. (2009). A qualitative investigation into why the motivation of massage therapy students changes over the course of their professional education. *International Journal of Therapeutic Massage & Bodywork*, 2(1), 3–7.

Ganji, R. (2019). Aromatherapy massage: A promising non-pharmacological adjuvant treatment for osteoarthritis knee pain. *The Korean Journal of Pain*, 32(2), 133–134.

Genik, L. M., McMurtry, C. M., Marshall, S., Rapoport, A., & Stinson, J. (2020). Massage therapy for symptom reduction and improved quality of life in children with cancer in palliative care: A pilot study. *Complementary Therapies in Medicine*, 48, 102263.

Gentile, D., Boselli, D., O'Neill, G., Yaguda, S., Bailey-Dorton, C., & Eaton, T. A. (2018). Cancer Pain Relief After Healing Touch and Massage. *Journal of Alternative and Complementary Medicine*, 24(9-10), 968–973.

Gönenç, I. M., & Terzioglu, F. (2020). Effects of massage and acupressure on relieving labor pain, reducing labor time, and increasing delivery satisfaction. *Journal of Nursing Research*, 28(1), e68.

Guzzetta, A., Baldini, S., Bancale, A., Baroncelli, L., Ciucci, F., Ghirri, P., et al. (2009). Massage accelerates brain development and the maturation of visual function. *The Journal of Neuroscience*, 29(18), 6042–6051.

Guzzetta, A., D'Acunto, M. G., Carotenuto, M., Berardi, N., Bancale, A., Biagioni, A., et al. (2011). The effects of preterm infant massage on brain electrical activity. *Developmental Medicine & Child Neurology*, 53(Suppl. 4), 46–51.

Haas, C., Best, T. M., Wang, Q., Butterfield, T. A., & Zhao, Y. (2012). In vivo passive mechanical properties of skeletal muscle improve with massage-like loading following eccentric exercise. *The Journal of Biomechanics*, 45(15), 2630–2636.

Haas, C., Butterfield, T. A., Abshire, S., Zhao, Y., Zhang, X., Jarjoura, D., & Best, T. M. (2013b). Massage timing affects postexercise muscle recovery and inflammation in a rabbit model. *Medicine & Science in Sports & Exercise*, 45(6), 1105–1112.

Haas, C., Butterfield, T. A., Zhao, Y., Zhang, X., Jarjoura, D., & Best, T. M. (2013a). Dose-dependency of massage-like compressive loading on recovery of active muscle properties following eccentric exercise: Rabbit study with clinical relevance. *British Journal of Sports Medicine*, 47(2), 83–88.

Hadfield, N. (2001). The role of aromatherapy massage in reducing anxiety in patients with malignant brain tumours. *International Journal of Palliative Nursing*, 7(6), 279–285.

Hall, H., Munk, N., Carr, B., Fogarty, S., Cant, R., Holton, S., et al. (2021). Maternal mental health and partner-delivered massage: A pilot study. *Women Birth*, 34(3), e237–e247.

Han, N. R., Moon, P. D., Yoou, M. S., Chang, T. S., Kim, H. M., & Jeong, H. J. (2018). Effect of massage therapy by VOSKIN 125+ painkiller(R) on inflammatory skin lesions. *Dermatologic Therapy*, 31(5), e12628.

Hand, M., Margolis, J., & Staffileno, B. A. (2019). Massage chair sessions: Favorable effects on ambulatory cancer center nurses' perceived level of stress, blood pressure, and heart rate. *Clinical Journal of Oncology Nursing*, 23(4), 375–381.

Happe, S., Peikert, A., Siegert, R., & Evers, S. (2016). The efficacy of lymphatic drainage and traditional massage in the prophylaxis of migraine: A randomized, controlled parallel group study. *Neurological Sciences*, 37(10), 1627–1632.

Harrison, T. M., Brown, R., Duffey, T., Frey, C., Bailey, J., Nist, M. D., et al. (2020). Effects of massage on postoperative pain in infants with complex congenital heart disease. *Nursing Research*, 69(5S Suppl. 1), S36–S46.

Hart, S., Field, T., Hernandez-Reif, M., Nearing, G., Shaw, S., Schanberg, S., et al. (2001). Anorexia nervosa symptoms are reduced by massage therapy. *Journal of Eating Disorders*, 9(4), 289–299.

Haun, J. N., Graham-Pole, J., & Shortley, B. (2009). Children with cancer and blood diseases experience positive physical and psychological effects from massage therapy. *International Journal of Therapeutic Massage & Bodywork*, 2(2), 7–14.

Hennenfent, B. R., & Feliciano, A. E. (1998). Changes in white blood cell counts in men undergoing thrice-weekly prostatic massage, microbial diagnosis and antimicrobial therapy for genitourinary complaints. *The British Journal of Urology*, 81(3), 370–376.

Hennenfent, B. R., Lazarte, A. R., & Feliciano, A. E., Jr. (2006). Repetitive prostatic massage and drug therapy as an alternative to transurethral resection of the prostate. *Medscape General Medicine*, 8(4), 19.

Hernandez-Reif, M., Field, T., Ironson, G., Beutler, J., Vera, Y., Hurley., J., et al. (2005). Natural killer cells and lymphocytes increase in women with breast cancer following massage therapy. *International Journal of Neuroscience*, 115(4), 495–510.

Hernandez-Reif, M., Field, T., Krasnegor, J., & Theakston, H. (2001). Lower back pain is reduced and range of motion increased after massage therapy. *International Journal of Neuroscience*, 106(3–4), 131–145.

Hildebrandt, P. (1991). Subcutaneous absorption of insulin in insulin-dependent diabetic patients. Influence of species, physico-chemical properties of insulin and physiological factors. *Danish Medical Bulletin*, 38(4), 337–346.

Hinds, T., McEwan, I., Perkes, J., Dawson, E., Ball, D., & George, K. (2004). Effects of massage on limb and skin blood flow after quadriceps exercise. *Medicine & Science in Sports & Exercise*, 36(8), 1308–1313.

Ho, S. S. M., Kwong, A. N. L., Wan, K. W. S., Ho, R. M. L., & Chow, K. M. (2017). Experiences of aromatherapy massage among adult female cancer patients: A qualitative study. *Journal of Clinical Nursing*, 26(23–24), 4519–4526.

Hoffmann, D. S., Dancing, D., & Rosenbaum, M. (2019). Massage and medicine: An interprofessional approach to learning musculoskeletal anatomy and enhancing personal wellness. *Academic Medicine*, 94(6), 885–892.

Holst, S., Lund, I., Petersson, M., & Uvnas-Moberg, K. (2005). Massage-like stroking influences plasma levels of gastrointestinal hormones, including insulin, and increases weight gain in male rats. *Autonomic Neuroscience: Basic and Clinical*, 120(1–2), 73–79.

Hong, C. Z. (2002). New trends in myofascial pain syndrome. *Zhonghua Yi Xue Za Zhi (Taipei)*, 65(11), 501–512.

Horner, P., Abshari, S., & Grove, C. (2020). Massage: An alternative approach to pain management. *Nursing*, 50(4), 17–19.

Hovind, H., & Nielsen, S. L. (1974). Effect of massage on blood flow in skeletal muscle. *Scandinavian Journal of Rehabilitation Medicine*, 6(2), 74–77.

Hsu, W. C., Guo, S. E., & Chang, C. H. (2019). Back massage intervention for improving health and sleep quality among intensive care unit patients. *Nursing in Critical Care*, 24(5), 313–319.

Hunt, E. R., Confides, A. L., Abshire, S. M., Dupont-Versteegden, E. E., & Butterfield, T. A. (2019). Massage increases satellite cell number independent of the age-associated alterations in sarcolemma permeability. *Physiological Reports*, 7(17), e14200.

Izgu, N., Metin, Z. G., Karadas, C., Ozdemir, L., Cetin, N., & Demirci, U. (2019). Prevention of chemotherapy-induced peripheral neuropathy with classical massage in breast cancer patients receiving paclitaxel: An assessor-blinded randomized controlled trial. *The European Journal of Oncology Nursing*, 40, 36–43.

Jackson, J. L., Fogerite, S. G., Glass, O., Bechard, E., Ali, A., Njike, V. Y., et al., (2019). Efficacy and safety of massage for osteoarthritis of the knee: A randomized clinical trial. *Journal of General Internal Medicine*, 34, 444.

James, H., Castaneda, L., Miller, M. E., & Findley, T. (2009). Rolfing structural integration treatment of cervical spine dysfunction. *Journal of Bodywork and Movement Therapies*, 13(3), 229–238.

Jeffs, E. (2006). Treating breast cancer-related lymphoedema at the London haven: Clinical audit results. *The European Journal of Oncology Nursing*, 10(1), 71–79.

Jones, J. F., Maloney, E. M., Boneva, R. S., Jones, A. B., & Reeves, W. C. (2007). Complementary and alternative medical therapy utilization by people with chronic fatiguing illnesses in the United States. *BMC Complementary and Alternative Medicine*, 7, 12.

Juberg, M., Jerger, K. K., Allen, K. D., Dmitrieva, N. O., Keever, T., Perlman, A. I. (2015). Pilot study of massage in veterans with knee osteoarthritis. *Journal of Alternative and Complementary Medicine*, 21(6), 333–338.

Kalichman, L. (2010). Massage therapy for fibromyalgia symptoms. *Rheumatology International*, 30(9), 1151–1157.

Kanitz, J. L., Reif, M., Rihs, C., Krause, I., & Seifert, G. (2015). A randomised, controlled, single-blinded study on the impact of a single rhythmical massage (anthroposophic medicine) on wellbeing and salivary cortisol in healthy adults. *Complementary Therapies in Medicine*, 23(5), 685–692.

Karagozoglu, S., & Kahve, E. (2013). Effects of back massage on chemotherapy-related fatigue and anxiety: Supportive care and therapeutic touch in cancer nursing. *Applied Nursing Research*, 26(4), 210–217.

Kargarfard, M., Lam, E. T. C., Shariat, A., Shaw, I., Shaw, B. S., & Tamrin, S. B. M. (2016). Efficacy of massage on muscle soreness, perceived recovery, physiological restoration and physical performance in male bodybuilders. *Journal of Sports Sciences*, 34(10), 959–965.

Kassolik, K., Andrzejewski, W., Dziegiel, P., Jelen, M., Fulawka, L., Brzozowski, M.,

et al. (2013). Massage-induced morphological changes of dense connective tissue in rat's tendon. *Folia Histochemica et Cytobiologica*, 51(1), 103–106.

Kassolik, K., Kurpas, D., Wilk, I., Uchmanowicz, I., Hyzy, J., & Andrzejewski, W. (2014). The effectiveness of massage in therapy for obturator nerve dysfunction as complication of hip joint alloplasty-case report. *Rehabilitation Nursing Journal*, 39(6), 311–320.

Kawabata, N., Hata, A., & Aoki, T. (2020). Effect of aromatherapy massage on quality of sleep in the palliative care ward: A randomized controlled trial. *Journal of Pain and Symptom Management*, 59(6), 1165–1171.

Kaye, A. D., Kaye, A. J., & Swinford, J., Baluch, A., Bawcom, B. A., Lambert, T. J., & Hoover, J. M. (2008). The effect of deep-tissue massage therapy on blood pressure and heart rate. *Journal of Alternative and Complementary Medicine*, 14(2), 125–128.

Kennedy, A. B., Cambron, J. A., Dexheimer, J. M., Trilk, J. L., & Saunders, R. P. (2018). Advancing health promotion through massage therapy practice: A cross-sectional survey study. *Preventive Medicine Reports*, 11, 49–55.

Khilnani, S., Field, T., Hernandez-Reif, M., & Schanberg, S. (2003). Massage therapy improves mood and behavior of students with attention-deficit/hyperactivity disorder. *Adolescence*, 38(152), 623–638.

Kim, I. H., Kim, T. Y., & Ko, Y. W. (2016). The effect of a scalp massage on stress hormone, blood pressure, and heart rate of healthy female. *The Journal of Physical Therapy Science*, 28(10), 2703–2707.

Kim, S. K., Min, A., Jeon, C., Kim, T, Cho, S., Lee, S. C., & Lee, C. K. (2020). Clinical outcomes and cost-effectiveness of massage chair therapy versus basic physiotherapy in lower back pain patients: A randomized controlled trial. *Medicine (Baltimore)*, 99(12), e19514.

Kim, S. R., Lee, T. Y., Kim, M. S., Lee, M. C., & Chung, S. J. (2009). Use of complementary and alternative medicine by Korean patients with Parkinson's disease. *Clinical Neurology and Neurosurgery*, 111(2), 156–160.

King, H. H. (2016). Japanese massage improves shoulder range of motion in elderly patients with late-stage Parkinson disease. *Journal of Osteopathic Medicine*, 116(10), 683–684.

Kinkead, B., Schettler, P. J., Larson, E. R., Carroll, D., Sharenko, M., Nettles, J., et al. (2018). Massage therapy decreases cancer-related fatigue: Results from a randomized early phase trial. *Cancer*, 124(3), 546–554.

Kobayashi, M., Kako, J., Kajiwara, K., Oosono, Y., & Noto, H. (2020). Response to "Effect of aromatherapy massage on quality of sleep in the palliative care ward: Randomized Controlled Trial." *Journal of Pain and Symptom Management*, 60(2), e106–e107.

Kong, L. J., Bannuru, R. R., Yuan, W. A., Cheng, Y., & Fang, M. (2011). Therapeutic massage on pain relief for fibromyalgia: A

systematic review and meta-analysis. *Arthritis & Rheumatology*, 63(10), S747.

Kozak, L., Vig, E., Simons, C., Eugenio, E., Collinge, W., & Chapko, M. (2013). A feasibility study of caregiver-provided massage as supportive care for Veterans with cancer. *The Journal of Supportive Oncology*, 11(3), 133–143.

Kshettry, V. R., Carole, L. F., Henly, S. J., Sendelbach, S., & Kummer, B. (2006). Complementary alternative medical therapies for heart surgery patients: Feasibility, safety, and impact. *The Annals of Thoracic Surgery*, 81(1), 201–205.

Kudo, Y., & Sasaki, M. (2020). Effect of a hand massage with a warm hand bath on sleep and relaxation in elderly women with disturbance of sleep: A crossover trial. *Japan Journal of Nursing Science*, 17(3), e12327.

Kukimoto, Y., Ooe, N., & Ideguchi, N. (2017). The effects of massage therapy on pain and anxiety after surgery: A systematic review and meta-analysis. *Pain Management Nursing*, 18(6), 378–390.

Kuriyama, H., Watanabe, S., Nakaya, T., Shigemori, I., Kita, M., Yoshida, N., et al. (2005). Immunological and psychological benefits of aromatherapy massage. *Evidence-Based Complementary and Alternative Medicine*, 2(2), 179–184.

Lacomba, M. T., Sánchez, M. J. Y., Goñi, A. Z., Merino, D. P., del Moral, O. M., Téllez, E. C., & Mogollón, E. M. (2010). Effectiveness of early physiotherapy to prevent lymphoedema after surgery for breast cancer: Randomised, single blinded, clinical trial. *British Medical Journal*, 340, b5396.

Lamas, K., Hager, C., Lindgren, L., Wester, P., & Brulin, C. (2016). Does touch massage facilitate recovery after stroke? A study protocol of a randomized controlled trial. *BMC Complementary and Alternative Medicine*, 16, 50.

Laosee, O., Sritoomma, N., Wamontree, P., Rattanapan, C., & Sitthi-Amorn, C. (2020). The effectiveness of traditional Thai massage versus massage with herbal compress among elderly patients with low back pain: A randomised controlled trial. *Complementary Therapies in Medicine*, 48, 102253.

Lasocki, S., Moncho, R., Bontemps, J., Verger, X., Tellier, A. C., Gergaud, S., et al. (2020). Massage therapy reduces arterial puncture-induced pain: The randomized cross-over bi-center TORREA study. *Intensive Care Medicine*, 46(1), 138–139.

Lavelle, E. D., Lavelle, W., & Smith, H. S. (2007). Myofascial trigger points. *Medical Clinics of North America*, 91(2), 229–239.

Lawrence, M. M., Van Pelt, D. W., Confides, A. L., Hunt, E. R., Hettinger, Z. R., Laurin, J. L., et al. (2020). Massage as a mechanotherapy promotes skeletal muscle protein and ribosomal turnover but does not mitigate muscle atrophy during disuse in adult rats. *Acta physiologica (Oxford, England)*, 229(3), e13460.

LeBlanc-Louvry, I., Costaglioli, B., Boulon, C., Leroi, A. M., & Ducrotte, P. (2002). Does mechanical massage of the abdominal wall after colectomy reduce postoperative pain and shorten the duration of ileus? results of a randomized study. *Journal of Gastrointestinal Surgery*, 6(1), 43–49.

Lee, Y. (2016). Principle study of head meridian acupoint massage to stress release via grey data model analysis. *Evidence-Based Complementary and Alternative Medicine*, 2016, 4943204.

Levine, E. G., & Silver, B. (2007). A pilot study: Evaluation of a psychosocial program for women with gynecological cancers. *Journal of Psychosocial Oncology*, 25(3), 75–98.

Linde, B., & Philip, A. (1989). Massage-enhanced insulin absorption—increased distribution or dissociation of insulin? *Diabetes Research*, 11(4), 191–194.

Lindgren, L., Rundgren, S., Winso, O., Lehtipalo, S., Wiklund, U., Karlsson, M., et al. (2010). Physiological responses to touch massage in healthy volunteers. *Autonomic Neuroscience: Basic and Clinical*, 158(1–2), 105–110.

Listing, M., Krohn, M., Liezmann, C., Kim, I., Reisshauer, A., Peters, E., et al. (2010). The efficacy of classical massage on stress perception and cortisol following primary treatment of breast cancer. *Archives of Women's Mental Health*, 13(2), 165–173.

Li, Q., Becker, B., Wernicke, B., Chen, Y., Zhang, Y., Li, R., et al. (2019). Foot massage evokes oxytocin release and activation of orbitofrontal cortex and superior temporal sulcus. *Psychoneuroendocrinology*, 101, 193–203.

Liu, F., Shen, C., Yao, L., & Li, Z. (2018). Acupoint massage for managing cognitive alterations in older adults: A systematic review and meta-analysis. *Journal of Alternative and Complementary Medicine*, 24(6), 532–540.

Liu, Y., Xu, S., Yan, J., Shen, G., Sun, W., Chew, Y., et al. (2004). Capillary blood flow with dynamical change of tissue pressure caused by exterior force. *Sheng Wu Yi Xue Gong Cheng Xue Za Zhi*, 21(5), 699–703.

Losito, J. M., & O'Neil, J. (1997). Rehabilitation of foot and ankle injuries. *Clinics in Podiatric Medicine and Surgery*, 14(3), 533–557.

Lucia, S. P., & Richard, J. F. (1933). Effects of massage on blood platelet production. *Proceedings of the Society for Experimental Biology and Medicine*, 31, 87.

Lucini, D., Malacarne, M., Solaro, N., Busin, S., & Pagani, M. (2009). Complementary medicine for the management of chronic stress: Superiority of active versus passive techniques. *Journal of Hypertension*, 27(12), 2421–2428.

Lyu, W. B., Gao, Y., Cheng, K. Y., Wu, R., & Zhou, W. Q. (2019). Effect of self-acupoint massage on blood glucose level and quality of life in older adults with type 2 diabetes mellitus: A randomized controlled trial. *Journal of Gerontological Nursing*, 45(8), 43–48.

MacDonald, G. (1998). Massage as a respite intervention for primary caregivers. *American Journal of Hospice and Palliative Medicine*, 15(1), 43–47.

MacDonald, G. (2014). Massage therapy in cancer care: An overview of the past, present, and future. *Alternative Therapies in Health and Medicine*, 20(Suppl. 2), 12–15.

Major, B., Rattazzi, L., Brod, S., Pilipović, I., Leposavić, G., & D'Acquisto, F. (2015). Massage-like stroking boosts the immune system in mice. *Scientific Reports*, 5, 10913.

Massingill, J., Jorgensen, C., Dolata, J., & Sehgal, A. R. (2018). Myofascial massage for chronic pain and decreased upper extremity mobility after breast cancer surgery. *International Journal of Therapeutic Massage & Bodywork*, 11(3), 4–9.

Mazlum, S., Chaharsoughi, N. T., Banihashem, A., & Vashani, H. B. (2013). The effect of massage therapy on chemotherapy-induced nausea and vomiting in pediatric cancer. *Iranian Journal of Nursing and Midwifery Research*, 18(4), 280–284.

McClurg, D., Hagen, S., Jamieson, K., Dickinson, L., Paul, L., & Cunnington, A. (2016a). Abdominal massage for the alleviation of symptoms of constipation in people with Parkinson: A randomised controlled pilot study. *Age Ageing*, 45(2), 299–303.

McClurg, D., & Lowe-Strong, A. (2011). Does abdominal massage relieve constipation? *Nursing Times*, 107(12), 20–22.

McClurg, D., Walker, K., Aitchison, P., Jamieson, K., Dickinson, L., Paul, L., et al. (2016b). Abdominal massage for the relief of constipation in people with parkinson: A qualitative study. *Parkinson's Disease*, 2016, 4842090.

McFeeters, S., Pront, L., Cuthbertson, L., & King, L. (2016). Massage, a complementary therapy effectively promoting the health and wellbeing of older people in residential care settings: A review of the literature. *International Journal of Older People Nursing*, 11(4), 266–283.

McNicol, K., Taunton, J. E., & Clement, D. B. (1981). Iliotibial tract friction syndrome in athletes. *Canadian Journal of Applied Sport Sciences*, 6(2), 76–80.

McQuillan, D. J. (2010). Massage therapy education online: Student satisfaction and achievement: Part I. *International Journal of Therapeutic Massage & Bodywork*, 3(2), 3–13.

Melillo, N., Corrado, A., Quarta, L., D'Onofrio, F., Trotta, A., & Cantatore, F. P. (2005). [Fibromyalgic syndrome: New perspectives in rehabilitation and management. A review]. *Minerva Medica*, 96(6), 417–423.

Menard, M. B. (2014). Choose wisely: The quality of massage education in the United States. *International Journal of Therapeutic Massage & Bodywork*, 7(3), 7–24.

Mercado, N. M., Collier, T. J., Sortwell, C. E., & Steece-Collier, K. (2017). BDNF in the aged brain: Translational implications for Parkinson disease. *Austin Neurology & Neurosciences*, 2(2), 1021.

Merchant, S. J., & Chen, S. L. (2015). Prevention and management of lymphedema after breast cancer treatment. *Breast Journal*, 21(3), 276–284.

Miake-Lye, I. M., Mak, S., Lee, J., Luger, T., Taylor, S. L., Shanman, R., et al. (2019). Massage for pain: An evidence map. *Journal of Alternative and Complementary Medicine*, 25(5), 475–502.

Miladinia, M., Baraz, S., Shariati, A., & Malehi, A. S. (2017). Effects of slow-stroke back massage on symptom cluster in adult patients with acute leukemia: Supportive care in cancer nursing. *Cancer Nursing*, 40(1), 31–38.

Mindell, J. A., Lee, C. I., Leichman, E. S., & Rotella, K. N. (2018). Massage-based bedtime routine: Impact on sleep and mood in infants and mothers. *Sleep Medicine*, 41, 51–57.

Miura, N., Akitsuki, Y., Sekiguchi, A., & Kawashima, R. (2013). Activity in the primary somatosensory cortex induced by reflexologic stimulation is unaffected by pseudo-information: A functional magnetic resonance imaging study. *BMC Complementary and Alternative Medicine*, 13, 114.

Miyahara, Y., Jitkritsadakul, O., Sringean, J., Aungkab, N., Khongprasert, S., & Bhidayasiri, R. (2018). Can therapeutic Thai massage improve upper limb muscle strength in Parkinson disease? An objective randomized-controlled trial. *Journal of Traditional and Complementary Medicine*, 8(2), 261–266.

Miyaji, A., Sugimori, K., & Hayashi, N. (2018). Short- and long-term effects of using a facial massage roller on facial skin blood flow and vascular reactivity. *Complementary Therapies in Medicine*, 41, 271–276.

Mizrak Sahin, B., Culha, I., Gursoy, E., & Yalcin, O. T. (2021). Effect of massage with lavender oil on postoperative pain level of patients who underwent gynecologic surgery: A randomized, placebo-controlled study. *Holistic Nursing Practice*, 35(4), 221–229.

Mok, E., & Woo, C. P. (2004). The effects of slow-stroke back massage on anxiety and shoulder pain in elderly stroke patients. *Complementary Therapies in Nursing & Midwifery*, 10(4), 209–216.

Momeni, M., Arab, M., Dehghan, M., & Ahmadinejad, M. (2020). The effect of foot massage on pain of the intensive care patients: A parallel randomized single-blind controlled trial. *Evidence-Based Complementary and Alternative Medicine*, 2020, 3450853.

Moraska, A. (2005). Sports massage: A comprehensive review. *Journal of Sports Medicine and Physical Fitness*, 45(3), 370–380.

Moraska, A. F., Hickner, R. C., Rzasa-Lynn, R., Shah, J. P., Hebert, J. R., & Kohrt, W. M. (2018). Increase in lactate without change in nutritive blood flow or glucose at active trigger points following massage: A randomized clinical trial. *Archives of Physical Medicine and Rehabilitation*, 99(11), 2151–2159.

Moraska, A. F., Stenerson, L., Butryn, N., Krutsch, J. P., Schmiege, S. J., & Mann, J. D. (2015). Myofascial trigger point–focused head and neck massage for recurrent tension-type headache: A randomized, placebo-controlled clinical trial. *The Clinical Journal of Pain*, 31(2), 159–168.

Morelli, M., Chapman, C. E., & Sullivan, S. J. (1999). Do cutaneous receptors contribute to the changes in the amplitude of the H-reflex during massage? *Electroencephalography and Clinical Neurophysiology*, 39(7), 441–447.

Morelli, M., Seaborne, D. E., & Sullivan, S. J. (1990). Changes in h-reflex amplitude during massage of the triceps surae in healthy subjects. *Journal of Orthopaedic & Sports Physical Therapy*, 12(2), 55–59.

Morelli, M., Seaborne, D. E., & Sullivan, S. J. (1991). H-reflex modulation during manual muscle massage of human triceps surae. *Archives of Physical Medicine and Rehabilitation*, 72(11), 915–919.

Morelli, M., Sullivan, S. J., & Chapman, C. E. (1998). Inhibitory influence of soleus massage onto the medial gastrocnemius h-reflex. *Electroencephalography and Clinical Neurophysiology*, 38(2), 87–93.

Morhenn, V., Beavin, L. E., & Zak, P. J. (2012). Massage increases oxytocin and reduces adrenocorticotropin hormone in humans. *Alternative Therapies in Health and Medicine*, 18(6), 11–18.

Mori, H., Ohsawa, H., Tanaka, T. H., Taniwaki, E., Leisman, G., & Nishijo, K. (2004). Effect of massage on blood flow and muscle fatigue following isometric lumbar exercise. *Medical Science Monitor*, 10(5), CR173–CR178.

Morikawa, Y., Takamoto, K., Nishimaru, H., Taguchi, T., Urakawa, S., Sakai, S., et al. (2017). Compression at myofascial trigger point on chronic neck pain provides pain relief through the prefrontal cortex and autonomic nervous system: A pilot study. *Frontiers in Neuroscience*, 11, 186.

Morris, C. R., Bowen, L., & Morris, A. J. (2005). Integrative therapy for fibromyalgia: Possible strategies for an individualized treatment program. *Southern Medical Journal*, 98(2), 177–184.

Moyer, C. A., Rounds, J., & Hannum, J. W. (2004). A meta-analysis of massage therapy research. *Psychological Bulletin*, 130(1), 3–18.

Munk, N. (2013). Case reports: A meaningful way for massage practice to inform research and education. *International Journal of Therapeutic Massage & Bodywork*, 6(3), 3–5.

Munk, N., Dyson-Drake, J., & Mastnardo, D. (2019). What should we do different, more, start and stop? Systematic collection and dissemination of massage education stakeholder views from the 2017 alliance for massage therapy educational congress. *International Journal of Therapeutic Massage & Bodywork*, 12(1), 29–39.

Murota, M., Iwawaki, Y., Uebaba, K., Yamamoto, Y., Takishita, Y., Harada, K., et al. (2016). Physical and psychological effects of head treatment in the supine position using specialized Ayurveda-based techniques. *Journal of Alternative and Complementary Medicine*, 22(7), 526–532.

Musial, F., & Weiss, T. (2014). The healing power of touch: The specificity of the "unspecific" effects of massage. *Forschende Komplementärmedizin*, 21(5), 282–283.

Nakano, H., Kodama, T., Ueda, T., Mori, I., Tani, T., & Murata, S. (2019). Effect of hand and foot massage therapy on psychological factors and EEG activity in elderly people requiring long-term care: A randomized cross-over study. *Brain Science*, 9(3), 54.

Nasiri, A., & Mahmodi, M. A. (2018). Aromatherapy massage with lavender essential oil and the prevention of disability in ADL in patients with osteoarthritis of the knee: A randomized controlled clinical trial. *Complementary Therapies in Clinical Practice*, 30, 116–121.

Nelson, N. L. (2015). Massage therapy: Understanding the mechanisms of action on blood pressure. A scoping review. *Journal of the American Society of Hypertension*, 9(10), 785–793.

Nelson, N. L., & Churilla, J. R. (2017). Massage therapy for pain and function in patients with arthritis: A systematic review of randomized controlled trials. *American Journal of Physical Medicine & Rehabilitation*, 96(9), 665–672.

Neu, M., Pan, Z., Workman, R., Marcheggiani-Howard, C., Furuta, G., & Laudenslager, M. L. (2014). Benefits of massage therapy for infants with symptoms of gastroesophageal reflux disease. *Biological Research for Nursing*, 16(4), 387–397.

Offenbacher, M., & Stucki, G. (2000). Physical therapy in the treatment of fibromyalgia. *Scandinavian Journal of Rheumatology*, 113, 78–85.

Okvat, H. A., Oz, M. C., Ting, W., & Namerow, P. B. (2002). Massage therapy for patients undergoing cardiac catheterization. *Alternative Therapies in Health and Medicine*, 8(3), 68–70, 72, 74–75.

Oumeish, Y. O. (2005). The cultural and philosophical aspects of pressure, massage, and touch healing as alternative therapies. *Skinmed*, 4(2), 93–100.

Pan, Y. Q., Yang, K. H., Wang, Y. L., Zhang, L. P., & Liang, H. Q. (2014). Massage interventions and treatment-related side effects of breast cancer: A systematic review and meta-analysis. *International Journal of Clinical Oncology*, 19(5), 829–841.

Park, J., Shim, J., Kim, S., Namgung, S., Ku, I., Cho, M., et al. (2017). Application of massage for ankle joint flexibility and balance. *The Journal of Physical Therapy Science*, 29(5), 789–792.

Pehlivan, S., & Karadakovan, A. (2019). Effects of aromatherapy massage on pain, functional state, and quality of life in an elderly individual with knee osteoarthritis. *Japan Journal of Nursing Science*, 16(4), 450–458.

Pepino, V. C., Ribeiro, J. D., Ribeiro, M. A., de Noronha, M., Mezzacappa, M. A., & Schivinski, C. I. (2013). Manual therapy for childhood respiratory disease: A systematic review. *Journal of Manipulative and Physiological Therapeutics*, 36(1), 57–65.

Perez, E. M., Carrara, H., Bourne, L., Berg, A., Swanevelder, S., & Hendricks, M. K. (2015). Massage therapy improves the development of HIV-exposed infants living in a low socio-economic, peri-urban community of South Africa. *Infant Behavior and Development*, 38, 135–146.

Perlman, A., Fogerite, S. G., Glass, O., Bechard, E., Ali, A., Njike, V. Y., et al. (2019). Efficacy and safety of massage for osteoarthritis of the knee: A randomized clinical trial. *Journal of General Internal Medicine*, 34(3), 379–386.

Perlman, A. I., Sabina, A., Williams, A. L., Njike, V. Y., & Katz, D. L. (2006). Massage therapy for osteoarthritis of the knee: Randomized controlled trial. *Archives of Internal Medicine*, 166(22), 2533–2538.

Pinar, R., & Afsar, F. (2015). Back massage to decrease state anxiety, cortisol level, blood pressure, heart rate and increase sleep quality in family caregivers of patients with cancer: A randomised controlled trial. *Asian Pacific Journal of Cancer Prevention*, 16(18), 8127–8133.

Piovesan, E. J., Di Stani, F., Kowacs, P. A., Mulinari, R. A., Radunz, V. H., Utiumi, M., et al. (2007). Massaging over the greater occipital nerve reduces the intensity of migraine attacks: Evidence for inhibitory trigemino-cervical convergence mechanisms. *Arquivos de Neuro-Psiquiatria*, 65(3A), 599–604.

Price, C. (2005). Body-oriented therapy in recovery from child sexual abuse: An efficacy study. *Alternative Therapies in Health and Medicine*, 11(5), 46–57.

Price, C. (2007). Dissociation reduction in body therapy during sexual abuse recovery. *Complementary Therapies in Clinical Practice*, 13(2), 116–128.

Qingguang, Z., Min, F., Li, G., Shuyun, J., Wuquan, S., Jianhua, L., & Yong, L. (2015). Gait analysis of patients with knee osteoarthritis before and after Chinese massage treatment. *Journal of Traditional Chinese Medical Sciences*, 35(4), 411–416.

Rafii, F., Ameri, F., Haghani, H., & Ghobadi, A. (2020). The effect of aromatherapy massage with lavender and chamomile oil on anxiety and sleep quality of patients with burns. *Burns*, 46(1), 164–171.

Rajendran, P. R., Thompson, R. E., & Reich, S. G. (2001). The use of alternative therapies by patients with Parkinson disease. *Neurology*, 57(5), 790–794.

Ranjbaran, M., Khorsandi, M., Matourypour, P., & Shamsi, M. (2017). Effect of massage therapy on labor pain reduction in primiparous women: A systematic review and meta-analysis of randomized controlled clinical trials in Iran. *Iranian Journal of Nursing and Midwifery Research*, 22(4), 257–261.

Rapaport, M. H., Schettler, P., & Breese, C. (2010). A preliminary study of the effects of a single session of Swedish massage on hypothalamic-pituitary-adrenal and immune function in normal individuals. *Journal of Alternative and Complementary Medicine*, 16(10), 1079–1088.

Rapaport, M. H., Schettler, P., & Bresee, C. (2012). A preliminary study of the effects of repeated massage on hypothalamic-pituitary-adrenal and immune function in healthy individuals: A study of mechanisms of action and dosage. *Journal of Alternative and Complementary Medicine*, 18(8), 789–797.

Ratajczak-Wielgomas, K., Kassolik, K., Grzegrzolka, J., Halski, T., Piotrowska, A., Mieszala, K., et al. (2018). Effects of massage on the expression of proangiogenic markers in rat skin. *Folia Histochemica et Cytobiologica*, 1(2), 83–91.

Richards, K. C. (1998). Effect of a back massage and relaxation intervention on sleep in critically ill patients. *American Journal of Critical Care*, 7(4), 288–299.

Rodriguez-Mansilla, J., Gonzalez-Lopez-Arza, M. V., Varela-Donoso, E., Montanero-Fernandez, J., Jimenez-Palomares, M., & Garrido-Ardila, E. M. (2013). Ear therapy and massage therapy in the elderly with dementia: A pilot study. *Journal of Traditional Chinese Medical*, 33(4), 461–467.

Rodriguez-Mansilla, J., Gonzalez-Sanchez, B., Torres-Piles, S., Martin, J. G., Jimenez-Palomares, M., & Bellino, M. N. (2017). Effects of the application of therapeutic massage in children with cancer: A systematic review. *Revista Latino-Americana de Enfermagem*, 25, e2903.

Rosenbaum, M. S., & Velde, J. (2016). The effects of yoga, massage, and reiki on patient wellbeing at a cancer resource center. *Clinical Journal of Oncology Nursing*, 20(3), E77–E81.

Roshanray, A., Rayyani, M., Dehghan, M., & Faghih, A. (2020). Comparative effect of mother's hug and massage on neonatal pain behaviors caused by blood sampling: A randomized clinical trial. *Journal of Tropical Pediatrics*, 66(5), 479–486.

Rosmiarti, M. R., & Murbiah. (2020). Reduction of labour pain with back massage. *Enfermería Clínica*, 30(Suppl. 5), 209–212.

Ruan, D., Li, J., Liu, J., Li, D., Ji, N., Wang, C., et al. (2019). Acupoint massage can effectively promote the recovery of gastrointestinal function after gynecologic laparoscopy. *Journal of Investigative Surgery*, 34(1), 91–95.

Rudnicki, J., Boberski, M., Butrymowicz, E., Niedbalski, P., Ogniewski, P., Niedbalski, M., et al. (2012). Recording of amplitude-integrated electroencephalography, oxygen saturation, pulse rate, and cerebral blood flow during massage of premature infants. *American Journal of Perinatology*, 29(7), 561–566.

Saetung, S., Chailurkit, L. O., & Ongphiphadhanakul, B. (2013). Thai traditional massage increases biochemical markers of bone formation in postmenopausal women: A randomized crossover trial. *BMC Complementary and Alternative Medicine*, 13(1), 69.

Sajedi, F., Kashaninia, Z., Hoseinzadeh, S., & Abedinipoor, A. (2011). How effective is Swedish massage on blood glucose level in children with diabetes mellitus? *Acta Medica Iranica*, 49(9), 592–597.

Sansone, P., & Schmitt, L. (2000). Providing tender touch massage to elderly nursing home residents: A demonstration project. *Geriatric Nursing*, 21(6), 303–308.

Satou, T., Chikama, M., Chikama, Y, Hachigo, M., Urayama, H., Murakami, S., et al. (2013). Effect of aromatherapy massage on elderly patients under long-term hospitalization in Japan. *Journal of Alternative and Complementary Medicine*, 19(3), 235–237.

Sawni, A. (2008). Attention-deficit/hyperactivity disorder and complementary/alternative medicine. *Adolescent Medicine: State of the Art Reviews*, 19(2), 313–326.

Schaub, C., Von Gunten, A., Morin, D., Wild, P., Gomez, P., & Popp, J. (2018). The effects of hand massage on stress and agitation among people with dementia in a hospital setting: A pilot study. *Association for Applied Psychophysiology and Biofeedback*, 43(4), 319–332.

Sefton, J. M., Dexheimer, J., Munk, N., Miccio, R., Kennedy, A. B., Cambron, J., et al. (2020). A research agenda for the massage therapy profession: A report from the massage therapy foundation. *International Journal of Therapeutic Massage & Bodywork*, 13(4), 42–46.

Sefton, J. M., Yarar, C., & Berry, J. W. (2012a). Massage therapy produces short-term improvements in balance, neurological, and cardiovascular measures in older persons. *International Journal of Therapeutic Massage & Bodywork*, 5(3), 16–27.

Sefton, J. M., Yarar, C., & Berry, J. W. (2012b). Six weeks of massage therapy produces changes in balance, neurological and cardiovascular measures in older persons. *International Journal of Therapeutic Massage & Bodywork*, 5(3), 28–40.

Sefton, J. M., Yarar, C., Berry, J. W., & Pascoe, D. D. (2010). Therapeutic massage of the neck and shoulders produces changes in peripheral blood flow when assessed with dynamic infrared thermography. *Journal of Alternative and Complementary Medicine*, 16(7), 723–732.

Sefton, J. M., Yarar, C., Carpenter, D. M., & Berry, J. W. (2011). Physiological and clinical changes after therapeutic massage of the neck and shoulders. *Manual Therapy*, 16(5), 487–494.

Shin, M. S., & Sung, Y. H. (2015). Effects of massage on muscular strength and proprioception after Exercise-induced muscle damage. *The Journal of Strength and Conditioning Research*, 29(8), 2255–2260.

Shoemaker, J. K., Tiidus, P. M., & Mader, R. (1997). Failure of manual massage to alter limb blood flow: Measures by doppler ultrasound. *Medicine & Science in Sports & Exercise*, 29(5), 610–614.

Shor-Posner, G., Hernandez-Reif, M., Miguez, M. J., Fletcher, M., Quintero, N., Baez, J., et al. (2006). Impact of a massage therapy clinical trial on immune status in young dominican children infected with HIV-1. *Journal of Alternative and Complementary Medicine*, 12(6), 511–516.

Shor-Posner, G., Miguez, M. J., Hernandez-Reif, M., Perez-Then, E., & Fletcher, M. (2004). Massage treatment in HIV-1 infected Dominican children: A preliminary report on the efficacy of massage therapy to preserve the immune system in children without antiretroviral medication. *Journal of Alternative and Complementary Medicine*, 10(6), 1093–1095.

Shourabi, P., Bagheri, R., Ashtary-Larky, D., Wong, A., Motevalli, M. S., Hedayati, A., et al. (2020). Effects of hydrotherapy with massage on serum nerve growth factor concentrations and balance in middle aged diabetic neuropathy patients. *Complementary Therapies in Clinical Practice*, 39, 101141.

Silva Gallo, R. B., Santana, L. S., Jorge Ferreira, C. H., Marcolin, A. C., Polineto, O. B., Duarte, G., & Quintana, S. M. (2013). Massage reduced severity of pain during labour: A randomised trial. *Journal of Physiotherapy*, 59(2), 109–116.

Silverdale, N., Wherry, M., & Roodhouse, A. (2019). Massage and reflexology for postoperative cancer cystectomy patients: Evaluation of a pilot service. *Complementary Therapies in Clinical Practice*, 34, 109–112.

Simons, D. G., & Mense, S. (2003). Diagnosis and therapy of myofascial trigger points. *Schmerz*, 17(6), 419–424.

Skillgate, E., Pico-Espinosa, O. J., Cote, P., Jensen, I., Viklund, P., Bottai, M., & Holm, L. W. (2020). Effectiveness of deep tissue massage therapy, and supervised strengthening and stretching exercises for subacute or persistent disabling neck pain. The Stockholm Neck (STONE) randomized controlled trial. *Musculoskeletal Science and Practice*, 45, 102070.

Sliz, D., Smith, A., Wiebking, C., Northoff, G., & Hayley, S. (2012). Neural correlates of a single-session massage treatment. *Brain Imaging and Behavior*, 6(1), 77–87.

Somani, S., Merchant, S., & Lalani, S. (2013). A literature review about effectiveness of massage therapy for cancer pain. *Journal of Pakistan Medical Association*, 63(11), 1418–1421.

Son, S. H., Lee, C. H., Jung, J. H., Kim, D. H., Hong, C. M., & Jeong, J. H. (2019). The preventive effect of parotid gland massage on salivary gland dysfunction during high-dose radioactive iodine therapy for differentiated thyroid cancer: A randomized clinical trial. *Clinical Nuclear Medicine*, 44(8), 625–633.

Sözen, K. K., & Karabulut, N. (2020). Efficacy of hand and foot massage in anxiety and pain management following laparoscopic cholecystectomy: A controlled randomized study. *Surgical Laparoscopy Endoscopy & Percutaneous*, 30(2), 111–116.

Stussman, B. J., Nahin, R. R., Barnes, P. M., & Ward, B. W. (2020). U.S. physician recommendations to their patients about the use of complementary health approaches. *Journal of Alternative and Complementary Medicine*, 26(1), 25–33.

Suoh, S., Donoyama, N., & Ohkoshi, N. (2016). Anma massage (Japanese massage) therapy for patients with Parkinson disease in geriatric health services facilities: Effectiveness on limited range of motion of the shoulder joint. *Journal of Bodywork and Movement Therapies*, 20(2), 364–372.

Supa'at, I., Zakaria, Z., Maskon, O., Aminuddin, A., & Nordin, A. (2013). Effects of Swedish massage therapy on blood pressure, heart rate, and inflammatory markers in hypertensive women. *Evidence-Based Complementary and Alternative Medicine*, 2013, Article ID 171852.

Suresh, S., Wang, S., Porfyris, S., Kamasinski-Sol, R., & Steinhorn, D. M. (2008). Massage therapy in outpatient pediatric chronic pain patients: Do they facilitate significant reductions in levels of distress, pain, tension, discomfort, and mood alterations? *Paediatric Anaesthesia*, 18(9), 884–887.

Sut, N., & Kahyaoglu-Sut, H. (2017). Effect of aromatherapy massage on pain in primary dysmenorrhea: A meta-analysis. *Complementary Therapies in Clinical Practice*, 27, 5–10.

Szuba, A. (2005). Literature watch. The addition of manual lymph drainage to compression therapy for breast cancer related lymphedema: A randomized controlled trial. *Lymphatic Research and Biology*, 3(1), 36–41.

Takamoto, K., Sakai, S., Hori, E., Urakawa, S., Umeno, K., Ono, T., & Nishijo, H. (2009). Compression on trigger points in the leg muscle increases parasympathetic activity of heart rate variability. *The Journal of Physiological Sciences*, 59(3), 191–197.

Taspinar, F., Aslan, U. B., Sabir, N., & Cavlak, U. (2013). Implementation of matrix rhythm therapy and conventional massage in young females and comparison of their acute effects on circulation. *Journal of Alternative and Complementary Medicine*, 19(10), 826–832.

Thanakiatpinyo, T., Suwannatrai, S., Suwannatrai, U., Khumkaew, P., Wiwattamongkol, D., Vannabhum, M., et al. (2014). The efficacy of traditional Thai massage in decreasing spasticity in elderly stroke patients. *Clinical Interventions in Aging*, 9, 1311–1319.

Törnhage, C. J., Skogar, O., Borg, A., Larsson, B., Robertsson, L., Andersson, L., et al. (2013). Short- and long-term effects of tactile massage on salivary cortisol concentrations in Parkinson disease: A randomised controlled pilot study. *BMC Complementary and Alternative Medicine*, 13, 357.

Tosun, B., Unal, N., Yigit, D., Can, N., Aslan, O., & Tunay, S. (2017). Effects of self-knee massage with ginger oil in patients with osteoarthritis: An experimental study. *Research and Theory for Nursing Practice*, 31(4), 379–392.

Toth, M., Marcantonio, E. R., Davis, R. B., Walton, T., Kahn, J. R., & Phillips, R. S. (2013). Massage therapy for patients with metastatic cancer: A pilot randomized controlled trial. *Journal of Alternative and Complementary Medicine*, 19(7), 650–656.

Trujillo, L. (1998). Trigger point relief. *Nurse Practitioner*, 23(2), 119.

Tsai, P. T., Chang, Y. C., & Chen, Y. W. (2016). Connective tissue massage accelerates recovery of facial nerve palsy after orthognathic surgery. *Journal of Dental Sciences*, 11(1), 107–109.

Tsao, J. C. (2007). Effectiveness of massage therapy for chronic, non-malignant pain: A review. *Evidence-Based Complementary and Alternative Medicine*, 4(2), 165–179.

Turan, N., & Ast, T. A. (2016). The effect of abdominal massage on constipation and quality of life. *Gastroenterology Nursing*, 39(1), 48–59.

Türkmen, H., & Oran, N. T. (2021). Massage and heat application on labor pain and comfort: A quasi-randomized controlled experimental study. *Explore*, 17(5), 438–445.

Tütün Yümin, E., Simsek, T. T., Sertel, M., Ankarali, H., & Yumin, M. (2017). The effect of foot plantar massage on balance and functional reach in patients with type II diabetes. *Physiotherapy: Theory and Practice*, 33(2), 115–123.

Urakawa, S., Takamoto, K., Nakamura, T., Sakai, S., Matsuda, T., & Taguchi, T. (2015). Manual therapy ameliorates delayed-onset muscle soreness and alters muscle metabolites in rats. *Physiological Reports*, 3(2), e12279.

Uysal, N., Kutluturkan, S., & Ugur, I. (2017). Effects of foot massage applied in two different methods on symptom control in colorectal cancer patients: Randomised control trial. *International Journal of Nursing Practice*, 23(3), e12532.

Van Dijk, W., Huizink, A. C., Muller, J., Uvnas-Moberg, K., Ekstrom-Bergstrom, A., & Handlin, L. (2020). The effect of mechanical massage and mental training on heart rate variability and cortisol in Swedish employees-a randomized explorative pilot study. *Frontiers in Public Health*, 8, 82.

Vernon, H., Humphreys, K., & Hagino, C. (2007). Chronic mechanical neck pain in adults treated by manual therapy: A systematic review of change scores in randomized clinical trials. *Journal of Manipulative and Physiological Therapeutics*, 30(3), 215–227.

von Stülpnagel, C., Reilich, P., Straube, A., Schäfer, J., Blaschek, A., Lee, S. H., et al. (2009). Myofascial trigger points in children with tension-type headache: A new diagnostic and therapeutic option. *Journal of Child Neurology*, 24(4), 406–409.

Walach, H., Guthlin, C., & Konig, M. (2003). Efficacy of massage therapy in chronic pain: A pragmatic randomized trial. *Journal of Alternative and Complementary Medicine*, 9(6), 837–846.

Wan, X. F., Tang, C. L., Zhao, D. D., An, H. Y., Ma, X., & Qiao, T. X. (2019). Therapeutic effect of massage on denervated skeletal muscle atrophy in rats and its mechanism. *Zhongguo Ying Yong Sheng Li Xue Za Zhi*, 35(3), 223–227.

Wändell, P. E., Arnlov, J., Nixon Andreasson, A., Andersson, K., Tornkvist, L., & Carlsson, A. C. (2013). Effects of tactile massage on metabolic biomarkers in patients with type 2 diabetes. *Journal of Metabolism and Diabetes*, 39(5), 411–417.

Wändell, P. E., Carlsson, A. C., Gafvels, C., Andersson, K., & Tornkvist, L. (2012). Measuring possible effect on health-related quality of life by tactile massage or relaxation in patients with type 2 diabetes. *Complementary Therapies in Medicine*, 20(1–2), 8–15.

Wang, Q., Zeng, H., Best, T. M., Haas, C., Heffner, N. T., Agarwal, S., & Zhao, Y. (2014). A mechatronic system for quantitative application and assessment of massage-like actions in small animals. *Annual Review of Biomedical Engineering*, 42(1), 36–49.

Warpenburg, M. J. (2014). Deep friction massage in treatment of radiation-induced fibrosis: Rehabilitative care for breast cancer survivors. *Journal of Integrative Medicine (Encinitas)*, 13(5), 32–36.

Waters-Banker, C., Dupont-Versteegden, E. E., Kitzman, P. H., & Butterfield, T. A. (2014). Investigating the mechanisms of massage efficacy: The role of mechanical immunomodulation. *Journal of Athletic Training*, 49(2), 266–273.

Weaver, M. S., Riley, B., Wolfe, A., Bace, S., & Wichman, C. (2018). Kneading acceptance: Experiential massage therapy education fosters nursing acceptance of massage therapy for pediatric patients. *Journal of Alternative and Complementary Medicine*, 24(11), 1128–1129.

Weerapong, P., Hume, P. A., & Kolt, G. S. (2005). The mechanisms of massage and effects on performance, muscle recovery and injury prevention. *Sports Medicine*, 35(3), 235–256.

Werner, R. (2010). The massage therapy foundation: Focus on education. *International Journal of Therapeutic Massage & Bodywork*, 3(2), 1–2.

Wikstrom, E. A., Song, K., Lea, A., & Brown, N. (2017). Comparative effectiveness of plantar-massage techniques on postural control in those with chronic ankle instability. *Journal of Athletic Training*, 52(7), 629–635.

Wiktorsson-Möller, M., Oberg, B., Ekstrand, J., & Gillquist, J. (1983). Effects of warming up, massage, and stretching on range of motion and muscle strength in the lower extremity. *The American Journal of Sports Medicine*, 11(4), 249–252.

Williams, N. A., Burnfield, J. M., Paul, S., Wolf, K., & Buster, T. (2019). Therapeutic massage to enhance family caregivers' wellbeing in a rehabilitation hospital. *Complementary Therapies in Clinical Practice*, 35, 361–367.

Wu, J., Yang, X., & Zhang, M. (2017). Massage therapy in children with asthma: A systematic review and meta-analysis. *Evidence-Based Complementary and Alternative Medicine*, 2017, 5620568.

Wu, J. J., Cui, Y., Yang, Y. S., Kang, M. S., Jung, S. C., Park, H. K., et al. (2014). Modulatory effects of aromatherapy massage intervention on electroencephalogram, psychological assessments, salivary cortisol and plasma brain-derived neurotrophic factor. *Complementary Therapies in Medicine*, 22(3), 456–462.

Yao, F., Ji, Q., Zhao, Y., & Feng, J. L. (2007). [Observation on therapeutic effect of point pressure combined with massage on chronic fatigue syndrome]. *Zhongguo Zhen Jiu*, 27(11), 819–820.

Yarar-Fisher, C., Sefton, J. M., & Pascoe, D. D. (2010). Therapeutic massage effects on skin and muscle blood flow. *Medicine & Science in Sports & Exercise*, 42(5).

Yeun, Y. R. (2017). Effectiveness of massage therapy for shoulder pain: A systematic review and meta-analysis. *The Journal of Physical Therapy Science*, 29(5), 936–940.

Young, J. D., Spence, A. J., Power, G., & Behm, D. G. (2018). The addition of transcutaneous electrical nerve stimulation with roller massage alone or in combination did not increase pain tolerance or range of motion. *Journal of Sports Science and Medicine*, 17(4), 525–532.

Yuan, S. L., Matsutani, L. A., & Marques, A. P. (2015). Effectiveness of different styles of massage therapy in fibromyalgia: Systematic review and meta-analysis. *Manual Therapy*, 20(2), 257–264.

Zainuddin, Z., Newton, M., Sacco, P., & Nosaka, Z. (2005). Effects of massage on delayed-onset muscle soreness, swelling, and recovery of muscle function. *Journal of Athletic Training*, 40(3), 174–180.

Zerkle, D., & Gates, E. (2020). The use of massage therapy as a nonpharmacological approach to relieve postlaparoscopic shoulder pain: A pediatric case report. *International Journal of Therapeutic Massage & Bodywork*, 13(2), 45–49.

Zhou, D., Wen, G., Rao, J., Zhao, W., & Zhang, D. (2020). Conditioning effect of traditional Chinese Medicine (TCM) Massage Therapy on lymphocyte immune function and physical and mental health symptoms in sub-healthy population. *Minerva Medica*, S0026(4806).

Zhou, Y., Wei, Y., Zhang, P., Gao, S., Ning, G., Zhang, Z., et al. (2007). The short-term therapeutic effect of the three-part massotherapy for insomnia due to deficiency of both the heart and the spleen—a report of 100 cases. *Journal of Traditional Chinese Medical*, 27(4), 261–264.

Zhu, Q., Li, J., Fang, M., Gong, L., Sun, W., & Zhou, N. (2016). Effect of Chinese massage (Tui Na) on isokinetic muscle strength in patients with knee osteoarthritis. *Journal of Traditional Chinese Medical Sciences*, 36(3), 314–320.

Zimmermann, A., Wozniewski, M., Szklarska, A., Lipowicz, A., & Szuba, A. (2012). Efficacy of manual lymphatic drainage in preventing secondary lymphedema after breast cancer surgery. *Lymphology*, 45(3), 103–112.

REVIEW AND APPLY YOUR KNOWLEDGE

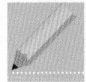

MATCHING ONE: CONCEPT REVIEW

Place the letter of the answer next to the number of the term or phrase that best describes it.

A. Cortisol
B. Dopamine
C. Electromyography
D. Hyperemia
E. Connective tissue effects of massage
F. Heart rate variability
G. Manual lymph drainage
H. Massage therapy
 I. Massage effects in persons with HIV and cancer
J. Lymphatic effects of massage
K. Psychological effects of massage
L. Serotonin

_____ 1. Reddened skin associated with increased blood flow.
_____ 2. Used to assess electrical activity in muscle.
_____ 3. Assessment used as a measure of autonomic nervous system function.
_____ 4. Reduced scar tissue formation, aided in the treatment for tendonitis and ligament injuries, and reduced pain and itching in burn scars.
_____ 5. Neurotransmitter regulating heart rate and blood pressure.
_____ 6. Complementary therapy with one of the highest physician referral rates.
_____ 7. Neurotransmitter regulating mood, appetite, sleep, and memory.
_____ 8. Increased killer T-cell levels and stimulates immune responses.
_____ 9. Reduced edema and increased lymphocyte levels.
_____ 10. A stress hormone.
_____ 11. Reduced anxiety, depression, and stress.
_____ 12. Commonly prescribed modality after breast cancer surgery.

MATCHING TWO: CONCEPT REVIEW

Place the letter of the answer next to the number of the term or phrase that best describes it.

A. Asthma
B. Endorphin
C. Pruritus
D. Eczema
E. Insulin
F. Cardiovascular effects of massage
G. Constipation
H. Mind-body connection
 I. Fibromyalgia
J. Peripheral arterial disease
K. Musculoskeletal effects of massage
L. Doppler

_____ 1. Neurotransmitter that reduces pain.
_____ 2. Increased range of motion.
_____ 3. Studies indicate massage improves this skin condition.
_____ 4. Interrelationship between physical health with the state of one's mind.
_____ 5. Massage may relieve pain and symptoms of this musculoskeletal or nervous system condition.
_____ 6. Massage reduced this gastrointestinal condition.
_____ 7. Instrument used to determine massage had no effect on blood flow within arteries.
_____ 8. Massage is effective for this respiratory condition, especially in children.
_____ 9. Massage may change the production and absorption of this hormone.
_____ 10. Medical term for itching.
_____ 11. Increased capillary flow rate and platelet count.
_____ 12. Massage slowed the progression of this disease through improved superficial circulation.

MULTIPLE CHOICE: TEST YOUR KNOWLEDGE

Place the letter of the answer next to the number of the term or phrase that best describes it.

_____ 1. What percentage of clients that discuss it with their physicians receive a massage recommendation?
  A. 15%
  B. 30%
  C. 50%
  D. 90%

_____ 2. Ongoing research on how to best teach massage is known as:
  A. pedagogy.
  B. promotion.
  C. integration.
  D. investigation.

_____ 3. The most recent research agenda for massage was updated by which group?
  A. American Massage Therapy Association
  B. Associated Bodywork and Massage Professionals
  C. Federation of State Massage Therapy Boards
  D. Massage Therapy Foundation

_____ 4. Decreased pain through massage of trigger points would be an effect on which system?
  A. Musculoskeletal
  B. Cardiovascular
  C. Lymphatic
  D. Endocrine

_____ 5. A literature review of massage on delayed-onset muscle soreness found massages' effect to be:
  A. clinically significant.
  B. clinically insignificant.
  C. greater than expected.
  D. lesser than expected.

_____ 6. An increased capillary flow rate would be an effect on which system?
  A. Musculoskeletal
  B. Cardiovascular
  C. Lymphatic
  D. Endocrine

_____ 7. One study has shown that manual lymphatic drainage may decrease the frequency of which condition?
  A. Migraines
  B. Constipation
  C. Eczema
  D. Excoriation

_____ 8. A decrease of stress, depression, and anxiety would be an effect on which system?
  A. Musculoskeletal
  B. Cardiovascular
  C. Nervous
  D. Lymphatic

_____ 9. A study by Li on foot massage showed an increase in _____ levels and activated regions of the brain associated with emotional touch.
  A. endorphin
  B. dopamine
  C. serotonin
  D. oxytocin

_____ 10. Which type of massage has shown promise in helping relieve symptoms of constipation?
  A. Reflexology massage
  B. Abdominal massage
  C. Thermotherapy
  D. Cryotherapy

_____ 11. Several studies have found massage to improve levels of focus, concentration, and functioning for patients with _____ disorders.
  A. migraine
  B. hyperactivity
  C. depressive
  D. respiratory

_____ 12. Research on fatigue and massage often focuses on improving which important factor of health?
  A. Diet
  B. Exercise
  C. Socialization
  D. Sleep

CRITICAL THINKING

Golden Opportunity

You have an opportunity to give a presentation on massage to a group of physicians. What would you say?

Answers can include but are not limited to:

Massage and other bodywork therapies have evolved over thousands of years, from a simple laying on of hands to the science-based healthcare of today. Throughout these years, massage has been shown to produce beneficial effects for clients. These effects can be specific, such as reduction of lower back pain, or more general such as an overall feeling of wellbeing. The continuing challenge for the profession is to improve our understanding of how massage produces physiologic changes in the body and how to use those changes to benefit our clients. With strong, evidence-informed knowledge, we can meet our goal of providing the best care possible.

Healthcare providers are more commonly including massage as part of an overall approach to address health concerns. Nineteen percent of clients who discussed massage with their healthcare providers received a massage referral, and 61% received a massage recommendation (American Massage Therapy Association [AMTA], 2017). Massage is one of the complementary therapies with the highest physician referral rates. Massage is also rated among physicians as the complementary therapy most likely to be beneficial and least likely to be harmful (Ernst, 1999). This positive outcome has been the result of new scientific knowledge elevating the overall standing of the massage profession in the healthcare, wellness, medical, and rehabilitation communities.

What should also be included are some of the effects of massage on the cardiovascular system, lymphatic system and immunity, musculoskeletal system, connective tissues, nervous system, endocrine system, internal organs, and other systems; psychological aspects; and whole-body effects.

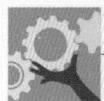

PROFESSIONAL PRACTICE
SOS

For the past few months, Adrienne has been having several health problems. Her physician referred her to Jeremy in hopes that massage would help her relax while waiting for test results. Adrienne explains to Jeremy she has pain in her neck and shoulders, as well as in her lower back. She sometimes feels lightheaded. She has digestive issues ranging from pain in the upper abdomen after eating, to constipation and diarrhea. Sometimes after she eats, she feels nauseated.

She also suspects she has plantar fasciitis because her feet hurt in the morning. During his assessment, Jeremy learns Adrienne works as an administrative assistant, sitting at a desk for 8 hours a day, plus an hour commute in either direction. Which techniques are suitable for Adrienne? Are there any cautions or contraindications to consider? Should Jeremy wait for Adrienne's test results before proceeding with massage? Why or why not?

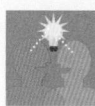

DISCUSSION
Complementary and Integrative Health

CIH stands for *complementary and integrative health*. The National Center for Complementary and Integrative Health (NCCIH) defines CIH as a group of diverse medical and healthcare systems, practices, and products used in conjunction with mainstream Western medicine. The NCCIH classifies CIH therapy into two groups: natural products (e.g., herbs, probiotics) and mind and body practices (e.g., yoga, massage, acupuncture).

Pick one area of CIH, and write a 75-word summary. Be sure to give examples. If available, post your reflections on an Internet-based discussion board monitored by your instructor.

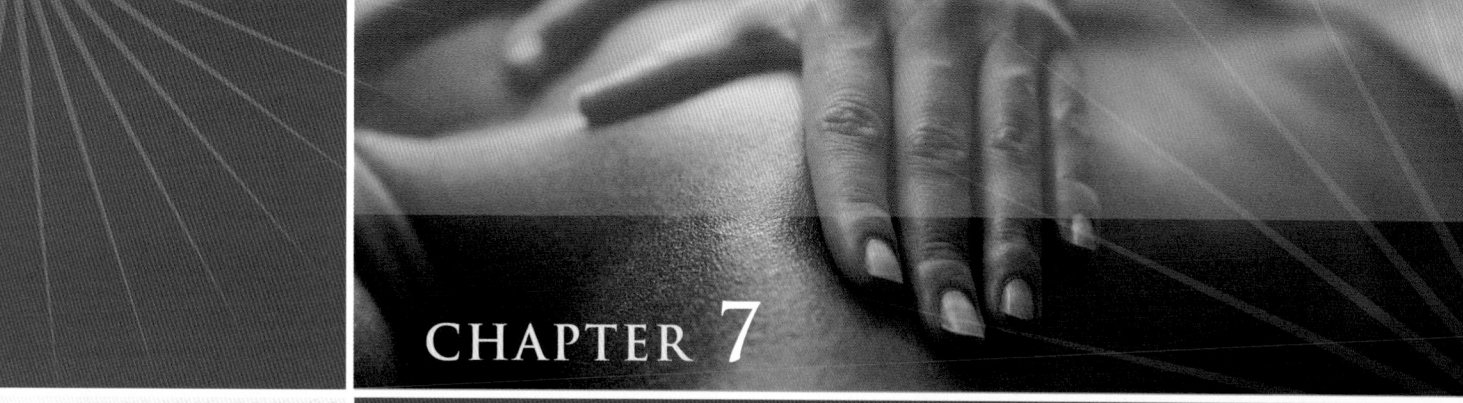

CHAPTER 7

Body Mechanics, Client Positioning, and Draping

The meaning of life is to find your gift. The purpose of life is to give it away.
—Pablo Picasso

LEARNING OBJECTIVES

After completing this chapter, the student should be able to:

1. Define body mechanics and state ways to prepare for the massage physically and mentally.
2. Discuss environmental factors and foot stances to help practitioners provide massage that is safe, energy-conserving, reduces stress and strain on their bodies, and delivers pressure that benefits the client.
3. State application principles and discuss body mechanics used when clients sit in a chair or lying on the floor.
4. Identify client positions and demonstrate use of bolsters for these positions.
5. Demonstrate appropriate draping techniques using sheets and towels, including accessing the abdomen, and while clients turn over on the massage table.

INTRODUCTION

In addition to specific massage techniques, foundations of giving massage are learning and applying effective body mechanics, client positioning, and draping. Effective body mechanics can help practitioners manage physical exhaustion, stress, and strain, both daily and cumulatively, over the span of a career while providing pressure beneficial to clients (Mohr, 2010; Turkeltaub et al., 2014). Using self-care techniques listed in Chapter 4 support the quest for obtaining and maintaining practitioner strength, stamina, and wellbeing. Client positioning helps them receive massage in ways that provide stability during pressure application and facilitate comfort and support through proper body alignment. Clients can receive massage in the prone, supine, side-lying, or seated positions with or without using positioning equipment such as bolsters and pillows. Draping ensures that the client maintains modesty and the professional maintains boundaries while providing warmth and feelings of security. Linens are used to cover the client as well as the massage table, and for positioning equipment such as face rests and bolsters for sanitation purposes.

BODY MECHANICS: PREPARATION, FOOT STANCES, AND APPLICATION PRINCIPLES

Body mechanics encompass the use of one's body that is safe, energy-conserving, and reduces physical stress and strain (Fairchild et al., 2017; Jonas, 2005). This can be accomplished by physical and mental preparation; managing fatigue; a proper workspace; appropriate settings and features of a massage table; wearing suitable attire; and using core stability, gravity, and body weight. Body mechanics also involve the use of foot stances that provide support, balance, and mobility. Effective body mechanics positively influence the massage, decrease practitioner fatigue, and help prevent massage-related injuries.

It is no secret that a 20-year-old massage practitioner is affected differently by giving massages compared with a 50-year-old massage practitioner. In fact, the median age of massage practitioners is 44 years old (American Massage Therapy Association [AMTA], 2020), so as you age, it is wise to adapt your body mechanics and techniques accordingly. Age, body height, shape, and size, previous injuries, or surgeries—they all play a role in determining ideal body mechanics. This concept, **ergonomics,** involves adapting the work to the worker.

Prepare Physically

Approximately 70% of massage practitioners experience work-related musculoskeletal pain (Greene & Goggins, 2006; Jang et al., 2006). Common pain locations are fingers and thumbs, wrists, elbows, and shoulders, followed by the neck and lower back (Albert et al., 2008; Greene & Goggins, 2006; Jang et al., 2006). Practitioners who work at least 6 hours a day or who attend to more than six clients per day are more likely to experience lower back pain (Sathya et al., 2016). Being female is also a risk factor for injury-related work loss, perhaps because females generally have less upper-body strength compared with males (Blau et al., 2013; Miller et al., 1993). Pain, fatigue, and injuries can have a major impact on a massage practitioner's income, and they may cause practitioners to leave the profession and seek less physically demanding employment (Mohr, 2010).

Blau and colleagues (2013) concluded that physical and mental exhaustion had the strongest relationship to work loss from massage-related injuries. This section will include suggestions for preparing physically and mentally while employing strategies that deliver the amount of pressure needed to maximize benefit to the client (Mohr, 2010; Turkeltaub et al., 2014). Prudden (1980) classifies massage as a strenuous occupation (see Table 4.1). To meet the physical demands of the profession, practitioners should follow these commonsense measures.

Participate in Regular Physical Activity

Types of physical activity, or exercise, are cardiorespiratory, resistance, flexibility, and neuromotor, and are discussed in Chapter 4. Recommendations by the American College of Sports Medicine (2011) are as follows. Cardiorespiratory exercise is 150 minutes (2 hours and 30 minutes) to 300 minutes (5 hours) a week of moderate-intensity, or 75 minutes (1 hour and 15 minutes) to 150 minutes (2 hours and 30 minutes) a week of vigorous-intensity physical activity, or an equivalent combination of moderate- and vigorous-intensity activity. Resistance exercise is 2 or 3 nonconsecutive days a week on all major muscle groups. Flexibility exercise is 2 or 3 days a week. Hold each stretch for 10 to 30 seconds to the point of tightness or slight discomfort. Repeat each stretch two to four times, accumulating 60 seconds for each stretch. Neuromotor exercise is 20 to 30 minutes, 2 or 3 days a week.

Eat a Healthy Balanced Diet

Half your plate should be vegetables and fruits, with the other half containing equal portions of whole grains and protein. Drink water, coffee, or tea. Skip sugary drinks, limit milk and dairy products to 1 to 2 servings a day, and limit juice to 1 small glass a day (Harvard School of Public Health [HSPH], 2011). Some health conditions warrant specialized diets; consultation with your healthcare provider is recommended to ensure optimal nutritional health. See Chapter 4 for more detailed information about nutrition.

Get Enough Rest and Sleep

Adults need 7 to 9 hours of sleep per night. Sleep allows the body to rest, recharge, and recover from the day's wear and tear activities (CDC, 2017). Although the amount of sleep is important, good sleep quality is also essential. Indicators of poor sleep quality include not feeling rested even after getting enough sleep, and repeatedly waking up during sleep. Rest and sleep are discussed in Chapter 4.

Warm-Up Before You Start

Consider performing warm-up activities shortly before the first massage, and perhaps repeating them throughout the workday. Warmups should start slowly and easily and include walking or low-intensity activities with the goal of increasing heart and breathing rates. After 5 to 10 minutes, focus on muscles and movements specific to the activity planned (Nadelen, 2010). Recommended activities are featured next. Keep in mind that a systematic review found weak evidence in support of warmups decreasing injury risks (Fradkin et al., 2006).

- **Squats and Lunges**. Maintain a straight spine, keep knees behind the toes, with much of the body's weight in the heels while knees and hips are flexing and extending during squats and lunges. Avoid deep bends if knee problems are present. A wall can be used for balance and support.
- **Over and Under the Fence**. Stand with feet together. Imagine a small fence alongside just below waist height. Step over the imaginary fence sideways by lifting the foot nearest the fence and swinging the foot up, over, and around the fence. Next, put your body weight onto the other foot and squat, then move or duck under the imaginary fence traveling in the same direction. Repeat, moving sideways, in the opposite direction.
- **Shoulder Circles**. Extend your arms out on either side of the body. Move the arms slowly in a circle at the shoulders without moving the elbows or wrists. Begin with small circles, then medium circles, and then larger circles. Repeat these movements in the opposite direction.
- **Wrist Circles**. Flex your elbows 90 degrees with hands in front of you. With your fingers relaxed and extended, circle wrists in one direction, and then reverse direction. Repeat wrist circles in both directions, but this time, close your hands into a fist.
- **Ankle Circles**. While sitting or standing, lift the foot off the ground. Move the ankle slowly in a circle, beginning with small circles, then medium circles, and then larger circles. Repeat these movements in the opposite direction. Perform the same sequence with the other ankle.
- **Spine Flexion and Extension**. While standing, reach overhead toward the ceiling. Flex the hips while bending forward, continuing these movements until the hands are touching or nearly touching the floor. Reverse the movement and, when you stretch the arms overhead, extend the spine slightly, holding this position for a few moments before returning to a neutral standing position with hands back down to the sides of the body. Slightly flex the knees during movements. Spine flexion and extension can be done while sitting in a sturdy chair.
- **Reach and Pull**. While standing and arms at your side, open palms. Next, pull your hands up to your chest while making a fist. Without stopping, reach overhead while extending your fingers and inhaling simultaneously. Reverse direction, bringing your arms back down. Close your hands as you pass your chest, and reopen them as they reach your sides, exhaling forcefully. Keep your pace slow and your movements graceful. Repeat several times but stop immediately if you become lightheaded.

Prepare Mentally

Mental fatigue was a significant risk factor correlated with injury-forced work reduction, just after physical exhaustion (Blau et al., 2013). Massage practitioners should prepare themselves mentally in ways that give their full attention to their clients through mindfulness.

Practice Mindfulness

Mindfulness is heightened self-awareness and focused attention given to present moments characterized by curiosity, openness, acceptance, and engagement (Bishop et al., 2004; Langer, 2000). When practitioners are mindful, they are aware of their external environment: this is **exteroception**, and when awareness is related to the internal environment is called **introception**. Introception includes the perception of physical sensations such as heartbeat, respiration, and physical discomfort. Introception related to body position is **proprioception**. Mindfulness and introception are needed so that massage practitioners can adjust during the massage when they notice physical discomfort in their body. For example, when a practitioner notices discomfort in the neck and shoulders or fatigue in one hand, they can change body position or use the opposite hand to apply the technique.

To become mindful, increase the awareness of your internal experiences (introception), and then shift your awareness to the external environment (exteroception). To increase awareness of the external environment, it helps to actively notice new things. When you notice new things, it puts you in the present. It makes you sensitive to context and perspective. Notice smells, sounds, lighting, and textures. With others, notice how they move, and pay attention to their facial expressions as they talk or while they listen. Mindfulness, awareness, and being curious about people promotes empathy (see Chapter 2 to learn more about nonverbal expressions of empathy).

Environmental Factors

To reduce injury risk and fatigue, and promote efficient body mechanics, evaluate and modify the workspace, including the area around the massage table, placement of the bolsters, flooring, and the massage table. A collection of recommendations is featured next (Abdallah et al., 2015; Anderson, 2018; Carley et al., 2017; Chaudhari, 2017; Greene & Goggins, 2008; Mohr, 2010; Muscolino, 2010).

Area Around the Massage Table

There should be at least 3 feet (1 meter) of open space around all sides of the table for practitioners to stand or sit comfortably in relaxed, efficient, and aligned posture while administering techniques. A workspace of 15 × 10 feet should provide ample room. Remove all unnecessary items from the workspace. If equipment such as hydrocollators or hot stone warming units are occasionally used, consider having them on a sturdy wheeled cart with handles to be moved into the workspace when needed.

Bolster Storage

Stow bolsters in easy-to-access locations between knee and waist height, so they can be accessed without bending or reaching. Store them in areas that do not create a fall risk.

Flooring

Prolonged standing on hard nonyielding surfaces (i.e., tile, stone, concrete, thin carpet over concrete) can contribute to fatigue and conditions such as varicose veins. If possible, perform massage on traditional wood flooring, on carpet with a cushioned backing, or on foam-backed vinyl flooring. Antifatigue mats can be placed around the table.

Massage Table Height

A correct table height allows practitioners to generate sufficient downward force while reducing strain on their bodies. Set the table height to the top of the practitioner's patellae. At this table height, the clients can easily transfer on or off the table. Because most practitioners work with a variety of clients with various widths or girths and use a variety of techniques during a single session and throughout the workday, an electric lift table is recommended—particularly for practitioners with full-time practices. The following guidelines apply for all table types, electric and nonelectric.

- Table height is *higher* when applying low-force, more detailed techniques while seated or standing or while applying techniques using pulling or decompressive forces such as traction.
- Table height is *lower* when applying downward force or compression to utilize gravity and body weight. A lower working height is recommended because most of the massage techniques involve compression.

Massage Table Width

Wider massage tables (≥31 inches) may be more appropriate for side-lying and larger clients. However, wider tables may promote uncomfortable working postures, as they encourage reaching when applying compression. If this situation occurs, ask the client to slide near the table edge toward the side on which you are standing, or opt for a narrower table (27 to 30 inches).

Massage Table Padding

Some practitioners prefer thin and firm padding, stating that less effort is required to apply compression. In contrast, some practitioners prefer soft and plush padding, stating it is easier to apply techniques between the table and the client, or beneath the client's body. Choose a table padding that suits your needs.

Massage Practitioner Attire

Clothing should allow freedom of movement and feel comfortable. However, avoid wearing clothing that is too loose-fitting or baggy, as practitioners may subconsciously lean back to keep clothes from brushing against the client during the massage, creating a less efficient body posture.

Additionally, practitioners may wear breathable or cooling fabrics to avoid overheating. However, research does not support the advantages of wearing synthetic cooling fabrics to improve endurance or compressive garments to reduce fatigue. Hands and wrists should be free of jewelry, and short sleeves are recommended, as many techniques incorporate the use of elbows and forearms. The best footwear for balance, performance, directional control, and productivity are slip-resistant enclosed shoes (i.e., covers all the foot, up to the ankle, without toe or heel holes), soft insoles, arch support, and a depression for the heel.

Foot Stances

For efficient body mechanics, massage practitioners use postures that provide stability, balance, and mobility. These goals are more easily achieved with appropriate foot stances. **Foot stances** are positions of the practitioner's feet used to provide a base of support while applying massage. **Base of support** refers to all points of contact on which an object rests. Each foot makes contact with the ground at three bony points, which include the (1) calcaneal tuberosity, (2) head of the first metatarsal, and (3) head of the fifth metatarsal. The three points make the shape of a triangle, which is the strongest and most stable geometric shape (Fig. 7.1). To ensure you are using all three bony points of contact, lift the toes from the ground while standing or sitting.

Keep in mind that your base of support changes as your body position changes. For example, as you reach to glide down a client's back, your balance changes, requiring a change in the base of support. To offset this imbalance, the

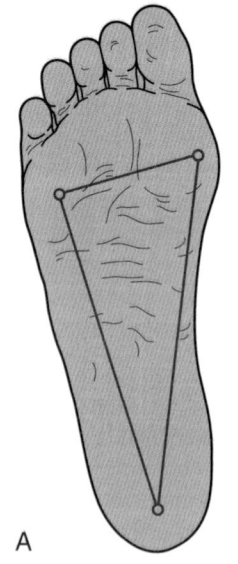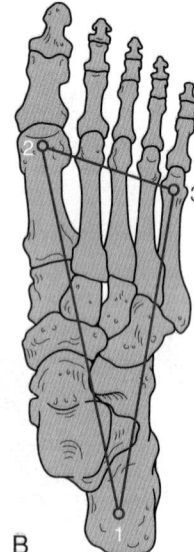

A   B

FIG. 7.1 Foot stances provide the practitioner's base of support with three points of contact with the ground on each foot. (A) Triangular-shaped base of support created by three points of contact on one foot. (B) Three bony points of contact include the calcaneal tuberosity (1); head of first metatarsal (2); and head of fifth metatarsal (3).

practitioner leans forward by bending one or both knees. This moves the base of support closer to the client's body. The practitioner can also widen the base of support by moving the feet further apart; this action also lowers the center of gravity and often further increases stability.

Common foot stances used by massage practitioners are the *archer stance* and the *horse stance* (Beck, 2016; Jonas, 2005). Which stance is used depends on the location and size of the target area(s) to be massaged, the length or excursion of the massage technique(s), the direction the practitioner's body must move to apply the technique(s), and the technique itself. The practitioner's feet and hands often mirror each other; when hand orientation changes, foot placement usually changes to match. In either stance, the hips and abdomen point in the direction of movement. This position helps keep the spine erect and not rotated.

Archer Stance

The **archer stance** is used when the target area(s) of the applied technique is toward one side of the practitioner's body. This stance provides a stable foundation while the practitioner moves or lunges forward or backward while administering more lengthy techniques. Feet are asymmetric and pointing in different directions. For these reasons, the archer stance is also the *staggered stance, asymmetric stance, bow stance,* or *lunge stance.* The foot pointing in the direction of movement is called the "lead" foot, and the foot pointing beneath the table is called the "trailing" foot. The

position of the lead foot is produced by external rotation of the hip; the degree of rotation is between 15 and 90 degrees, depending on the length of the technique the practitioner is using. The associated knee is usually flexed. Feet are hip distance apart or wider. The spine is erect, shoulders relaxed and hips pointing toward the direction of movement, like you are an archer (Fig. 7.2). During technique application, the majority of movement is produced in the lower extremities to move the hands forward rather than flexing the spine and extending the elbows. Lengthy techniques require the practitioner to step forward to reach distal target areas. To accomplish this, lift the trailing foot and place it behind the lead foot. Shift the body weight to the trailing foot momentarily while you step forward with the lead foot. During the step forward, avoid pushing against the client to maintain balance. Done properly, the client will not detect the step forward.

Horse Stance

The **horse stance** is used when the target area(s) of the applied technique is directly in front of the practitioner's body. This stance allows the practitioner to stand in place while administering techniques directly in front of them. Feet are symmetric and pointing in the same direction, usually beneath the massage table. Distance between the feet varies slightly, usually just wider than hip width. Both knees are slightly flexed, and hips are laterally rotated slightly and pointing in the direction of movement, like you are riding on a horse. The practitioner's spine is erect, and shoulders

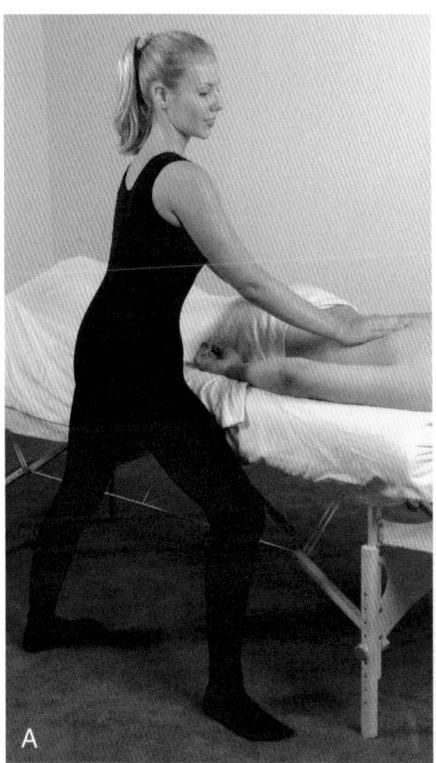 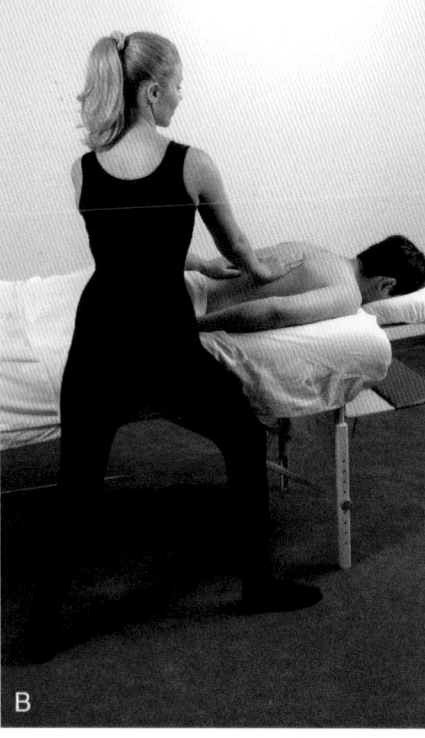 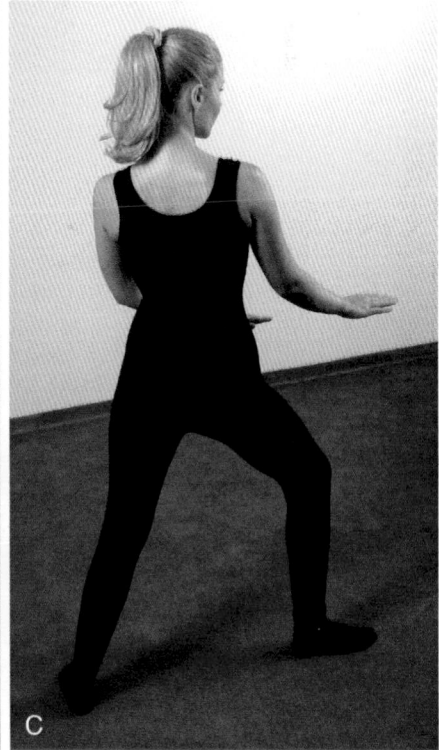

FIG. 7.2 Practitioner in the archer stance. Feet in the archer stance are pointing in different directions with one foot pointing in the direction of movement (*lead foot*) and the other foot pointing beneath the massage table (*trailing foot*). (A) Lateral view. (B) Posterior view. (C) Posterior view without the massage table.

relaxed (Fig. 7.3). As the practitioner's hands move laterally (side to side) or anteriorly and posteriorly (front to back), the practitioner's weight shifts alternately from one foot to the other foot and back to support hand movements. The horse stance is also called the *parallel stance, symmetric stance,* or *warrior stance.*

Application Principles

Once you have prepared physically and mentally, tended to environmental factors, and understand foot stances, apply the following key principles to reduce wear and tear on your body. Because physical exhaustion and fatigue had the strongest relationship to work reduction from massage-related injuries, practitioners should manage these while providing pressure that benefits clients. A few application principles derived from a variety of reliable sources (Blau et al., 2013; CDC, 2020; Fairchild et al., 2017; Greene & Goggins, 2008; Maughan, 2003; Mohr, 2010; Sathya et al., 2016). These principles include engaging the core, stacking the joints, and combining body weight and gravity when applying force, use a variety of techniques, perform some techniques while seated, stay hydrated, rest between clients, and keep a consistent, reasonable workload.

Engage the Core

Core stability is the ability to control the position and motion of the trunk, which allows for optimum production and transfer of force and stabilization during the massage. The core is postural muscles, most of which are centrally located. Core muscles include:

- Muscles of the abdomen
- Muscles of the back or spine, and pelvic floor
- Muscles of the hips and knees (glutes, hamstrings, quads)

Use the following phrases to help you remember the aforementioned structures and how to engage them while administering massage techniques (Kibler et al., 2006; King, 2000).

- **Suck It**. Contract your abdominal muscles, or suck and pull them in toward your spine.
- **Tuck It**. Tilt your pelvis posteriorly to tuck it beneath you.
- **Drop It**. Flex the hips and knees slightly to lower the body.

Engaging the core has several advantages for massage practitioners. Larger and stronger muscles create a stable base as limbs move. The core serves as the generator or "engine"; small changes that occur in the core translate into changes in distal joints, similar to the cracking at the end of a whip. When practitioners rely on core-generated force, distal joints in the wrists and hands are free to deliver skillfully applied techniques. This strategy also helps reduce practitioner fatigue, physical strain, and injury risk.

Stack the Joints

Practitioners should position themselves close to and above the application area and arrange the joints vertically as much as possible when applying compression—this may require

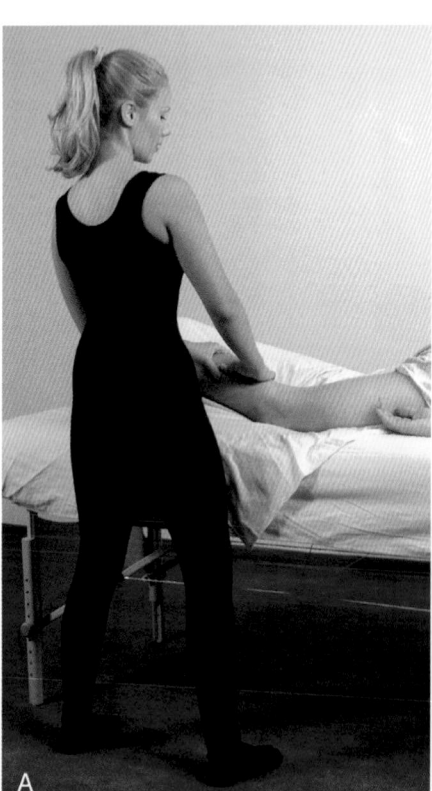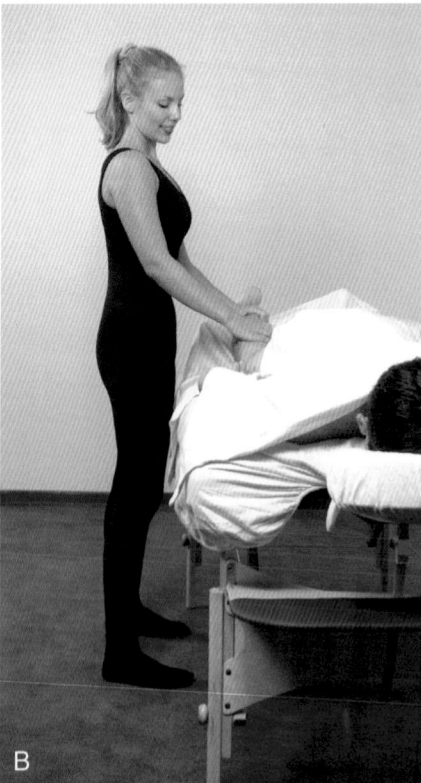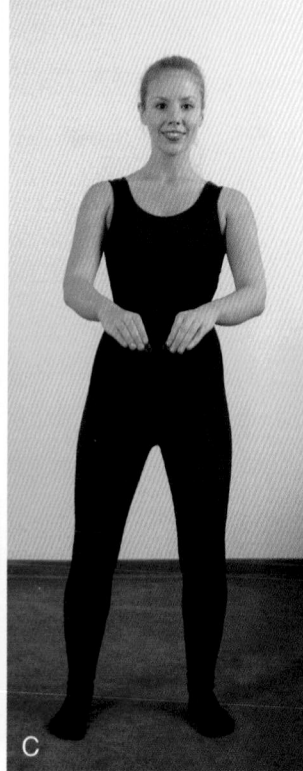

FIG. 7.3 Practitioner in the horse stance. Feet in the horse stance are pointing in the same direction, usually beneath the massage table. (A) Posterolateral view. (B) Lateral view. (C) Anterior view without the massage table.

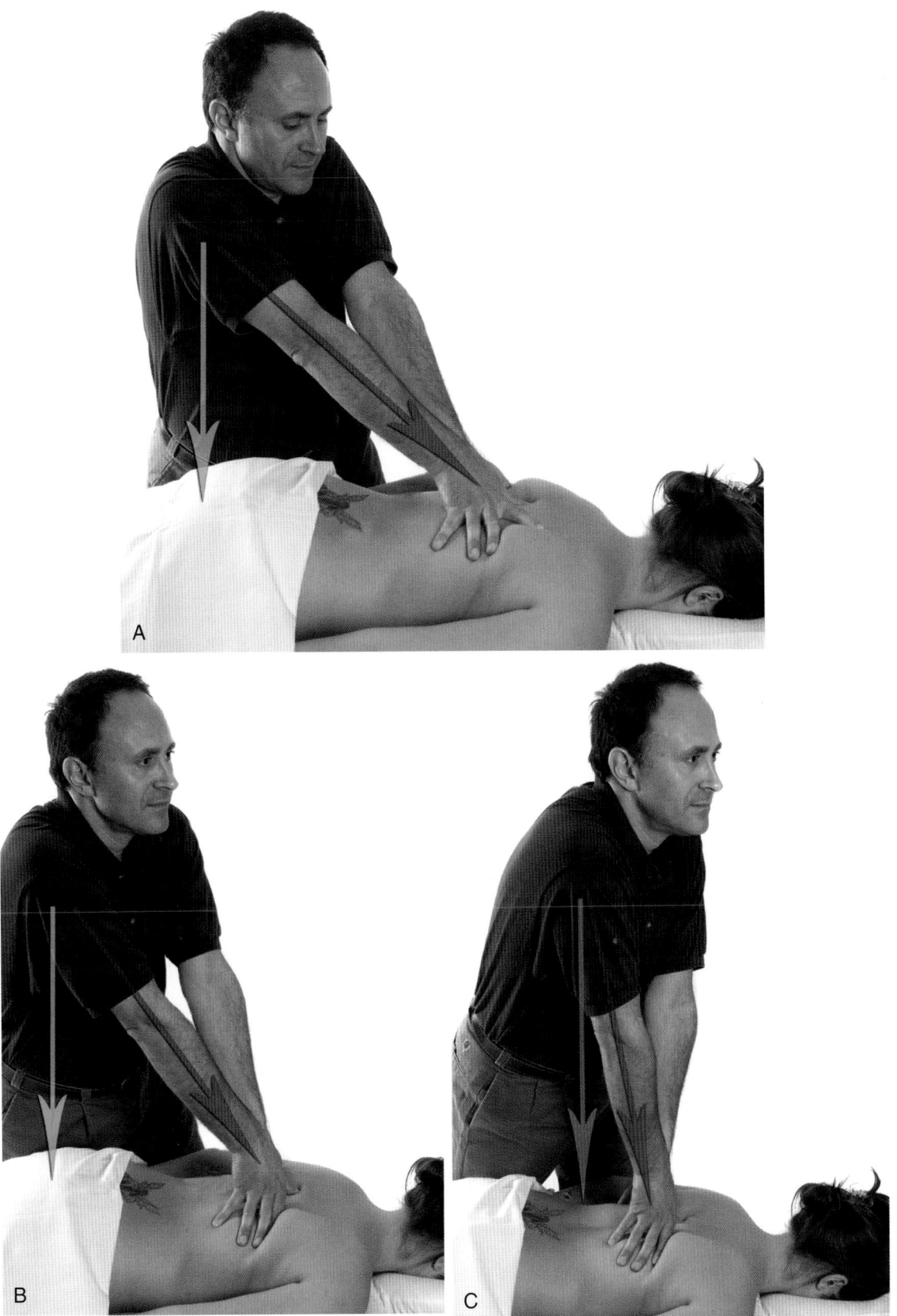

FIG. 7.4 Relationships between table height, gravity *(green arrow)*, and practitioner use of body weight during compression *(purple arrow)* during massage with client laying on (A) a high-height massage table, (B) a medium-height massage table, and (C) a lower-height massage table. Note that the lower-height massage table allows efficient use of gravity and body weight when applying compression. (From Muscolino, J. E. [2009]. *The muscle and bone palpation manual.* St. Louis: Mosby).

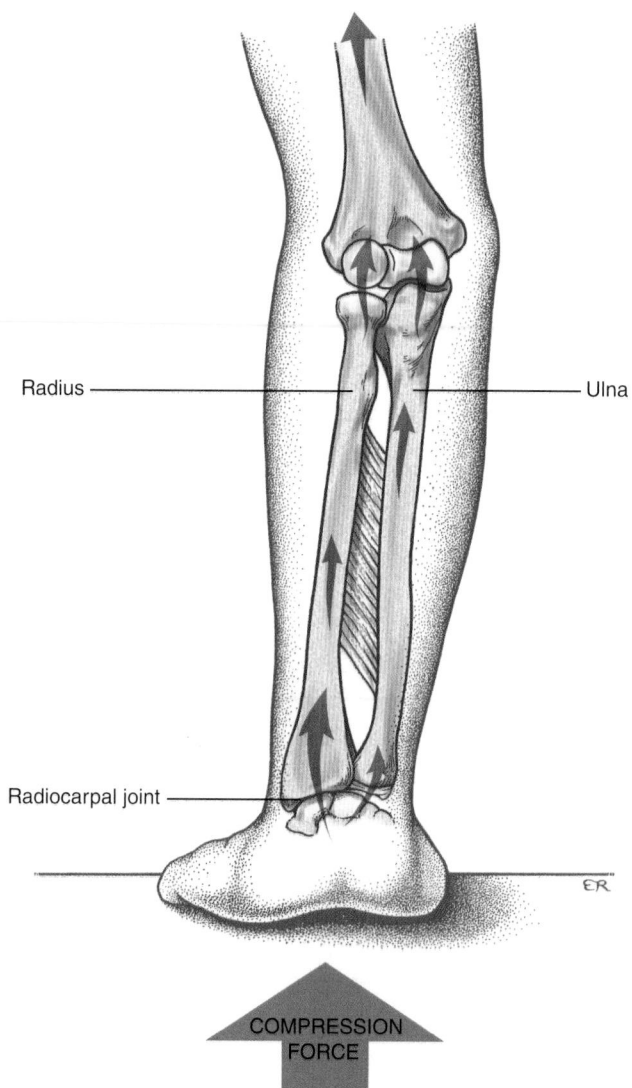

Radius

Ulna

Radiocarpal joint

COMPRESSION FORCE

FIG. 7.5 Compression force through the hand should be transmitted via the radiocarpal joint primarily through the radius to take advantage of its wide distal end. This force then crosses the elbow and is directed toward the shoulder.

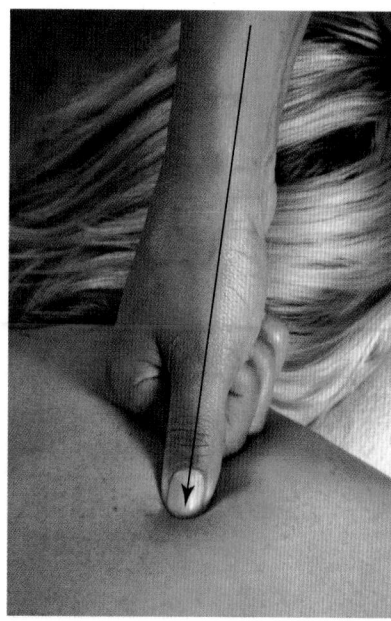

FIG. 7.6 Maintain wrists and finger joints as vertically as possible. If needed, brace the thumb behind a closed fist for joint stability.

a lower-height table (Fig. 7.4). Mohr (2010), Braun and Simonson (2013) call this vertical position "stacking the joints." Once the joints are stacked, the practitioner transfers their weight into the client's soft tissues. While massaging a client in a side-lying position, adjust your body for the best possible use of body weight, which may include using a stool, squatting, or kneeling on the floor.

Compression applied with the forearm should be transmitted with the proximal ulna while keeping the working limb's wrist and hand relaxed. Compression applied with the hand should be transmitted at the radiocarpal joint primarily through the radius located on the left side of the wrist. This strategy takes advantage of the wide distal end of the radius (Fig. 7.5). Compression force applied with the fingers should be transmitted through vertically stacked joints. If needed, support the interphalangeal joint of the thumb behind a closed fist to maintain joint stability (Fig. 7.6). You can use products designed to protect the finger joints.

When applying traction, direct force away from the client's body by pulling. This can be accomplished by positioning the practitioner's body weight distal to the application area. For example, decompress the client's right hip by standing at the foot of the table and grasping the client's right lower extremity above the ankle while leaning back. During the lean, the practitioner's spine should be erect with the core engaged, and the feet positioned in the archer stance. The practitioner's hands should be at a comfortable height during traction application—not reaching too far up or down. In addition, be sure the floor has a nonslip surface.

Use Body Weight and Gravity When Applying Force

Force is a push or pull upon an object resulting from one object's interaction with another. Massage techniques involve application of forces, which cause the client's body to move (if it can move) and soft tissue's to be displaced. Because most massage techniques involve the application of compression, practitioners should use gravity and their body weight instead of muscular contraction. This reduces the risk of physical exhaustion, fatigue, and injury. Types of physical forces and their application in massage techniques are in Chapter 8.

Gravity is the force that pulls objects toward the center of the earth. **Center of gravity** is the exact center of an object's mass (also called *center of mass*). The center of gravity for an average person is in the lower abdomen when standing in an anatomic position. The center of gravity is lower for females because of larger hip mass, and higher for males because of larger shoulder mass.

Position your center of gravity as close as possible to the area of the client's body where you will apply compression. This will allow more efficient use of gravity and practitioner body weight, which will reduce muscular effort and fatigue

(Fairchild et al., 2017). A shorter distance between the center of gravity and the ground is associated with increased balance and stability. Flexing your hips and knees slightly will lower your center of gravity.

Use a Variety of Techniques

Alternate intensive hands-on techniques (e.g., deep tissue, pressure point work) with less intensive hands-on techniques (e.g., passive range-of-motion, Trager). Also, supplement techniques that require little or no hand use (e.g., hydrotherapy, ashiatsu, polarity, reiki).

Perform Some Techniques While Seated

Approximately 25% of the massage should be spent seated; this can reduce fatigue. The client's face, neck, feet, or hands can be massaged while seated, as these areas require less downward force. Practitioners should position their feet in stances similar to those used while standing (see section titled "Foot Stances" for more information).

Stay Hydrated

Drinking water while working reduces the risk of dehydration. Dehydration can lead to fatigue, headaches, constipation, decreased performance, mood changes, unclear thinking, and cause the body to overheat.

To avoid a massage-related injury and ensure career longevity, apply all the body mechanics principles for every massage (Box 7.1).

Rest Between Clients

If possible, leave a minimum of 15 minutes between clients to rest, stretch, drink water, walk around, and mentally "let

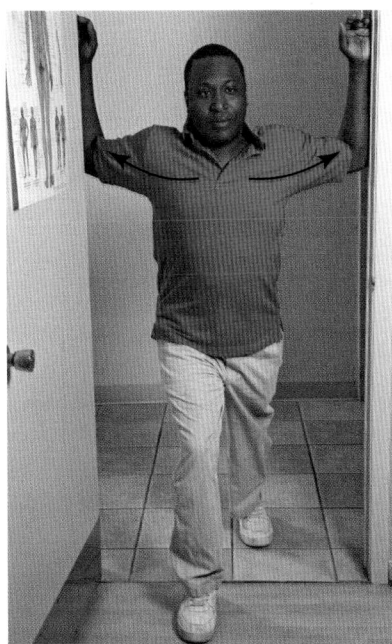

FIG. 7.7 A minimum of 15 minutes is recommended between clients so massage practitioners can rest, stretch, mentally "let go" of the previous client, and be ready for the next one.

go" of the previous client and get ready for the next one. This timeframe allows the practitioner's body to rest and recover from the physicality of massage application (Fig. 7.7).

Keep a Consistent, Reasonable Workload

Try to keep a consistent workload from day-to-day and week-to-week, as sudden increases in physical activity may lead to painful symptoms. Avoid working more than 6 hours a day or on more than six clients a day, as increased hours or clients were associated with a higher risk of lower back pain among massage practitioners.

> *You know the rule: If you are falling, dive. Do the thing that has to be done.*
>
> **—Joseph Campbell**

Body Mechanic Modifications for Clients Sitting or Lying on the Floor

Many of the same body mechanics used while massaging clients lying on a massage table are also applicable when clients are sitting in a chair or lying on a floor mat. Warm up before the session, wear appropriate attire, have ample space around the chair or floor mat, monitor your body with mindful awareness, and adjust when needed. The hips and abdomen should face the direction of movement. Keep the spine erect and use gravity and body weight when applying compression.

For clients in a chair, use the lunge position to apply compression. For clients on the floor, most practitioner postures involve sitting on the heels with knees together or with knees apart. From this position, the practitioner can rise to apply compression. Other positions include crawling, squatting, and lunging. *Crawling* is a natural way of moving around a client lying on a mat. *Squatting* is a posture from

---

BOX 7.1

Body Mechanics Quick Check

Answering the following questions will help you determine correct body mechanics during the massage and what areas might need improvement:

1. Am I prepared physically? Did I warm up before the massage?
2. Am I prepared mentally? Do I feel relaxed and focused?
3. Do I have ample workspace?
4. Is my table height appropriate?
5. Am I wearing appropriate and comfortable attire?
6. Are both feet planted firmly on the ground? Am I using the right foot stance?
7. Is my spine aligned and my core engaged? Is my head erect and not looking down at my hands?
8. Are my joints stacked and my wrists straight? Are my thumbs and fingers supported while applying direct pressure?
9. Am I using gravity and body weight when applying pressure?
10. Am I using a variety of techniques during the massage?
11. Is a stool nearby?
12. Am I staying hydrated and rested between clients?

If you answered *no* to one or more of these questions, then you may be at risk for stress, strain, and injury resulting from poor body mechanics.

which the practitioner can move into other positions easily. *Lunging* is essentially modified squatting and provides a posture to easily reach certain parts of the client's body.

As mentioned previously, practitioners who "stand" while working are at risk for upper extremity pain in the fingers and thumbs, wrists, elbows, and shoulders. Thai massage practitioners who knelt on the floor while working are at risk for pain in the lower back, upper back, and neck (Chumnanya et al., 2013). This suggests that different working postures (i.e., standing vs. kneeling) are correlated with different predispositions of body pain.

CLIENT POSITIONING

Client positioning ensures comfort through proper body alignment, allowing the client to receive a massage in ways that promote stability and enhance the practitioner's body mechanics. Most clients lie down in a **recumbent position**, which usually involves positioning equipment, such as bolsters, strategically placed for client comfort. Client positioning can be modified to address conditions such as gastroesophageal reflux disease (GERD) and respiratory difficulties, further facilitating client comfort. The health questionnaire and interview prior to the massage will help determine which body positions are appropriate and which to avoid. For example, a client in advanced pregnancy requires different positions during the massage as compared with nonpregnant clients. Clients with edema in the feet or lower back discomfort may require bolstering to elevate the lower extremities. Regardless of which positions are selected, always ask the client, "How can you become even more comfortable?" This question allows fine-tuning of client positions to address comfort needs. The primary client positions are:

- **Prone**. Lying with the back or posterior surface of the body facing upward and the chest or anterior surface of the body facing downward (i.e., lying face down).
- **Supine**. Lying with the chest or anterior surface of the body facing upward and the back or posterior surface of the body facing downward (i.e., lying face up). The supine position is the 180-degree contrast to the prone position.
  - **Semireclining**. A modified supine position in which the torso is elevated. In heathcare settings, a semireclining position is called the **Fowler position**, classified according to the degree torso elevation. A *low Fowler* is between 15 and 30 degrees. A *semi-Fowler* is between 30 and 45 degrees. A *standard Fowler* is between 45 and 60 degrees. A *high (full) Fowler* is between 60 and 90 degrees.
- **Side-lying**. Lying on the side, usually with hips and knees flexed. This position is also called the *lateral recumbent position*; left or right lateral recumbent position refers to on which side the client lies.
- **Seated**. Sitting down, usually with the torso erect and knees bent with glutes or buttocks supported.

Bolsters

Bolsters are pillows or cushions of various sizes and densities used for supporting the client in the prone, supine, side-lying,

and seated positions. Sheets, blankets, or towels can be rolled up or stacked and used as bolstering devices. Bolsters should not be on the table as clients transfer on and off its surface. In addition, avoid lifting the client when inserting or removing bolsters, as this can increase the risk of lower back injury of the practitioner.

The most commonly used bolstering device is a tubular-shaped cushion of approximately 26 inches in length and 6 to 8 inches in diameter. Bolsters are usually covered with the same fabric used on massage tables such as polyurethane or vinyl. Cover bolsters with a clean cloth such as a pillowcase or slide the bolster beneath the table drape—avoid contact between the bolster fabric and the client's skin. As mentioned previously, stow bolsters in an easy-to-access location between the practitioner's knee and waist height, so they can be lifted without bending or reaching; do not leave bolsters in areas that could potentially create a fall risk.

Prone Position

When clients are in the prone position, bolsters are placed in front of the ankles with the ankles about hip distance apart (Fig. 7.8). A bolster should be high enough so that the client's toes do not touch the tabletop. A face rest can be used to keep the client's cervical spine in a neutral position. If the face rest frame is adjustable, consider allowing the client to determine the degree of this angle (Fig. 7.9). First, unlock the cams and ask the client to pull the face rest frame up to the face to a comfortable position. Next, lock the cams in place as the client holds the face rest stationary.

Clients with large or tender breasts may require additional supports, such as cushions placed above, below, or between the breasts. This may necessitate adjustment of the face rest frame above the level of the tabletop (Fig. 7.10). Clients with lower back pain may require a pillow under the abdomen or hips to reduce excessive lumbar spine curvature. An arm shelf can be used for client comfort. Alternatively, a linen-draped stool placed under the face rest can serve as an arm shelf.

Supine Position

In the supine position, bolsters are placed behind the cervical spine and the knees, with the knees about hip distance apart (Fig. 7.11). A higher knee bolster (i.e., 8 inches) may be needed if the client is experiencing lower back discomfort.

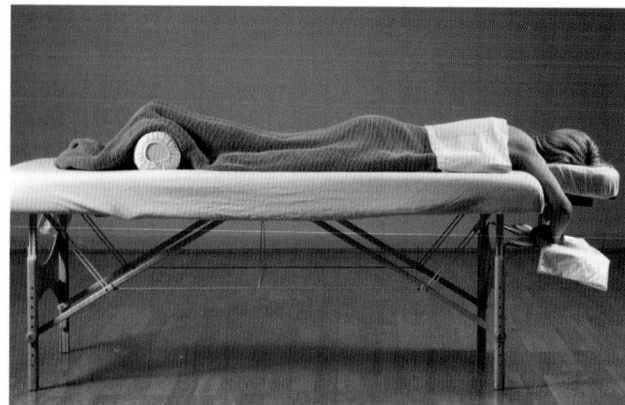

FIG. 7.8 Prone-lying client using a face rest, an arm shelf, and a bolster placed in front of the ankles.

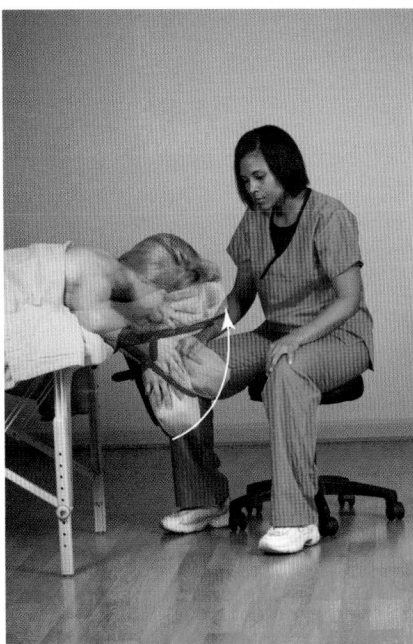

FIG. 7.9 Prone-lying client moving the face rest frame into a comfortable position before the practitioner locks the cams into place.

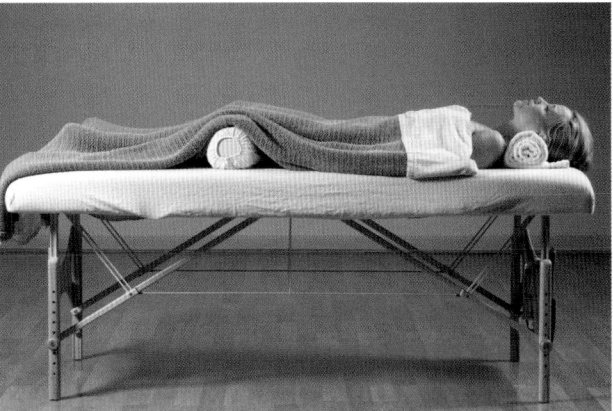

FIG. 7.11 Supine-lying client using a bolster placed behind the knees and a rolled-up towel placed beneath the cervical spine.

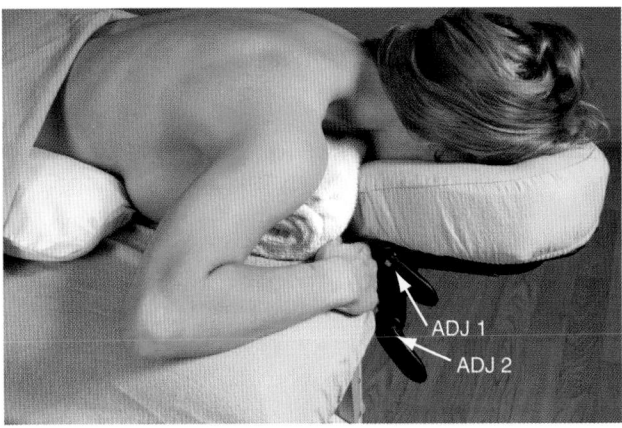

FIG. 7.10 Prone-lying client with cushions placed above and below the breasts with face rest frame adjusted above the level of the massage table.

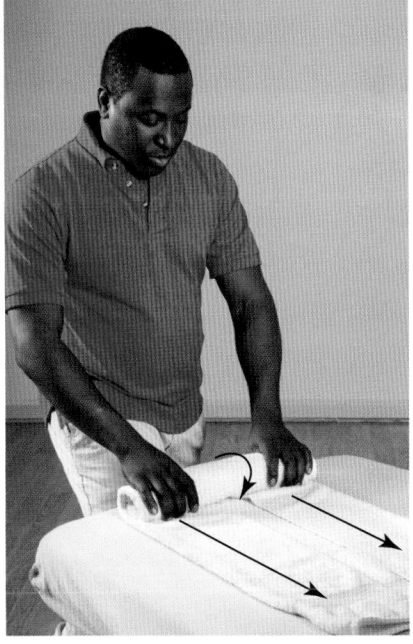

FIG. 7.12 Practitioner rolling up bath-size towel for use as a cervical pillow. Note the 1-inch gap down the center of the towel, which will provide a space for the cervical spinous processes. The thicker sides of the rolled towel provide support for muscles in the lamina grooves of the cervical spine.

The cervical spine should be in a neutral position with a slight anterior curvature. A rolled-up towel slipped into a pillowcase can be used as a neck bolster. When preparing a towel roll, bring the two long edges toward the center, leaving a 1-inch gap down its center. Next, roll the towel from the bottom edge (Fig. 7.12). This will create space for the cervical spinous processes. The thicker sides of the towel roll provide support for muscles in the lamina groove. Rolling or unrolling the towel adjusts its height.

Semireclining Position

Ways to achieve the semireclining position include (1) using a specially designed massage table (Fig. 7.13); (2) using a wedge-shaped bolster (Fig. 7.14); or (3) several pillows may be stacked to create an incline. For the latter option, use two pillows at the base, with a single pillow on top. This incline begins at the client's hips rather than midback.

Side-Lying Position

Be sure the table is devoid of pillows as the client transfers onto the table. Ask the client to lie on their side. If the client is pregnant, has acid reflux, or any respiratory condition that affects breathing, the left side is best. After the client lies on their side, place a pillow beneath the client's head. The wrist and hand of the client's lower arm can also rest on this pillow. Next, the client's upper elbow and wrist rests on another pillow placed in front of the chest, and the knee and ankle of the client's upper leg rests on a pillow placed in front of the knees. The height of the client's supported arm and leg should be at or near the same height

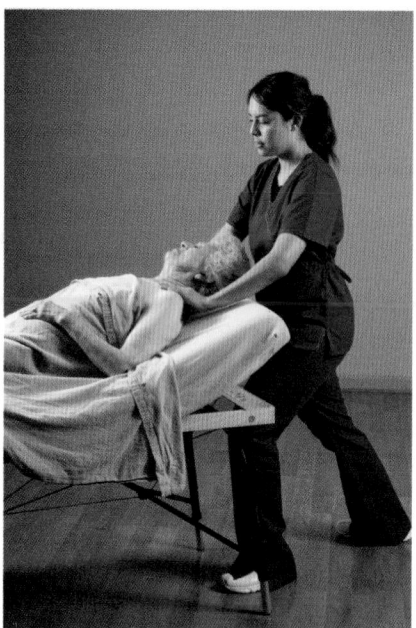

FIG. 7.13 Client in a semireclining position using a specially designed table.

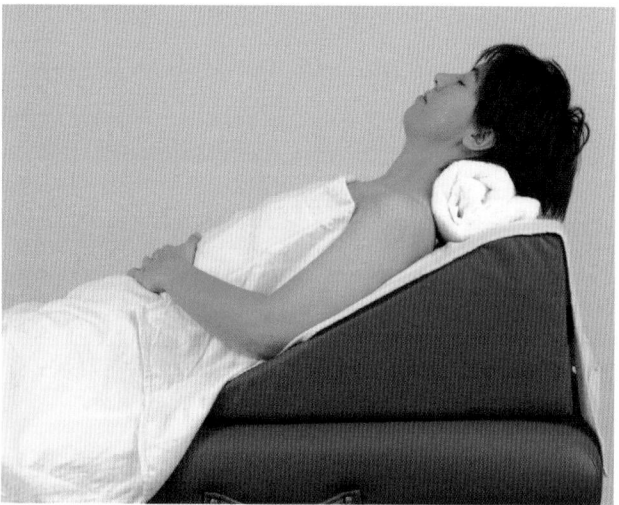

FIG. 7.14 Client in a semireclining position using a wedge-shaped bolster.

(e.g., shoulder, elbow, and wrist at the same height; hip, knee, and ankle at the same height) (Fig. 7.15). A small pillow or towel roll can be placed beneath the ankle of the lower leg. When pillow placement is complete, the client's spine will be in a neutral position and not rotated. When repositioning the client to lie on their other side, remove all pillows except the one beneath the head. Ask the client to move toward the center of the table before changing positions. Replace the pillows if continuing with the massage. Remove all pillows before the client transfers off the table.

Seated Position

The seat supporting the client may be a sturdy four-legged chair, a bed, a wheelchair, or a specially designed massage

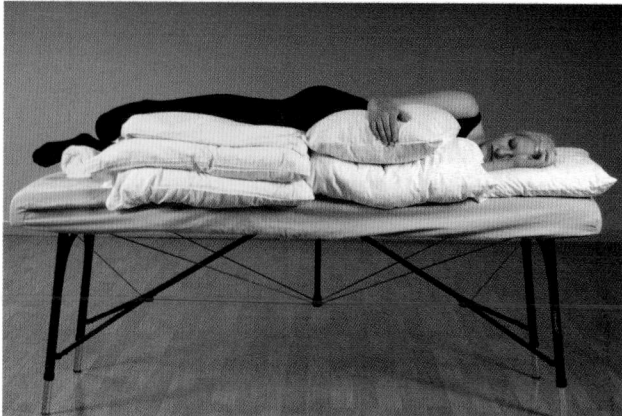

FIG. 7.15 Client in a side-lying position with pillows placed beneath the head, the upper extremity, and the lower extremity.

chair (Fig. 7.16A). A *tripod position* helps ensure the client's body has support during the seated massage and promotes easy breathing. The three parts of the tripod in the seated position are the:

1. Feet on the floor;
2. Buttocks on the chair seat or bed; and
3. Hands or elbows on the thighs (see Fig. 7.16B) or a table (see Fig. 7.16C).

An unsupported seated position is not recommended, as the client may tire easily from providing counterbalance. If using a bedside table with casters, lock them so the table is stationary and does not move during the massage. Devices that sit or clip to a tabletop may also be used (see Fig. 11.21). Chapter 15 discusses massage while the client is in a seated position.

Avoid Assisting Clients Off the Massage Table

Assisting clients off the massage table is discouraged for several reasons. First, it puts massage practitioners at risk for injury. There is a growing body of research on healthcare worker injuries related to lifting or assisting patients. An article on patient handling published by the Occupational Safety and Health Administration or OSHA (n.d.) states, "One major source of injury to healthcare workers is musculoskeletal disorders (MSDs). In 2017, nursing assistants had the second highest number of cases of MSDs. There were 18,090 days away from work cases, which equates to an incidence rate of 166.3 per 10,000 workers, more than five times the average for all industries." The article goes on to state, "These injuries are due in large part to overexertion related to repeated manual patient handling activities, often involving heavy manual lifting associated with transferring and repositioning patients …."

Second, movements required to assist clients off the table may cause the drape to fall and expose a partially or totally naked client. Lastly, physically assisting a client off the table often requires the client to grab or hold onto the practitioner, which may lead to allegations of non-massage inappropriate contact and sexual harassment (Richard et al., 2020). Hence, not assisting a client off the table serves the

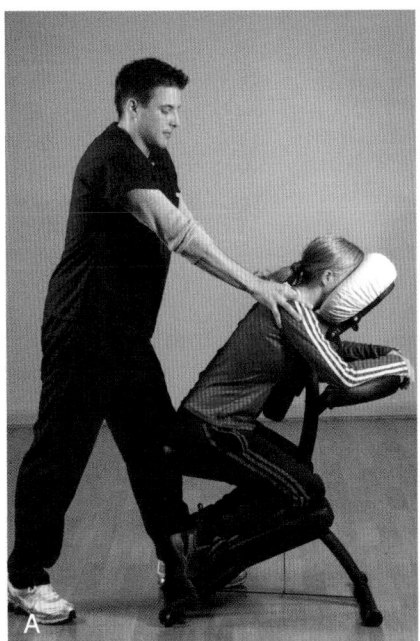 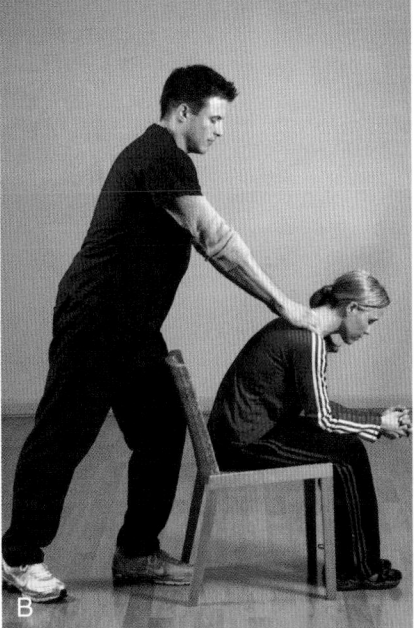 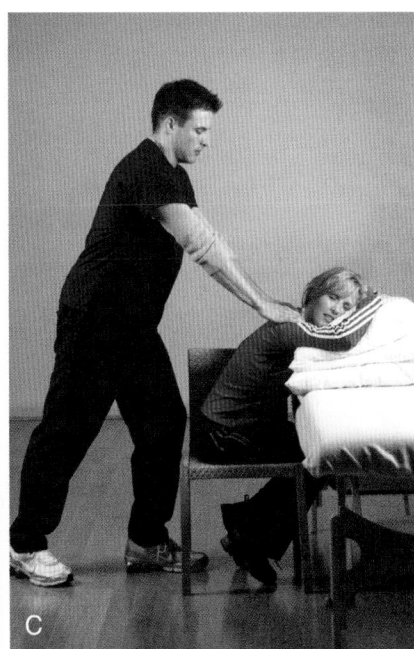

FIG. 7.16 Client in a seated position using (A) a massage chair; (B) a sturdy four-legged chair with elbows resting on the thighs; (C) a table for upper body support.

dual interests of supporting the practitioner's safety and the client's privacy.

How you do anything is how you do everything.
~ **Martha Beck**

DRAPING

Draping involves using linens or similar fabrics to cover the client's body, the massage table, and table accessories. Examples of linens used for draping include sheets and pillowcases, blankets, or towels. *Linens* is a term used to describe frequently used fabric goods such as bedding, tablecloths, and towels, and has been adapted for use in massage and other professions. Linens must be clean and fresh smelling before use, and laundered before they are reused. Massage linens are discussed in Chapter 3, and disinfection protocols are discussed in Chapter 9.

Massage practitioners must use functional draping during the massage and comply with the client's request to remain partially or fully clothed under the drape. The purpose of draping is to provide (1) a protective barrier between equipment and the client's skin; (2) client modesty, emotional privacy, and feelings of comfort and security, as most clients are fully or partially undressed while receiving massage; (3) client warmth; and (4) professionalism and boundaries. In fact, many massage practitioners consider the client drape to signify a physical boundary.

The drape(s) must be sufficient to ensure the genitals, gluteal cleft, and chest/breast areas are covered. The student/faculty member/practitioner must maintain the draping, and massage or body movements should never uncover the genitals, gluteal cleft, or chest/breast areas. This section features gender-neutral draping methods.

During the massage, uncover only the treatment area while leaving adjacent areas covered. For example, during a back massage, uncover the back and keep the buttocks and lower extremities covered. Re-cover that area after completing the massage before uncovering the next treatment area.

Use the anchor method to secure the sheet covering the client as they roll to change positions (described next). Inform the client that the sheet is being secured before asking them to change positions. If the client becomes accidentally uncovered during this process, the practitioner should look away while recovering the exposed area. Looking away demonstrates respect for the client's privacy.

Sheet Draping

Sheets are the most commonly used fabric in a massage practice. A minimum of two sheets are used: one sheet covers the massage table, and one sheet covers the client. If a flat rather than a fitted sheet covers the table, ensure that the edges of the sheet do not touch the floor. Drape the sheet used to cover the client on top of the first sheet and fold the top corners back to show the bottom sheet. This lets the client know there are two sheets. Before the massage begins, ask the client to undress after you leave the room, position themselves between the sheets, and cover themselves with the top sheet before you return to the room.

Accessing the Abdomen

When accessing the abdomen for abdominal massage, use a king-size pillowcase or a bath-size towel to cover the chest area. Hold the top edge of the pillowcase or towel at the level of the client's clavicles while pulling the top sheet down to the level of the iliac crests—this should expose the client's abdomen. Fanfold the pillowcase or towel from the bottom edge until it reaches the xiphoid process. After abdominal massage, re-drape the abdomen with the top sheet.

Client Turning Over

Remove all bolsters from the massage table. If clients are lying prone and using the face rest, ask them to move down on the table until their head is out of the face rest. Keep clients covered as they move down the table. It is helpful to have the client's arms beneath the top sheet and the feet uncovered to prevent becoming entangled in the sheet while the client turns over.

Anchoring Method. Anchor the sheet edge nearest you by leaning on it using your thigh. This secures the sheet to the edge of the massage table. Reach across and grasp the sheet along the opposite table edge with both hands. Lift the sheet up to form a tent (Fig. 7.17). Instruct the client to turn over. The top sheet remains in contact with the client's skin as they turn over to prevent the feeling of draft or air space. If the client is now supine, place covered bolsters beneath the cervical spine and knees. If the client is now lying prone, instruct them to move up to use the face rest and place a covered bolster beneath their ankles.

Side-Lying Client and Sheet Draping

Cover the side-lying client with a sheet. Use the bolstering recommendations for side-lying clients featured in the "Client Positioning" section of this chapter. Proceed with the massage, uncovering the treatment area and re-covering it when the massage to that area is complete. Use a towel folded in half lengthwise to help secure the sheet when the back is undraped (Fig. 7.18). The practitioner can be seated while massaging the client's back (see Fig. 7.18B). When massaging the client's upper extremity resting on the pillow, tuck the sheet beneath the treatment area (see Fig. 7.18C). For massage of the lower extremities resting on the table, tuck the sheet beneath the pillow (see Fig. 7.18D). When massaging the lower extremities resting on the pillow, tuck the sheet underneath the thigh (see Fig. 7.18E).

Towel Draping

Towels are thicker and heavier compared with sheets because towels are made from terrycloth, which is ideal for absorbing water after bathing. However, do not cover the table or table accessories such as bolsters and face rests with towels, as they can leave pit-like compression marks on a client's skin.

A minimum of two towels are used: One towel covers the client's torso, and one towel covers the client's pelvis and lower extremities (Fig. 7.19). Place the towels on the sheet covering the massage table. Instruct the client to undress, lie prone on the table, and use one towel to cover the hips or buttocks area. When you enter the room, use the other towel to cover the client's back. Rotate the bottom towel 90 degrees so it drapes across the lower extremities. To do this, grasp the bottom corner of the towel closest to you with your lower hand (hand nearest the foot of the table) and the top corner of the towel on the opposite side of the table with your upper hand (hand nearest the head of the table). Pull these corners apart until you feel a slight traction. While maintaining traction and keeping the center of the towel over the client's hips, rotate the towel 90 degrees. The towel should now cover the lower extremities.

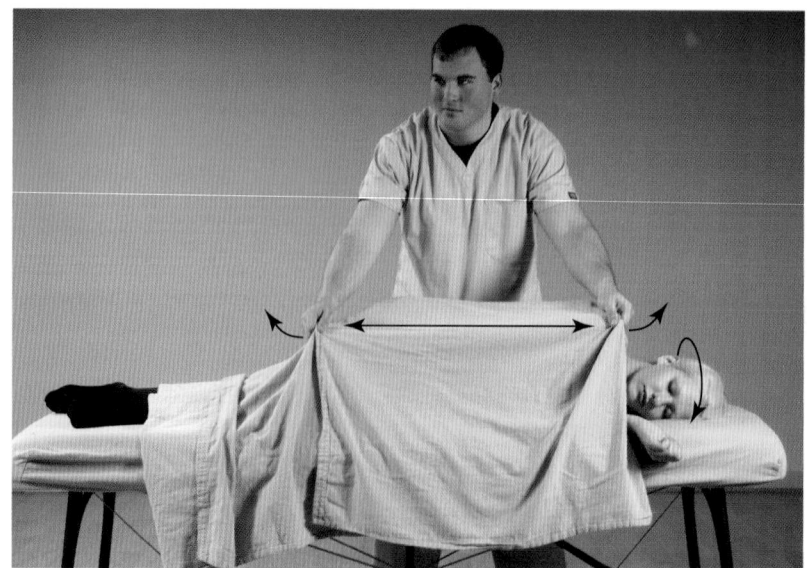

FIG. 7.17 Client turning from a supine position to a prone position while the practitioner lifts the sheet to form a tent. Note that the client's arms are beneath the top sheet and the feet are uncovered as they may become entangled in the sheet while the client is turning.

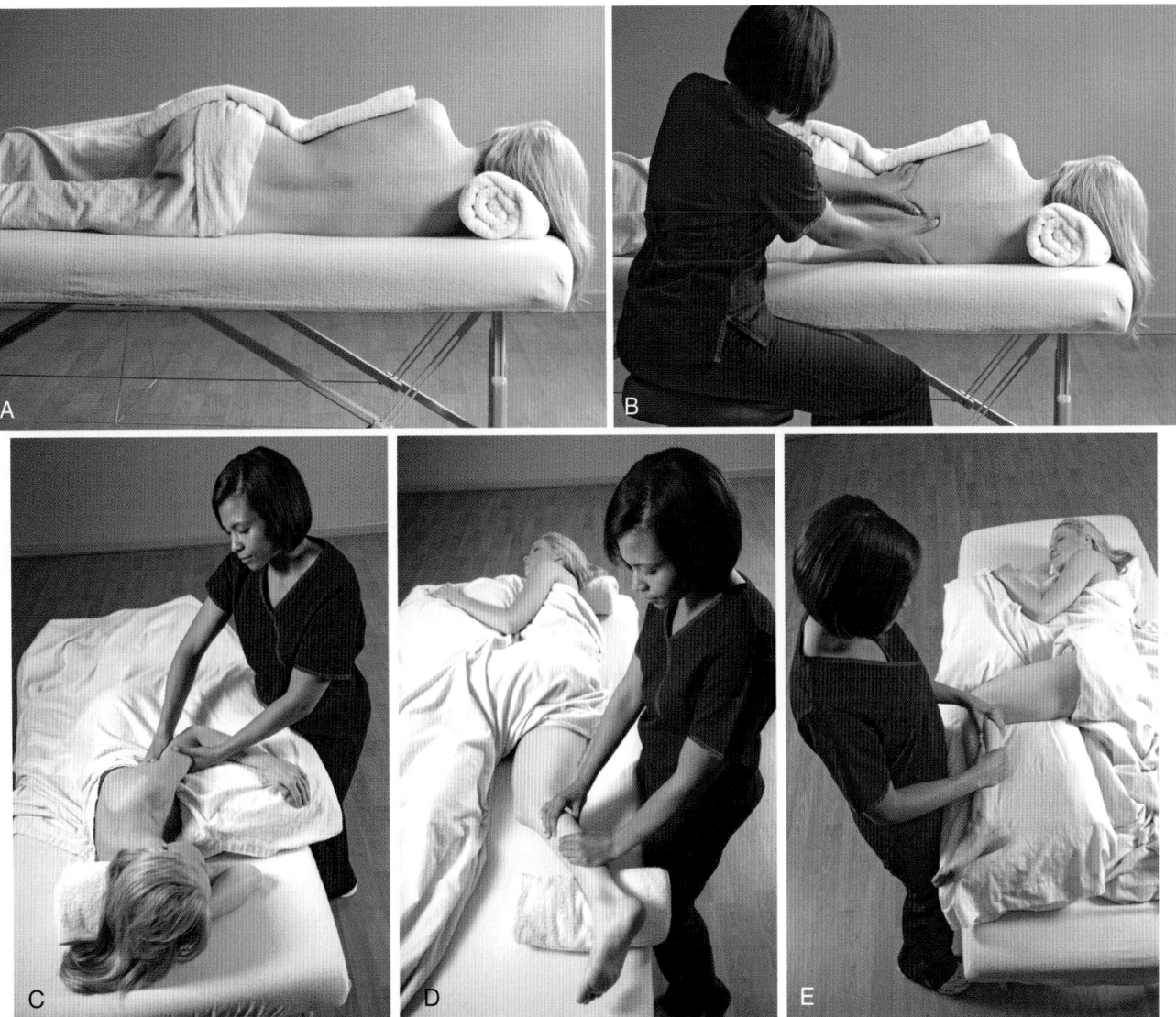

FIG. 7.18 Side-lying sheet draping. (A) Client with back exposed while a folded towel secures the sheet. (B) Practitioner massaging client's back while sitting on a stool. (C) Client's upper extremity resting on the pillow with the sheet tucked beneath the treatment area. (D) Right lower extremity resting on the table with the sheet tucked beneath the nearby pillow. (E) Left lower extremity resting on the pillow with the sheet tucked beneath the thigh.

Accessing the Abdomen

A bath-sized towel is used to cover the chest area during abdominal massage (Fig. 7.20). After abdominal massage, re-cover the abdomen by holding the top edge of the towel with one hand and pulling the bottom edge of the towel with the other hand. Continue pulling the towel until it unfolds (see Fig. 7.20). A king-size pillowcase can also be used instead of a folded towel when accessing the abdomen.

Client Turning Over

Remove all bolsters from the table before asking the client to turn over. If the client is prone and using a face rest, ask them to move down the table until the head is off the face rest. Keep the client covered as they move down. Next, rotate the lower towel so both towels are parallel to each other. Use the anchor method by leaning on the towel edges nearest using your thigh. This secures the edge of towels to the table. Reach across and grasp the top corner of the top towel with your upper hand (hand nearest the head of the table) and near the lower corner of the top towel and upper corner of the bottom towel with your lower hand (hand nearest the foot of the table). Lift the corners of the towel to form a tent. Instruct the client to turn over. The towels remain in contact with the client's skin as they turn to prevent the feeling of draft or air space. Return the bottom towel to the T formation with the towel covering the client's pelvis and lower extremities (Fig. 7.21). If your client is lying supine, place covered bolsters beneath the client's cervical spine and knees. If clients are lying prone, instruct them to move up to take advantage of the face rest and then place a covered bolster beneath their ankles.

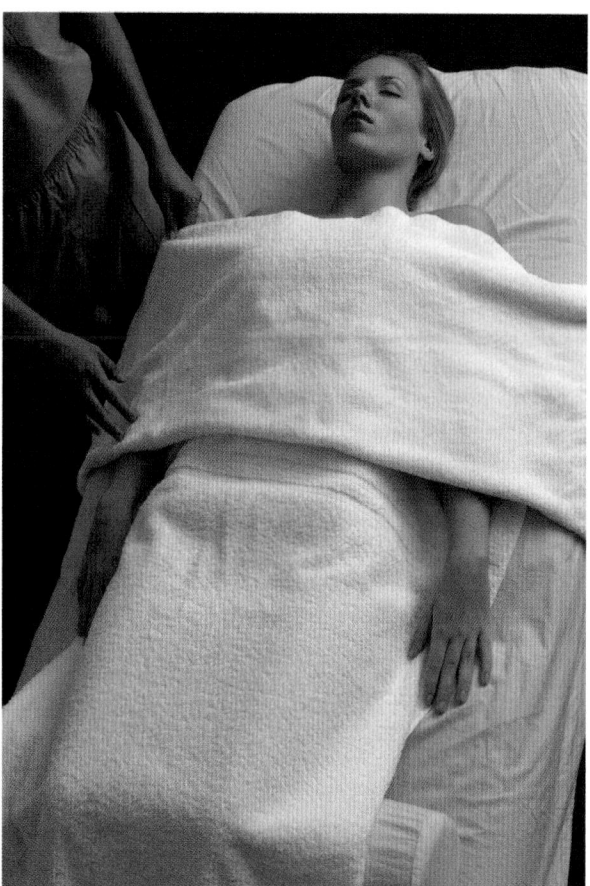

FIG. 7.19 Supine-lying client with two towels; one towel covers the client's torso and one towel covers the client's pelvis and lower extremities.

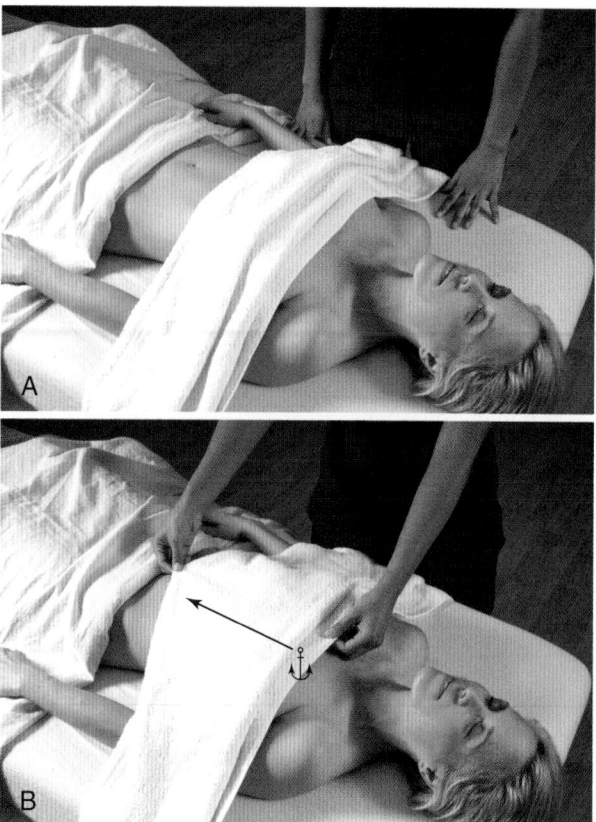

FIG. 7.20 Accessing the abdomen. (A) A folded towel is used to cover the chest area during abdominal massage. (B) After abdominal massage, recover the abdomen by holding the top edge of the towel with one hand and pulling the bottom edge of the towel with the other hand. Continue pulling the towel until it is unfolded.

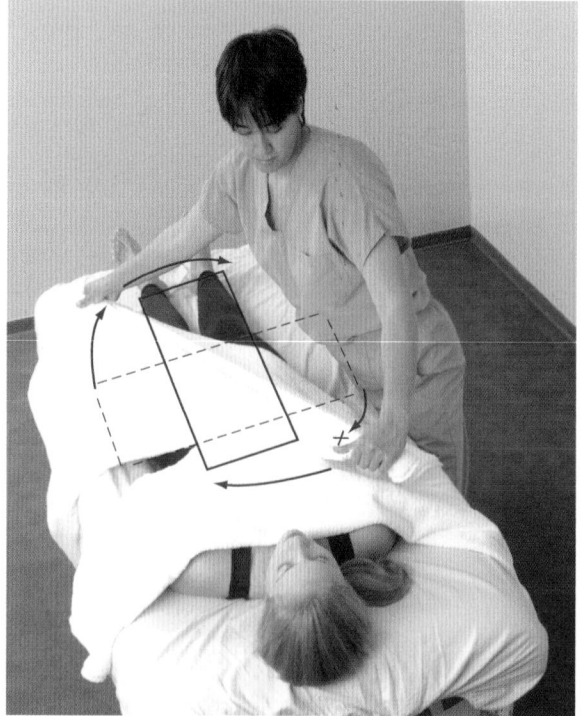

FIG. 7.21 After the client has turned from prone to supine or supine to prone, position the towel so it covers the client's pelvis and lower extremities.

HARRY HARLOW

I think we can all agree moms are important, especially to their babies! In the middle of the 20th century, there was a drive toward less contact, touch, and nurturing for babies and small children, referred to as "independence parenting." Harry Harlow set out to answer some important questions about the physical and psychologic importance of mothers. As a researcher, he worked with baby rhesus monkeys to figure this out. His work to this day is highly controversial, but it has been influential in the world of psychology as he attempted to further shed light on the "nature versus nurture" debate.

Harry Harlow Israel was born in 1905 in Fairfield, Iowa. He transferred to Stanford University in 1924, where he initially struggled as an English

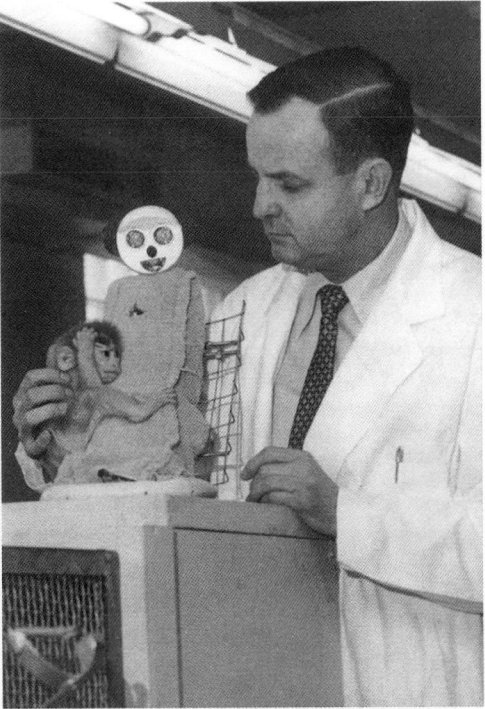

Courtesy Harlow Primate Laboratory, University of Wisconsin, Madison, Wisconsin.

major student. He changed his major to psychology and became one of the most well-known psychologists of his time. After obtaining his PhD in 1930, he changed his name to Harry Harlow in response to the anti-Semitic sentiment of the time, despite the fact his family was not Jewish.

Harlow became a professor at the University of Wisconsin-Madison, where he created the first primate laboratory in the world. Approximately 40 students earned PhDs under his tutelage at this groundbreaking facility. Most famously, he provided baby rhesus monkeys with wire mothers and cloth-covered wire mothers to see which they preferred. Because they preferred the "mother" with a soft covering, he demonstrated that "maternal" bonding involves more than simply feeding. The baby monkeys behaved more bravely if they had a soft maternal figure to return to, even if she was inanimate.

Harlow was married three times: first to Clara Mears, then to child psychologist Margaret Kuenne, then again to Clara Mears after the death of his second wife. Harlow died in Tucson, Arizona, in 1981.

His primate laboratories provided important insights into maternal-infant bonding, the importance of peer groups, and the effects of isolation. However, his research was criticized by many for being unethical. In fact, many of the experiments he performed influenced the ethical regulations we have today. Nonetheless, several important findings came out of his research:

1. Mothers and fathers can both provide the most vitally important aspects of nurturing for little ones, and nurturing extends beyond feeding.
2. Poor or absent bonding with a caregiver can result in not only psychologic, but also physical distress, such as poor digestion.
3. Social stress such as isolation from peer groups results in panic disorder.

Keep in mind, these are primate studies. We know basic science studies, including animal studies, cannot automatically be applied to human beings. Nonetheless, Harlow's research provided some important ideas to consider regarding human psychology. His research provides a look at the importance of touch and connection. Of all the many benefits of massage, touch and connection are what we do best.

So far as love or affection is concerned, psychologists have failed in their mission. The little we know about love does not transcend simple observation, and the little we write about it has been written better by poets and novelists.

—Harry Harlow

E-RESOURCES

http://evolve.elsevier.com/Salvo/MassageTherapy

- Chapter challenge
- Flash cards
- Technique videos
- Additional information

REFERENCES

Abdallah, S. J., Krug, R., & Jensen, D. (2015). Does wearing clothing made of a synthetic "cooling" fabric improve indoor cycle exercise endurance in trained athletes? *Physiological Reports*, 3(8), e12505.

Albert, W. J., Currie-Jackson, N., & Duncan, C. A. (2008). A survey of musculoskeletal injuries amongst Canadian massage therapists. *Journal of Bodywork and Movement Therapies*, 12(1), 86–93.

American College of Sports Medicine. (2011). Quantity and quality of exercise for developing and maintaining cardiorespiratory, musculoskeletal, and neuromotor fitness in apparently healthy adults: Guidance for prescribing exercise. *Medicine and Science in Sports and Exercise*, 43(7), 1334–1359.

American Massage Therapy Association (AMTA). (2020). *Massage profession research report: Who is practicing massage therapy?* Retrieved from https://www.amtamassage.org/publications/massage-profession-research-report/.

Anderson, R. B. (2018). Improving body mechanics using experiential learning and ergonomic tools in massage therapy education. *International Journal of Therapeutic Massage and Bodywork*, 11(4), 1–9.

Beck, M. (2016). *Theory and practice of therapeutic massage* (6th ed.). Boston: Cengage Learning.

Bishop, S. R., Lau, M., Shapiro, S., Carlson, L., Anderson, N. D., Carmody, J., et al. (2004). Mindfulness: A proposed operational definition. *Clinical Psychology: Science and Practice*, 11(3), 230–241.

Blau, G., Monos, C., Boyer, E., Davis, K., Flanagan, R., Lopez, A., & Tatum, D. S. (2013). Correlates of injury-forced work reduction for massage therapists and bodywork practitioners. *International Journal of Therapeutic Massage and Bodywork*, 6(3), 6–13.

Braun, M. B., & Simonson, S. J. (2013). *Introduction to massage therapy* (3rd ed.). Philadelphia: Lippincott Williams and Wilkins.

Carley, P., Lachowski, S., & Mullin, E. (2017). Floor mats and insoles: Workplace considerations for safe dynamic standing. *Journal of Bones and Muscle Study*, 1, 1–8.

Centers for Disease Control and Prevention (CDC). (2017). *How much sleep do I need?* Retrieved from https://www.cdc.gov/sleep/about_sleep/how_much_sleep.html.

Centers for Disease Control and Prevention (CDC). (2020). *Get the facts: Drinking water and intake*. Retrieved from https://www.cdc.gov/nutrition/data-statistics/plain-water-the-healthier-choice.html.

Chaudhari, A. (2017). *Study reveals compression tights don't help runners reach finish line*. Retrieved from https://wexnermedical.osu.edu/mediaroom/pressreleaselisting/compression-tights.

Chumnanya, M., Perngparn, U., & Sayorwan, W. (2013). Health problem from working as Thai traditional massage therapists in Thailand. *Journal of Health Research*, 2(2), 119–122.

Fairchild, S. L., O'Shea, R. K., & Washington, R. D. (2017). *Pierson and Fairchild principles and techniques of patient care* (6th ed.). St Louis: Elsevier.

Fradkin, A. J., Gabbe, B. J., & Cameron, P. A. (2006). Does warming up prevent injury in sport? The evidence from randomised controlled trials? *Journal of Science and Medicine in Sport*, 9(3), 214–220.

Greene, L., & Goggins R. W. (2006). *Musculoskeletal symptoms and injuries among experienced massage and bodywork professionals* (pp. 48–58). Massage & Bodywork. Retrieved from https://nohandsmassage.com/wp-content/uploads/2017/03/Six_Studies_Worldwide-Copyright-GerryPyves.pdf.

Greene, L., & Goggins, R. W. (2008). *Save your hands! The complete guide to injury prevention and ergonomics for manual therapists* (2nd ed.). Florida: Body of Work Books.

Harvard School of Public Health. (2011). *Health eating plate*. Retrieved from https://www.hsph.harvard.edu/nutritionsource/healthy-eating-plate/.

Jang, Y., Chi, C. F., Tsauo, J. Y., & Wang, J. D. (2006). Prevalence and risk factors of work-related musculoskeletal disorders in massage practitioners. *Journal of Occupational Rehabilitation*, 16(3), 425–438.

Jonas, W. B. (Ed.). (2005). *Mosby's dictionary of complementary and alternative medicine*. St. Louis: Elsevier.

Kibler, W. B., Press, J., & Sciascia, A. (2006). The role of core stability in athletic function. *Sports Medicine*, 36(3), 189–198.

King, M. A. (2000). Core stability: Creating a foundation for functional rehabilitation. *International Journal of Athletic Therapy and Training*, 5(2), 6–13.

Langer, E. J. (2000). Mindful learning. *Current Directions in Psychological Science*, 9(6), 220–223.

Maughan, R. J. (2003). Impact of mild dehydration on wellness and on exercise performance. *European Journal of Clinical Nutrition*, 57(Suppl. 2), S19–S23.

Miller, A. E., MacDougall, J. D., Tarnopolsky, M. A., & Sale, D. G. (1993). Gender differences in strength and muscle fiber characteristics. *European Journal of Applied Physiology and Occupational Physiology*, 66(3), 254–262.

Mohr, E. G. (2010). Proper body mechanics from an engineering perspective. *Journal of Bodywork and Movement Therapies*, 14, 139–151.

Muscolino, J. (2010). *Body mechanics: Working from the core* (pp. 72–76). Massage Magazine. Retrieved from https://www.learnmuscles.com/wp-content/uploads/2016/08/WorkingFromCore2.pdf.

Nadelen, M. D. (2010). *American College of Sports Medicine: Basic injury prevention concepts*. ACSM Fit Society, spring newsletter. Retrieved from https://www.shapeamerica.org/publications/resources/teachingtools/coachtoolbox/upload/Fit-Society-Spring-2010-Issue.pdf.

Prudden, B. (1980). *Pain erasure: The Bonnie Prudden way*. Lanham, MD: M. Evans & Company.

Richard, M. E., O'Sullivan, L. F., & Peppard, T. (2020). Sexual harassment of massage therapists by their clients. *The Canadian Journal of Human Sexuality*, 29(2), 205–211.

Sathya, P., Ramakrishnan, K. S., & Gowda, H. (2016). Prevalence of musculoskeletal problems in masseuse. *International Journal of Therapies & Rehabilitation Research*, 5(5), 140–148.

Turkeltaub, P. C., Yearwood, E. L., & Friedmann, E. (2014). Effect of a brief seated massage on nursing student attitudes toward touch for comfort care. *Journal of Alternative and Complementary Medicine*, 20(10), 792–799.

United States Department of Labor's Occupational Safety and Health Administration (OSHA). (n.d.). *Healthcare: Safe patient handling*. Retrieved from https://www.osha.gov/healthcare/safe-patient-handling.

REVIEW AND APPLY YOUR KNOWLEDGE

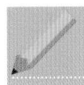 **MATCHING ONE: CONCEPT REVIEW**
Place the letter of the answer next to the number of the term or phrase that best describes it.

A. Force
B. Body mechanics
C. Bolsters
D. Archer
E. Physical exhaustion
F. Core of the body
G. Higher
H. Lower
I. Horse
J. Center of gravity
K. Warm-up activities
L. Base of support

_____ 1. Factor found to strongly contribute to loss of work from massage-related injuries.
_____ 2. Point at the exact center of an object's mass; in the average person, it is in the lower abdomen when standing in an anatomic position.
_____ 3. Table height used for applying compression to use gravity and body weight.
_____ 4. All points of contact on which an object rests.
_____ 5. A push or pull upon an object resulting from one object interacting with another.
_____ 6. Group of musculoskeletal structures that include the muscles of the abdomen, spine, hips, and pelvic floor.
_____ 7. Pillows or cushions of various sizes and densities used for supporting clients in the prone, supine, side-lying, and seated positions.
_____ 8. Stance used when the target area(s) of the massage technique is directly in front of the practitioner's body.
_____ 9. Stance used when the target area(s) of the massage technique is toward the side and not directly in front of the practitioner's body.
_____ 10. Low-intensity movements performed before the first massage, and perhaps repeated throughout the workday.
_____ 11. Table height used when applying small, detailed, low-force techniques while seated or standing or while applying traction.
_____ 12. Encompasses the use of one's body in a manner that is safe, energy-conserving, and reduces physical stress and strain.

 MATCHING TWO: CONCEPT REVIEW
Place the letter of the answer next to the number of the term or phrase that best describes it.

A. Mindfulness
B. Posterior tilt
C. Stance
D. Fowler
E. Draping
F. Core stability
G. Prone
H. Seated
I. Semireclining
J. Side-lying
K. Supine
L. Client positioning

_____ 1. Term to describe the semireclining position used on patients in healthcare settings and classified according to the degree of elevation.
_____ 2. Position in which the client is lying face down.
_____ 3. A modified supine position in which the torso is elevated.
_____ 4. Using linens or similar fabrics to cover the client's body, the massage table, and table accessories.
_____ 5. Position in which the client lies on their side, usually with the hips and knees flexed.
_____ 6. Position of the pelvis to help stabilize the core.
_____ 7. Positions of the practitioner's feet used to provide the practitioner's base of support during the massage.
_____ 8. Position in which the client's torso is usually erect, knees are bent, and buttocks supported.
_____ 9. Position in which the client is lying face up or on the back.
_____ 10. Heightened self-awareness and focused attention given to present moments.
_____ 11. Involves helping the client receive massage in ways that promote stability and provide comfort through proper body alignment.
_____ 12. Ability to control the position and motion of the trunk, allowing for optimum production and transfer of force and motion.

MULTIPLE CHOICE: TEST YOUR KNOWLEDGE

Place the letter of the answer next to the number of the term or phrase that best describes it.

_____ 1. The concept of adapting the work to the worker describes:
   A. mechanics
   B. ergonomics.
   C. efficiency.
   D. accommodations.

_____ 2. Approximately ____ of massage practitioners experience work-related pain.
   A. 20%
   B. 50%
   C. 70%
   D. 90%

_____ 3. The recommended amount of moderate-intensity physical activity for healthy adults ages 18 to 65 is a minimum of _____ minutes for ____ days a week.
   A. 20/3
   B. 30/3
   C. 20/5
   D. 30/5

_____ 4. The recommended amount of sleep that adults ages 18 to 64 should get is between _____ hours of sleep a night.
   A. 5 to 7
   B. 6 to 8
   C. 7 to 9
   D. 8 to 10

_____ 5. Awareness of one's thoughts, feelings, and sensations related to the external environment is called:
   A. mindfulness.
   B. exteroception.
   C. introception.
   D. proprioception.

_____ 6. Practitioners should leave a minimum of ____ of open space around all sides of the table.
   A. 1 foot
   B. 2 feet
   C. 3 feet
   D. 4 feet

_____ 7. Table height should be set _____ when applying ____ force when applying more detailed techniques while seated.
   A. higher/low
   B. higher/downward
   C. lower/low
   D. lower/downward

_____ 8. The table consideration that makes it easier to apply techniques beneath the client's body is:
   A. firm padding.
   B. plush padding.
   C. wider table.
   D. narrower table.

_____ 9. The stance in which the feet are pointing in the same direction is the:
   A. archer stance.
   B. bow stance.
   C. lunge stance.
   D. horse stance.

_____ 10. The stance that provides a stable foundation for administering more lengthy techniques is the:
   A. archer stance.
   B. horse stance.
   C. warrior stance.
   D. symmetric stance.

_____ 11. A semireclining position that elevates a person's torso between 45 and 60 degrees describes a:
   A. low Fowler.
   B. semi-Fowler.
   C. standard Fowler.
   D. high Fowler.

_____ 12. Bolsters are placed in front of the ankles in the _____ position.
   A. prone
   B. supine
   C. side-lying
   D. seated

CRITICAL THINKING

I'm Fine

You have noticed a classmate's body mechanics beginning to slip. When you mention this to the classmate, they say they feel more comfortable than when they were trying to use the postures and movements taught in class. How would you respond to this?

Answers can include but are not limited to:

Performing massage is very physical. Like anything physical, proper form is the foundation of success. Body mechanics are not something learned once. They require the massage practitioner to continually check in with their own body to correct inefficient and possibly injurious postures and movements. Habitual postures and movements may feel more comfortable at first than the new methods involved in efficient body mechanics. However, in the long run, if efficient body mechanics are not used, the massage practitioner will experience fatigue, loss of strength, and most likely an injury, especially when doing multiple massages in a row.

PROFESSIONAL PRACTICE

The Bachelorette

Nikki's clientele are athletes who have sports-related injuries. In most cases, she massages the targeted area while seated. Today is a busy day for Nikki. In addition to five half-hour sessions, Nikki's sister hired her to provide relaxation massage to her three bridesmaids. Fifteen minutes into the first massage, Nikki notices she is having a difficult time controlling her pressure, causing discomfort in her upper back and neck. By the middle of the second session, Nikki's lower back is hurting, too. Why do you think Nikki is having a hard time adjusting her body mechanics? Is there a difference in body mechanics when using a table over a chair? Do longer sessions make body mechanics more challenging? What suggestions might you offer Nikki to improve her body posture?

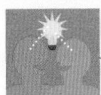

DISCUSSION

Is My Back Straight?

Do an honest self-assessment of your posture and your body mechanics while performing massage. What do you think your strengths are? Where do you think you could improve? What can you do to prevent injury? If available, post your reflections on an Internet-based discussion board monitored by your instructor.

CHAPTER 8

Massage Techniques, Mobilizations, Stretches, Endangerment Sites, and Contraindications

LEARNING OBJECTIVES

After completing this chapter, the student should be able to:

1. Define massage, types of massages, and massage techniques and their characteristics.
2. Outline the side effects of massage, endangerment sites, adverse events, physical forces, and massage technique application.
3. Discuss massage contraindications.
4. Describe and perform basic massage techniques, including effleurage, petrissage, friction, compression, tapotement, and vibration, as well as their variations.
5. Describe and perform passive range of motion, mobilizations, and stretches.

http://evolve.elsevier.com/Salvo/MassageTherapy

INTRODUCTION

Massage therapy is the manipulation of soft tissue using compression and decompression/traction for clinical, therapeutic, and palliative purposes, as well as for wellness and self-care purposes (DeDomenico, 2007; Ernst et al., 2006). A **massage practitioner** is a trained individual who practices massage. Massage has been used worldwide for thousands of years in many cultures. The history of massage is discussed in Chapter 1. The most significant influence on the massage profession was made by Pehr Henrik Ling (1776 to 1839) from Sweden. Ling developed his own system of massage and passive and active movements called "gymnastics" after accepting a position at the University of Lund in Sweden in 1804. His system of massage and movements was called the Swedish Movement Cure, or Ling system. Swedish massage was the term used to describe the massage component of Ling's system (Calvert, 2002). Although massage has evolved, massage techniques taught today have their roots in Ling's system. Swedish massage is also called *European massage* or *classic massage.*

Although massage has many benefits, which are discussed in Chapter 6, the primary benefits are reductions in symptoms such as pain, depression, and anxiety, and improvements in function, sleep, and quality of life. Clients continue to receive massage because of the positive outcomes they receive, which are often immediate. Another important reason is the client-practitioner relationship, which they believe contributes to positive outcomes. Elements of the massage valued most by repeat clients are the pleasant unhurried atmosphere of the massage setting; firm, confident, and appropriate touch; and rapport with the practitioner who they feel is caring, knowledgeable, skilled, competent, and genuinely interested in their wellbeing (Smith et al., 2009a, 2009b). Massage is also good for practitioners, as they reported reductions in anxiety after giving a massage (Jensen et al., 2012).

TYPES OF MASSAGE

Based on the definition of massage, we can categorize massage into two main types—wellness massage and clinical massage.

- **Wellness massage.** Wellness massage is used as self-care to reduce stress, promote relaxation, improve function, and decrease pain and muscle soreness unrelated to diagnosed medical conditions. Clients can receive massage at any time in their lives at their discretion, without a prescription or medical referral. Wellness massage is often full-body or area-focused, as directed by the client. The length of a session is based on a list of services posted by individual massage practitioners or by massage establishments such as spas, hotels, resorts, cruise lines, beauty salons, or health clubs. Medical settings, which will be discussed next, may also offer wellness massage. Most massage clients use massage for general health, wellness, relaxation, and stress reduction (American Massage Therapy Association [AMTA], 2021; Sundberg et al., 2017).

- **Clinical massage.** Clinical massage is used as healthcare to help rehabilitate patients who have sustained injuries, manage diagnosed medical conditions and their treatments or complications, and manage issues related to surgery. Clinical massage can also refer to the practice settings where massage services are provided, such as hospitals, physical therapy clinics, physical rehabilitation clinics, chiropractic clinics, sports clinics, military clinics, and hospice care facilities. Clients can receive massage based on medical directives or prescriptions, and treatment goals are condition-related. The length of a session is based on published procedural codes (called CPT for current procedural terminology), often 15 minutes per code, applied to a specified area. Practitioners may utilize orthopedic assessments to determine the best course of treatment. The recipients of these services are usually referred to as patients. Clinical massage is discussed in Chapter 14.

The vast majority of clients receive wellness massage compared with clinical massage (AMTA, 2021). In both types of massage, information is gathered on an intake form and clients are screened for contraindications. Clients are usually positioned on a table, and the practitioner utilizes body stances or body mechanics to deliver techniques in ways that maximize benefits to the client and minimize risk of self-injury. Techniques, procedures, and client positions may be modified depending on the client's condition and level of comfort.

MASSAGE TECHNIQUE TERMINOLOGY AND CHARACTERISTICS

Historically, terms used to describe massage techniques were broad and nonspecific, such as *rubbing* or *friction.* Specific terminology related to massage techniques emerged during Ling's time. Since then, early physicians and practitioners largely use French terms, which include:
- Effleurage
- Petrissage
- Friction
- Tapotement
- Vibration
- Compression

"Swedish" massage techniques use "French" terms because French was the international language during this time. English became the international language after World War II, but the use of French terms remains an integral part of the massage culture. These terms are used to describe massage in state laws and legislation; they are used by allied practitioners such as nurses, chiropractors, and physical therapists, as well as in professional scientific literature such as research studies. They are also used in procedural codes and in healthcare when billing for clinical massage services provided in medical settings.

Many French massage terms have their English counterparts—*gliding* or *stroking* for effleurage; *kneading* or *rolling* for petrissage; *rubbing* for friction; *percussion* for tapotement; and *shaking* for vibration. Each massage technique has several variations (Table 8.1). In addition, these techniques are used when applying either wellness

TABLE 8.1 Massage Techniques and Their Variations

TECHNIQUE	VARIATIONS
Effleurage (*stroking, gliding*)	One-hand
	Two-hand
	Alternate hand
	Nerve stroke (*feathering*)
Petrissage (*kneading*)	One-hand
	Two-hand (*fulling, broadening*)
	Alternate hand
	Skin rolling
Friction	Superficial warming (*sawing, towel friction*)
	Rolling
	Wringing
	Transverse (*cross-fiber*)
	Chucking (*parallel*)
	Circular
Compression (*ischemic*)	One-hand
	Two-hand
	Alternate hand
Tapotement (*percussion*)	Tapping (*raindrops*)
	Pincement
	Hacking (*quacking*)
	Cupping
	Pounding (*rapping*)
	Clapping (*slapping*)
	Diffused
Vibration (*shaking*)	Fine
	Jostling (*fluffing*)

massage or clinical massage, as they are effective in helping clients achieve their goals (Cherkin et al., 2011; Romanowski et al., 2012).

When applying massage techniques, there are several characteristics they all possess, such as pressure or the application of force, direction of pressure, excursion, rate, rhythm, duration, and frequency (DeDomenico & Wood, 1997). Many characteristics can be modified depending on a client's preference and desired outcome. For example, pressure can be light, moderate, or deep.

Pressure

In massage, **pressure** is the application of gliding or nongliding force. As we learned in Chapter 7, *force* is essentially a push or a pull. Pushing, or downward pressure, is called compression and pulling, or upward pressure, is called decompression or traction. The direction of downward force is between 45 and 90 degrees to help spread tissue fibers in taut muscles, tendons, or ligaments. When we apply pressure or force, the client's body will move if it can move, and tissues will be displaced or deformed. How much the tissue deforms depends on several factors, such as the amount of pressure used, properties of the soft tissue (i.e., viscoelasticity), and temperature of the tissue. When applying pressure, be mindful of the size of the area used to apply pressure.

- A wider or broader area may be experienced as comfortable (e.g., forearm).

- A narrower or smaller area may be experienced as uncomfortable (e.g., fingertip).

Pressure is determined objectively by a weight scale and is measured in pounds (i.e., lbs.). Pressure is determined subjectively by descriptive or numeric scales and is measured using adjectives (e.g., light, moderate/medium, deep) or numbers (e.g., 0, 5, 10). Regardless of the level of pressure applied, the practitioner must always be within the client's parameters of comfort (minimally painful or not painful). Let us look more closely at the three main types of pressure (Walton, 2010).

Light/Gentle Pressure (0 to 3)

Light pressure is thought to displace superficial adipose tissue and fascia. The skin is not displaced, or it is only slightly displaced. The practitioner administers light pressure by using only the weight of their arms and hands, not by leaning their body weight into the client's tissue. Hand strength is used only for contouring around body curves and angles, as well as over bony prominences and endangerment sites. Light pressure is used to apply lubricant, to introduce touch and pressure at the beginning of the massage, and to conclude the massage. Light pressure, also called *superficial pressure*, is appropriate for palliative outcomes, for clients who are frail, or who have reduced bone density (e.g., osteoporosis). Very light pressure may be used over endangerment sites (e.g., anterior neck [anterior/posterior cervical triangles], posterior knee [popliteal area]).

Medium/Moderate Pressure (4 to 7)

Medium or moderate pressure attempts to displace superficial muscle and its fascial layers. As pressure is applied, adjacent joints may move (i.e., the hip may rotate while applying upward pressure along the lower extremity). The practitioner administers medium/moderate pressure by using their upper body and upper extremity strength and transfers their body weight into the client's tissues by leaning. Moderate hand strength is needed for select massage techniques (e.g., petrissage, friction).

Moderate pressure is used for wellness massage and is frequently regarded as a pleasurable experience. Indeed, massage recipients preferred pressure of 6 to 7 on a 10-point pressure scale and these same recipients stated they were more likely to continue to receive massages for self-care (Koren & Kalichman, 2018; Turkeltaub et al., 2014). Moderate pressure has been found to reduce stress and pain, enhance immune function, and promote weight gain in infants. Furthermore, moderate pressure stimulates the relaxation response (parasympathetic nervous system) through increased vagal nerve activity. This promotes production of the hormone oxytocin which, in turn, decreases the production of the stress hormone cortisol and/or vice versa (Field, 2019; Field et al., 2010). In contrast, light touch can elicit a sympathetic "stress" response.

Deep/Heavy Pressure (8 to 10)

Deep pressure attempts to move deeper muscles and their fascial layers as well as tendons and ligaments. As with moderate/medium pressure, adjacent joints may move. The practitioner administers deep pressure by using their upper body and lower extremity strength and transfers their body weight into the client's tissues by leaning. Substantial hand strength or force is required, and one hand may be braced by the other to deliver deep pressure. The practitioner often uses the bony elements of their fingertips, knuckles, forearms, or elbow to apply pressure and reach the bones of the massaged area—this strategy helps the practitioner apply deep pressure with less effort.

Deep pressure is used by practitioners who offer **deep tissue massage**, the use of deep pressure to reduce tension. Deep pressure is also called strong pressure or high-intensity pressure and is associated with methods such as structural integration or Rolfing, and trigger point therapy. Some define deep tissue massage as the application of massage techniques that reaches a client pain pressure threshold by applying more pressure (Koren & Kalichman, 2018). Clients who receive deep pressure, especially over endangerment sites, are more likely to experience side effects and/or adverse events (AEs).

Massage Side Effects

A massage **side effect** is a non-harmful and unintended but predictable effect that occurs after the session. The most common side effect associated with massage is soreness. However, this soreness did not prevent clients from performing normal activities at home or at work. Soreness affects approximately 10% of massage clients, beginning ≤12 hours after the session and lasting ≤36 hours. Other less common side effects include increased discomfort, bruising, headaches, and fatigue (Cambron et al., 2007).

Endangerment Sites and Adverse Events

Endangerment sites are areas containing structures that are vulnerable to injury from applied pressure because they are not well protected by bones and muscles. Examples of structures that can be injured are nerves, blood vessels, organs, and glands. Only very light pressure, or no pressure, should be used over endangerment sites to prevent AEs. Endangerment sites are also called *cautionary sites* or *areas of caution.*

Adverse events (AEs), or *adverse effects,* are rare (<1%) but serious massage-related injuries; they may not be apparent until a few days later or even longer. Disc herniation, neurologic compromise, spinal cord injury, dissection of the carotid arteries, and others are the main AEs of massage (Yin et al., 2014). AEs often require medical treatment and can cause varying degrees of temporary or permanent disability.

Endangerment sites include the anterior neck, the abdomen, the costovertebral angle (CVA) of the lower back, the armpit (axillary area), and the posterior knee (popliteal area). The most serious AEs have been associated with pressure applied to the neck area (Ernst, 2003; Koren & Kalichman, 2018; Posadzki & Ernst, 2013). These areas and various related AEs case reports are listed next.

Anterior Neck (Anterior and Posterior Cervical Triangles)

The anterior neck is a four-sided region delineated by the anterior margins of the trapezius muscle (at the level of the vertebral transverse processes), the inferior border of the mandible, and the superior borders of the clavicles (Fig. 8.1). This region contains the posterior and anterior triangles of the neck. The *posterior cervical triangle* of the neck is bordered by the anterior margin of the trapezius, the superior border of the clavicle, and the sternocleidomastoid muscle. The *anterior cervical triangle* is bordered by the side of the lower border of the mandible, the midline of the

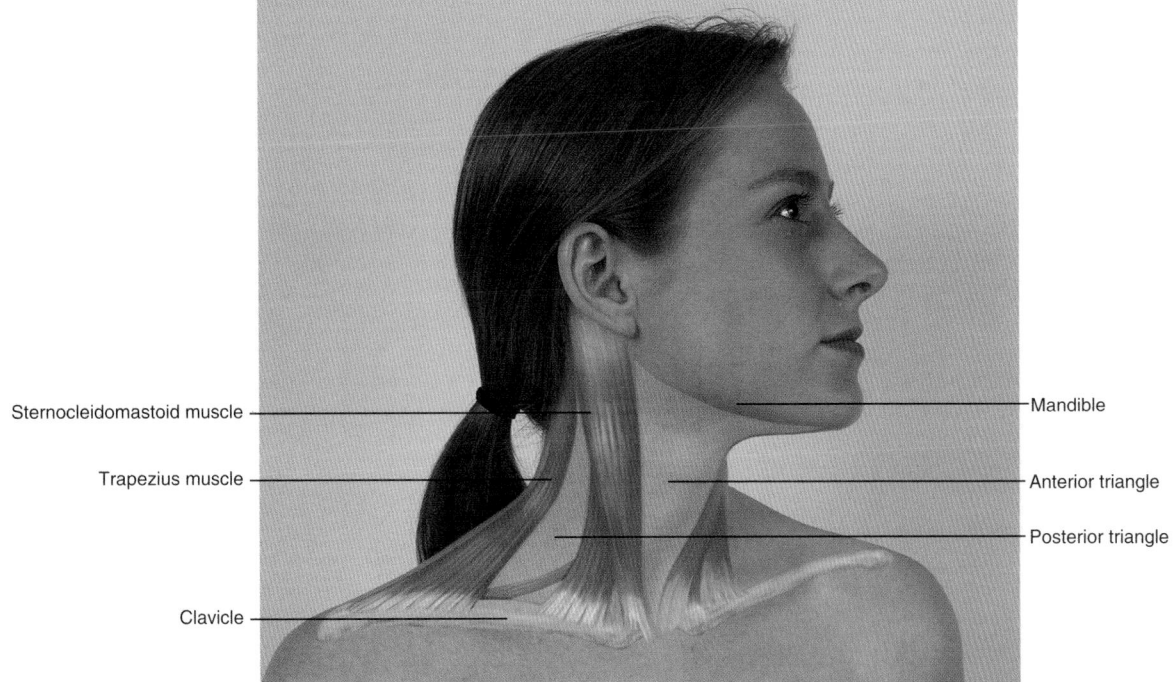

FIG. 8.1 Endangerment site: anterior and posterior cervical triangles within the anterior neck. (From Forbes, H., & Watt, E. [2021]. *Jarvis's physical examination and health assessment* [3rd ed.]. Australia: Elsevier.)

body, and the sternocleidomastoid muscle. The anterior neck contains structures vulnerable to damage from pressure such as the thyroid gland, carotid arteries, jugular veins, vagus nerve, spinal accessory nerve, and the brachial plexus.

Anterior neck massage has caused vascular and neurologic AEs, including arterial dissection, jugular vein thrombosis (Chakrapani et al., 2008; Dutta et al., 2018; Elliott & Taylor, 2002; Foster, 2015; Grant & Wang, 2004; Kaur et al., 2017; Liu et al., 1993; Wada et al., 2005), brachial plexus injury, and spinal accessory neuropathy (Aksoy et al., 2009; Chang et al., 2015; Kitisomprayoonkul, 2018; Schrader & Ross, 2008). Case reports of cervical cord injury from neck massage have been reported and involved disc herniation and nerve compression evidenced by magnetic resonance imaging (Cheong et al., 2012; Lee et al., 2011). The most serious adverse effects were associated with neck massage (Posadzki & Ernst, 2013).

Abdomen
The abdomen is bordered by the diaphragm superiorly and the pelvis inferiorly. The abdomen contains abdominopelvic organs and blood vessels, and deep pressure is contraindicated in this region. AEs related to deep pressure were a liver hematoma, a cystic rupture and bladder hemorrhage, small bowel hemorrhage, and displacement of a urethral stent (Chen et al., 2013; Kerr, 1997; Mufarrij & Hitti, 2011; Trotter, 1999). Furthermore, increasing numbers of individuals in the United States have abdominal aortic aneurysms and most are asymptomatic. Therefore you cannot rely on prior diagnosis before avoiding deep, penetrating pressure over the abdomen.

Costovertebral Angle (Lower Back)
The CVA is an acute angle on either side of the lower back between the twelfth rib and the vertebral column. This area contains the kidneys, which are two bean-shaped organs that filter blood and produce urine. The kidneys are behind the protective peritoneum (i.e., retroperitoneally) and are loosely suspended in fat and connective tissues. Forceful or heavy tapotement or percussion is contraindicated in this area.

Axilla (Armpit Area)
The armpit or axilla is a triangular-shaped area under the arm. It is bordered by the latissimus dorsi posteriorly, the pectoralis major anteriorly, and the chest wall inferiorly about the level of rib 5. The axilla contains structures vulnerable to damage from deep pressure, such as the brachial artery, axillary artery and vein, cephalic vein, and nerves of the brachial plexus.

Popliteal Area (Posterior Knee)
The popliteal area is a diamond-shaped space behind the tendons of the semimembranosus and semitendinosus muscles (medial) and the tendons of biceps femoris (lateral), which form the superior borders. The medial and lateral heads of the gastrocnemius form the inferior borders. The popliteal artery and vein, tibial nerve, and the peroneal nerve are located here.

Physical Forces and Technique Application
Massage introduces physical or mechanical forces into the body by the application of pressure and decompression or traction. Massage techniques can utilize one or more forces, and these forces can be modified by factors such as the amount, direction, and duration of pressure. Types of physical force include compression, tension, bending, shearing, and torsion (Fig. 8.2).

- **Compression**. Pressing force, usually by pushing downward (e.g., effleurage). Tapotement and vibration also use compressive forces (e.g., tapping, hacking, cupping, pounding, clapping, jostling).

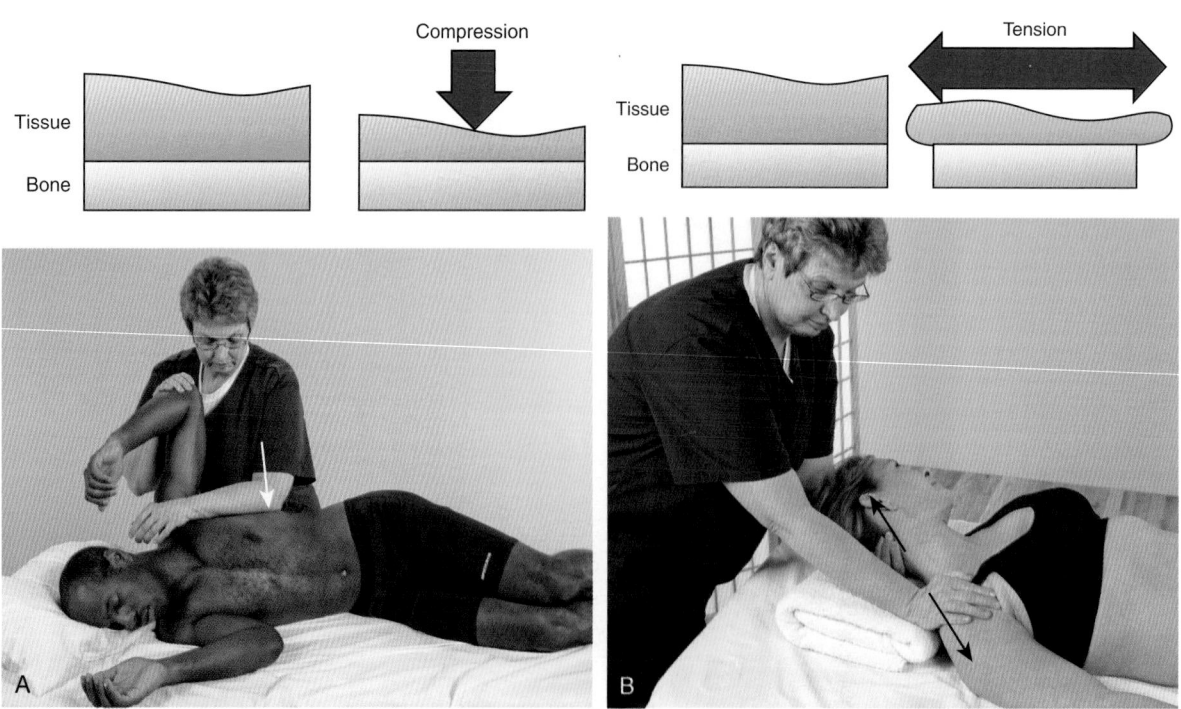

FIG. 8.2 (A–E) Physical forces and their relationship to massage techniques. (A) Compression and effleurage. (B) Tension and stretching.

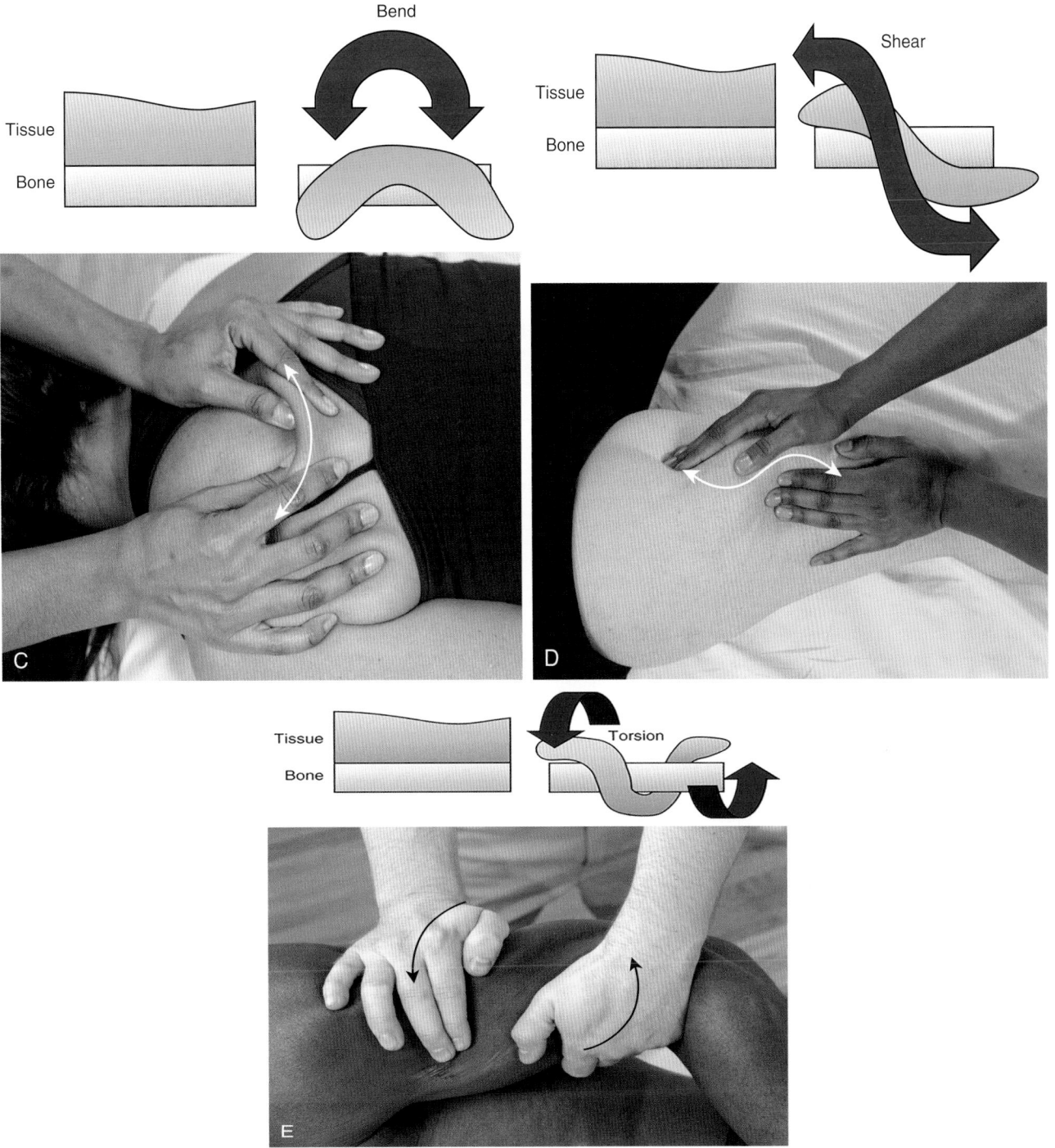

FIG. 8.2, CONT'D (C) Bending and skin rolling petrissage. (D) Shearing and skin rolling petrissage. (E) Torsion and ocean wave petrissage. (From Fritz, S. [2017]. *Mosby's fundamentals of therapeutic massage* [6th ed.]. St. Louis: Mosby.)

- **Tension**. Elongating or lengthening force, usually by pulling an object in opposite directions (e.g., stretching). Passive range of motion and myofascial techniques use tensile forces (e.g., pin and stretch, cross-hand stretch).
- **Bending**. Compressive and tension forces are combined, usually by pushing (squeeze) and pulling (lifting) tissues in a C shape (e.g., petrissage). This action compresses the central region and stretches outer regions. Skin rolling, fulling, and pincement use bending forces.

- **Shearing**. Sliding force, usually by compressing and gliding two surfaces against each other in the same or opposite directions (e.g., friction). This action may produce heat, but excessive amounts may cause tissue irritation. Several friction and petrissage variations use shearing forces (e.g., superficial, transverse, chucking, skin rolling).
- **Torsion**. Twisting or rotational force, usually by compressing and moving tissues in the same or opposite directions (e.g., petrissage). Several variations of

petrissage and friction apply torque to soft tissues (e.g., fulling, ocean waves, wringing, rolling).

Direction and Excursion

Most physicians and practitioners advocate for the **centripetal** (toward the center) direction of massage movements with pressure applied "from below upward" in the direction of venous and lymphatic circulation (DeDomenico & Wood, 1997). Unidirectional pressure is important for techniques such as effleurage and petrissage, and less important for techniques such as friction and compression.

Excursion is the distance traveled. Excursion ranges from the length of the palpable taut band, muscle, or muscle group (e.g., quadriceps, hamstrings), the length of a bone (e.g., humerus, tibia), the length of a limb (e.g., upper extremity, lower extremity), or area (e.g., back). Some massage techniques travel the length of the entire body.

Rate and Rhythm

Rate is the number of times or speed that massage techniques are repeated. Rate is often described as slow, moderate, or rapid/fast. The length of the technique often determines the speed of delivery. In general, effleurage is applied slowly—petrissage, friction, tapotement, and vibration are applied more rapidly. Slow techniques tend to be more calming and relaxing while quick techniques tend to be more stimulating. Slow techniques are more suitable for pretreatment palpatory assessments, transitions between techniques and areas of the body, and posttreatment palpatory reassessment.

Rhythm is the pattern or regularity of applied techniques. Rhythmical repetitions are preferred as they are more predictable to the client. Techniques should be applied without hesitancy or irregularity. The time between the end of one technique and the beginning of the next should be uninterrupted. The massage session should begin slowly and end slowly (Wood, 1974).

Duration and Frequency

As mentioned previously, the duration (length of the session) and frequency (how often sessions are received) are determined by the reasons why the massage is administered (wellness vs. clinical reasons). The session length and frequency for wellness massages are determined by the client based on the list of services posted by the massage establishment (i.e., 30-, 60-, to 90-minute sessions received weekly, monthly, quarterly, or as needed).

The session length and frequency for clinical massages are determined by medical directives or prescriptions and by limits of the procedural codes used. Other factors that may influence session duration and frequency include third-party payers such as insurance companies, and award or settlement limits related to legal claims.

Sequence and Routine

Sequence is the order in which techniques are arranged during the session. In general, techniques are repeated in structured multiples of three (e.g., 3, 6, 9, 12) until the desired

---

> ### BOX 8.1
>
> #### General Guidelines for Massage
>
> - Practice hand hygiene before and after each massage.
> - Protect yourself by using good body mechanics.
> - Promote client comfort by providing a restful environment and bolsters.
> - Base treatment plans on client goals.
> - Screen clients for contraindications.
> - Work deeply enough to reduce tension, but not so deep that you cause tension and pain.
> - Glide lightly over bony prominences and endangerment sites.

> ### BOX 8.2
>
> #### Factors That May Inhibit Client Relaxation
>
> - Strange or new surroundings
> - Fear of unknown treatments
> - Unpleasant odors
> - Excessive noise
> - Bright lights or total darkness
> - Cold, drafty rooms
> - Fear of undressing/lack of privacy
> - Shortness of breath or other breathing difficulties
> - Inadequate or uncomfortable support, draping, or positioning

Adapted from DeDomenico, G. (2007). *Beard's massage: Principles and practice of soft tissue manipulation* (5th ed.). Philadelphia: Saunders.

effect is achieved. This number is recommended as the first technique administration introduces a new or novel stimulus; during the second administration, it is recognized and no longer novel; and the third administration is predictable, which helps clients to relax (Buckle, 2014).

Routines are the sequence of techniques within a session. Most massage sessions are tailored to address the client's goals. Massage routines will vary according to your training and requirements set forth by the setting in which you are practicing, or by the client's preferences, treatment goals, and health condition (Box 8.1). Rely on experienced instructor(s) to properly demonstrate each technique, to model techniques, and to guide your practice. Sample massage routines focusing on relaxation have been developed by several massage professionals and can be accessed on the Internet (Chaumont, 2018; Schacter, 2021). A sample routine is also available on Evolve.

Relaxation is an important component to treatment effectiveness. Practitioners should take proactive measures to promote relaxation and eliminate factors that may cause anxiety for clients receiving massage (Box 8.2).

Tracking Client Responses

Good tracking skills are essential as they allow massage practitioners to work with awareness and sensitivity. **Tracking** is the ability to notice and respond to changes that a client experiences during the session. Notice the client's facial expressions; watch for changes in breath (i.e., in the belly when supine or the lumbar region when prone); or a subtle flinch or wince from a technique applied too forcefully or quickly. Listen for modulations in voice tone or cadence. With each new technique introduced, palpate whether the muscles are tightening or relaxing. Can you tell if pressure is adequate or too deep? Watch for signs such as a squint, a grimace, or the hands or feet being clenched.

Tracking combines careful observation of a client's moment-to-moment responses to technique with your willingness to adjust and change your work accordingly. Developing tracking competency can be summed up by asking yourself, "What can I do, in this moment, to bring my client into a deeper state of relaxation?" Critical to this process is being mindful and paying attention. Mindfulness allows practitioners to be present and engaged with clients in a way that promotes their feeling nurtured. When a client winces presumably in pain, the practitioner may be applying too much pressure. When this happens, lighten the pressure and work at or below the client's pain threshold. Massage that is continuously painful produces muscle guarding and additional spasms rather than relaxation. If there is pain, the client does not gain.

MASSAGE CONTRAINDICATIONS

For healthy clients, massage practitioners have a wide range of techniques used safely. However, some clients have conditions or have undergone medical treatments that may represent contraindications. A **contraindication** is a condition that could be aggravated by the application of massage. Situations that may represent contraindications include the presence of allergies, diseases and their complications, surgeries, recent injuries, the use of devices such as pacemakers, and the use of certain medications or their administration routes, such as transdermal patches or chemotherapy access ports. The presence of a contraindication is usually determined during the intake process, but this determination can also occur during the session. Contraindications can be absolute or local. The following are some examples of how to manage contraindications:

- Your client cannot receive a massage that day (absolute contraindication).
- Your client can receive massage, but an area of the body is avoided (local contraindication).
- Your client can receive massage with a few treatment, procedural or positional modifications.

Absolute Contraindications

Absolute contraindications are conditions that make receiving a massage absolutely inadvisable. Examples of absolute contraindications include the following situations:

- Contagious disease.
- Widespread infection or systemic inflammation, often indicated by fever: measured body temperature of 100.4°F (38°C) or higher (Centers for Disease Control and Prevention [CDC], 2017). Fever is also called pyrexia.
- Client in a state of medical emergency.

When a client has an absolute contraindication, massage is not advised and should be postponed. When the client's condition resolves or is released by the healthcare provider who managed the medical emergency, the client can then receive massage. Do not expect a written release from the healthcare provider, as this is not a standard medical procedure; the provider generally ceases to continue treatment and allows the client to return to their normal routines. First aid measures for medical emergencies are discussed in Chapter 9.

When you, the practitioner, are ill or experiencing signs and symptoms of the flu such as sneezing, coughing, fever, general body aches, sore throat, and/or a runny or stuffy nose, you may be a reservoir in the chain of infection. In these cases, canceling appointments or arranging for a fellow practitioner to take your place is preferred. The CDC (2021) recommends you stay home and not return to work until you have been fever-free for 24 hours without the use of fever-reducing drugs such as ibuprofen or acetaminophen.

Local Contraindications

A **local contraindication** is a condition that makes receiving massage to a local area of the body inadvisable. Massage can be administered to other areas of the body while avoiding the localized area where massage is contraindicated. The following are potential areas of local contraindication:

- Recently injured areas.
- Acutely inflamed areas.
- Endangerment sites mentioned previously.
- Areas containing medicated transdermal patches, chemotherapy ports, pacemakers, hormonal implants, or other medical devices.
- A lump, lesion, suspicious mole, warts, localized rash, or enlarged lymph nodes.

Too often we underestimate the power of a touch, a smile, a kind word, a listening ear, an honest compliment, or the smallest act of caring, all of which have the potential to turn a life around.
—Leo Buscaglia

EFFLEURAGE

Effleurage is the application of gliding movements that follow the contours of the body. The term effleurage (ef-flur-ahzh) originates from the French verb *effleurer,* meaning "to flow" and "to glide". Effleurage is also called *stroking* or *gliding*. Variations include one-hand, two-hand, alternate hand, and nerve stroke. Effleurage movements may be linear or circular.

Effleurage is commonly used to begin the massage session, apply or reapply lubricant, introduce touch and pressure to the client, assess tissues before treatment, and to reassess tissues after treatment. Effleurage can also be used when transitioning between different massage techniques and can provide overall continuity to the session. Effleurage can be used to conclude a body region or end the massage session. Research related to effleurage is on Evolve.

Technique

After skin is lubricated, apply movements with the hands (fingers, thumbs) or forearms, with the deeper or heavier pressure applied centripetally, or inferior from below moving upward, and less pressure applied centrifugally, or from above moving downward. Keep hands or forearms in constant contact with the client's skin when changing directions. Keep thumbs and fingers together during technique application if possible. Deeper pressure can be applied by leaning to transfer body weight into the client's tissues. Generally, deep pressure is applied more slowly and by using a broader base of physical contact (e.g., use the heel of the hand instead of fingertip). Stack the joints by arranging them vertically as much as possible during deep pressure application. The practitioner's hips and abdomen and pelvis, neck, and head should face the direction of movement.

One-Hand Effleurage

One hand (finger, thumb) is used to apply downward pressure (Fig. 8.3). When applying deep pressure centripetally on an extremity, anchor and/or traction the wrist or ankle distally so the extremity remains stationary as centripetal pressure is applied (Fig. 8.4).

Hands may be stacked to increase pressure (Fig. 8.5). The forearm can be used to apply deep pressure effleurage (Fig. 8.6). Deep effleurage can be applied on a muscle or muscle group while simultaneously lengthening the muscle (Fig. 8.7).

Two-Hand Effleurage

Two-hand effleurage uses both hands gliding simultaneously on the skin. The hands may move together in the same direction or in different directions. Two-hand effleurage is used to perform heart-shaped effleurage over the back, neck, and shoulders in one continuous movement (Fig. 8.8). Two-hand effleurage can be used up the leg and thigh (Fig. 8.9) or up the forearm and arm.

Alternate Hand Effleurage

During alternate hand effleurage, one hand begins the movement and lifts off the client's skin as the other hand

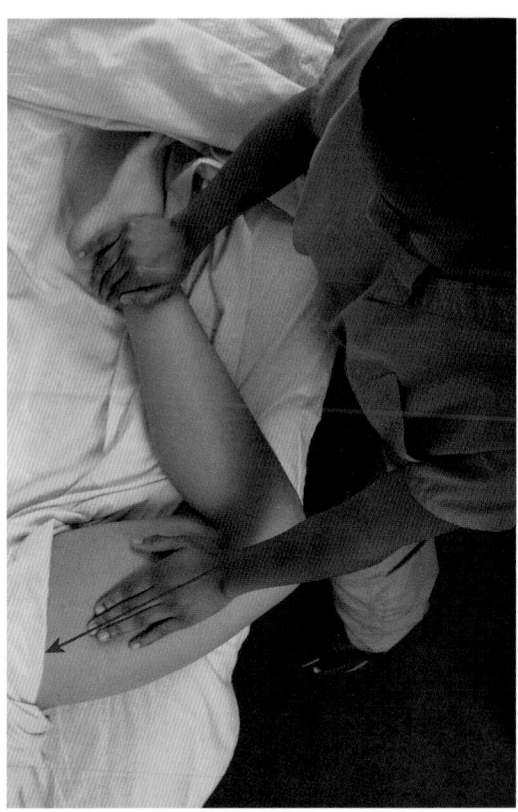

FIG. 8.4 One-hand effleurage. An open hand is used to apply pressure to the lateral thigh while the opposite hand anchors the ankle to the massage table.

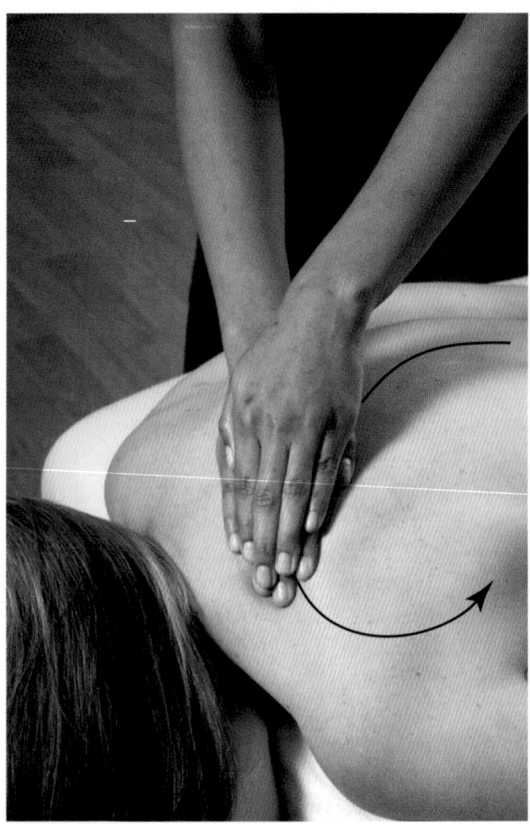

FIG. 8.5 One-hand effleurage. The hands are stacked to increase pressure while one hand is contact with the skin.

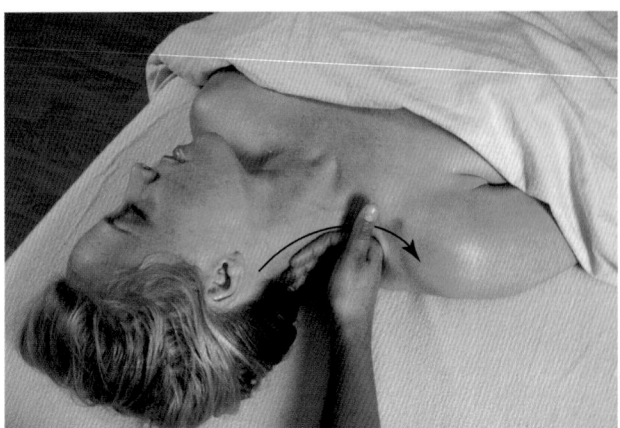

FIG. 8.3 One-hand effleurage. The knuckles of one hand are used to apply pressure to the upper trapezius.

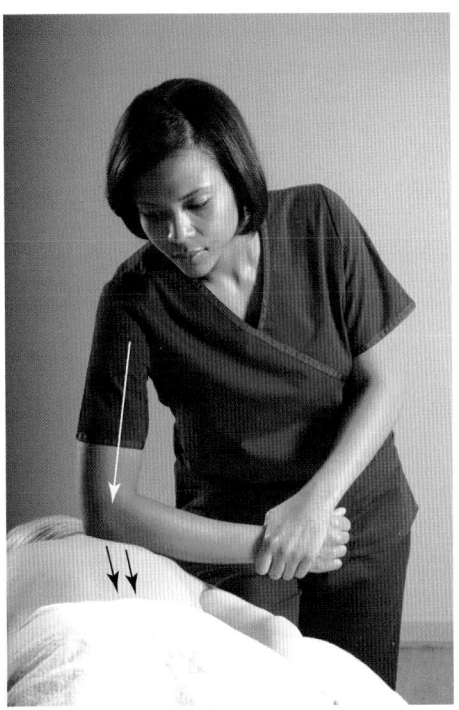

FIG. 8.6 One-hand effleurage. The forearm near one hand can be used to apply pressure on the back.

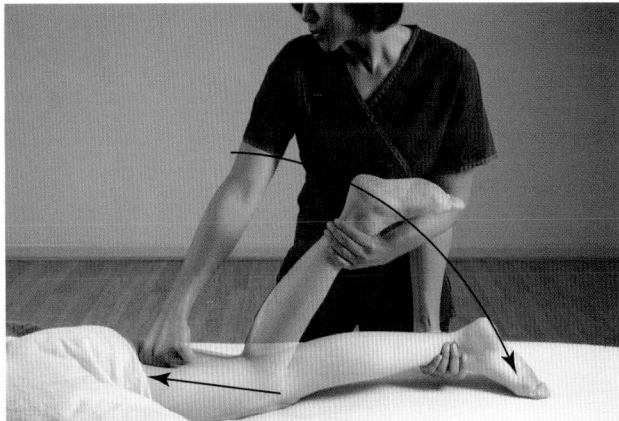

FIG. 8.7 One-hand effleurage. The knuckles of one hand can be used to apply pressure to the hamstrings while the other hand simultaneously lengthens the muscle by passively extending the knee.

repeats the movement, beginning from behind the lifted hand, while remaining in continuous contact during each repetition (Fig. 8.10). The practitioner may use the thumbs or fingers (Fig. 8.11). Alternate hand effleurage can be applied in a circular direction, with one hand moving in a circle and the other hand moving in a half-circle or crescent shape (Fig. 8.12).

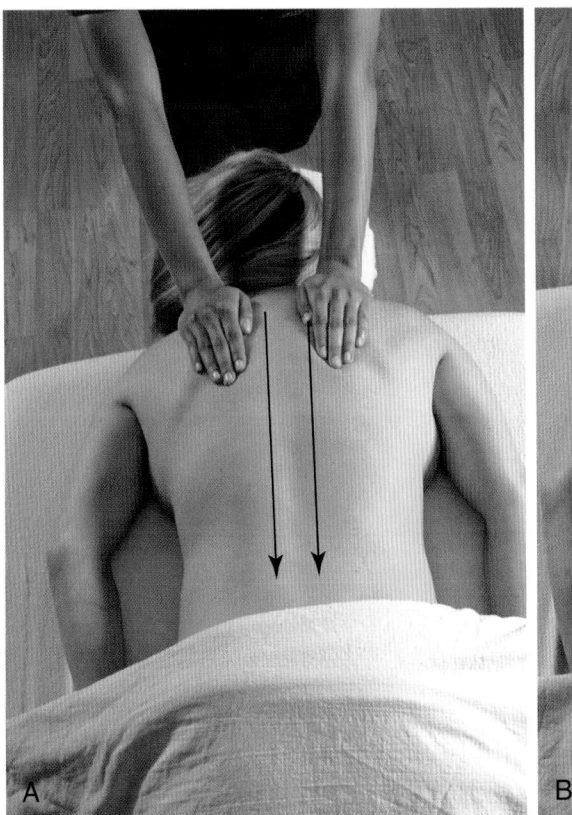

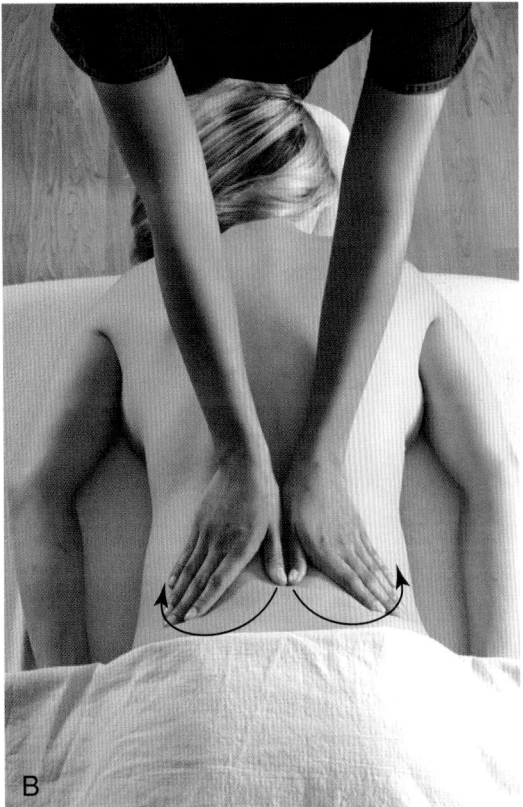

FIG. 8.8 Two-hand effleurage. Two hands move simultaneously to apply pressure to the back. (A) Hands start at the top of the shoulders and move down the back. (B) Hands move down the back to the base of the spine.

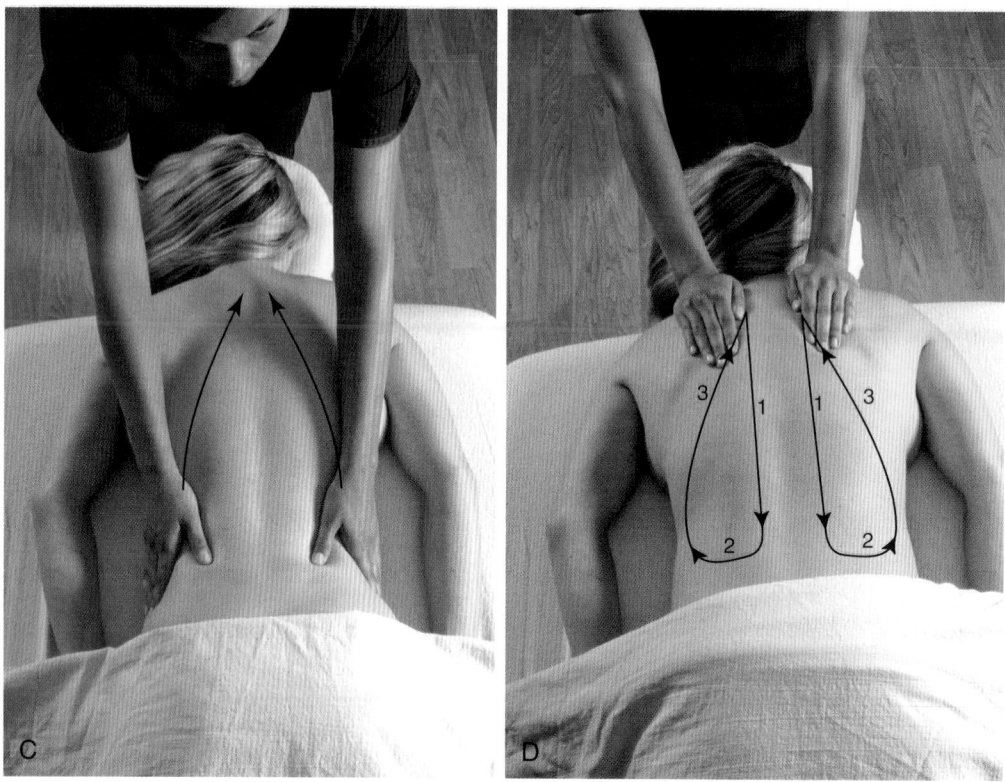

FIG. 8.8, CONT'D (C) Hands move up the sides of the back. (D) Hands return to their original position at the top of the shoulders.

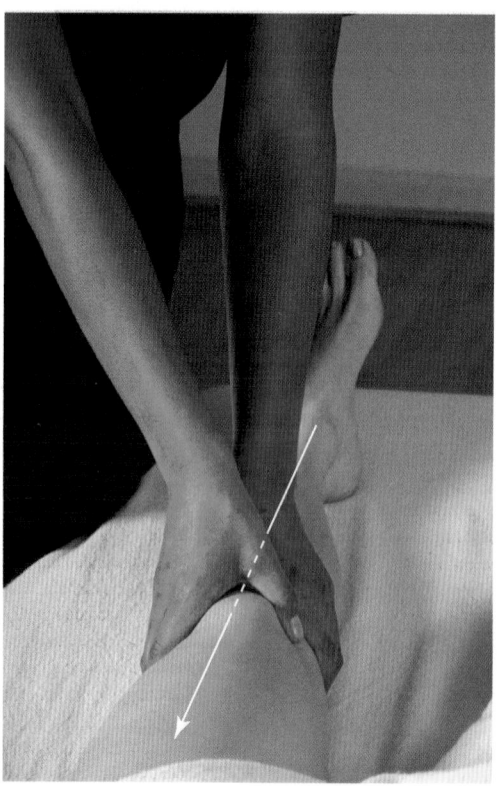

FIG. 8.9 Two-hand effleurage. Two hands move simultaneously to apply pressure to the anterior thigh. Keep thumbs and fingers together during technique application, if possible.

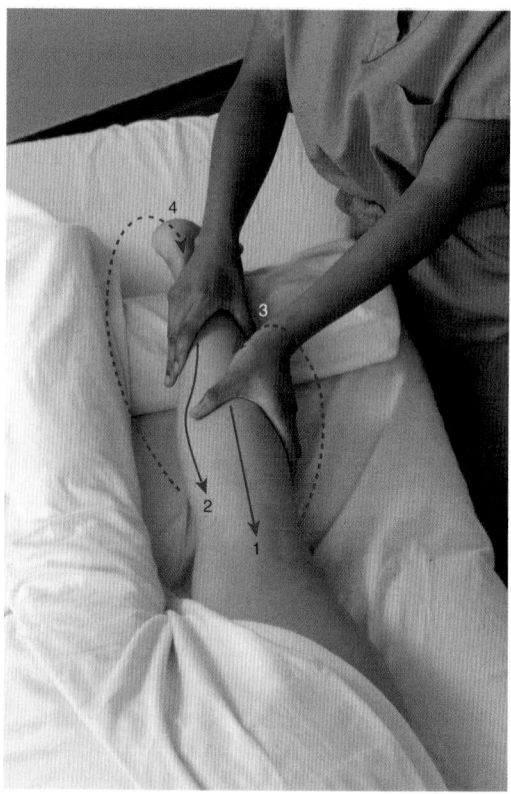

FIG. 8.10 Alternate hand effleurage. Two hands alternating to apply pressure on the calf. Keep thumbs and fingers together during technique application, if possible.

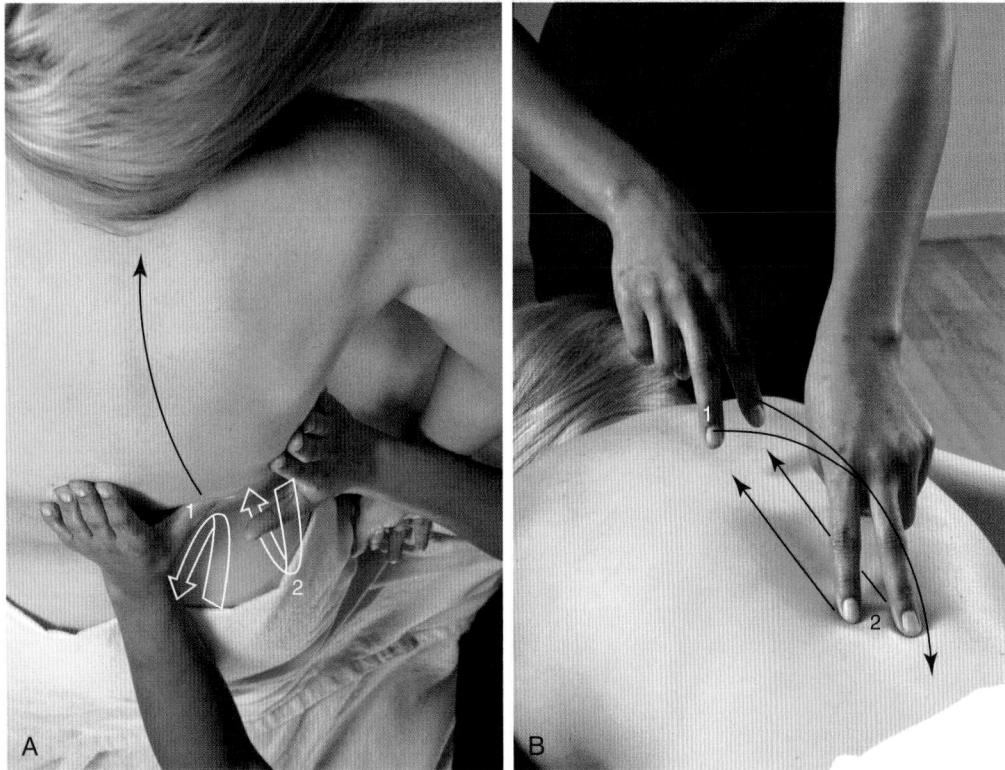

FIG. 8.11 Alternate hand effleurage. Two thumbs (A) and two fingertips alternating (B) to apply pressure over the paraspinal muscles.

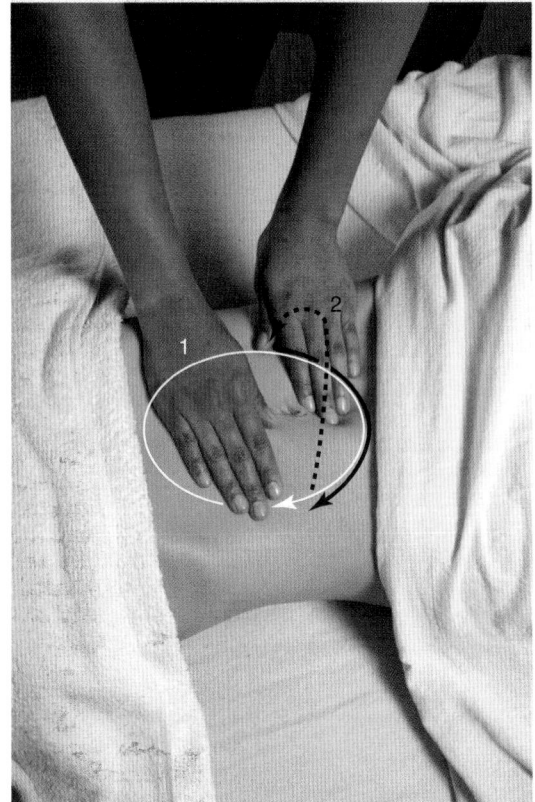

FIG. 8.12 Alternate hand effleurage. Two hands alternating to apply circular pressure on the abdomen.

Nerve Stroke

Nerve stroke, or *feathering*, uses light pressure applied with the weight of the fingers or hands as they glide down the body. Avoid rapidly applied light pressure because it may produce goose bumps or feel ticklish to the client. The direction of pressure is down the body (Fig. 8.13). The technique may be applied to bare skin, over the drape, or over clothing during sports or seated massage.

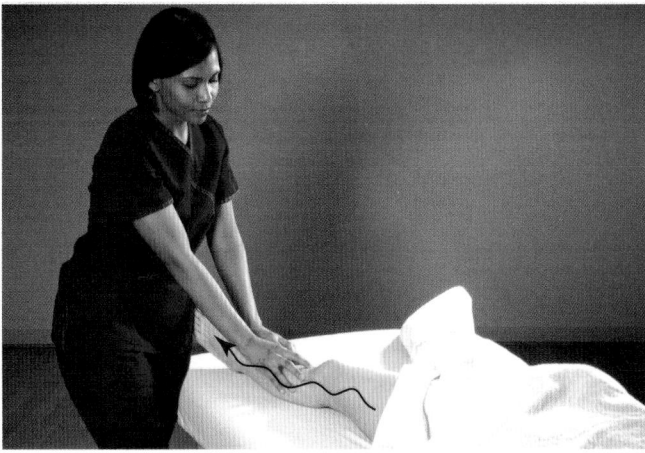

FIG. 8.13 Nerve stroke. One or two hands used to apply light pressure down the lower extremity.

PETRISSAGE

Petrissage involves compression, lifting or decompression, and then releasing soft tissues, such as skin and muscle. The term petrissage (peh-tre-sahzh) comes from the French verb *petrir*, meaning "to mash" or "to knead". Petrissage is also called *kneading*. Two types of pressure are superficial and deep. Superficial pressure targets skin and underlying tissues; deep pressure targets muscles. Several variations of petrissage are one-hand, two-hand, alternate hand, and skin rolling. Research related to petrissage is on Evolve.

Technique

Undrape the area and lightly lubricate the skin if needed. For superficial petrissage, grasp the skin and underlying tissue firmly and lift vertically. Compress the tissues by squeezing them and then releasing them. The lifted and compressed tissue can be rolled over muscle and bone using one hand or two hands moving either simultaneously or alternately.

For deep petrissage, grasp the muscle or muscle group firmly and lift vertically using a rolling motion. Next, compress the lifted tissue by squeezing it. Then release pressure while maintaining contact with the skin. The grasp-lift-compress-release sequence is repeated with the same hand or opposite hands moving simultaneously or alternately. Keep thumbs and fingers together during technique application if possible. Although pressure is applied vertically to muscle fibers, movements are still applied centripetally, with the greatest pressure applied when the hand is engaged with the lowest part of the limb (DeDomenico & Wood, 1997). Most deep petrissage applications merit the use of the entire palmar surface of the hand with significant hand strength required. If the treatment areas contain lots of body hair, use linear movements rather than small, circular movements, as the latter can cause hair to tangle. Additional lubricant may be needed in this circumstance.

One-Hand Petrissage

For one-hand petrissage, use one hand to compress, lift, and release the tissue repeatedly (Fig. 8.14). This variation is well-suited for smaller muscular areas such as the arms, forearms, or shoulders (Fig. 8.15).

Two-Hand Petrissage

Use two hands simultaneously to compress, lift, and release the tissue repeatedly. Two-hand petrissage can be applied with the heels of two hands while fingers are interlaced (Fig. 8.16), or two hands can move simultaneously in opposite directions while compressing and lifting tissues (Fig. 8.17). Two hands can be used to grasp, lift, and compress the tissue while moving it laterally; this is called *fulling* or *broadening* (Fig. 8.18).

Skin Rolling

Skin rolling is a superficial petrissage technique that compresses and lifts the skin, then moves or rolls the lifted skin across adjacent areas. The skin should be unlubricated or lightly lubricated. The rolling action is much like

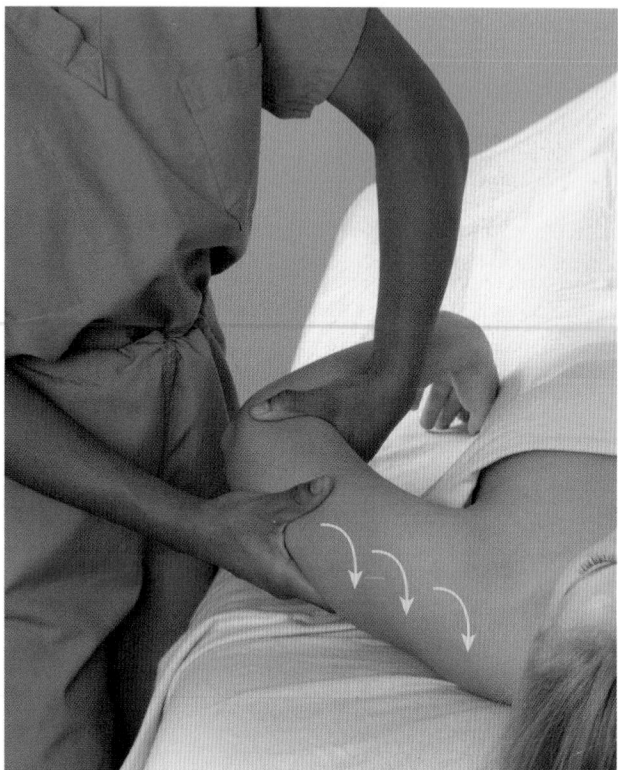

FIG. 8.14 One-hand petrissage. One hand is used to compress, lift, and release tissues of the posterior arm.

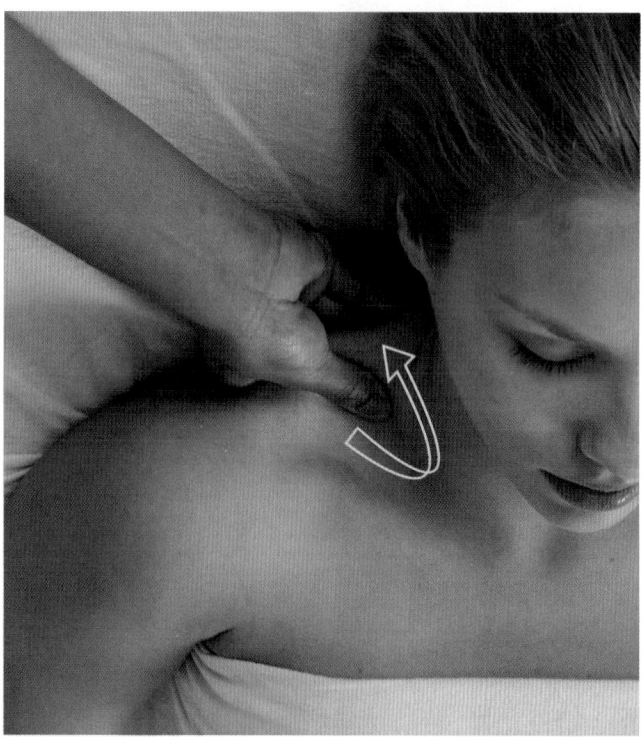

FIG. 8.15 One-hand petrissage. Fingers and thumb of one hand are used to compress, lift, and release the upper trapezius.

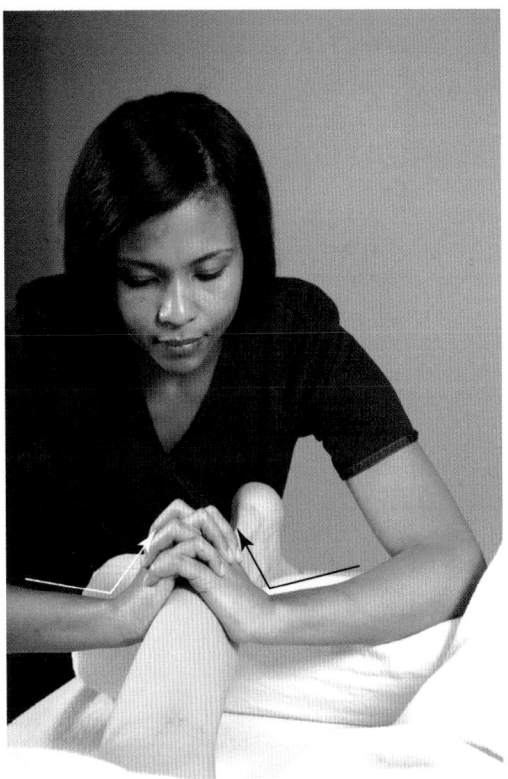

FIG. 8.16 Two-hand petrissage. Two hands are used to compress, lift, and release tissues on the posterior leg or calf.

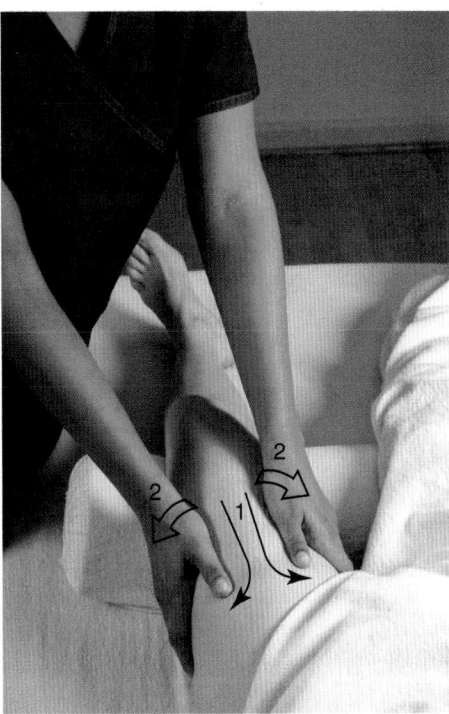

FIG. 8.18 Two-hand petrissage. Two hands are used to compress, lift, and release tissues on the anterior thigh. The hands move in opposite directions.

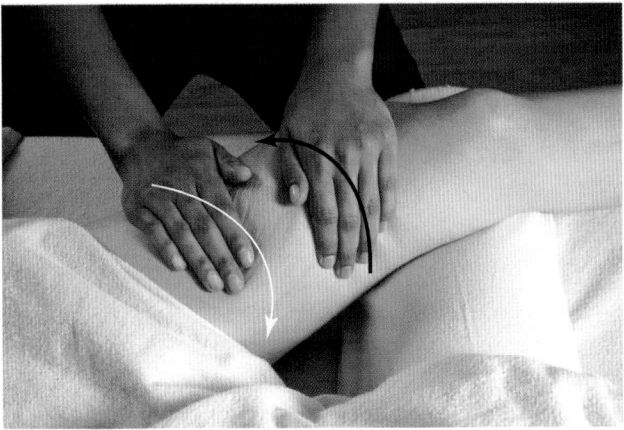

FIG. 8.17 Two-hand petrissage. Two hands are used to compress, lift, and release tissues on the anterior thigh. The hands move in opposite directions.

rolling a pencil between the practitioner's fingers and thumb (Fig. 8.19). Because underlying tissues such as superficial fascia are randomly arranged, skin rolling movements should be applied in several directions (e.g., transverse, diagonal). Skin can also be compressed, lifted, and held stationary for a few moments (Fig. 8.20). Skin rolling may be uncomfortable for the client, so use light pressure, gradually increasing pressure while working at or below the client's pain threshold.

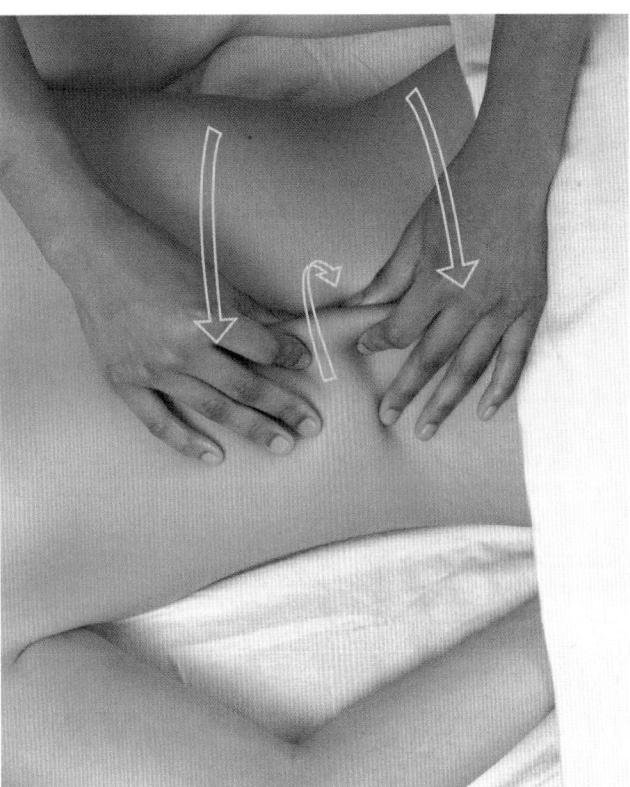

FIG. 8.19 Skin rolling petrissage. Skin is compressed and lifted between two fingers and thumbs, then moved or rolled across adjacent areas.

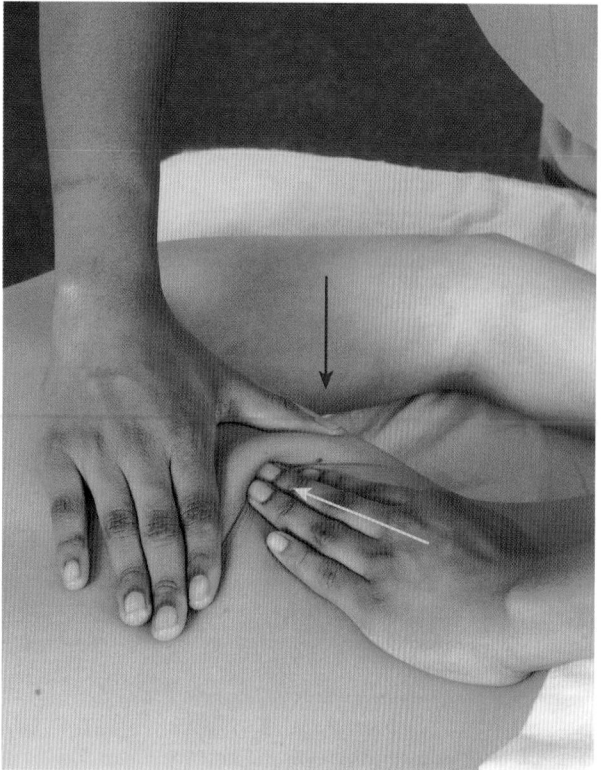

FIG. 8.20 Skin rolling petrissage. Skin is compressed and lifted between the fingers of one hand and the thumb web of the other hand, then repeated in adjacent areas.

Alternate Hand Petrissage

During alternate hand petrissage, two hands perform the compress, lift, and release sequence alternately, rather than simultaneously (Fig. 8.21). Do not lose contact with the skin while switching hands.

FRICTION

Friction involves rubbing one body surface against another while maintaining constant and equal pressure in all directions. The term friction (frik-shon) comes from the French term *frictionner,* meaning "to rub". Movements may be linear or circular. Unlike effleurage, in which pressure is unequal when applied in two or more directions (centripetal = deeper pressure), friction involves equal pressure in all directions. These movements can produce heat and may stimulate therapeutic inflammation. Research related to friction is on Evolve. Types of pressure are superficial and deep.

- **Superficial friction**. The practitioner's hands slide over the client's skin. Variations of superficial friction are *superficial warming, rolling,* and *wringing.*
- **Deep friction**. The practitioner's hands do not slide across the client's skin but rather take the skin with it, allowing the force to be transmitted directly to the deep tissues, including tendons and ligaments. Deep friction can help muscle, tendon, and ligament lesions heal quickly and completely, and can decrease adhesions at the injury site, thereby increasing tissue mobility and assisting in the repatterning of scar tissue itself. Variations of deep friction are *transverse* or *cross-fiber, chucking,* and *circular.*

Technique

Friction can be applied to bare skin, through the drape, or through clothing. When friction is applied to bare skin, the skin should be lubricant-free or lightly lubricated. Movements are back and forth in a linear or circular direction.

During *superficial friction*, the practitioner's hands glide briskly over the client's skin. Movements are back and forth in a linear or circular direction.

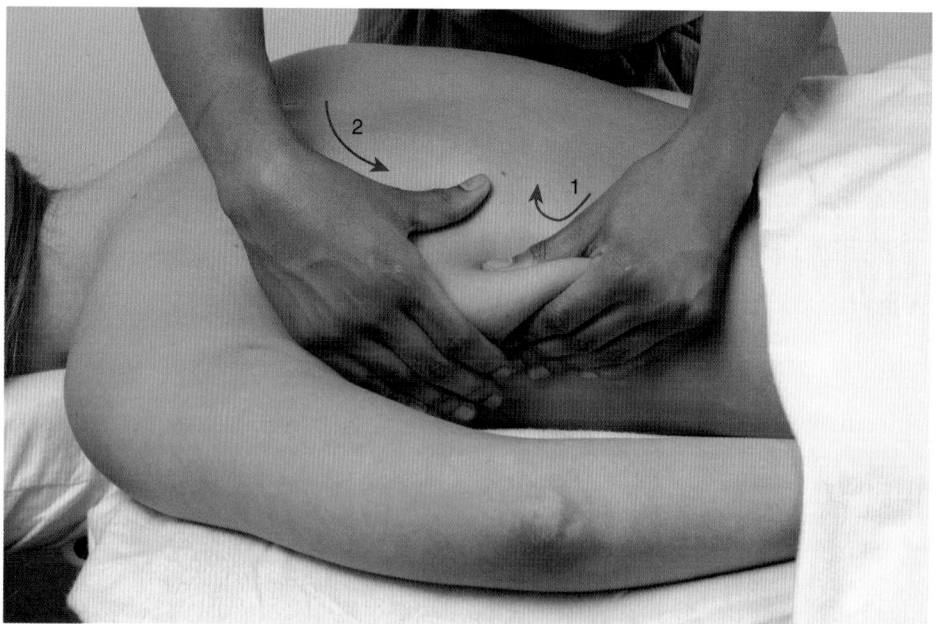

FIG. 8.21 Alternate hand petrissage. Two hands are alternating to apply compression, lifting, and releasing movements on the lateral aspect of the back.

During *deep friction*, the practitioner moves the client's skin over the underlying tissue layers. The practitioner's hand and the client's skin move together as a single unit. Pressure should be moderate, between 4 and 7 on a 10-point pressure scale.

Superficial Warming Friction

Place one or two hands on the client's skin, fingers held together firmly. Move hand(s) briskly up and down or in a circular direction. If two hands are used, they can move in the same or in opposite directions (Fig. 8.22). The fingertips, knuckles, heel of hand, or ulnar surface of one or two hands may also be used (Fig. 8.23). The latter variation is called *sawing* (Fig. 8.24). Superficial warming friction can be applied with a towel on bare skin, also called *towel friction*.

Rolling Friction

Compress the tissues firmly using two hands, fingers extended. Move the hands back and forth in opposite directions quickly. These movements will "roll" or rotate tissues around the underlying bone(s) (Fig. 8.25). Keep both hands in constant contact as you compress and roll in a fashion that produces a mild amount of opposing traction between your left and right hands. Begin the technique at the distal end of the extremity, and then proceed proximally. The client can assist by holding the extremity in a stable position. To apply this technique on the fingers or toes, compress the tissue with fingertips instead of the entire hand.

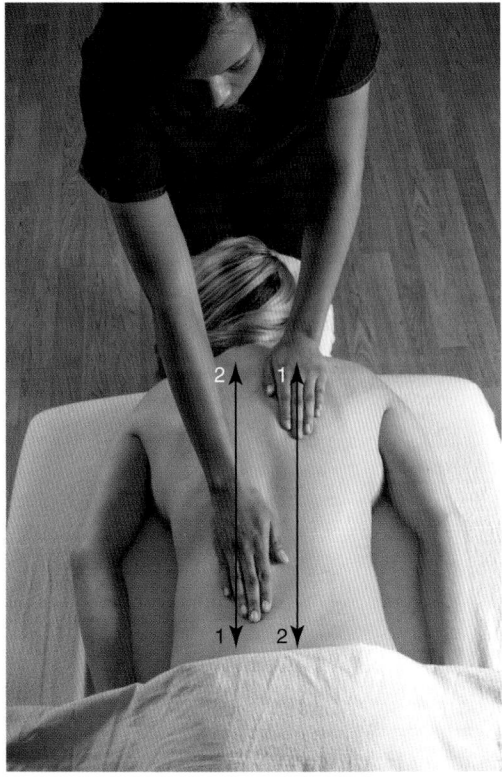

FIG. 8.22 Superficial warming friction. Two hands move rapidly over the skin to generate warmth.

Wringing Friction

Compress lightly lubricated skin with two hands, fingers wrapped around and molded to the extremity. Begin "wringing" or moving your hands back and forth in opposite directions quickly (Fig. 8.26). Keep both hands in constant contact as you grip and twist in a fashion that produces a mild amount of opposing traction between your left and right hands. As in rolling friction, begin the technique at the distal end of the extremity, and then proceed proximally. The client can assist by holding the extremity in a stable position. To apply this technique on the fingers or toes, compress the tissue with fingertips instead of the entire hand. Wringing friction is performed vigorously, as though squeezing water from a washcloth.

Transverse Friction

Transverse friction is also called *cross-fiber friction*. This technique was popularized by Cyriax (1984) and is occasionally referred to as *Cyriax friction massage*. Place the thumb, fingertips, or heel of hand on the treatment area and compress (Fig. 8.27). Move the client's skin back and forth over the treated fibers at right angles or perpendicular to the tissue fibers (Fig. 8.28).

Chucking Friction

Place the thumb or fingertips on the treatment area and compress. Move the client's skin back and forth over the treated fibers parallel to the tissue fibers. Chucking can be performed with one hand while the other hand supports the treated area or extremity (Fig. 8.29). Chucking friction is also known as *parallel friction*.

Circular Friction

Place the thumb or fingertips on the treatment area and compress. Move the client's skin over the treatment area in a circular direction (Fig. 8.30). Circular friction can be applied around joints and bony areas.

COMPRESSION

Compression is a non-gliding technique of pressure application. The term compression comes from the French *compresser*, which means "to press" or "to squeeze". Two types of compression are sustained and rhythmic. Sustained compression was once called *ischemic compression*—Travell and Simons (1998) coined the term because the skin initially blanches pale or becomes ischemic on removal of pressure before becoming hyperemic and pinkish-red. Variations of compression include *one-hand*, *two-hand*, and *alternate hand*.

Technique

Compression can be applied to bare skin, through the drape, or through clothing. When compression is applied to bare skin, the skin should be lubricant-free or lightly lubricated. During sustained compression, place your fingers, thumb, knuckle, heel of hand, fist, forearm, or elbow on the client's

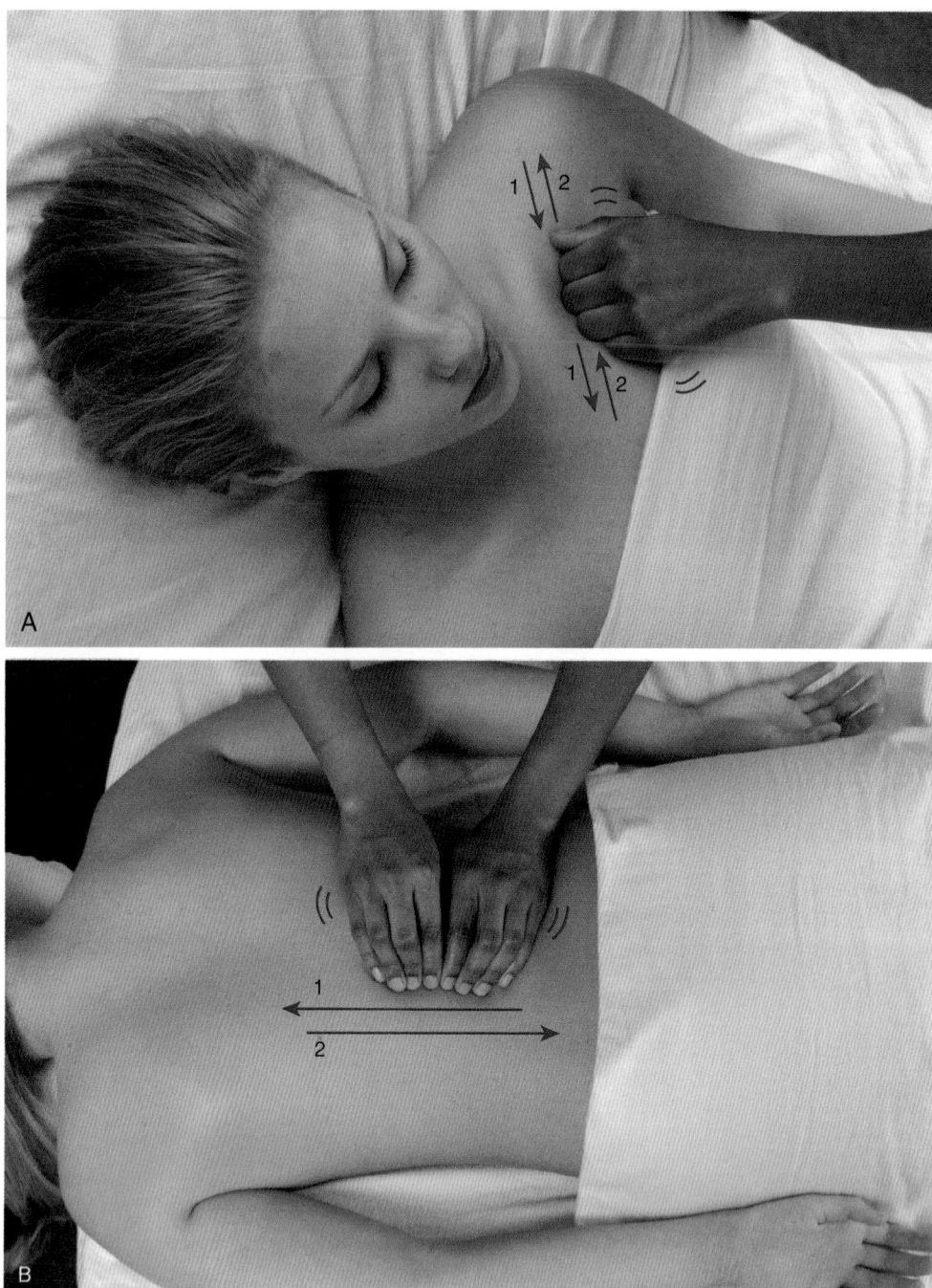

FIG. 8.23 Superficial warming friction. The knuckles of one hand are used to apply pressure on the pectoralis major muscle below the clavicle (A). The fingertips of two hands are used to apply pressure up and down the paraspinal muscles (B).

skin and compress toward an underlying bone. Pressure is maintained for 10 to 20 seconds (Gatterman, 2011). Sustained compression can be combined with other techniques such as jostling. For example, compress a tender area within a muscle while shaking a nearby joint.

For rhythmic compression, pressure is regularly applied by pressing and releasing pressure. Tissues can be compressed with the heel of the hand, fist, or forearm. As you sink into the tissue, try to land softly yet firmly like a cat.

After a brief moment, spring the hands up and off the tissue. Focus on a rhythmic sinking, landing, and springing back out. Rhythmic compressions resemble a "pumping action" and may cause the client's body to rock back and forth. As the client's body rocks back, compress it again to repeat the rocking motion—like pushing someone on a swing. Rhythmic compressions applied rapidly at shorter intervals tend to be more stimulating. Conversely, they are more relaxing or calming when applied slowly at longer intervals.

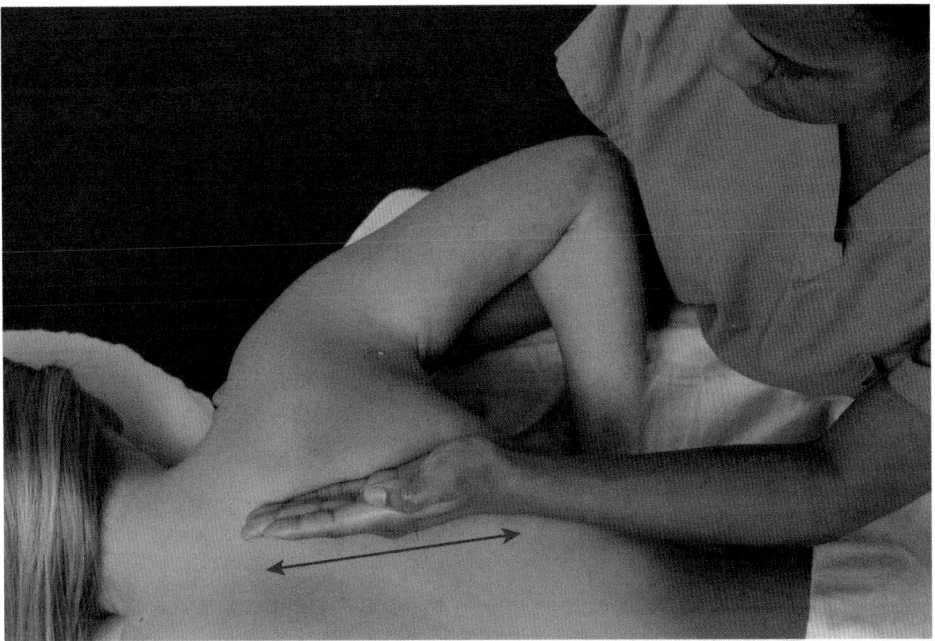

FIG. 8.24 Superficial warming friction. The ulnar surface of one hand is used to apply pressure along the medial border of the scapula.

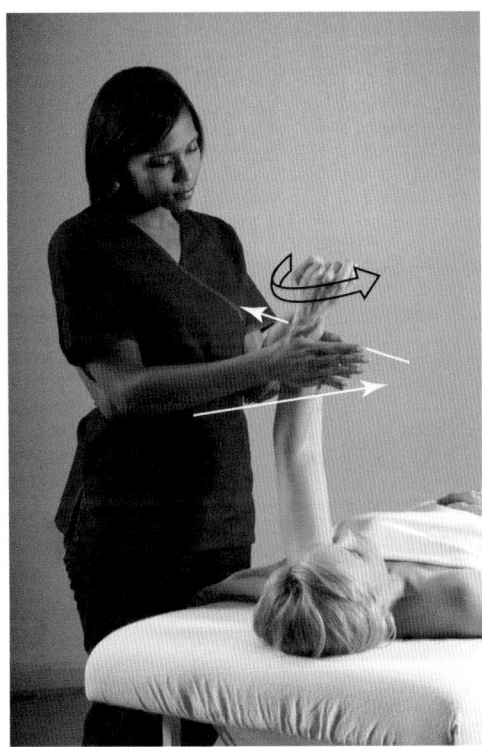

FIG. 8.25 Rolling friction. Two hands are used to apply rolling friction on the forearm.

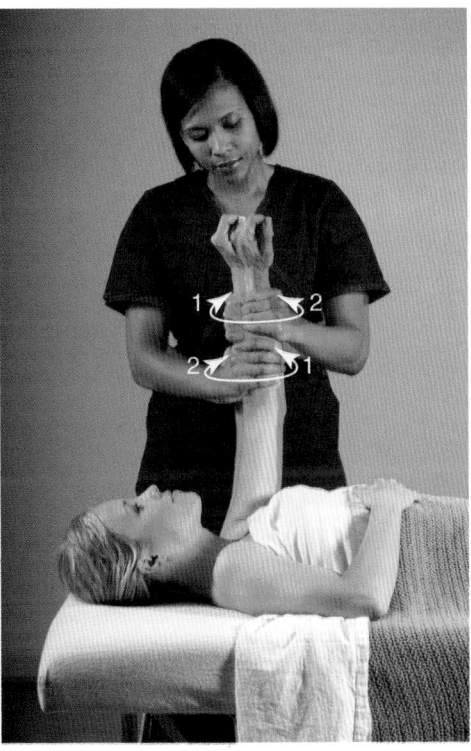

FIG. 8.26 Wringing friction. Two hands are used to apply wringing friction on the forearm.

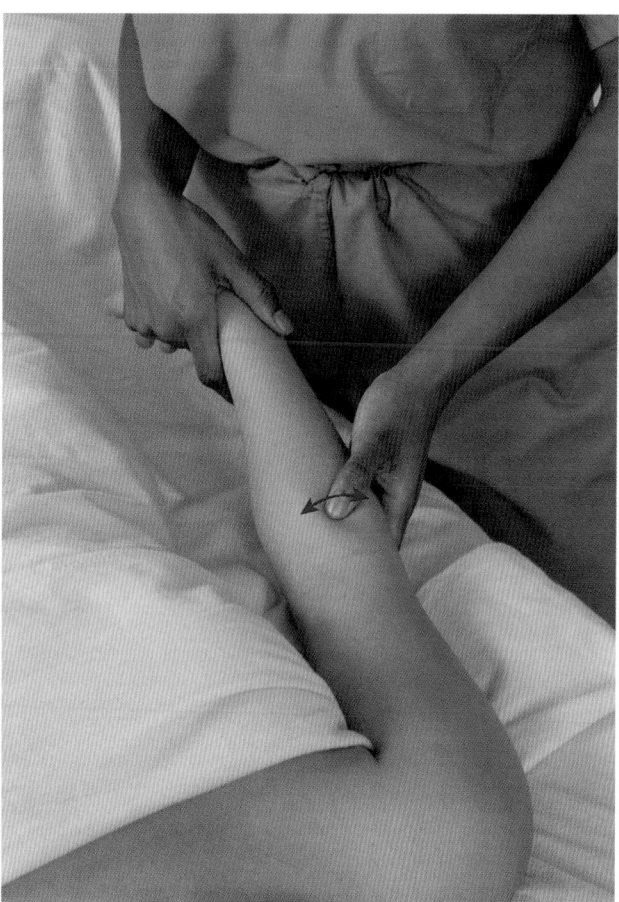

FIG. 8.27 Transverse friction. The thumb of one hand is used to apply transverse friction on the forearm.

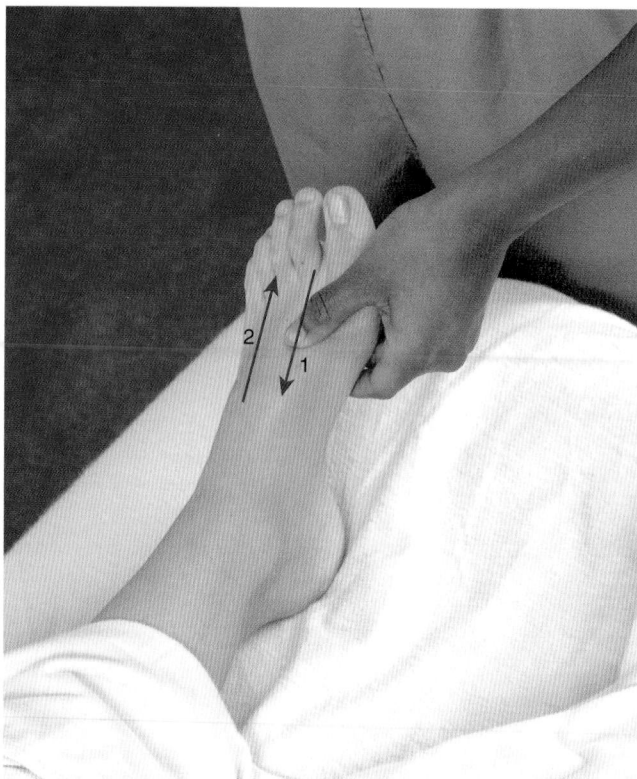

FIG. 8.29 Chucking friction. The thumb of one hand is used to apply chucking friction between the metatarsals.

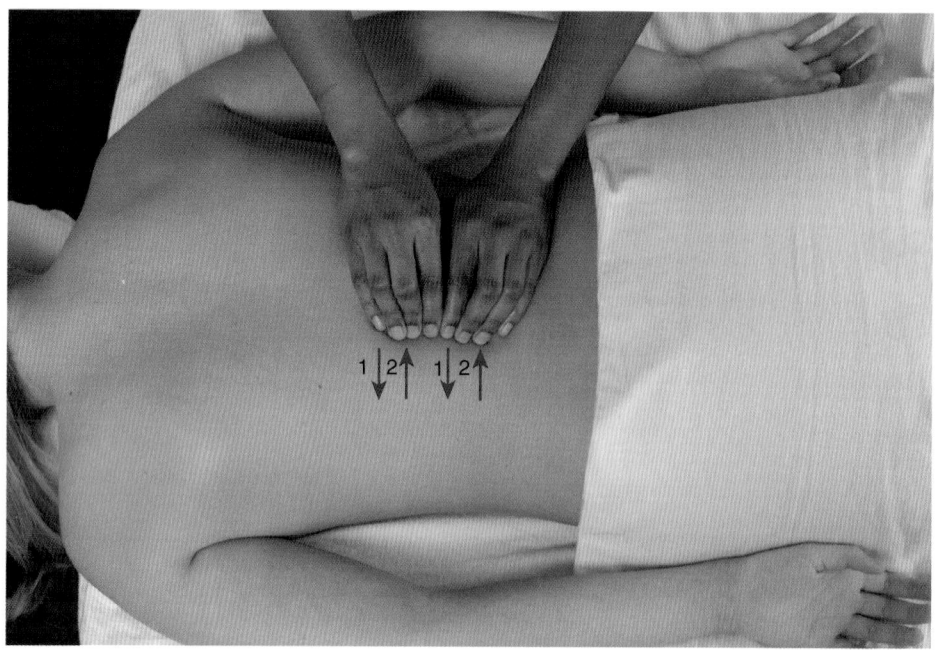

FIG. 8.28 Transverse friction. Fingertips of two hands are used to apply transverse friction over the paraspinal muscles.

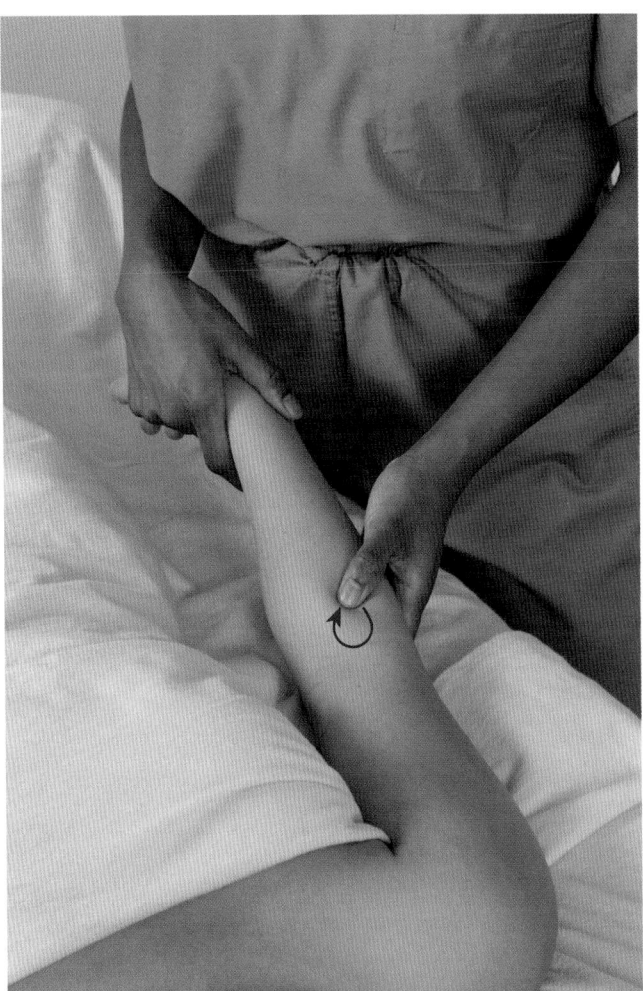

FIG. 8.30 Circular friction. The thumb of one hand is used to apply circular friction on the forearm.

One-Hand Compression

For one-hand compression, use one hand to compress the tissue (Fig. 8.31). Hands may be stacked to increase pressure (Fig. 8.32).

Two-Hand Compression

For two-hand compression, use two hands simultaneously to compress the tissue.

Alternate-Hand Compression

For alternate-hand compression, two hands are used to apply pressure, but at different times. Alternate hand compression is used to apply rhythmic compression.

> *Often the hands will solve a mystery that the intellect has struggled with in vain.*
>
> **—C. G. Jung**

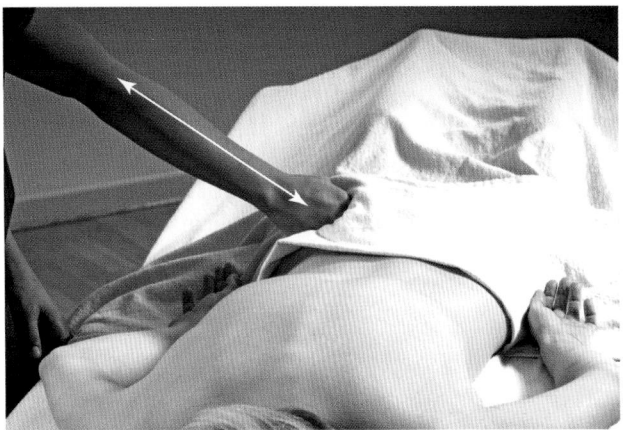

FIG. 8.31 One-hand compression. The fist of one hand is used to apply compression to the hip.

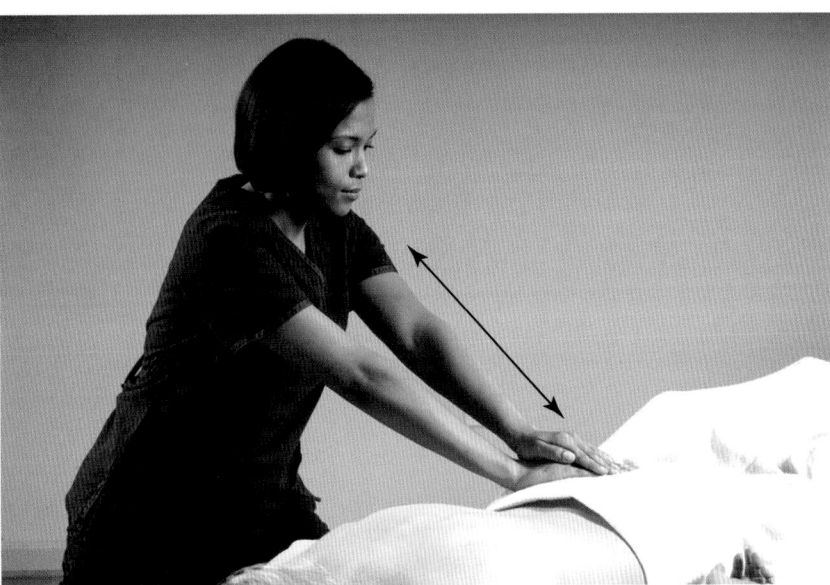

FIG. 8.32 One-hand compression. Hands are stacked to increase pressure while one hand is in contact with the skin.

TAPOTEMENT

Tapotement is a repetitive striking motion. The term tapotement (tap-ot-mon) is a derivation of an Old French term, *taper*, meaning "a light blow", which, in turn, was derived from the Anglo-Saxon term *taeppa*, meaning "to tap", in the sense of draining fluid from a cavity. At first, this word origin may seem peculiar, but interestingly, cupping tapotement is still used by respiratory practitioners and nurses to loosen and expel phlegm in the lungs within the chest cavity. Tapotement is also called *percussion* because it is like beating a drum. The synonym percussion comes from the Latin term *percussio*, which means "a striking." Types of tapotement include *tapping, pincement, hacking, cupping, pounding, clapping,* and *diffused.* Each variation uses a different part of the practitioner's hands, such as the fingertips, ulnar surface of an open palm or closed fist, knuckles of the closed fist, edges of a cupped hand, or palm of an open hand. Research related to tapotement is on Evolve.

Technique

Strike the client's skin with one or two hands and remove the hand(s) quickly. The motion is similar to hands bouncing off the client. When two hands are used, they can move simultaneously or alternately. Tapotement can be applied to bare skin, through the drape, or through clothing. When performed over bare skin, inform the client about the possibility of loud noises accompanying some tapotement variations such as cupping. Tapotement can be applied gently or vigorously by varying delivery speed and pressure. Light tapotement is more relaxing and calming while forceful or vigorous tapotement is more stimulating. Use light tapotement over thin tissue or delicate areas such as the face. Vigorous tapotement is more appropriate for muscular areas such as the back, hips, thighs, and calves.

Tapping

Use fingertips of one or two hands to strike the skin alternatively or simultaneously. Fingers can be held apart or together (Fig. 8.33). Use the finger pads when tapping lightly for a variation called *raindrops*. Light tapping is suitable over parts of the face or the scalp (Fig. 8.34).

Pincement

Use the tips of several fingers and thumb to strike, grasp, lift, and release the skin (Fig. 8.35). This action is like plucking facial tissue from a tissue box. Light pincement is suitable over the scalp and can include gentle lifting of the hair. Some textbooks classify pincement as petrissage because of its lifting action.

Hacking

Hacking is achieved with the ulnar surfaces of one or two hands. When both hands are used, palms face each other to strike the skin simultaneously or alternately. The action involves flicking the hands rhythmically up and down in rapid succession. Wrists should be flexible, and fingers slightly spread apart before applying the flicking motions (Fig. 8.36).

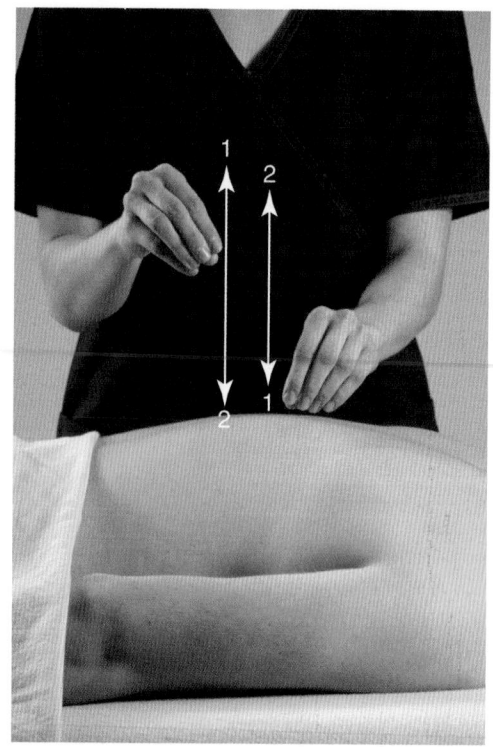

FIG. 8.33 Tapping tapotement. Fingertips of both hands are used to tap the skin on the back.

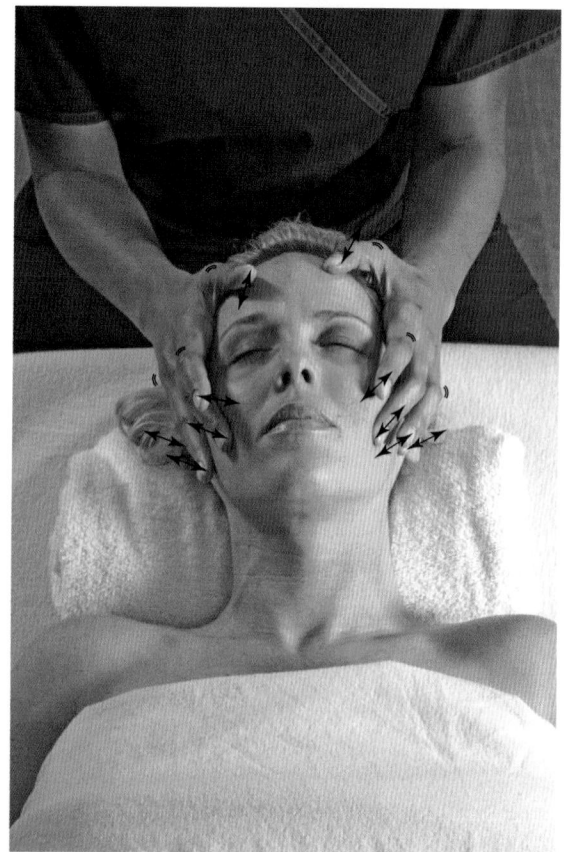

FIG. 8.34 Tapping tapotement (raindrops). Fingertips of both hands are used to gently tap the skin on the face.

As the skin is struck, the momentum of this action causes each finger to contact the finger below, which can produce a vibratory effect. A variation of hacking, called *quacking,* is applied using two hands moving simultaneously. The hands face each other with fingertips touching (palms do not touch), and the air moving from the hands after the strike makes a "quacking" sound (Fig. 8.37).

Cupping

During cupping, edges of one or two downwardly facing cupped hands strike the skin in quick succession (Fig. 8.38). As cupped hands are brought down in quick succession, a vacuum is created, which ceases when the hands are lifted. The sound should be hollow, similar to horse hooves striking the ground. The client is asked to take a deep breath, and

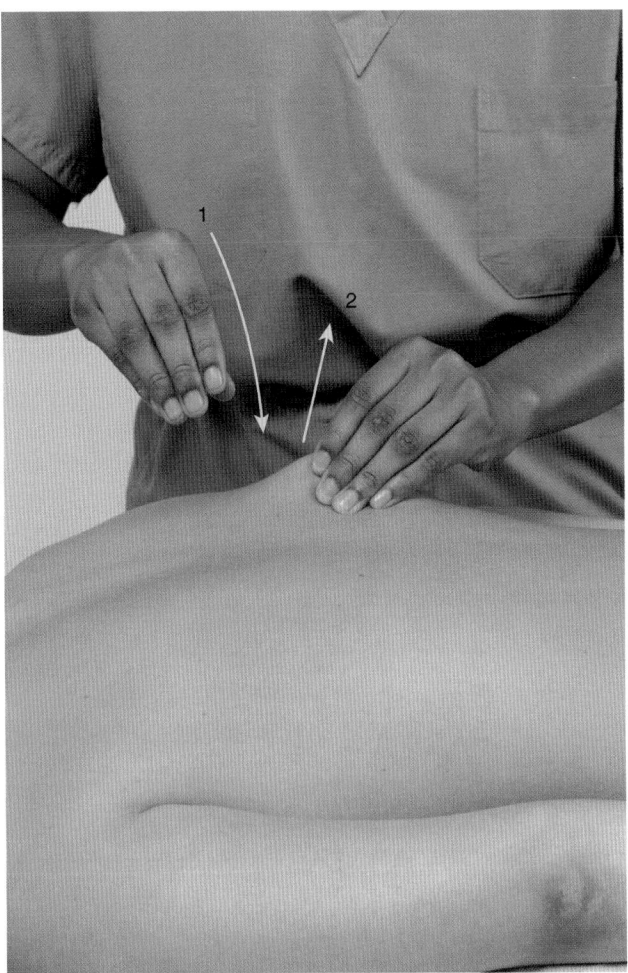

FIG. 8.35 Pincement tapotement. Tips of the fingers and thumbs of both hands are used to strike, grasp, lift, and release the skin on the back.

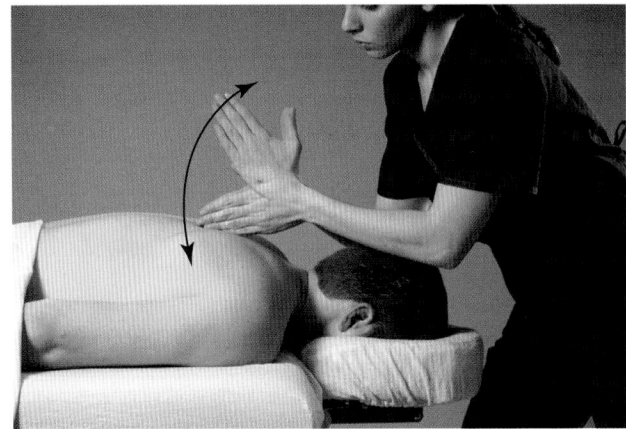

FIG. 8.37 Hacking tapotement (quacking). Two hands are used and as air moves from the palms after they strike the skin, a quacking sound may be heard.

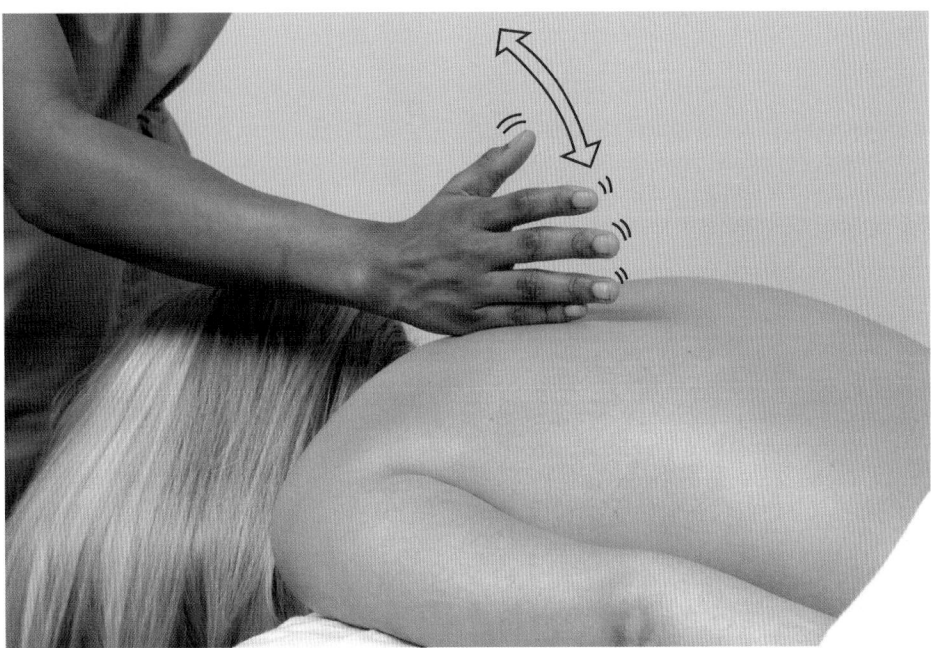

FIG. 8.36 Hacking tapotement. The ulnar surface of one hand is used on the back along the paraspinal muscles.

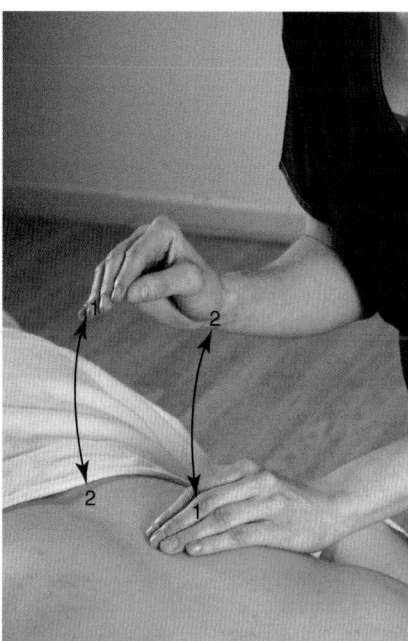

FIG. 8.38 Cupping tapotement. The edges of one or two downwardly facing cupped hands striking the skin in quick succession, which can make a hollow sound like horse hooves striking the ground.

cupping begins upon the exhalation (Wood, 1974). Cupping tapotement specifically is part of postural drainage and percussion (PD&P), an airway clearance technique used on the back and chest to loosen mucus in the lungs so it can be removed by coughing. PD&P is discussed in *Mosby's Pathology for Massage Professionals*. Furthermore, cupping tapotement is different from "cupping therapy," which uses the placement of plastic, silicone, or glass cups on the skin to create negative pressure through suction. Cupping therapy is discussed in Chapter 14.

Pounding

Use the ulnar sides of a loose fist to strike the skin (Fig. 8.39). Pounding can be applied on large, muscular areas such as the back, thighs, and hips. A variation of pounding, called *rapping,* uses the knuckles of a loose fist to strike the skin as if knocking on a door (Fig. 8.40).

Clapping

Clapping is accomplished with the fingers and palms open and downwardly facing to strike the skin. Fingers are held together firmly. The action is a rhythmic, quick, repetitive motion and is relatively noisy and dynamic. Clapping is also called *slapping* (Fig. 8.41). Light clapping directed upward is suitable over the sides of the face.

Diffused

For diffused tapotement, lay a relaxed hand, palm up or down, over the client's skin and strike the back of this hand with the other hand positioned in a loose fist (Fig. 8.42). Drag the relaxed hand across the skin instead of lifting the

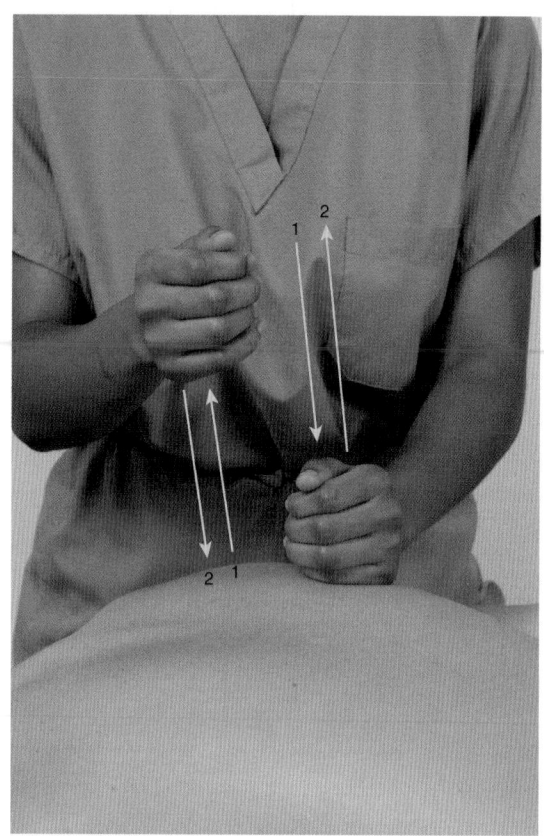

FIG. 8.39 Pounding tapotement. The sides of loose fists are used to strike the skin.

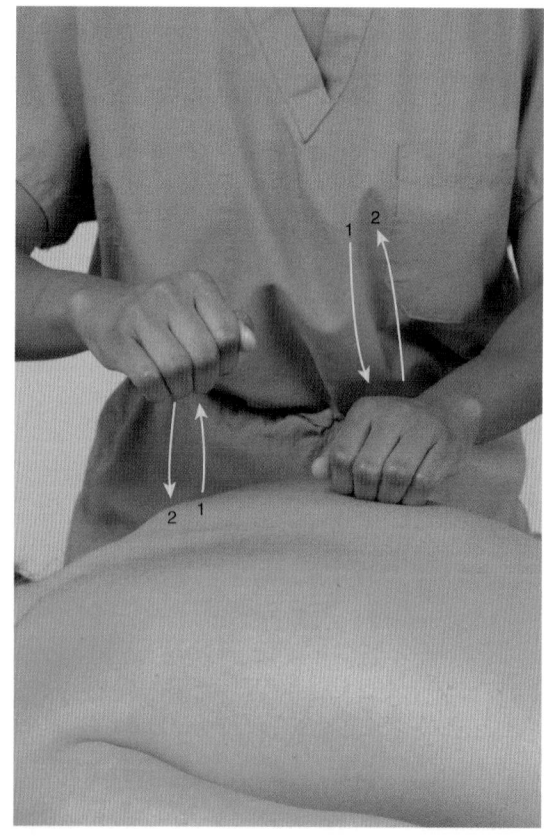

FIG. 8.40 Pounding tapotement (rapping). The knuckles of loose fists are used to strike the skin.

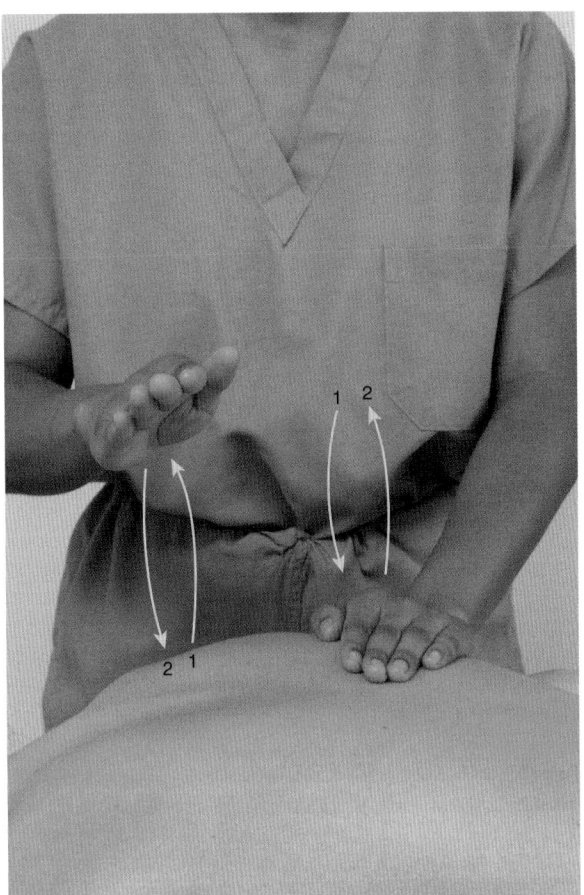

FIG. 8.41 Clapping tapotement. Fingers are held together firmly with palms open and downward facing, then the hands gently strike the skin.

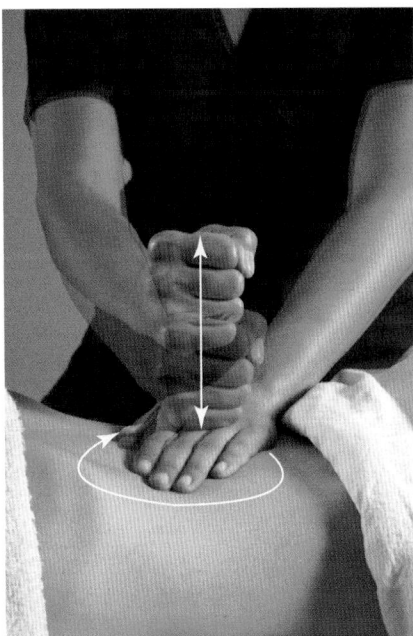

FIG. 8.42 Diffused tapotement. A relaxed hand is placed on the skin while the other hand strikes the back of the relaxed hand.

hand to move to the next treatment area. Gently applied, diffused tapotement is suitable over the abdomen.

VIBRATION

Vibration is a shaking or trembling motion. The term vibration comes from the French *vibrer,* which means "to shake". Variations of vibration include *fine vibration* and *jostling*.

Technique

Vibration can be applied to bare skin, through the drape, or through clothing. When vibration is applied to bare skin, the skin should be lubricant-free or lightly lubricated. Vibrational movements are back and forth or up and down and can be applied rapidly or slowly. Vibration can be applied with the fingertips, the full hand, or an electrical vibration device.

Fine Vibration

For fine vibration, compress the skin slightly with the fingers or hand(s) before applying vibrational movements. Tissues can be lifted while compressed and vibrated. The hand can remain in one location or may move across the skin (Fig. 8.43). If two hands are used, the palms can face each other, as in praying, or can be stacked one on top of the other (Fig. 8.44). Fine vibration differs from tapotement because contact between the client's skin and the practitioner's hands is maintained during the application, unlike

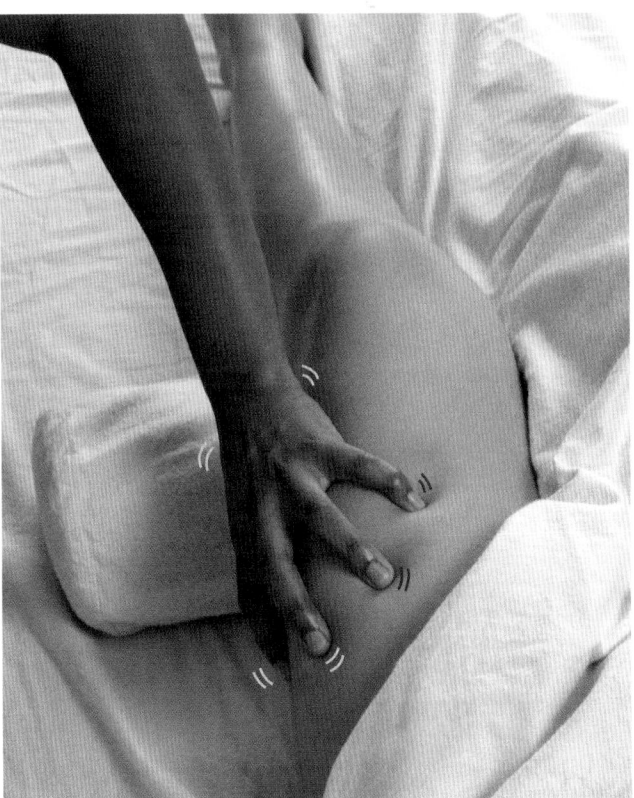

FIG. 8.43 Fine vibration. The skin is compressed slightly with one hand before applying vibratory movements.

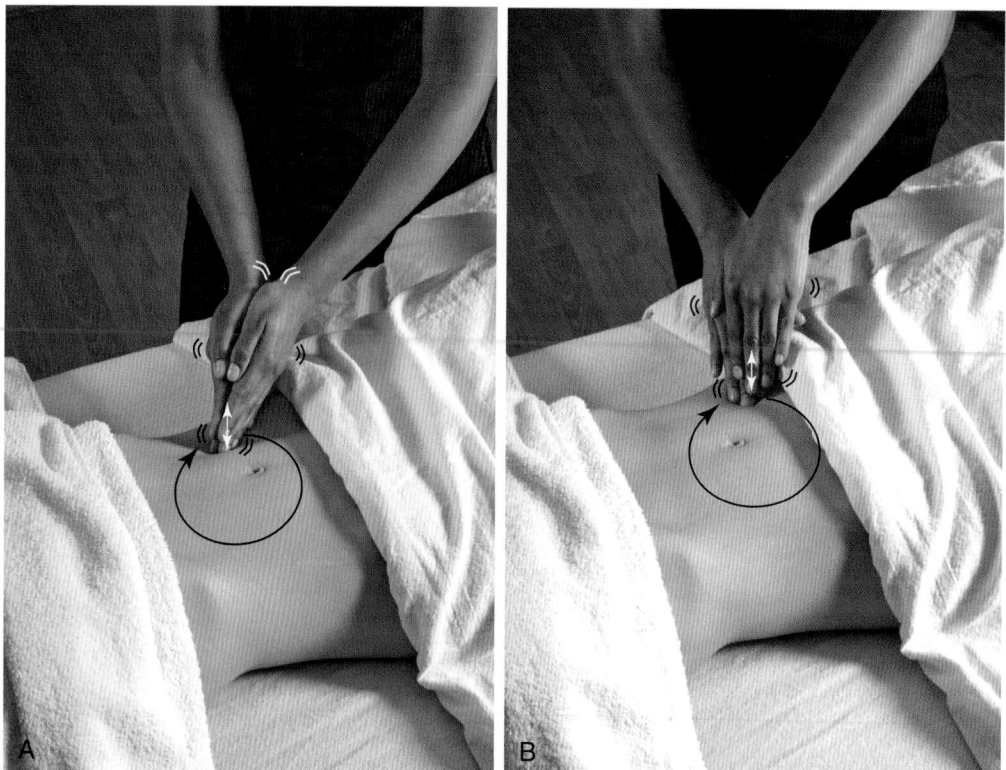

FIG. 8.44 Fine vibration. Fingertips of two hands apply vibratory movements with the palms facing each other (A) or stacked on top of each other (B).

tapotement, where contact between the client's skin and the practitioner's hands is broken as hands are lifted between strikes.

An electrical device can be used to apply fine vibration. Avoid moving the device over bony prominences. Because prolonged use of an electrical device to deliver vibration can be irritating, limit its use to several minutes. If the device is corded, be sure the cord is not in a location that could create a fall risk. In addition, ensure the cord does not touch the client while in use.

Jostling

During jostling, grasp the muscles, joint, or extremity and shake vigorously (Fig. 8.45). Traction or decompression of

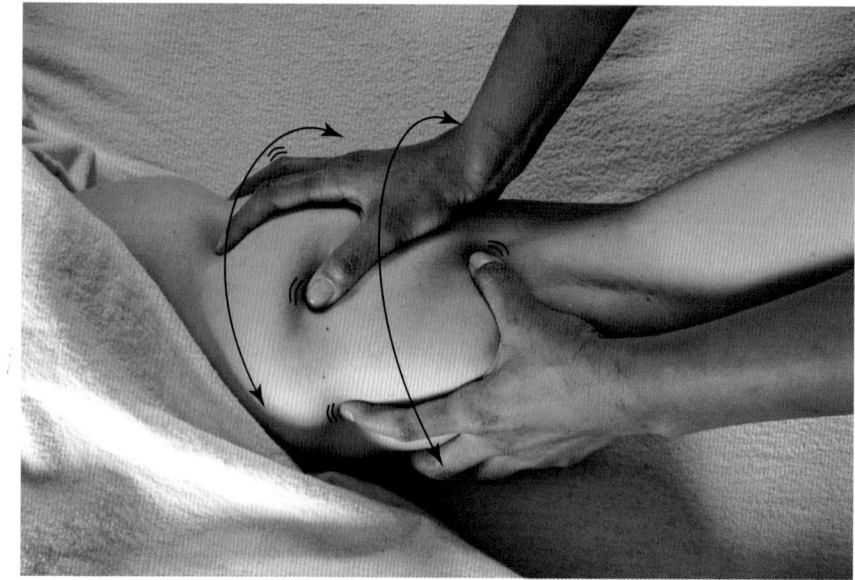

FIG. 8.45 Jostling vibration. Tissues are grasped with two hands and shaken vigorously.

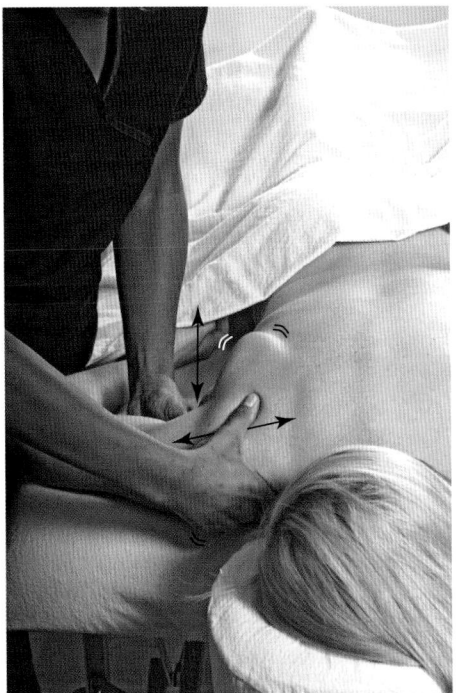

FIG. 8.46 Jostling vibration. Traction or decompression of the proximal joint is applied during the vibratory movements.

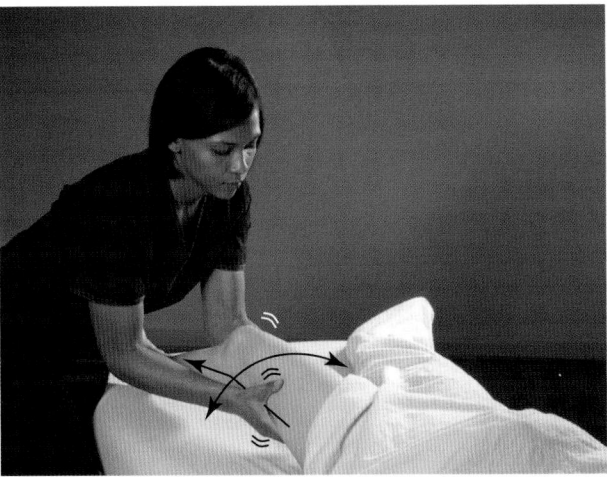

FIG. 8.47 Jostling (fluffing). An extremity can be gently lifted and released while applying manual traction to the proximal joint(s).

the proximal joint(s) can be applied during jostling vibration (Fig. 8.46). A variation of jostling is *fluffing,* which involves gently lifting and releasing the limb while applying manual traction to the proximal joint (Fig. 8.47).

The humble improve.

—Wynton Marsalis

PASSIVE RANGE OF MOTION: MOBILIZATIONS AND STRETCHING

Massage practitioners may use mobilizations and stretching techniques to passively move the client's body through their available range of motion (ROM). These techniques provide additional treatment options and can be applied before, during, or after the massage. Passive ROM can also be applied exclusively and not as part of a massage session.

Description

Range of motion is the amount of motion that occurs when one segment of the body moves in relation to another segment of the body. For example, the left hip moves 90 degrees in flexion while the rest of the body does not move. Normal ROM has been documented and is often expressed in degrees of a circle (e.g., 90 degrees). ROM is influenced by how bones, muscles, and ligaments are arranged to allow motion. ROM is affected by health, disease, body mass, physical activity, deformity, age, and gender, with females generally having greater ROM than males.

Although ROM is discussed here and in Chapters 4 and 14, the passive ROM routine featured in this chapter is intended as self-care and part of wellness massage, not orthopedic pre- or post-assessments during clinical massage (Chapter 14). Several types of movements are passive and active. Active ROM includes both active assisted and active resistance.

- **Passive range of motion (PROM).** Movement produced by external forces without voluntary contraction. Examples of external forces include movements produced by another individual, an object such as a machine or belt, gravity, or by another part of the person's own body. During PROM during a session, the client is relaxed and passive while the practitioner performs the movements on the client.
- **Active range of motion (AROM).** Movement produced by voluntary contraction, wherein the clients themselves move the limb or body part. During AROM, the client performs the movement (i.e., joint mobilization, stretch) described or demonstrated by the practitioner. Active movements can be performed with assistance or against resistance.
  - **Active assisted range of motion (AAROM).** Movement produced by voluntary contraction while the practitioner assists and physically guides the motion in the same direction the client is moving.
  - **Active resisted range of motion (ARROM).** Movement produced by voluntary contraction while the practitioner applies resistance to the client's motion. Active resisted movements, also called *resisted range of motion*, are used in a variety of clinical massage techniques such as proprioceptive neuromuscular facilitation, as well as muscle energy techniques (postisometric relaxation, and reciprocal inhibition), as discussed in Chapter 14.

PROM can be applied as mobilizations or as stretches (International Federation of Orthopaedic Manipulative Physical Therapists [IFOMPT], 2016). Research related to joint mobilizations and stretching is on Evolve. The differences between mobilizations and stretches are discussed next.

- **Mobilizations**. These occur with passively moving a joint without a manual thrust at the end of available PROM. In contrast, *manipulations* are high-velocity, low-amplitude manual thrusts applied at the end of available PROM. A significant difference between mobilizations and manipulations is the inclusion of a manual thrust at the end range of available PROM. In fact, to distinguish between the two techniques, some professions use the term *nonthrust manipulations* to describe mobilizations and *thrust manipulations* to describe manipulations. **NOTE**: *Thrust manipulations* are outside of massage scope of practice.
- **Stretching**. This occurs when passively positioning muscle attachments as far apart as possible to elongate the muscle in the direction opposite of its action. Several clinical massage methods that incorporate stretching are featured in Chapter 14.
  - **Pin and stretch**. This is used to stretch a region of muscle between a pinned point and the muscle attachment. The practitioner uses their hand or forearm to press and "pin" a muscle against the underlying bone, which prevents the stretch from spreading to areas of muscle beyond the pinned point. The smaller the pinpoint, the more precise the stretch. However, smaller pinpoints tend to be uncomfortable for the client—larger pinpoints are usually more comfortable. The size of the area or length of the muscle may dictate the size of the pinpoint (thumb/fingertip vs forearm). Pin and stretch can be performed passively or actively.

Technique

The routine in this chapter includes mobilizations and stretches with clients in prone and supine positions. They should be performed on both sides of the body when applicable. Because this section contains movement terminology that has not yet been discussed, it is highly recommended you refer to Chapters 19 to 21 when encountering an unfamiliar term (e.g., flexion, rotation).

Mobilizations and stretches are best applied on unlubricated skin and while the client is wearing active wear such as gym shorts, sweats, leggings, tights, and a tee shirt. If the client is unclothed and draped, secure the drape before initiating the movements and maintain the drape during the movements. Describe or demonstrate the movements before administering them on the client.

- Apply a slight manual traction before the movement begins.
- Begin the movement as the client exhales.
- For mobilizations, perform full ROM three times.
- For stretches, stop when you detect a little tension in the targeted muscle. Maintain the stretch for 10 to 30 seconds. Repeat the stretch three times.

Joints sounds, called **crepitus,** may occur during movement. These sounds are described as creaking, cracking, grating, crunching, or popping sounds. Crepitant sounds are thought to be caused by tiny bubbles of nitrogen forming in synovial fluid, which sometimes burst when the joint is stretched (Brakke, 2016; Nelsen, 2015). These sounds are common and normal during joint movement. Crepitus may also occur in joints affected by diseases such as osteoarthritis (OA) or rheumatoid arthritis (RA). Crepitus is also used to describe any noise originating in the body, including flatulence released by the digestive tract, and lungs crackling from respiratory disease.

CAUTION: Some passive movements that involve lifting the client off the massage table increases the risk of practitioner injury, especially back injury. Factors that influence the risk of injury during lifting include:

1. Presence of a lower back disorder in the practitioner.
2. The level from which the lift will be made, called vertical lift orientation.
3. The distance from the practitioner's spine to the center of the load, called horizontal reach.
4. Trunk-twist angle during the lift.

Other factors include how often the lift occurs and how long the load is lifted and held (Occupational Safety and Health Administration [OSHA], 2015). An online calculator assessing risk factors has been developed by the Ohio Bureau of Worker's Compensation (n.d.) and can be found at https://www.bwc.ohio.gov/employer/programs/safety/liftguide/liftguide.aspx. These factors alone do not determine the risk of back injury. Massage practitioners should assess their injury risk and determine if a technique is safe for them or whether it should be avoided during the session.

Contraindications

PROM is contraindicated when motion may disrupt the healing process, such as in a recent or unhealed dislocation, unhealed fracture, or after surgical procedures involving muscles, tendons, ligaments, joints, vertebral discs, or skin until they are completely healed. Contraindications also include the presence of bone or joint inflammation, infection, injury, or malignancy including bone cancer, osteoporosis, or any condition causing bone frailty, as well as hypermobile joints, or joints prone to separation or subluxation (Cameron, 2018).

NECK

Movements of the neck are flexion, extension, lateral flexion, and rotation. PROM of the neck includes neck circles, neck lateral flexion with and without rotation, and neck forward flexion (Table 8.2). These techniques are performed while the client is supine. Follow the technique guidelines listed in the previous section when applying mobilizations and stretches.

Neck Rotation

Place one hand on the client's forehead and begin neck rotation by moving the head away from you. Using the fingertips of the opposite hand, compress the tissues in the cervical laminar groove while rotating the neck toward you. Repeat the sequence up to six times on both sides of the neck (Fig. 8.48).

TABLE 8.2 Passive Range of Motion: Mobilizations and Stretches	
AREA	**TECHNIQUE**
Neck	Neck rotation
	Neck lateral flexion
	Neck lateral flexion with rotation
	Neck forward flexion
Wrists and hands	Flip wrist
	Interlace fingers and mobilize wrist
	Metacarpal scissors
	Pull and circumduct fingers
Shoulders	Arm pull (shoulder traction)
	Shoulder circles
Spine	Spinal rotation I
	Spinal rotation II
	Spinal rotation III
	Spinal rotation IV
Hips and knees	Leg pull (hip traction)
	Leg rock
	Hip clock stretch
	Hip circles
	Glute, hamstring, and calf stretch
	Adductor stretch
	Quadriceps stretch
	Iliopsoas and quadriceps stretch
Ankles and feet	Ankle mobilization
	Calf stretch
	Metatarsal scissors
	Pull and circumduct toes

Neck Lateral Flexion

Place one hand on the side of the client's head and pull the head toward the near shoulder while the other hand stabilizes the client's far shoulder (Fig. 8.49). Repeat the stretch on both sides of the neck.

Neck Lateral Flexion With Rotation

Place one hand on the side of the client's head and rotate the neck laterally until the client's head is facing away from you. Next, pull the client's head toward you while the other hand stabilizes the client's far shoulder (Fig. 8.50). Repeat the stretch on both sides of the neck.

Neck Forward Flexion

Place one or two hands on the base of the client's skull and lift the head toward the chest in forward flexion (Fig. 8.51). If both hands are used, the forearms can be crisscrossed at the base of the client's skull before lifting the head off the table.

WRISTS AND HANDS

Wrist movements are abduction, adduction, flexion, and extension. PROM of the wrist and hand are flip wrist, interlace fingers and mobilize wrist, metacarpal scissors, and pull and circumduct fingers.

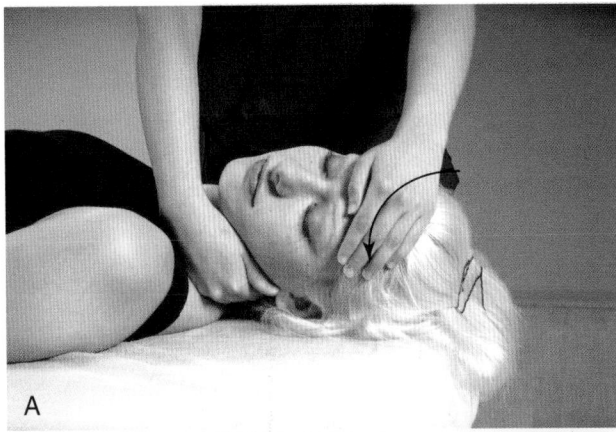

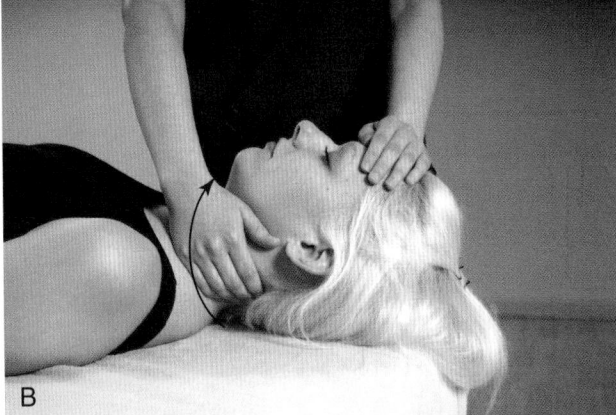

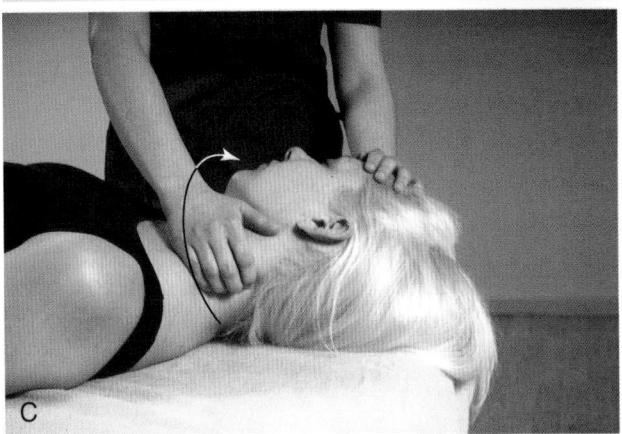

FIG. 8.48 Neck rotation. Place one hand on the forehead. Rotate the neck by moving the head away from you (A). Use the fingertips of the opposite hand to compress the tissues in the cervical laminar groove (B) while rotating the head and neck toward you (C).

Flip Wrist

Lightly grip above and below two sides of the client's wrist using the thumbs and index fingers of two hands. Flip the wrist up and down using your fingers (Fig. 8.52). Repeat the mobilization up to six times on both wrists.

Interlace Fingers and Mobilize Wrist

Lightly grip the client's proximal wrist with one hand and interlace your fingers in the client's fingers with the other hand. Move the client's wrist into flexion, extension, abduction, and

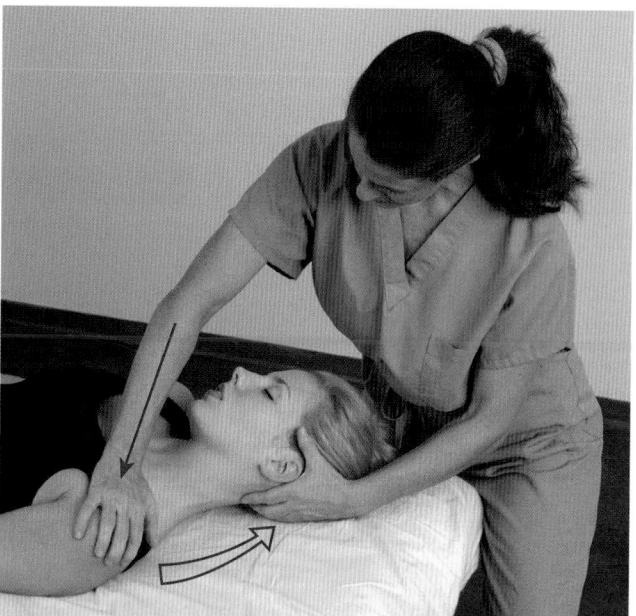

FIG. 8.49 Neck lateral flexion. Place one hand on the side of the client's head and pull the head toward the near shoulder while the other hand stabilizes the far shoulder.

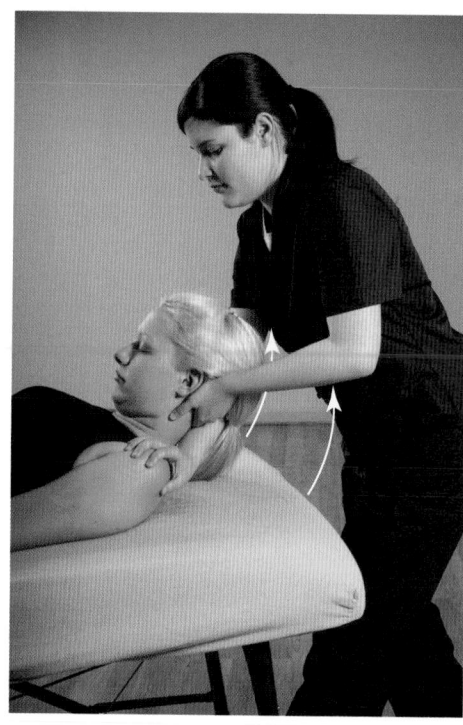

FIG. 8.51 Neck forward flexion. Place one hand on the base of the skull and lift it up and toward the chest. The other hand can stabilize the shoulder.

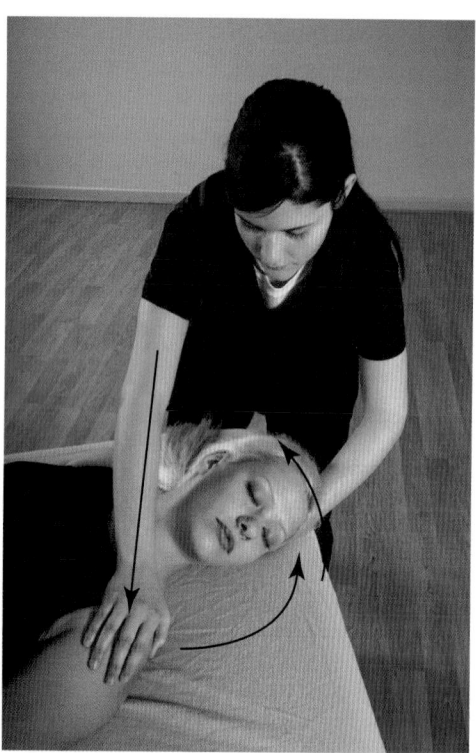

FIG. 8.50 Neck lateral flexion with rotation. Place one hand on the side of the head, rotate the neck laterally with the head facing away from you, then pull the client's head toward you while stabilizing the far shoulder.

adduction (Fig. 8.53). Repeat the mobilization up to six times on both wrists.

Metacarpal Scissors

Using two hands, lightly grip the dorsal and palmar surfaces of the client's hand at the distal ends of the metacarpal bones. Move adjacent metacarpals upward and downward in a scissor-like motion up to six times. Reapply these movements between each pair of metacarpal bones (Fig. 8.54). Repeat the mobilization on both hands.

Pull and Circumduct Fingers

Lightly grip the client's proximal wrist with one hand. With the other hand, gently pull and circumduct each of the client's fingers (Fig. 8.55). Circumduction is applied in both directions (i.e., clockwise and counterclockwise). Repeat the pull and circumduction movements on all fingers. Repeat the sequence on both hands.

SHOULDERS

Movements of the shoulders are flexion, extension, adduction, abduction, rotation, and circumduction. PROM of the shoulders are arm pulls or shoulder traction and shoulder circles and feature flexion, extension, adduction, abduction, rotation, and circumduction.

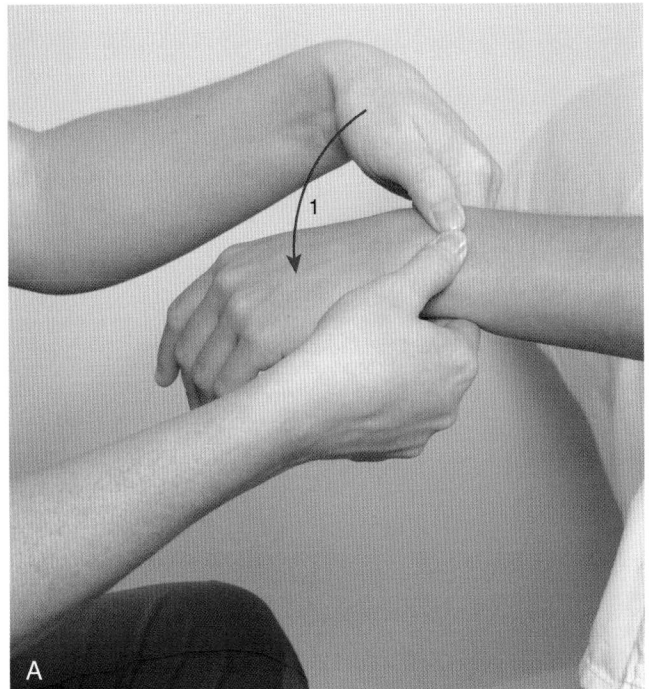

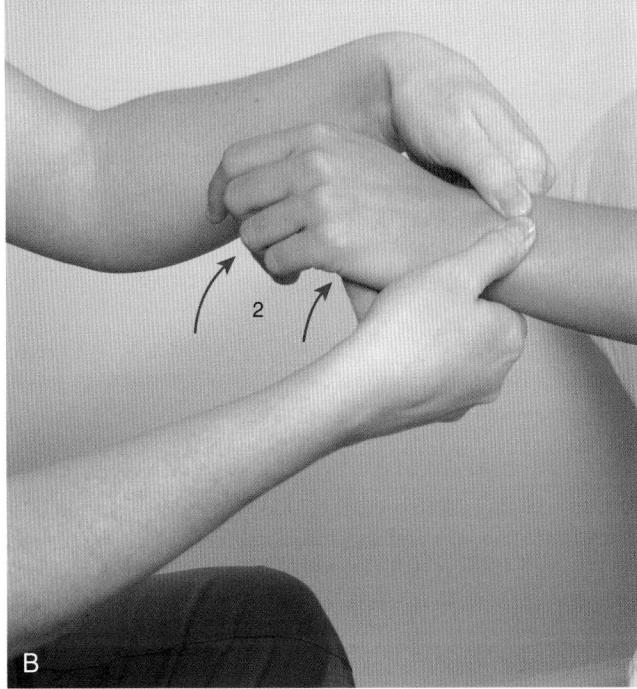

FIG. 8.52 Flip wrist. Lightly grip above and below both sides of the wrist using the thumbs and index fingers of both hands. Flip the wrist down into flexion (A) and up into extension (B).

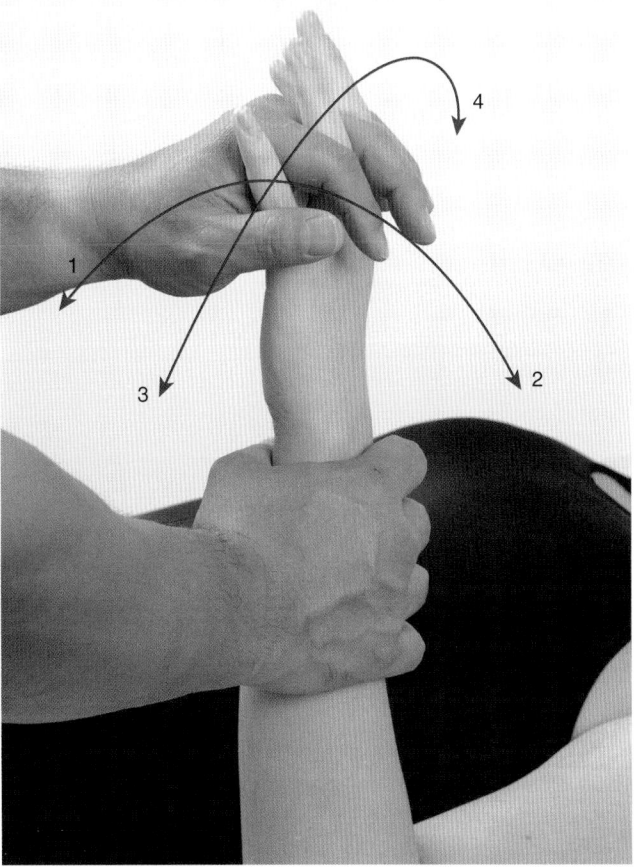

FIG. 8.53 Interlace the fingers and mobilize the wrist into flexion, extension, abduction, and adduction.

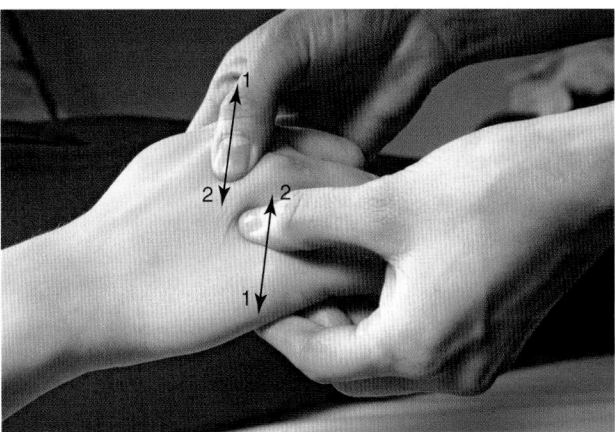

FIG. 8.54 Metacarpal scissors. Move the adjacent metacarpal bones upward and downward in a scissor-like motion.

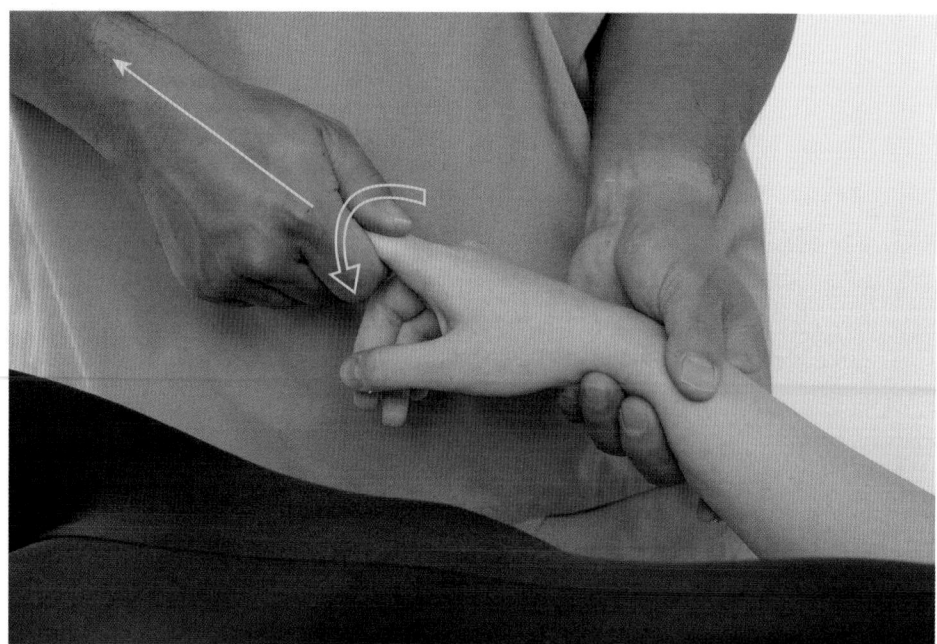

FIG. 8.55 Pull and circumduct the fingers.

Arm Pull (Shoulder Traction)

This technique consists of four parts that are repeated on both sides of the body:

1. While standing tableside near the client's hip, lightly grasp the client's proximal wrist and apply gentle, intermittent traction by pulling on and releasing pressure (Fig. 8.56A). Keep the client's upper extremity parallel to the client's torso during the movement. Pull and release up to six times.
2. While standing several feet from the tableside, lightly grasp the client's proximal wrist and apply gentle intermittent traction by pulling on and releasing pressure. The shoulder will be abducted 90 degrees (see Fig. 8.56B). Keep the client's upper extremity perpendicular to the client's torso during the movement. Pull and release up to six times.
3. While standing tableside, horizontally adduct the client's shoulder by moving the client's upper extremity across the chest. Sustain this position for a few seconds (see Fig. 8.56C).
4. While standing several feet from the tabletop, lightly grasp the client's proximal wrist and apply gentle intermittent traction by pulling on and releasing pressure (see Fig. 8.56D). Keep the client's upper extremity parallel to the client's torso during the movement. Pull and release up to six times.

Shoulder Circles

While standing tableside, use your top hand, lightly grasp the client's proximal wrist and apply gentle traction by pulling on the arm inferiorly. While maintaining traction, lift the client's arm toward the ceiling and then over the client's head (Fig. 8.57A). Return the client's arm to the starting position by bending their elbow with your other hand. Now,

using two hands (one hand grasping the wrist and the other grasping the elbow), move the client's upper extremity downward to their side (see Fig. 8.57B). Release the grasp on the elbow approximately midway down the returning arc. Repeat the circular-shaped mobilization up to six times and the entire sequence on both sides of the body.

SPINE

Movements of the spine are largely rotational and are listed as spinal rotations I through IV. Spinal rotations are also called *spinal twists*.

Spinal Rotation I

While standing tableside, use your bottom hand to anchor the client's far hip and use your top hand to lift and pull the client's far shoulder toward you to rotate the spine (Fig. 8.58). The client's upper extremity can remain relaxed by their side (see Fig. 8.58A), or the client's fingers can be interlaced behind their posterior neck (see Fig. 8.58B). Repeat the movement on both sides of the body.

Spinal Rotation II

With the client's near knee flexed and the foot placed on the lateral side of the far knee, push the near knee across the client's body as your top hand lifts and pulls the client's far shoulder toward you to rotate the spine (Fig. 8.59). Repeat the movement on both sides of the body.

Spinal Rotation III

While standing tableside, use your top hand to anchor the client's far shoulder and use your bottom hand to pull the far flexed knee across the client's body and downward to rotate

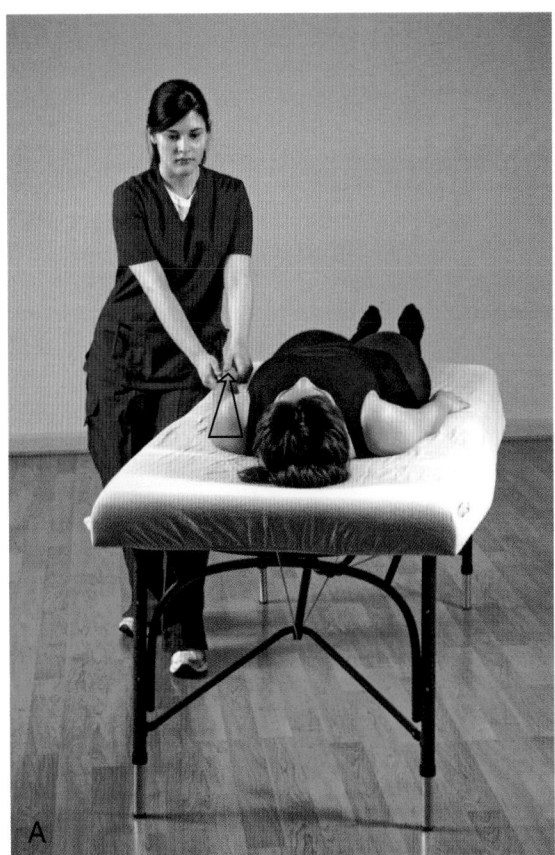

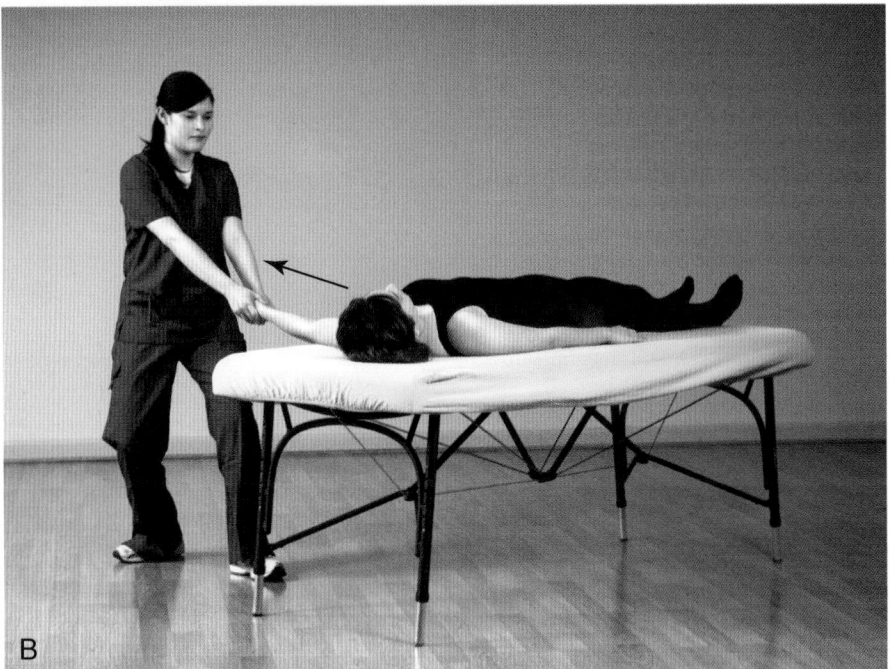

FIG. 8.56 Arm pull. Pull the arm down the client's side using intermittent traction (A). Pull the arm away from the client using intermittent traction (B).

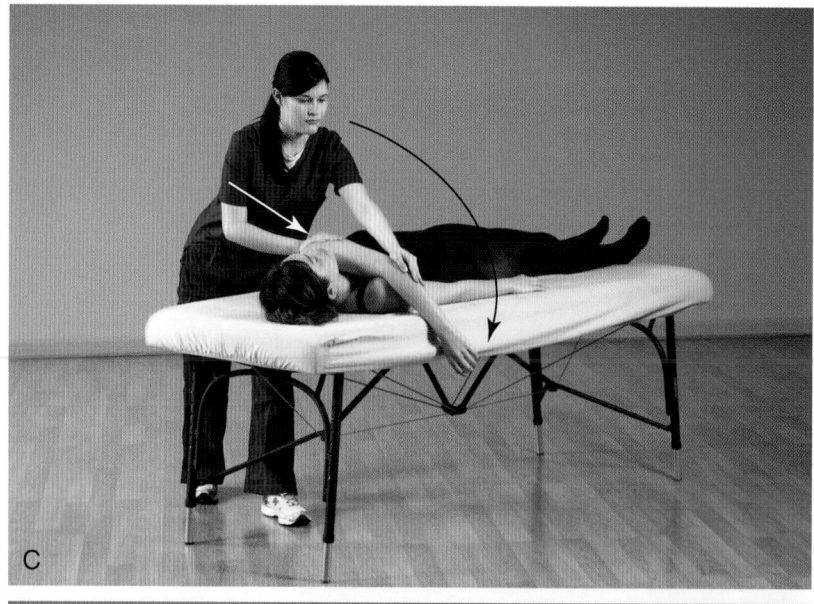

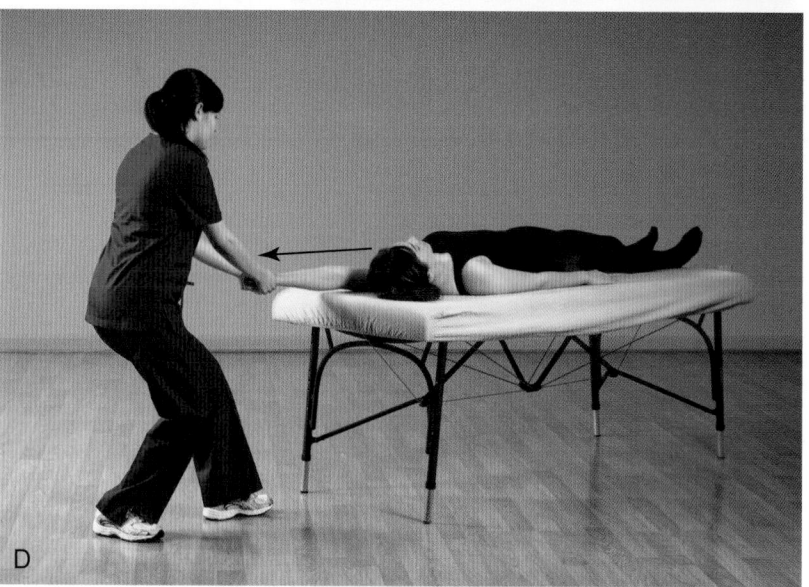

FIG. 8.56, CONT'D Pull the arm across the chest (C). Pull the arm up over the client's head using intermittent traction (D).

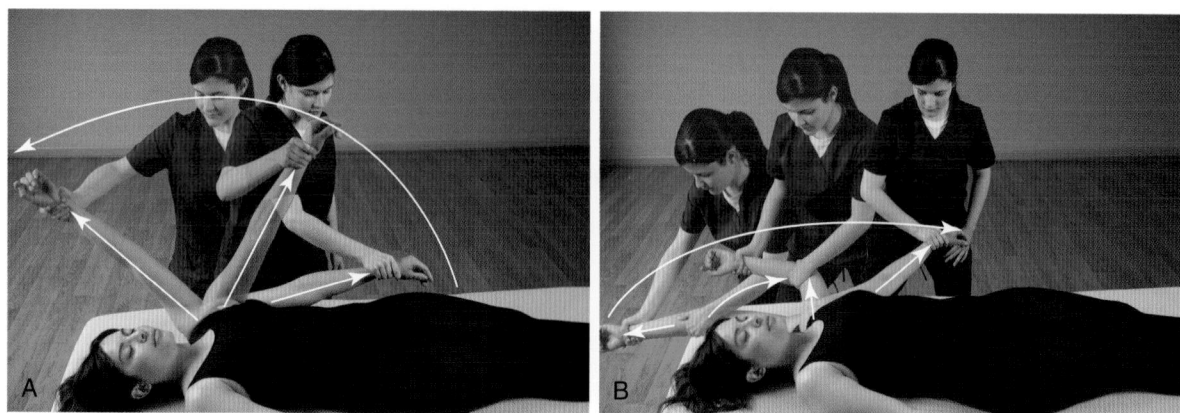

FIG. 8.57 Shoulder circles. Pull the arm over the client's head (A). Pull the arm down to the client's side (B).

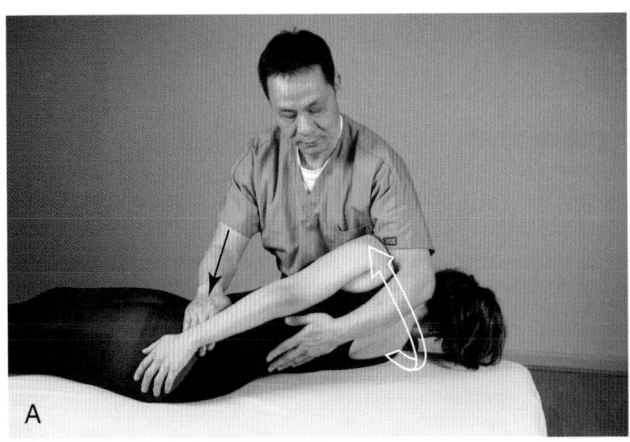 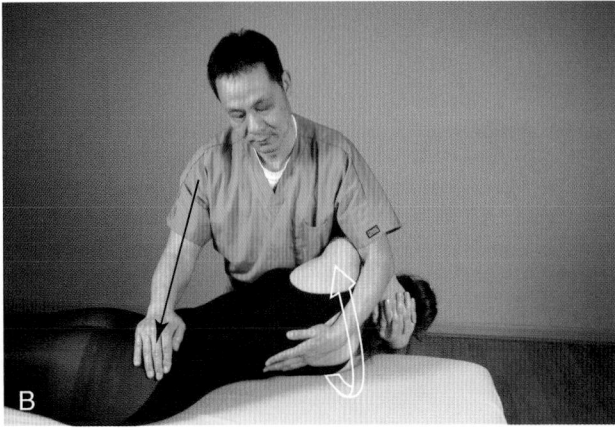

FIG. 8.58 Spinal rotation I. Anchor the far hip and pull the far shoulder up and toward you (A). The client's hands can be placed behind their head with fingers interlaced (B).

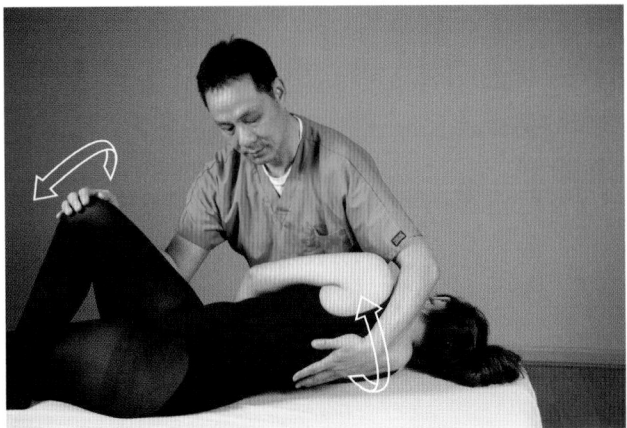

FIG. 8.59 Spinal rotation II. Push the near knee away from you as you pull the far shoulder up and toward you.

the spine (Fig. 8.60). Repeat the movement on both sides of the body.

Spinal Rotation IV

While standing tableside, use your top hand to anchor the client's near shoulder and your bottom hand to push the near flexed knee across the client's body away from you and downward to rotate the spine (Fig. 8.61). Repeat the movement on both sides of the body.

HIPS AND KNEES

Hip movements are flexion, extension, adduction, abduction, rotation, and circumduction. Knee movements are flexion and extension. PROM of the hips and knees are leg pull (hip traction), leg rock, hip clock stretch and circles, hip flexion and hyperextension, adductor stretch, and knee flexion or heel to hip.

Leg Pull (Hip Traction)

While standing a short distance from the foot of the table, lightly grasp the client's proximal ankle and apply gentle

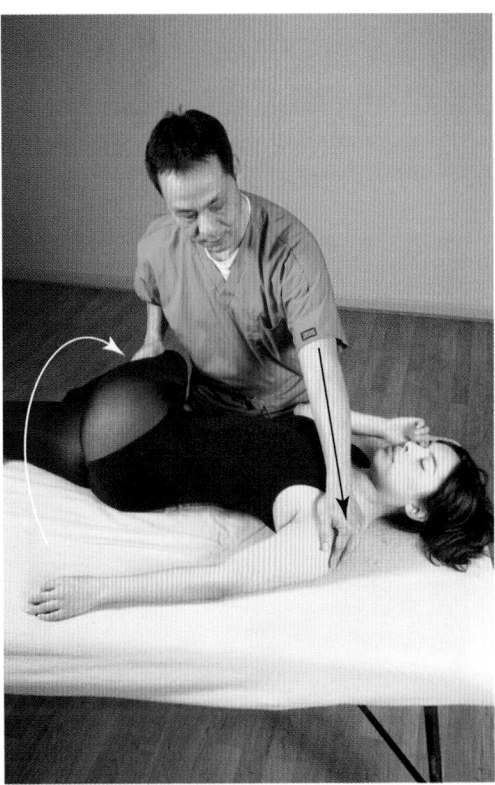

FIG. 8.60 Spinal rotation III. Anchor the far shoulder and pull the far knee toward you and down.

intermittent traction by pulling on and releasing pressure (Fig. 8.62). Pull and release up to six times. Repeat the sequence on both sides of the body.

Leg Rock

While standing tableside, place your top hand above and your bottom hand below the client's near knee. Rotate the hip by rocking the lower extremity back and forth (Fig. 8.63). Repeat the mobilization up to six times on both sides of the body.

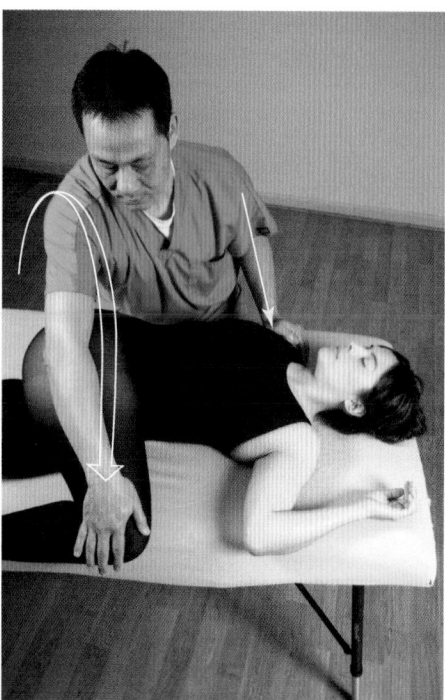

FIG. 8.61 Spinal rotation IV. Anchor the near shoulder and push the near knee away from you and down.

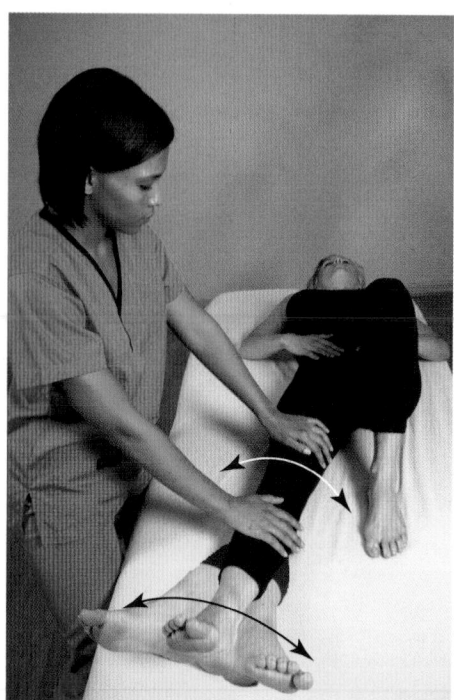

FIG. 8.63 Leg rock. Rotate the hip by rocking the lower extremity back and forth.

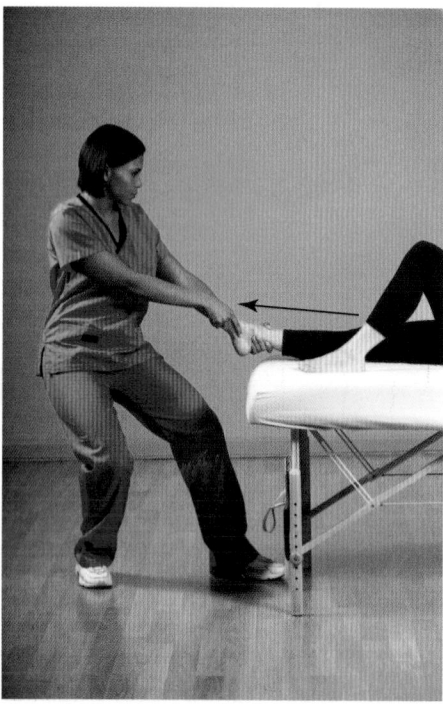

FIG. 8.62 Leg pull. Grasp the proximal ankle with one hand and the foot with the other hand and apply gentle intermittent traction.

Hip Clock Stretch

While standing tableside, place your top hand on the lateral side of the client's flexed knee. The hip is also flexed. Place your bottom hand on the plantar surface of the near foot, palm facing the client's foot. Using the image of a clock,

push the near knee to a 10 o'clock position, then a 12 o'clock position, and then a 2 o'clock position to apply the stretching motions (Fig. 8.64). Repeat the mobilization up to six times on both sides of the body.

Hip Circles

After completing the hip clock stretch, mobilize the hip by moving the flexed knee in a circle while the hip is flexed (Fig. 8.65). Repeat the mobilization up to six times on both sides of the body.

Glute, Hamstring, and Calf Stretch

While standing tableside, use your bottom hand, positioned at the posterior surface of the proximal near ankle, to flex the client's near hip. Use your top hand, placed at the anterior surface of the proximal near knee, to maintain knee extension moving the lower extremity toward the trunk to stretch the glutes and hamstrings (Fig. 8.66A). **CAUTION**: Do not apply this technique if the client has lumbar disc pathology. A calf stretch can be added by using the bottom hand to dorsiflex the client's near ankle (see Fig. 8.66B). Repeat the stretches on both sides of the body.

Adductor Stretch

While standing tableside, place your bottom hand over the client's far anterior superior iliac spine and apply moderate downward pressure to anchor the hip while applying moderate downward pressure on the medial aspect of the near flexed knee to stretch the adductors. The near hip is also flexed and outwardly rotated (Fig. 8.67). Repeat the stretch on both sides of the body.

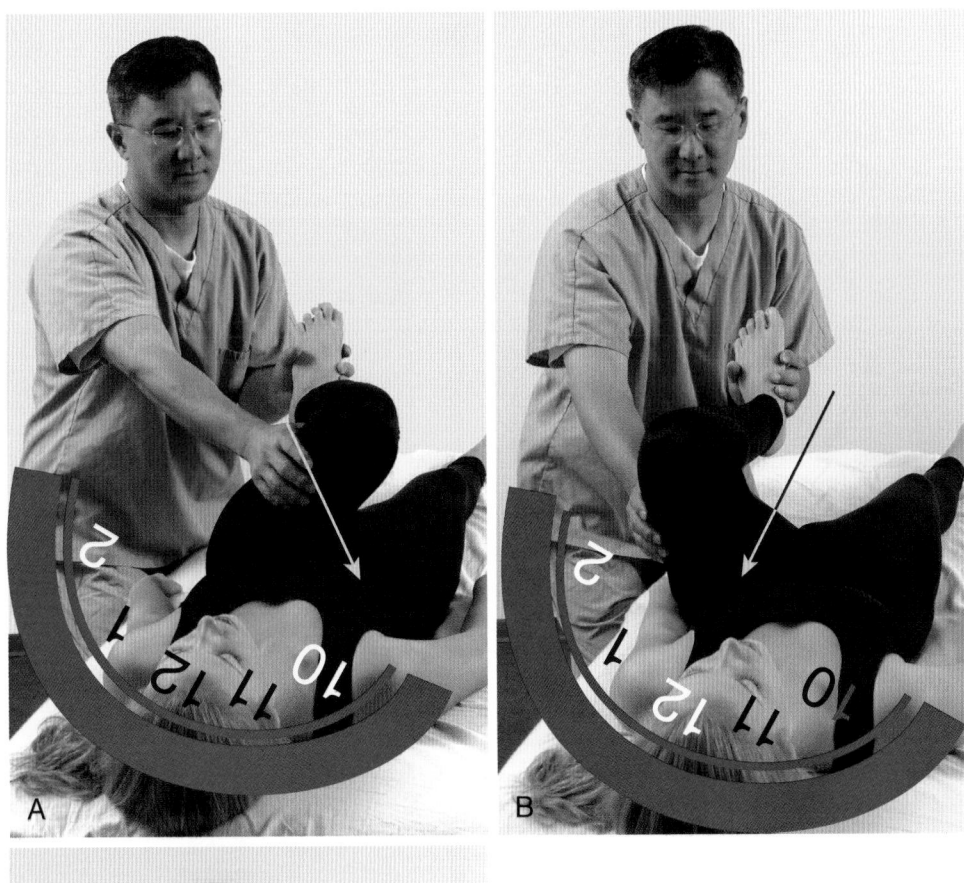

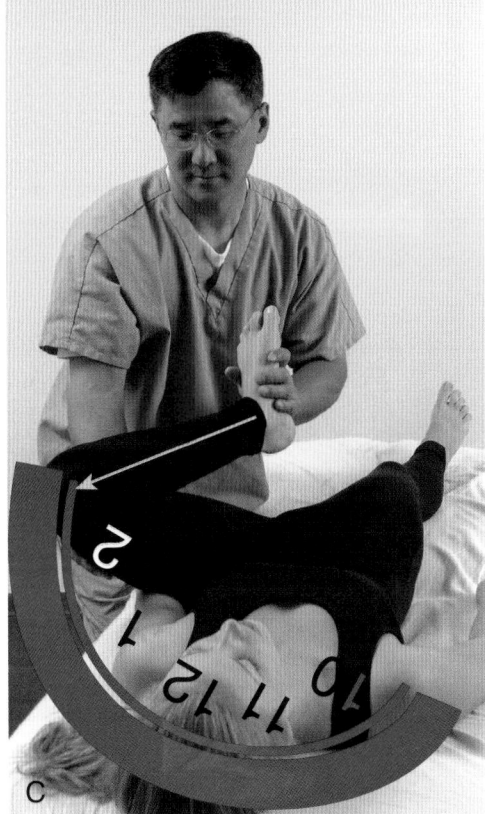

FIG. 8.64 Hip clock stretch. Using the image of a clock, stretch the hip muscles by pushing the near knee to a 10 o'clock position (A), then to 12 o'clock (B), and then to 2 o'clock (C).

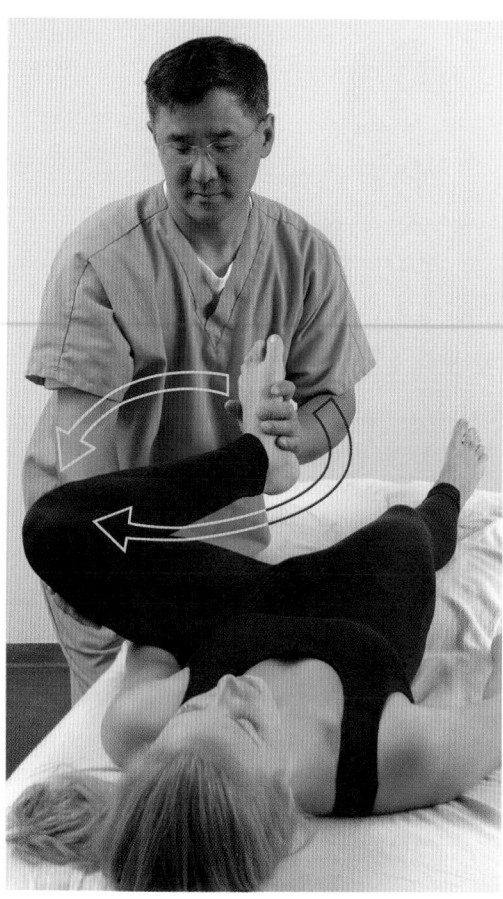

FIG. 8.65 Hip circles. Mobilize the hip by moving the flexed knee in a circle.

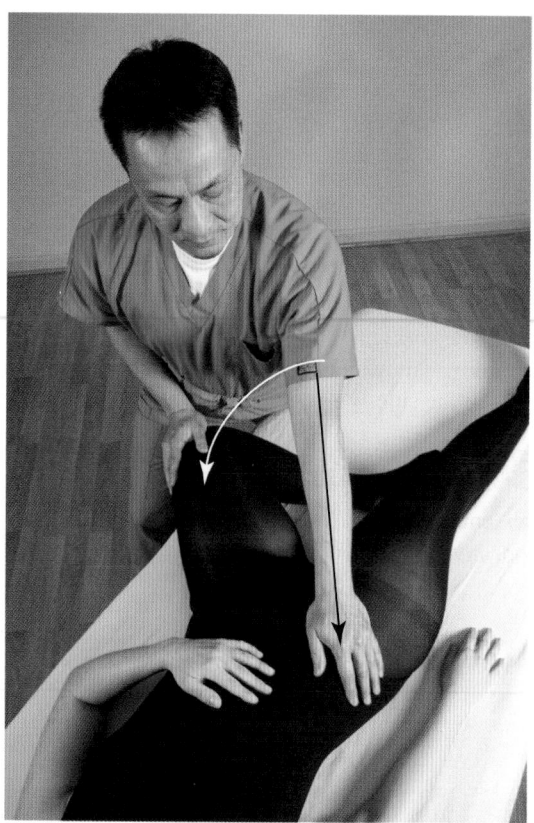

FIG. 8.67 Adductor stretch. Place your bottom hand over their anterior superior iliac spine and gently press downward while applying moderate downward pressure on the knee with the other hand.

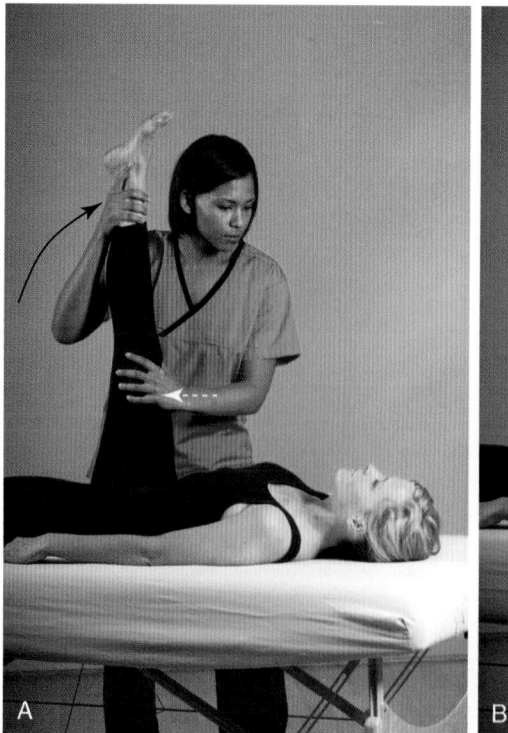
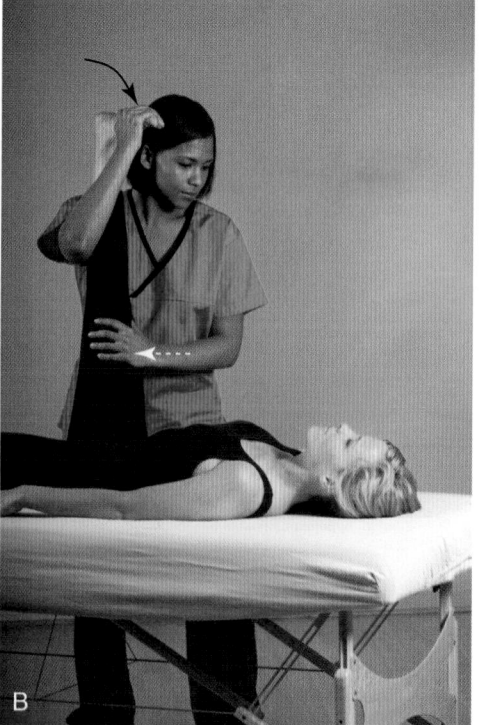

FIG. 8.66 Glute, hamstring, and calf stretch. Lift the lower extremity toward the trunk to stretch the glutes and hamstrings (A). Stretch the calf by dorsiflexing the ankle (B).

Quadriceps Stretch

While standing tableside, place your top hand over the client's back and use your bottom hand positioned on the anterior surface of the near ankle to flex the knee and stretch the quadriceps (Fig. 8.68). Repeat the stretch on both sides of the body.

Iliopsoas and Quadriceps Stretch

While standing tableside, place your top hand over the client's back and use your bottom hand to lift the near thigh off the table to hyperextend the hip and stretch the iliopsoas and the quadriceps (Fig. 8.69). Repeat the stretch on both sides of the body. This stretch can also be performed while the client is in the side-lying position.

ANKLES AND FEET

Movements of the ankles and feet are plantar flexion, dorsiflexion, inversion, and eversion. PROM movements of the ankle and foot are ankle mobilization, calf stretch, metatarsal scissors, and pull/circumduct toes.

Ankle Mobilization

While standing at the foot of the table, use one hand to stabilize the heel and the other hand to move the ankle into plantar flexion and dorsiflexion (Fig. 8.70). Repeat the movements up to six times on both sides of the body.

Calf Stretch

While standing at the foot of the table, use one hand to stabilize the heel and the other hand to dorsiflex the ankle by pushing on the ball of the foot to stretch the calf muscles (Fig. 8.71). Repeat the stretch on both sides of the body.

Metatarsal Scissors

Using two hands, lightly grip the dorsal and plantar surfaces of the client's foot at the distal ends of the metatarsal bones. Move adjacent metatarsals upward and downward in a scissor-like motion up to six times. Reapply these movements between each pair of metatarsal bones (Fig. 8.72). Repeat the sequence on both feet.

Pull and Circumduct Toes

Lightly grip the client's foot with one hand. With the other hand, gently pull and circumduct each of the client's toes (Fig. 8.73). Circumduction is applied in both directions (i.e., clockwise and counterclockwise). Repeat the pull and circumduction movements on all toes. Repeat the sequence on both feet.

E-RESOURCES

http://evolve.elsevier.com/Salvo/MassageTherapy

- Chapter challenge
- Flash cards
- Technique videos

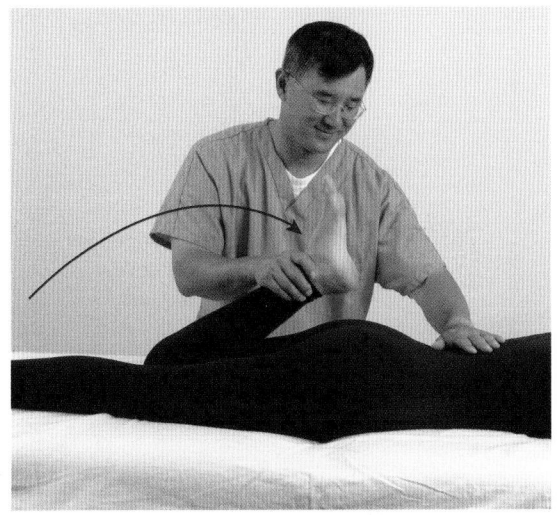

FIG. 8.68 Quadriceps stretch. Flex the knee to stretch the quadriceps.

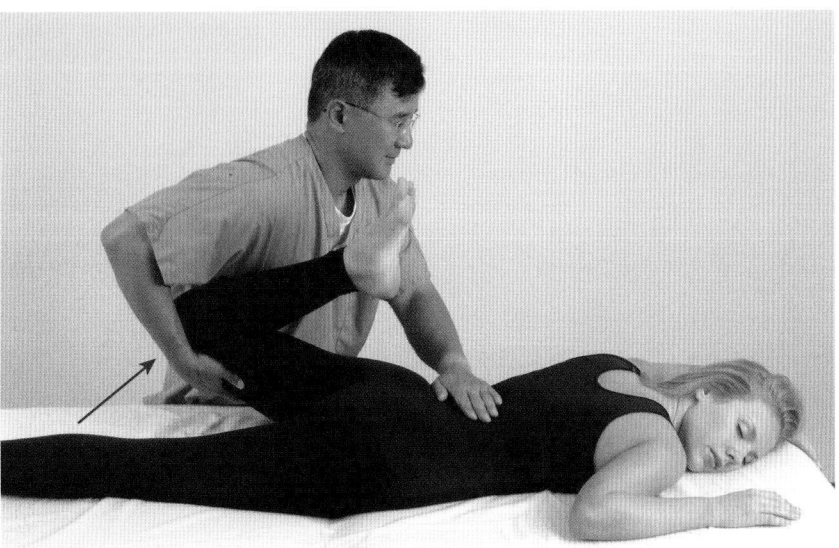

FIG. 8.69 Iliopsoas and quadriceps stretch. Lift the near thigh off the table with one hand and stabilize the lower back with the other hand.

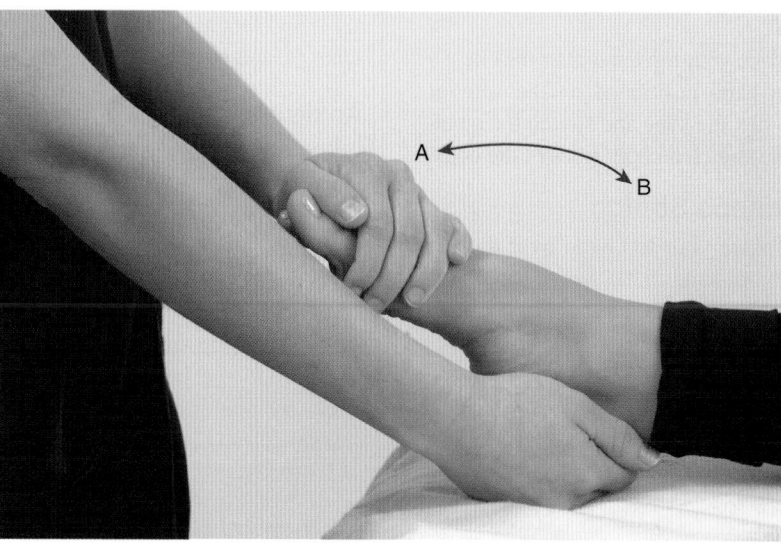

FIG. 8.70 Ankle mobilization. Use one hand to stabilize the heel and the other hand to move the ankle into plantar flexion (A) and dorsiflexion (B).

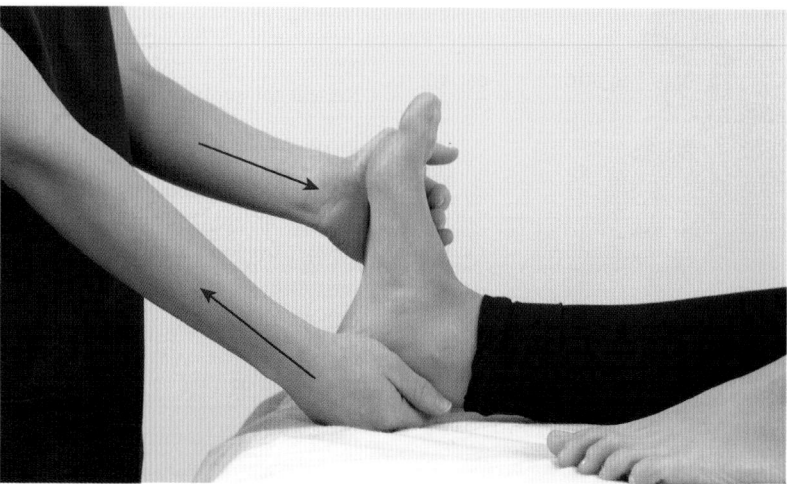

FIG. 8.71 Calf stretch. Use one hand to stabilize the heel and the other hand to dorsiflex the ankle by pushing on the ball of the foot forward.

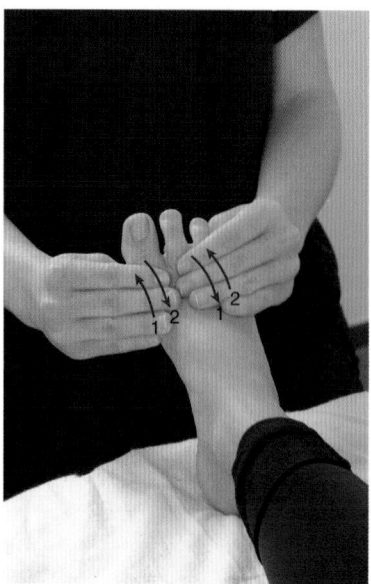

FIG. 8.72 Metatarsal scissors. Move the adjacent metatarsal bones upward and downward in a scissor-like motion.

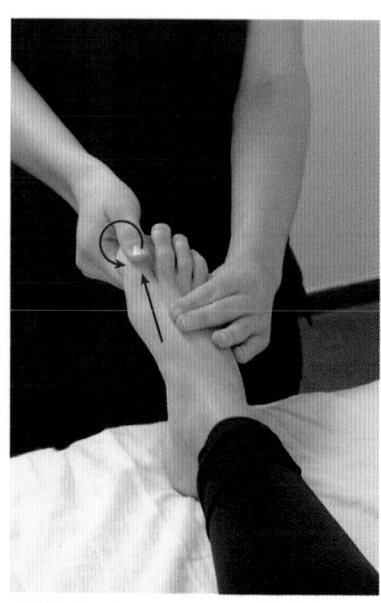

FIG. 8.73 Pull and circumduct toes.

JAMES HENRY CYRIAX

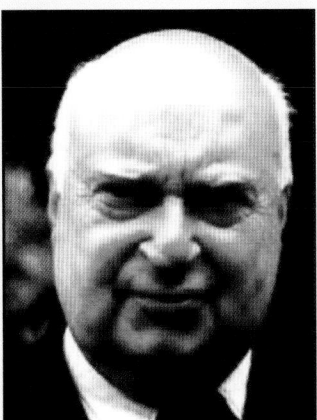

The medical field, like any other, has its share of divergent views, arguments, and controversies. Those with strong views and unusual methods can often be extremely polarizing figures. Time may smooth controversies surrounding these individuals because scientific advancements either confirm these theories or prove them to be wrong. However, some people develop theories that are strongly contested even now, and the debate rages on. James Cyriax is called the father of orthopedic medicine. It is up to the physicians and scientists of the future to decide whether the title is an insult or an honor.

Cyriax was born in London to a father and mother who had both studied medicine. His mother's family often used exercise and tissue manipulation for treatment of musculoskeletal disorders, which was unorthodox at the time. James Cyriax followed in his parents' footsteps, attending St. Thomas's Hospital Medical School in London, and began working in the St. Thomas's Hospital Department of Orthopedic Surgery as soon as he received his license to practice.

Far from limiting himself to surgical interventions and segregating massage and tissue manipulation into an entirely separate sphere, Cyriax instead brought orthopedics and tissue manipulation together under one roof and coined the term *orthopedic medicine* to describe this different focus. In 1938, he transformed the massage department into the very first department of orthopedic medicine and transformed the massage done there from an art to a science.

Cyriax developed a four-step system for diagnosing soft tissue dysfunction. In his *Textbook of Orthopedic Medicine,* he outlines the following:

- Active motion: patient moves the body part in question on their own.

- Passive motion: practitioner moves the patient's body without the patient's assistance.
- Resisted contractions: patient attempts to move the body in a particular way while the practitioner provides resistance against this motion.
- Palpation: practitioner uses his or her hands to examine the affected area.

Although diagnosis is outside of massage therapy's scope of practice, massage practitioners still widely use these four assessment techniques to develop an appropriate protocol. Notes from these assessments can also be passed along to the client's primary physician (with the client's permission, of course), which can help the physician make a diagnosis more quickly and accurately.

In fact, this use of his assessments in a massage practice would undoubtedly please Cyriax, who was a great believer in deep massage techniques, both on their own and in conjunction with physical therapy. To him, massage was to the muscles as mobilization was to the joints. Both have their place in the field of orthopedic medicine.

Although all this sounds very impressive now, orthopedic medicine never gained popular acceptance during James Cyriax's life. He was never elected a fellow of the British Royal College of Physicians because of the controversial nature of his work. Even now, there are a wide variety of opinions on the validity of his theories, and the individualized and hands-on nature of the work makes it difficult to study. Even so, manual therapy, muscle-specific treatments, and orthopedic assessments are now a part of the healthcare landscape thanks to Cyriax's work. Whether new research affirms or refutes his claims, nobody can doubt the great good he has done for the world of massage.

REFERENCES

Aksoy, I. A., Schrader, S. L., Ali, M. S., Borovansky, J. A., & Ross, M. A. (2009). Spinal accessory neuropathy associated with deep tissue massage: A case report. *Archives of Physical Medicine and Rehabilitation, 90*(11), 1969–1972.

American Massage Therapy Association (AMTA). (2021). *Massage profession research report*. Retrieved from: https://www.amtamassage.org/publications/massage-profession-research-report/.

Brakke, R. (2016). *What is crepitus?* Retrieved from: https://www.arthritis-health.com/types/general/what-crepitus.

Buckle, J. (2014). *Clinical aromatherapy: Essential oils in healthcare* (3rd ed.). St Louis: Elsevier Health Science.

Calvert, R. (2002). *The history of massage.* Rochester, VT: Healing Art Press.

Cambron, J. A., Dexheimer, J., Coe, P., & Swenson, R. (2007). Side-effects of massage therapy: A cross-sectional study of 100 clients. *Journal of Alternative and Complementary Medicine, 13*(8), 793–796.

Cameron, M. H. (2018). *Physical agents in rehabilitation: An evidenced-based approach to practice.* St. Louis: Elsevier.

Centers for Disease Control and Prevention (CDC). (2017). *Definitions of signs and symptoms for reportable illnesses.* Retrieved from: https://www.cdc.gov/quarantine/air/reporting-deaths-illness/definitions-symptoms-reportable-illnesses.html.

Centers for Disease Control and Prevention (CDC). (2021). *Guidance for school administrators to help reduce the spread of infection.* Retrieved from: https://www.cdc.gov/flu/school/guidance.htm.

Chakrapani, A. L., Zink, W., Zimmerman, R., Riina, H., & Benitez, R. (2008). Bilateral carotid and bilateral vertebral artery dissection following facial massage. *Angiology, 59*(6), 761–764.

Chang, C. Y., Wu, Y. T., Chen, L. C., Chan, R. C., Chang, S. T., & Chiang, S. L. (2015). Massage-induced brachial plexus injury. *Physical Therapy, 95*(1), 109–116.

Chaumont, C. (2018). *60 minute sample Swedish massage routine.* Retrieved from; https://lamassageschool.wordpress.com/2018/04/18/60-minute-sample-swedish-massage-routine/#more-35.

Chen, H. L., Wu, C. C., & Lin, A. C. (2013). Small bowel intramural hematoma secondary to abdominal massage. *The American Journal of Emergency Medicine, 31*(4), 758.

Cheong, H. S., Hong, B. Y., Ko, Y. A., Lim, S. H., & Kim, J. S. (2012). Spinal cord injury incurred by neck massage. *Annals of Rehabilitation Medicine, 36*(5), 708–712.

Cherkin, D. C., Sherman, K. J., Kahn, J., Wellman, R., Cook, A. J., Johnson, E., et al. (2011). A comparison of the effects of 2 types of massage and usual care on chronic low back pain: A randomized, controlled trial. *Annals of Internal Medicine, 155*(1), 1–9.

Cyriax, H. J. (1984). *Cyriax's illustrated manual of orthopaedic medicine.* Oxford: Butterworth-Heinemann.

DeDomenico, G. (2007). *Beard's massage: Principles and practice of soft tissue manipulation* (5th ed.). Philadelphia: Elsevier Saunders.

DeDomenico, G., & Wood, E. C. (1997). *Beard's massage* (4th ed.). Philadelphia: WB Saunders.

Dutta, G., Jagetia, A., Srivastava, A. K., Singh, D., Singh, H., & Saran, R. K. (2018). "Crick" in neck followed by massage led to stroke: Uncommon case of vertebral artery dissection. *World Neurosurgery, 115,* 41–43.

Elliott, M. A., & Taylor, L. P. (2002). "Shiatsu sympathectomy": ICA dissection associated with a shiatsu massager. *Neurology, 58*(8), 1302–1304.

Ernst, E. (2003). The safety of massage therapy. *Rheumatology (Oxford), 42*(9), 1101–1106.

Ernst, E., Pittler, M. H., Wider, B., & Boddy, K. (2006). *The desktop guide to complementary and alternative medicine* (2nd ed.). Edinburgh: Elsevier Mosby.

Field, T. (2019). Social touch, CT touch and massage therapy: A narrative review. *Developmental Review, 51,* 123–145.

Field, T., Diego, M., & Hernandez-Reif, M. (2010). Moderate pressure is essential for massage therapy effects. *The International Journal of Neuroscience, 120*(5), 381–385.

Foster, J. (2015). *How a massage can cause a stroke: It happened to Elizabeth. Here she warns of a danger beauty therapists don't know about.* Daily Mail. http://www.dailymail.co.uk/femail/article-3343681/How-massage-cause-stroke-happened-Elizabeth-warns-danger-beauty-therapists-don-t-know-about.html.

Gatterman, M. I. (2011). *Whiplash: A patient-centered approach to management.* St Louis: Elsevier.

Grant, A. C., & Wang, N. (2004). Carotid dissection associated with a handheld electric massager. *Southern Medical Journal, 97*(12), 1262–1263.

International Federation of Orthopaedic Manipulative Physical Therapists (IFOMPT). (2016). *Educational standards in orthopaedic manipulative therapy.* Retrieved from: http://www.ifompt.org/site/ifompt/IFOMPT%20Standards%20Document%20definitive%202016.pdf.

Jensen, A. M., Ramasamy, A., Hotek, J., Roel, B., & Riffe, D. (2012). The benefits of giving a massage on the mental state of massage therapists: A randomized, controlled trial. *Journal of Alternative and Complementary Medicine, 18*(12), 1142–1146.

Kaur, J., Singla, M., Singh, G., & Singh, G. (2017). Frequent neck massage leading to bilateral anterior cerebral artery infarction. *BMJ Case Reports, 2017,* bcr2017222169.

Kerr, H. D. (1997). Ureteral stent displacement associated with deep massage. *WMJ: Official Publication of the State Medical Society of Wisconsin, 96*(12), 57–58.

Koren, Y., & Kalichman, L. (2018). Deep tissue massage: What are we talking about? *Journal of Bodywork and Movement Therapies, 22*(2), 247–251.

Kitisomprayoonkul, W. (2018). Brachial plexus injury after massage: A case report. *Journal of Thai Rehabilitation Medicine, 28*(1), 21–23.

Lee, T. H., Chiu, J. W., & Chan, R. C. (2011). Cervical cord injury after massage. *American Journal of Physical Medicine & Rehabilitation, 90*(10), 856–859.

Liu, J. S., Tsai, T. C., & Chang, Y. Y. (1993). Extracranial internal carotid artery dissection secondary to neck massage: Visualization of mural hematoma by MRI. *Gaoxiong yi xue ke xue za zhi = The Kaohsiung Journal of Medical Sciences, 9*(5), 322–327.

Mufarrij, A. J., & Hitti, E. (2011). Acute cystic rupture and hemorrhagic shock after a vigorous massage chair session in a patient with polycystic kidney disease. *The American Journal of the Medical Sciences, 342*(1), 76–78.

Nelsen, E. (2015). *Why do your knuckles pop?* Retrieved from https://www.youtube.com/watch?v=IjiKUmfaZr4.

Occupational Safety and Health Administration (OSHA). (2015). *OSHA procedures for safe weight lifting when manually lifting.* Retrieved from https://www.osha.gov/laws-regs/standardinterpretations/2013-06-04-0.

Ohio Bureau of Worker's Compensation. (n.d.). *Lifting guidelines.* Retrieved from https://info.bwc.ohio.gov/wps/portal/gov/bwc/for-employers/safety-and-training/safety-education/Lifting-guidelines.

Posadzki, P., & Ernst, E. (2013). The safety of massage therapy: An update of a systematic review. *Focus on Alternative and Complementary Therapies, 18*(1), 27–32.

Romanowski, M., Romanowska, J., & Grześkowiak, M. (2012). A comparison of the effects of deep tissue massage and therapeutic massage on chronic low back pain. *Studies in Health Technology and Informatics, 176,* 411–414.

Schacter, E. (2021). *Beginner massage therapy sequence.* Retrieved from https://elanschacter.com/beginner-massage-therapist-sequence/.

Schrader, A., & Ross, M. A. (2008). Spinal accessory neuropathy following massage: Case report. *AANEM: Clinical Neurophysiology, 119,* e51.

Smith, J. M., Sullivan, S. J., & Baxter, G. D. (2009a). Massage therapy services for healthcare: A telephone focus group study of drivers for clients' continued use of services. *Complementary Therapies in Medicine, 17*(5–6), 281–291.

Smith, J. M., Sullivan, S. J., & Baxter, G. D. (2009b). The culture of massage therapy: Valued elements and the role of comfort, contact, connection and caring. *Complementary Therapies in Medicine, 17*(4), 181–189.

Sundberg, T., Cramer, H., Sibbritt, D., Adams, J., & Lauche, R. (2017). Prevalence, patterns, and predictors of massage practitioner utilization: Results of a US nationally representative survey. *Musculoskeletal Science & Practice, 32,* 31–37.

Travell, J. G., & Simons, D. (1998). *Myofascial pain and dysfunction, the trigger point manual* (2nd ed.). Baltimore: Lippincott Williams and Wilkins.

Trotter, J. F. (1999). Hepatic hematoma after deep tissue massage. *The New England Journal of Medicine, 341*(26), 2019–2020.

Turkeltaub, P. C., Yearwood, E. L., & Friedmann, E. (2014). Effect of a brief seated massage on nursing student attitudes toward touch for comfort care. *Journal of Alternative and Complementary Medicine, 20*(10), 792–799.

Yin, P., Gao, N., Wu, J., Litscher, G., & Xu, S. (2014). Adverse events of massage therapy in pain-related conditions: A systematic review. *Evidence-Based Complementary and Alternative Medicine: eCAM, 2014,* 480956.

Wada, Y., Yanagihara, C., & Nishimura, Y. (2005). Internal jugular vein thrombosis associated with shiatsu massage of the neck. *Journal of Neurology, Neurosurgery, and Psychiatry, 76*(1), 142–143.

Walton, T. (2010). *Medical conditions and massage therapy: A decision tree approach.* Baltimore: Lippincott Williams and Wilkins.

Wood, E. C. (1974). *Beard's massage: Principles and techniques* (2nd ed.). Philadelphia: WB Saunders.

REVIEW AND APPLY YOUR KNOWLEDGE

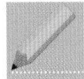

MATCHING ONE: CONCEPT REVIEW

Place the letter of the answer next to the number of the term or phrase that best describes it.

A. Compression
B. Excursion
C. Transverse friction
D. Effleurage
E. Friction
F. Mobilization
G. Nerve stroke
H. Petrissage
I. Rhythm
J. Centripetal
K. Tapotement
L. Vibration

_____ 1. Refers to the pattern or regularity of the applied massage technique.

_____ 2. Distance a massage technique travels over the body.

_____ 3. Massage technique of gliding movements following the contours of the client's body.

_____ 4. Massage technique using light pressure applied with the weight of the fingers or hands as they glide down the body.

_____ 5. Shaking or trembling massage technique.

_____ 6. Massage technique involving compression, lifting or decompression, and then releasing of soft tissues.

_____ 7. Massage technique of rubbing one body surface over another while maintaining constant and equal pressure in all directions.

_____ 8. Massage technique that moves the client's skin back and forth over the treated fibers at right angles or perpendicular to the tissue fibers.

_____ 9. Massage technique using repetitive striking motions.

_____ 10. Direction massage techniques such as effleurage are applied.

_____ 11. Movements applied to a joint complex without a manual thrust at the end of available passive range of motion.

_____ 12. Non-gliding technique of pressure application.

MATCHING TWO: CONCEPT REVIEW

Place the letter of the answer next to the number of the term or phrase that best describes it.

A. Pressure
B. Active
C. Diffused
D. Pincement
E. Pin and stretch
F. Hacking
G. Massage
H. Passive
I. Range of motion
J. Effleurage
K. Stretching
L. Skin rolling

_____ 1. Tapotement performed by laying a relaxed hand, palm down, over the client's skin and striking the back of this hand with the other hand positioned in a loose fist.

_____ 2. Movements produced by external forces without voluntary muscle contraction.

_____ 3. Manipulation of soft tissue using compression and decompression/traction for clinical, therapeutic, and palliative purposes and for wellness and self-care purposes.

_____ 4. Tapotement performed with the ulnar surfaces of one or two hands.

_____ 5. Amount of motion that occurs when one segment of the body moves in relationship to another segment of the body.

_____ 6. Superficial petrissage that compresses and lifts the skin, then moves lifted skin across adjacent areas.

_____ 7. Application of gliding or non-gliding force.

_____ 8. Passively positioning muscle attachments as far apart as possible to elongate the muscle in the direction opposite of its action.

_____ 9. Techniques that concentrate a stretch to a region of muscle.

_____ 10. Movements produced by voluntary muscular contraction; clients move the limb or body part themselves.

_____ 11. Tapotement using the tips of several fingers and thumb to strike, grasp, lift, and release the skin.

_____ 12. Massage technique commonly used to begin the session, to apply or reapply lubricant, to introduce touch and pressure to the client, to assess tissues before treatment, and to reassess tissues after treatment.

MULTIPLE CHOICE: TEST YOUR KNOWLEDGE

Place the letter of the answer next to the number of the term or phrase that best describes it.

_____ 1. Which type of massage is used for self-care to reduce stress and promote relaxation?
   A. Wellness
   B. Clinical
   C. Sports
   D. Medical

_____ 2. Massage techniques largely use _____ terms.
   A. Swedish
   B. French
   C. Italian
   D. Russian

_____ 3. Gliding is another term for which technique?
   A. Effleurage
   B. Petrissage
   C. Friction
   D. Tapotement

_____ 4. Percussion is another term for which technique?
   A. Effleurage
   B. Petrissage
   C. Friction
   D. Tapotement

_____ 5. An unintended but predictable effect that occurs after a session is called a:
   A. Side effect
   B. Adverse event
   C. Endangerment site
   D. Cautionary site

_____ 6. Of all the endangerment sites, the most serious adverse effects were associated with which area?
   A. Abdomen
   B. Axilla
   C. Neck
   D. Popliteal

_____ 7. Which describes a lengthening force, usually achieved by pulling objects in opposite directions?
   A. Compression
   B. Tension
   C. Bending
   D. Shearing

_____ 8. The ocean waves technique is an example of which type of physical force?
   A. Tension
   B. Bending
   C. Shearing
   D. Torsion

_____ 9. What is the number of times or speed that massage techniques are repeated and described as slow, moderate, or rapid/fast?
   A. Excursion
   B. Rhythm
   C. Rate
   D. Frequency

_____ 10. In general, techniques are structured in multiples of:
   A. Two
   B. Three
   C. Four
   D. Five

_____ 11. The ability to notice and respond to changes in a client's experience is called:
   A. Sequence
   B. Routine
   C. Tracking
   D. Duration

_____ 12. Which of the following describes an absolute contraindication?
   A. Recently injured area
   B. Acutely inflamed area
   C. Medical device
   D. Contagious disease

CRITICAL THINKING

It's All in the Wrist

What do you think about learning massage techniques as part of a routine? Do you think it is more useful to learn the individual techniques and put them together in your own routine, or to learn a standard routine first, then individualize it as you gain more experience?

Answers can include but are not limited to:

Some students learn better by having a set routine in which they learn the techniques. Once they have mastered the routine, they feel more confident branching out into creating their own routines. Other students find a standard routine too confining and will become bored using it, which can inhibit their learning process. They may find that learning the individual techniques first, then combining them in creative ways, can be more fulfilling.

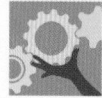

PROFESSIONAL PRACTICE

After the Accident

Margaret is a recent graduate from massage school and has begun her practice at a chiropractic clinic. Margaret massages the patients before their chiropractic adjustments. Mark was involved in a car accident and is Margaret's next client. It is his first massage. Mark explains he is having some residual dizziness from the head injury he sustained from being rear-ended. He has been cleared for massage by his physician. What techniques would be most appropriate for Margaret to perform on Mark?

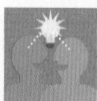

DISCUSSION

Effects of Massage Techniques

There are numerous published studies on the effects of massage. But what do we know about individual massage techniques? Using an Internet-based search engine, locate studies examining the effects of specific massage techniques. Use traditional and modern terms and keywords (i.e., effleurage and gliding) in your search. If available, post your reflections on an Internet-based discussion board monitored by your instructor. Post a link to any studies you locate.

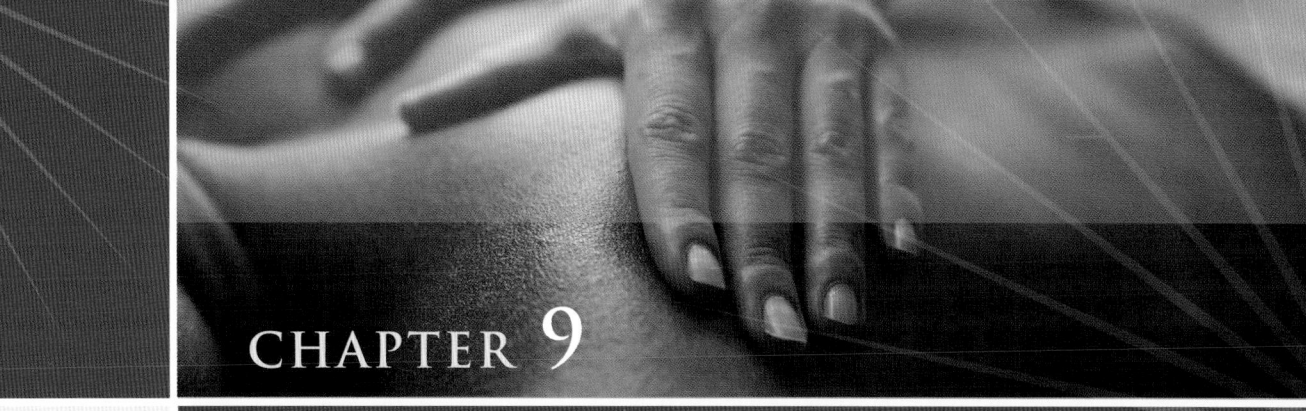

CHAPTER 9

Concepts of Disease, Standard Precautions, Transmission-Based Precautions, Disinfection Procedures, and Emergency Preparedness

All of life is a constant education.
—Eleanor Roosevelt

LEARNING OBJECTIVES

After completing this chapter, the student should be able to:

1. Define vocabulary terms used to discuss disease.
2. Identify types of diseases and disorders.
3. Describe the chain of infection and processes of disease transmission.
4. Summarize standard precautions and transmission-based precautions.
5. Discuss disinfecting procedures for surfaces, objects, and laundry.
6. State what to do in medical emergencies such as choking, hypoglycemia, stroke, heart attack, and seizures.

INTRODUCTION

Massage is one of the safest, least intrusive, and most effective treatments for reducing pain and stress and for increasing quality of life. However, clients are susceptible to infection or experience medical emergencies such as hypoglycemia or a heart attack. To reduce the risk of infection, massage practitioners need a system of infection control to protect clients and themselves and to minimize disease transmission. These measures include hand hygiene, use of personal protective equipment, and disinfection procedures. Hippocrates, the father of Western medicine, is frequently quoted as saying physicians should "do no harm." Likewise, massage practitioners across the globe must adopt policies of impeccable cleanliness and adherence to standard and transmission-based precautions to safeguard against infection. Although chances are low clients will have a medical emergency, it is best to be prepared.

Both students and practitioners must continually check for the newest and most updated medical and procedural information available. Although the Internet contains valuable information, it also contains much misinformation, hearsay, and personal opinion. Trust only reliable, authoritative sources such as state or federal agencies, professional journals, and seminars and their associated websites. The following agencies provide vast amounts of information on health and disease:

- World Health Organization (http://www.who.int/en)
- United States Department of Health and Human Services (http://www.hhs.gov)
- National Institutes of Health (http://www.nih.gov)
- Centers for Disease Control and Prevention (CDC) (http://www.cdc.gov)

INTRODUCTION TO DISEASE: VOCABULARY

Massage practitioners seek to improve the health and well-being of their clients through massage. Regardless of your work setting or methods you use, you will encounter clients who have diseases or medical conditions and who are under medical supervision. You need to be familiar with basic terminology frequently used when discussing diseases and infection control measures such as standard precautions. The importance of vocabulary fluency cannot be overstated, as words are the currency of communication. A robust vocabulary improves all areas of communication, including speaking, listening, reading, and writing.

Disease is a condition of abnormal function involving anatomic structures or body systems. Diseases are characterized by a recognizable set of signs and symptoms, which can be caused by heredity and genetics; infection status; lifestyle choices, including diet and physical activity; and environmental factors, including exposure to ultraviolet (UV) radiation and air pollutants, water, and soil. Diseases are diagnosed by physicians or other medical experts according to standardized diagnostic codes. In contrast to disease, **illness** is defined as the feeling of ill health a person identifies themselves, often based on self-report. Illness may represent a minor or temporary problem or may indicate severe health problems, which may necessitate a referral to a medical practitioner.

Pathology is the study of disease and includes causes (etiology), effects, and typical behaviors resulting from disease. Pathology also includes the examination of body tissue samples for forensic or diagnostic purposes. **Diagnosis** is the process of identifying a disease and includes evaluation of signs and symptoms, medical and surgical histories, physical examination, laboratory tests, and other procedures. *Differential diagnosis* distinguishes a disease from others that possess similar signs and symptoms. **Prognosis** involves predicting how a disease will progress and chances of recovery based on the person's condition and the usual course of the disease.

Signs and Symptoms

Diseases display signs and symptoms. **Signs** are objective and can be measured and observed by others and include swelling, rash, fever, jaundice, and high blood pressure. **Symptoms** are subjective and apparent only to the individual, and include headache, back pain, nausea, fatigue, and anxiety. *Clinical manifestation* is a collective term that describes both signs and symptoms. A syndrome is a group of signs and symptoms that characterize or suggest an underlying disease or increases the risk of disease development. An example is metabolic syndrome, which suggests type 2 diabetes mellitus and increased risk of heart and kidney diseases. *Asymptomatic* describes the absence of symptoms. People are often asymptomatic in the early stages of cancer and viral infections, including human immunodeficiency virus (HIV), hepatitis C virus (HCV) infections, and some cases of the novel coronavirus (COVID-19).

Etiology and Risk Factors

Etiology is the cause or origin of disease. A single causative factor may be present, or it may be multifactorial and include predisposing factors or risk factors, the nature of the etiologic agents, and the route the pathogen used to invade the body. Etiologic agents include pathogens, such as viruses or bacteria, congenital defects, inherited or genetic disorders, immunologic dysfunctions, metabolic imbalances, degenerative changes, malignancies, nutrient deficiencies, or trauma. A disease with unknown causes or origins is called **idiopathic**.

Risk factors increase or decrease the chances of getting a disease. Two types of risk factors are modifiable and nonmodifiable. *Nonmodifiable risk factors* cannot be changed, such as a person's age, family history, and race. *Modifiable risk factors* can be changed, such as lifestyle, including tobacco use, food choices and amounts, and levels of physical activity. Age as a risk factor can increase or decrease the chance of disease acquisition. For example, infants are more susceptible to respiratory diseases. Certain types of leukemia are more common in children. Older adults are more

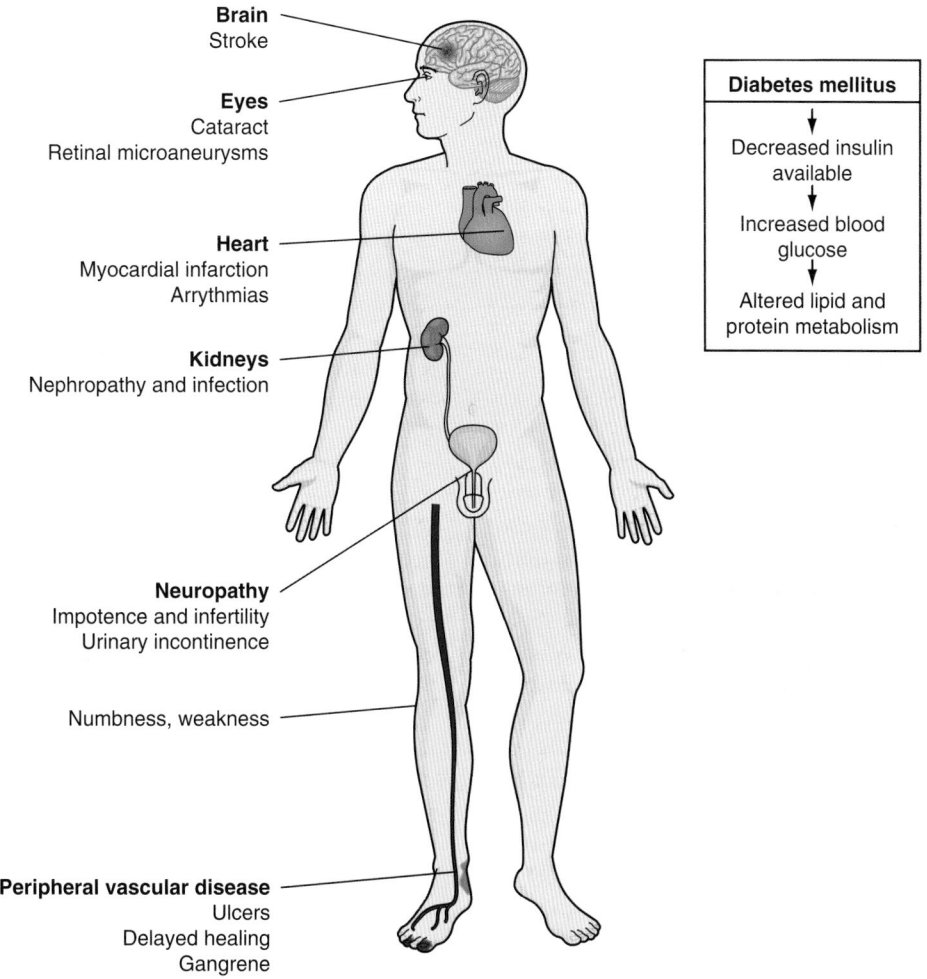

FIG. 9.1 Disease complications of diabetes mellitus. (From VanMeter, K., & Hubert, R. [2014]. *Gould's pathophysiology for the health professions* [5th ed.]. Louis: Saunders.)

likely to have Alzheimer's disease and osteoarthritis. Complications during pregnancy increase in females age 40 years and older. Lifestyle risk factors can increase heart disease, certain cancers, and sexually transmitted diseases or infections, to name a few.

Disease Complications

Diseases also may have **complications**, which are conditions arising as a disease progresses. Examples of complications are congestive heart failure developing after a heart attack, and peripheral neuropathy developing after a diagnosis of diabetes (Fig. 9.1). Some disease complications are also called *secondary diseases*.

Local and Systemic Diseases

Diseases can be described by their degree of involvement. A **local disease** affects one area of the body. An example of a local disease is athlete's foot, a fungal infection usually confined to the feet. A **systemic disease** is distributed throughout the body. An example is systemic lupus erythematosus, an autoimmune disease affecting the skin, joints, nervous system, kidneys, lungs, and other organs.

Disease Outbreaks: Endemics, Epidemics, and Pandemics

A **disease outbreak** is disease occurrence of more than what is normally expected within a community, a geographic area, or a season. Disease outbreaks may last for a few days, weeks, or several years. An **endemic** is a disease that occurs regularly in particular regions or populations. Malaria is an endemic in parts of Africa, and chickenpox is an endemic that occurs regularly among young children. These diseases are always present in the area or population, but in relatively low numbers. **Epidemics** are disease outbreaks affecting many individuals at about the same time, and often spread to one or more communities. The severe acute respiratory syndrome (SARS) epidemic of 2003 took the lives of nearly 800 people. Unlike endemics, epidemics eventually subside. **Pandemics** are epidemics that spread across many regions, often worldwide. The COVID-19 pandemic has caused over 6 million deaths worldwide as of June 2022. The HIV/acquired immunodeficiency syndrome (AIDS) pandemic is one of the deadliest in history, with a worldwide death toll of approximately 33 million as of December 2020.

Acute and Chronic Diseases

Acute diseases occur suddenly, persist for a brief time (<3 months), and then resolve or, in some cases, cause death. An example of an acute disease is gastroenteritis or "stomach flu," with accompanying vomiting, diarrhea, and abdominal pain. **Chronic diseases** have an insidious onset, gradual increase in signs and symptoms, and last for a longer time, perhaps for a lifetime. An example of a chronic disease is osteoarthritis. *Subacute diseases* have characteristics somewhere between acute and chronic. An example of a subacute disease is asthma.

Morbidity, Incidence, Prevalence, and Mortality

Morbidity involves the departure from a state of physiologic or psychologic wellbeing. It includes acute and chronic diseases, illnesses, injuries, and disabilities. A person can have a morbidity or multiple morbidities at the same time, which are called comorbidities. An example of a comorbidity is a diagnosis of diabetes in addition to a diagnosis of hypertension or high blood pressure. One morbidity may lead to another morbidity. For example, a person with diabetes may later be diagnosed with kidney disease. Treatments for morbidities may cause additional morbidities. For example, a person undergoing chemotherapy for cancer may develop chemotherapy-induced peripheral neuropathy.

Morbidity rate is the number of persons who are diseased, ill, injured, or disabled within a population or region. Two ways to measure morbidity frequency are incidence and prevalence. **Incidence** is the number of new cases of a given condition within a population per unit of time, usually a calendar year. For example, an estimated 1.5 million new cases of diabetes were diagnosed among people aged 18 years or older in 2018. **Prevalence** is the number of all existing cases (new and old) of a given condition within a population per unit of time. For example, an estimated 34.1 million people aged 18 years or older had diabetes in 2018.

Mortality is the condition of being dead. **Mortality rate** is the number of deaths within a population or region. Both morbidity and mortality rates are expressed mathematically; the number of cases divided by the total population. For example, if there are 25 lung cancer deaths in one year in a population of 30,000, mortality rates for this population are 83 per 100,000.

TYPES OF DISEASES AND DISORDERS

As mentioned previously, **diseases** are conditions of abnormal function involving anatomic structures or body systems. Diseases can be classified by how they were acquired or how they developed. Types of diseases include *autoimmune*, *cancer*, *deficiency*, *degenerative*, *genetic*, *infectious*, and *metabolic*. **Disorders** are disruptions of normal body function and may not involve a structural change. Two types of disorders are *congenital* and *traumatic*. The terms disorder and disease are often used interchangeably.

Congenital Disorders

Congenital disorders present at or before birth. These disorders may be caused by genetic abnormalities, by a maternal diet deficient in nutrients, or by the mother's habits while the baby is in utero, such as drug, alcohol, or tobacco use. Other causes of congenital abnormalities include fetal exposure to radiation, poisons, and disease-causing organisms, such as rubella, or oxygen deprivation of the baby before or during birth. Examples of congenital disorders include cerebral palsy, cleft palate or lip, and spina bifida. Some congenital disorders are not recognized until years after birth or, in some cases, never. About 3% of babies are born with congenital defects in the United States each year.

Many individuals with congenital disorders, chronic diseases, or debilitating conditions, such as cancer, experience tremendous strain on their finances and may have limited access to massage by a licensed provider. Give these individuals and their families the gift of massage by teaching caregivers how to massage their loved ones. A good way to connect with caregivers is through various support groups. Teach gentle techniques and convey the same precautions to the caregivers that licensed practitioners follow, such as avoiding skin lesions and areas containing medical devices such as ports.

Traumatic Disorders

Traumatic disorders involve injury to the body often from violence or accidents. Examples of traumatic disorders are open wounds, fractures, sprains, spinal cord and brain injuries, and head injuries. Traumatic disorders can be cumulative, resulting from continuous body movements over an extended period. The latter, which are also called cumulative traumatic disorders, repetitive stress injuries, or repetitive motion disorders, can lead to degenerative diseases mentioned later in this section. In the United States, injury accounts for over 150,000 deaths and over 3 million nonfatal injuries per year. The most common causes of traumatic injury are automobile accidents, unhelmeted motorcycle or bicycle accidents, physical assaults, and falls.

Autoimmune Diseases

Autoimmune diseases are marked by an inappropriate or excessive immune response. The body mistakenly attacks and destroys healthy tissue. Examples of autoimmune diseases are rheumatoid arthritis (synovial membrane destruction), systemic lupus erythematosus (connective tissue destruction), and multiple sclerosis (brain and spinal cord nerve sheath destruction).

Periods of remission and exacerbation characterize many autoimmune diseases. **Remissions** are periods when signs and symptoms disappear or diminish significantly. **Exacerbations** are periods when signs and symptoms worsen or become more severe. Periods of exacerbation are also called flare-ups or relapses. During disease exacerbation, massage is postponed or only slowly applied using light pressure (3 on a 10-point pressure scale).

Approximately 23.5 million Americans have an autoimmune disease. They are more common among females, and among Black/Hispanic/Latinx people.

Cancerous Diseases (Cancer)

Cancer is characterized by growth of abnormal cells possessing uncontrolled cell division, lack programmed cell death, and can accumulate into masses or tumors. Cancer can spread or metastasize, which is the ability to invade other tissues of the body. An estimated 1,735,350 new cases of cancer were diagnosed in the United States and 609,640 people died from the disease in 2018. The most common cancers are breast, cancer, lung cancer, prostate cancer, colorectal cancer, melanoma of the skin, bladder cancer, non-Hodgkin lymphoma, kidney cancer, uterine cancer, leukemia, pancreatic cancer, thyroid cancer, and liver cancer.

Deficiency Diseases

Deficiency diseases are caused by lack of an essential nutrient in the individual's diet or by the inability to digest and absorb a particular nutrient properly. This deficiency typically interferes with the body's growth, development, and metabolism. Examples of deficiency diseases are scurvy, caused by a deficiency of vitamin C (ascorbic acid); pernicious anemia is caused by inadequate absorption of vitamin B12 from a lack of intrinsic factor secretions from the stomach's lining. Vitamin B12 is necessary for the absorption of iron from the digestive tract into the blood. B12 is critical to red blood cell formation. Less than 10% of the U.S. population is deficient in vitamins A and D, folate, iron, or iodine.

Degenerative Diseases

Degenerative diseases involve tissue breakdown caused by overuse or occur naturally because of the aging process. Examples of degenerative diseases are osteoporosis (bone degeneration), osteoarthritis (joint degeneration), and Alzheimer and Parkinson diseases (neurodegeneration). More than 5 million Americans live with Alzheimer disease, and at least 500,000 Americans live with Parkinson disease, although some estimates are much higher.

Genetic Diseases

Genetic diseases are caused by abnormalities in the genetic code. Genes are the cell's hereditary units and are arranged in a single file along chromosomes in the nucleus. Each gene codes for a single protein and provides the physical makeup of each individual. Genetic diseases can be passed from one generation to the next or the result of spontaneous mutation. Examples of genetic diseases are sickle cell anemia (affects the blood's hemoglobin molecule), Down syndrome (three instead of two chromosomes 21), and cystic fibrosis (produces abnormally thick respiratory and digestive secretions).

Metabolic Diseases

Metabolic diseases occur when metabolism fails, causing the body to have too much or too little of an essential substance, such as hormones. Metabolic diseases develop when organs become diseased or do not function properly. For example, when the adrenals produce excess amounts of the hormone cortisol, Cushing disease can develop. When the pancreas produces insufficient amounts of the hormone insulin, diabetes can develop.

Infectious Diseases

Infectious diseases, or infections, are caused by pathogens. A **pathogen** is a biologic agent capable of causing infectious disease. Examples of pathogens are viruses, bacteria, fungi, protozoa, prions, and pathogenic animals. Plant resins can cause diseases, such as contact dermatitis from poison ivy. Signs and symptoms of local infection are swelling, heat, redness, pain, pus, and enlarged lymph glands. Signs and symptoms of widespread infection are fever, headaches, body aches, fatigue, and loss of appetite.

Lower respiratory infections are the leading cause of death from infection, accounting for almost 80% of all infectious disease mortality. Death rates by diarrheal infections were the second-leading cause of death, and the only infectious disease mortality that increased since 2000. These diseases accounted for about 7% of infectious disease deaths. After respiratory and diarrheal infections, HIV/AIDs are the most common causes of death by infectious disease.

Healthcare–associated infections (HAIs) are acquired while a person is receiving healthcare for another condition. HAIs are associated with healthcare delivery in all settings, including hospitals, surgical centers, infusion or dialysis centers, long-term care facilities, and home healthcare. The previous term was *nosocomial infections*; both terms are often used interchangeably. However, the term HAI reflects the inability to determine where the infection was acquired, because individuals can be exposed to pathogens outside the healthcare setting, before receiving healthcare, or while moving from one setting to another within the healthcare delivery system. At any given time, one in 25 inpatients has an HAI. The most common HAI in hospitals are urinary tract infections related to catheter use. Other common HAIs include surgical site infections, pneumonia, *Clostridium difficile* (*C. diff.*) and methicillin-resistant *Staphylococcus aureus* (MRSA) infections. *C. diff* is a bacterium causing colitis with symptoms ranging from fever, diarrhea, and abdominal pain. MRSA is a bacterium resistant to the effects of many common antibiotics. Symptoms of MRSA include a red, swollen, warm, tender area; it may look like a pus-filled pimple or boil and may progress to an open area of skin that drains fluid. In severe cases, the person may have systemic symptoms, including fever. To prevent the transmission of *C. diff.* and MRSA infections, wash hands before and after leaving a healthcare facility and practice contact precautions when with someone who has these infections or symptoms of these infections (see the following sections for established handwashing and contact precaution protocols). Alcohol-based hand rubs/sanitizers should only be used if soap and clean water are unavailable as they do not eliminate all pathogens, including *C. diff* bacterium and harmful chemicals, such as pesticides.

CHAIN OF INFECTION: THE PROCESS OF DISEASE TRANSMISSION

The **chain of infection** is a model used to explain infectious disease transmission and uses a six-linked chain that includes: (1) a pathogen; (2) a reservoir or source; (3) a portal of exit; (4) a mode of transmission; (5) a portal of entry to a new host; and (6) a host's susceptibility to infection (Fig. 9.2). Each link plays an important role and can be broken through various

means of infection control, such as standard precautions and transmission-based precautions (featured later).

Pathogens are the first link in the chain. As mentioned previously, **pathogens** are biologic agents capable of causing infections. Examples of pathogens are viruses, bacteria, fungi, protozoa, prions, and pathogenic animals (Fig. 9.3). **Viruses** are nonliving entities that depend on a host cell for growth and replication. Viruses, a type of organic parasite, attach to the plasma membrane of a host cell and inject their own genetic materials into the cell. These materials travel to and enter the nucleus of the host cell. The host cell reads the viral deoxyribonucleic acid (DNA) and makes viruses instead of the cell's usual proteins. Once the host cell is filled, the cell explodes, releasing the newly made viruses. Each viral fragment can travel to and infect other host cells. Examples of viral infections are the common cold, influenza, HIV infection, measles, mumps, rabies, herpes simplex, and severe acute respiratory disease caused by coronavirus. **Bacteria** are single-cell organisms; they can be spherical, spiral, or rod-shaped; and appear singly or in chains. Most bacteria are not pathogenic, and some can be used to process foods such as bread, yogurt, and wine. Helpful bacteria, or probiotics, occur as natural flora in the gastrointestinal (GI) tract and aid digestion. Examples of bacterial infections are boils, impetigo, tuberculosis, gastroenteritis, and strep throat.

Fungi include molds, yeast, and dermatophytes called tinea. Only a few fungi are pathogenic (Candida albicans,

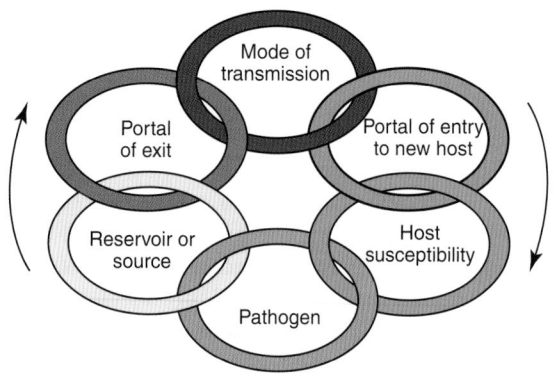

FIG. 9.2 Chain of infection. (From Perry, A., & Potter, P. [2014]. *Clinical nursing skills and techniques* [8th ed.] St. Louis: Mosby.)

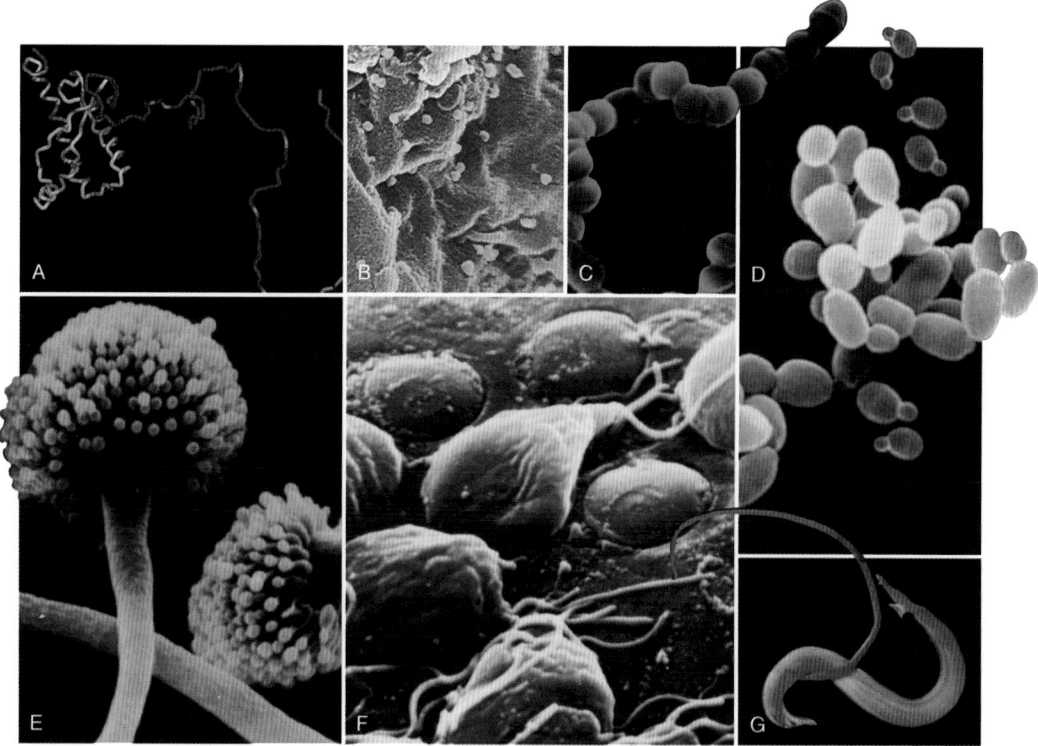

FIG. 9.3 Pathogens. (A) Prion (cause of Creutzfeldt-Jakob disease). (B) Virus (human immunodeficiency virus [HIV] causing acquired immunodeficiency syndrome [AIDS]). (C) Bacteria (Streptococcus bacterium causing strep throat and other bacterial infections). (D) Fungi (cause of many urogenital tract infections). (E) Fungi (causes aspergillosis infections, most involving the respiratory tract). (F) Protozoa (cause of many cases of traveler's diarrhea). (G) Pathogenic animals (parasitic worm causing schistosomes or snail fever). (From Patton, K., Thibodeau, G. [2015]. *Anatomy & physiology* [9th ed.]. St. Louis: Mosby.)

dermatophytes). Warm, moist environments promote their growth. Examples of fungal infections are thrush, ringworm, and athlete's foot. **Protozoa** are the simplest form of animal life and include amoebas, flagellates, sporozoans, and many other forms. Examples of protozoal infections are trichomoniasis, amoebic dysentery, African sleeping sickness, and malaria. **Prions** are proteinaceous infectious particles that can affect the central nervous system; these infections are currently untreatable and fatal. Diseases caused by prions include bovine spongiform encephalopathy (mad cow disease) and Creutzfeldt–Jakob disease. **Pathogenic animals** live on or within a host, depend on it for nourishment and replication, and can cause diseases called infestations. Examples of pathogenic animals are intestinal worms, lice, and scabies.

A **reservoir** is the second link and is the person or environment (soil, water) where pathogens live and reproduce, or depend on for its survival. Reservoirs can also be animals, such as rodents.

A **portal of exit**, the next link, is the pathway pathogens use to leave a reservoir. Respiratory infections often exit through the nose or mouth. GI infections exit through the colon, and sexually transmitted infections exit through the urethra or genitalia. The most common portal of exit is contact with unclean human hands.

Next is the **mode of transmission**, or transfer of pathogens by contact (direct and indirect), through vehicles, such as food or water, or by vectors, such as insects or animals to spread pathogens between two or more hosts. The word vehicle and vector both come from Latin words meaning "carrier."

- **Contact Transmission**. This type of transmission involves some form of touch. There are two forms of contract transmission. Contact transmission is the most common method of disease transmission.
  - **Direct Contact**. Contact with a person or animal. Many diseases spread through direct contact transmission, including conjunctivitis (pink eye) and herpes simplex (cold sores). Direct contact transmission includes sexual acts; examples include human papilloma virus (HPV) and HIV infections.
  - **Indirect Contact**. Contact with a **fomite**, which is a contaminated object or material, such as faucet handles, doorknobs, or clothing. Indirect contact transmission, also called *fomite transmission*, occurs when an infected person coughs or sneezes, and spreads infected droplets into the surrounding area. The noninfected individual must be within 6 feet, or 2 m; if not, it is called airborne transmission (a type of vehicle transmission; see the next section). Most respiratory tract diseases are spread by indirect contact.
- **Vehicle Transmission** occurs when pathogens transmit through a common vehicle or source, such as food, water, air, and in some cases, blood distributed by transfusion services. Vehicle transmission can be foodborne, waterborne, or airborne.
  - **Foodborne Transmission**. Food containing pathogens gets consumed because they were either transferred to or not destroyed during preparation or storage. For example, failing to wash the hands after handling raw meat or

after using the toilet, and then preparing or serving meals can cause foodborne diseases. An example of foodborne disease is Salmonella poisoning associated with chicken, eggs, beef, raw cashews, and other foods.
- **Waterborne Transmission**. This occurs from bathing, washing, drinking, or ingesting food prepared with water containing pathogens. Sewage is often a source of contamination. Some cases of cholera and dysentery are examples of diseases caused by waterborne transmission.
- **Airborne Transmission**. This occurs when pathogens travel on dust particles or small respiratory droplets that become aerosolized when an infected person sneezes or coughs. A noninfected person can inhale the infected droplets, or they can land on their eyes, nose, and mouth. Examples of diseases that may result from airborne transmission are tuberculosis, chicken pox, measles, and swine flu.
- **Vector Transmission** uses a vector to spread pathogens between two or more hosts. Most vector-borne diseases are transmitted by animal bites, insect stings, or tissue infestation. Examples of diseases from vector transmission are malaria, Lyme disease, and Rocky Mountain spotted fever.

The **portal of entry** is the next link and is the route pathogens use to enter a new host after transmission has occurred. Portals of entry are similar to the portals of exit (e.g., nose, mouth).

The final link in the chain is the **host susceptibility** or how vulnerable an individual is to developing infection after exposure to pathogens. The future host is the next person exposed to the pathogen. Pathogens may spread to another person but do not develop into an infection if the person's immune system can fight it off. The very young, older people and people who have a disease or illness, or who are immunocompromised or immunosuppressed, such as those with diabetes, HIV infection, and those receiving medications that reduce immunity, such as chemotherapy, are among the most vulnerable to infection.

Infection and Inflammation

If pathogens overcome the host's immune response, infection occurs. The host now becomes a reservoir for future disease transmissions. Or they may become an asymptomatic "carrier" during the incubation period, being the next "mode of transmission" to another "susceptible host." The **incubation period** is the time interval between initial exposure to pathogens and the first appearance of disease signs and symptoms. This is more common in viral infections. The length of incubation periods varies. For example, the incubation period for influenza and the common cold is 1 to 3 days. The incubation for chickenpox is 14 to 16 days.

After the incubation period, some infections include a **prodromal period**, where the host begins to experience signs and symptoms of disease from immune response activation. For example, a person with herpes simplex infection may experience itching, burning, or tingling in the affected area before a blister-like skin rash appears. Other signs and symptoms seen during the prodromal period are fever and inflammation.

Inflammation is a protective response to tissue damage resulting from a variety of causes, including infection and trauma. The body attempts to wall off, destroy, and digest bacteria and dead or foreign tissue. Vascular changes allow fluid to leak into the area, which contains chemicals that stimulate phagocytic activity by white blood cells (WBCs). Exudate (pus) may appear in wounds and neighboring lymph nodes may enlarge. These processes reduce or prevent the spread of infection. Next, the body begins to clean up the affected area, and begins the repair and replacement processes of damaged or destroyed tissue. Widespread or systemic inflammation is marked by fever, headaches, body aches, fatigue, malaise, and loss of appetite. The inflammation related to soft tissue injuries is discussed in Chapter 14.

Tests may be administered during this time, such as blood and urine tests, stool samples, and throat swabs that may reveal infection or other types of disease.

Treatment of Disease

After initial tests and physical exams are completed, diagnosis can be established, with appropriate treatments or interventions implemented. For infections, treatment often consists of antivirals, antibiotics, antifungals, and antiparasitics. Many infections, such as colds, will resolve on their own. Some substances have been shown to prevent or shorten the duration of infection, such as cranberry juice, Echinacea, garlic, ginseng, vitamins C and D, and zinc.

Treatment goals may be curative, to control symptoms, to be supportive, or may be a combination of these. Therapeutic interventions may include methods including drugs to reduce pain, physical rehabilitation, counseling for mental health issues, patient education, surgical procedures, and preventive measures. The massage practitioner should encourage active participation in the treatment plan.

The Centers for Disease Control and Prevention (2016) recommends certain vaccines be used to reduce the risk of acquiring or spreading vaccine-preventable diseases in healthcare settings. Recommended vaccines include hepatitis B; influenza (flu); measles, mumps, rubella (MMR); chickenpox (varicella); tetanus, diphtheria, and pertussis (Tdap); meningococcal; and COVID-19.

A musician must make music, an artist must paint, a poet must write, if he is to be ultimately at peace with himself.
~ **Abraham Maslow**

PRECAUTIONS TO PREVENT TRANSMISSION OF INFECTIOUS AGENTS: STANDARD AND TRANSMISSION-BASED PRECAUTIONS

There are two tiers of precautions to prevent the transmission of infectious agents: standard and transmission-based precautions. **Standard precautions** are minimum infection control practices to prevent occupational transmission of disease. These apply to all clients/patients regardless of suspected or confirmed infection or colonization status (CDC, 2018). Colonization is the presence of pathogens on

a body surface (e.g., skin, GI, or respiratory tract) without causing disease. **Transmission-based precautions** are practices used in addition to standard precautions. They are only applied to patients/clients who are infected or colonized with pathogens that can be transmitted by droplet or airborne transmission or by contact with skin or contaminated surfaces. Transmission-based precautions apply when standard precautions alone are not enough to break the chain of infection. Infection control principles are applicable in all care settings, including spas, clinics, hospitals, private practices, and client residences.

Using infection control measures on all patients was first recommended in the mid-1980s, mostly in response to the HIV epidemic and reports of HIV infections occurring through needlesticks and contact with skin contaminated with blood. The term originally used to describe these measures was universal precautions. In 1987, the CDC implemented another set of guidelines aimed at avoiding direct physical contact with "all moist and potentially infectious body substances," even if blood was not visible. In 1996, isolation precautions were added, and universal precautions became standard precautions. In 2007, respiratory hygiene/cough etiquette was added to combat widespread respiratory infections during this time, namely influenza and SARS. Infection control guidelines will continue to evolve over time. Basic principles of standard precautions include:

- Effective and timely hand hygiene.
- Appropriate use of personal protective equipment (PPE).
- Respiratory hygiene/cough etiquette.
- Proper cleaning and disinfecting or sterilizing of contaminated environmental surfaces and shared electronic equipment, such as tablets, touch screens, keyboards, and mice. Next are terms used when discussing infection control.
- **Cleaning.** Removal of adherent visible soil, blood, and other substances, usually with soap (i.e., detergent), water, and friction. Cleaning may involve the use of heat (warm to hot water).
- **Disinfection.** Use of chemicals to destroy pathogens and may include heat. Disinfection kills most bacterial spores.
- **Sterilization.** Destruction of all microorganisms, pathogenic and nonpathogenic, and can be achieved through heat, chemicals, irradiation, high pressure, and other means.
- **Sanitation.** Removal of impurities and harmful agents to promote health and safety, and usually refers to the environment (e.g., soil, water). Sanitation does not indicate a specific level of cleanliness.

Three categories of transmission-based precautions include contact precautions, droplet precautions, and airborne precautions. They are grouped according to the route of transmission used by the infectious agent.
- **Contact Precautions.** These methods reduce or prevent transmission of pathogens that spread by direct or indirect contact. Contact precautions require the use of barriers, such as gloves and disinfecting of contaminated surfaces.
- **Droplet Precautions.** These methods reduce or prevent transmission of pathogens transmitted by respiratory droplets generated by speaking, coughing, or sneezing.

Droplets may spray as far as 3 feet. Droplet precautions require the use of respiratory hygiene/cough etiquette; mask use may also be required.

- **Airborne Precautions**. These methods reduce or prevent transmission of pathogens transmitted by the airborne route, such as measles, chickenpox, and tuberculosis. These require postponing massage (i.e., absolute contra-indications) for the duration of infection while the risk of airborne transmission exists.

Precautions may be combined for diseases that have multiple modes of transmission. For example, massage businesses implemented both contact and droplet precautions to protect their staff and the public from COVID-19. These precautions included wearing face masks, social distancing (distance of 6 feet or 2 m), limiting the number of people in common areas, and increasing the time between clients for cleaning and disinfecting of massage rooms.

Hand Hygiene

Hand hygiene is a general term for cleaning or disinfecting the hands by handwashing (washing with soap and water) or by alcohol-based hand rubs (foam or gel). Authorities prefer the term hand "rubs" over "sanitizers" to emphasize the physical action of rubbing the hands together after applying the product. Hand hygiene is the best infection control measure because the primary source of disease transmission is contact with human hands. Situations requiring hand hygiene include:

- Before and after treating each client.
- Before and after eating.
- After removing gloves.
- After using the toilet.
- After touching contaminated instruments, equipment, and surfaces (including rubbish) with bare hands.
- After nose blowing, sneezing, or coughing.
- When hands are visibly soiled.

No jewelry, except a simple ring (band), should be worn during hand hygiene procedures. Hand and wrist jewelry may interfere with disinfection and the skin may not dry properly following handwashing (Cimon & Featherstone, 2017; Moolenaar et al., 2000).

After hand hygiene procedures, protect you and others by limiting opportunities for "touch contamination" while providing client care. This includes not touching your face (e.g., adjusting your glasses, rubbing your nose, moving hair out of your face and behind your ear), and avoiding unnecessary contact with massage room surfaces, such as light switches, door handles, and cabinet knobs. Avoid wearing loose fitting clothing, watches, bracelets, dangling necklaces, or hair styles that may touch the client's body. Shirt sleeve length should be mid-arm or higher so you can easily use the forearms to apply massage techniques.

Handwashing is the best way to clean your hands. Use alcohol-based hand rubs when soap and clean water are not available.

Handwashing Procedure

Use the following procedure when handwashing with soap and water (Fig. 9.4). Push up shirt sleeves if needed. Stand close to the sink but far enough away so clothing does not touch the sink/counter or become wet from splashing water.

- Wet hands and forearms with running water. Keep the hands lower than the elbows (see Fig. 9.4A). This prevents water and germs from running down the arms and onto garments.
- Apply soap.
- Rub hands together and over the forearms briskly (see Fig. 9.4B). Include areas between the fingers and under the nails. Do this for at least 20 seconds. This is about the time it takes to sing or hum the "Happy Birthday" song from beginning to end twice.
- Rinse the area thoroughly to remove germs and dirt suspended in the lather (see Fig. 9.4C).
- Dry the area thoroughly with a clean paper towel (see Fig. 9.4D). Drying is essential because germs are less likely to spread from dry skin.
- Use a paper towel to turn off the water faucet (see Fig. 9.4E). If possible, use the same towel to touch surfaces between the sink and the massage room, including the massage room doorknob.
- Discard the paper towel.

Liquid soap is preferred over bar soap because the latter can become contaminated by direct contact with unclean surfaces. Paper towels are preferred over electric air dryers because paper towels dry hands more efficiently, remove bacteria more effectively, and cause less washroom contamination (Huang et al., 2012). Frequent handwashing may cause skin to become dry and chapped, which provides an opening for pathogens, so regular use of hand moisturizer is also recommended.

Handwashing is required for removing massage lubricants and other massage-type products from the practitioner's hands after treating clients. Massage lubricants create a barrier over the skin, making alcohol-based hand rubs less effective (CDC, 2021b). If hands are not covered with massage products or visibly soiled, hand hygiene with alcohol-based hand rubs can be used before and after direct contact with a client, before gloving or after removing gloves, and after touching objects in the client's vicinity.

Alcohol-Based Hand Rubs Procedure

Use the following procedure when using hand rub solutions, which should contain at least 60% alcohol.

- Dispense the recommended amount of product into the palm of one hand.
- Rub hands together and continue rubbing onto forearms, making sure all surfaces are covered with the product.
- Continue rubbing until the skin is dry (rinsing not required). Do not wipe wet products off your hands.

Personal Protective Equipment

Personal protective equipment (PPE) items are worn (usually gloves, masks, and gowns) to create a barrier, to reduce or prevent transmission of pathogens when someone requires a contact precaution, or as source control to prevent disease transmission through respiratory secretions, which are spread when speaking, coughing, or sneezing. Diseases

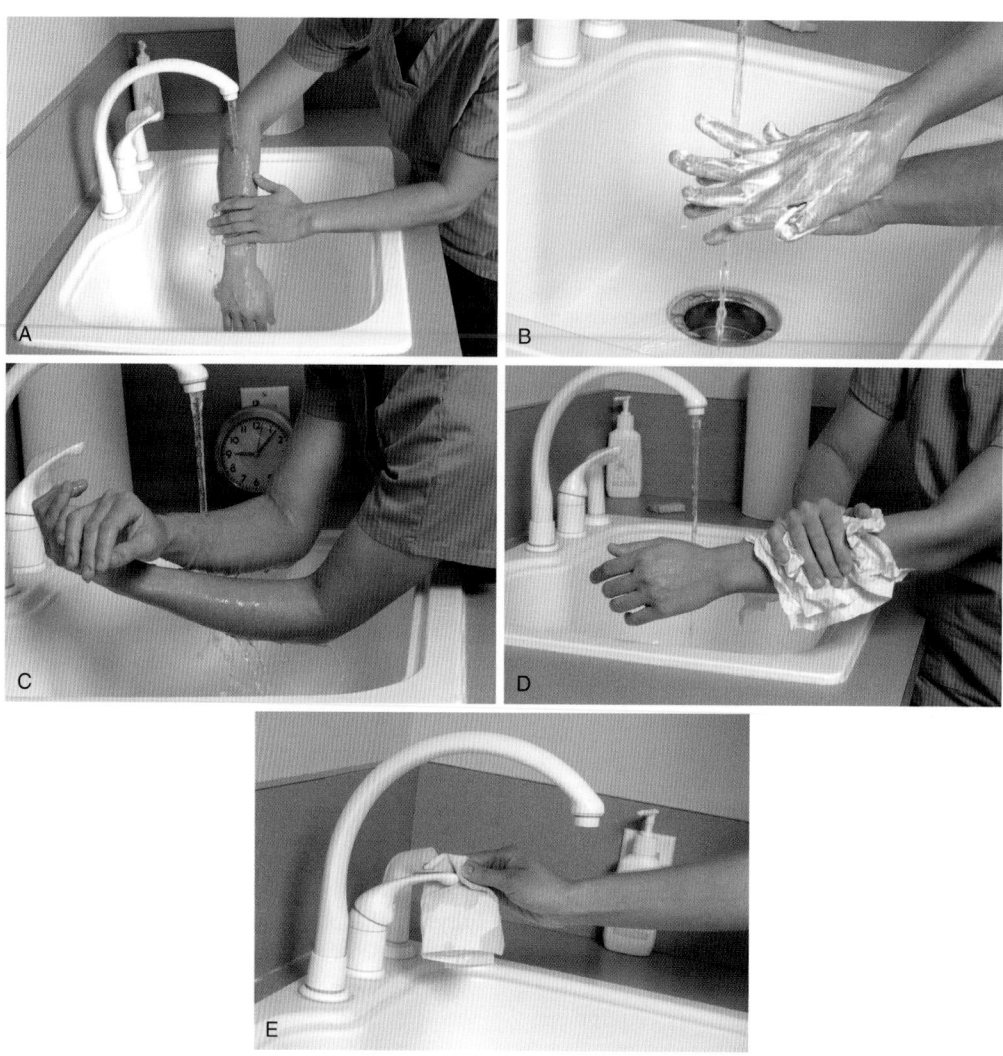

FIG. 9.4 Handwashing. (A) Wet hands and forearms. (B) Generate lather. (C) Rinse thoroughly. (D) Dry with a clean paper towel. (E) Turn off valve with same paper towel.

such as COVID-19 are spread through respiratory secretions by infected individuals who are asymptomatic.

PPE is also used when the practitioner has nonintact skin on the hands and when touching mucous membranes inside the mouth, such as while assessing or treating temporomandibular disorders (opportunistic pathogens, such as herpes simplex virus and candida are found in the mouth and can be transmitted to the hands). If the practitioner is unsure of the presence of cuts on their hands, the area should be wiped with alcohol. If it stings, the skin is open. In this case, gloves or similar PPE should be worn. Avoid long nails and artificial nails, and hand/wrist jewelry, as these increase the risk of glove tears and promote the colonization of healthcare-associated infections (Cimon & Featherstone, 2017; Moolenaar et al., 2000).

Nitrile gloves are currently the most popular glove of choice. Most facilities have eliminated or limited latex products because of latex allergy concerns. Also, nitrile gloves can be used with oil- or water-based massage products. If using latex gloves, be sure the client does not have a latex allergy. Massage products must be water-based because oil and oil-based products break down latex, making the gloves sticky, misshapen, and ineffective as a protective barrier.

Disposable gloves should be available in all treatment areas and placed near the massage table to prevent putting them on too early. Once gloves are on (called *donning*), limit opportunities for "touch contamination," such as those discussed in the prior section. Gloves should fit the user's hands comfortably; not too loose or too tight, as gloves used while performing massage will likely be worn for an hour or longer. Wearing gloves is not a substitute for hand hygiene.

When removing gloves (called *doffing*), use a method that avoids contamination from the glove surface (Fig 9.5). A recommended method follows (CDC, 2021a).
- With both hands gloved, pinch or grasp and hold the outside of one glove; do not touch bare skin.
- Peel the glove downward from your wrist to your fingertips, turning the glove inside out. Tilt your hand away from your body (see Fig 9.5A).
- When removed, hold the inside-out glove in your gloved hand.
- With your ungloved hand, slide your fingers under the wrist of the remaining glove; do not touch the outside surface of the glove (Fig. 9.5B).

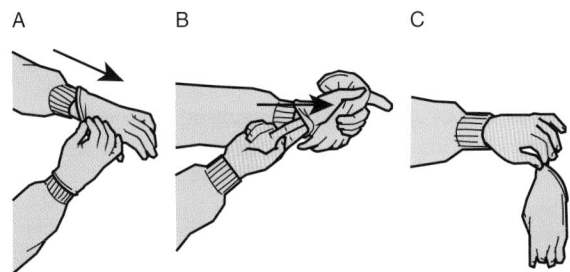

FIG. 9.5 Glove removal. Pinch the outside of one glove and peel it downward from wrist to fingertips, turning it inside out (A). Slide the fingers of the ungloved hand under the wrist of the remaining glove and peel it off (B). Discard the gloves (C). (From Stromberg, H. [2021]. *deWit's medical-surgical nursing* [4th ed.]. St. Louis: Saunders.)

- Peel off the second glove downward from your wrist to your fingertips, turning it inside out while pulling it away from your body; leave the first glove inside the second glove.
- Discard the gloves in the nearest appropriate receptacle (see Fig. 9.5C).

Perform hand hygiene immediately after glove removal and before touching any objects or surfaces or providing care to the same or another client.

Respiratory Hygiene and Cough Etiquette

Respiratory hygiene and cough etiquette help to reduce or prevent transmission of pathogens spread by droplet or airborne transmission. Respiratory hygiene and cough etiquette include the following:

- Cover the mouth and nose with a tissue when coughing or sneezing.
- Promptly dispose of used tissues.
- If you do not have tissues, cover your nose and mouth with your arm, sleeve, or elbow (not your hands) when coughing or sneezing.
- Wash hands after contact with respiratory secretions.

All facilities should provide tissues and no-touch receptacles for their disposal. Other measures may include using a mask, depending on the policies of the facility where services are provided.

DISINFECTING PROCEDURES FOR SURFACES, OBJECTS, AND LAUNDRY

Contaminated surfaces, reusable objects, or laundry must be disinfected before they are reused. Contamination occurs when these items come into contact with blood, blood-tinged saliva, infected skin, or respiratory fluids. Occupational exposure to breast milk does not pose any infection risk to the practitioner unless it is ingested. Uncontaminated equipment and supplies do not require special disinfecting procedures, only cleaning procedures. Cleaning is required before disinfecting if particles are on the surfaces, as they interfere with the disinfection process.

Hard Surfaces

Use a disinfectant registered with the Environmental Protection Agency (EPA). An EPA registration number will be

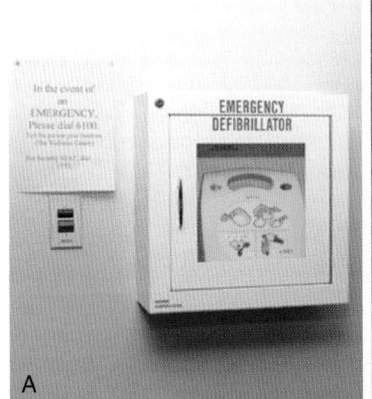
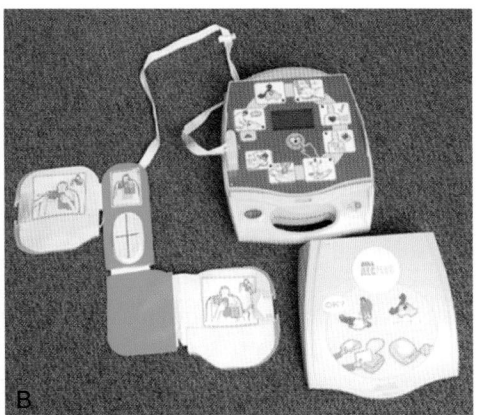
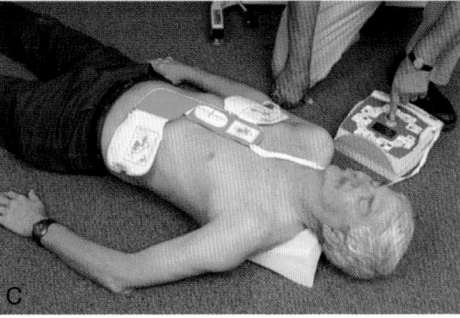

FIG. 9.6 (A) Wall-mounted automated external defibrillator (AED) unit. (B) AED training unit. (C) Demonstration of the application of an AED unit. (From Gould, B., & Dyer, R. [2011]. *Pathophysiology for the health professions* [4th ed.]. Philadelphia: Saunders.)

listed on the product label. Follow the instructions on the label to ensure safe and effective use of the product. Many products recommend ensuring the area is well-ventilated, wearing gloves during the disinfection process, and keeping the surface wet for a period of time (CDC, 2021c).

Diluted household bleach solution may also be used. Read the label to see if the bleach is intended for disinfection. Some bleach, such as those formulated for safe use on colored clothing or for whitening, may not be suitable for disinfection. Never mix bleach with ammonia or any other cleaner. To make a bleach solution, mix:

- 5 tablespoons (1/3 cup) of bleach per gallon of water, or
- 4 teaspoons of bleach per quart of water.

Bleach solutions will be effective for disinfection for up to 24 hours. Alcohol solutions or alcohol-based wipes of at least 70% alcohol can also be used.

- Work from "clean to dirty" to reduce the spread of infectious material; clean the areas farthest from the contaminated area, working toward the most contaminated area.
- Allow to air dry.
- Remove and discard gloves and paper towels in the nearest appropriate receptacle.
- Perform hand hygiene before touching any surfaces.
- Wear eye protection while diluting to protect your eyes in case the solution splashes.

Shared Electronic Equipment

For electronic equipment, such as tablets, touch screens, keyboards, and mice, consider using a wipeable cover on these items. For cleaning and disinfecting, follow the manufacturer's instructions. If no guidance is provided, use alcohol-based wipes or sprays containing at least 70% alcohol. Allow to air dry.

Soft Surfaces

For soft surfaces, such as carpeted floors, rugs, and drapes, use the following protocol. You can also disinfect soft surfaces with an EPA-registered disinfectant approved for porous surfaces.

- Clean the surface using soap and water, or cleaner appropriate for use on these surfaces.
- Launder items (if possible) according to the manufacturer's instructions. Use the warmest water setting and dry items completely.

Removing Vomit From Surfaces Before Disinfection

Use the following procedure when removing vomit from surfaces.

- Ask individuals within a 25-foot radius of the vomit to leave the contaminated area and wash their hands. Block entry into the contaminated area while cleaning and disinfecting.
- While wearing PPE, such as disposable gloves, place paper towels over the vomit, then carefully remove the towels and their contents. If you expect the vomit may splash, wear a disposable mask, and a cover gown or apron.
  - Do not vacuum the material.

- Work from clean to dirty; clean the areas farthest from the contaminated areas, working toward the most contaminated area.
- For carpet or upholstery, use absorbent materials, such as kitty litter or baking soda to absorb liquid before removing it with paper towels.
- Dispose of the soiled paper towels and used PPE in plastic garbage or biohazard bag.
- Place contaminated laundry in a separate plastic bag for transport to laundry or discard.
- Wash the surfaces in the contaminated area with soapy water. Rinse thoroughly with clean water, and wipe dry with paper towels. Steam cleaning is recommended for carpet and upholstery.
- Next, disinfect contaminated surfaces.
- Wash and dry your hands.

Reusable Objects

Use the following procedure when disinfecting contaminated reusable objects, such as massage tools.

- Immerse objects in one of the following for the specified length of time:
  - 70% isopropyl alcohol for 5 minutes.
  - 3% hydrogen peroxide for 30 minutes.
  - 1:10 solution of household bleach and water for 5 minutes.
- Allow the objects to air dry.

Some practitioners enclose their massage tools in plastic wrap before use and discard the used wrap afterward. Perform hand hygiene after removing and discarding the used plastic wrap.

Laundry

Use the following procedure to disinfect contaminated laundry, such as sheets, face rest covers, bolster covers, towels, blankets, and clothing (CDC, 2021b).

- While wearing gloves, roll laundry so the used surface is inside. Transport the laundry to the washroom and place it in the washing machine tub, avoiding contact between the laundry and other surfaces, such as your uniform. Do not shake out used laundry before washing.
  - If unable to wash contaminated laundry immediately or if the washing machine tub is unavailable, place contaminated laundry in a clothes basket, hamper, or disposable plastic bag labeled "Contaminated Laundry Only." Wash and dry these items as soon as possible. Contaminated items can be washed with noncontaminated items (CDC, 2021b).
- Remove and discard gloves and wash your hands.
- Add the amount of detergent and bleach listed in the washing machine owner's manual. The bleach amount ranges from {1/2} cup to 1{1/4} cup. Use the bleach dispenser if the machine has one, and do not exceed the maximum capacity of the bleach dispenser.
- Select the "sanitize" cycle on the washing machine, if available. Otherwise, select the warmest water setting and the longest wash setting. The CDC (2015) recom-

mends wash water should be at least 160°F (71°C) and washed for a minimum of 25 minutes.

- Select the "sanitize" cycle on the dryer, if available. Otherwise, select the highest temperature setting and dry items completely. The CDC recommends air should be approximately 170°F (76°C).
- Use the protocol under "Hard Surfaces" to clean and disinfect clothes baskets or hampers.

Consider having several labeled baskets or hampers for different types of laundry, such as clean, soiled, and contaminated. As an alternative, use different colors to denote which basket contains clean, soiled, or contaminated laundry.

I happen to feel that the degree of a person's intelligence is directly reflected by the number of conflicting attitudes she can bring to bear on the same topic.

~ Lisa Alter

EMERGENCY PREPAREDNESS

Emergency preparedness is the process of providing first and immediate responses during health or medical emergencies to minimize loss of life. Agencies such as the American Red Cross and the American Heart Association (AHA) offer training and certification programs in basic life support or first aid measures. These courses include how to administer cardiopulmonary resuscitation (CPR) and how to use an automated external defibrillator (AED) in a safe, timely, and effective manner. Even if your state or municipality does not require you to be current in CPR/AED certification, it is a good idea for you to do just in case you have a client with a medical emergency. Next are steps to take during emergencies.

- **Step 1: Ensure Scene Safety**. When you encounter an incident and it appears someone needs help, check the scene for any hazards. A *hazard* is anything that can cause harm. You cannot provide help if you become injured. If you arrive at the scene of a road traffic collision, look for smoke, fire, fallen power lines, or movement of vehicles. Stay out of harm's way and warn others.
- **Step 2: Check for Responsiveness**. Check for responsiveness to determine if the person needs help or if they are simply resting. If they are unresponsive, not breathing, or only gasping, get help by calling 911.
- **Step 3: Call 911**. If others are nearby, tell someone to call 911. Because many are likely to be in a state of panic, identify the person and give clear instructions such as "Call 911 now" instead of "Call for help." Tell them to hurry—time is critical.

If you are alone with an adult who has signs of cardiac arrest, call 911 and get an AED, if one is available (see Fig. 9.6). If the person is an infant or a child 1 to 8 years of age, do not leave them until you have provided first aid measures. For example, if a child is unresponsive, check the brachial pulse on the upper arm closest to you for 5 to 10 seconds. If there is no pulse, provide 1 to 2 minutes of CPR and then call 911.

When calling 911, give the following information:

- What the emergency is or what is happening now.
- Precise location of the emergency. When indicating the location of the person(s) or emergency, street addresses are preferred over names of office buildings.
- Condition of the person(s) if known, starting with the most serious and ending with the least.
- Pertinent medical history, if known.
- The age of the person(s), if possible. Some areas have special pediatric units, and they may be called out if the dispatcher knows the person is a child. If there is more than one person, state how many people are injured/ill.

Do not end the call unless instructed to do so by the dispatcher. You may be asked to meet the rescuers and direct them to the scene. Some dispatchers give first aid instructions over the phone, such as how to perform CPR or how to use an AED. Early use of an AED or other defibrillation device improves outcomes related to heart attacks. Emergency medical units average 7 minutes from the time of a 911 call to arrival on scene, but this time increases in rural areas.

It is advisable for the massage practitioner to have a first-aid kit available for minor emergencies. You can purchase a preassembled kit or assemble your own. A simple kit might include adhesive bandages and antiseptic solution, such as isopropyl alcohol.

In the next sections, we will look at first aid measures for clients who are choking, who may be in insulin shock related to hypoglycemia, who are experiencing a stroke or heart attack, or who are having a seizure. After the emergency has ended and your client has received proper medical care, write an incident report of the event. Look on Evolve for this and other important forms (see the Resources section in Chapter 10).

Choking

Choking occurs when the trachea is blocked, and the affected person cannot breathe. Choking may occur when a person is talking while eating or inhaling while swallowing. Choking is the fourth-leading cause of unintentional injury death. Of the 5,051 people who died from choking in 2015, 2,848 were older than 74 (National Safety Council [NSC], 2017). In massage environments, choking is more likely when the client has a mint or piece of gum in the mouth while lying supine and talking.

First, confirm the person is choking. A person who is coughing and can speak is not choking, so encourage the person to cough. The person is likely choking if they cannot cough or speak, has difficulty breathing or cannot breathe, and has a bluish tint of the lips and nails (Mayo Clinic, 2017). If the person is choking, use the Heimlich maneuver, or abdominal thrusts, to help open a suddenly obstructed trachea.

First Aid Measures for Choking

Follow these measures when someone is choking:

1. Send someone to call 911.
2. Help the victim stand and put your chest against their back.

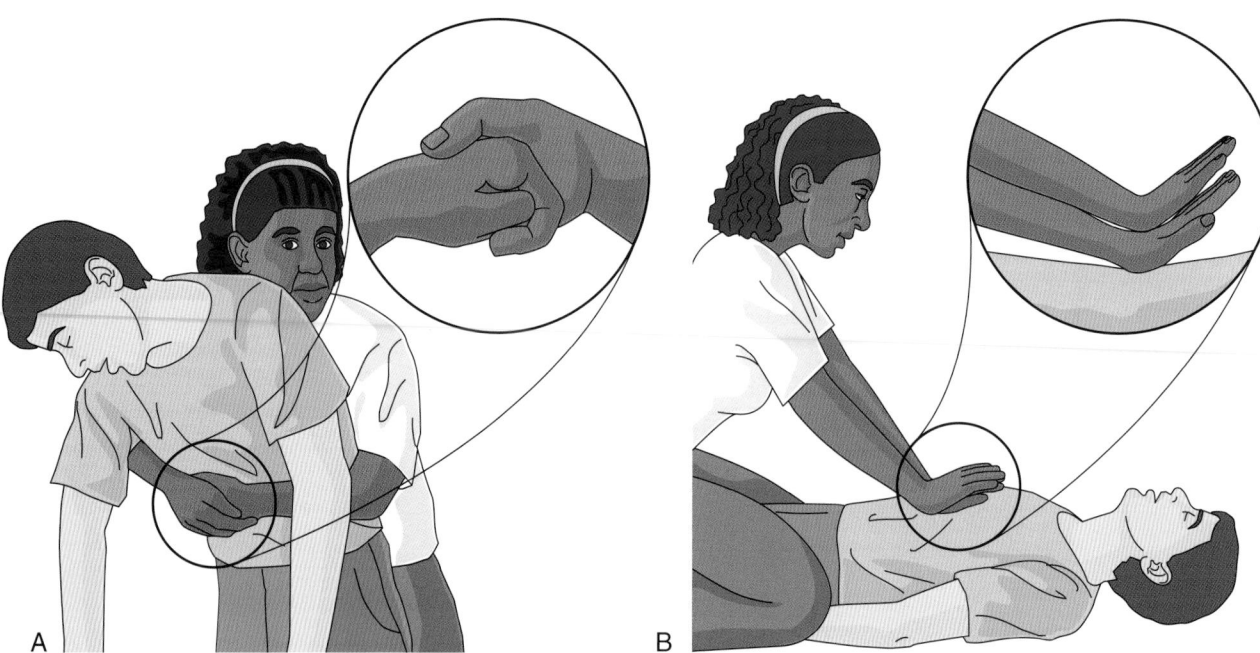

A

With the conscious victim standing or sitting, place your fist between the victim's lower rib cage and navel. Wrap the palm of your hand around your fist. A quick inward, upward thrust expels the air remaining in the victim's lungs, and with it the foreign body. If the first thrust is unsuccessful, repeat several thrusts in rapid succession until the foreign body is expelled or until the victim loses consciousness.

B

With the unconscious victim lying supine, straddle the victim's thighs. Place one hand on top of the other as shown, with the heel of the bottom hand just above the victim's navel. Quickly thrust inward and upward, toward the victim's head.

FIG. 9.7 Heimlich maneuver performed while choking person is standing or sitting (A) or is lying supine (B).

3. Wrap your arms around the victim's waist. Make a fist with your dominant hand and place it thumb-side down against the victim's upper abdomen, above the navel and below the xiphoid process. Cover your fist with your other hand (A). **NOTE**: If you cannot reach around the victim or if the victim is pregnant, compress the sternum, or breastbone, between the victim's breasts (B) (Fig. 9.7).

4. Apply five quick abdominal thrusts inward and slightly upward with your fist, like you are trying to lift the victim off the ground. These thrusts should cause air in the lungs to be expelled and dislodge the object. **NOTE**: Do not squeeze the rib cage, because you could break a bone; confine the force of the thrusts to your hands.

5. Repeat the thrusts until the object dislodges or the victim becomes unresponsive.

NOTE: If the victim is or becomes unresponsive, check the carotid pulse on the side of the neck closest to you for 5 to 10 seconds. If no pulse, lower them to the ground, expose the chest, and begin chest compressions. Continue chest compressions until EMTs arrive.

Hypoglycemia

Hypoglycemia is abnormally low blood glucose levels, usually below 70 mg/dL. Hypoglycemia, also called an insulin reaction, is a complication of diabetes mellitus, especially Type 1. It occurs most frequently with insulin therapy, and is associated with injecting too much prescribed insulin, late or skipped meals, or overexertion in physical activity. Although hypoglycemia can occur in Type 2, it is mild and infrequent among this population (diabetes mellitus is discussed in Chapter 24). Symptoms of hypoglycemia include:

- Confusion
- Disorientation
- Irritability
- Lack of muscular coordination
- Slurred speech (resembles drunkenness)
- Inability to respond to verbal commands
- Visual disturbances
- Tremors
- Cold clammy skin

If left untreated, hypoglycemia can develop into insulin shock (also called insulin reaction), which can lead to coma and death.

First Aid Measures for Hypoglycemia

Glucose is the preferred treatment for conscious individuals experiencing symptoms of hypoglycemia. Follow the 15-15 rule. Consume glucose or sugar equal to 15 g of carbohydrates (carbs). Rest for 15 minutes. If symptoms have not abated, consume 15 more g of carbs. Once symptoms abate, consume a meal or snack (such as crackers with cheese or peanut butter) to prevent recurrence of hypoglycemia. Use a blood glucose meter to check levels, if possible. This procedure does not harm the hyperglycemic person but could potentially save the life of a hypoglycemic person.

Examples of foods equal to 15 g of carbs are:
- 4 ounces of fruit juice.
- 5 to 6 ounces (about 1/2 can) of regular soda (not diet soda).
- 7 to 8 gummy or regular Life Savers.
- 1 tablespoon of honey, sugar, or jelly.

To prevent aspiration, fluids should not be forced. The unconscious/unresponsive person needs immediate medical attention. Call 911 (American Diabetes Association [ADA], 2019; Joslin Diabetes Center [JDC], 2019).

Stroke

A **stroke** is a sudden disruption in cerebral blood flow from an occluded or ruptured blood vessel leading to irreversible brain damage or, in some cases, death. Early signs include facial drooping or numbness, arm weakness or numbness, instability, speech difficulties, and visual disturbances. Early recognition of these signs is vital to a person receiving immediate medical attention. The acute care principle is "time is brain." To remember the early signs of a stroke and what to do, use an acronym such as F-A-S-T-E-R.
- **F**ACE. Ask the person to smile. Does one side of the face droop and the smile uneven?
- **A**RM. Ask the person to raise both arms. Does one arm drift downward or is immobile?
- **S**TABILITY. Does the person have trouble standing upright or walking?
- **T**ALKING. Ask the person to repeat a simple phrase, such as "The sky is blue." Is the speech slurred or are they difficult to understand?
- **E**YES. Does the person have difficulty seeing out of one eye or one side of the room? Do they have double vision?
- **R**EACT. If you observe any signs of stroke mentioned above, call 911 immediately. Tell them the time when any signs first appeared. This information helps EMTs determine the best treatment.

Other acronyms for stroke signs include F-A-S-T for face, arm, speech, and time and B-E-F-A-S-T for balance, eyes, face, arm, speech, and time.

First Aid Measures for Stroke

The "R" in the acronym F-A-S-T-E-R stands for REACT and is the first aid measure—call 911.

Heart Attack and Cardiac Arrest

A **heart attack**, or **myocardial infarction** (MI), occurs when blood flow to the heart is suddenly disrupted from a blocked or occluded vessel. Every year, approximately 735,000 Americans have a heart attack. Of these, 525,000 are a first-ever heart attack, and 210,000 occur in people who have had a heart attack previously. Sudden death occurs in approximately 25% of cases, usually from arrhythmias. Those who do survive (75%) have an increased risk for a second MI, cardiogenic shock (failure of the cardiovascular system to deliver enough oxygen), stroke, thromboembolism

(vessel occlusion or blockage from a blood clot), rupture of the infarcted area, or aneurysm.

MIs can lead to **cardiac arrest**, sudden cessation of the heartbeat, affecting blood flow to the brain and other vital organs. Other conditions that can disrupt heart rhythm and cause cardiac arrest are coronary heart disease, congestive heart failure, cardiomyopathy, and ventricular fibrillation (v-fib), a type of arrhythmia. Using certain recreational drugs can cause sudden cardiac arrest, even in otherwise healthy people. Cardiac arrest can cause death if not treated within minutes. Some signs and symptoms of heart attack are (American Heart Association [AHA], 2016):
- Chest pain lasting more than a few minutes. This pain may be described as crushing, burning, viselike, heaviness, or fullness.
- Discomfort in other areas of the upper body, such as one or both arms, shoulder, neck, jaw, or upper abdomen.
- Shortness of breath with or without chest pain.
- Other signs are profuse sweating, nausea, and dizziness or lightheadedness.

First Aid Measures for Heart Attack/Cardiac Arrest

If the person complains of chest pain lasting more than a few minutes, especially with other signs and symptoms listed here, call 911.

If the person becomes unconscious and/or nonresponsive, they may be in cardiac arrest. The person can die unless the normal heart rhythm returns, so take immediate action (AHA, 2017). The acute care principle is time is muscle—heart muscle, in this case.
- If you are *alone*, call 911 and get an AED yourself, if one is available. Use as directed.
- If you are *not alone*, yell for help and tell someone nearby to call 911. Tell the person or another bystander to bring you an AED if there is one on hand. Tell them to hurry as time is of the essence. Use as directed.

Check to see if the person is breathing. If the person is not breathing or only gasping, begin chest compressions until an AED arrives or while waiting for EMS. Ideally, lay the person on a firm surface, such as the floor or the ground. CPR is applied best skin to skin.

1. Place the heel of one hand on the center of the person's chest. Place the other hand on top of the first hand with fingers interlaced.
2. Push down into the chest hard and fast. Push down at least 2 inches at a rate of 100 to 120 pushes a minute. Allow the chest to return to a normal position after each push. Be sure elbows are locked and your shoulders are directly over your hands. Do not break contact between compressions.
3. Continue chest compressions until the person starts to breathe or move, until an AED arrives, or until someone with more advanced training takes over, such as an EMS team member.

Know how to differentiate between a hypoglycemic event, a panic attack, and a heart attack. Hypoglycemia will resolve quickly after ingesting a sugar source. The intensity of a panic attack will promptly decrease once the person is distracted. Signs and symptoms of a heart attack will increase with measures used to resolve hypoglycemia or a panic attack. If the client is having a heart attack, call 911.

Seizures

Seizures are episodes of uncontrolled and excessive electrical activity in the brain, resulting in a sudden change of behavior and level of consciousness. The event is described as a *lightning storm in the brain*. A seizure may be subtle and consist of abnormal sensations, or it may produce overt involuntary repetitive movements and loss of consciousness. Epilepsy is a term used to describe recurrent seizures. The two main types of seizures are focal or partial and generalized.

- **Focal (Partial) Seizures**. Seizure activity is limited to a single area of the brain. These represent 60% of cases. Focal seizures fall into two categories.
  - **Focal Seizures Without Loss of Consciousness**. These types of seizures do not cause a loss of consciousness. They may change the way things look (including flashing lights), feel, smell, taste, or sound. They may also result in involuntary movements or abnormal sensations such as dizziness or electricity.
  - **Focal Seizures With Impaired Awareness**. These types of seizures involve a change or loss of consciousness or awareness. The person may have a blank stare or perform repetitive movements, such as hand rubbing, smacking or chewing, or start walking in circles.
- **Generalized Seizures**. These involve a more diffuse area of the brain and are seen in approximately 30% of cases. Two types of generalized seizures are absence and tonic-clonic.
  - **Absence Seizure (Petit Mal)**. These involve a brief loss of awareness and often some transient facial movements (see "Signs and Symptoms") lasting for up to 10 seconds. Then the previous activity is resumed, and the person has no memory of what occurred during the seizure.
  - **Tonic-Clonic Seizure (Grand Mal)**. These produce an intermittent contract-and-relax pattern in muscles and are associated with a loss of consciousness. During the *tonic phase*, general tone increases, and muscular contraction begins. If the person is standing, the seizure will often cause them to fall to the ground. A cry may be heard as the thoracic and abdominal muscles contract, forcing air out of the lungs. This phase lasts approximately 10 seconds (Fig. 9.8). The *clonic phase* is the classic manifestation of alternating contraction and relaxation of muscles. The person may have increased salivation (foaming of the mouth); bowel and bladder incontinence may occur. These contractions gradually subside in several minutes; the person is then confused, weak, and drowsy and has no memory of the event. The postseizure period is called the *postictal state* and can last from several minutes to several hours.

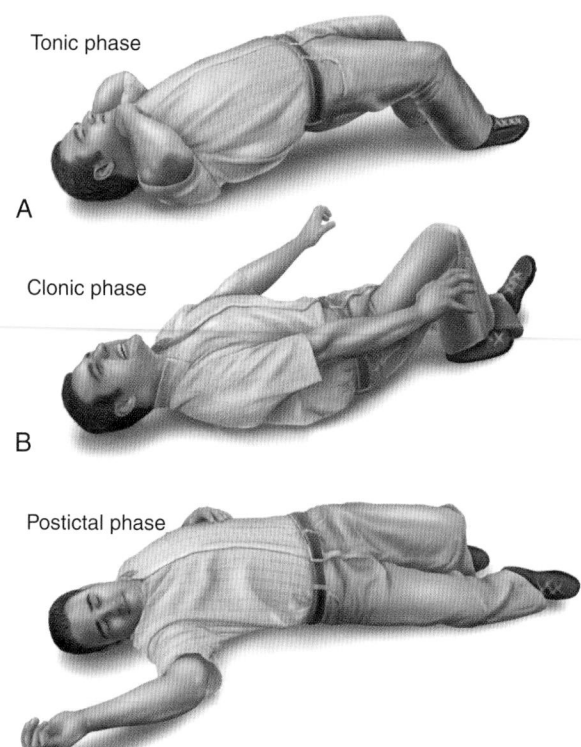

Tonic phase

A

Clonic phase

B

Postictal phase

C

FIG. 9.8 Tonic-clonic seizure. (A) The tonic phase is characterized by increased tone and muscular contraction lasting approximately 10 seconds. (B) The clonic phase is the classic presentation of alternating contraction and relaxation of muscles, which gradually subside in several minutes. (C) The postictal phase is the recovery phase after the seizure. (From Black, J. [2009]. *Medical-surgical nursing: Clinical management for positive outcomes* [8th ed.]. St. Louis: Saunders.)

First Aid Measures for Seizures

If the client appears to be having a seizure, follow these measures. Every situation will be different.

1. Stay calm. If possible, time the length of the shaking phase of the seizure.
2. Gently place the person on the floor (if possible).
3. Place a cushion or soft jacket under the person's head to keep it inclined; this prevents the head from banging the floor during the shaking phase. Roll the person onto their side. This will allow saliva to fall out of the mouth instead of blocking the airway, causing the person to choke.
4. Remain with the person until the seizure has ended.

   After the seizure has ended, place them in the recovery position if possible (Fig. 9.9). If you think the person may have a spinal injury, do not move them (Epilepsy Society, 2018; National Health Service [NHS], 2018).

- With the person lying on their back, kneel on the floor at their side.
- Extend the arm nearest you at a right angle to their body with their palm facing up.
- Take their other arm and fold it so the back of their hand rests on the cheek closest to you and hold it in place (see Fig. 9.9A).

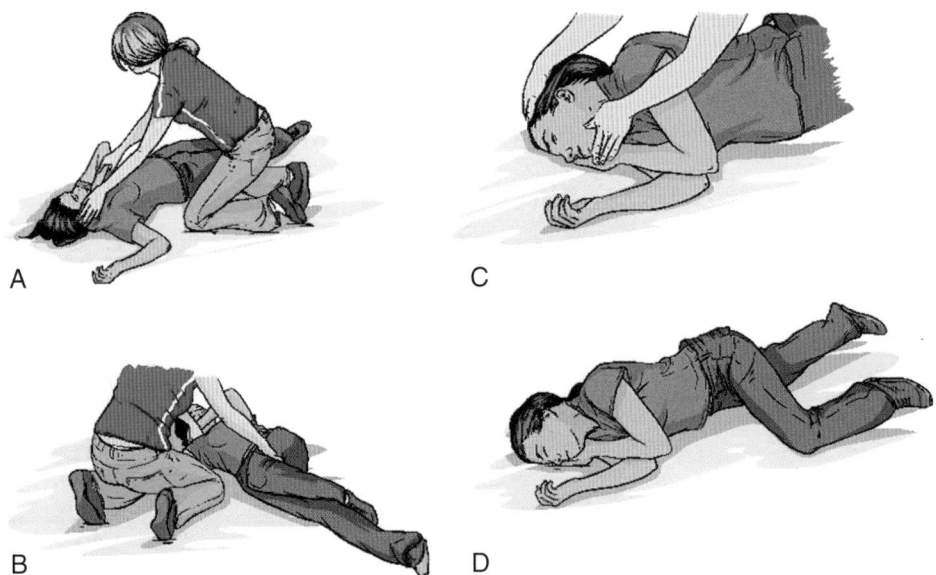

FIG. 9.9 The recovery position. (A) Extend the arm nearest you and take their other arm and fold it so the back of their hand rests on the cheek closest to you, and hold it in place. (B) Bend the knee and carefully roll the person onto their side. (C) Open their airway by gently tilting their head back and lifting their chin. (D) Person in the recovery position.

- Use your free hand to bend the person's knee farthest from you to a right angle.
- Carefully roll the person onto their side by pulling on the bent knee. If the person is pregnant, roll them onto the left side (see Fig. 9.9B).
- Their bent arm should be supporting the head, and their extended arm will stop you from rolling them too far.
- Be sure their bent leg is at a right angle.
- Open their airway by gently tilting their head back and lifting their chin, and check that nothing is blocking their airway (see Fig. 9.9C).

Help the person back to normal awareness by asking a few simple questions, such as what is their name and the location. Use a calm and reassuring voice. The postseizure period is called the postictal period and can last from several minutes to several hours.

Ensure the client is safe. If they have bitten their tongue or cheek, those areas may be sore. If the person experienced incontinence, be sensitive and helpful and provide aid if needed. The person may feel tired, confused, and have no memory of the event. They may also complain of a headache or general muscle soreness.

Call 911 in the following cases:
- It is the person's first seizure or if you do not know.

- If the seizure lasts more than 5 minutes or immediately repeats, or if the person cannot be awakened after the seizure.
- If the person is injured or vomits during the seizure.
- If the person has a medical condition such as diabetes, heart disease, congestive heart failure, or is pregnant.
- Inform EMTs how long the seizure has lasted, and symptoms exhibited.
  Things to avoid during or after a seizure:
- Do not restrain the person; this may provoke an aggressive response.
- Do not put anything in the person's mouth. You may get bitten.
- Do not give the person water, food, or medicine until the seizure is over and they are alert.

E-RESOURCES

http://evolve.elsevier.com/Salvo/MassageTherapy
- Chapter challenge
- Flash cards
- Technique videos
- Additional information

DAVID LAUTERSTEIN

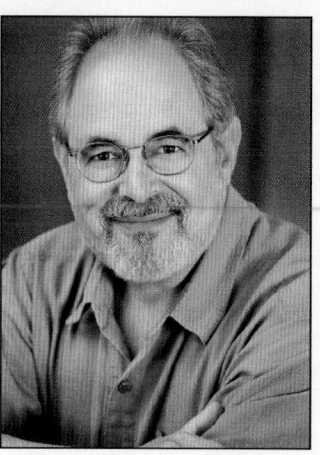

"Wow, that's really deep," people sometimes say about a philosophical conversation or a bit of poetry. But what does that mean, really? It pushes relentlessly on your brain until you agree? That it is painful to think about? Of course not. Some of the deepest ideas are the most subtle as well—just a slight adjustment in perspective changes everything. David Lauterstein sees deep massage the same way. The deepest massage, not always the most aggressive massage, can sometimes involve very gentle touch, but the effects are far more than skin deep.

Lauterstein was born in Chicago in 1947 into a household steeped in music. He began studying guitar at age 13 and went on to study Indian music and music composition at the University of Illinois. In 1964, he attended a Bob Dylan concert in which Dylan broke a guitar string and asked, "Anyone out there have a string or a guitar?" The 16-year-old Lauterstein carried his guitar everywhere, so he walked up to the stage and handed it to Dylan. The artist complimented the guitar and played the rest of the concert with it.

It was while pursuing graduate studies in composition in Munich, Germany, in 1972 Lauterstein started to become frustrated with the educational system for its exclusive focus on the education of the mind. Awareness of the body, emotions, and any other nonmental aspect of the human experience was left to develop on its own. For answers, Lauterstein turned to Gestalt psychotherapy and yoga. A series of Rolfing sessions further convinced him the body itself should be respected as a source of knowledge and wisdom.

Lauterstein studied massage at the Bodymind Center in Chicago, learning from James Hackett and Bob King, and graduating in 1979. He became certified in structural bodywork in 1982.

That same year, Lauterstein became an instructor of anatomy and deep tissue massage at the Chicago School of Massage Therapy. He also studied craniosacral therapy, an extremely subtle form of bodywork using no more pressure than the weight of a nickel resting on the skin. He was struck by how profoundly clients were affected by this very gentle touch, compared with the stiffening and guarding that can often occur in response to the more aggressive bodywork often associated with the term deep tissue massage. In response, Lauterstein changed the name for what he taught from deep tissue to deep massage, to help people understand the true depth of a massage is not measured by how far you can wedge your thumb under someone's scapula. His later study of zero balancing (another very subtle form of bodywork) further developed the ideas behind deep massage.

In 1989, Lauterstein and his fellow teacher John Conway co-founded the aptly named Lauterstein-Conway Massage School in Austin, Texas. Known for its innovative curriculum, the school is still in operation today.

Lauterstein has published two books. His latest book, *The Deep Massage Book: How to Combine Structure and Energy in Bodywork,* explains the art and science of deep massage he has been teaching for over 30 years. He has also recorded an album of massage music. *Roots and Branches,* published in 2009, was recorded as Lauterstein performed live music during massage sessions in the studio itself.

Lauterstein teaches deep massage and zero balancing at his own school and travels to teach throughout the United States and United Kingdom. He has been given several prestigious awards, including being named the Jerome Perlinski Teacher of the Year by the American Massage Therapy Association in 2012 and Educator of the Year by the Alliance for Massage Therapy Education in 2013. He was inducted into the Massage Therapy Hall of Fame in 2010.

Are you a deep thinker? You can absolutely put this to work for you as a massage practitioner. David Lauterstein proves it can be done.

REFERENCES

American Diabetes Association (ADA). (2019). *Standards of medical care in diabetes—2019 abridged for primary care providers*. Retrieved from https://clinical.diabetesjournals.org/content/37/1/11.

American Heart Association (AHA). (2016). *Warning signs of a heart attack*. Retrieved from https://www.heart.org/en/health-topics/heart-attack/warning-signs-of-a-heart-attack.

American Heart Association (AHA). (2017). *Emergency treatment of cardiac arrest*. Retrieved from https://www.heart.org/en/health-topics/cardiac-arrest/emergency-treatment-of-cardiac-arrest.

Centers for Disease Control and Prevention (CDC). (2015). *Parameters of the laundry process*. Retrieved from https://www.cdc.gov/infectioncontrol/guidelines/environmental/background/laundry.html.

Centers for Disease Control and Prevention (CDC). (2016). *Recommended vaccines for healthcare workers*. Retrieved from https://www.cdc.gov/vaccines/adults/rec-vac/hcw.html.

Centers for Disease Control and Prevention (CDC). (2018). *Standard precautions*. Retrieved from https://www.cdc.gov/oral-health/infectioncontrol/summary-infection-prevention-practices/standard-precautions.html.

Centers for Disease Control and Prevention (CDC). (2021a). *Healthcare providers: Glove use*. Retrieved from https://www.cdc.gov/handhygiene/providers/index.html.

Centers for Disease Control and Prevention (CDC). (2021b). *Cleaning and disinfecting your facility*. Retrieved from https://www.cdc.gov/coronavirus/2019-ncov/community/disinfecting-building-facility.html.

Centers for Disease Control and Prevention (CDC). (2021c). *COVID-19: Cleaning and disinfecting your home*. Retrieved from https://www.cdc.gov/coronavirus/2019-ncov/prevent-getting-sick/disinfecting-your-home.html.

Cimon, K., & Featherstone, R. (2017). *Jewellery and nail polish worn by healthcare workers and the risk of infection transmission: A review of clinical evidence and guidelines.* Canadian Agency for Drugs and Technologies in Health. Retrieved from https://www.ncbi.nlm.nih.gov/pubmed/29533568.

Epilepsy Society. (2018). *Step-by-step recovery position*. Retrieved from https://www.epilepsysociety.org.uk/step-step-recovery-position#.Xid9wchKiSR.

Huang, C., Ma, W., & Stack, S. (2012). The hygienic efficacy of different hand-drying methods: A review of the evidence. *Mayo Clinic Proceedings*, 87(8), 791–798.

Joslin Diabetes Center. (2019). *How to treat a low blood glucose*. Retrieved from https://www.joslin.org/info/how_to_treat_a_low_blood_glucose.html.

Mayo Clinic. (2017). *Choking: First aid*. https://www.mayoclinic.org/first-aid/first-aid-choking/basics/art-20056637.

Moolenaar, R. L., Crutcher, J. M., San Joaquin, V. H., Sewell, L. V., Hutwagner, L. C., Carson, L. A., et al. (2000). A prolonged outbreak of Pseudomonas aeruginosa in a neonatal intensive care unit: Did staff fingernails play a role in disease transmission? *Infection Control & Hospital Epidemiology*, 21(2), 80–85.

National Health Service (NHS). (2018). *Recovery position*. Retrieved from https://www.nhs.uk/conditions/first-aid/recovery-position/.

National Safety Council (NSC). (2017). *Choking*. Retrieved from https://www.nsc.org/home-safety/safety-topics/choking-suffocation.

REVIEW AND APPLY YOUR KNOWLEDGE

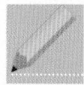

MATCHING ONE: CONCEPT REVIEW

Place the letter of the answer next to the number of the term or phrase that best describes it.

A. Chronic
B. Acute
C. Nosocomial
D. Inflammation
E. Exacerbation
F. Incubation period
G. Personal protective equipment
H. Idiopathic
I. Pathogen
J. Reservoir
K. Standard precautions
L. Virus

_____ 1. Nonliving entities that depend on a host cell for growth and replication.

_____ 2. Diseases that occur suddenly and persist for a brief period of time (<3 months), and then resolve or, in some cases, cause death.

_____ 3. Disease with an unknown cause or origin.

_____ 4. Biologic agent capable of causing infectious disease.

_____ 5. Diseases that have an insidious onset, gradually increase in signs and symptoms, and last for a longer period of time, perhaps for a lifetime.

_____ 6. Minimum infection control measures used to prevent disease transmission.

_____ 7. Term that can be used for infections that were acquired while a person was receiving healthcare for another condition.

_____ 8. Items worn to reduce or prevent transmission of pathogens; examples include gloves, masks, and gowns.

_____ 9. Period of an autoimmune disease in which signs and symptoms worsen or become more severe.

_____ 10. Term to describe the second link in the chain of infection, also known as the source.

_____ 11. Protective response to tissue damage resulting from a variety of causes, including infection and trauma.

_____ 12. Time interval between initial exposure to pathogens and the first appearance of disease signs and symptoms.

MATCHING TWO: CONCEPT REVIEW

Place the letter of the answer next to the number of the term or phrase that best describes it.

A. Bleach
B. Disposable gloves
C. Twenty
D. Seizure
E. Heart attack
F. Heimlich
G. Human hands
H. Hypoglycemia
I. Emergency preparedness
J. Stroke
K. Contact precautions
L. Massage lubricant

_____ 1. Providing first and immediate responses during certain situations to minimize loss of life.

_____ 2. Primary source of disease transmission is contact with _____.

_____ 3. Minimum number of seconds lather should be rubbed into your hands, forearms, and elbows during hand washing.

_____ 4. Procedures used to reduce the risk of spreading infection caused by contact transmission.

_____ 5. Condition for which a diabetic client would need honey or another substance containing sugar.

_____ 6. Include this product in the water when washing contaminated linens.

_____ 7. 911 should be called if this lasts more than 5 minutes.

_____ 8. Maneuver that may dislodge an object from the trachea if a person is choking on it.

_____ 9. "Time is muscle" is the acute care principle for persons experiencing this type of medical emergency.

_____ 10. Creates a barrier between hand sanitizer and the skin, making hand sanitizer less effective.

_____ 11. Worn while disinfecting contaminated surfaces or handling contaminated linens.

_____ 12. "Time is brain" is the acute care principle for persons experiencing this type of medical emergency.

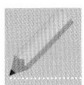

MULTIPLE CHOICE: TEST YOUR KNOWLEDGE

Place the letter of the answer next to the number of the term or phrase that best describes it.

_____ 1. Which describes a condition of abnormal function involving anatomic structures or body systems?
   A. Disease
   B. Illness
   C. Pathology
   D. Disorder

_____ 2. What is the term for the origin or cause of a disease?
   A. Pathology
   B. Etiology
   C. Diagnosis
   D. Prognosis

_____ 3. Secondary diseases are sometimes also called:
   A. risk factors.
   B. clinical manifestations.
   C. complications.
   D. symptoms.

_____ 4. Which of the following describes a disease outbreak that spreads worldwide?
   A. Idiopathic
   B. Endemic
   C. Epidemic
   D. Pandemic

_____ 5. Which describes the number of deaths within a population or region?
   A. Morbidity rate
   B. Mortality rate
   C. Incidence
   D. Prevalence

_____ 6. Cushing syndrome is an example of which type of disease?
   A. Autoimmune
   B. Deficiency
   C. Infectious
   D. Metabolic

_____ 7. Examples are viruses, bacteria, fungi, protozoa, prions.
   A. Pathogens
   B. Reservoirs
   C. Cancers
   D. Portals

_____ 8. Malaria is caused by which type of pathogen?
   A. Virus
   B. Bacteria
   C. Protozoa
   D. Prion

_____ 9. Which mode of transmission spreads pathogens through an animal bite?
   A. Contact
   B. Vehicle
   C. Waterborne
   D. Vector

_____ 10. Destruction of all microorganisms through use of heat, chemicals, irradiation, or high pressure is:
   A. cleaning.
   B. disinfection.
   C. sterilization.
   D. sanitation.

_____ 11. The use of a mask during massage is an example of a:
   A. universal precaution
   B. contact precaution.
   C. droplet precaution.
   D. Massage precaution.

_____ 12. Facial drooping and speech difficulties are signs of a:
   A. seizure.
   B. stroke.
   C. myocardial infarction.
   D. hypoglycemic episode.

CRITICAL THINKING

Forget Something?

You work in a massage office with a bathroom of multiple toilet stalls. As you are washing your hands, you see your next client exiting a stall, then leave without washing hands. What do you do?

Answers can include but are not limited to:

Explain to the client the importance of handwashing for infection control for both massage practitioners and clients, then request the client to wash their hands. The client may or may not be open to hearing the information. It is important to remain professional and to not be "preachy." Another option is to not say anything to the client about washing hands. Instead, tell the client the treatment will start with freshening up the hands and feet, and use hand sanitizer on the client's hands and feet.

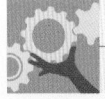

PROFESSIONAL PRACTICE

Seize the Day

Moxie is a middle-aged female who recently had her second child. During her early twenties, she began having anxiety attacks with mild seizures. Her physician prescribed medication to control her seizures. While she was pregnant, she discontinued the medication as directed by her obstetrician. Her doctor told her to remain off the medication until she stopped nursing.

Many of Moxie's discomforts were alleviated with massage, and she enjoyed them twice a month. During today's appointment, Moxie was unusually tired. Chantell entered the room and asked Moxie a few questions. Moxie replied in single syllables. After about 5 minutes, Chantell asked Moxie to comment on the pressure. Moxie did not answer. Chantell asked again. She looked down at Moxie and saw her eyes were moving rapidly under her closed lids. Because Chantell had done an in-depth client intake, she knew about Moxie's history of seizures. Not ever seeing one in the past, Chantell assumed Moxie was experiencing a seizure.

What should Chantell do? How might Moxie feel coming out of the seizure? If Moxie's seizure had been physical, how might Chantell respond? If Chantell had called emergency services, what information should she provide?

DISCUSSION

Antibacterial Soap

Find the answer to the question, "Is antibacterial soap more effective than regular soap at killing germs?" You can ask authoritative persons, such as a physician or pharmacist, or use an Internet-based search engine. If you find nonscholarly sources, confirm their source of information, such as a peer-reviewed journal or person in the medical profession. Include any known benefits and risks from use of antibacterial products. If available, share your findings on an Internet-based discussion board monitored by your instructor.

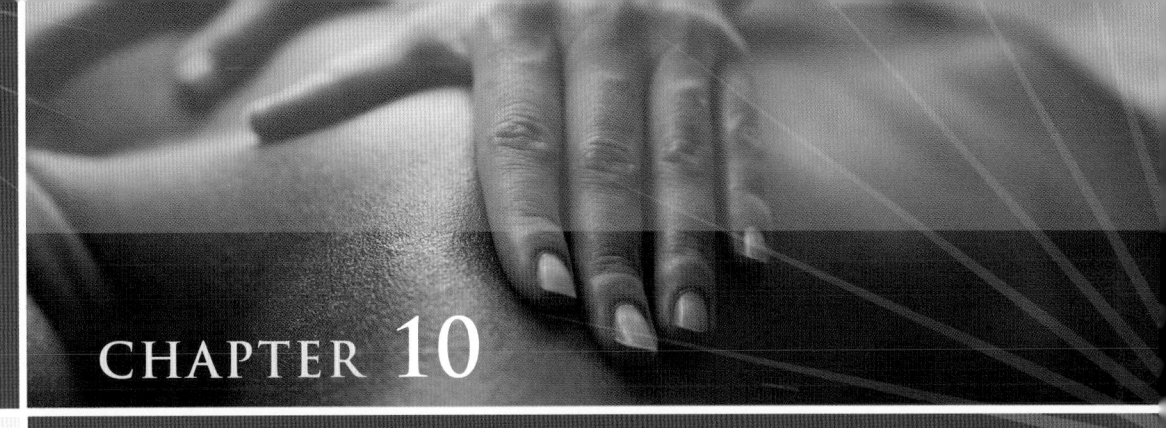

CHAPTER 10

Professional Standards: Scope of Practice, Standards of Care, Assessments, Documentation, Informed Consent, Treatment Planning, and Referrals

LEARNING OBJECTIVES

After completing this chapter, the student should be able to:

1. Discuss the scope of practice and standards of care.
2. Describe massage-related assessments and documentation.
3. Conduct client health assessments using an intake form and client interview.
4. Define informed consent and state benefits and potential risks related to massage.
5. Explain treatment planning and the importance of evidence in a massage practice.
6. Utilize standardized client documentation formats and explain how to refer a client to a healthcare provider for medical evaluation.

http://evolve.elsevier.com/Salvo/MassageTherapy

INTRODUCTION

Massage practitioners manipulate soft tissues using pressure and traction to facilitate a variety of client outcomes such as reduction of pain, stress, anxiety, and depression and improved function. During the massage, the time spent with each client is limited and structured. Within this time frame, the practitioner decides which activities will occur for the client to have a safe and satisfactory outcome, which may be based on the following factors:

- Information gathered on a completed client intake form, the client's primary healthcare provider, and the client's caregivers (if applicable).
- Treatment goals stated by the client.
- Client's preferences, including time and financial restraints.
- Review of previous treatment plans.
- Parameters set by third-party payers, such as insurance companies.
- Assessments performed by the practitioner or other healthcare providers.
- The practitioner's training and experience.
- The best available evidence (research).
- Standards of care and scope of practice as defined by professional organizations and regulatory agencies.

After the massage, the client's responses or outcomes of those actions are noted. These tasks are captured within client documents which must be maintained in confidence and securely stored. These tasks reflect the massage practitioner's commitment to client care and professionalism.

Massage practitioners may be part of a healthcare team assembled according to the client's needs, as well as the skill and expertise of individual members. Members of the healthcare providers may include:

- Physicians and surgeons.
- Nurse practitioners and physician assistants.
- Osteopathic and chiropractic physicians.
- Physical, occupational, and respiratory therapists.
- Mental health counselors.
- Dieticians.
- Massage practitioners.

This chapter will examine the process of collecting client information, obtaining consent, developing an individualized treatment plan, and ways to communicate with the client's healthcare provider when a medical referral is indicated. This plan is the organizational framework and forms the basis for planning current sessions and influences future sessions. The treatment plan is essentially the strategy used to help the client achieve their treatment goals. Because this process includes dialogue via an interview, treatment planning also enhances communication, rapport, and trust. This chapter also includes documentation procedures.

SCOPE OF PRACTICE AND STANDARD OF CARE

Massage practitioners are expected to understand and operate within their scope of practice. **Scope of practice** are professional activities that can be performed legally by members of a licensed profession and the context in which these activities can be applied. Scope of practice is defined by state law or the practice act. Approximately 49 states and territories regulate the massage profession in some form to ensure safe and competent practitioners are the only ones practicing on the public (Federation of State Massage Therapy Boards [FSMTB], 2021). Codes of ethics and standards of practice are discussed in Chapter 2.

Delegation is the assignment of a task or task completion from one person to another person. The delegated task must be within the scope of practice identified by state law. For example, a healthcare provider cannot delegate tasks such as the application of topical prescriptive products unless this task is part of the delegatee's scope of practice. For massage practitioners, this restriction includes not only facilities offering massage services but also care provided in the practitioner's home office or client's residence. In protection of your license and current position, communicate your scope of practice if asked to provide a service outside the scope.

Scope of Practice: What's In

Activities often permitted under a massage practitioner's scope of practice may include the following:

- Assessment by client subjective self-report (e.g., intake form, interview), by practitioner observation and measurement (e.g., range of motion, posture, gait, swelling).
- Documentation of assessments, treatment plans and their outcomes, and progress reports.
- Obtaining consent for treatment.
- Use of manual techniques, including effleurage (gliding), petrissage (kneading), tapotement (percussion), vibration, and friction by use of fingers, hands, forearms, elbows, knees, and feet.
- Use of mechanical appliances and handheld instruments that duplicate or complement massage techniques.
- Passive movements of stretching and joint mobilizations.
- Energetic methods using physical contact or noncontact.
- Use of lubricants, essential oils, powders, liniments, and similar preparations.
- Use of physical agents such as hot and cold applications (e.g., packs, stones), hydrotherapy, and nonprescription topical products (e.g., muds, clays, salts, sugars).
- General nonspecific suggestions and recommendations for self-care and health promotion or health maintenance activities, including but not limited to self-massage, self-administered hydrotherapy, movement and stretching activities, stress reduction, and stress management techniques.
- Consultation with other service providers.

Scope of Practice: What's Out

Massage practitioners cannot provide services or apply techniques that require a separate license to practice, such as psychotherapy, chiropractic or osteopathic procedures, physical or occupational therapy, or any branch of medicine, unless they have the appropriate state license. If you are trained in a particular technique or method (e.g., ear candling, herbalism), you cannot provide the service unless it is in your legally defined scope of practice. Those who provide services outside their scope may be in violation of state law.

Bear in mind that massage practitioners who are licensed in other occupations (e.g., nursing, cosmetology) should refrain from wearing "two hats" simultaneously. For example, when operating in the capacity of a massage practitioner, provide only those services within that scope of practice. When operating as a non-massage professional, provide only those services within that scope of practice. In addition, all professions have their own standards of care and codes of ethics (e.g., codes of ethics for licensed mental health counselors are different from codes of ethics for massage practitioners); the profession with the strictest code of ethics prevails and becomes the standard of conduct for all professional activities for the dually licensed massage practitioner.

The following is a list of activities commonly outside of a massage practitioner's scope of practice:

- Acupuncture
- Manual thrusts at the end range of available passive range of motion as performed in chiropractic, osteopathic, or naturopathic procedures (may be described as high-velocity and low-amplitude joint manipulations)
- Ultrasound, electrotherapy, laser and microwave therapy, injection therapy, diathermy, and transdermal electrical nerve stimulation
- Dietary and nutritional counseling
- Therapeutic exercise
- Cosmetology or specific procedures to beautify the skin
- Depilation, waxing, hair extractions, and electrolysis
- Colonic irrigation and other methods of internal hydrotherapy
- Ear candling
- Herbalism
- Homeopathy
- Naturopathy
- Diagnosis of diseases or injuries
- Psychotherapy, hypnotherapy, counseling, or related practices or procedures
- Recommending, prescribing, dispensing, administering, applying, or modifying prescription and over-the-counter drugs
- Intentional use of techniques to evoke an emotional response in the client
- Genital, intra-anal, or intravaginal contact or manipulation.

Standard of Care

Standard of care is the degree and level of care given by similarly trained and qualified individuals who are in the same or similar line of work or work setting (Moffett & Moore, 2011). The standards define and direct professional responsibilities or duties, and all practitioners are expected to meet the standards. Standards of care are important for several reasons.

They provide consistency so all clients receive the same quality care. They promote the best possible outcomes while minimizing the risk of harm. They also provide an objective standard to evaluate differences between standard and substandard care if unsafe practices are suspected. And they guarantee professionals are held accountable for their decisions and actions. Standards of care are established by leading organizations and outlined in standard-setting documents.

ASSESSMENT AND DOCUMENTATION

Assessment is a systematic process of gathering information in order to make informed decisions about treatment. An assessment gives you a deeper understanding of the client's condition, helps you formulate professional judgments, and serves as the foundation of the treatment plan. Assessment includes client self-reporting of health status via an intake form, stress or pain levels through the various use of scales, a client interview, and visual, palpatory, and physical assessments conducted by the practitioner. Some assessments reveal the presence of contraindications or the need for a referral. A **contraindication** is a condition that could be aggravated by the application of massage. Contraindications can be absolute or local and are briefly discussed next (see Chapter 8 for a full discussion).

- **Absolute Contraindications**. Conditions that make receiving a massage absolutely inadvisable. In these cases, massage is postponed until the condition resolves.
- **Local Contraindications**. Conditions that make receiving a massage to a local area inadvisable. Massage can be administered to other areas of the body while avoiding the area locally contraindicated.

Documentation is the process of collecting, confirming, and recording information. Systematic collection and review of previously recorded client information help practitioners evaluate past treatment decisions, which sharpens the practitioner's critical thinking skills. *Critical thinking* is the process of analyzing, evaluating, interpreting, or synthesizing information and applying creative thought to form an argument, solve a problem, or reach a conclusion. Treatment modifications are made according to the client's response if previous actions did not meet the client's expectations.

Documentation is the "gold standard" of admissible evidence in legal proceedings. Documentation verifies client information disclosed and the type of treatment the client received. Adequate and accurate documentation also supports payment reimbursement, improves the quality of client care, and demonstrates to the public that the practitioner followed accepted standards of care. As in all professional settings, "if it isn't documented, it didn't happen." Certainly, relying on memory is poor record keeping. Furthermore, many state licensing and certification boards require systematic and ongoing documentation, which may be used in review proceedings and licensing or certification determinations. In many states, practitioners are required to collect and maintain documentation for each client.

In the early 1900s, paper-based documentation became part of routine practice and the most common form of documentation until the late 20th century when documentation became digitized. This practice was slow to implement and met with resistance as some healthcare providers were more comfortable with paper and the conversion to a digital format was costly. As computers and digital information became more widely available, electronic health records (EHRs) became more common. EHRs are efficient, as test results are quickly available and easily shared with other members of the healthcare team. Complementary and integrative healthcare providers are often mandated to use EHR formats, and affordable options are emerging for small practices.

The type of documentation and the amount of information the massage practitioner is required to collect or has access to, will differ depending on how the facility views the massage practitioner's role. Some practitioners will use paper documents that may or may not be scanned into an electronic record, and some practitioners will use electronic documents exclusively. Documents should include the signatures of the person who completed the form and when the information was recorded. Essential documents are discussed next.

- **Intake Form**. Completed by the client and updated annually or when client information changes.
- **Consent Form**. Completed by the client and updated when the treatment changes.
- **Treatment Plan**. Completed by the practitioner documenting the initial session, subsequent session modifications, or as required by state law.

Information on intake forms and consent forms should contain uncomplicated language understood by the average adult, and use an easy-to-read font style and point size. Low or limited health literacy are associated with poor health outcomes. **Health literacy** is the capacity of an individual to obtain, communicate, and understand health information and services when making decisions. The average American adult's reading level is about the ninth grade (DuBay, n.d.). Populations most negatively affected by health illiteracy and reading barriers are older adults, individuals with disabilities, immigrant populations, minorities, and low-income. Language barriers can be reduced by using language translation software or mobile device applications (apps). The client may also bring a support person to act as an interpreter.

Tips for Documenting

Tips and suggestions for documenting are next. These suggestions apply more to handwritten records.

- Write legibly. Documentation which cannot be read and understood by others is worthless.
- If a client document spans multiple pages, ask the client to initial each page in the lower-right-hand corner that does not specifically request a signature.
- Use commonly accepted medical terms and abbreviations. Appendix A contains a list of abbreviations, acronyms, and symbols.
- Avoid massage jargon (e.g., circulatory massage, energy work) which may be misunderstood or dismissed as meaningless by non-massage professionals.
- If working in a facility, only use abbreviations on the facility's approved list.
- If working independently, include a legend for clarity. Different disciplines may use abbreviations in varying ways, and this leads to confusion.
- Draw a line from the end of the handwritten note to the end of the blank space, and insert your initials at the end of the line. This line will fill blank spaces and prevent later alterations or additions made to the client's chart.
- Use blue or black ink, and correct errors with a single line and initials. Do not erase or use correction fluid and tape.
- Use direct quotes with appropriate quotation marks when applicable, stating exactly what the client said.
- Record facts (i.e., what is observed or heard) and professional judgments made based on these facts.

Factual Documenting

Massage practitioners have a duty to factually communicate and document. False documentation can place blame or liability on previous service providers or create contrived events in the client's records. For example, you walk into a room and find the client lying unconscious on the floor between the massage table and the door leading to the toilet. How would you document this?

1. The client fell off the table and was found on the floor unconscious.
2. The client fell on the floor on his way to the toilet. He was knocked unconscious.
3. The client was found on the floor beside the massage table. The bolster must not have been secured and he tripped, hitting his head, and rendering himself unconscious.
4. The client was found on the floor next to the massage table. The client was unconscious.

The correct answer in the list is "4" because it states the facts without speculation.

It is important you do not promise or assure the client of an improbable positive outcome. "Promise to cure" laws are explicit, and healthcare providers are held accountable in civil lawsuits if there has been a promise for a cure or a guaranteed positive outcome did not come to fruition.

Who Maintains Client Records?

Client records, including billing files, are maintained by the office manager and stored on the property where services were provided. This includes spas, clinics, and massage franchises. If copies of a client's files are needed for legal evidence, a formal request can be made to the facility and a subpoena may be required. Unauthorized removal may be grounds for legal action by the facility and disciplinary action by a state licensing board.

How Long Are Client Records Kept?

Client records are kept for at least as long as the statute of limitations for malpractice claims. The time frame varies from state to state; generally, it is 2 years but could be as long as 6 years after the last date of service. State medical associations and insurance carriers are the best resources for this information. A minimum of 4 years from the termination of the professional relationship is recommended by the National Certification Board for Therapeutic Massage and Bodywork (NCBTMB, 2017).

Safeguarding Client Information

Massage practitioners have a professional duty to safeguard clients' personal, health, and medical information and keep up to date with changes related to privacy laws dictated by state and federal agencies. This includes all information written, spoken, recorded, or electronically stored that pertains to the past, present, or future care of clients.

One method used to safeguard client information is the *double lock rule*. If client information is on paper, secure paper documents behind two locks such as a locked fireproof file cabinet inside a locked office. If client information is digitized, secure electronic files behind two locks such as a passcode-protected computer program or cloud-based storage accessed through a passcode-protected digital device. In addition, if services are provided onsite such as in residential settings, client files are secured within a locked mobile transport case and in a locked vehicle.

Digital devices must be fitted with a firewall to protect client information from hackers. Do not allow unauthorized individuals to use or "play" on digital devices containing client information.

Back up electronically stored client files routinely onto a passcode-protected external storage device or utilize a reputable web-based file storage company. This way, you will have access to client information in the event of a technological malfunction.

When replacing digital devices containing client information, completely wipe the hard drive before you sell or donate them. Simply erasing the hard drive after transferring files does not provide adequate protection of client information, as it does not completely remove data called metadata. Consider consulting an information technologist or appropriate company for the most up-to-date secure methods, as information technology is constantly changing.

Most privacy guidelines are derived from federal legislation, including the **Health Insurance Portability and Accountability Act of 1996** (HIPAA), and the **Patient Protection and Affordable Care Act** of 2010.

HIPAA was created by the Department of Health and Human Services (DHHS) to protect clients' rights and targets the storage, transmission, and dissemination of personal health information. A misconception exists about whether HIPAA applies only to health insurance agencies, probably because the term health insurance is in the title of the act. However, HIPAA guidelines apply to all healthcare providers, including employees, volunteers, trainees, independent contractors, and business associates, to whom client information has been distributed. Massage practitioners must ensure their actions are HIPAA-compliant. Violating client

privacy is a serious offense with repercussions that may include federal or state legal indictments, lawsuits, loss of state licensure, termination from an organization, and loss of the client's trust. Invasion of privacy includes compromising client information through social media, unencrypted transmission, discussing client information in common areas, disclosing client information to family or friends, misplaced documents, and improperly storing or disposing of documents. Protected client identifiers are as follows:

- Partial or full names.
- Geographic subdivisions smaller than a state, including street address, city, county, precinct, and zip code (except for the first three digits of a zip code).
- All dates directly related to the client, including admission date, discharge date, date of birth, date of death, date of diagnosis, date of service, and age.
- Phone numbers.
- Fax numbers.
- Email addresses.
- Social Security numbers.
- Medical record numbers.
- Health plan identification and beneficiary numbers.
- Account numbers.
- Certificate/license numbers.
- Vehicle identifiers and serial numbers, including license plate numbers.
- Device identifiers and serial numbers.
- Web Universal Resource Locators (URLs).
- Internet Protocol (IP) addresses.
- Biometric identifiers, including finger, palm, retina, and voiceprints.
- Facial photographs or comparable images, such as identifying birthmarks, scars, and tattoos.
- Any other unique identifying number, characteristic, or codes.

HIPAA laws protecting client information extend to social media platforms. Common social media HIPAA violations include posting pictures or videos of clients without written consent, posting information that could allow clients to be identified, posting gossip about clients, and sharing pictures or videos taken inside a facility in which clients or client records are visible. Posting restrictions include private groups within social media platforms. Box 10.1 contains information regarding the safeguarding of client information.

Releasing Client Information

Client health and medical information can only be released to a third-party if the client authorizes the release by signing and dating a **document release form**. This form includes the client's name, the name and address of the institution maintaining the client's information, and the name and address of the institution receiving the information. The form also includes an expiration period. Release only the information listed on the form. If the client is a minor, a parent or legal representative must sign the client's release form. An example of a document release form is on Evolve.

BOX 10.1

Safeguarding Client Information: Guidelines for Massage Practitioners

- Obtain written or verbal consent from each client before treatment.
- Keep the appointment book and all client records out of view.
- Protect electronic client files by assigning passwords to anyone who has access to them. Computers connected electronically to the Internet must be fitted with a firewall to protect information from hackers.
- Obtain written client consent before dispensing any material such as newsletters, facsimile (FAX) referrals, greeting cards, or email, or leaving text or voice messages.
- Place confidentiality notices on all facsimiles and emails. Remind the client that although these notices may defer viewing, the messages may not be secure.
- Store paper copies of client files in a locked fireproof cabinet and restrict access.
- Create a client information sheet outlining how you intend to use the information obtained from the client, how this information will be maintained and stored, and under what circumstances this information will be disclosed, as well as how the practitioner will obtain permission for such incidences, how copies can be obtained by the client of their files, how long these files will be kept once the client is released, and how these records will be destroyed. Give a copy of this document to each client. Go over each item with the client, asking them to sign and date a separate statement that they received the notice of privacy policies.
- When talking on the telephone, do not use the caller's name if anyone else can hear the conversation.
- If you have a computer in your office, ensure the screen is out of view or shows a screen saver when clients or unauthorized individuals are nearby.

Prescriptions and Insurance Claims

The public has direct access to massage services meaning no prescription is required. However, a prescription may be issued by authorized prescribers which include medical and chiropractic physicians, physician assistants, and nurse practitioners to help their patients recover from personal injuries (PIs) and occupational injuries after accidents. In these cases, the cost of massage services may be paid or reimbursed by third-party payers such as insurance companies. These situations often require a prescription. Massage practitioners who wish to work under prescriptive orders or file insurance claims must follow legal parameters, policies, and procedures.

A **prescription** is authorization and instructions from a medical practitioner for drugs, procedures (e.g., physical or massage therapy), or devices (e.g., hearing aids, eyeglasses). Prescriptions often include the patient's name, the patient's diagnostic code, the date written, the name and address of the prescribing provider, and other legal requirements such as a registration number. Diagnostic codes are listed in the **International Classification of Disease** (ICD), a comprehensive database used in healthcare and research to classify and monitor incidence and prevalence rates of diseases, disorders, and injuries. ICD codes always include the edition number. For example, ICD-10 is listed when the code came from the 10th edition.

Prescriptions for procedures also list the procedural code, or CPT code. CPT stands for **current procedural terminology** and is a list of codes used to report medical services and procedures administered to patients. CPT codes are issued by the American Medical Association and arranged according to their specialty. Most CPT codes associated with massage are under "Therapeutic Procedure" or "Manual Therapy" and include massage techniques such as effleurage, petrissage, and/or tapotement (compression, percussion). CPT codes also change over time, so always consult the most recently published list. Prescriptions may also state the *strength* of massage or length of time of each session or its *dosage* such as twice a week for 6 weeks. Most sessions are administered in 15-minute units. There are restrictions regarding how many times a code can be used within a day. The practitioner may provide 30 minutes of treatment using two different codes. A prescription may instruct the massage practitioner to evaluate and treat the client at their own discretion, or state specific techniques or methods used, such as cupping therapy or myofascial techniques. At the end of the prescribed period, the patient returns to the prescriber for reevaluation.

Most insurance claims are filed electronically. Some filing systems use a health insurance claim form called *CMS 1500*, which was created by the Healthcare Financing Administration to standardize claim processing. If unable to prepare and submit all required documentation yourself, a medical billing company may be used to do this for you. Insurance companies pay for "medically necessary" procedures and products. Therefore, documentation such as assessments made before and after the massage is needed to indicate any progress. FDAR charting discussed later in the chapter features a progress report. Some practitioners write progress reports like formal letters and include the following sections:

1. Introductory paragraph, recapping the original prescription.
2. Summary of initial treatment goals.
3. Special tests used such as orthopedic assessments and their results.
4. Summary of sessions and their outcomes.
5. Any remaining treatment goals and specific strategies to reach these goals.
6. Request for additional sessions, if needed.
7. Closing with an offer to provide more information upon request.

Progress reports may be sent directly to the prescriber or may be given to the patient to deliver to the prescriber during the next appointment.

INTAKE FORM

The intake form is the form used to collect the client's personal and contact information, health and medical information, and massage information such as past experiences and pressure preferences. The client may provide information about chronic diseases, cancer, infectious diseases, cardiovascular and neurologic conditions, musculoskeletal conditions, injuries, allergies, bruising risks, pregnancy, surgeries and medical procedures, and medication use, which may also affect treatment planning. The intake form, also called the health history form or health questionnaire, is completed by the client during the initial appointment (Fig. 10.1). Some practitioners email the intake form to clients before the initial appointment or have these forms available as downloadable documents on a website.

During the client interview conducted in subsequent sessions, ask the client about changes in their health or medical status and update the intake form when needed. The client should complete a new intake form annually, such as at their first appointment in the next calendar year or the anniversary of their initial appointment.

Pain and Stress Level Assessments

Pain is an unpleasant sensory and emotional experience associated with, or resembling, actual or potential tissue damage (International Association for the Study of Pain [IASP], 2020). Pain relief is the second most common reason clients seek massage; stress reduction and relaxation are the top reasons (American Massage Therapy Association [AMTA], 2020). If pain reduction is a treatment goal, pain is assessed before and after treatment to determine the client's response to the massage. Pain and Stress level assessment scales can be incorporated into the intake form (Fig. 10.2). Characteristics of pain can be recorded using visual analog scales, numeric rating scales, verbal descriptor scales, and Wong-Baker FACES scales. A body diagram can be used to record pain locations. These methods are popular because they are quick and easy to administer, are easily understood, and provide quantifiable data.

Stress is the body's response to any demand placed on it which triggers sympathetic arousal or the stress response. If stress reduction is a treatment goal, stress levels are assessed before and after treatment to determine the client's response to the massage. Visual, numeric, and verbal descriptive scales can be easily modified to gather information about a client's stress level. These scales are discussed next.

- **Visual Analog Scale (VAS)**. This consists of a straight horizontal or vertical line with the endpoints to measure extreme limits such as no pain and the worst pain possible (Fig. 10.3). The client is asked to mark their pain level on the line between the two endpoints.
- **Numeric Rating Scale (NRS)**. This consists of a line of numbers between 0 and 10, with 0 representing no pain and 10 representing the worst pain possible (Fig. 10.4). The client is asked to mark which number best represents their pain intensity.

- **Verbal Descriptor Scale (VDS)**. This uses a series of descriptive phrases such as mild, moderate, severe, and worst (Fig. 10.5). The client is asked to mark which phrase best describes their pain intensity.
- **Wong-Baker FACES Scale (WBS)**. This shows a series of faces ranging from a happy face at 0, which represents no hurt, to a sad crying face at 10, which represents hurts worst (Fig. 10.6). The client is asked to choose the face that best represents their pain intensity. This scale can be used for individuals who have difficulty using numeric or verbal scales, including children and clients with language barriers or cognitive deficits.
- **Body Diagram**. This is an outline of a body and the client is asked to indicate where the pain is experienced. Combining pain scales with body diagrams are popular in a massage practice and the client can indicate the location and the nature of pain or discomfort (Fig. 10.7).

Gathering information about the client's pain and stress levels will help you decide which areas to focus on, which areas to avoid, which techniques to use, or whether the massage should be postponed. Severe pain is an absolute contraindication in which massage is postponed. In these cases, a referral to the client's primary healthcare provider for evaluation may be needed before a massage can be administered (see the section on Referring Clients to Their Healthcare Providers for Medical Evaluation later in this chapter). Pain and pain theories are discussed in more detail in Chapter 14.

Completing the Intake Form

While the client is completing the form, be available for questions. If the client is unable to complete the form, obtain the information verbally. Some practitioners prefer to ask the client all queries and record the information on the intake form. It also provides an opportunity to ask the client questions and obtain clarification immediately during the interview. In these cases, write down the client's responses on the form and place your initials next to the main entry when the writing on the form is your own and not the client's.

When the client returns the form, ensure it is completed and contains a dated signature. Make a note of prescriptions, and third-party payers such as insurance companies, which may require additional information or specific forms. Do not leave the completed form unattended. Afterward, place their information in a secure location away from unauthorized individuals.

THE CLIENT INTERVIEW

During the interview, you will review the completed form and ask the client specific questions, if needed. This process helps you gain a greater insight into the client's health and problems for which they are seeking help. The interview gives you additional pieces of the puzzle. The interview also

---

Massage Intake Form

Personal Information

Name _____   Phone (day) _____ (evening) _____

Preferred Name _____   Preferred Pronouns _____

Address _____   City/State/Zip _____ DOB* _____

Occupation _____   Employer _____

Email _____   Primary Physician _____

Emergency Contact _____   Relationship _____ Phone _____

How did you hear about us?_____

Medical Information

Are you taking any medications?   ☐ yes   ☐ no

  If yes, please list names and how administered: _____
  _____

Are you currently pregnant?   ☐ yes   ☐ no

  If yes, how far along? _____

  Any high risk factors? _____

Do you suffer from chronic pain?   ☐ yes   ☐ no

  If yes, please explain_____

  What makes it better? _____
  _____

  What makes it worse? _____
  _____

Have you had any injuries?   ☐ yes   ☐ no

  If yes, please list: _____

Please indicate any of the following that apply to you.

☐ Cancer   ☐ Infection
☐ Bulging/herniated disk ☐ Disabilities or impairments
☐ Arthritis   ☐ Heart attack
☐ Diabetes   ☐ Seizures
☐ Surgeries   ☐ Blood clots
☐ Bruise easily   ☐ Recent injury (≤72 hr)
☐ Neuropathy   ☐ Aged ≥65

Explain any conditions you have marked above:

_____
_____
_____
_____

Massage Information

Have you had a professional massage before? ☐ yes ☐ no

What type of massage are you seeking?

    ☐ Relaxation   ☐ Therapeutic/Palliative

Other _____

What pressure do you prefer?

    ☐ Light   ☐ Medium   ☐ Deep

Do you have any allergies or sensitivities?   ☐ yes ☐ no

    Please explain _____

Are there any areas (feet, face, abdomen, etc.) you do not want massaged?   ☐ yes   ☐ no

    Please explain _____

What are your goals for this treatment session?

_____

Please circle any areas of discomfort

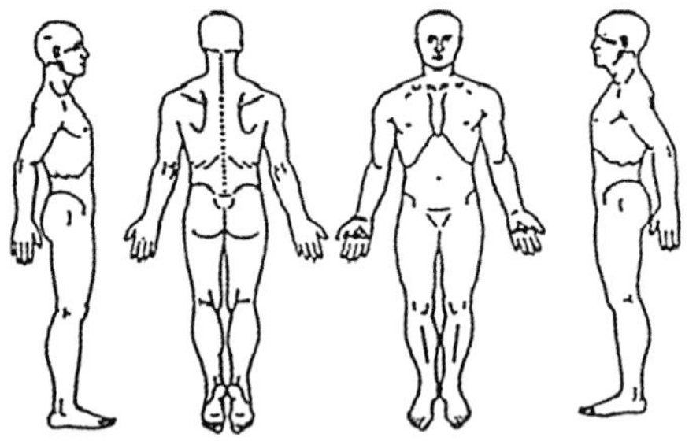

By signing below you agree to the following.
I have completed this form to the best of my ability and knowledge and agree to inform my therapist if any of the above information changes at any time.

Client Signature _____ Date _____

Practitioner Signature _____ Date _____

FIG. 10.1 Health questionnaire or massage intake form used to gather a client's personal, medical, and massage information. (Courtesy mymassageworld.com.)

helps you screen for contraindications and recognize the need for adaptations, such as hypoallergenic lubricants or a side-lying position.

The interview is an essential component of the health assessment and is used to establish or maintain communication and rapport. **Communication** is the act of exchanging information by encoding and decoding verbal and nonverbal messages within a defined cultural, physiological, relational, and perceptual context. Communication helps to express thoughts, ideas, and feelings. Whether we are using words or not, we are also communicating nonverbally through eye contact, body stance, and space. **Rapport** is the emotional bond that people experience when concerns, feelings, and ideas are mutually expressed.

Client Intake Form

Mary Smith, LMT, BCTMB
1234 Front Street, Anytown WA 00000
123-456-7890

Name: _____ Phone: ( ) _____-_____

Address: _____

City: _____ State: _____ Zip: _____ Date of Birth: _____

E-Mail: _____

Occupation: _____ Referred by: _____

In case of emergency: _____ Phone: ( ) _____-_____

Treatment goal(s): _____

Medical & Surgical Information; Pain/Stress: Pre- & Post-treatment measures

❑Yes ❑No Have you ever had professional massage?	Indicate by circling pain or stress and their levels. "0" is no stress/pain. "10" is the worst stress/pain ever experienced.
❑Light ❑Medium ❑Deep What is your pressure preference?	
❑Yes ❑No Do you have any medical conditions?	Stress or pain level BEFORE massage.
❑Yes ❑No Are you taking medications?	0 1 2 3 4 5 6 7 8 9 10
❑Yes ❑No Have you ever had surgery?	Stress or pain level AFTER massage.
❑Yes ❑No Do you have environmental or product allergies?	0 1 2 3 4 5 6 7 8 9 10

Notes: _____
_____
_____
_____
_____

PLEASE READ THE FOLLOWING INFORMATION AND SIGN WHERE INDICATED.

While massage has numerous benefits, there are inherent massage-related risks, such as bruising, increased pain, or soreness lasting a few days, which do not disrupt activities of daily living. However, there are also reported rare, harmful effects from massage such as damage to nerves, glands, organs, and blood vessels. To reduce these risks:

- I have stated all known medical conditions and answered questions honestly;
- I will keep the massage practitioner updated as to any changes in my health; and
- I will promptly communicate any pain or discomfort experienced during the session(s).

I understand massage should not be construed as substitute for medical examination and I should consult an appropriate health care provider for mental or physical ailments. I further understand massage practitioners are not qualified to perform spinal manipulations, diagnose, or prescribe.

Finally, I understand any illicit or sexually suggestive remarks or conduct will result in immediate termination of the session, and I will be liable for payment of the scheduled appointment.

I have read and agree to comply with all above terms, and consent to treatment acknowledging above-stated risks.

_____   _____   _____
Signature of person completing this form   Date   Therapist initials

---

Information and Suggestions

☻ Prior to massage, remove all jewelry. Pull long hair back with a clip.

☻ As a rule, massage is given while you are unclothed. We provide a top sheet. You may choose to wear undergarments or a swim suit if you prefer. This is YOUR massage and you should feel as comfortable as possible.

☻ During your massage, give feedback regarding pressure (more or less) and point out ticklish areas.

☻ Feel free to ask any questions about the procedure. We want you to be well-informed and comfortable.

FIG. 10.2 Health questionnaire or massage intake form with pain and stress numeric rating scale.

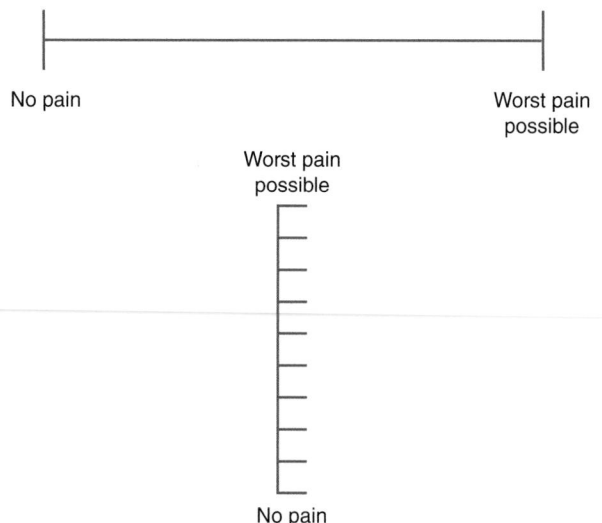

FIG. 10.3 Visual analog scale: A straight horizontal or vertical line with the endpoints can be used to measure extreme limits from no pain and the worst pain possible. The scale can be modified to measure stress levels. (From Cameron, M. [2018]. *Physical agents in rehabilitation* [5th ed.]. St Louis: Elsevier.)

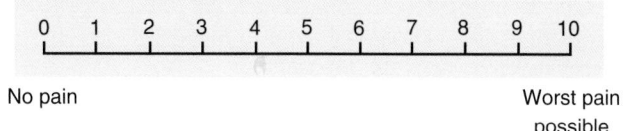

FIG. 10.4 Numeric rating scale: A line of numbers between 0 and 10 can be used to measure extreme limits with 0 representing no pain and 10 representing the worst pain possible. The scale can be modified to measure stress levels. (From Cameron, M. [2018]. *Physical agents in rehabilitation* [5th ed.]. St Louis: Elsevier.)

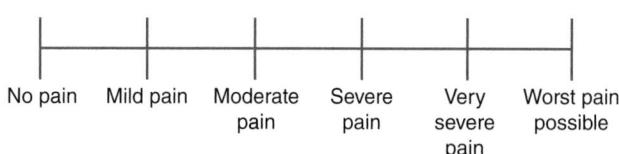

FIG. 10.5 Verbal descriptor scale: A series of descriptive phrases such as mild, moderate, severe, and worst pain possible can be used to measure pain levels. The scale can be modified to measure stress levels. (From Cameron, M. [2018]. *Physical agents in rehabilitation* [5th ed.]. St Louis: Elsevier.)

Effective communication is one of the most valuable skills a practitioner can acquire and it involves undivided attention, listening, observing or seeing, compassion or feeling, and critical thinking (Fig. 10.8). Develop and maintain a professional demeanor that conveys genuine caring, empathy, respect, safety, and trust, and that respects appropriate boundaries. Practitioners who are distant and cold in their communications are unlikely to facilitate a positive connection with clients. Conversely, an overly friendly style may be perceived as intrusive and disrespectful. Good rapport facilitates clear communication and promotes cooperation, which may lead to client satisfaction and continued patronage. For these reasons, the attending practitioner should be the one conducting the client interview.

Greetings and Interview Logistics

Greet the client by smiling, making eye contact, and stating a greeting that includes the client's name. Then, introduce yourself and state your title. Next, escort the client to the interview area. The area should be private, comfortable, at a pleasant room temperature, ventilated, well lit, and free of distractions and interruptions. The seating should be at a relatively close proximity; no more than 6 feet apart. Ensure the area is private during oral disclosures and cannot be overheard. This level of privacy may require soundproof walls or partitions and/or a white noise device. The latter is used to protect privacy by masking sounds.

Face the client at eye level during the interview (Fig. 10.9). This position facilitates conversation and fosters trust and goodwill. Inquire about the client's reasons for receiving a massage.

Use a variety of question types during the interview, including exploratory, reflective, open-ended, and close-ended questions. **Exploratory questions** help practitioners gain a deeper understanding of the client's health and preferences. **Reflective questions** confirm the client's response was received and understood. Reflective questions give the client an opportunity to reflect and clarify information if the practitioner misunderstood the meaning of the client's message. **Open-ended questions** offer little restriction when answering. **Close-ended questions** are more precise and require affirmative, denial, or specific answers such as "yes," "no," or "the right shoulder." Remain neutral to the client's responses and do not imply they said something "right" or "wrong." Avoid leading questions suggesting a certain answer.

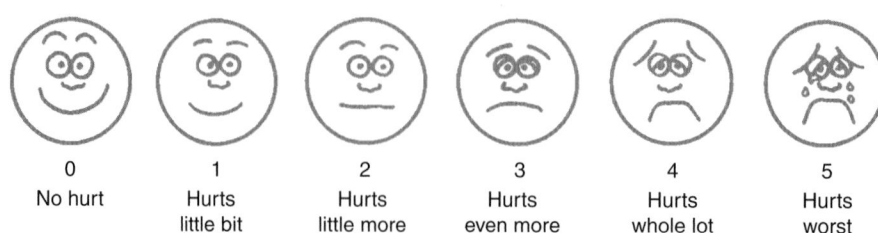

FIG. 10.6 Wong-Baker FACES pain rating scale: A series of faces, numbers, and descriptive phrases ranging from a happy face at 0 or no hurt, to a sad crying face at 10 for hurts worst. (From Cameron, M. [2018]. *Physical agents in rehabilitation* [5th ed.]. St Louis: Elsevier.)

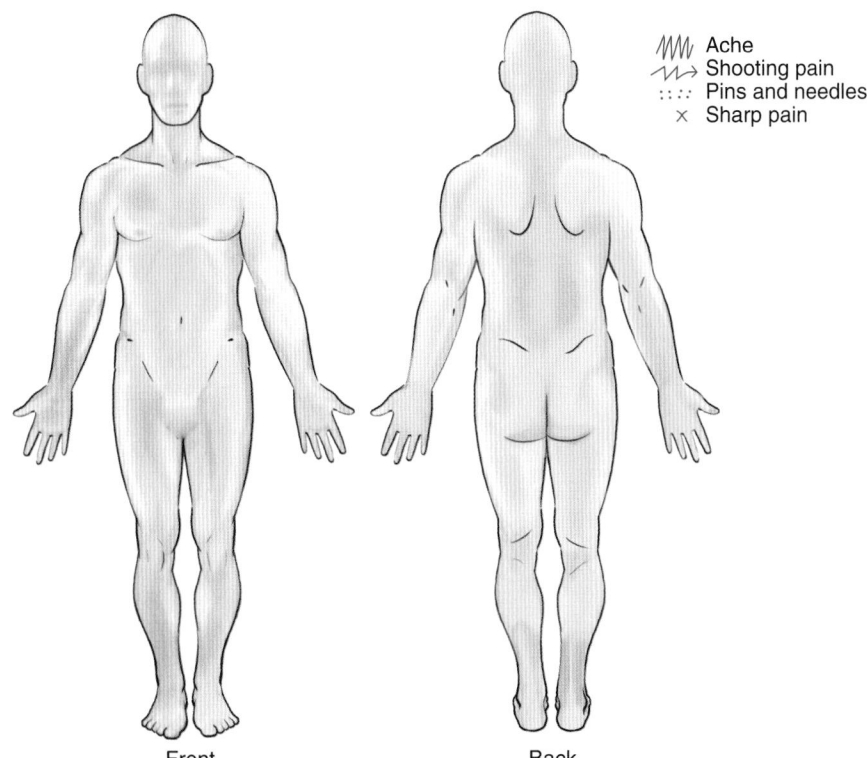

FIG. 10.7 Body diagram: An outline of the human body can be used to indicate the location and characteristics of a client's pain or discomfort. (From Cameron, M. [2018]. *Physical agents in rehabilitation* [5th ed.]. St Louis: Elsevier.)

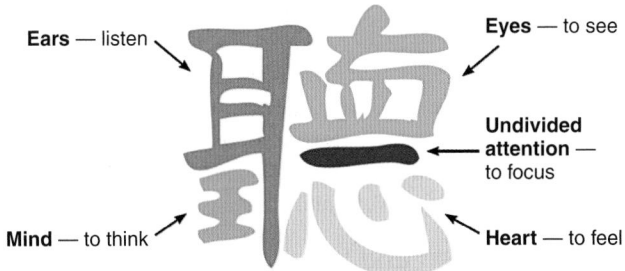

FIG. 10.8 Chinese calligraphy depicting effective communication strategies to promote rapport. (From Salvo, S. [2016]. *Massage therapy: Principles and practice* [5th ed.]. St Louis: Mosby.)

Keep conversation centered on the client's health and problems related to massage. Guide the conversation back if it strays to unrelated topics. To ensure all relevant information for the assessment was gathered, end the interview with an open-ended question such as, "Is there anything else you would like to tell me I have not already asked?" Interview skills develop with continued practice.

Be cognizant of the length of the interview, as most clients, new or established, want to spend the appointment time receiving a massage. Set aside 5 to 7 minutes of time to gather assessments relevant to the treatment plan. A healthy client seeking a relaxation massage will not require a lengthy interview. In contrast, a client with coexisting medical conditions, recent injury, or usual or unexplained symptoms may require a lengthier interview and perhaps special tests or orthopedic assessments (see Chapter 14). If a lengthy intake is part of your paid services, let clients know upfront so they will not be surprised when an hour session results in a 20-minute intake and a 40-minute massage.

PPALM is a mnemonic acronym to remember key assessment questions to ask during the interview. Parts of the mnemonic are

- **P: P**urpose or focus of the massage
- **P: P**ain
- **A: A**llergies and skin conditions
- **L: L**ifestyle, including occupation and physical activity
- **M: M**edical and surgical information.

Purpose/Massage Focus

Ask the client the purpose or focus of the massage. Is it stress reduction or relaxation? Is it pain reduction? A combination of the two? Begin with an open-ended question, such as, "What is your primary goal for today's session?" If this question does not elicit an answer, use a more direct or close-ended question, such as, "Do you need pain relief or stress relief today?" If the massage is provided for therapeutic or palliative reasons, or if the practitioner is working in a healthcare setting, the purpose of the massage is often dictated by the client's physician or healthcare provider managing the client's condition, injury, or disease. The client may also have a prescription for massage. These are retained as part of the client record.

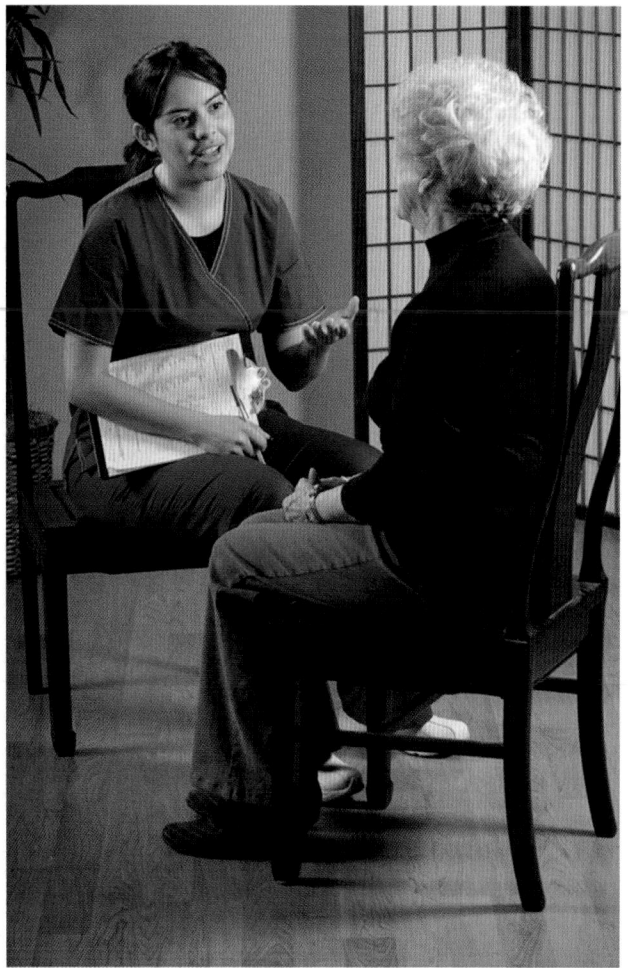

FIG. 10.9 Practitioner seated facing the client at eye level during the interview. (Salvo, S. [2016]. *Massage therapy: Principles and practice* [5th ed.]. St Louis: Mosby.)

Pain

If the client is seeking pain relief, the practitioner can ask questions related to the acronym OPPQRST (Fig. 10.10). OPPQRST stands for the following:

- **O: O**nset—ask "When did it start?"
- **P: P**rovocative—ask "What makes it worse?"
- **P: P**alliative—ask "What makes it better?"
- **Q: Q**uality—ask "How would you describe your pain?"
- **R: R**adiation—ask "Does the pain radiate?"
- **S: S**ite—ask "Where does it hurt?"
- **T: T**iming—ask "How often does it hurt?"

Provocative pain may be explored further by asking "Does it affect your work, sleep, or recreational activities?" "Does it hurt more during movement, during rest, or when you feel anxious?" Timing may be explored further by asking, "Does it hurt more first thing in the morning or at the end of your day?" "How long has it been there?" "Is it there all the time?" These types of questions will give the practitioner clues as to whether the pain is related to physical stress, psychosocial stress, or sustained body postures while sitting or sleeping.

Keep principles of health literacy in mind when speaking with clients. For example, use common terms (e.g., collarbone) along with scientific terms (e.g., clavicle) as you discuss or touch areas on your body containing relevant anatomic structures. *Be sure and read* Chapter 14 *on Clinical Massage if pain management or physical rehabilitation is the primary reason your client is seeking massage as this chapter includes valuable information.*

When asking clients to describe the quality of their pain, you can use the descriptive, numeric, or visual scales mentioned previously. The same scale can be used to keep track of increases and decreases in pain by recording the client's pain levels after the massage and before and after subsequent sessions.

Lifestyle: Occupation and Physical Activity

Ask about the client's occupation and the types of physical activities they participate in regularly. Answers to these questions may uncover potential areas of muscle tension. Use the information in Table 4.1 titled "Types of Occupations, their Activity Levels, and Related Areas of Pain."

Client Allergies and Skin Conditions

Ask about allergies. The practitioner always considers the client's skin reaction to products used. Inquire about past skin reactions from chemicals in laundry detergents and

O	P	P	Q	R	S	T
Onset	**Provocative**	**Palliative**	**Quality**	**Radiation**	**Site**	**Timing**
Ask the client:	Ask the client:	Ask the client:	Ask the client:	Ask the client:	Ask the client:	Ask the client:
• When did it start?	• What makes it worse?	• What makes it better?	• How would you describe the pain?	• Does the pain radiate?	• Where does it hurt?	• How often does it hurt?

FIG. 10.10 Pain questions using OPPQRST.

eliminate contact with linens washed in the detergent identified, if applicable. Also, inquire about allergies to latex and wool. Shea butter contains a latex/protein that people with type B Latex allergies might react to (Grier, 2012). If the client is allergic to these, they may have allergic reactions to shea butter or lanolin, respectively. In these cases, avoid products containing these ingredients and use a hypoallergenic product. Avoid latex gloves on clients who have latex allergies. If the client mentions they have severe allergic reactions such as respiratory distress, ask if the client is carrying an epinephrine auto-injector, such as an EpiPen, and where it is in case it is needed.

Ask your client about skin conditions. Skin conditions that are not bothersome (e.g., psoriasis and eczema) may be overlooked on the client intake form. Noncontagious skin conditions can often benefit from a lubricated massage if the affected skin is not broken. See Chapter 22 for more information about dermatologic pathologies.

Medical and Surgical Information

Ask about current medical conditions and related signs and symptoms—find out your client's experience with the disease. If you are unfamiliar with a particular disease or disorder, look it up in this textbook or a reliable information source.

Inquire about how the client is managing any medical conditions, such as medications. If the client is taking medications, ask about medication side effects and routes of administration and factor this information into the treatment plan (see Chapter 3 of *Mosby's Pathology for Massage Professionals* for more information).

Ask about any past surgeries. Surgical considerations are in Chapter 14.

Massage Experience

It is also helpful to ask the client about their past experiences with massages. If a regular client, ask about responses to recent sessions. If a new client, ask if they have ever received a massage and, if so, ask about massage preferences including pressure preferences. Use this information during treatment planning.

Body Language and Nonverbal Communication

Some client communication is nonverbal. For example, the way a client answers a question, their tone, volume, enthusiasm, apprehension, frustration, and body movements convey meaning behind spoken language. James Borg, author of *Body Language: 7 Easy Lessons to Master the Silent Language*, stated human communication is 93% body language, and much of it is expressed nonverbally. Ways body language manifests itself include (1) facial expressions such as grimaces, frowns, puckers, rapid blinking, yawning, and eye contact; (2) gestures such as making fists, fidgeting, looking up or down or side to side; (3) mannerisms and idiosyncrasies such as tapping fingers while talking or twirling strands of hair when anxious; (4) vocal cues such as hmm and uh-huh, as well as sounds such as sighs, grunts, and groans; and (5) posture and position in relation to others (i.e., when one individual is positioned higher than another, either while sitting or standing, which may imply the higher person is more important or has more power than the other).

Remember the client is also "reading" your body language, consciously or subconsciously. You may be perceived as insincere if you speak in a way implying the client is important but behave in a way conveying a different message as you glance at your mobile phone or rifle through papers as if bored or a hurry. How will clients react if your body language says you are tired when you greet them, distracted during the interview, or impatient to start the treatment? Nonverbal messages are often less conscious and are therefore perceived as more honest. Some linguists argue nonverbal behavior such as gestures and body movements are primitive forms of speech, whereas verbal language takes thought and puts it into linear digital form, that is, a sentence. Gestures and body movements can display instantaneous thought.

CONSENT FORM

The consent form is the form signed by the client giving consent to receive a procedure. The overarching principle is called **informed consent**, permission given by a client to receive treatment after they have been informed of all relevant facts. Items on the consent form include, but are not limited to, the practitioner qualifications, procedural details such as products, techniques, draping, potential benefits and risks or adverse effects of treatment, cost of services, scope of practice, office policies, client rights, and protection of client privacy. Clients may feel vulnerable when undressed and draped or when lying down, so discussions need to take place when clients are appropriately dressed and seated or standing to permit eye contact.

Three essential elements of informed consent include:
- **Full Disclosure of Information.** Individuals must be adequately informed about the treatment they are subjecting themselves to, including potential benefits and risks associated with treatment.
- **Voluntary Nature of the Decision.** The decision to receive treatment must be voluntary. Restated, individuals should not be pressured or coerced into making treatment decisions.
- **Competency of the Individual.** Individuals must be competent to express their decisions about treatment. Individuals must be capable of understanding the information presented and the consequences of those decisions. A non-competent individual, such as a child, may receive treatment if the parent or legal representative gives consent on the non-competent individual's behalf.

In most states, individuals 18 years old and older can legally consent to therapeutic procedures such as medical and/or psychiatric treatments. Age of consent for nontherapeutic or procedures such as those received in spas and some private practice settings is usually 16, but this age varies from state to state and is determined by the age a new driver can receive a driver's license. Also, an individual under the age of 18 is no longer considered a minor if married, pregnant, is a parent themselves, or is legally emancipated.

Responsible parties must explain services and treatments clearly, without technical or confusing terms, before the client signs the consent form. This responsibility might include describing procedures and answering questions in the client's preferred language using translation software or applications. As stated in the previous section on health literacy, forms are written at appropriate reading levels for all clients, which is currently between eighth- and ninth-grade levels. Moreover, clients must be notified if new information emerges which might affect treatment.

Be mindful of the client's cultural or religious practices which may affect treatment such as products used or services provided. For example, it may be inappropriate for a client to be touched by someone of the opposite sex without certain conditions being met, such as the presence of a spouse or other appropriate person. Next is a discussion of content areas within the informed consent document.

Practitioner Qualifications

Inform the client of the practitioner's qualifications such as formal education, knowledge accumulation from professional development (also called continuing education), areas of specialization, state licenses or board certificates held, and professional affiliations such as membership in trade organizations.

Procedural Details

Discuss procedures, techniques, and methods used. If the client has never received a massage before, spend time explaining procedures because they will not have previous experiences from which to draw. Procedures include disrobing, how the client's personal items are stored and secured, draping procedures, and the location of toilets. Clients have varying levels of comfort with disrobing, so allow clients to remain partially clothed if it is their wish. Discuss massage methods used such as myofascial and lymphatic massage. Discuss the importance of communication and feedback during massage, especially with applied pressure not exceeding the client's pain threshold. Pain threshold is the *minimum intensity* perceived as painful. In contrast, pain tolerance is the *maximum intensity* perceived as painful and any more would be unbearable and intolerable. Pain threshold and pain tolerance levels are subjective experiences unique to each individual.

Discuss the use of handheld tools such as stones, cups, or scraping instruments used to apply massage techniques, or materials such as hot or cold packs used to apply hydrotherapy. If massage lubricants are used, have ingredient lists available if they are requested by the client.

Potential Benefits

Discuss potential benefits of massage and other methods used during treatment to help clients achieve their goals.

Past scientific investigations found massage lowered stress, reduced stress perception, increased relaxation, reduced lower back pain, reduced jaw pain, decreased arthritis pain and stiffness, reduced tension headache pain, decreased fatigue, reduced anxiety and depression, decreased heart rate and blood pressure, increased joint range of motion, accelerated recovery after muscle injuries, supported tendon injury healing, decreased delayed-onset muscle soreness, improved scar formation, reduced adhesion-related pain, improved sleep quality, and reduced sleep difficulties.

Potential Risks: Side Effects and Adverse Effects

Massage is not entirely risk-free (Posadzki & Ernst, 2013). An essential aspect of the consent process is the disclosure of potential risks such as side effects. Also, disclose rare but harmful adverse events. The main adverse events associated with massage are disc herniation, neurologic compromise, spinal cord injury, and dissection of the carotid arteries (Yin et al., 2014). Side effects and adverse events were discussed in Chapter 8.

If tools or methods are used (e.g., silicone cups, elastic tape, instrument assisted soft tissue mobilization [IASTM]), their potential benefits and risks (such as bruising or skin rash) must be included in the consent process.

Scope of Practice

Include a statement about the legally defined scope of practice and explain massage practitioners do not diagnose or provide services for which a separate license is required, including medicine, chiropractic, physical, or occupational therapy, podiatry, and cosmetology. Some consent forms include a statement indicating if services needed to fulfill the client's treatment goals are beyond the scope of practice, a referral to an appropriate provider can be made.

Office Policies

Disclose fees for services and forms of payment accepted. Include your policy for insufficient fund transactions. Discuss policies for canceled or missed appointments.

Client Communication and Information Use

Ask clients how they prefer to be contacted (e.g., phone, text, email). A client communication form is on Evolve. Inform clients how you prefer to be contacted and how to schedule future appointments.

Let clients know how copies of their files can be obtained (e.g., document release form), how long these files are kept once treatments are complete or services discontinued (e.g., 4 years minimum is recommended by the NCBTMB [2017]), and how these records will be destroyed at this time (e.g., shredded). Disclose circumstances in which client information can be released without prior client authorization. These include consultations, medical emergencies, court proceedings, insurance filing and billing, collections, complaints, and suspected child or elder abuse.

Rights of Refusal

The client has the right to refuse unwanted treatment or if they feel unsafe, even with prior consent. The client can request a technique be modified if they feel the pressure is too deep or too light. The client also has the right to request a technique be stopped or simply not performed.

The practitioner can also refuse treatment of an area or postpone treatment if the client has contraindications, expresses sexual comments or makes sexual advances after being asked to stop, or makes the practitioner feel unsafe.

Client Gives Consent

After a competent client or client legal representative has been adequately informed of the relevant facts related to treatment, the client can voluntarily consent. Give the client or legal representative the opportunity to ask questions and receive answers before obtaining a dated signature on the consent form. Some practitioners ask the client to initial each section within the consent form. Keep the original signed and dated form and give the client a copy of the form for their records.

TREATMENT PLANNING

Treatment planning is the documented process by which the practitioner or healthcare team plans an appropriate treatment or course of treatment for a client. The treatment plan, also called the session note, paints a picture of what occurred during client-practitioner interactions. There is a movement toward *evidence-informed practice (EIP)*, a problem-solving approach used when making treatment decisions that integrate relevant evidence, the client's preferences, and the practitioner's professional expertise. EIP is discussed in Chapter 5. The treatment plan also takes into account information gathered on the completed intake form and during the client interview, standards of care, client safety and safe practice procedures, and scope of practice. **NOTE**: Postsurgical and soft tissue injury massage modifications are in Chapter 14.

The Role of Evidence

Evidence, in this context, includes research articles found in scholarly and academic literature such as peer-reviewed journals. Most practitioners use Internet search engines to locate relevant research. Search engines use keywords to retrieve articles by looking for these words within the title, abstract, or body of the published work. Be sure to check the web address or URL (Uniform Resource Locator) as this suggests the credibility of the source. First, look at the three-letter extension. In the United States, common extensions of credible websites are .edu for educational websites, .gov for governmental websites, and .org for organizational websites. Try to avoid .com and .net, as these are often commercial websites published by for-profit businesses. If a .com site mentions a research study, search for the original study.

Although all research evidence is valuable, some studies are given more "weight" when informing a treatment plan.

The evidence ranking system is often denoted by a pyramid, with the strongest evidence at the peak and the weakest evidence at the wide base (see Fig. 5.3). Higher levels indicate stronger evidence and that bias was less likely to influence the results of the study. Lower levels indicate weaker evidence and that bias could have influenced the study's results.

Treatment Planning and Evidence-Informed Practice: PICO

Practitioners of EIP often use a framework, called PICO, to form a question about a specific client problem and search for relevant evidence via the Internet that will help the client achieve the desired treatment outcome. The results of the search are collected and organized into a data table (see Table 10.1), and the strength of the evidence (e.g., systematic reviews [SR] and randomized control trials) is noted, as well as if two or more studies yield similar outcomes. If the Internet search does not yield sufficient results, the practitioner may refine the question, conduct another Internet search, or consider an alternative treatment. Once the search is complete, the practitioner blends the client's preferences and their professional expertise and formulates an appropriate treatment plan. The treatment plan is implemented, and its outcome is evaluated for effectiveness. PICO stands for:

- **P: Patient/Client or Population**. Who is the patient (client) or population of interest?
- **I: Intervention**. What intervention is being considered? Massage is very likely the intervention, but there may be others such as reflexology, aromatherapy, acupressure, and hydrotherapy.
- **C: Comparison or Control**. Are alternative interventions being considered? C is not always needed in the PICO method. If the practitioner has additional training and expertise such as yoga or personal training, other interventions may be considered, which may be provided by the massage practitioner or may require referral to other service providers.
- **O: Outcome of Interest**. What is the desired outcome(s)? Is it symptom reduction such as decreased pain? Increased function such as range of motion? Stress reduction or relaxation? A client may request multiple outcomes, which are included in PICO.

Some formulae include one or more Ts, which may stand for time element, type of question, or type of study. Not all questions can be answered using the PICO method and evidence may not be available to inform your treatment plan. In these cases, the practitioner may rely more heavily on their professional expertise, including past treatment decisions, and their outcomes.

Formulating an Evidence-Informed Treatment Plan: A Step-by-Step Approach

Here are the six steps of creating an evidence-informed treatment plan mentioned previously.

1. Identify the problem.
2. Formulate a question using P-I-C-O.

TABLE 10.1 Example of a Data Table

Citation	Outcome, Intervention, and Notable Details
Wasserman et al. (2016). Chronic caesarian section scar pain treated with fascial scar release techniques: A case series.	Thirty minutes of scar tissue massage improved pressure tolerance and scar mobility, and decreased premenstrual pain Four sessions administered over 2 weeks Techniques included scar stretching until release of tissue tension was felt by practitioner Case series (Level 4)[a]
Wasserman et al. (2018). Soft tissue mobilization techniques are effective in treating chronic pain following cesarean section: a multicenter randomized clinical trial.	Thirty minutes of soft tissue mobilization over the abdomen reduced abdominal pain pressure threshold and improved scar mobility Four sessions were administered over 3 weeks Techniques included skin stretching and skin rolling Randomized control trial (Level 1)[a]
Kelly et al. (2019). Soft tissue mobilization techniques in treating chronic abdominal scar tissue: A quasi-experimental single-subject design.	Thirty minutes of soft tissue mobilization over the abdomen reduced abdominal pain pressure threshold Four sessions were administered over 4 weeks Techniques included skin stretching and skin rolling Case series (Level 4)[a]
Wasserman et al. (2019). Wasserman, J. B., Copeland, M., Upp, M., & Abraham, K. (2019). Effect of soft tissue mobilization techniques on adhesion-related pain and function in the abdomen: A systematic review.	Soft tissue mobilization reduced adhesion-related pain in post-surgical and nonsurgical cases Techniques included massage and myofascial release Most sessions were 15–30 min administered once or twice weekly for 6–8 weeks Systematic reviews (Level 1)[a]

[a]Strength of the evidence.

3. Search for, collect, evaluate, and synthesize the evidence.
4. Create a treatment plan by integrating evidence, client preferences, and practitioner expertise.
5. Implement the plan.
6. Evaluate the outcome.

Let's look at one example of how to create an evidence-informed treatment plan for after a C-section procedure. If you use a general Internet search engine such as Google, include the word "research" to your list of keywords to get the kind of search results you need. Remember to focus on studies on websites with the extensions .edu, .gov, and .org.

Step 1: Identify the Problem
A client who delivered a child by cesarean (C) section a year ago wants to reduce adhesion-related pain with massage.

Step 2: Formulate a Question Using P-I-C-O
"Does massage (intervention) reduce adhesion-related pain (outcome) after a C-section in postpartum females (population)?"

Step 3: Search for, Collect, Evaluate and Synthesize the Evidence
When searching for evidence on the Internet, you might use keywords such as adhesions, abdominal, childbirth, postpartum, cesarean, and surgery for P (patient/population), massage, myofascial release, and friction for I (intervention), and pain for O (outcome). Add the keyword research if using Google or general Internet search engines. Table 10.1 provides an example of a data table.

Next, synthesize the evidence. Four studies found that 15 to 30 minutes of abdominal massage techniques was effective at reducing pain and improving function. Most studies administered four sessions over 2 to 4 weeks and included techniques of skin stretching and skin rolling around and along the scar. The other study was an SR, which analyzed several studies, and found massage and myofascial release effective. Sessions averaged 15 to 30 minutes in length and were administered once or twice a week for 6 to 8 weeks in total.

Step 4: Create a Treatment Plan by Integrating Evidence, Client Preferences, and Practitioner Expertise
Fifteen to 30 minutes of abdominal massage using skin stretching, skin rolling, and deep perpendicular pressure along the C-section scar will be administered to the client during the session. The client will be encouraged to schedule one to two sessions per week for a total of 4 to 8 weeks.

Step 5: Implement the Plan
Stated above.

Step 6: Evaluate the Outcome
The practitioner used a numeric scale to measure levels of pain pre- and post-treatment and recorded the outcome. In this case, pain levels went from a numeric value of 7 to a value of 4 after four weekly sessions. Visual or descriptive scales can also be used to evaluate the outcome.

If the client exhibits or discloses any of the following conditions, it may be related to an underlying unidentified pathologic process. Encourage the client to seek evaluation from their primary healthcare provider.
- Unexplained weight loss.
- Abnormal bleeding from any orifice.
- Unexplained inflammation.
- Shortness of breath.
- Unexplained persistent fatigue.
- Changes in body function (sleep, eating, bowel, etc.).

Home Care

Unless restricted by scope of practice in the state in which you will be or are licensed, you can suggest home care activities to help clients achieve their goals. Teaching client activities that improve outcomes is an important part of treatment planning and empowers them to take control of their own health. These self-care activities are done between scheduled appointments. Suggest an activity that would fit easily into the day and would tie into something the client does daily. For example, suggest sleeping with the cervical spine in a neutral position to reduce neck pain.

For stress management, recommend diaphragmatic breathing or progressive muscle relaxation. Progressive muscle relaxation is based upon the practice of tightening one muscle group at a time for 5 to 10 seconds followed by a relaxation phase of 10 to 20 seconds before tensing another muscle group. For pain management and improved function, perhaps suggest self-massage, applications of heat, and body movements such as joint mobilizations and stretching.

When teaching body movements, explain and demonstrate the movement, ask the client to mirror the movement back to you, and ensure the client is doing it correctly. If body movements are performed bilaterally, ask the client to complete the movement on both the left and right sides of the body.

Subsequent Sessions

Prepare for the client's subsequent sessions by reviewing your past treatment plans. Begin the interview by asking about responses to the prior massage. If the client sought pain management, ask about any changes (better or worse) in the frequency, intensity, or duration of pain. If the client sought stress management, ask if an increase in relaxation and a decrease in anxiety occurred.

Update the client record by asking if there are any changes in the client's health status since the last session. Finally, inquire about goals for today's session. Answers to these questions will help you decide if the last session was well received and whether the treatment plan should be repeated or if modifications are needed.

Help Clients Achieve Their Goals

Keep the client's treatment goals clearly in mind. It is difficult to know, given the variable of client response, how often and how many massages may be needed to achieve the client's desired results. In general, the initial period consists of frequent sessions, tapering off as symptoms subside and goals are achieved. Goals expressed in functional terms (i.e., massage needed to increase ROM in the right shoulder) are necessary when documenting client progress.

Ideally, you hope to see an increase in flexibility and ROM and a decrease in the frequency and severity of symptoms, most notably pain.

Remind the client about self-care activities they can do at home such as ice packs, stretching, and self-massage, so that the client takes responsibility for maintaining progress.

Realize that a 100% return of function and complete freedom from pain is not possible in all cases. Sometimes 50% improvement is tremendous progress. The purpose of massage is to benefit the client and meet their needs, not to meet the expectations of the practitioner. A practitioner who is mindful of this is truly a professional.

TREATMENT PLAN DOCUMENTATION FORMATS

Popular treatment plan formats are SOAP notes and FDAR notes and contain the client's focus or treatment goal, subjective and objective information, the treatment provided, and the outcomes of the treatment. Which format is used often depends on the facility or business where massage services are provided or the practitioner's preference. Important factors to consider when choosing a documentation format are (1) does it collect all relevant information and (2) does it allow ease of use?

Subjective information is obtained from the client, written or spoken. It is based on or influenced by opinions, attitudes, feelings, and beliefs the client has about pain and stress, and other symptoms. When recording subjective information, include brief quotes the client makes regarding the location and when symptoms started, their duration, what makes it better or worse, what has been done to treat it until now, and the results of those treatments.

Objective information the practitioner observes or measures and can be verified. This can include range of motion, measuring the circumference of a swollen ankle, behaviors made by the client such as holding the right hip while walking or grimacing while raising the arm overhead, and other signs.

If a client states their height and weight the information is subjective. If the practitioner uses a tape measure and a scale to determine the client's height and weight, the information is objective. Keep in mind if the client tells you of any test results, this would be regarded as subjective information. If the client gives you a document containing test results, the document would be regarded as objective information.

SOAP Notes

SOAP notes are a task-oriented approach to documentation and were originally designed to be used by medical doctors. Over time, SOAP notes were adopted by other healthcare providers (Fig. 10.11). SOAP stands for:

- **S: <u>S</u>ubjective**. Record subjective data.
- **O: <u>O</u>bjective**. Record objective data.
- **A: <u>A</u>ssessment**. Record the diagnostic code provided by the client's healthcare provider and a summary of the session. Originality, this section was the physician's diagnosis.
- **P: <u>P</u>lan**. Record plan of care such as frequency and focus of future massage sessions, and any home care or referrals.

SOAP NOTES

Client: __John Doe__   Therapist: __Mary Therapist, LMT__

Date: __5/10/12__ Session Type: __SW/DT/MFR__ Duration: __60 min__

Pre-Massage Pain Scale
0 --------------------⑦-- 10
None   Severe

S
Information from client

Ct. c/o Ⓡ sh. Ⓟ 2° yard work
Rec't surgery @ Ⓛ ACL
~ 1 week; seeks ↓Ⓟ + ☰

O
Assessment by therapist

↓AROM @ Ⓡ AC joint; ☰ @ Ⓡ trap
TP's @ Ⓡ mid- + post. delts; ct.
prefers MFR @ Ⓡ ↑trap, Fx @
Ⓡ delts

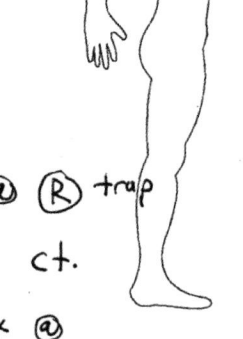

Right   **Front**

A
Summary of session

FB SW w/o Ⓛ knee 2° contra;
DT @ Ⓡ sh. girdle, conc. MFR
@ Ⓡ ↑trap, Fx @ Ⓡ mid +
post delts. ↑PROM post sess,
Δ Ⓟ from 7 to 3

Back   **Left**

P
Treatment plan

↑H₂O intake post sess; return for
60 min sess @ 2 weeks.
HW: AROM Ⓡ sh, stretches +
    moist heat after work

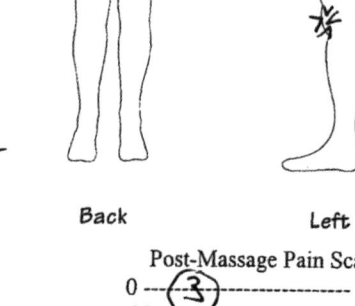

Post-Massage Pain Scale
0 --③---------------- 10
None   Severe

Mary Therapist

FIG. 10.11 Sample SOAP note. This SOAP note includes a numeric pain scale and a body diagram.

The weakness of SOAP notes is inconsistencies on what the "A" and the "P" mean. Some sources say assessment as others say analysis of subjective and objective data. "P" might mean the procedure a client received or the session summary. Other flaws are the inability to document changes over time and SOAP does not explicitly integrate time into its framework.

FDAR Notes

FDAR notes, or focus notes, are a problem-oriented approach used by most healthcare providers. FDAR focuses on a client's specific treatment goal, subjective and objective data, actions taken to address the goal, and the client's response (Fig. 10.12). FDAR stands for:

- **F: Focus**. Record the reason for seeking massage or treatment goals.

- **D: Data**. Record subjective and objective data gathered to conduct pre-massage assessments. Scientific data from research relevant to treatment planning can also be included in this section.

- **A: Action**. Record the action taken to address the client's treatment goals or session summary. This can include home care and referrals, or these can be recorded as a separate entry.

- **R: Response**. Record the client's response to the action performed by the practitioner or the post-massage assessments.

Information is organized into three columns. The first or left column contains the date and the times of pre- and post-massage assessments. The second or middle column contains the client focus. The third or right column contains the progress notes which include data (subjective and objective)

FDAR NOTES

Client name: John Doe   Practitioner name: Mary Smith, LMT

Date/Time	Focus	Progress Notes
Date: 4/1/19 Time: 10:00	Reduction of pain from tension headache	D: Stress or (pain) level BEFORE massage. No stress/pain is "0" and the worst stress/pain you have ever experienced is "10." 0 1 2 3 4 5 6 (7) 8 9 10 Reports dull pain at left temple and base of skull bilaterally
		A: Massage with emphasis on upper back, shoulders, posterior neck, and suboccipital regions of head. Heat pack applied to posterior neck for 10 min
Time: 11:00		R: Stress or (pain) level AFTER massage. 0 1 2 (3) 4 5 6 7 8 9 10 Client states "I feel much better." Ms

Date/Time	Focus	Progress Notes
Time:		D: Stress or pain level BEFORE massage. No stress/pain is "0" and the worst stress/pain you have ever experienced is "10." 0 1 2 3 4 5 6 7 8 9 10
		A:
Time:		R: Stress or pain level AFTER massage. 0 1 2 3 4 5 6 7 8 9 10

FIG. 10.12 Sample F-DAR note.

or pre-massage assessments, the action performed, and the client's response or post-massage assessments. Draw a line from the end of the handwritten note to the end of the blank space, and insert your initials at the end of the line in the response section. This line will fill blank spaces and prevent later alterations or additions made to the client's chart. Pain or stress scales can be inserted into the progress note section.

Other Formats: APIE, SOAPIER, and CARE

Other client documentation formats include APIE, SOAPIER, and CARE. APIE arose from the nursing profession and provides an opportunity to evaluate care and decide if modifications are needed. In APIE, the assessment section contains subjective and objective data, as well as the client's diagnosis. Assessment addresses the practitioner's pretreatment conclusions. The plan or treatment plan section states what should be done today and in the near future to address the client's goals. This section is written before the massage begins. The implementation section contains the methods and techniques used during the session. This section is written after the massage. Finally, the evaluation section is the practitioner's determination of the treatment outcome to date. Evaluation addresses the practitioner's posttreatment conclusions.

SOAPIER notes are a combination of SOAP and APIE. SOAPIER stands for subjective, objective, assessment, plan, implementation, evaluation, and review.

CARE stands for condition, action, response, and evaluation. C is the condition of the client, A is the action taken by the practitioner, R is the response of the client to the action taken by the practitioner, and E is the evaluation of the procedure. CARE notes are completed after the session and represent what was done (practitioner action), why it was done (client condition), and how the client responded to the session. The fourth section, Evaluation, is optional and is used to document observations, recommendations, or questions arising from the session.

REFERRING CLIENTS TO THEIR HEALTHCARE PROVIDERS FOR MEDICAL EVALUATION

A **referral** is an act of recommending services or products to help clients achieve treatment goals. When a client presents with signs and symptoms of a possible condition or when a diagnosed condition worsens, it is vital that massage practitioners make a prompt referral to their healthcare provider for medical evaluation. Effective communication between service providers improves client care, strengthens relationships between allied care professions, and promotes the model of complementary and integrative healthcare advocated by the National Institutes of Health (2017).

The practitioner must demonstrate a sensible evidence-informed approach when making a referral, and there needs to be clear documentation of the decision-making process. This type of documentation supports professional behavior

in case the practitioner is accused of behaving unprofessionally or unethically. Documentation includes details about the treatment the client received and its rationale, signs and symptoms that caused concern, what was discussed with the client such as the importance of medical evaluation to exclude their causes, and their dates. If the client chooses not to seek a medical opinion, this should be documented as well.

There are three main methods by which a massage practitioner can refer a client to their healthcare provider to discuss observations and to express concerns.
1. Ask the client to be the communicator.
2. Call the practice or clinic and speak to the client's healthcare provider or a staff member.
3. Write a letter to the client's healthcare provider.

Client as Communicator

The most common method is to ask the client to communicate with the healthcare provider. In this scenario, the client is instructed to make an appointment and explain the signs and symptoms causing the massage practitioner's concern. The healthcare provider then decides if testing is needed so the presence of a problematic condition can be omitted or confirmed. This is a good option as long as the client understands the necessary information and can communicate effectively.

Calling the Clinic

Another method is calling the practice or clinic of the client's healthcare provider. This is the preferred method of communication if the situation is somewhat urgent or if there is a matter of some complexity that needs to be discussed. Many healthcare providers are happy to discuss a problem concerning one of their patients over the telephone. It is a normal practice for healthcare providers to return telephone calls related to their practice at a particular time of the day. Also, keep in mind the healthcare provider you are speaking with may be the person on-call and not know the client, so be able to provide enough detailed information so they can make informed professional decisions about how to proceed.

Writing a Letter

A letter is an appropriate method of referring a client in non-urgent situations. A letter can also precede or accompany the client who has made an appointment with a healthcare provider. However, letter writing is the most time-consuming method for both the massage practitioner and the client's healthcare provider—this process involves typing, editing, possible printing, and sending. Referral letters should be confined to less than one page in length. Be sure the letter has a heading that includes the name of the referring massage practitioner, professional titles and qualifications, address, telephone numbers, fax number, e-mail address, and website address. The date of the referral is also listed.

When communicating with a healthcare provider about a shared patient/client, the practitioner needs to inform the client in advance about the content of the letter or conversation and ensure the client has given consent to their information about to be disclosed to a third-party.

Referral Letter: Structure and Content

Information in the referral letter includes:

- Client identifiers such as their full name, date of birth, and physical address.
- A brief one-sentence statement of the reason for the referral.
    - For example, "I would appreciate if you would assess Mrs. Smith, who is 33 years old and in her second trimester of pregnancy, presents with facial and widespread edema, and complains of recurrent severe headaches and occasional spots before her eyes."
- A brief historical synopsis of key events related to the situation including:
    - Symptoms described by the client with their dates.
- Signs noted by the practitioner during health assessments with their dates.
- Summary of medications the client is currently taking, if applicable.
- List of relevant lifestyle factors, such as smoking and occupational factors, such as what the client does for a living which might have impacted the situation.
- If appropriate, description of how the client has been treated and how they have responded to massage.

E-RESOURCES

http://evolve.elsevier.com/Salvo/MassageTherapy

- Chapter challenge
- Flash cards
- Technique videos
- Additional information
- Downloadable forms

MILTON TRAGER

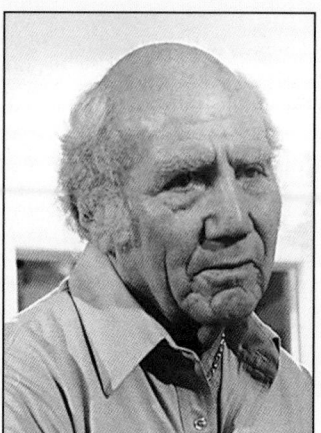

Breathe. It is such a simple action, is it not? We breathe all day, every day. We breathe in our sleep. We sigh and snore and snort and sing. Eventually, we quit breathing for good, and we die. Breath is one of the most fundamental components of life, and yet we usually ignore it unless something has gone wrong. But for Milton Trager, one breath triggered a lifetime of work that was simultaneously revolutionary and as natural as breathing.

Trager was born in 1908 and had an unremarkable childhood. He dropped out of high school and lied about his age to get a job in the post office. It was hard work and could have been the first of many such back-breaking jobs had it not been for the health tip posted for employees one day. The paper instructed him to breathe deeply. He obeyed. At that moment, Trager became aware of his body for the first time. He later said of that moment, "It was the beginning of me."

Inspired, Trager began his personal journey into the world of physical wellbeing. He started working out at the beach, getting stronger, and practicing acrobatics as he listened to the constant rush of the waves. He took up boxing, working with a trainer to develop his skills, strength, and agility. One day, he offered to give his trainer a massage and discovered he had a natural talent for easing aches and pains. He went home to massage his father, who suffered from sciatica. There, too, he was successful.

Trager enlisted with the Navy Medical Corps, then decided to pursue the study of medicine. Unfortunately, there was no medical school in the United States that would accept a 42-year-old student. Determined to earn his credentials anyway, Trager and his wife moved to Guadalajara, Mexico, where he completed medical school.

Upon moving back to the United States, Trager found it very difficult to establish a medical practice but finally settled in Honolulu, Hawaii. He continued to develop his approach, which consists of nonintrusive movements designed to calm the body and gently encourage it to function in a healthier, more mobile, and pain-free way. Some of these movements include holding and gently rocking the body in a pattern reminiscent of the waves Trager once listened to on the beach as a young man.

Although trained in medicine, Trager never felt such training was necessary to practice as he did. Instead, the Trager approach places great emphasis on the importance of what has been called *hook-up,* or a degree of focus enabling the practitioner to be extremely sensitive to the body's cues. This skill can be taught to anyone, not only those with extensive training in the medical sciences.

The recipient's mental state is also given its due in the Trager approach. Trager developed the idea of "mentastics" (a portmanteau of "mental" and "gymnastics"), which are gentle movement exercises helping a client re-experience positive mental shifts experienced during a session. Mentastics can be done anywhere and does not require a practitioner's assistance. This helps healthier patterns take hold in the client's life.

The Trager Institute was founded in 1980, and Trager continued to share his approach until his death in 1997. Today practitioners all over the world use the Trager approach and mentastics movement education to help clients break free of negative physical and mental patterns and achieve their full potential.

REFERENCES

American Massage Therapy Association (AMTA). (2020). *Massage profession research report*. Retrieved from https://www.amtamassage.org/scr/Operating-Your-School/Massage-Profession-Research-Report—-Schools-Version.html.

DuBay, W. H. (n.d). *Know your readers*. Retrieved from http://www.impact-information.com/impactinfo/literacy.htm.

Federation of State Massage Therapy Boards (FSMTB). (2021). *States that regulate massage*. Retrieved from https://www.fsmtb.org/consumer-information/regulated-states/.

Grier, T. (2012). Is there cross-reactivity between shea butter and natural rubber latex? American Latex Allergy Association, Alert Newsletter.

International Association for the Study of Pain (IASP). (2020). *IASP announces revised definition of pain*. Retrieved from https://www.iasp-pain.org/publications/iasp-news/iasp-announces-revised-definition-of-pain/.

Moffett, P., & Moore, G. (2011). The standard of care: Legal history and definitions: The bad and good news. *The Western Journal of Emergency Medicine, 12*(1), 109–112.

National Certification Board for Therapeutic Massage and Bodywork (NCBTMB). (2017). *Standards of practice: Standard of confidentiality*. Retrieved from https://www.ncbtmb.org/standards-of-practice/.

Posadzki, P., & Ernst, E. (2013). The safety of massage therapy: An update of a systematic review. *Focus on Alternative and Complementary Therapies, 18*(1), 27–32.

Yin, P., Gao, N., Wu, J., Litscher, G., & Xu, S. (2014). Adverse events of massage therapy in pain-related conditions: A systematic review. *Evidence-Based Complementary and Alternative Medicine: eCAM, 2014*, 480956.

REVIEW AND APPLY YOUR KNOWLEDGE

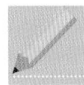 **MATCHING ONE: CONCEPT REVIEW**

Place the letter of the answer next to the number of the term or phrase that best describes it.

A. Assessments
B. Documentation
C. Informed consent
D. Delegation
E. Document release form
F. Standard of care
G. Objective
H. Action
I. Scope of practice
J. Subjective
K. Treatment planning
L. Double lock

_____ 1. Information obtained from the client and is based on or influenced by their opinions, attitudes, feelings, and beliefs.

_____ 2. Level and type of care a reasonably competent and skilled professional provides who has similar training and works under similar circumstances.

_____ 3. A way to safeguard client information is by applying the _____ rule.

_____ 4. The process of collecting, confirming, and recording information.

_____ 5. Documented process in which the practitioner or healthcare team plans an appropriate treatment or course of treatment for a client.

_____ 6. Document used by companies or individuals to legally share client information with a third party.

_____ 7. Permission given by a client to receive treatment after being made aware of all relevant facts related to treatment.

_____ 8. In FDAR notes, what the letter "A" represents.

_____ 9. Assessment-based information that is measurable and verifiable.

_____ 10. Assignment of a task or task completion from one person to another person.

_____ 11. Evaluations of an individual's health status, stress or pain levels, levels of function pre- and post-treatment, and presence of possible massage contraindications.

_____ 12. Activities and procedures that can be performed legally by members of a licensed profession.

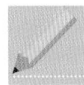 **MATCHING TWO: CONCEPT REVIEW**

Place the letter of the answer next to the number of the term or phrase that best describes it.

A. Verbal descriptor scale
B. Referral
C. Acupuncture, psychotherapy
D. Visual analog scale
E. Home care
F. Close-ended
G. Response
H. Rapport
I. Open-ended
J. Health literacy
K. PICO method
L. Communication

_____ 1. Process used to develop a question by identifying client characteristics or problems, desired treatment outcomes, and interventions that are being considered to achieve the desired treatment outcome.

_____ 2. Activities outside a massage practitioner's scope of practice.

_____ 3. Act of exchanging information through verbal and nonverbal messages.

_____ 4. Emotional bond that people experience when concerns, feelings, and ideas are mutually expressed.

_____ 5. Questions with little restriction when answering.

_____ 6. Series of descriptive phrases such as mild, moderate, and severe to measure pain or stress levels.

_____ 7. Activities performed by the client between scheduled appointments.

_____ 8. Act of recommending services or products to help clients achieve treatment goals.

_____ 9. A straight horizontal or vertical line with the endpoints used to measure extreme limits of pain or stress.

_____ 10. Degree to which an individual has the capacity to obtain, communicate, and understand basic health information and services in order to make appropriate decisions.

_____ 11. Questions that require affirmative, denial, or specific answers.

_____ 12. In FDAR notes, what the letter "R" represents.

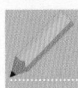

MULTIPLE CHOICE: TEST YOUR KNOWLEDGE

Place the letter of the answer next to the number of the term or phrase that best describes it.

_____ 1. Which of the following provides an objective measure to evaluate differences between standard and substandard care if unsafe practices are suspected?
   A. Scope of practice
   B. Standard of care
   C. Treatment planning
   D. Health literacy

_____ 2. Which of the following is commonly *within* a massage practitioner's scope of practice?
   A. Cosmetology
   B. Chiropractic manipulations
   C. Hydrotherapy
   D. Extractions

_____ 3. Which form is completed by the client and must be updated when the treatment changes?
   A. Document release
   B. Treatment plan
   C. Intake
   D. Consent

_____ 4. The National Certification Board for Therapeutic Massage and Bodywork recommends a minimum of ___ years for recordkeeping.
   A. 2
   B. 4
   C. 6
   D. 8

_____ 5. Prescriptions for massage are typically administered in ___ minute units.
   A. 5
   B. 10
   C. 15
   D. 50

_____ 6. The most common reason clients seek massage is for:
   A. stress reduction.
   B. pain reduction.
   C. improved range of motion.
   D. enhanced sleep.

_____ 7. The "M" in PPALM refers to which of the following?
   A. Medical and surgical history
   B. Massage therapy
   C. Maternal status
   D. Manual lymphatic drainage

_____ 8. Which assessment scale can be used with children or clients with language barriers?
   A. Visual analog
   B. Numeric rating
   C. Verbal descriptor
   D. Wong-Baker FACES

_____ 9. A type of question that confirms a client's response and gives them an opportunity to clarify is a _____ question.
   A. exploratory
   B. reflective
   C. open-ended
   D. close-ended

_____ 10. The "A" in PPALM refers to which of the following?
   A. Action
   B. Assessment
   C. Accommodation
   D. Allergy

_____ 11. Which is the minimum intensity perceived as painful?
   A. Pain threshold
   B. Pain management
   C. Side effect
   D. Adverse effect

_____ 12. Using the FDAR notes method, in which section would a practitioner record the subjective information gathered during the client interview?
   A. Focus
   B. Data
   C. Action
   D. Response

CRITICAL THINKING

I Just Want a Massage

John is a new client and has arrived about 3 minutes before his massage is scheduled to start. You hand him a health history form and ask him to fill it out. He glances quickly at the form and says he doesn't want to and it shouldn't be necessary because he "just wants a massage." How should you proceed?

Answers can include but are not limited to:

Explain to John the health history form is a requirement for your office's record-keeping policies. You may also explain they are required by law if, in fact, your municipality or state massage law requires it. In addition, health history forms give you valuable information you need to perform a treatment customized to his needs. Many conditions require special massage modifications, and you may end up causing him harm if you do not have all the information you need.

Sometimes clients do not want to fill out forms because they may have literacy or visual issues, which they may find embarrassing to speak about. You could say, in the interests of time and wanting to make sure there is adequate time for the massage, you could fill out the form while you do a verbal intake with him.

Occasionally, clients will refuse to fill out health history forms because they may be seeking illicit massage; they do not want any record of them being in your office. Having a health history form is a deterrent for these types of people.

PROFESSIONAL PRACTICE

Scar Tactics

Rebecca is scheduled for a 90-minute massage. On her intake form, she indicates she had surgery on her left anterior knee about 7 years ago. The scar appears hypertrophic (elevated). Rebecca says the knee does not bother her and you can massage it. During the massage, you think the scar could have adhesions. Rebecca is dozing, and you don't want to disturb her so you decide to just start applying cross-fiber friction to the area. Within a minute the scar looks paler and the surrounding skin, in contrast, looks quite reddened. In addition, the scar is swollen and more hypertrophic than it was previously. Rebecca looks at the area and becomes really upset at the appearance. What would have been the best and most ethical approach with Rebecca before the massage started? How would you explain this tissue reaction to Rebecca? Is this type of massage out of your scope of practice? What should you do next?

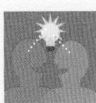

DISCUSSION

HIPAA

HIPAA stands for the Health Insurance Portability and Accountability Act. It outlines privacy standards for healthcare providers.

Use the Internet to find out if HIPAA applies to massage practitioners in your state. Do you agree with the ruling? Why or why not? Does HIPAA apply to professions or to situations? Be specific, and use current, reliable resources to support your answer. What do you feel are the three most important regulations for a massage practice? Why do you feel these are most important?

Some suggested websites are the U.S. Department of Health and Human Services (http://www.hhs.gov) (click Regulations then Health Information Privacy [HIPAA]) and the Centers for Disease Control and Prevention (http://www.cdc.gov) (type in HIPAA under SEARCH).

CHAPTER 11

It is only with the heart that one can see rightly. What is essential is invisible to the eye.

—Antoine de Saint-Exupéry

Special Populations: Massage for Pregnant and Postpartum Clients, Infants, Children, Adolescents, Aging Adults, and Those With Visual, Hearing, and Mobility Impairments

LEARNING OBJECTIVES

After completing this chapter, the student should be able to:

1. Define special populations, disability, and quality of life.
2. Discuss pregnancy massage, state modifications for spa hydrotherapy, and high-risk pregnancies by trimester, for childbirth and the postpartum period.
3. Discuss massage modifications for infants, children, and adolescents.
4. Describe aging and its physiologic effects by body systems with their associated diseases.
5. Identify massage modifications for aging adults and clients with visual, hearing, and mobility impairments, as well as mandatory reporting.

http://evolve.elsevier.com/Salvo/MassageTherapy

INTRODUCTION

Special populations are groups of individuals who are disadvantaged, vulnerable, and/or at risk for harm. Causative or contributory risk factors include physical or cognitive limitations, a life stage, or unique life circumstances that restrict an individual's rights and privileges. Special populations may be individuals who have one or more chronic illnesses, are disabled, have impairments, or require more-than-the-usual healthcare services and/or specialized healthcare services.

A **disability** is an impairment or condition that makes it more difficult for a person to participate in one or more major life activities. Major life activities include, but are not limited to, caring for oneself, performing manual tasks, seeing, hearing, eating, sleeping, walking, standing, lifting, bending, speaking, breathing, learning, reading, concentrating, thinking, communicating, and working. The **Americans with Disabilities (ADA) Act** of 1990 prohibits discrimination of individuals with disabilities and guarantees that these individuals have the same opportunities as nondisabled individuals. This legislation requires most business to provide reasonable access and accommodations for these clients. Indeed, removing architectural barriers improves accessibility for all clients. Examples of removing barriers include a parking with a space for a wheelchair lift, ramps instead of steps at an entrance or within its serving/selling space, aisles wide enough to accommodate mobility devices, lower counters, or restrooms with enough space to allow for mobility devices. Examples of accommodations for clients with visual, hearing, and mobility impairments are discussed later in the chapter. Information regarding tactical athletes (military personnel, first responders) can now be found in Chapter 14.

Aday (1991) states that there are several types of vulnerabilities among special populations: physical, psychological, and social. Special populations with *physical vulnerabilities* include pregnant females and infants; children; the elderly; the chronically, seriously, and terminally ill; the disabled; and those dealing with serious physical injury. Special populations with *psychological vulnerabilities* consist of people with chronic mental conditions, such as schizophrenia, bipolar disorder, and major depression; those with a history of alcohol and/or substance abuse; those who are suicidal; those who are prone to homelessness; and those subjected to major emotional trauma. Special populations with *social vulnerabilities* are persons living in abusive or neglectful families; the homeless; immigrants; minorities; refugees; subcultures such as LGBTQ+ communities; individuals living in poverty or who are economically disadvantaged; and those who are institutionalized. This chapter will address the special population with physical vulnerabilities.

Massage can improve quality of life, especially among special populations. **Quality of life** (QL) is the perception people have regarding their position in life in the context of their culture and value systems, and the degree to which they are able to participate in and enjoy life events. QL has several measurable domains (World Health Organization [WHO], n.d.b):

- **Physical**. This includes energy and fatigue, pain and discomfort, sleep and rest, sexual activity, and somatosensory functioning.
- **Psychological**. This includes bodily image and appearance, positive and negative feelings, self-esteem, and cognitive ability (thinking, learning, memory, concentration).
- **Independence**. This includes mobility, activities of daily living (ADLs), dependence on medicine and medical aids, and the capacity to work.
- **Relational**. This includes interpersonal relationships, social support, and social roles, such as being a provider or caregiver.
- **Environmental**. This includes financial resources, personal and professional freedom, transportation, physical safety, healthcare and social services (access and quality), home and work environments, opportunities to acquire new information and skills, opportunities for and participation in recreation and leisure activities, and physical environment (pollution, noise, traffic, climate).
- **Spiritual/Religious/Personal Beliefs**. This is highly individualized, and there is no single facet of this QL domain.

QL definitions can help us determine which human needs are being met and which are unmet. Massage can improve QL through feelings of comfort, improved mood, reduced stress, enhanced relaxation, decreased pain, improved function, and social connection through compassionate and safe touch.

PREGNANCY MASSAGE

Pregnancy massage is the modification of techniques and body positions to meet the needs of clients as they undergo changes during pregnancy and the postpartum period. Massage is the most used complementary and integrative service among pregnant clients (Field, 2010; Wang et al., 2005). Pregnancy-induced lower back pain is the most common reason pregnant clients receive massage—hip, shoulder, and neck pain and improved mental health are also reasons pregnant clients receive massage (Fogarty et al., 2019). The American Pregnancy Association (n.d.c) encourages the use of massage during pregnancy. Research related to massage during pregnancy and the postpartum period is on Evolve.

The benefits of pregnancy massage can extend to the expectant parent's relationship with the co-parent. Consider inviting co-parents to pregnancy massage sessions and teaching them massage techniques that can be performed at home. Limit techniques that are taught to light effleurage\ petrissage and convey the same precautions licensed practitioners follow, such as avoiding skin lesions. Invite co-parents to make loving statements to both the pregnant client and unborn child or children—this may promote family bonding (Latifses et al., 2005). Family bonding strengthens the shared love and responsibility of new life, which belongs to all parents.

Pregnancy Massage and Spa Hydrotherapy

Pregnant clients can safely engage in sitting in hot baths (104°F [40°C]) or hot/dry saunas (158°F [70°C]) at 15% relative humidity) for up to 20 minutes irrespective of pregnancy stage (Ravanelli et al., 2018). Temperatures or time frames exceeding these guidelines may result in damage to the unborn child. This is also discussed in Chapter 12.

Pregnancy Massage, Essential Oils, and Topical Cannabidiol Products

The use of essential oils appears to be safe during pregnancy, as there have been no reports of abnormal or aborted fetuses from the use of essential oils, either by inhalation or by topical application (Buckle, 2014). In fact, a 70-minute aromatherapy massage using lavender in a 2% solution administered every other week for 20 weeks reduced stress (i.e., reduced salivary cortisol levels) and improved immunity (i.e., increased salivary IgA levels) (Chen et al., 2017). In addition, using cannabidiol (CBD) products, including topical applications, in any form during pregnancy or while breastfeeding is not recommended (U.S. Food and Drug Administration [FDA], 2019). This caution includes topical applications. There is currently no evidence that suggests using these products is safe during this developmentally important time in a person's life.

Massage and High-Risk Pregnancy

High-risk pregnancy is where complications, including disease and death of the mother, the developing baby, or both are more likely. Risk factors include maternal age (<15 and >35 years); carrying multiple babies (twins, triplets, or higher-order multiples); preexisting conditions such as hypertension and human immunodeficiency virus (HIV) infection; and pregnancy-related conditions such as preeclampsia and placenta previa.

Maternal age and carrying multiple babies do not require special massage modifications. However, some pregnancy-related conditions do require modifications (Stillerman, 2008). These conditions and their massage modifications are found in the second and third trimester sections of this chapter.

MASSAGE DURING THE FIRST TRIMESTER

The first trimester is the first 14 weeks of pregnancy. Modifications are made for miscarriage signs and symptoms, deep vein thrombosis (DVT), types of morning sickness, and breast changes.

Miscarriage (Spontaneous Abortion)

Miscarriage is a noninduced embryonic or fetal death, or passage of conception products before 20 weeks of gestation. Approximately 20% to 30% of females with confirmed pregnancies experience vaginal bleeding during this timeframe, and half of these pregnancies spontaneously abort. Incidence rate in all pregnancies is likely higher because some miscarriages are mistaken for late menstruation. In contrast, stillbirth is fetal death after 20 weeks of gestation.

Signs and symptoms of miscarriage are abdominopelvic pain and cramping, vaginal bleeding or spotting, and discharge of tissue. Approximately 90% of miscarriages progress without treatment, but miscarriage can take several weeks. Medications and surgical procedures can be used to help expel uterine contents once miscarriage is confirmed.

Massage and Miscarriage

Massage should be postponed if the client is experiencing signs or symptoms of miscarriage (abdominopelvic pain or cramping, vaginal bleeding or spotting, discharge of tissue), and a referral should be made to the obstetrician or healthcare provider managing the pregnancy. **NOTE:** This restriction is applicable to all trimesters of pregnancy. As the time after miscarriage can be emotionally and physically taxing; a relaxing and nurturing massage is recommended.

There has been an erroneous belief that massage and foot reflexology may cause miscarriage or premature labor and, therefore, put providers at risk for malpractice lawsuits and other litigious events (Embong et al., 2015; Stillerman, 2021). However, there is no scientific evidence that suggests that massage or foot reflexology causes miscarriage or premature labor. In fact, massage and foot reflexology are safe during all trimesters of pregnancy (Fogarty et al., 2019). Agren and Berg (2006) investigated the effects of massage on severe nausea and vomiting among pregnant females in their first and second trimesters; no adverse events were reported. Females with a history of miscarriage are more likely to use complementary and integrative healthcare services such as massage (Huberty et al., 2018).

Furthermore, denying massage services to clients who are pregnant or breastfeeding, or who have recently given birth may be in violation of antidiscrimination laws. Although denying massage services to this population is not explicitly prohibited under current federal law, standards are evolving. Pending federal legislation regarding the Equality Act (2021) would prohibit discrimination on the basis of sex, sexual orientation, gender identity, pregnancy, childbirth, or related medical conditions. If enacted, discrimination against this population would be unlawful, even if the service provider was acting with good intention. Furthermore, denying services to pregnant clients could also be considered unethical, as it violates principles of autonomy or decisional authority, justice, and nondiscrimination.

Deep Vein Thrombosis

DVT is a thrombus or blood clot within a deep vein, usually in the legs (from knee to ankle). Thrombophlebitis occurs when the clot causes inflammation. Because of decreased clot-dissolving properties during pregnancy and increased clot-producing factors, pregnant clients are at a greater risk, five to six times higher, of developing DVT. This risk remains until 10 weeks after childbirth. Typical signs and symptoms of DVT are unilateral leg swelling (may include the ankle and foot), heat, redness or noticeable discoloration, pain, and tenderness. Left-sided DVT is more common during pregnancy than right-sided DVT (Chan et al., 2010).

The most life-threatening acute complication of DVT is *pulmonary embolism* (PE), a partial or complete blocked artery in the lungs. PE may progress to pulmonary hypertension, which may lead to heart failure. DVT/PE affects an estimated 900,000 people each year in the United States. *Venous thromboembolism* (VTE) is a collective term for DVT and PE. VTE and DVT are often used interchangeably.

Massage and Deep Vein Thrombosis

In pregnant clients diagnosed with DVT, avoid the affected lower extremity (e.g., local contraindication). For all other pregnant clients, look for signs and symptoms of DVT (unilateral leg swelling, heat, redness or noticeable discoloration, pain, tenderness). If present, avoid massage to the affected lower extremity. Lastly, a prompt referral should be made to the client's healthcare provider for possible medical testing.

Massage is safe for clients who have or are suspected of having DVT if precautions are taken, such as DVT screening and avoidance of the affected limb (Ng et al., 2018). Case reports have revealed the importance of DVT assessment in expediting DVT diagnosis and treatment (Mallory et al., 2018). **NOTE**: These guidelines are applicable for in all trimesters and continue until 10 weeks postpartum. Leg massage in persons with DVT has been linked to previous adverse events (Behera et al., 2018; Crump & Paluska, 2010; Jabr, 2007; Lim et al., 2009).

Morning Sickness and Hyperemesis Gravidarum

Morning sickness is nausea with or without vomiting during pregnancy. Morning sickness, also called *nausea and vomiting of pregnancy* (NVP), affects approximately 75% of pregnant clients. The term "morning sickness" can be misleading, as nausea can occur any time of the day or night. Morning sickness can begin as early as day 10; it is most prevalent during the first trimester but can occur throughout pregnancy.

Hyperemesis gravidarum (HG) is severe and uncontrollable nausea and vomiting during pregnancy. HG can cause electrolyte imbalance, dehydration, reduced maternal kidney function, and may have adverse fetal consequences. Some cases of HG require hospitalization. Signs and symptoms include severe nausea and vomiting, food aversion, weight loss of 5% or more of pre-pregnancy weight, headaches, dizziness, and decreased urination due to dehydration.

Massage and Morning Sickness/Hyperemesis Gravidarum

Massage is indicated and may reduce symptom severity. A semireclining (semi or standard Fowler), or upright (high Fowler) position while the client is supine will help reduce nausea (Fathi et al., 2014). Avoid techniques that cause the client to rock or shake, because excessive body motion may worsen nausea (Kloter et al., 2019). Consider having a disposable emesis bag in the massage room in case it is needed.

Breast Changes

Breasts undergo changes during pregnancy. Fat accumulates and blood supply increases, causing breasts to enlarge. These changes begin by week 8 of pregnancy. In the third trimester, breasts may leak colostrum (early breast milk) in preparation for their job of providing nourishment. Breasts become heavier and tender. Some clients notice visible veins on their breasts during pregnancy.

Massage and Breast Changes

Position the client for comfort while lying prone if breast tenderness is present. You may offer a cylindrical pillow to be placed under, above, or between the breasts, depending on which position is most comfortable. If a rolled-up towel is used, place it in a pillowcase or beneath the sheet to reduce or prevent terrycloth compression marks on the client's skin. If breast bolstering devices are used, adjust the face rest frame above the level of the table. Several massage table manufacturers offer breast recesses or comfort cushions, which lie on the tabletop. Alternatively, you may use a side-lying position. If the client elects to wear a bra during the massage, modify massage technique to work around the bra.

MASSAGE DURING THE SECOND TRIMESTER

Weeks 15 to 28 make up the second trimester of pregnancy. Many discomforts of the first trimester resolve, and the mother-to-be begins to feel more energetic. While first-time mothers will likely begin to feel the baby move between weeks 18 and 22, this may happen earlier for those who have had previous advanced pregnancies. Modifications for the second trimester are supine hypotensive syndrome, preterm labor, preeclampsia, gestational diabetes, and placenta previa.

Supine Hypotensive Syndrome

Supine hypotensive syndrome is a drop in blood pressure caused by compression of the pregnant uterus against major abdominal blood vessels. The normal anterior curve of the lumbar spine causes it to move toward the abdominopelvic cavity where the enlarging uterus is located. Between the lumbar spine and the pregnant uterus are the inferior vena cava and the abdominal aorta. Gravity keeps the pregnant uterus off these blood vessels when the mother is upright. In the supine position, the uterus may rest against the lumbar spine and compress these blood vessels under its weight. As a result, there is a decrease in venous return from the lower extremities to the maternal heart, causing hypotension. This situation also reduces cardiac output, sometimes by 30%

to 40%. Reduced cardiac output may decrease blood flow to the placenta and cause fetal distress and death to both mother and baby (De-Giorgio et al., 2012). Supine hypotensive syndrome is also called *aortocaval compression syndrome*. Signs and symptoms include dizziness, light-headedness, shortness of breath, pallor, nausea, and agitation; these are usually transient and resolve with a change in positioning.

Massage and Supine Hypotensive Syndrome

To prevent supine hypotensive syndrome, use the left lateral tilt or side-lying positions beginning from week 22 of pregnancy, or earlier if the pregnant client is "showing" (McMahon et al., 2009).

For the left lateral tilt, place a small cushion beneath the right hip while the client is supine in a semireclining position (Fig. 11.1). This position moves the uterus off the abdominal blood vessels and reduces the risk of supine hypotensive syndrome (Fig. 11.2).

For the side-lying position, ask your client to lie on the left side. The American Pregnancy Association (n.d.a) recommends the left side because it helps blood travel from the heart to the placenta and prevents the enlarged and heavy uterus from putting pressure on the liver. Furthermore, there is a connection between those in late pregnancies who slept supine or on their right sides and stillbirth (Gordon et al., 2015; Heazell et al., 2018; Stacey et al., 2011). Although body positions used while sleeping many hours are not the

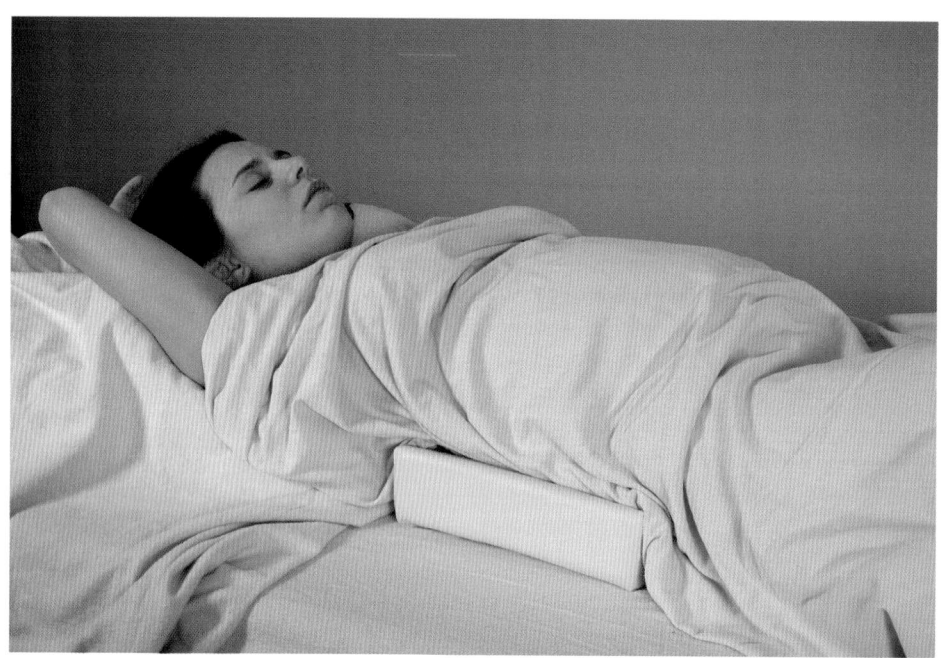

FIG. 11.1 Left lateral tilt: Pregnant clients lying supine should be in a semireclining position with a cushion placed under the right hip. This helps reduce the risk of supine hypotensive syndrome.

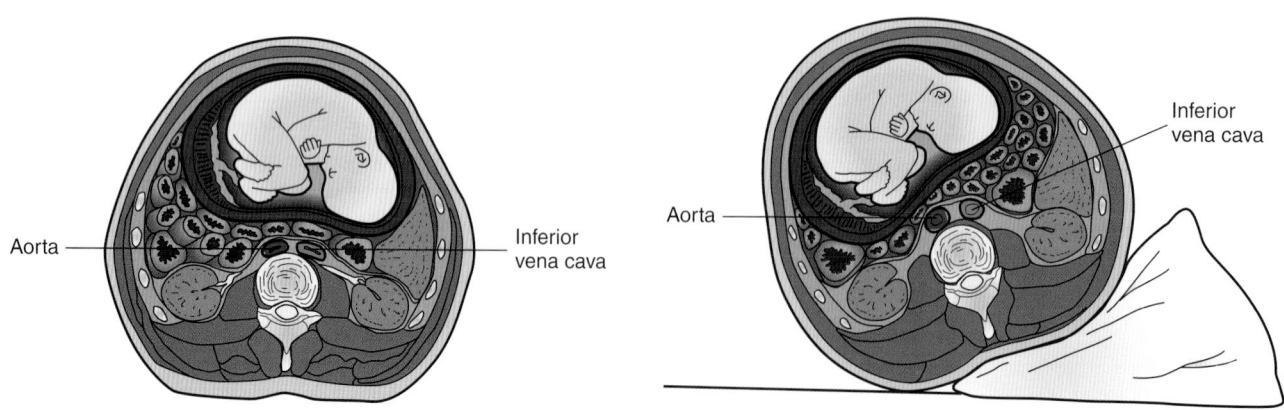

FIG. 11.2 Supine hypotensive syndrome: A supine position may lead to supine hypotensive syndrome, a drop in blood pressure caused by compression of the pregnant uterus against major abdominal blood vessels (*right image*). Place a cushion under the right hip to make use of a left lateral tilt position to reduce the risk of supine hypotensive syndrome (*left image*). (From Lowdermilk, D., Cashion, M. C., & Perry, S. [2012]. *Maternity and women's healthcare* [10th ed.]. St Louis: Mosby.)

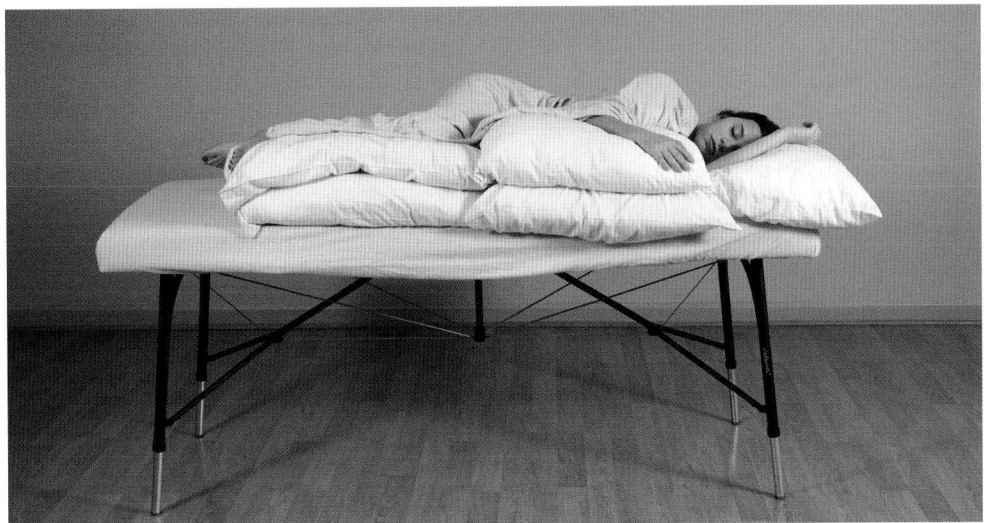

FIG. 11.3 Side-lying position: Pregnant client supported by pillows and cushions.

same as body positions used when receiving a 30-, 60-, or 90-minute massage, it appears the left side is the safest choice for the unborn.

Next, ask the client to slide backward until the hips and shoulders are approximately 4 inches from the table edge. Placing your hands at the appropriate distance helps the client know when to stop sliding back. This client position accomplishes two things. First, it is easier for the practitioner to massage the client's back when it is closer to the table's edge. Second, it provides extra room in front of the client for support pillows placed on the tabletop.

Place the first pillow beneath the client's head. The client's wrist can rest on this pillow. The next pillow is placed in front of the client's chest for the upper arm (arm not lying directly on the table). The next pillow is used for the client's upper leg (leg not lying directly on the table). Ensure that the upper and lower extremities are at the same height (e.g., shoulder, elbow, and wrist at same height— hip, knee, and ankle at same height) (Fig. 11.3). A small pillow or towel roll can be placed below the opposite ankle. The client's spine should be in a neutral position and not rotated once supportive cushions are in place. A supported side-lying position also stabilizes the client and is less likely to roll forward or backward as pressure is applied during the massage. Remove all pillows at the end of the massage before asking the client to get up and get dressed. **NOTE**: These positional modifications are also used in the third trimester.

In addition, several manufacturers offer massage tables with pregnancy recesses or specially designed bolstering systems that lie on the tabletop (Fig. 11.4). These options allow pregnant clients in their second or third trimester to lie safely in the prone position and reduce the risk of supine hypotensive syndrome. A seated position may also be used in the second and third trimesters (Fig. 11.5).

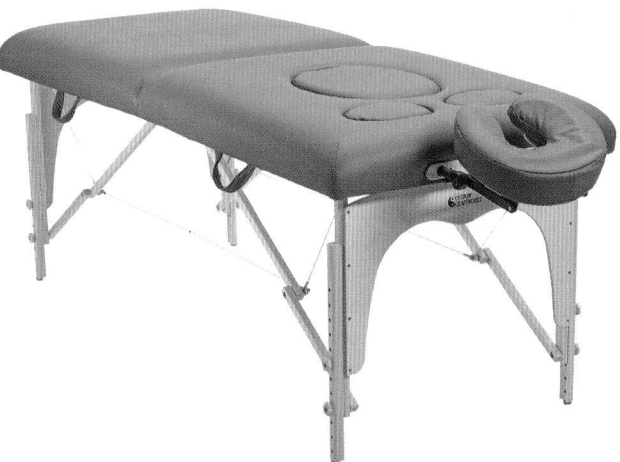

FIG. 11.4 Pregnancy massage table: These tables often have recesses that permit pregnant clients to lie in the prone position.

Preterm Labor

Preterm labor involves regular uterine contractions that result in changes in cervical size (dilation) or its length (effacement) after week 20 of gestation and before week 37. In some cases, the female has contractions but cannot feel them; they are evident only with a fetal monitor. Preterm labor is also called *premature labor*. In some cases, preterm labor causes preterm (premature) birth. The earlier preterm birth occurs, the greater the health risk for the newborn. Health risks are greatest for babies born before week 34. Most premature babies (called *preemies*) need skilled care in the neonatal intensive care unit (NICU). Once preterm labor is confirmed, medication or surgical procedures may slow down uterine contractions. These procedures may delay birth for several hours or days. During this time period, drugs such as corticosteroids may be administered to help the baby's lungs mature before childbirth.

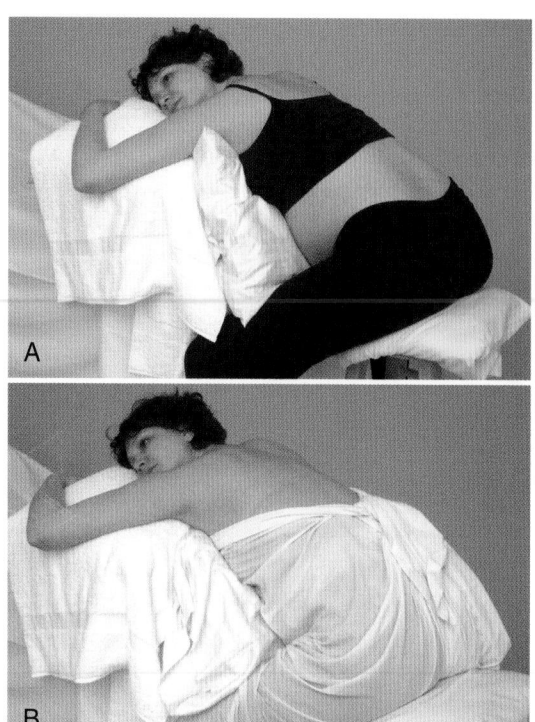

FIG. 11.5 Seated position: Pregnant clients in the second and third trimester can receive seated massage while clothed (A) or disrobed using a secured drape (B). (From Stillerman, E. [2008]. *Prenatal massage: A textbook of pregnancy, labor and postpartum bodywork.* St Louis: Mosby.)

Massage and Preterm Labor

Massage should be postponed if the client is in preterm labor. Massage administered regularly during pregnancy may reduce the risk of preterm labor. Follow all standards of care related to pregnancy massage. The overall effect should be relaxing and nurturing. Massage can be taught to the client's co-parent or caregiver (e.g., client's friend or parent) and administered to the pregnant client at home. In the event of preterm birth, infant massage should be taught to the new parents to promote parent–child attachment behaviors (Shoghi et al., 2018).

Preeclampsia

Preeclampsia is persistent high blood pressure and protein in the urine during pregnancy. Preeclampsia usually develops after 20 weeks of gestation in females with previous blood pressure readings in the normal range. This condition resolves after childbirth. In rare cases, preeclampsia develops earlier than 20 weeks. If left untreated, preeclampsia can lead to serious, even fatal, complications for the mother and unborn. Preeclampsia occurs in 5% to 8% of all pregnancies. Preeclampsia is more common in first pregnancies, those with many prior pregnancies, those who are young or of advanced maternal age, and those who are pregnant with more than one baby. Pregnancy-induced hypertension and toxemia are outdated terms for preeclampsia. Postpartum preeclampsia, a rare condition, develops within 48 hours of childbirth, but it can develop as long as 6 weeks after childbirth.

Eclampsia and HELLP syndrome are complications of preeclampsia. *Eclampsia* is the presence of preeclampsia and seizures. *HELLP syndrome,* a severe form of preeclampsia, stands for **H**emolysis (destruction of red blood cells), **E**levated **L**iver enzymes, and **L**ow **P**latelet count.

The classic triad of symptoms includes hypertension (>140/90 mm Hg), sudden weight gain with generalized edema particularly noticeable in hands, feet, and face (anasarca), and protein in the urine (proteinuria). Some pregnant females with the beginning of severe preeclampsia or impending eclampsia experience severe headaches, and/or changes in vision (spots before the eyes [floaters]).

Massage and Preeclampsia

Massage should be postponed while the client has preeclampsia. In addition, screen the client for preeclampsia starting at week 20. If you notice generalized or widespread edema, severe headaches, and visual disturbances, postpone the massage, and make a referral to the obstetrician or healthcare provider who is managing the pregnancy. **NOTE**: This restriction is applicable for the third trimester.

Gestational Diabetes Mellitus

Gestational diabetes mellitus (GDM) is diabetes that develops during pregnancy in females who did not already have diabetes. Like other types of diabetes, GDM causes high blood sugar (hyperglycemia). GDM occurs between 2% and 10% of pregnancies in the United States annually, and it is more common among females who are obese, are of advanced maternal age, who have a family history of diabetes, and who are non-White. If GDM is not well controlled, it can lead to complications including excessive fetal growth, preeclampsia, preterm birth, and infant respiratory distress syndrome. GDM usually occurs in the second trimester, and most maternal healthcare providers screen for the condition between 24 and 28 weeks of pregnancy, or earlier if risk factors are present. Females diagnosed with GDM have a 50% chance of developing type 2 diabetes mellitus later in life. Most pregnant females are asymptomatic, whereas others experience excessive urination, excessive thirst, and excessive hunger. Malaise and blurred vision may also be present.

Massage and Gestational Diabetes Mellitus

Massage should be postponed until the condition is well managed (determined by the healthcare provider). When cleared for massage, follow all standards of care related to pregnancy massage.

Ask if the client carries a blood glucose meter and, if so, where it is in case it is needed during a possible hypoglycemic episode. Some clients with type 2 diabetes mellitus require insulin by injection. Avoid vigorous massage over sites of recent injection for 24 hours because this may increase absorption rates (Berger et al., 1982; Linde, 1986) and thereby decrease blood glucose levels, possibly causing hypoglycemia. In addition, Tosun et al. (2019) found injection site complications were significantly more common in those who massaged the area after injection. See Chapter 24 for more information about diabetes mellitus. First aid measures for hypoglycemia are discussed in Chapter 9.

Placenta Previa

Placenta previa occurs when the placenta partially or totally covers the cervix, the passageway between the uterus and the vagina. Normally, the placenta grows into the upper part of the uterine wall, away from the cervix. Placenta previa occurs in approximately one in 200 pregnancies. The most common sign of placenta previa is painless vaginal bleeding that is bright red. Some females also experience contractions with vaginal bleeding. In some cases, bleeding does not begin until labor starts and the cervix dilates.

Massage and Placenta Previa

Massage should be postponed until the condition has been resolved or the child is born, and the mother has fully recovered.

MASSAGE DURING THE THIRD TRIMESTER

The third trimester begins from week 29 leading up to birth, which is around week 40. As the baby grows, postural changes in the mother are evident. As a reminder, use a left side-lying position or left lateral tilt position while in the supine position during the third trimester. Discussions in this section include relaxin, gastroesophageal reflux disease, heartburn, lower back pain, uterine ligament pain, edema in the legs, ankles, and feet, varicose veins, and stretch marks.

Relaxin

Relaxin is a hormone that alters the properties of connective tissues by activating collagenase, an enzyme that breaks down collagen and reduces its strength. Relaxin is produced by the ovaries (corpus luteum) and the placenta during pregnancy. In males, relaxin is produced by the prostate and is present in semen. After intercourse, relaxin in semen enhances sperm motility and fertilization. In pregnant females, relaxin relaxes the uterine wall to promote implantation and reduce the risk of miscarriage or premature birth. Toward the end of pregnancy, relaxin helps the cervix relax and dilate, and relaxes pelvic ligaments to assist in childbirth.

Pregnant females have 10 times more relaxin compared with nonpregnant females, and the effects of relaxin remain in the body for 4 to 6 months after childbirth. Relaxin has a slight effect on all joints in the body, which may make them hypermobile. Some clients experience instability or clumsiness while walking; others report pelvic girdle pain from ligament laxity.

Massage and Relaxin

Because of the effects of relaxin on connective tissues, joint mobilizations may need slight modifications, such as supporting beneath the joint with one hand while mobilizing the joint with the other hand. Avoid manual traction of lower extremities, because it may cause separation and pain over the sacroiliac and pubic symphysis joints. This restriction remains in place for 4 to 6 months after childbirth.

Gastroesophageal Reflux Disease and Heartburn

Gastroesophageal reflux disease (GERD) is the periodic regurgitation of gastric contents into the esophagus. The main symptom of GERD is **heartburn** or a burning sensation in the chest or epigastrium behind the sternum. While this feeling is experienced in the area of the heart (hence the name heartburn), it is not related to the heart. This sensation worsens when lying down. Heartburn is also called *indigestion*.

Pregnancy hormones such as relaxin and progesterone relax the lower esophageal sphincter (LES), allowing gastric juice to enter the esophagus. In addition, an enlarged uterus puts pressure on the stomach and pushes its contents into the esophagus. Heartburn most often occurs 30 to 60 minutes after eating or at night. Between 30% and 50% of pregnant individuals have heartburn.

Massage and Gastroesophageal Reflux Disease/ Heartburn

If the client has heartburn, the client should wait 3 hours after consuming a meal before lying down for a massage. Discuss this with your client and consider scheduling the massage appointment accordingly. A semireclining position while supine reduces heartburn symptoms (Mayo Clinic, 2018). A seated position can also be used.

Lower Back Pain and Uterine Ligament Pain

Lower back pain affects between 50% and 70% of pregnant clients during the third trimester. This type of pain is often associated with postural changes such as leaning backward while standing and walking to compensate for the increased abdominal girth. Leaning backward may cause the pelvis to tilt anteriorly, placing strain on the lumbar spine and pelvic joints. Ligaments become softer and stretch due to the presence of relaxin, as mentioned previously.

Sudden, sharp, or jabbing pain can occur from overstretched uterine ligaments during the second or third trimester. Sudden movements can cause these ligaments to tighten quickly and then relax after a few seconds. Uterine ligaments most often involved are the round and broad ligaments.

- **Round ligament.** This arises from the anterolateral surface of the uterus, passes through the groin, enters the labia majora, and terminates at the mons pubis. The round ligament is situated between layers of the broad ligament discussed next. Stretching of the round ligament can refer pain to the groin, abdomen, and/or anterior thigh.
- **Broad ligament.** This is a wide double-layer section of peritoneum that extends laterally from the uterus,

surrounds the ovaries and fallopian tubes, and connects to the walls and floor of the pelvis. Stretching of the broad ligament can refer pain to the lumbar and/or gluteal regions.

Massage and Lower Back/Uterine Ligament Pain

Massage is indicated and was found to reduce back pain in pregnant clients (Field, 2010). Spend massage time on the lower back, the lumbosacral area, and the gluteal area. **NOTE**: If lower back pain is severe or does not subside after the massage, refer the client to the healthcare provider, as this pain may be related to a medical condition such as kidney infection or preterm labor.

If clients experience sudden pain related to uterine ligaments while repositioning or getting on or off the massage table, suggest they lie back slowly and remain there until the pain subsides. After a few moments, ask them to try moving again, but more slowly.

Edema in the Legs, Ankles, and Feet

Edema, or swelling, may occur in the legs, ankles, and feet from several factors: (1) fluid volume increases up to 50% during this time, (2) the enlarged uterus compresses vessels and impairs circulation of blood and lymph in the lower extremities, and (3) pregnancy hormones may contribute to swelling. As legs, ankles, and feet swell, the person may experience feelings of heaviness or tightness, as well as aching or discomfort in the affected or adjoining areas. Edema tends to be more severe at the end of the day and during summer months.

Massage and Edema in the Legs, Ankles, and Feet

For localized edema, place the affected area on cushions to raise it above the level of the heart. Use light pressure effleurage, applied centripetally, and skin stretching. Massage proximal to the affected area first and then proceed distally (e.g., massage the thigh, then the leg, then the ankle, and the foot last) as lymph moves toward the groin in the lower extremities. The recommended pressure to move lymph is approximately 5 g of pressure or about the weight of a nickel. **NOTE**: Mild swelling of the legs, ankles, and feet during pregnancy is normal and not a contraindication for massage. However, widespread swelling requires a referral made to the client's obstetrician or healthcare provider managing the pregnancy as it could indicate preeclampsia. Unilateral leg swelling, especially in the presence of heat, redness, pain, and tenderness, also requires a referral as it could indicate DVT. See prior sections for preeclampsia and DVT.

Varicose Veins

Varicose veins are enlarged veins caused by incompetent vascular valves. Once enlarged, they tend to remain. Pregnant clients may develop varicose veins or find that varicose veins that were present before pregnancy worsen. Factors contributing to varicose veins during pregnancy are increased blood volume combined with decreased blood return—an enlarged uterus compresses blood vessels and impairs blood flow. The compression also increases the pressure in veins within the lower extremities. These factors add to the burden on an already compromised venous system. In addition, progesterone relaxes smooth muscle in blood vessels and dilates peripheral blood vessels, which contributes to the development of varicose veins. Signs and symptoms of varicose veins develop gradually. The person may notice feelings of fatigue or achiness in the legs at the end of the day. The ankles may swell, and there may be leg cramping at night. As the condition progresses, veins appear as bluish-purple lines in the skin, are bulbous and tortuous, and feel hard to the touch. The area may itch. Signs and symptoms worsen after sitting or standing for prolonged periods.

Massage and Varicose Veins

Avoid the affected area during pregnancy and for 10 weeks postpartum because of the increased risk of blood clots within veins.

Stretch Marks

Stretch marks are indented lines or bands from overstretched skin. These are caused by rapid expansion of connective tissue, which leads to skin thinning and atrophy. They can occur from advanced pregnancy and are more common on the abdomen, breasts, hips, buttocks, and thighs. Approximately 50% of pregnant females acquire stretch marks. The likelihood and severity of stretch marks depend on genetic factors, the degree of skin stress from weight gain, and elevated levels of cortisone; the latter weakens elastin fibers within the skin. Stretch marks begin as painless pink, red, purple, reddish brown, or dark brown marks on the skin, depending on skin color; these marks later fade to a silvery color and some appear glossy. Stretch marks may be slightly depressed and have a texture different from normal skin.

Massage and Stretch Marks

Use light pressure over stretch marks, as they are weaknesses in the skin. An example of light pressure is 3 on a 10-point pressure scale. Massage will not reduce or minimize stretch marks because they are not caused by a buildup of collagen as occurs in scar tissue.

MASSAGE, CHILDBIRTH, AND THE POSTPARTUM PERIOD

Childbirth is the process of delivering the baby, placenta, membranes, and umbilical cord to the outside world. There are three stages of childbirth: dilation of the cervix, expulsion of the baby, and expulsion of the placenta. The first stage, often called *labor*, begins with the onset of uterine contractions and continues until the cervix has dilated to approximately 10 cm (4 inches). Rupture of the amniotic sac often occurs during this stage. Next, the uterus contracts and the fetal journey down the vagina begins, which marks the second stage of childbirth. Finally, uterine contractions help expel the placenta or *afterbirth*. Uterine contractions also constrict blood vessels torn during childbirth and delivery to help prevent hemorrhage. Childbirth is also called *parturition* or *labor and delivery*. The time period before childbirth is called the *prenatal period*. The time period that includes both before and after childbirth is called the *perinatal period*. The **postpartum** is the time frame after childbirth and extends for approximately 6 weeks.

The American Pregnancy Association (n.d.b) supports the use of postpartum massage, listing some of the benefits as reduced swelling; increased relaxation; improved sleep; and lowered levels of anxiety, depression, and pain. *Lochia* is the vaginal discharge after childbirth containing blood, mucus, and uterine tissue. Lochia discharge typically continues for 2 to 8 weeks.

Vaginal Childbirth

Vaginal childbirth occurs when the baby, placenta, membranes, and umbilical cord are delivered out of the mother's vagina. Vaginal deliveries make up approximately 69% of childbirths in the United States (CDC, 2021). Most women are discharged and go home 24 to 48 hours after an uncomplicated vaginal delivery.

Massage and Vaginal Childbirths
Massage can begin after vaginal childbirth once the client is medically stable. Medical stability occurs when vital signs such as pulse, temperature, and blood pressure are within normal limits; the client is conscious and comfortable; and the prognosis is good to excellent. Position the client for comfort, which may include extra support for the breasts while in the prone position. The client may elect to leave on undergarments because of the use of menstrual products, such as pads or tampons, because of lochia discharge. Keep disposable menstrual products available in your office for client use.

Cesarean Childbirth

Cesarean childbirth, or *C-section*, is a surgical removal of the baby, placenta, membranes, and umbilical cord through an incision in the abdominal wall (Fig. 11.6). Reasons for cesarean delivery include: multiple babies or a baby who is too large; breech presentation; complications during labor or problems with the placenta; and presence of a maternal viral infection (to prevent transmission to the baby during childbirth). The pregnant person may or may not go into labor. Cesarean deliveries make up approximately 31% of childbirths in the United States (CDC, 2021). Most women are discharged and go home 3 days after an uncomplicated cesarean childbirth. There have been quite a few scientific investigations on the effects of massage after C-section surgery. Results of these investigations are found on Evolve in Chapter 11.

Massage and Cesarean Childbirths
Massage can begin after surgery once the client is medically stable. Communicate with the patient care coordinator if the client is still under medical supervision and follow their directives.

Position the client for comfort. A side-lying position may be needed to avoid pressure on areas containing the recent incisions and drain tubes. Because the client will likely be using menstrual products such as pads for several weeks after childbirth, the client may choose to leave on undergarments. Keep disposable menstrual products available in your office for client use. Avoid vigorous massage techniques on the lower extremities (thighs and legs) for 12 weeks after surgery because of increased risk of blood clots or venous thromboembolism (Kuznar, 2010; Sweetland et al., 2009).

The area near the incisions is avoided until sutures or staples are removed, the area is dry, not moist or open, and into the remodeling (maturation) phase. This may take up to 8 weeks after surgery. See Chapter 14 for more information on tissue healing and scar maturation. Furthermore, the area around the incision should not be manipulated in a way that places stress on it while it is healing. Once the incision is healed, surgical scar tissue massage can begin. Use skin rolling near and directly over the scar with or without lubricant. Massage tissues in several directions (circular, vertical, and horizontal) because scar tissue is arranged haphazardly. Begin with light pressure and progress to deeper pressure. Ask the client about pressure sensitivity and adjust it according to the client's pain tolerance. Discontinue scar tissue massage and refer the client to their healthcare provider if the scar is redder, warmer, or more painful upon subsequent sessions (Moffitt Cancer Center [MCC], 2008).

Clients Who Are Breastfeeding

Breastfeeding, also called *nursing*, is feeding a child with milk from lactating breasts. The breasts undergo many changes during pregnancy and the lactation period. Initially, the breasts may be sore and enlarged as the breastfeeding begins after childbirth. Fluid may leak from breasts between feedings.

Most infants start out breastfeeding (84%), but only about half of infants (58%) are breastfed at 6 months of age (CDC, 2021b). Medical conditions limiting or restricting breastfeeding are rare. However, people who breastfeed

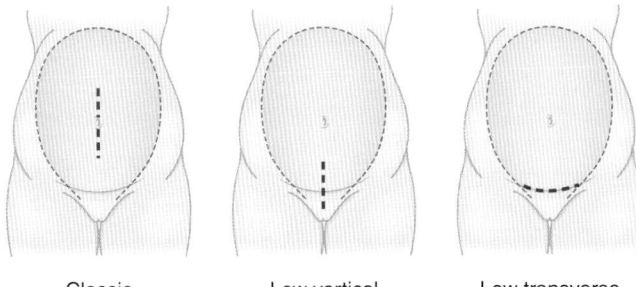

| Classic | Low vertical | Low transverse |

FIG. 11.6 Cesarean childbirth: Types of incisions include a classic, low vertical, and low transverse. (From Stillerman, E. [2008]. *Prenatal massage: A textbook of pregnancy, labor and postpartum bodywork*. St Louis: Mosby.)

should refrain from smoking and should limit consumption of alcohol and coffee.

Massage and Breastfeeding

Offer the nursing mother water before and after the massage, as increased fluid intake is required during this time. If the client is wearing a bra during the massage, modify massage techniques to work around the bra. Breasts may be sore and tender, and the client may feel more comfortable in a side-lying position during the massage. Several options can be used to help make the client more comfortable while lying prone. For more information, see the section on breast changes earlier in this chapter. Spend time massaging the back, neck, shoulders, and arms, which may be tight and sore from holding the baby during feedings. **NOTE:** The CDC does not list breast milk as a body fluid requiring special handling precautions, such as disinfection procedures. The exception is frequent exposure, such as persons who work in a milk bank (CDC, 2022).

> *It is through our hands that we speak to the child. That we communicate. Touch is the child's first language, understanding comes long after feeling.*
> —**Frederick Leboyer**

INFANT MASSAGE

Infant massage involves modifications of massage techniques and body positions to meet the needs of the child and the child's family (newly born to age 3). Infant massage can be taught to parents and caregivers who provide the massage, or it can be provided by a massage practitioner or other qualified individual. The framework of infant massage is to promote parent–child interaction, which facilitates understanding, builds trust, and promotes attachment, the latter of which helps the child feel safe, secure, and protected.

When instructing parents or caregivers, the massage practitioner uses a doll to demonstrate massage techniques while the parent/caregiver performs the massage on the infant (Fig. 11.7). Parents and caregivers are taught how to provide a full-body infant massage and to identify behaviors that suggest the child is engaged (receptive to massage) or disengaged (at which time infant massage should be postponed). Research related to infant massage is on Evolve.

Practice Setting

The room should be warm and without drafts. Natural light or low light is best, as bright light may overstimulate the child. Soft background music can be played. However, the child's favorite music is often the parent's or caregiver's voice talking in a high-pitched voice, humming, or singing a lullaby. Place all massage supplies within reach.

Body Positions

The child's position during massage depends on age (e.g., 4 vs. 8 months), developmental stage (e.g., not crawling versus crawling), and personal preference. The child can

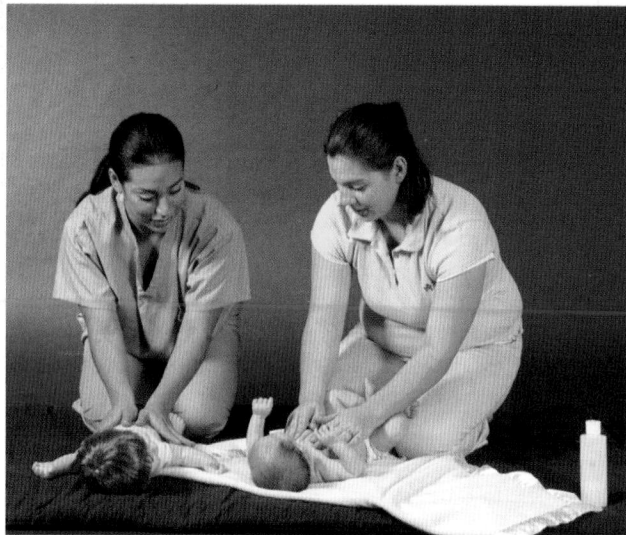

FIG. 11.7 Infant massage: The instructor uses a doll to demonstrate massage techniques while the parent or caregiver massages the infant.

receive massage while draped across the parent's lap, while lying beside the parent or between the parent's knees, while being held in the arms of one parent while the other parent massages, while lying on the floor in front of the parent while they sit on their heels, while nursing, or while being held by the parent. Regardless of which position is used, never leave the baby unattended.

Techniques

Postpone massage until approximately 45 minutes after infant feedings to reduce the risk of vomiting. Use food-grade oils, such as jojoba, apricot, coconut, safflower, and olive in small amounts. Inevitably, the infant's hand covered with oil will end up in their mouth. Avoid scented and peanut or almond oils because they may cause allergic reactions in sensitive babies. Keep the oil bottle closed when not in use, because it can be knocked over by a parent or squirming baby. Cover nonmassaged areas. Infant massage sessions are typically short in duration, perhaps 10 to 15 minutes. Mostly effleurage and petrissage are used; techniques should be modified, refined, or even created according to the baby's response. The most important thing is that the parent enjoys time with the child and uses techniques the child enjoys.

CHILD AND ADOLESCENT MASSAGE

Massage can be provided to children aged 3 years and into adolescence. The parent or guardian and minor child/adolescent are all present during treatment planning and discussions of policies and procedures. Use terms the child/adolescent understands.

In most states, the age of consent for nontherapeutic/self-care procedures is 16 years. This age is determined by the age a new driver can receive a driver's license in the state where massage services are provided. Individuals 18 years of age and older can legally consent to medical or therapeutic procedures. The parent or legal guardian must grant consent for children/adolescents who cannot grant consent for themselves. However, massage is inappropriate on a minor child/adolescent who does not want it even with parental/guardian consent. Touch is a powerful experience, one that cannot be undone. The potential for influencing the attitude and acceptance of touch cannot be underestimated. How touch is given, and how the child/adolescent receives it, may determine whether the child/adolescent becomes a person who views touch, especially massage, as nurturing, positive, and beneficial, or as something to be avoided. Research related to massage for children and adolescents is on Evolve.

Practice Setting

Follow state guidelines regarding massage of minors. When working with younger children, consider having a few toys such as finger puppets, simple puzzles, stickers, and crayons and paper in the office. To build rapport with younger children, interact with them while they play with these items. Consider asking parents to bring a blanket, toy, or stuffed animal to the appointment, which will remain with the child during the entire session. To build rapport with older children and adolescents, ask them about their favorite music, food, miniseries, movies, or video games.

For younger children, massage room lighting should be bright and not as dark as massage room lighting for adults. Darkly lit rooms may cause younger children to become anxious, especially if they fear darkness. Older children and adolescents may have unique lighting preferences. They may bring their own music downloaded on their mobile phones and want to listen to their own music during the massage. If the child is using earphones or earbuds, suggest only one side be used so they can respond to questions and comments during the massage.

It is recommended a parent or guardian remains in the room during the massage for children under 16. If the parent or guardian elects not to be in the room, the massage room door should remain open during the massage, preferably with the parent or guardian within view.

When working with adolescents going through puberty, females are getting accustomed to menstrual cycles, and males may be dealing with spontaneous erections. Adolescents who are menstruating may be embarrassed with the thought of having an accident or bleeding through during their massage. In these cases, offer to reschedule or place an extra towel beneath them. Because spontaneous erection may cause embarrassment, consider having the top drape bunched up in the groin area and using a blanket of heavier-weight material over the sheet drape. If an erection occurs, ask the child questions about mundane topics, such as school, sports, or favorite foods.

Body Positions

Positioning for massage administration is child-directed. The child may feel more comfortable with a blanket on the floor, be totally fine on the massage table, or content sitting in a comfy chair. Have plenty of pillows, blankets, a comfy chair, and extra floor space to accommodate a range of preferences.

Techniques

Children should wear loose clothing during the massage rather than disrobe completely. Younger children and children with developmental delays may not understand the importance of the top drape and fling it off without warning, leaving the practitioner with an exposed child on the table. If the child is receiving massage for therapeutic reasons such as injury rehabilitation or sports-related issues, suggest athletic-type shorts and a tank top with a sports bra for female children. Drape your clothed minor client just as you would other clients.

Use oil-free lotion or cream on adolescents, as they may have varying degrees of acne, and oil-based products are not recommended.

When working with younger children, consider demonstrating what massage is like on the item they brought with them, on a parent or caregiver, or on the child's forearm. Allow children to direct the massage, which helps them feel empowered and more relaxed about the session. In a child-directed session, the practitioner may find themselves using a finger puppet during the massage while telling stories or pretend making a pizza using gliding and kneading techniques.

The duration of the massage depends on many factors, including the child's age, developmental stage, and attention span. A 3-year-old toddler may receive a 15-minute session and a 10-year-old child may receive a 45- to 60-minute session.

AGING ADULTS: GERIATRIC MASSAGE

Geriatric massage is the modification of massage techniques and body positions to meet the needs of older and aging adults. Geriatric massage takes into account physical, psychologic, and socioeconomic factors. The process of aging is a series of biologic changes that follow a natural progression from birth through maturity to old age and death. Aging occurs over the life span of all living things. Health plays a role in how old a person becomes, as do genetics. People whose parents or grandparents live to old age seem to have a better chance of living long lives themselves.

Old age is a life stage determined by three factors—chronologic age, changes in social roles, and changes in functional capacities. Sixty-five years old is the chronologic age considered by most developing countries as the beginning of old age and when an individual is considered a senior citizen (WHO, n.d.a). Changes in social roles include occupational retirement and eligibility for pension benefits. Changes in functional capacities include physical and sensory declines, such as changes in muscles and joints, decreased neural response time, and impairments of vision, hearing, and mobility.

How do young, middle-aged, and older individuals view old age? A survey published by the Pew Research Center (2009) found a generation gap in response to the question of when old age begins. Survey respondents who were 29 years of age and younger viewed people 60 years of age as old. Middle-aged respondents (aged 30 to 64 years) indicated it was closer to 70 years, and respondents 65 years and older do not believe they are getting older until they reach 74 years. The average of all answers from the 2969 respondents was 68 years old, just 3 years later than the chronologic age published by the WHO. Currently, 23% of males and 15% of females aged 65 years and older are found in the labor force; projections are that by 2022, this will increase to 27% of males and 20% of females in the same age group.

Medication use increases with age. Some 85% of adults 65 years and older report they are currently taking prescription drugs. More than half of adults 65 years and older (54%) report taking four or more prescription drugs (Kirzinger et al., 2019). This population accounts for approximately 30% of nonprescription drug use in the United States. Commonly used drugs (both prescription and nonprescription) in this age group are: (1) cardiovascular agents, (2) antihypertensives, (3) analgesics, (4) antiarthritic agents, (5) sedatives, tranquilizers, and antidepressants, and (6) laxatives and antacids.

Older adults receive the least amount of touch of all age groups in Western healthcare systems. In a study by Barnett (1972), the age group touched least in medical environments was individuals 66 to 100 years of age. However, the use of touch and physical closeness may be the most important way to communicate to ill and aged people that they are important as human beings (Montagu, 1986). Research indicates social connection is a key component of health and happiness in older adults, and an ongoing relationship with a massage practitioner can be a significant part of life because of the focused attention received from a caring and compassionate person while during massage.

The aging population presents us with unique challenges. There is an increased incidence of disease, medication use, impairment, and disability. Some older clients are active and robust, whereas others are sedentary and frail. The massage practitioner must take these and many other factors into consideration when formulating a treatment plan; this may include modifying techniques and the time of day or duration of the session. This population often faces lifestyle and emotional changes, such as retirement, lower income, and loss of loved ones. In fact, some practitioners offer discounts to older adults because some are on a reduced fixed income. In addition, older clients may be living at home or in residential care facilities, which may necessitate an outcall. Even though people 65 and older comprise the smallest massage consumer group by age, they receive the most massages (American Massage Therapy Association [AMTA], 2021).

"Old age ain't no place for sissies," said Bette Davis. As Lohman (2001) points out, neither is providing massage to older adults, but "yet it is as rewarding as it is demanding." It requires genuine interest in their lives, getting over squeamishness about body functions and physical decline, being willing to enter the institutional world of older adults, and treating them with dignity, irrespective of their eccentricities or circumstances.

Every client will be different; every session will be different, even if it is the same client seen each week. As stories are shared, some clients need to cry, some need to express anger, some need to complain, and others need to convey their fears. Provide the space for the clients to express their feelings with your attitude of compassion. A half-hour of respectful, attentive touch helps the client feel valued. Research related to older adults and massage is on Evolve.

I'm not 70, I'm 18 with 52 years of experience.
—Anonymous

Aging: Physiologic Effects and Associated Diseases

As mentioned previously, aging is a series of biologic changes that follow a natural progression from birth through maturity to old age and death. Although many aspects of aging are universal, the process is unique to each person, and just as there are no typical 40-year-olds, there are no typical 70-year-olds. The average life expectancy in the United States is approximately 78 years.

Life expectancy for females is 81.2 years and 76.4 years for males, a difference of 4.8 years. The longest documented human lifespan is 122 years 164 days (Jeanne Calment, Arles, France, 1875–1997). **Senescence** is the period of life from old age to death.

According to the National Council on Aging (n.d.), approximately 92% of older adults report having at least one chronic disease, and 77% report having at least two. The four most common chronic diseases of older adults are heart disease, cancer, stroke, and diabetes. Osteoporosis and neurodegeneration such as Parkinson disease (PD) and Alzheimer disease (AD) are also seen in this population (Fig. 11.8). However, it is important to separate the irreversible process of aging from the often-reversible processes of disease. Many physiologic and structural changes are a normal part of aging, such as those seen in joints, blood vessel walls, and the brain. Degenerative changes may predispose older adults to certain diseases and conditions, and, conversely, diseases may accelerate the aging process. Body systems are featured next, with age-related changes listed. Diseases and conditions common in older populations are featured in *italics*.

Aging and the Musculoskeletal System

Age-related changes in bone include the loss of bone density and increased susceptibility to fractures. This change begins between 30 and 40 years of age. With each successive decade, bones become more porous and fragile. Females can lose approximately 8% of bone mass each decade after age

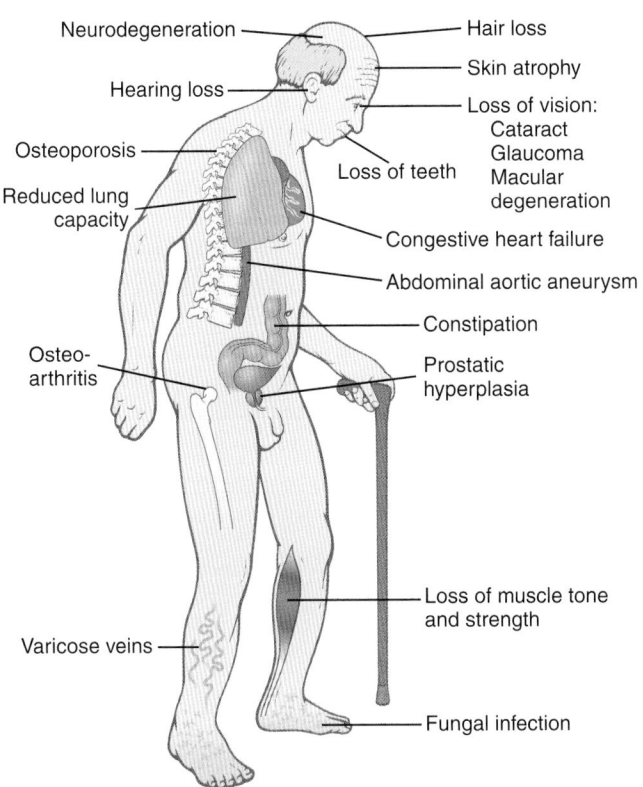

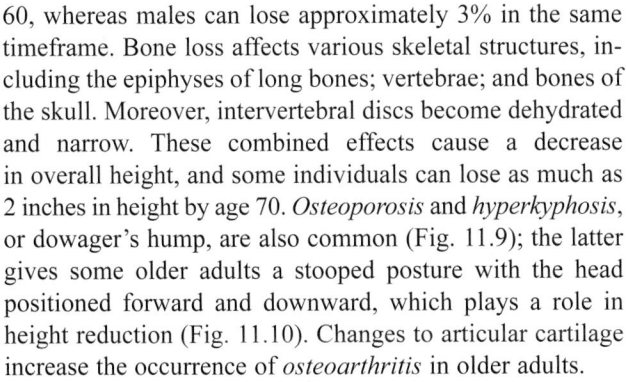

FIG. 11.8 Common diseases and conditions affecting older adults. (From Damjanov, I. [2017]. *Pathology for the health professions* [5th ed.]. St Louis: Elsevier.)

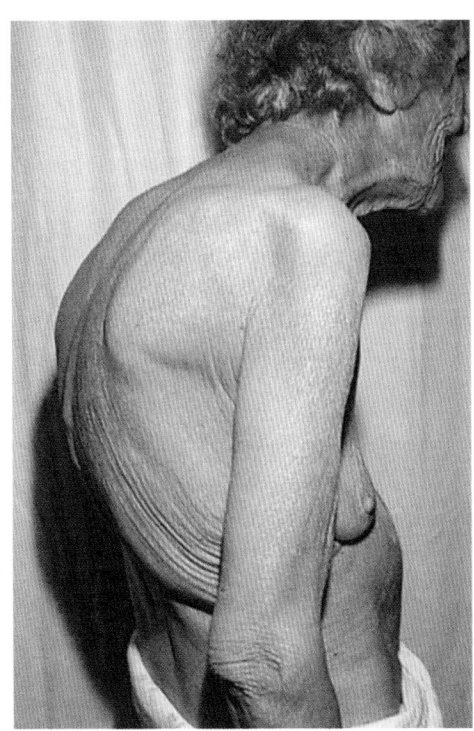

FIG. 11.9 Osteoporosis and hyperkyphosis: These can cause a stooped posture and a head position that is forward and downward, which contributes to a reduction in height. (From Kamal, A., & Brockelhurst, J. [1992]. *Color atlas of geriatric medicine* [2nd ed.]. St Louis: Mosby.)

60, whereas males can lose approximately 3% in the same timeframe. Bone loss affects various skeletal structures, including the epiphyses of long bones; vertebrae; and bones of the skull. Moreover, intervertebral discs become dehydrated and narrow. These combined effects cause a decrease in overall height, and some individuals can lose as much as 2 inches in height by age 70. *Osteoporosis* and *hyperkyphosis*, or dowager's hump, are also common (Fig. 11.9); the latter gives some older adults a stooped posture with the head positioned forward and downward, which plays a role in height reduction (Fig. 11.10). Changes to articular cartilage increase the occurrence of *osteoarthritis* in older adults.

Loss of muscle tone, strength, and endurance is typically seen in older adults and is related to a decrease in physical activity. Grip strength decreases, making it more difficult to perform routine tasks such as opening a jar or turning a key. Loss of muscle tone, muscle mass, and muscle strength resulting from age-related inactivity is called *sarcopenia;* the condition causes muscles to appear smaller, looser, and flattened (Fig. 11.11). Sarcopenia is linked to severe osteoporosis, as well as disabilities, and may prevent a person from living an independent life. With aging, ligaments and tendons become less elastic, which reduces flexibility. Other musculoskeletal diseases common in older adults are *rheumatoid arthritis*, *bursitis*, and *gout*. Many older adults experience instability in walking and may depend on a walking stick, a multi-footed cane, or a walker for assistance.

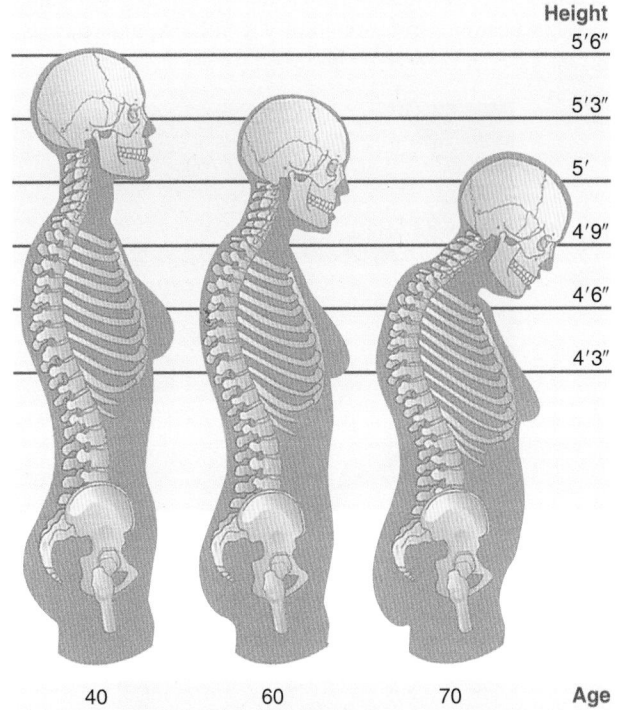

FIG. 11.10 Decreases in height over time: This is a common consequence of aging. (From Mahan, L., & Escott-Stump, S. [2008]. *Krause's food and nutrition therapy* [12th ed.]. St Louis: Saunders.)

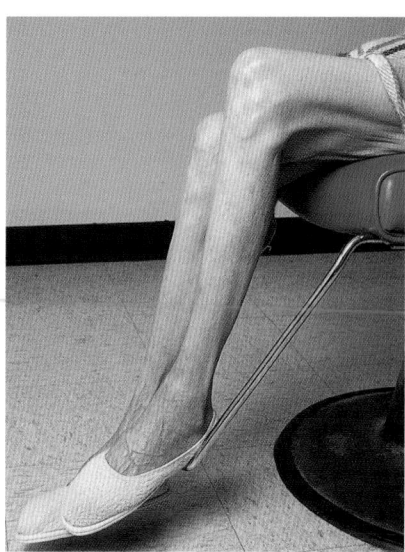

FIG. 11.11 Sarcopenia: Loss of muscle tone, muscle mass, and muscle strength is common in inactive older adults. (From Sorrentino, S. [2017]. *Mosby's textbook for nursing assistants* [9th ed.]. St Louis: Elsevier.)

Aging and the Integumentary System

Skin begins to lose elasticity, is less supple, and becomes thinner and more fragile, due to the loss of collagen—especially in sun-exposed areas of the body, thereby increasing the risk of skin damage. Skin also heals more slowly after damage, thus increasing the risk of infection.

Wrinkles or "crow's feet" may appear on the face, and the skin on the neck may sag (Fig. 11.12). Facial shaving becomes more difficult for men due to sagging/wrinkling. The skin becomes thin, rough, dry, and flaky, and may itch

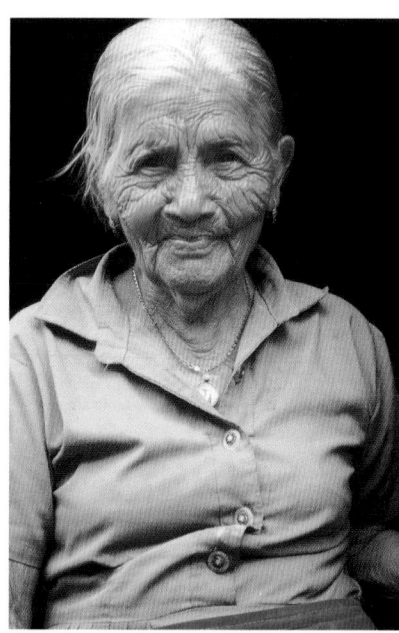

FIG. 11.12 Aging skin: Wrinkling and sagging are common signs. (From Copstead, L., & Banasik, J. [2012]. *Pathophysiology* [4th ed.]. St Louis: Saunders. Photograph by L Copstead.)

from reduced glandular activity and decreased circulation. Skin pigmentation increases, especially on sun-exposed areas, such as the face and forearms. Increased pigmentation can cause *senile lentigo*, or age/liver spots (Fig. 11.13). *Seborrheic keratosis*, *actinic keratosis*, and *seborrheic dermatitis* are also more common in older adults.

The amount of subcutaneous tissue and underlying fat decreases with age and can often be seen in the eye sockets, in the hollows below the clavicles, and in the back of the hands. This reduction in fat also decreases the body's ability to regulate internal temperature, which can lead to cold intolerance. There is an increased risk of decubitus ulcers in older adults who are immobile. Capillary walls become

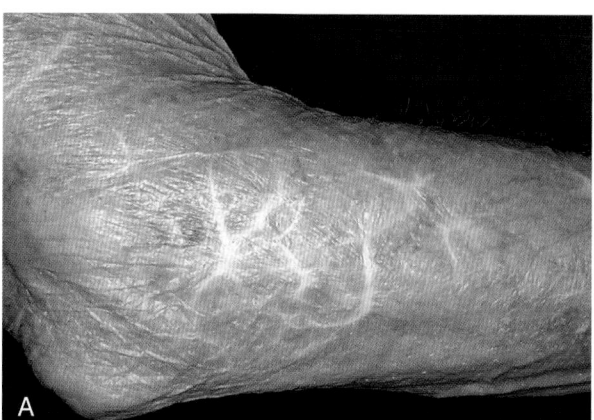

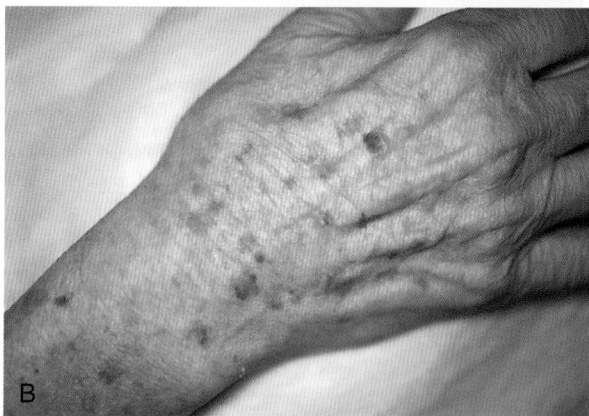

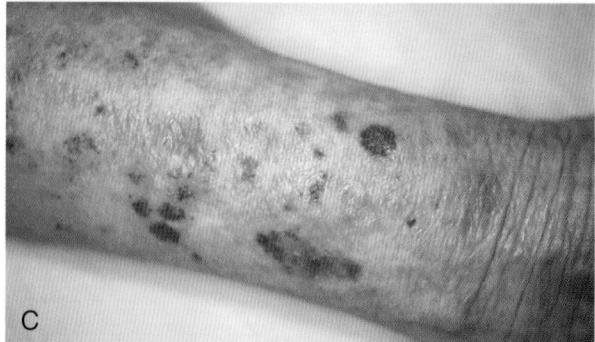

FIG. 11.13 Aging skin: Thin, frail, rough, and flaky skin are common (A). Increased pigmentation may cause senile lentigo or age/liver spots (B) and senile purpura (C). (From Stillerman, E. [2016]. *Modalities for massage and bodywork* [2nd ed.]. St Louis: Elsevier.)

increasingly fragile and may rupture from minor trauma, leading to a type of bruising called *senile purpura* (see Fig. 11.13C). Skin cancers are also more common, including *basal* and *squamous cell carcinomas.*

Hair color fades and begins to turn gray. The number of hair follicles decreases, reducing hair thickness on the scalp, pubis, and axilla. Hairs in the nose and ears may become thicker and more noticeable. Some females experience facial hair growth, especially after menopause. Pattern hair loss in both males and females tends to be hereditary. Nails grow more slowly and may become thick, rough, and more brittle. Nail surfaces may contain lines or ridges. Fungal infections of the feet and toenails become more common (Fig. 11.14).

Aging and the Nervous System

Nerve cells in the central nervous system (CNS) and peripheral nervous system (PNS) begin to degenerate, and cerebral blood flow decreases. Neural changes in the areas of the brain responsible for balance and coordination, coupled with reduced nerve cell conduction rate, can result in decreased reflexes, slowed response time, and unsteady gait. These may increase the risk of injury from slips and falls. Nerve cell degeneration contributes to diseases such as AD and PD, which are more common in the aging population. Cerebrovascular changes seen in older adults contribute to transient ischemic attacks and stroke. Some older individuals note an increase in pain sensitivity, whereas others note a decrease.

Changes in vision and hearing occur with age. Lenses in the eyes become larger and less elastic, which contributes to

presbyopia, the inability to read or see nearby objects. Presbyopia affects depth perception, which further increases the risk of injury from slips and falls. Night vision is also impaired. Most older adults wear glasses to improve vision. The surface of the eye may develop a white, gray, or bluish ring around the cornea called *arcus senilis* (Fig. 11.15). Ocular pathologies also contribute to loss of vision and include *cataracts, glaucoma,* and *age-related macular degeneration* (Fig. 11.16).

Ear canals become thinner and eardrums become thicker. Ear wax may accumulate, which contributes to age-related hearing loss. Many older adults find it difficult to discriminate between different sounds, especially in noisy environments. Hearing loss is usually greater for high-pitched sounds, which makes it difficult to hear the ringing of a phone, a doorbell, or the voices of children or adult females. Hearing loss can cause *tinnitus,* or the perception of noise or ringing in the ears. Tinnitus affects 20% to 30% of older populations. Some older adults use hearing aids to improve hearing.

Aging and the Endocrine System

In general, endocrine glands continue to produce adequate levels of important hormones throughout life. There are a few exceptions. Ovarian function ceases, reducing levels of estrogen and progesterone. This reduction stimulates menopause and contributes to osteoporosis. Studies indicate that decreased levels of estrogen also affect cardiovascular function, memory, and cognition. Thyroid hormone production decreases, increasing the risk of *hypothyroidism.* This reduces metabolism in older adults and contributes to cold intolerance. Pancreatic function also decreases with age, increasing the incidence of *hypoglycemia* and *type 2 diabetes mellitus* and diabetic complications, such as diabetic retinopathy (see Fig. 11.16).

Aging and the Reproductive System

In females, *menopause* occurs as levels of estrogen and progesterone decline and ovarian function ceases. In the United States, females generally reach menopause between the ages of 48 and 55 years; the median age is 51 years. When factoring life expectancy, females spend approximately one-third of their lives in menopause. Several

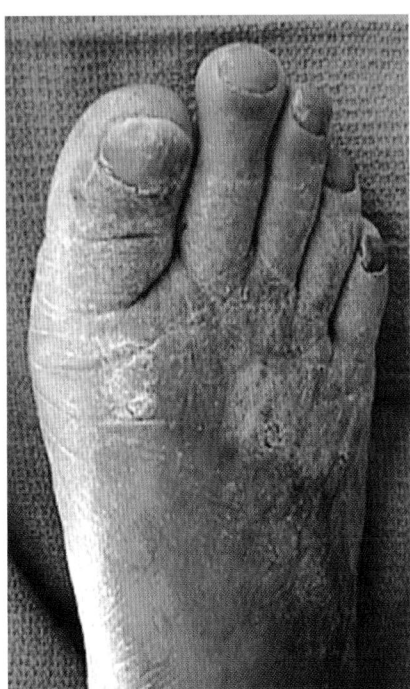

FIG. 11.14 Fungal infection of the foot and toenails: These are more common in older adults. (From Stillerman, E. [2016]. *Modalities for massage and bodywork* [2nd ed.]. St Louis: Elsevier.)

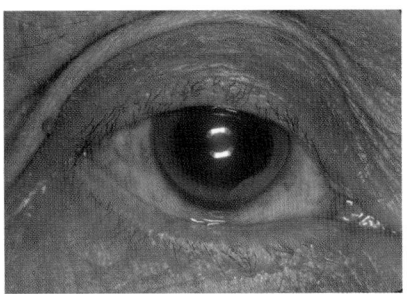

FIG. 11.15 Eye appearance changes: Some aging adults develop a white, gray, or bluish ring around the cornea called arcus senilis. (From Palay & Krachmer, Primary Care Ophthalmology, 2005).

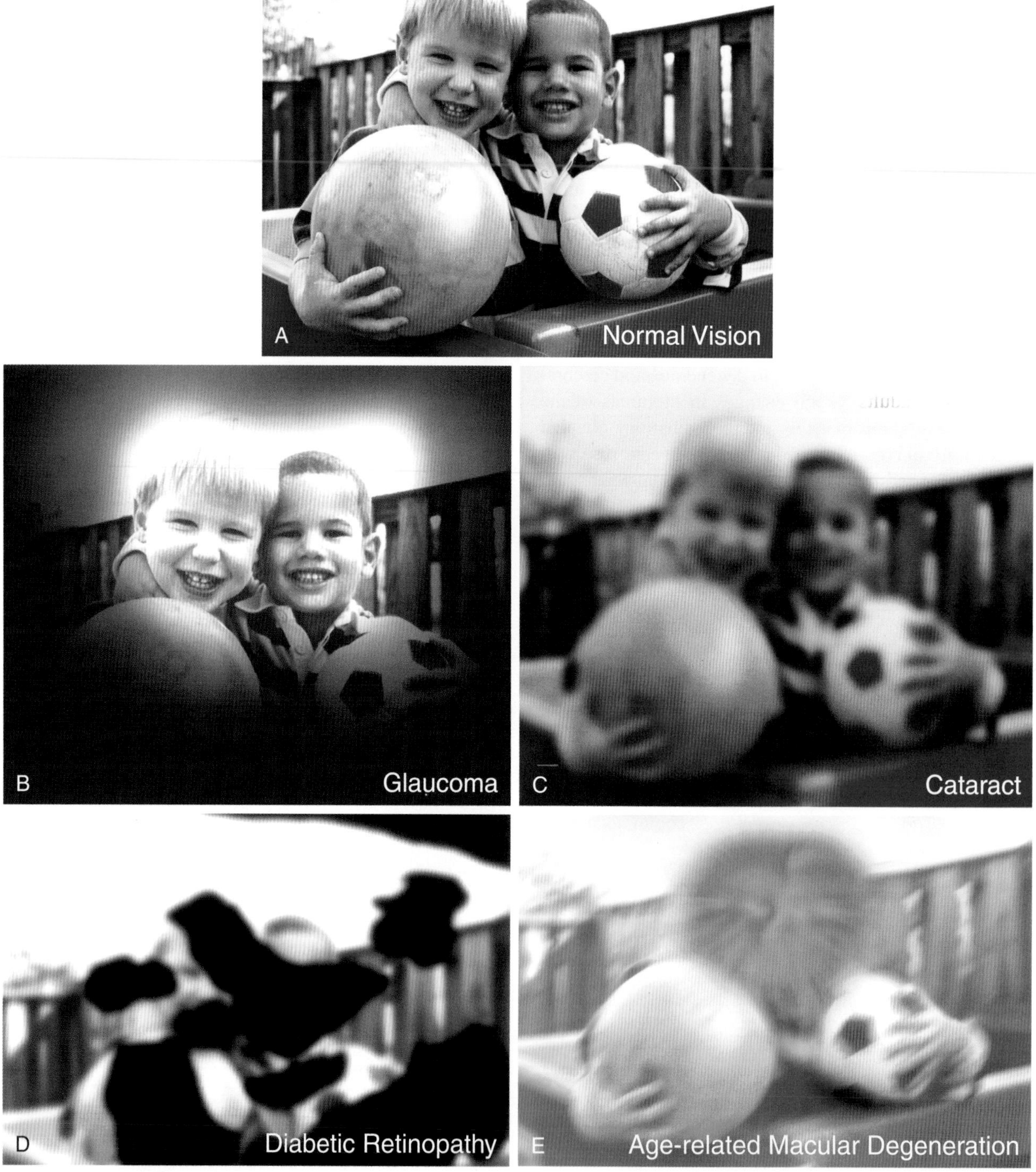

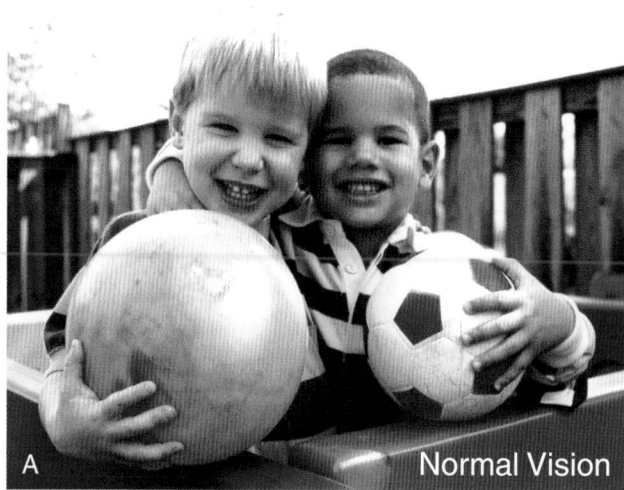

FIG. 11.16 Ocular pathologies: Normal vision (A). Vision affected by glaucoma (B), by cataracts (C), by diabetic retinopathy (D), and by age-related macular degeneration (E). (From Touhy, T. A., & Jett, K. F. [2016]. *Ebersole and Hess' toward healthy aging* [9th ed.]. St Louis: Elsevier.)

significant changes occur with menopause. There is a loss of bone density, which may lead to osteoporosis. Reproductive organs and their related tissues begin to flatten and atrophy. This leads to a loss of breast fullness. *Vaginal infections* are more prevalent, as these tissues become dry, fragile, and more easily irritated; aging females do not produce as many natural fluids that help keep the vagina naturally cleansed. Other reproductive conditions and diseases more common in older females are *pelvic organ prolapse* and *breast cancer*.

In males, testosterone continues to be produced until their late 80s. There are some changes in the size and firmness of the testes. The prostate commonly enlarges with age, leading to *benign prostatic hyperplasia (BPH)*. Problems related to an enlarged prostate include increased urinary urgency, hesitancy in starting flow, weak urine stream, post-voiding dribbling, and incomplete bladder emptying, which then leads to urinary frequency. Prostate cancer is also more prevalent in older males.

Aging and the Cardiovascular System

Several significant changes occur in the heart and blood vessels with aging. The heart may enlarge, which reduces cardiac output and increases the risk of *congestive heart failure*. The endothelium, or internal lining, of blood vessels loses elasticity and is less responsive to postural changes. This, along with the changes in cardiac output, increases the likelihood of varicosities in the lower extremities.

Many older adults experience dizziness and loss of balance related to a sudden drop in blood pressure when moving from a lying down or sitting position to an upright or standing position; this is called *orthostatic (postural) hypotension (OH)*. During OH, systole drops at least 20 mm Hg and diastole drops at least 10 mm Hg within 3 minutes of sitting up or standing. OH is caused by gravity-induced blood pooling in the lower extremities. This pooling reduces venous return, causing a sudden decrease in cardiac output and a subsequent drop in blood pressure. Instances of OH are also called *dizzy spells*. Dizziness and loss of balance can also occur from vision or hearing impairments, or be side effects of medication.

Arterial plaque may accumulate in older adults, causing arteries to narrow and thicken. These changes contribute to *hypertension*, *coronary* and *carotid artery diseases*, and *abdominal aortic aneurysms*. *Anemia* is common and its prevalence increases with age. The most common causes of anemia in older adults are iron deficiency and chronic disease. Cerebrovascular changes seen in older adults contribute to *transient ischemic attacks* and *stroke*. Weakness of the valves in the rectal veins can lead to *hemorrhoid*s.

Aging and the Lymphatic System/Immunity

The main effect of aging on the lymphatic system is a reduction in the amount of body fluids, particularly intracellular fluids. Whereas plasma and extracellular volume remain somewhat constant, intracellular fluid decreases, which increases the risk of dehydration in older adults. Inactivity, as well as a decline in kidney function and cardiovascular function, increases the risk of edema, especially in the lower extremities. The immune response is slower and weaker in older adults. This increases the risk of many diseases, including autoimmune diseases, influenza, shingles, and cancer.

Aging and the Respiratory System

With aging, changes are seen throughout the respiratory system. Lung capacity reduces as tissues in the airways and in alveoli lose elasticity. The number of capillaries surrounding alveoli also decreases, which interferes with gas exchange. Arthritic changes are common in older adults and alter the size, shape, and functionality of the ribcage. Osteoporosis and complications of this disease, such as hyperkyphosis or dowager's hump, cause changes in the ribcage of females. Costal cartilage begins to calcify and become more rigid, reducing the mobility of the ribcage. These changes contribute to the reduction of lung capacity seen in older adults, as well as an increased risk of secretions pooling in the lower lobes of the lungs (Fig. 11.17). Many elderly people have chronic postnasal drainage. The number of cilia in the upper respiratory tract decreases, and the cilia's ability to trap and remove debris declines. As vocal cords become less elastic, voice quality also changes. This leads to alterations in pitch, creating a more tremulous voice. Respiratory diseases commonly seen in older adults are *chronic obstructive pulmonary diseases*, such as *bronchitis* and *emphysema*, *influenza*, and p*neumonia*.

Aging and the Gastrointestinal System

In aging, there is often a decrease in saliva production in the oral cavity, which leads to dry mouth. Medications may contribute to this condition. There is also a risk of losing teeth from periodontal disease or gum recession from the loss of periodontal bonds holding teeth in place. These structural changes limit not only the types of foods eaten,

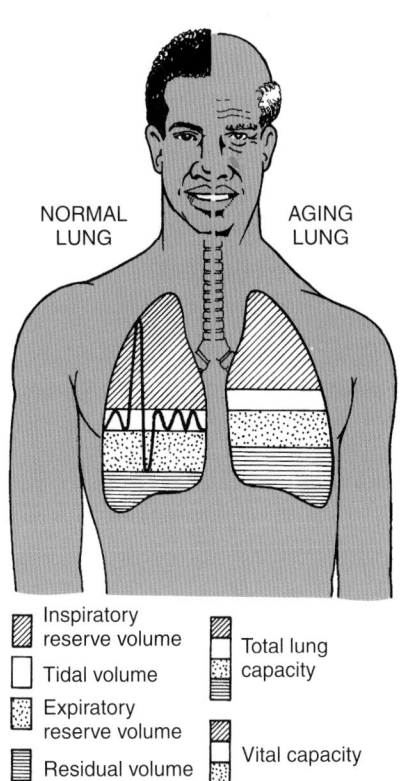

FIG. 11.17 Reduced lung capacity: This is often noted in older adults. (From McCance, K., & Huether, S. [2015]. *Pathophysiology: The biological basis for disease in adults and children* [7th ed.]. St Louis: Elsevier.)

but the amounts of food consumed, because tooth loss alters the way individuals bite and chew. Good oral hygiene can slow these changes. In fact, it is no longer considered normal for older adults to lose their teeth, which was common in the past.

The tone of sphincter muscles decreases. A lack of tone in the lower esophageal sphincter increases the risk of *gastroesophageal reflux disease (GERD)*; lack of tone in the anal sphincter increases the risk of *fecal incontinence*. Gastric glands begin to atrophy, which decreases the amount of substances assisting processes of digestion and absorption. These effects often contribute to malnutrition and anemia. A generalized reduction of muscle tone also occurs along the entire gastrointestinal (GI) tract, which reduces peristaltic activity, slows digestion, and increases the likelihood of constipation and the incomplete elimination of feces during a single bowel movement.

Other diseases of the GI tract commonly seen in older adults include *peptic ulcers*, *diverticulosis*, *diverticulitis*, *colon cancer*, and *hemorrhoids*. Bowel problems are observed to be the cause of much anxiety and may reduce quality of life in these individuals.

Aging and the Urinary System

The kidneys decrease in size from approximately 400 g at age 40 to 250 g by age 80. Even with the decrease in size, the kidneys are usually able to adequately perform vital functions to meet the body's needs. The bladder also decreases in size; this reduces bladder capacity, or the amount of urine the bladder can hold before the person experiences the urge to void. Some older individuals have an overactive bladder, causing it to contract before the bladder is full. To aggravate the problem, loss of muscle tone in the pelvic floor can impair voluntary control of the external urethral sphincter muscle. All these factors can lead to urinary urgency and urinary frequency, which are common in older adults. Other conditions seen in older adults include a decrease in the urinary stream, incomplete or unsuccessful voiding, and continuous dribbling of urine. In males, this can be caused by *benign prostatic hyperplasia (BPH)*, an enlarged prostate, which compresses and narrows the urethra as it passes through the gland. Urinary pathologies common in older individuals include *urinary incontinence (UI)*, *urinary tract infections (UTIs)*, and *chronic kidney failure*. UTIs can cause sudden confusion or delirium in older adults and people with dementia.

Practice Setting

The best time to schedule massage sessions may be during daylight hours. Older clients may prefer not to drive their vehicles after sunset because of impaired night vision and increased sensitivity to glare.

Ensure that lighting is adequate while the client is moving through the office and massage room, that all throw rugs are secured to the floor, and that there are no cords in the walking path. Age is considered a major risk factor for falls. People 75 years of age and older have the highest rate of falls, and one in three individuals over the age of 65 fall each year.

Arrange office furniture so that the client can move around without difficulty. Adequate space is needed between furniture and walls so that a client using a cane or walker can easily pass (32 inches are recommended by the ADA) (Fig. 11.18); this arrangement will also accommodate a client who is "furniture walking" without a walker or cane. Furniture should be stable enough to support the weight of the client and not move if the client leans on it.

Allow plenty of time for filling out of intake and consent forms. Assist the client with filling out the forms if needed. Reduce noise levels in the room where the client interview is conducted. Read Box 11.1 titled Communication, Aging, and Massage for suggestions when communicating with older adults.

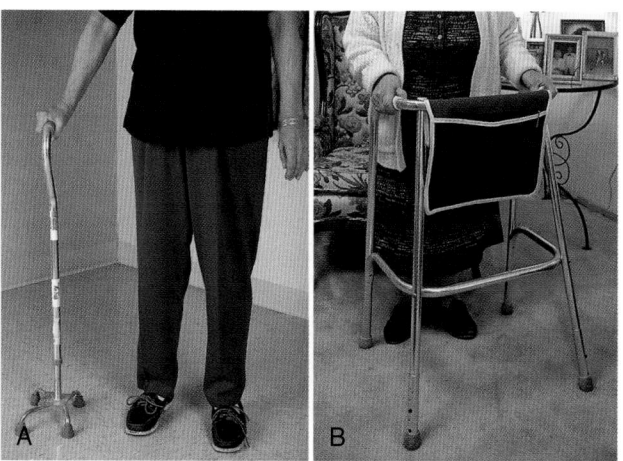

FIG. 11.18 Mobility devices: Quad canes (A) and walkers (B) may be used to increase mobility and promote safety in older adults. (From Sorrentino, S. A. [2017]. *Mosby's textbook for nursing assistants* [8th ed.]. St Louis: Elsevier.)

BOX 11.1

Communication, Aging, and Massage

Do	Don't
Identify yourself	Assume the person knows who you are
Address the client using the name they desire (Mrs. Smith vs. Betty)	Use "baby talk" or patronizing names, such as "sweetie" or "honey"
Speak clearly and slowly in a normal tone of voice	Shout
Get to know the person	
	Make generalizations about older adults
Listen with empathy	Pay too much attention to tasks and forget about the person
	Ignore non-verbal messages
Pay attention to body language—yours and theirs	

Modified from Wold, G. H. (2019). *Basic geriatric nursing* (7th ed.). St Louis: Mosby.

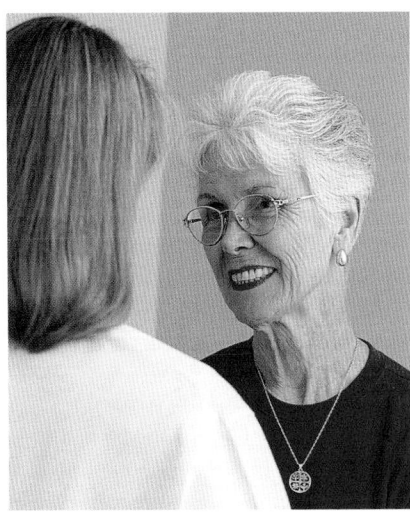

FIG. 11.19 Client intake: Query the client about health conditions, impairments, disabilities, and medication use during the intake. (From Stillerman, E. [2016]. *Modalities for massage and bodywork* [2nd ed.]. St Louis: Elsevier.)

Asking about health conditions is important because 92% of older adults report having at least one chronic condition and 77% report having at least two. Inquire about limitations from impairments or disabilities (see later sections on impairments). Query the client about medication use, methods of administration (e.g., oral, injected, etc.), and any medication side effects they may be experiencing (Fig. 11.19).

Provide unobstructed passage to and from the massage table. Allow ample time for tasks, such as removing and donning clothing, and getting on and off the massage table. Assist in the removal of any eyeglasses or hearing aids and the placement of walkers and canes if needed. At the conclusion of the session, replace these items.

If the client has cold intolerance, provide comfort measures, such as a warm blanket, an electric table warmer, raising the room temperature, or a combination of these. If using an electric table warmer, turn it on before the client arrives to warm the table surface and turn it off when the client is on the table, because some older adults have poor thermal regulation.

Sometimes it is best to perform the massage at the client's residence rather than at the practitioner's office. Space is often limited, so inquire before bringing a portable massage table. Instead, massage clients where they are most comfortable, which may be their bed, recliner, or wheelchair.

Determine Client Robustness or Frailty

Gillick (1996) describes a robust older person as physically vigorous, mentally acute, a fount of wisdom and experience for family and friends, and busy accomplishing all the things they never had the time to undertake. Robust older clients are likely to have at least one chronic disease, but it is well-managed and does not limit most activities. Gillick describes frail older individuals as having more than one

health problem and impairment in multiple domains. A frail older client may be physically weak; more vulnerable to stressors, such as heat, cold, infection, and injury from falling; and may be more prone to dependency. Not every older individual will become frail, but the risk of frailty increases with age and is more common in females than males.

It is useful to identify if an older client is robust or frail by applying Fried's frailty criteria (Fried et al., 2001). A score of 2 or less suggests the client is robust. A score of 3 or more suggests the client is frail. Although Fried's criterion is the most commonly used tool to determine frailty, other tools may be preferred by the practitioner or the facility where the practitioner is working. Fried's frailty criteria are as follows:

1. Slow walking speed;
2. Muscle weakness evidenced by weak handgrip and sarcopenia;
3. Self-reported exhaustion;
4. Low level of physical activity; and
5. Underweight or unintentional weight loss.

Slow Walking Speed

Pay attention to how fast or slowly the client walks. Frail clients walk more slowly and may appear unstable or fearful while walking. A slow walking speed may also indicate AD and poor cardiovascular health. Robust clients have a faster-paced walking speed and a steady gait.

Muscle Weakness Evidenced by Weak Handgrip and Sarcopenia

Ask the client to shake and squeeze your hand. Weak handgrip strength can indicate frailty, poor health, and increased dependency on others for ADLs. Robust clients have a strong handshake and good grip strength. Handgrip strength usually correlates with leg strength. Robust clients have good muscle tone and resultant muscle strength. Look at and palpate muscles of the lower extremities. Are they of adequate size and firm, or small and flattened? The latter is a sign of sarcopenia: a loss of muscle tone, muscle mass, and muscle strength from age-related inactivity (see Fig. 11.11).

Self-Reported Exhaustion

Ask the client about their energy level. Frail clients may say they are often tired, have low energy, are fatigued, or have no pep or get-up-and-go. They may look fatigued. Energy levels may also be determined by how clients describe their lifestyle during the intake. Frail clients will report spending much of their time at their residence. Robust clients may report participation in activities such as fishing or gardening, or share stories about vacations they have taken recently or plan to take.

Low Level of Physical Activity

Ask the client about the types and amounts of physical activity in which they participate. A strong indicator of a client's health is the level of physical activity and the client's reports of regular exercise and routine tasks, such as caring for neighbors or family members. Low levels of physical activity are an indicator of frailty.

Underweight or Unintentional Weight Loss

Ask the client if they have experienced recent weight loss and if it was intentional through means of diet and/or exercise. Although most clients will not know their body mass index (BMI), underweight BMI is defined as 18.5 kg/m^2 or less. Robust clients experience normal age-related weight loss of approximately 0.25 to 0.50 pound per year beginning around age 65 to 70 resulting from changes in hormones regulating appetite and satiety and decreases in basal metabolic rates.

- **Robust (≤2).** Clients who have two or less frailty criteria are classified as robust. Robust clients require few, if any, age-related massage modifications.
- **Frail (≥3).** Clients who have three or more frailty criteria are classified as frail. Frail clients may require varying degrees of modification, including fewer changes in position and slowly applied light pressure.

Body Positions for Elderly Clients

Use a massage table that can be lowered to 18 to 24 inches, such as an electric-lift or hydraulic table. This will help clients get on or off the table safely and more easily. The specific height to which the table is lowered is determined by the client's actual height. If the practitioner does not have an electric-lift or hydraulic table, consider using a sturdy, stable stepstool the client can use to get on and off the table safely. A wider table (≥33 inches) is preferred so that the client easily can change body positions while on the table. To reduce the risk of falls, be sure your table is barrier-free and devoid of pillows and bolsters while the client transfers on and off the table.

Ask the client in which positions they sleep at night and reproduce these positions when possible, which may include side-lying positions. Have at least six cushions or pillows available for positioning.

Many older clients are uncomfortable while prone. Dental appliances may make the prone position uncomfortable, even when a soft face rest cushion is used. In these cases, avoid the prone position or limit time in the prone position. Some clients, especially those with GERD or congestive heart failure, may be uncomfortable lying supine.

In these situations, use a semireclining (semi or standard Fowler), or upright (high Fowler) position. Avoid using a massage chair, because it may be difficult for an older client to get on and off of these chairs. If a seated position is needed, use a sturdy regular chair. Do not massage older clients on the floor, because it may be difficult for them to get down to and up off the floor.

Some disorders make it difficult for the client to lie flat comfortably prone or supine (e.g., advanced osteoporosis with hyperkyphosis, PD). In these situations, a side-lying position may be needed. Also consider limiting the number of times the client changes positions and allow more time

for positional changes if moving is difficult, as can occur among individuals with PD or mobility impairments. See the later section for more information on how to modify the massage for clients who have mobility impairments.

Because of the high frequency of dizziness and loss of balance owing to OH from sudden changes in position among this population, ask the client to arise from the massage table in three stages; (1) sit up on the table for 1 minute; (2) sit on the side of the table with legs dangling for 1 minute; and (3) stand with care, holding onto the edge of the table or another non-movable object for 1 minute.

Geriatric Massage Techniques

Factor any medications and medical conditions, such as osteoporosis and frailty, into the treatment plan. If the client is frail, use slowly applied light pressure. An example of light pressure is 3 on a 10-point pressure scale.

Aging skin is often thin and delicate. When using massage lubricants, use adequate amounts to reduce friction, because friction may injure the skin of older clients. Use of deep tissue products should be avoided because they absorb quickly and do not provide adequate glide over the client's skin. Skin lesions, in general, are more common in older adults. Although many of these skin conditions are not life-threatening (e.g., age spots, senile purpura, seborrheic dermatitis), they may cause disfigurement, perceived by the client as unattractive, and may be a source of embarrassment, anxiety, and psychosocial distress. When working with these clients, display loving kindness, acceptance, empathy, and nonjudgment.

Gentle passive range of motion (PROM), such as mild rocking, should be applied for frail older clients. Avoid forceful spinal mobilizations (including PROM of the cervical region) because of decreased bone density and compromised intervertebral joints.

As foot problems are common in older adults, inspect the client's feet, even if you do not massage them. Look for signs and symptoms, such as discoloration, bone deformities, and thick toenails. Physical limitations and visual impairments make it difficult for an older individual to inspect their own feet. If the client is wearing socks or slippers, ask for permission before removing them and replace them afterward. If you massage the feet and use lubricant, do not place lubricant between the toes, because lubricant may contribute to bacterial infections. Avoid unhealthy or suspicious areas and bring them to the attention of the client or client's caregiver.

Although the session may be 1 hour, the actual treatment or hands-on time may be shorter, sometimes 45 minutes. Respect the client's slower pace rather than maximizing massage time.

More time may be needed for comfort measures, such as using the toilet, drinking water, and arranging pillows and blankets. Your client may like to share a personal story with you. Make time for that. This may require more time between scheduled appointments.

When the session is complete, replace the client's eyeglasses, socks, or slippers and anything else you removed before the massage began. If you lowered the massage room lights, raise them before you leave the room. Remind the client to arise slowly from the massage table to reduce the risk of OH from sudden changes in position (the three stages mentioned previously).

CLIENTS WITH VISUAL IMPAIRMENTS

Visual impairment is a decreased capacity to see, and the impairment cannot be corrected by usual means, such as eyeglasses or contact lenses. The term blindness is reserved for a complete or near-complete loss of vision. Visual impairment may interfere with ADLs such as driving, reading, socializing, and walking. Common causes of visual impairment are presbyopia and ocular diseases such as glaucoma, cataracts, diabetic retinopathy, and age-related macular degeneration (see Fig. 11.16). Approximately 14 million Americans aged 12 years and older have visual impairments; 20.5 million people aged 40 years and older have cataracts, as do 5.3 million people aged 18 years and older.

Practice Setting

Announce your presence when you enter the room where the client awaits. Begin by addressing the client by name, and then state your name. When transferring the client from one area to another, stand in front or toward the client's left. This allows the client to touch your right elbow and follow. State any directional changes ahead of time, such as when you turn to enter a different room. Use descriptive words, such as straight, forward, left, and right. Avoid vague words, such as over there, here, this, and that. Describe room surroundings using the face of a clock. For example, say, "There is a table at 2 o'clock," instead of, "There is a table in front of you." Keep equipment and supplies in the same place and explain any changes to the client during subsequent sessions. When handing objects such as clipboards or bottles of water to clients, touch the back of their hand with the object so they can easily grab it.

The best reading fonts are sans-serif, such as Verdana, Arial, or Tahoma. Use black text on a white or yellow background. If a digital device such as a tablet is used, set the zoom feature to 200%. For paper documents, 16- to 18-point or a larger font is best. When enlarging printed materials using a copy machine, select 160% to 175% from the enlargement menu. This will increase the contents of an 8.5 × 11-inch page to an 11 × 17-inch page. Regardless of which reading format you choose (digital or print), provide adequate lighting for the client.

If the client has an assistant, acknowledge the assistant, but direct all conversation to the client. If the client has a service animal, do not touch, make eye contact with, talk to, feed, or distract the animal in any way. A distracted animal is not paying attention to its job, and its disabled human

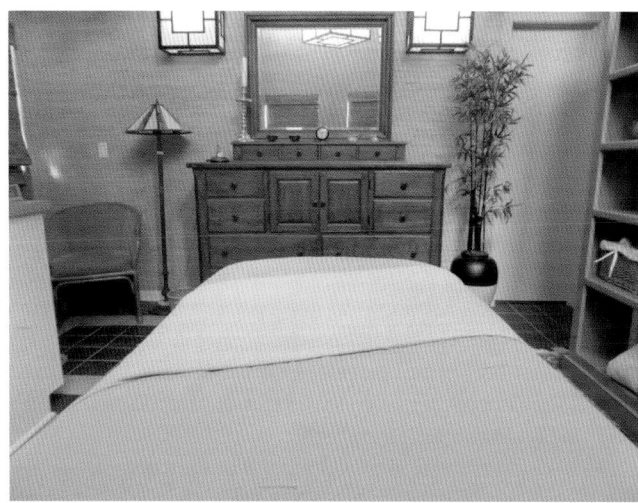

FIG. 11.20 Massage table linens: Consider using linens of contrasting color to help clients with visual impairments distinguish between the two sheets more easily.

handler could very well be injured. Even while resting, the animal is still working. In fact, many handlers do not give out their animal's name to avoid the possibility of the animal becoming distracted by hearing its name. If you are standing or walking alongside a person who has an assistant or service animal, be sure to stand or walk on the opposite side of the assistant or service animal.

Use linens of contrasting color (Fig. 11.20). These will help clients who are visually impaired distinguish between two sheets on the massage table more easily. Let the client know when the massage session is complete. If room lights were dimmed before the massage, increase light levels before you exit the massage room. This is applicable to any client and not only those who are visually impaired.

CLIENTS WITH HEARING IMPAIRMENTS

Hearing impairment, or hearing loss, is the decreased capacity to hear, and may occur in one or both ears. The term deafness is reserved for little or no hearing. In children, hearing impairment may affect the ability to learn a spoken language. Common causes of hearing impairment include advancing age, exposure to noise, ear trauma, and ear infections. Approximately 37.2 million people aged 18 years and older have hearing loss. One in three people who are 60 years of age and older have mild hearing loss, and half of those older than age 85 have significant hearing loss. Approximately 30% of people aged 70 and older wear hearing aids to improve hearing.

Practice Setting

Announce your presence and gain the client's attention before you speak. Eye contact is considered a sign of attention. Waving a hand in the person's direction or tapping a person lightly on the shoulder or arm are acceptable ways of gaining attention. Position yourself in relation to the impairment because one ear may function better than the other. Stand or sit near the client and remove objects that obstruct the client's view of you. This includes not holding your hands in front of your mouth, because seeing your mouth as you speak provides helpful visual cues. Maintain eye contact, speak in a normal tone of voice, do not shout, and do not chew gum. Only 10% of people who are hearing-impaired lip read, partly because lip reading is a difficult skill to master. Therefore, do not assume the client can lip read. Even if the client can lip read, enunciate clearly but do not exaggerate lip movements. Use facial expressions and body language to clarify your verbal message. Demonstrate your message as much as possible.

Hearing aids make sounds louder, but they do not clarify the meaning of what is heard, so observe the facial expressions and body language of the client to help determine whether your message was understood. Keep your language simple and succinct. If a word is not understood, use a different word. If the client is struggling with verbal communication, try written communication. In fact, written communication may be more effective for clients who are hearing-impaired.

Techniques

If the client is wearing hearing aids during the massage, avoid moving your hands close to the ears. Objects near the device may produce feedback (an uncomfortable squeaking noise). Let the client know when the massage session is complete. Consider establishing a nonverbal communication method before beginning the massage. For example, ask the client to raise a hand if they are experiencing discomfort from a massage technique, which will be responded to immediately. A 5-point pressure scale can be used and indicated by the number of fingers extended on a raised hand. In this situation, one extended finger represents light pressure, and five fingers represent deep pressure.

CLIENTS WITH MOBILITY IMPAIRMENTS

Mobility impairment is the decreased capacity to move or use one or more of the extremities, or a lack of strength needed to walk, grasp objects, or lift objects. Individuals affected by mobility impairment or who have disabilities may use wheelchairs, quad canes, crutches, walkers, or motor scooters to aid mobility (see Fig. 11.18). Reasons for their use include aging, disease (arthritis, chronic obstructive pulmonary disease), congenital disorder (spina bifida, muscular dystrophy), inactivity, obesity, and injury (spinal cord injury, stroke). While some disabilities are temporary, such as those incurred while healing from surgery, others are long term.

Thirteen million people in the United States use mobility aids, and lack of or limited mobility is the most common disability among older Americans.

Practice Setting

The first consideration is how the client will enter your office. Most municipalities require businesses to be barrier-free and wheelchair accessible. If your office is not compliant (e.g., a home office in a historical district), schedule a home visit or perform the massage offsite in a location with proper client access.

Include a rest period before the intake, as the client may be fatigued from using the mobility aid. Some clients who use mobility aids take prescribed medications that have accompanying side effects such as drowsiness. In addition, as the wheelchair or mobility device is part of the client's body space, avoid leaning on the device/wheelchair and move it only when asked. If the client appears to require your assistance, offer it. Respond to a "no, thank you" graciously if your offer for assistance is declined.

During the intake, sit down so both of you are at the same eye level. If the client is unable to speak clearly, ask family members or caregivers for the best communication method. Possible methods used to communicate include raising a finger or blinking the eyes once to indicate "yes," raising two fingers or closing eyes to indicate "no," or using an alphabet board. Ask the client to describe the degree of limitation they experience. This information will help you determine any modifications.

Techniques

Adapt the massage to the client if mobility devices such as a wheelchair are used. You can place pillows on a massage table onto which the client can lean forward while sitting in the chair, or use a face rest device that clips on to a table (Fig. 11.21). Use a tripod position to ensure the client's body is supported during a seated massage. The three parts of the tripod are the client's: (1) feet on the floor, (2) buttocks on

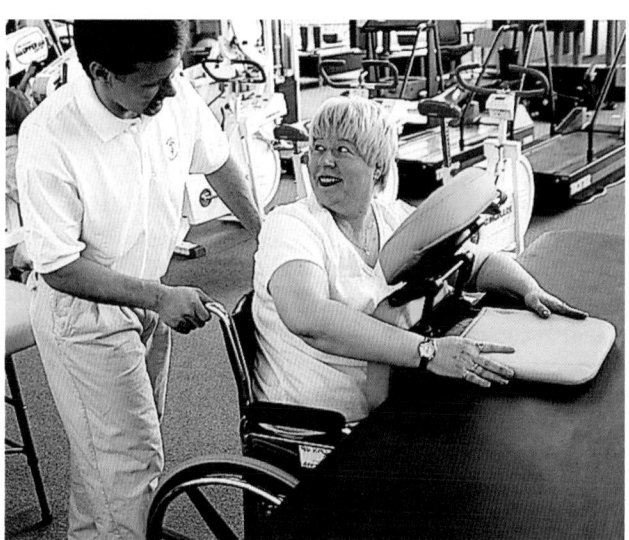

FIG. 11.21 Wheelchair modification: A face rest device that clips onto a table can be used to massage a client who is seated in a wheelchair. (From Salvo, S. [2016]. *Massage therapy: Principles and practice* [6th ed.]. St Louis: Elsevier.).

the chair, and (3) hands or elbows on a supportive surface, such as a table or their own thighs. An unsupported seated position is not recommended because the client may tire easily from providing counterbalance. Be sure the chair wheels are locked before the massage begins.

Clients may elect to use the massage table. Clients who use a wheelchair know how to transfer, or move, into and out of the chair. If you are providing massage in a healthcare facility, ask the floor supervisor to locate a qualified person for assistance with transfer when needed. If the client has cold intolerance, provide comfort measures such as a warm blanket, an electric table warmer, raising the room temperature, or a combination of these. If using an electric table warmer, turn it on before the client arrives to warm the table surface, and turn it off when the client is on the table because some clients have poor thermal regulation.

Be sure to address tension in the shoulders, chest, arms, and forearms. These areas are often tense because of the amount of upper body strength needed to use mobility devices. Generally speaking, the longer a client has been inactive, the greater the risk of reduced bone density and DVT or blood clots in deep veins in the legs. If the client has areas of reduced bone density, decrease the amount of applied massage pressure and avoid forceful PROM. If the client has been diagnosed with DVT, avoid the affected lower extremity (e.g., local contraindication). Otherwise, look for signs and symptoms of DVT, such as unilateral leg swelling, heat, redness or noticeable discoloration, pain, and tenderness. If present, avoid massage to the affected lower extremity (thigh and leg). Massage has been found to be safe when precautions, such as screening for DVT and avoiding the affected limb, are taken (Ng et al., 2018).

Local massage is contraindicated over areas at risk for decubitus ulcer formation among individuals who are wheelchair-bound. At-risk areas are over the scapula, sacrum, ischial tuberosities, popliteal areas, and plantar surfaces of the feet. Decubitus ulcers (pressure sores) are discussed in Chapter 22. Anything that looks suspicious needs to be reported to the client and/or the client's caretaker.

THE DUTY TO PROTECT: MANDATORY REPORTING

Mandatory reporting is a legislative mandate that applies to individuals who have regular contact with vulnerable populations (i.e., children, dependent adults, the elderly) to file a report with protection services when abuse or neglect (including self-neglect) is observed or suspected. This mandate is called the *Duty to Protect*. Approximately 4% to 6% of older populations are abused physically, psychologically, or financially. Neglect accounts for about 14% of complaints in nursing homes.

Know the requirement for mandatory reporting in the state where you are working or plan to work. A document titled Mandatory Reports of Child Abuse and Neglect is available from the Child Welfare Information Gateway (www.childwelfare.gov). Similar information about the duty to report elder abuse can be obtained from the National Center on Elder Abuse at https://ncea.acl.gov/. Follow the links to State Resources in the state in which you practice.

If you suspect neglect or physical abuse through observations of bruises (especially bilateral bruising that might suggest grabbing), black eyes, welts, broken eyeglasses, or marks indicating restraints, report your observations to your supervisor if you work in a spa or medical setting. In these cases, the supervisor is responsible for making the report. If you are a sole practitioner, contact your local protection services or an eldercare hotline (800-677-1116). When reporting, include all known information about the suspected neglect or abuse, along with your contact information. In most states, reports are made anonymously with no repercussions, called *immunity for good faith reporting*.

If a dependent or older adult discloses abuse or neglect to you directly, reassure them that you believe what was said, and that you will take steps to help. Contact the applicable protection agency as soon as possible. If the practitioner has reason to suspect someone is in immediate danger, the practitioner should call 911.

Mandated reporters are not required to, and in no circumstances, serve as investigators. However, information such as photographs may be taken in support of the report, which may be used during an investigation. Avoid asking the client questions to try get to the bottom of the allegation. In addition, avoid informing the client's family about the report.

E-RESOURCES

http://evolve.elsevier.com/Salvo/MassageTherapy

- Chapter challenge
- Flash cards
- Additional information

TINA ALLEN

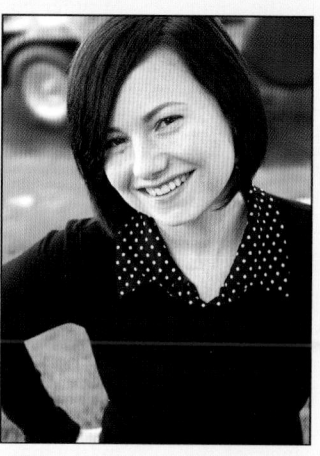

Kids—if you are the type who loves them, what is your first instinct when there are children in your vicinity? Whether you are a pick-them-up-and-throw-them-in-the-air type, a snuggle-with-a-picture-book type, or simply a high-fiver, your answer probably involves touch. People have been snuggling, hugging, and providing nurturing touch to children since the dawn of time. Animals do it, too. How we bathe, carry, and feed our children changes from culture to culture, but the overwhelming similarities are clear: Nothing is more universal than caring touch.

Tina Allen says, "It is my belief that with nurturing, compassion, and touch, children will develop and reach their full potential." Her mission is to reach every corner of the globe to provide nurturing touch and teach others to do the same. Allen believes infant massage is "the property of the world" and teaches her evidence-based, safe, and professional techniques while honoring the many traditions of touch found in history and around the world.

This mission is no side gig; it is Allen's life. She lives in a tour bus with her husband and son, and travels throughout the United States and Canada teaching multiple variations of pediatric massage. Topics covered in her workshops range from infant massage training for parents, to advanced training for children with autism spectrum disorders, cerebral palsy, and other illnesses that affect children. Her courses provide techniques that can be applied by all kinds of caregivers and health professionals, not just massage practitioners.

To accomplish her goals, Allen founded Liddle Kidz Foundation Global, through which she regularly organizes groups of professional volunteers to travel to other parts of the world providing outreach to vulnerable infants, children and their caregivers. Employing the use of stickers, smiles, interpreters, and lots of gesturing, Allen and her team overcome language and cultural barriers to provide and teach nurturing touch to improve the lives of children and caregivers alike. Each program Allen devises is designed to create sustainable change in the long term. Caregivers receive training so that nurturing touch can continue even after Allen and her team of ambassadors have left. During two such humanitarian trips, efforts of the team were captured on film to create the groundbreaking short documentaries *Liddle Kidz in Japan,* a documentary film about pediatric massage in Japan following the tsunami and *Liddle Kidz in Vietnam,* a documentary film about pediatric massage for orphaned children.

Allen managed the first U.S. comprehensive pediatric massage program at Children's Hospital Los Angeles, where she trained volunteer massage practitioners and medical professionals to work with hospitalized rehabilitation patients and medically complex infants, as well as children with retinoblastoma, spina bifida, and cerebral palsy. She has developed pediatric massage programs at numerous hospitals and health centers throughout the country and acts as a consultant on the development of comprehensive pediatric massage programs for several medical programs and hospitals.

Allen is the go-to expert in the field of pediatric massage and has appeared on Public Broadcasting Service (PBS), National Broadcasting Company (NBC), and The Learning Channel (TLC). She has also been the subject of numerous print interviews and articles, and writes regularly for major massage publications in the United States and Canada. Allen was inducted into the Massage Hall of Fame in 2009 and named the Massage Therapy Foundation Performance Health Humanitarian of the Year in 2012. Allen's first book, *A Modern-Day Guide to Massage for Children,* was published in 2013 and provides families and professionals with an illustrated, easy-to-follow guide to incorporating nurturing touch into the lives of children.

REFERENCES

Aday, L. A. (1991). *At risk in America: The health and healthcare needs of vulnerable populations.* San Francisco, CA: Jossey-Bass.

Agren, A., & Berg, M. (2006). Tactile massage and severe nausea and vomiting during pregnancy: Women's experiences. *Scandinavian Journal of Caring Sciences, 20*(2), 169–176.

American Massage Therapy Association (AMTA). (2021). *Massage profession research report.* Retrieved from https://www.amtamassage.org/publications/massage-profession-research-report/.

American Pregnancy Association. (n.d.a). *Best sleeping positions during pregnancy.* Retrieved from https://americanpregnancy.org/healthy-pregnancy/pregnancy-health-wellness/sleeping-positions-while-pregnant/.

American Pregnancy Association. (n.d.b). *Postpartum massage.* Retrieved from https://americanpregnancy.org/healthy-pregnancy/first-year-of-life/postpartum-massage/.

American Pregnancy Association. (n.d.c). *Prenatal massage.* Retrieved from https://americanpregnancy.org/healthy-pregnancy/is-it-safe/prenatal-massage/.

Barnett, K. (1972). A survey of the current utilization of touch by health team personnel with hospitalized patients. *International Journal of Nursing Studies, 9*(4), 195–209.

Behera, C., Devassy, S., Mridha, A. R., Chauhan, M., & Gupta, S. K. (2018). Leg massage by mother resulting in fatal pulmonary thromboembolism. *Medico-Legal Journal, 86*(3), 146–150.

Berger, M., Cüppers, H. J., Jörgens, V., & Berchtold, P. (1982). Absorption kinetics and biologic effects of subcutaneously injected insulin preparation. *Diabetes Care, 5*(2), 77–91.

Buckle, J. (2014). *Clinical aromatherapy: Essential oils in healthcare* (3rd ed.). Philadelphia: Elsevier Science.

Centers for Disease Control and Prevention (CDC). (2020). *Breastfeeding report cards.* Retrieved from http://www.cdc.gov/breastfeeding/data/reportcard.htm.

Centers for Disease Control and Prevention (CDC). (2021). *Birth data.* Retrieved from https://www.cdc.gov/nchs/fastats/delivery.htm.

Centers for Disease Control and Prevention (CDC). (2022). *Breastfeeding: Frequently asked questions.* Retrieved from https://www.cdc.gov/breastfeeding/faq/index.htm

Chan, W. S., Spencer, F. A., & Ginsberg, J. S. (2010). Anatomic distribution of deep vein thrombosis in pregnancy. *CMAJ, 182*(7), 657–660.

Chen, P. J., Chou, C. C., Yang, L., Tsai, Y. L., Chang, Y. C., & Liaw, J. J. (2017). Effects of aromatherapy massage on pregnant women's stress and immune function: A longitudinal, prospective, randomized controlled trial. *Journal of Alternative and Complementary Medicine, 23*(10), 778–786.

Crump, C., & Paluska, S. A. (2010). Venous thromboembolism following vigorous deep tissue massage. *The Physician and Sportsmedicine, 38*(4), 136–139.

De-Giorgio, F., Grassi, V. M., Vetrugno, G., d'Aloja, E., Pascali, V. L., & Arena, V. (2012). Supine hypotensive syndrome as the probable cause of both maternal and fetal death. *Journal of Forensic Sciences, 57*(6), 1646–1649.

Embong, N. H., Soh, Y. C., Ming, L. C., & Wong, T. W. (2015). Revisiting reflexology: Concept, evidence, current practice, and practitioner training. *Journal of Traditional and Complementary Medicine, 5*(4), 197–206.

Equality Act. (2021). *HR. 5, 117th Congress.* Retrieved from https://www.congress.gov/bill/117th-congress/house-bill/5?q=%7B%-22search%22%3A%5B%22pregnancy+discrimination%22%5D%7D&s=1&r=8.

Fathi, M., Nikbakht Nasrabadi, A., & Valiee, S. (2014). The effects of body position on chemotherapy-induced nausea and vomiting: A single-blind randomized controlled trial. *Iranian Red Crescent Medical Journal, 16*(6), e17778.

Field, T. (2010). Pregnancy and labor massage. *Expert Review of Obstetrics & Gynecology, 5*(2), 177–181.

Fogarty, S., McInerney, C., Stuart, C., & Hay, P. (2019). The side effects and mother or child related physical harm from massage during pregnancy and the postpartum period: An observational study. *Complementary Therapies in Medicine, 42*, 89–94.

Fried, L. P., Tangen, C. M., Walston, J., Newman, A. B., Hirsch, C., Gottdiener, J., et al. (2001). Frailty in older adults: Evidence for a phenotype. *The Journals of Gerontology. Series A, Biological Sciences and Medical Sciences, 56*(3), 146–156.

Gillick, M. R. (1996). *Choosing medical care in old age: What kind, how much, when to stop.* Cambridge, MA: Harvard University Press.

Gordon, A., Raynes-Greenow, C., Bond, D., Morris, J., Rawlinson, W., & Jeffery, H. (2015). Sleep position, fetal growth restriction, and late-pregnancy stillbirth: The Sydney stillbirth study. *Obstetrics & Gynecology, 125*(2), 347–355.

Heazell, A., Li, M., Budd, J., Thompson, J., Stacey, T., Cronin, R. S., Martin, B., Roberts, D., Mitchell, E. A., & McCowan, L. (2018). Association between maternal sleep practices and late stillbirth: Findings from a stillbirth case-control study. *BJOG, 125*(2), 254–262.

Huberty, J., Matthews, J., Leiferman, J. A., & Lee, C. (2018). Use of complementary approaches in pregnant women with a history of miscarriage. *Complementary Therapies in Medicine, 36*, 1–5.

Jabr, F. (2007). Massive pulmonary emboli after legs massage. *American Journal of Physical Medicine & Rehabilitation, 86*(8), 691.

Kirzinger, A., Neuman, T., Cubanski, J., & Brodie, M. (2019). *Data note: Prescription drugs and older adults.* Retrieved from https://www.kff.org/health-reform/issue-brief/data-note-prescription-drugs-and-older-adults/

Kloter, E., Gerstenberg, G., Berenyi, T., Gollmer, B., Flüger, C., Klein, U., et al. (2019). Treatment of hyperemesis gravidarum with anthroposophic complex therapy in 3 case reports. *Complementary Therapies in Medicine, 44*, 14–17.

Kuznar, W. (2010). Increased risk of thromboembolism 12 weeks after surgery. *American Journal of Nursing, 110*(3), 17.

Latifses, V., Estroff, D. B., Field, T., & Bush, J. P. (2005). Fathers massaging and relaxing their pregnant wives lowered anxiety and facilitated marital adjustment. *Journal of Bodywork and Movement Therapies, 9*(4), 277–282.

Lim, D., Jayanthi, H., Money-Kyrle, A., & Ramrakha, P. (2009). Massaging the outcome: An unusual presentation of pulmonary embolism. *BMJ Case Report*, bcr01.2009.1505.

Linde, B. (1986). Dissociation of insulin absorption and blood flow during massage of a subcutaneous injection site. *Diabetes Care, 9*(6), 570–574.

Lohman, J. S. (2001). Massage for elders: An ever-growing opportunity. *Massage Therapy Journal, 40*(3), 60–79.

Mallory, M. J., Hauschulz, J. L., Do, A., Dreyer, N. E., & Bauer, B. A. (2018). Case reports of acupuncturists and massage therapists at Mayo Clinic: New allies in expediting patient diagnoses. *Explore, 14*(2), 149–151.

Mayo Clinic. (2018). *Heartburn.* Retrieved from http://www.mayoclinic.org/diseases-conditions/heartburn/basics/lifestyle-home-remedies/con-20019545.

McMahon, M., Fenwick, A., Banks, A., & Dineen, R. A. (2009). Prevention of supine hypotensive syndrome in pregnant women undergoing computed tomography: A national survey of current practice. *Radiography, 15*(2), 97–100.

Moffitt Cancer Center (MCC). (2008). *Managing your scar.* Retrieved from https://moffitt.org/media/1086/managing_your_scar.pdf.

Montagu, A. (1986). *Touching: The human significance of the skin* (3rd ed.). New York: HarperCollins.

National Council on Aging. (n.d.). *Health aging facts.* Retrieved from https://www.ncoa.org/news/resources-for-reporters/get-the-facts/healthy-aging-facts/.

Ng, A. H., Francis, G. J., Sumler, S. S., Liu, D., & Bruera, E. (2018). The efficacy and safety of massage therapy for cancer inpatients with venous thromboembolism. *Journal of Integrative Oncology, 7*, 203.

Pew Research Center. (2009). *Growing old in America: Expectation vs reality.* Retrieved from http://www.pewsocialtrends.org/2009/06/29/growing-old-in-america-expectations-vs-reality/.

Ravanelli, N., Casasola, W., English, T., Edwards, K. M., & Jay, O. (2018). Heat stress and fetal risk. Environmental limits for exercise and passive heat stress during pregnancy: A systematic review with best evidence synthesis. *British Journal of Sports Medicine, 53*(13), 799–805.

Shoghi, M., Sohrabi, S., & Rasouli, M. (2018). The effects of massage by mothers on mother-infant attachment. *Alternative Therapies in Health and Medicine, 24*(3), 34–39.

Stacey, T., Mitchell, E. A., & Zuccollo, J. M. (2011). Association between maternal sleep practices and risk of late stillbirth: A case-control study. *BMJ, 342*, d3403.

Stillerman, E. (2008). *Prenatal massage: A textbook of pregnancy, labor, and postpartum bodywork.* St Louis: Mosby.

Stillerman, E. (2021). *Top 7 tips for working with pregnant massage clients.* Retrieved from https://www.massagemag.com/elaine-stillermans-top-7-tips-for-working-with-pregnant-massage-clients-129938/

Sweetland, S., Green, J., Liu, B., de González, A. B., Canonico, M., Reeves, G., et al. (2009). Duration and magnitude of the postoperative risk of venous thromboembolism in middle aged women: Prospective cohort study. *BMJ, 339*, b4583.

Tosun, B., Cinar, F. I., Topcu, Z., Masatoglu, B., Ozen, N., Bağçivan, G., et al. (2019). Do patients with diabetes use the insulin pen properly? *African Health Sciences, 19*(1), 1628–1637.

U. S. Food and Drug Administration. (2019). *What you should know about using cannabis, including CBD, when pregnant or breastfeeding*. Retrieved from https://www.fda.gov/consumers/consumer-updates/what-you-should-know-about-using-cannabis-including-cbd-when-pregnant-or-breastfeeding.

Wang, S. M., DeZinno, P., Fermo, L., William, K., Caldwell-Andrews, A. A., Bravemen, F., et al. (2005). Complementary and alternative medicine for low-back pain in pregnancy: A cross-sectional survey. *Journal of Alternative and Complementary Medicine, 11*(3), 459–464.

World Health Organization. (n.d.a). *Working definition of an older elderly person*. Retrieved from http://www.who.int/health-info/survey/ageingdefnolder/en/.

World Health Organization. (n.d.b). *WHOQOL: Measuring quality of life*. Retrieved from https://www.who.int/tools/whoqol.

REVIEW AND APPLY YOUR KNOWLEDGE

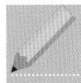 **MATCHING ONE: CONCEPT REVIEW**
Place the letter of the answer next to the number of the term or phrase that best describes it.

A. Deep vein thrombosis
B. First
C. Disability
D. Infant massage
E. Preeclampsia
F. Special populations
G. Relaxin
H. Left lateral tilt
I. Supine hypotensive syndrome
J. Third
K. About week 22
L. High-risk

_____ 1. Condition of persistent high blood pressure and protein in the urine during pregnancy.
_____ 2. Pregnancy trimester in which heartburn, lower back pain, and feet swelling are more prevalent.
_____ 3. Pregnancy more likely to have complications for the mother, the developing baby, or both.
_____ 4. Client position to reduce the risk of supine hypotensive syndrome during pregnancy.
_____ 5. Group of individuals who are disadvantaged, vulnerable, and/or at risk for harm.
_____ 6. When to begin using positional modifications to prevent supine hypotensive syndrome during pregnancy.
_____ 7. A drop in blood pressure caused by compression of the pregnant uterus against major abdominal blood vessels.
_____ 8. Hormone altering the properties of connective tissues.
_____ 9. Modifications of massage techniques and body positions to meet the needs of the child and the child's family.
_____ 10. An impairment or condition that makes it more difficult for the person to participate in one or more major life activity.
_____ 11. Pregnancy trimester in which morning sickness and miscarriage are more prevalent.
_____ 12. Vascular condition pregnant females are at a higher risk for developing because of decreased clot-dissolving properties and increased clotting-producing factors.

MATCHING TWO: CONCEPT REVIEW
Place the letter of the answer next to the number of the term or phrase that best describes it.

A. 16 years old
B. 65 years old
C. Edema
D. Pregnancy massage
E. Fried's Frailty Criteria
F. Visual impairments
G. Geriatric massage
H. Mandatory reporting
I. Mobility impairment
J. Ischial tuberosities
K. Orthostatic hypotension
L. Sarcopenia

_____ 1. Loss of muscle tone and strength from age-related inactivity.
_____ 2. Method used to determine whether an older client is robust or frail.
_____ 3. Dizziness experienced from a drop in blood pressure after moving from a lying down or sitting position to an upright or standing position.
_____ 4. Possible locations of decubitus ulcers among chair-bound clients.
_____ 5. Modifications of massage techniques and body positions to meet the needs of older and aging adults.
_____ 6. Age a person can legally consent to nontherapeutic/self-care procedures in most states.
_____ 7. Legislative requirement to individuals who have regular contact with vulnerable populations (children, dependent adults, elderly) to file a report with protection services when abuse or neglect (including self-neglect) is observed or suspected.
_____ 8. Decreased capacity to see that cannot be corrected by usual means, such as eyeglasses or contact lenses.
_____ 9. Modifications of massage techniques and body positions to meet the needs of clients as they undergo changes during pregnancy and the postpartum period.
_____ 10. Swelling that may occur in the legs, ankles, and feet during pregnancy.
_____ 11. Chronologic age marking the beginning of old age in most developing countries.
_____ 12. Decreased capacity to move or use one or more of the extremities, or a lack of strength needed to walk, grasp objects, or lift objects.

MULTIPLE CHOICE: TEST YOUR KNOWLEDGE

Place the letter of the answer next to the number of the term or phrase that best describes it.

_____ 1. Which Quality of Life domain includes transportation and opportunities to participate in recreation and leisure activities?
   A. Psychological
   B. Physical
   C. Relational
   D. Environmental

_____ 2. The most common reason pregnant clients receive massage is:
   A. lower back pain.
   B. shoulder pain.
   C. carpal tunnel syndrome.
   D. relaxation.

_____ 3. The first trimester refers to the first ____ weeks of pregnancy.
   A. 10
   B. 14
   C. 16
   D. 22

_____ 4. The safest position for the unborn beginning on about week 22 is:
   A. prone.
   B. supine.
   C. left side-lying.
   D. right side-lying.

_____ 5. When do most cases of gestational diabetes mellitus develop?
   A. First trimester
   B. Second trimester
   C. Third trimester
   D. Postpartum

_____ 6. What pregnancy-related hormone may make body joints hypermobile?
   A. Relaxin
   B. Oxytocin
   C. Dopamine
   D. Serotonin

_____ 7. Which is the recommended method for infant massage?
   A. Practitioner massages infant with parent participation
   B. Practitioner massages infant while parent observes
   C. Practitioner demonstrates on doll while parent observes
   D. Practitioner demonstrates on doll while parent massages infant

_____ 8. Inquiring about medication use for clients 65 or older is important, as ____% report taking prescription drugs.
   A. 30%
   B. 50%
   C. 60%
   D. 85%

_____ 9. Which aging-related condition causes a stooped posture and can make it uncomfortable to lie prone?
   A. Hyperkyphosis
   B. Sarcopenia
   C. Tinnitus
   D. Hypertension

_____ 10. Practitioners working on aging clients are encouraged to inspect their ____ for suspicious areas or injury.
   A. hands
   B. scalp
   C. feet
   D. abdomen

_____ 11. Which is the best instruction to guide a client with visual impairments to the massage table?
   A. The table is over there.
   B. The table is right in front of you.
   C. The table is at 2 o'clock.
   D. The table is a few steps to the right.

_____ 12. A practitioner that works in a medical setting that suspects a patient has been abused should:
   A. Call 911
   B. Report the observation to a supervisor
   C. Report the observation to a local hotline
   D. Report the observation to the patient's family

CRITICAL THINKING

The Best Laid Plans

Kimberly and Rochelle are just about ready to graduate from massage school. They are discussing what types of settings in which they would like to practice massage. Rochelle says because she can't afford to open her own office right away, she'll be applying at a local franchise. Kimberly says that she'd never work at a franchise because clients who go there can "have all sorts of things wrong with them," and she doesn't want to deal with that. Instead, she plans to work only on clients who are in peak physical condition, like athletes. What is the best way for Rochelle to respond to Kimberly?

Answers can include but are not limited to:

Very few people are in peak physical condition, including athletes. Many times, athletes are dealing with injuries. In addition, athletes usually have a health and fitness team already in place; it is difficult for a new massage practitioner with little experience to break into the sports massage field.

It is more realistic for new massage practitioners to be open to working on all types of clients. This will give the massage practitioner a great deal of experience and a better chance to build a stable client base, which is key to career longevity. Generally, almost every client is dealing with some issue, whether it be physical, mental, emotional, or even spiritual. The most successful massage practitioners are those who can work with a diverse clientele.

Finally, in some locations it is illegal to not work on certain clients; it is viewed as discrimination. Plus, the massage practitioner may not know if a client has a challenge that requires special consideration until the client arrives for the appointment. The massage practitioner telling clients directly that they cannot work on them creates awkward and unprofessional situations that, again, may be illegal.

PROFESSIONAL PRACTICE

Amyo-... What?

Your first client of the day is Stephanie. She arrives in a wheelchair looking fatigued. During the health assessment, she indicates she has a condition called amyotrophic lateral sclerosis. You are unfamiliar with this condition. How do you proceed? Include questions you would ask the client in your response, and list specific modifications for a client in a wheelchair.

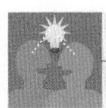

DISCUSSION

Pregnancy

Pregnancy is one of the most challenging times in our lives; whether it's trying to get pregnant, trying to keep from getting pregnant, physical and emotional changes during pregnancy, and life-altering experiences of a new baby in the house after childbirth. This discussion forum highlights the world of pregnant couples and identifies ways to improve the quality of client care. If you were or are pregnant, what was it like? Ask a friend, classmate, or family member if you do not have firsthand experience. If available, post your reflections on an internet-based discussion board monitored by your instructor.

I would like to thank Kim Corpus and JoEllen Sefton for their past contributions on this chapter.

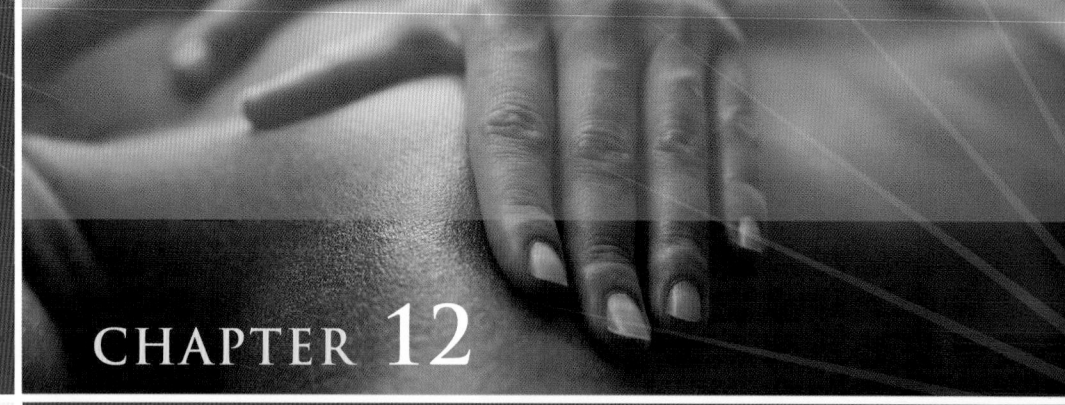

CHAPTER 12

Hydrotherapy: Clinical Applications, Spa Applications, and Spa Procedures

Nothing on earth is as weak and yielding as water, but for breaking down the firm and strong, it has no equal.

—Lao Tzu

LEARNING OBJECTIVES

After completing this chapter, the student should be able to:

1. Define hydrotherapy and explain the physical properties of water.
2. Discuss clinical cryotherapy, its beneficial effects and uses, contraindications and adverse effects, and various application methods.
3. Discuss clinical thermotherapy, its beneficial effects and uses, contraindications and adverse effects, and various application methods.
4. Define spa hydrotherapy, contraindications and safety issues, and state various application methods.
5. Identify various spa therapies and their application methods.

http://evolve.elsevier.com/Salvo/MassageTherapy

INTRODUCTION

Hydrotherapy is the use of water in any of its forms for health promotion or treatment of various diseases and conditions. Heat and cold are temperature aspects of hydrotherapy and are given specialized names of *cryotherapy* and *thermotherapy*. Like massage, hydrotherapy is one of the most widely used treatment systems in the world. For centuries, cultures have enjoyed the benefits of water. It has been used to obtain and maintain health, manage pain, and treat physical and emotional ailments. Water has also been an essential component in religious rituals and healing rites (e.g., baptism). Hippocrates advised both hot and cold bathing, and this was the first recorded use of contrast bathing. Hydrotherapy is also known as *water therapy*, *water cure*, and *balneotherapy* (Mooventhan & Nivethitha, 2014).

Both ancient Grecians and Romans believed water had healing properties. The Romans integrated water into their social and political life, building temples and baths near natural springs. Later, Grecians built public baths in conjunction with gymnasiums to facilitate sound bodies and sound minds. Bath temperatures were adjusted to meet the needs of individual bathers and achieve desired outcomes. In the Grecian city Sparta, laws were passed making frequent bathing mandatory.

Father Sebastian Kneipp (1821–1897), from Wörishofen, Bavaria, in western Germany, is regarded as the father of hydrotherapy. Kneipp possessed exceptional knowledge and skill in using water to heal the ailments affecting members of his community. These treatments, known collectively as *Kneipp therapy,* are still used today at world-class spas. Key components of Kneipp therapy are herbal and mineral baths, as well as cold or alternating hot and cold treatments administered by water, stones, or pebbles. Father Kneipp published his only book on hydrotherapy, *My Water Cure*, in 1886.

Drs. George Henry Taylor (1829–1899) and Charles Fayette Taylor (1827–1899) used "water cures" as part of their treatment regimen at the Remedial Hygienic Institute in New York City, which opened in 1856. The Institute was an orthopedic center specializing in the Ling system of massage and exercise.

In the late nineteenth century, areas of natural springs became popular destinations across Europe and later in the United States. These were the beginnings of the modern-day health spas, a place where people came to relax and rejuvenate. Sanitariums were established as a type of health resort where individuals could go to regain health after a long-term illness such as tuberculosis or polio. The most famous US sanitariums were in Hot Springs, AR; Saratoga Springs, NY; and White Sulfur Springs, WV. John Harvey Kellogg (1852–1943) was the director of the Battle Creek Sanitarium in Michigan where both massage and "water cures" were a central aspect of the health regimen (see Chapter 1). Water is still used today in clinics, spas, and wellness centers across the globe.

Water can be used in all three of its physical states—solid, liquid, and vapor—to rehabilitate and relax clients and improve their quality of life. Water can be applied to clients with or without immersion. Methods range from superficial heating or cooling by topical applications to edema control. Wellness and self-care uses of water are common in spa practices and include the use of spa tubs, steam and sauna chambers, and showering methods. Complementary agents such as soaps, minerals such as salts and clays, plant essences, essential oils, aromatics, and seaweed can be added to water to enhance its properties or to produce additional effects. **Thalassotherapy** is the external use of seawater specifically. The term thalassotherapy comes from the Greek word for sea. Spa treatments that incorporate thalassotherapy are seawater baths and body wraps. Aromatherapy is discussed in Chapter 3.

WATER: PHYSICAL PROPERTIES

Water has physical properties to help fulfill client goals. These properties include solvency, heat transference, and hydrostatic pressure. Water is extremely adaptable and can mold itself to any container or vessel. Properties of water such as buoyancy, resistance, and cleanliness will not be included as they are aligned with water exercise and wound care, which are often out of a massage practitioner's scope of practice.

Solvency

Water is a universal solvent and can dissolve more substances than any other liquid. It is an excellent medium for water-soluble agents such as baking soda (sodium bicarbonate), Epsom salt (magnesium sulfate), or sea salt (sodium chloride) for mineral baths. Milk or insoluble agents such as plant essences and herbs can be added to water to create milk baths or herbal baths, respectively.

Epsom salt takes its name from a bitter saline spring at Epsom in Surrey, England, where the salt was originally produced. Soaking in a warm bath containing Epsom salts is occasionally recommended to reduce muscle aches and pains. However, benefits appear to be related to soaking in heated water rather than the salt additive (Laliberte, 2019).

Heat Transference

Heat transfers from a warmer area to a cooler area. When one object or area is heated, it interacts with the cooler object/area, transferring heat in the process. Heat transfer will continue until the temperature between the two objects or areas is equal. Heat can be transferred to, from, or within the body by conduction, convection, radiation, evaporation, or conversion. Subcutaneous fat may serve as an insulation against the penetrating effects of cold or heat and heat transference may be significantly impaired in people who are overweight or obese (Petrofsky et al., 2009; Prentice, 1982).

- **Conduction.** Transfer of heat between objects or substances that are in direct contact with each other. Water has a high thermal conductivity and transfers heat 25 times faster than air at the same temperature. Nonmoving warm/hot water, hot packs, and paraffin baths transfer heat by conduction.

- **Convection**. Transfer of heat by circulating currents of water or air between a warmer object or substance and a cooler object or substance. Principles of conduction and convection are similar—the warmer object/substance interacts with the cooler object/substance and heat is transferred. Whirlpool baths transfer heat by convection.
- **Radiation**. Transfer of heat through heat rays. Infrared heat lamps transfer heat by radiation.
- **Evaporation**. Transfer or loss of heat when a liquid changes into a gas or vapor. Vapocoolant sprays are ethyl chloride that induce evaporative cooling when applied to the skin.
- **Conversion**. Transfer of a nonthermal form of energy (e.g., mechanical, electrical, chemical) into heat in the body. For example, ultrasound is a mechanical form of energy that converts to heat as the vibration and friction of molecules in the tissue generate heat. Use of ultrasound is often outside of a massage practitioner's scope of practice. Some types of instant cold packs work by conversion, initiating chemical reactions when cells in the pack are broken.

Hydrostatic Pressure

Hydrostatic pressure is pressure exerted by a fluid on an immersed object. According to Pascal's law, a fluid exerts equal pressure on an object at a given depth, and the pressure will increase as water depth increases. Because hydrostatic pressure increases at greater depths, a vertical position with the feet immersed most deeply will produce the best hydrostatic effects. Hydrostatic pressure can increase venous circulation and reduce peripheral edema and has effects similar to compressive bandages and garments. Urine output also increases because of hydrostatic pressure. When a body is immersed for 1 hour, urination increases by 50%. In fact, part of the edema reduction effects attributed to water's hydrostatic pressure is because of its impact on kidney function (Cameron, 2018).

CLINICAL CRYOTHERAPY

Cryotherapy is the therapeutic use of cold. Cryotherapy may be applied by a massage practitioner, by other qualified providers, or by properly instructed clients as part of home care. Ways to apply cryotherapy in clinical settings include cold packs, ice massage, cryokinetics, cryostretch, and the contrast method.

Clinical Cryotherapy: Beneficial Effects and Uses

Cryotherapy exerts its effects by influencing changes in blood flow; managing edema; and decreasing nerve conduction velocity, which reduces pain and spasticity. **NOTE**: Cryotherapy is no longer recommended during the acute phase of soft tissue injury because it interrupts or delays the inflammatory cascade (Mirkin, 2021; Scialoia & Swartzendruber, 2020). The *inflammatory cascade* is a process that increases the delivery of oxygen and blood flow to aid in healing and recovery following an injury. Ice can be used to reduce pain and swelling while in the subacute phase after acute inflammation has resolved. During this time, limit ice application to 10 minutes or less and for no more than 6 hours total.

Changes in Blood Flow

Cold application alters blood flow by causing immediate vasoconstriction. This initial response to cold is consistent and well-documented. Vasoconstriction continues for approximately 15 to 20 minutes. Blood flow effects are greater if cold applications are repeated twice—10 minutes off and 10 minutes on for two more application cycles—than for a single 20-minute application of cold (Karunakara et al., 1999; Weston et al., 1994).

Cold-induced vasodilation may occur when application exceeds 20 minutes or when tissue temperature reaches approximately 50°F (10°C). This effect was first noted by Lewis (1930) and called the *hunting response*. However, this response was later found to be inconsistent. Cold-induced vasodilation is more likely to occur in the distal areas of the body such as the fingers and toes.

Decreases Pain and Spasticity

Cold application can reduce edema applications may reduce pain and spasticity by increasing the pain threshold and pain tolerance, by providing counterirritation via gate control mechanisms, and by reducing nerve conduction velocity (Algafly & George, 2007; Ernst et al., 1994; Park et al., 2014; Singh et al., 2001; Zankel, 1966). Cold was more effective than heat to reduce pain (Benson & Copp, 1974). However, Garra and colleagues (2010) stated differences between cold and heat in their pain-reducing effects were similar, and therefore the choice to use cold or heat should be based on client or practitioner preference and on application availability.

Reduces Edema

Cold application can reduce edema associated with trauma or acute injury, especially when combined with compression and elevation. During elevation, the affected area is positioned above the level of the heart (Quillen et al., 1982).

Clinical Cryotherapy: Contraindications and Adverse Effects

There are several contraindications and reported adverse events associated with cyrotherapy (Cameron, 2018; Day, 1974).

- Cold intolerance.

- Cold hypersensitivity.
  - This reaction is characterized by smooth, slightly elevated patches that are redder or paler than surrounding skin and may be accompanied by severe itching called *cold-induced urticaria.*
- Very young or very old clients because of poor thermoregulation.
- Clients who have a diminished capacity to communicate.
- Areas of impaired or compromised circulation (e.g., hands or feet in clients with conditions such as Raynaud disease or peripheral arterial disease).
- Areas of nerve damage or compromised sensation, such as hands or feet, in clients with peripheral neuropathy.
- Open wounds, rashes, or previous cold injury.

A few adverse effects have been reported, including prolonged vasoconstriction and ischemia, which resulted in tissue damage. Excessive exposure to cold may also cause temporary or permanent nerve damage. To avoid these, limit the duration of cold application to 20 minutes with tissue temperature maintained above 59°F (15°C).

Clinical Cryotherapy: Procedures and Application Methods

Cryotherapy can be applied using a variety of methods, including cold gel or ice packs, ice massage, cold towel friction, cryokinetics, cryostretch, and the contrast method. Different methods cool superficial tissues at different rates and depths. For example, ice packs cooled skin faster than cold gel packs at the same initial temperature (Kanlayanaphotporn & Janwantanakul, 2005).

During cold application of any method, the client usually experiences a sequence of sensations including (1) feeling of intense cold, (2) burning, (3) stinging or aching, and (4) numbness or analgesia. These sensations are thought to correspond to the activation of thermoreceptors and nociceptors followed by blocking sensations caused by gate control mechanisms (Cameron, 2018).

Cryotherapy Procedure

A recommended cryotherapy procedure is:
1. Assess the client and determine whether cryotherapy is an appropriate and safe intervention.
2. Select the cryotherapy method.
3. Explain the procedure, reasons the treatment was selected, and sensations the client is expected to feel (e.g., cold, burning, stinging/aching, numbness/analgesia), and potential adverse events.
4. Obtain consent. Age of consent is 18 for clinical procedures and 16 for self-care and spa procedures. Check with applicable regulatory agencies.
5. Apply the cryotherapy method for up to 20 minutes.
6. Assess the client's response and treatment outcome.
7. Document the procedure including treatment details such as:
   - Type of treatment.

- Why treatment was administered.
- Application area.
- Position of the client.
- Temperature of the water or agent.
- Duration of application.
- Client's response or treatment outcome.

Cold Gel Packs and Ice Packs

Cold gel packs are strong vinyl pouches filled with gel composed of silica or a mixture of saline and gelatin. Cold packs are available in a variety of sizes and conform to the contours of the body because the gel remains semisolid at temperatures that normally freeze water to ice (Fig. 12.1). Cold packs can be made by filling a plastic bag with a 4:1 ratio mixture of water and rubbing alcohol cooled in a freezer. The alcohol prevents water from freezing solid, so pack contents remain pliable.

Ice packs are plastic bags filled with ice or icy water. For home use, clients can fill a plastic bag with ice or use a package of frozen vegetables such as peas. Use a barrier, such as a pillowcase or several paper towels, between the pack and the treatment area.

Ice Massage

Ice massage combines ice with friction massage. Often the ice is frozen water in a foam or paper cup. A wooden tongue

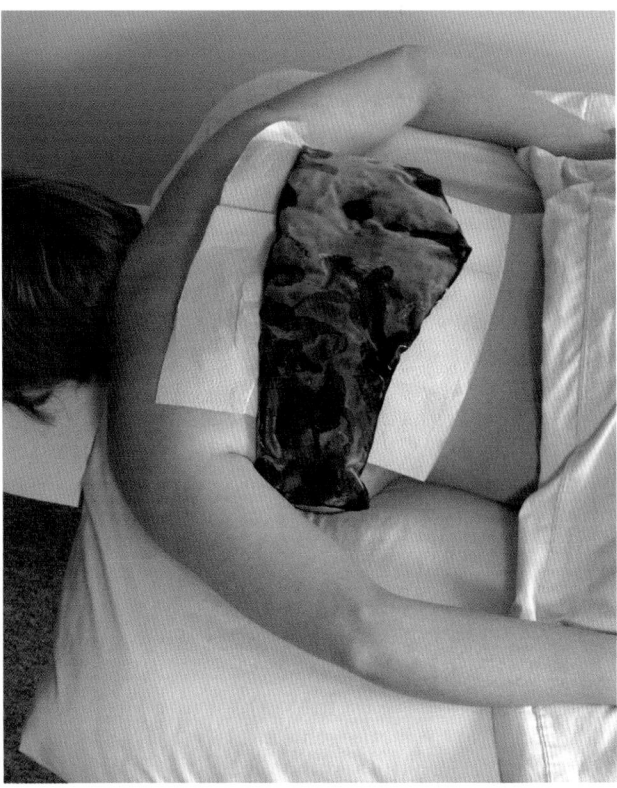

FIG. 12.1 Cold gel pack. Cold packs are available in a variety of sizes and conform well to the contours of the body because the gel remains semisolid.

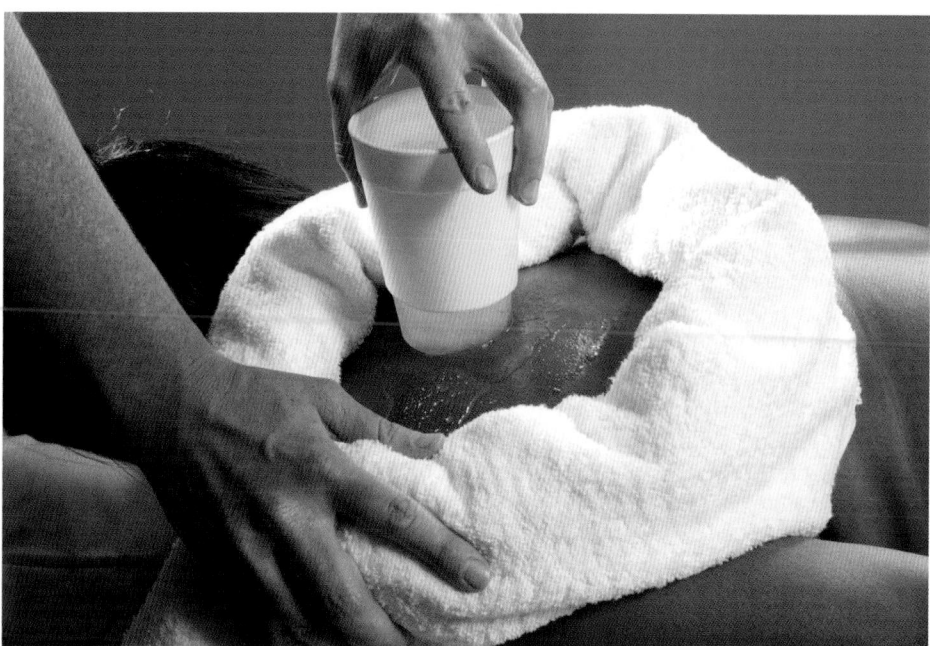

FIG. 12.2 Ice massage combines ice with friction massage. A towel is placed under the treatment area to absorb the water from melting ice.

depressor can be inserted into the water before freezing and can later serve as a handle. Tear the top edges or bottom portion of the cup to expose the ice. Rub the ice on the client's skin using continuous friction movements while holding the cup edge or wooden handle. Place a towel under the treatment area or a rolled-up towel around the area to absorb the water from melting ice (Fig. 12.2).

Cold-Towel Friction

Cold-towel friction, also called *cold-mitten friction*, combines ice application with friction massage (Fig. 12.3). During treatment, the client may stand, sit, or lie down on a water-resistant stool or surface. To apply cold-towel friction, dip two small towels into icy water. Do not wring the excess water from the towels. Apply the cold, wet towels to the client's skin. Move them back-and-forth using friction movements. The movements should be quick with moderate pressure. After 15 to 30 seconds, redip the towels in the icy water and repeat the friction movements. Dry the treatment area with a terrycloth using the same friction movements. Repeat this sequence 3 times.

Cryokinetics and Cryostretch

Cryokinetics combines cold application with joint mobilizations. **Cryostretch** combines cold application before stretching. Once analgesia has been achieved with ice application, passive or active movements can begin using the protocol guidelines listed in Chapter 8.

Contrast Method

The **contrast method** combines cold and heat in the same treatment. Cold can be applied at the same time as heat on

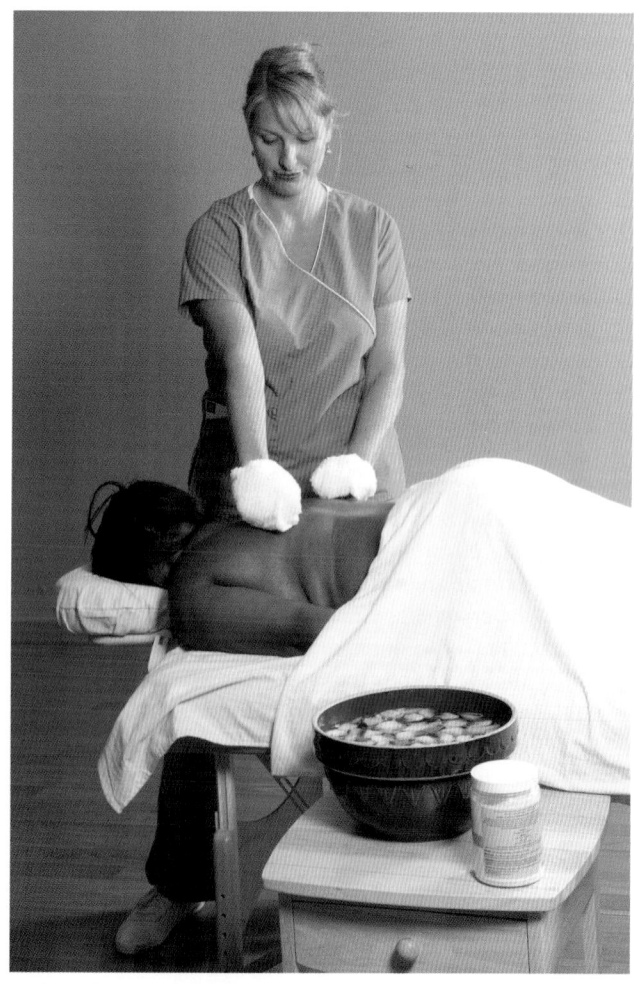

FIG. 12.3 Cold-towel friction. Dip two small towels into icy water, then apply friction.

adjacent areas such as the anterior thigh and posterior thigh. Cold and heat can also be applied alternately.

CLINICAL THERMOTHERAPY

Thermotherapy is the therapeutic use of heat. Thermotherapy may be applied by a massage practitioner, by other qualified providers, or by a properly instructed client as part of home care. Electric heating pads are not recommended for client home use unless they turn off automatically after a designated timeframe or have a manual "on" switch held down to deliver heat. These features protect the client from burning if they fall asleep while using the device. Ways to apply thermotherapy in clinical settings include hot packs, paraffin baths, and the contrast method.

Clinical Thermotherapy: Beneficial Effects and Uses

Thermotherapy exerts its effects by increasing superficial blood flow; decreasing nerve conduction velocity, which reduces pain and spasticity; increasing collagen extensibility, which increases range of motion (ROM); and decreasing joint stiffness.

Increases Blood Flow
Heat stimulates vasodilation, causing an increase in superficial blood flow to the area of application (Wyper & McNiven, 1976). Vasodilation is thought to be stimulated by increased parasympathetic output and decreased smooth muscle contraction in vessel walls.

Decreases Pain
Superficial heat applications decrease pain. Analgesic effects may occur by stimulation of thermoreceptors, which may reduce pain by gate control mechanisms. Pain may also be reduced by the psychologic experience of comfort, which may promote relaxation and reduce pain (Benson & Copp, 1974; Malanga et al., 2015; Mayer et al., 2005; Michlovitz et al., 2004; Yildirim et al., 2010). When comparing heat and cold to reduce pain, Garra and colleagues (2010) noted their similar effects and recommend that the decision on which approach to use should be based on client or practitioner preference and on application availability.

Increases Collagen Extensibility
Heat increases collagen extensibility in tissues when temperatures are maintained at 104°F to 113°F (40°C to 45°C) for 5 to 10 minutes. Collagen is a protein found in connective tissues and is abundant in tendons, ligaments, and skin (Lehmann et al., 1970, 1974; Lentell et al., 1992; Warren et al., 1971; Warren et al., 1976).

Increases Range of Motion/Flexibility and Decreases Stiffness
Heat increased ROM, improved flexibility, and decreased joint stiffness, especially when combined with movement. These effects are thought to be the result of increased collagen extensibility mentioned in the previous paragraph. Movements (e.g., stretching, joint mobilizations) should be performed during and immediately after heat application or the effects of prior heating will be lost (Funk et al., 2001; Knight et al., 2001; Lentell et al., 1992; Nakano et al., 2012; Petrofsky et al., 2013; Usuba et al., 2006; Yildirim et al., 2010).

Clinical Thermotherapy: Contraindications and Adverse Effects

There are several contraindications and reported adverse events associated with thermotherapy (Cameron, 2018; Magness et al., 1970; Schmidt et al., 1979).
- Recent or potential hemorrhage.
- Deep vein thrombosis or blood clots.
- Cardiac insufficiency.
- Very young or very old clients because of poor thermoregulation.
- Clients who have a diminished capacity to communicate.
- Areas of impaired or compromised circulation (e.g., the hands or feet of clients with conditions such as Raynaud disease or peripheral arterial disease).
- Areas of nerve damage or compromised sensation, such as the hands or feet of clients with peripheral neuropathy.
- Edema or lymphedema.
- Malignant tumor.
- Acute injury or inflammation.
- Metal in the area.
- Over open wounds, skin rashes, previous burn injuries, or metal objects such as piercings or titanium markers.
- Medical implanted devices, including pellets.
- Over areas where topical liniments or other topical agents have recently been applied, including prescription and nonprescription medications.

Adverse effects have been reported, including burns and fainting related to orthostatic hypotension. Skin can be burned if heat is applied too long, when the heating agent is too hot, or when the client does not have sufficient protective response. Skin can be burned at temperatures of 113°F (45°C) after 60 minutes and at 115°F (46°C) after 7½ minutes, so temperatures of heat application and duration should always be maintained below these levels (Cihoric et al., 2015; Sapareto & Dewey 1984). **NOTE:** Mun and colleagues (2012) found hot packs were the most common cause of contact burns in clinical settings, with the leg the most common injury site, followed by the foot and ankle. Individuals with diabetes mellitus had the highest correlation to contact burns from clinical uses of thermotherapy. Limit the amount of time a hot pack remains on areas below the knee to 10 minutes for this population.

The client may become dizzy, especially when moving to an upright position. This is called orthostatic hypotension (OH) and is from a sudden decrease in blood pressure related to peripheral vasodilation. Dizziness may lead to fainting. To reduce the risk of OH, ask the client to arise from the massage table in three stages: (1) sit up on the table for 1 minute; (2) sit on the side of the table with legs dangling for 1 minute; and (3) stand with care, holding onto the edge of the table or other non-movable object for 1 minute.

Clinical Thermotherapy: Procedures and Application Methods

Thermotherapy may be applied using a variety of methods, including hot packs, paraffin baths, and the contrast method. The contrast method was discussed in a previous section. During heat application, your client will experience the sensation of warmth. Discontinue treatment immediately if the client feels overheated, is in pain, or has discomfort. If applying massage to increase ROM, movements such as stretching should be applied during or immediately after heat application, or tissue extensibility effects will be lost. In addition, the client should be provided with a means of calling for assistance if the practitioner or other team members are not in the immediate vicinity.

Thermotherapy Procedure

A recommended thermotherapy procedure is:
1. Assess the client and determine whether thermotherapy is an appropriate and safe intervention for the client.
2. Select the thermotherapy method.
3. Explain the procedure, reasons why the treatment was selected, and sensations the client is expected to feel (warmth), and potential adverse events.
4. Obtain consent.
5. Apply the thermotherapy method. Temperatures and duration of treatment depend on the application method.
6. Assess the client's response and treatment outcome.
7. Document the procedure (see prior section for documentation details).

Hot Packs

Hot packs made for commercial use are pouches filled with bentonite (a type of clay) heated in a thermostatically controlled, stainless-steel water cabinet. Most professionals use a water cabinet called a *hydrocollator* (Fig. 12.4). Water temperature within the hydrocollator is usually between 158° F and 167°F (70°C and 75°C). The packs take approximately 2 hours to heat and 30 minutes to reheat between applications. Once heated, the packs are removed, wrapped in six to eight layers of dry terrycloth or a specially designed cover, then placed on the treatment area. More layers can be added if the client is feeling too much warmth, or layers can be reduced if the client does not feel enough warmth. Remove the pack after 15 to 20 minutes. Be sure the unit is in a location away from clients because touching the heating unit may burn the skin.

Chemical heating pads are made from a variety of materials that become warm once exposed to air or when the two materials blend once an inner seal is broken. These pads can maintain their temperature for 1 to 8 hours. Most chemical heating pads are single-use only. Electric heating pads are

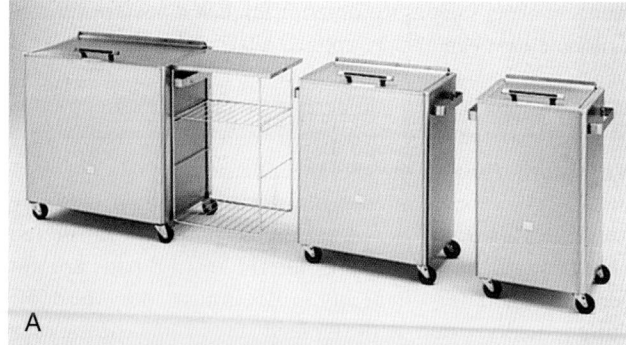

A

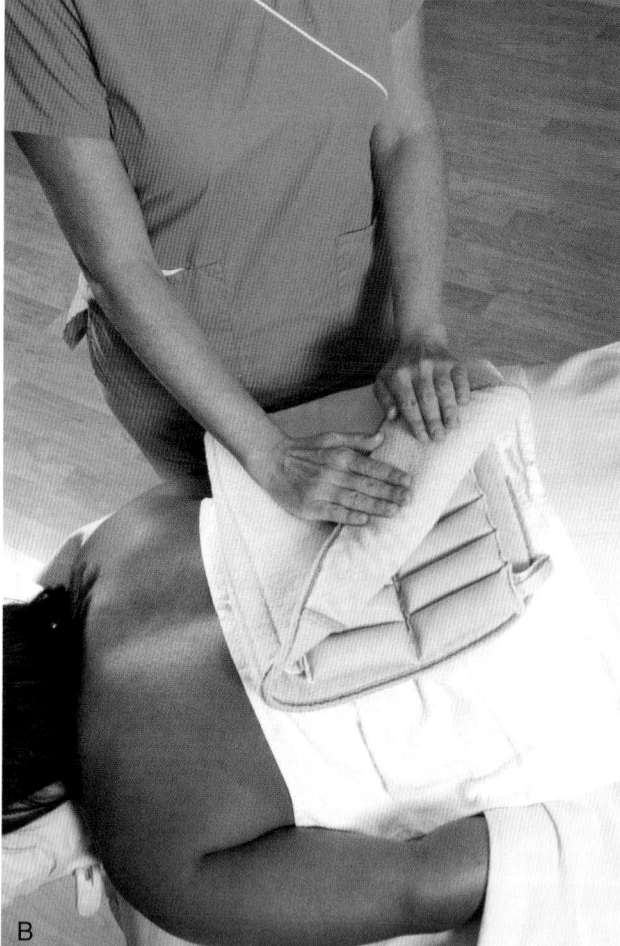

B

FIG. 12.4 Hot packs. Most professionals use a water cabinet called a hydrocollator to heat and store hot packs (A). Once heated, the packs are removed, wrapped in six to eight layers of dry terrycloth or a specially designed cover, and then placed on the treatment area (B). (A, From TouchAmerica, Hillsborough, NC.)

plugged-in devices and are not recommended for clinical use because the pads do not cool naturally after application and therefore can burn the skin.

Paraffin Bath

Paraffin bath is the dipping of a limb into a heated mixture of paraffin wax and mineral oil in a 6:1 or 7:1 ratio of wax to oil. Paraffin is an excellent insulator, so when applied, the heat penetrates deeply instead of being lost to the air. Paraffin is heated and stored in a thermostatically controlled container maintaining temperatures between 124°F and 126°F (52°C to 57°C). Follow the manufacturer's recommendations listed in the owner's manual for unit usage and safety precautions. Paraffin is suited for irregularly contoured areas of the body such as the hands, elbows, feet, and knees. Paraffin applications are also performed in nontherapeutic settings such as spas and salons.

Remove all jewelry from the treatment area before paraffin is applied to the skin. To use the dip-wrap method on the hands, ask the client to spread the fingers apart and dip the hand into the paraffin as far as possible without touching the bottom or the sides of the container because these areas may be hotter than the paraffin (Fig. 12.5). Remove the hand from the wax after a few seconds. Keep the hand over the container so any excess wax can drip into it. Repeat the dip-remove sequence until the area is opaque and skin can no longer be seen through the wax. Advise the client to avoid moving the fingers during treatment, as this action may crack the wax coating. Wrap the client's hand in a plastic bag or wax paper, and then in a towel or terrycloth mitt. Allow the wax to cool. This will take approximately 10 to 15 minutes. Remove the wax coating and discard. Modify the procedure for the elbows, feet, and ankles. Another method is to dip a paintbrush into the paraffin and then spread it on the skin. For sanitary reasons, used paraffin should not be returned to the container.

SPA: INTRODUCTION

A **spa** is a place where water treatments and other services are administered to encourage relaxation and rejuvenation of the mind and body. The origin of the word *spa* is uncertain. Some scholars believe it is derived from the Walloon (Wallonia, Belgium) phrase *espa,* meaning "fountain."

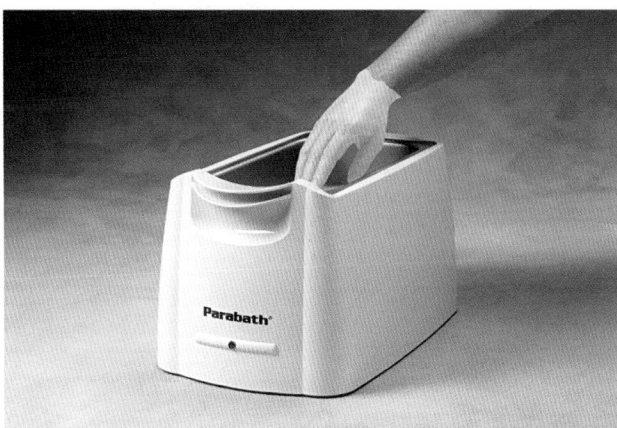

FIG. 12.5 Paraffin bath. Dipping of a limb into a heated mixture. Paraffin is heated and stored in a thermostatically controlled container. (From Cameron, M. H. [2018]. *Physical agents in rehabilitation* [5th ed.]. St. Louis, MO: Saunders.)

Others believe it comes from the letters S-P-A scribbled on marble walls of the ancient public baths of Rome. This translates from the Latin *sanus per aqua,* meaning "healing through water" or "cure of water." In the sixteenth century, people traveled to the town of Spa, Belgium, to "take the waters" to rest, retreat, find lost health, preserve vitality, and rejuvenate, which also may be where the word originated.

Today, there are several different types of spas: day spas, medical spas, hotel or resort spas, and destination spas.
- **Day Spa**. These offer services on a day-use basis. Salon services, such as hair, nails, and skin treatments, are available along with massage services.
- **Medical Spa**. A type of day spa integrating medical esthetics and spa services. Medical spas often offer Botox injections, laser treatments, and skin resurfacing procedures.
- **Hotel or Resort Spa**. These are within a hotel or resort and usually offer day spa services.
- **Destination Spa**. Clients come here to relax, rejuvenate, or improve their lifestyle choices. The length of stay varies from a weekend to several weeks or longer. Education is often a central theme of destination spas.

Spa Hydrotherapy: Contraindications and Safety

Take steps to reduce the risks of slips and falls, electrical shock, and the spread of infection. Use nonslip walking surfaces and hand grip bars next to the entrance and exit areas in wet areas. Provide nonslip shoes or sandals for clients. Spa equipment located outdoors should not be used during storms.

Apply the cryo- and thermotherapy contraindications mentioned previously when spa therapies include hot or cold water. Long hair should be secured or tucked in a cap when clients enter tubs or pools because it may become trapped in water pumps.

Use a thermometer to check water temperature before a client enters the water. If needed, adjust the water temperature by adding cooler or warmer water until the desired temperature is achieved. Water temperature may range from cold to very hot.
- **Cold**. 55°F to 65°F (12°C to 18°C)
- **Cool**. 65°F to 80°F (18°C to 26°C)
- **Tepid**. 80°F to 95°F (26°C to 35°C)
- **Warm**. 95°F to 99°F (35°C to 37°C)
- **Hot**. 99°F to 104°F (37°C to 40°C)
- **Very Hot**. 104°F to 110°F (37°C to 43° C)

If tubs are not drained between usages, use a filter or disinfecting agents to kill water-borne pathogens. Be sure wet areas are well-ventilated as clients with asthma and other respiratory disorders may be sensitive to chemical fumes. All chemicals used to sanitize pool water should be kept in original containers and in a locked cabinet. Ozonators, which use ozone to clean the water, may also be used.

NOTE: Pregnant clients can safely engage in sitting in hot baths (up to 104°F, 40°C,) or hot/dry saunas (up to 158°F, 70°C; 15% relative humidity) for up to 20 minutes irrespective of pregnancy stage (Ravanelli et al., 2018). Temperatures or timeframes exceeding these guidelines may result in damage to the unborn.

Spa Procedures and Application Methods

Spa hydrotherapy may be used exclusively or combined with spa procedures and application methods, including whirlpool baths, sauna and steam baths, Vichy and Swiss showers, exfoliations, body wraps, underwater massage, aqua stretch, Watsu, floatation therapy, Swedish and Turkish shampoos, cold plunge, Shirodhara, and hot stone massage. Discontinue treatment immediately if the client feels uncomfortably cold or warm or experiences any pain or discomfort. In addition, the client should be provided with a means of calling for assistance if the practitioner or other team members are not nearby.

Recommended Protocol

A recommended spa procedure is:

1. Check the temperature of the unit to ensure safe administration.
2. Assess the client and determine whether the spa method is appropriate and safe.
3. Explain the procedure and instruct clients how to enter the tub, tank, cabinet, or wet table.
4. Obtain consent. Age of consent for self-care and spa procedures is 16 compared with 18 for clinical procedures. Check with applicable regulatory agencies
5. Ask clients to shower with soap before entering tubs or pools.
6. Offer clients towels, robes, or other needed items.
7. Apply the method.
8. Assess the client's response and outcome. Provide a rest area and drinking water to cool down after treatments, including heat immersion such as whirlpools, saunas, or steam baths.
9. Document.
   When documenting, include treatment details such as:
   - Type of treatment.
   - Position of the client.
   - Temperature of the unit.
   - Duration of application.
   - Client's response or treatment outcome.

Whirlpool Bath

A **whirlpool bath** is a bath in a tub containing heated water that is continuously circulated. Jets along the sides and sometimes bottom of the tub are connected to a pump circulating the water. The pressure and direction of the jets connected to the water pump can often be adjusted (Fig. 12.6). Whirlpool tubs are also called *spa tubs* or *hot tubs*. Water temperature is maintained by a heating element and the water is sanitized for multiple uses. The temperature of the water ranges between 99°F and 104°F (37°C and 40°C). The

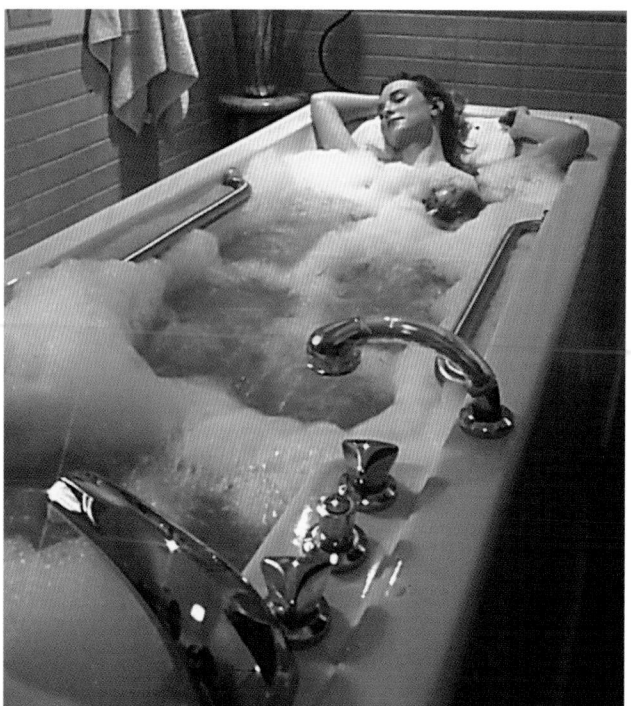

FIG. 12.6 Whirlpool bath. The tub containing heated water is continuously circulated. (Courtesy Golden Ratio, Emigrant, MT.)

length of time the client remains in the tub is between 15 and 20 minutes.

Give me the power to create a fever, and I shall cure any disease.

—Hippocrates

Sauna Bath

A **sauna bath** is a dry heat bath received in a wood-lined room or cabinet. Radiant heat can be provided by hot stones (Finnish sauna) or by infrared light bulbs (modern sauna). In Finnish saunas, water can be poured on the hot stones to increase heat and humidity and promote sweating. Water can also be poured on the bather to reduce body temperature and cool down. In most saunas, humidity is between 10% and 20% with temperatures around 175°F at head level and bathing times are 20 to 30 minutes in duration (Laukkanen, 2018). Benefits of sauna bathing can be achieved at a temperature of 160°F; sauna temperature should never exceed 195°F. **NOTE**: Avoid consuming alcoholic beverages 1 to 2 hours before entering the sauna as it may lead to hypotension and increased risk of fainting or other accidents (Laukkanen, 2018; Ylikahri et al., 1988).

Steam Bath

Steam bathing is a vapor bath taken in a ceramic-tiled room, cabinet, or canopy. The air temperature of most steam baths is between 105°F and 120°F (40.5°C and 50°C) and bathing times are 15 to 20 minutes in duration. Advise the client to shower before steam bathing. After a steam bath, individuals should cool down for a few minutes by resting in a normal-temperature room and drinking two to four 8-ounce glasses of water (Laukkanen, 2018). Because of the dense air, clients with respiratory disorders should avoid steam baths in an enclosed room because it may be difficult to breathe easily. In these circumstances, use a steam cabinet or canopy because the client's head remains out of the steam bath during treatment.

Vichy and Swiss Showers

Two popular shower techniques offered at some spas are *Vichy showers* and *Swiss showers.*

- **Vichy Shower**. Warm water sprayed over a client lying on a shallow table. Most often, the shower contains multiple downward-facing showerheads situated along a horizontal water pipe running the length of the table (Fig. 12.7). Vichy showers originated in Vichy, France.
- **Swiss Shower**. Warm water sprayed over a client standing or sitting in a shower stall. The shower stall contains multiple vertically wall-mounted and horizontally ceiling-mounted showerheads (Fig. 12.8). Swiss showers originated in Switzerland.

> *The cure for anything is salt water—sweat, tears, or the sea.*
>
> **—Isak Dinesen**

Exfoliations: Scrubs, Polishes, and Dry Brushing

Exfoliation procedures use grainy products or items such as brushes, loofahs, or textured cloth and superficial friction (light to medium/moderate pressure) to exfoliate the skin.

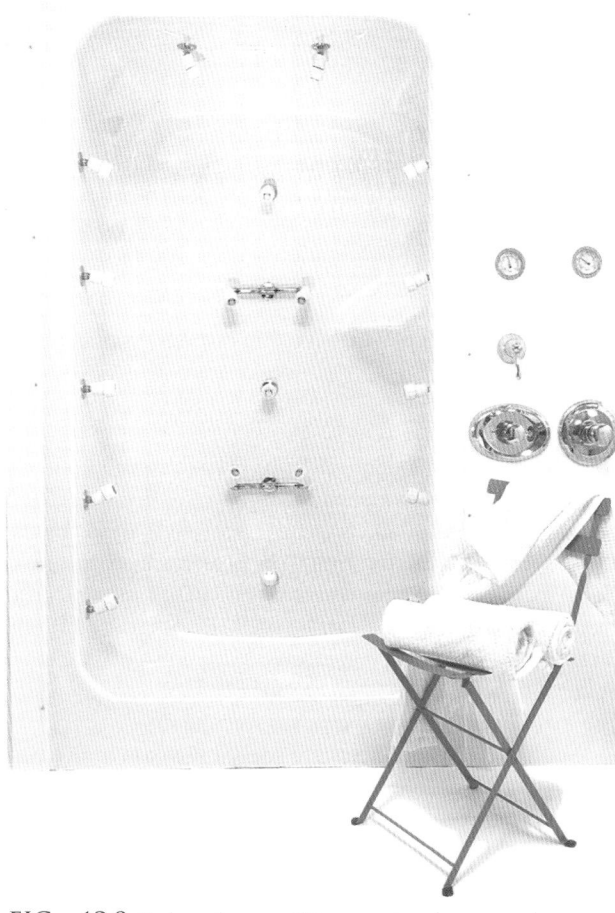

FIG. 12.8 Swiss shower. Warm water is sprayed over a client from multiple showerheads. (Courtesy TouchAmerica, Hillsborough, NC.)

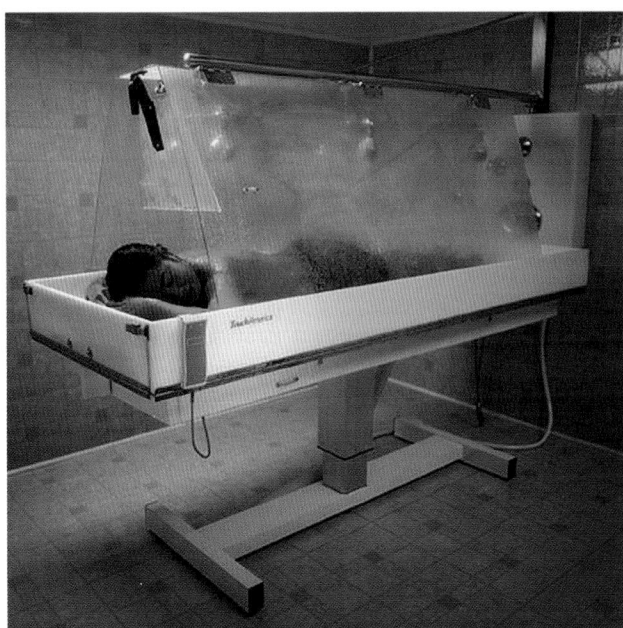

FIG. 12.7 Vichy shower. Warm water is sprayed over a client while they lie on a shallow table. (Courtesy TouchAmerica, Hillsborough, NC.)

Exfoliation procedures are usually described as scrubs or polishes.

- **Body Scrub**. This uses a coarse, grainy product such as salt (non-iodized), sugar, cornmeal, coffee, ground herbs, nuts, or seeds.
- **Body Polish**. This uses a fine, grainy product usually blended with a crème-based product. This type of product is also called a *gommage.*

Products can be removed with water or a warm damp towel stored in an electric hot towel warmer (Fig. 12.9). The damp towel can be scented with essential oils. Body glow was the term previously used because the skin "glowed" during and immediately after treatment from superficial vasodilation.

A natural bristle brush or loofah sponge can be used to exfoliate the skin. Exfoliation procedures can be combined with other massage and spa services or as a stand-alone service. *Garshana*, an Ayurvedic dry brush treatment, may be performed with a loofah, wool gloves, raw silk, or textured cotton. **NOTE**: Avoid using deep pressure over recently shaved or waxed skin as this can cause skin irritation. In addition, avoid exfoliation

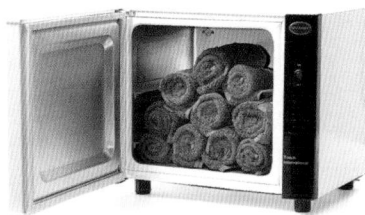

FIG. 12.9 Damp towels can be stored in an electric hot towel until ready to use.

procedures on clients who have thin or fragile skin such as the elderly.

Body Wraps

A **body wrap** is the application of products to the client's body, which is then wrapped in large wet or dry sheets and blankets. Applied products include seaweed, algae, muds, clays, fango (Italian for "mud" but can include peat and clays), paraffin, parafango (paraffin and mud), volcanic ash, charcoal, and honey and can be scented with essential oils (Fig. 12.10). The client can receive a dry brush massage, an immersion bath, steam bath, or sauna before the body wrap. The main types of body wraps are wet and dry.

- **Wet Sheet Wrap**. Sheets are soaked in warm to hot water; wring them out before wrapping the body.
  - **Herbal Wrap**. This uses sheets that are soaked in herbal tea.
- **Dry Sheet Wrap**. Dry sheets are used to wrap the body.

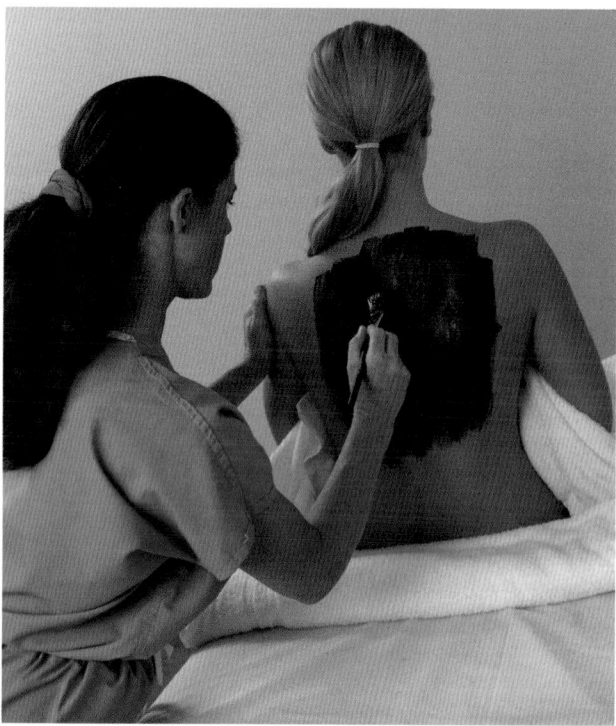

FIG. 12.10 Body wrap. Mud or other products can be applied before a body wrap.

To prepare the table for the body wrap, place a towel lengthwise at the head of the table; this will later serve as the collar of the wrap. Be sure that sheets, thermal blankets, and other layers are lined up at the head of the table and tucked between the folded towel. Lay the wet or dry sheet over the Mylar foil sheet (Fig. 12.11).

During the body wrap, the wet or dry sheet and blankets are wrapped tightly around the client, keeping the face exposed (Fig. 12.12). Place a bolster behind the knees. Gentle massage techniques can be administered while the client is in the wrap. **NOTE**: If the client experiences claustrophobia-related anxiety while in the body wrap, loosen the fabric around their neck and shoulders. If this does not relieve anxiety, place the client's arms on top of the wrap for the duration of treatment, or discontinue treatment.

Remove the products after the body wrap with warm, wet towels or by using a shower (Vichy, Swiss, regular shower, or hand-held hose). A moisturizer can be applied to the client's skin as a final step.

Underwater Massage, Aqua Stretch, and Watsu

These methods combine massage, movement, or pressurized water and immersion. The client wears a bathing suit during the session. Water temperatures are between 97°F to 101°F (36°C to 38°C).

- **Underwater Massage**. During this procedure, the client lies in a bath-sized tub of water while the practitioner holds a hose with an adjustable spray nozzle and massages the client with a stream of pressurized water.
- **Aqua Stretch**. During aqua stretch, the practitioner stands in about 3 feet of water and supports the client in various positions while applying passive and active-assisted stretching and myofascial techniques. Floatation devices are often used.
- **Watsu**. During Watsu (a term derived from "water shiatsu"), the practitioner stands in about 3 feet of water and helps the client float, sometimes with the aid of floatation devices. Techniques include the shiatsu, compression, joint mobilizations, stretching, and deep breathing. A biography of Harold Dull, the originator of Watsu, is in this chapter.

Floatation Therapy

In **floatation therapy**, a client floats in a foot or less of warm salt water within a dark, soundproof tank. Most sessions are between 60 and 90 minutes. A shower is recommended before to help keep the water clean and again afterward to rinse off the salt water. Floatation therapy was developed by John Lilly who used it to research the effects of isolation and sensory deprivation on creativity. Floatation is also spelled *flotation*.

Swedish and Turkish Body Shampoos

Body shampoos are gentle scrubbing of the client's skin using a cloth or brush dipped in warm, soapy water. Body shampoos may be administered indoors or outdoors while

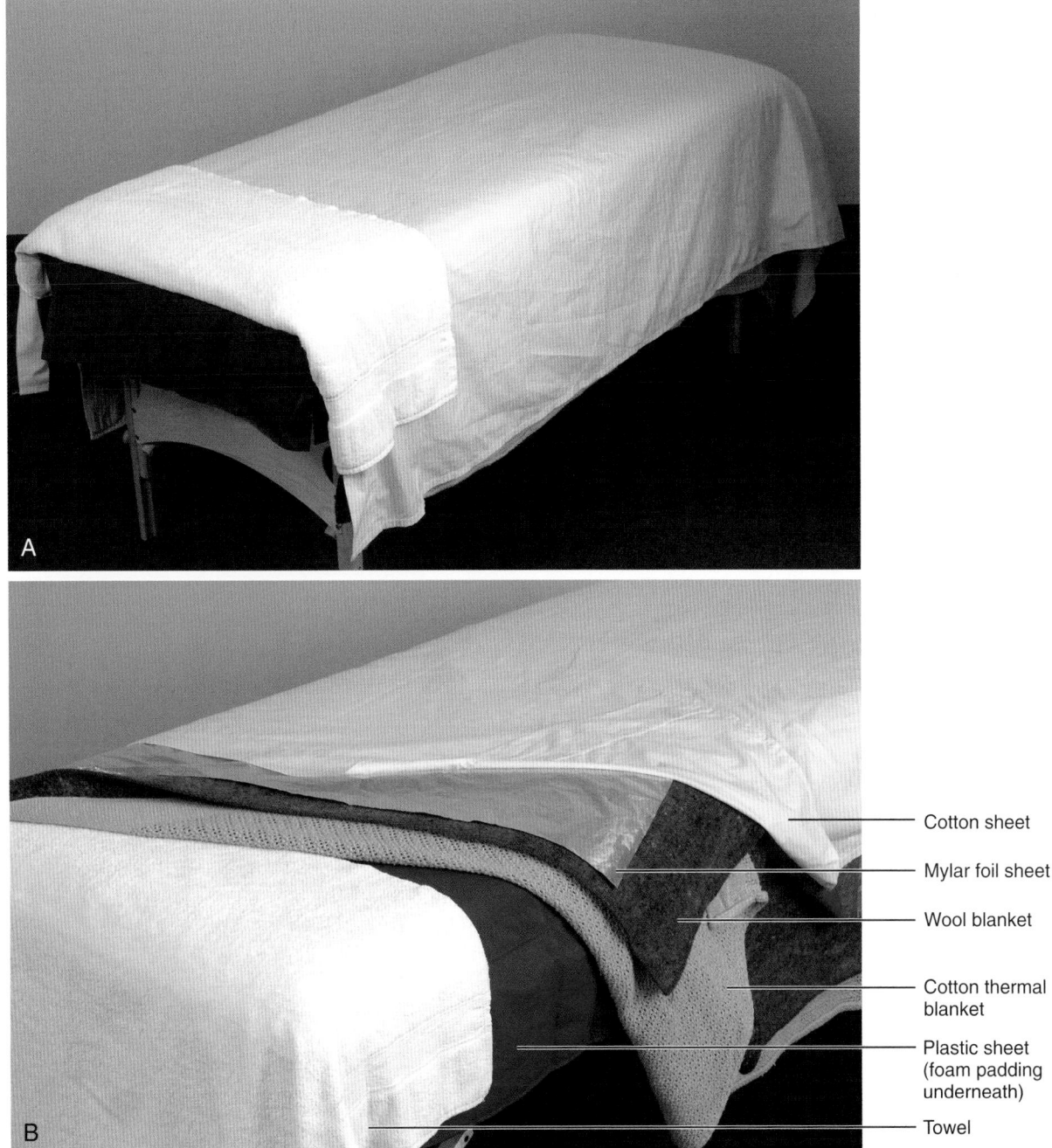

FIG. 12.11 Body wrap. (A) Table set up for body wrap. (B) Bottom edge pulled back to reveal layering.

the client stands, sits on a water-resistant stool, or lies on a wet table. Soap lather can be removed with a shower, hand-held hose, or a pail of water poured over the client's skin. The main difference between a Swedish and a Turkish shampoo is the water temperature of the final rinse.

- **Swedish Shampoo.** A Swedish shampoo includes pouring a pail of hot water at 105°F (40°C) over the client's skin as the final rinse.
- **Turkish Shampoo.** A Turkish shampoo includes pouring a pail of tepid water at 90°F (32°C) as a final rinse after the hot pail pour of 105°F (40°C).

Cold Plunge

A **cold plunge** is a brief submersion in a pool or tub of cold water. The temperature of the water ranges between 45° and 55°F (7° and 12°C) and the client can remain in the water up to 3 minutes. The plunge can follow a warm to hot water immersion bath, a sauna, or a steam bath.

Shirodhara

Shirodhara is an Ayurvedic treatment where a steady stream of warm oil pours over the client's forehead. During the procedure, the client lies on a table while warm oil flows

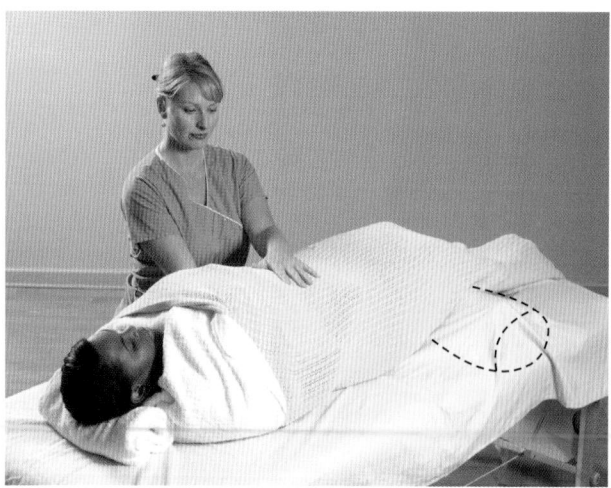

FIG. 12.12 Body wrap. Sheets and blankets are wrapped tightly around the client's body, keeping the face exposed. A bolster can be used under the knees and gentle massage techniques can be administered while the client is in the wrap.

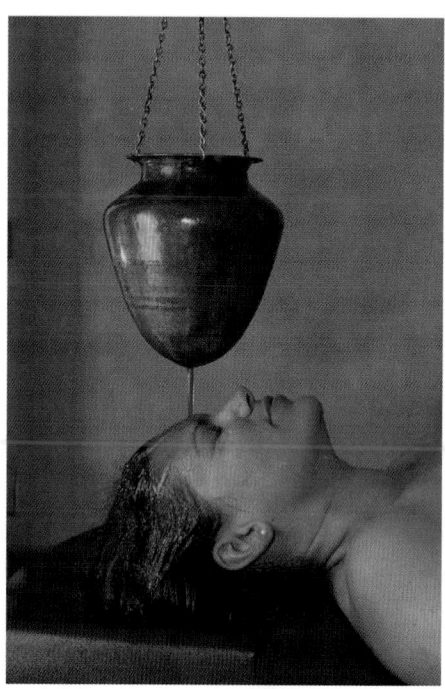

FIG. 12.13 Shirodhara. During the procedure, the client lies on a table while warm oil flows in a steady stream from a vessel positioned above the forehead.

from a vessel positioned above the forehead (Fig. 12.13). Shirodhara is usually combined with other spa treatments, such as body wraps or massage, but is suitable as a stand-alone service.

Hot Stone Massage

Hot stone massage uses smooth, flat heated stones placed on the skin or used as hand-held massage tools. Cold stones can also be used. Basalt is recommended for hot stones, and marble is recommended for cold stones. Stones of various sizes are used for different areas of the body. For example, larger stones are used for the back and smaller stones for between the toes. Hot stone massage gained in popularity because of Mary Nelson, who coined the term *LaStone therapy*. **NOTE:** Hot stones and the heating unit can burn the skin. The water temperature to heat the stones is between 130°F and 140°F (54° and 60°C) Use two insulating layers, such as a folded sheet, between the hot stones and the client's skin. Never place a hot stone beneath the client, even with insulating layers as the client's weight increases heat transfer and risk for burns. Practitioners have also burned themselves on hot stones.

E-RESOURCES

http://evolve.elsevier.com/Salvo/MassageTherapy
- Chapter challenge
- Flash cards

HAROLD DULL

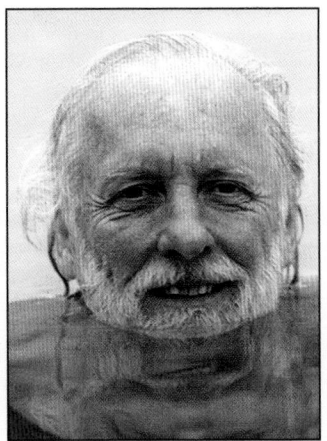

There can be a tremendous amount of pressure to be "original," to do something nobody else has thought of. It can be paralyzing—this feeling that everything you have in mind has surely been tried before. But do not panic. Some of the most original ideas (in massage and in all areas of life) come from combining concepts already well known in new and interesting ways. Harold Dull is a perfect example of someone who has done exactly that and created one of the most unique modalities in massage today.

Born in 1935 in Seattle, Dull grew up interested in absolutely everything. He hoped to study physics, prelaw, or philosophy but ended up studying poetry instead and became a writer. Happy with life as a poet but never content without exploring new things, Dull began studying Zen shiatsu in San Francisco after receiving his first professional massage. He then traveled to Japan, where he studied under the expert guidance of Shizuto Masunaga.

It was upon returning to the United States that Dull had his brilliant idea: Why not combine shiatsu, as practiced in Japan, with hot spring therapy? And Watsu was born.

In Watsu, a combination of the words "water" and "shiatsu," the practitioner uses traditional shiatsu massage techniques, stretching, joint mobilization, and flotation to help the client relax. It is performed in water around 4-feet deep that has been heated to the body's natural temperature. The warm water helps the client to experience weightlessness and ease of movement while also allowing the practitioner to reposition the client with ease. The water and the massage combine to create a uniquely nurturing environment. Dull believes the feeling of caring acceptance is one of the greatest values of Watsu. He states it is "the unconditional acceptance that is so powerful. So many injured people are treated as less than what they once were."

Dull taught Watsu to massage practitioners and others around the world, and the world has certainly taken notice. For his work, Dull received the International Aquatics Award from the United States Water Fitness Association, was honored at the National Aquatic Exercise Conference in Japan, and in 1998 he received the Tsunami Spirit Award from the Aquatic Therapy and Rehab Institute.

The art of poetry involves taking images and words, things used by people every day, and combining them to form something beautiful. Quite naturally, it was the poet Harold Dull who thought to unite the properties of shiatsu with those of a relaxing soak in a hot spring. The next time you are worried others are already doing everything under the sun, ask yourself if there is any way to combine what you already know. Not sure if your idea could work? There is only one way to find out.

REFERENCES

Algafly, A. A., & George, K. P. (2007). The effect of cryotherapy on nerve conduction velocity, pain threshold and pain tolerance. *British Journal of Sports Medicine*, *41*(6), 365–369.

Benson, T. B., & Copp, E. P. (1974). The effects of therapeutic forms of heat and ice on the pain threshold of the normal shoulder. *Rheumatology and Rehabilitation*, *13*(2), 101–104.

Cameron, M. H. (2018). *Physical Agents in Rehabilitation: An Evidence-Based Approach to Practice* (5th ed.). St Louis: Elsevier Health Sciences.

Cihoric, N., Tsikkinis, A., van Rhoon, G., Crezee, H., Aebersold, D. M., Bodis, S., et al. (2015). Hyperthermia-related clinical trials on cancer treatment within the ClinicalTrials.gov registry. *International Journal of Hyperthermia*, *31*(6), 609–614.

Day, M. J. (1974). Hypersensitive response to ice massage: Report of a case. *Physical Therapy*, *54*(6), 592–593.

Ernst, E., & Fialka, V. (1994). Ice freezes pain? A review of the clinical effectiveness of analgesic cold therapy. *Journal of Pain and Symptom Management*, *9*(1), 56–59.

Funk, D., Swank, A. M., Adams, K.J., & Treolo, D. (2001). Efficacy of moist heat pack application over static stretching on hamstring flexibility. *The Journal of Strength & Conditioning Research*, *15*(1), 123–126.

Garra, G., Singer, A. J., Leno, R., Taira, B. R., Gupta, N. Mathaikutty, B., et al. (2010). Heat or cold packs for neck and back strain: A randomized controlled trial of efficacy. *Academic Emergency Medicine*, *17*(5), 484–489.

Kanlayanaphotporn, R., & Janwantanakul, P. (2005). Comparison of skin surface temperature during the application of various cryotherapy modalities. *Archives of Physical Medicine and Rehabilitation*, *86*(7), 1411–1415.

Karunakara, R. G., Lephart, S. M., & Pincivero, D. M. (1999). Changes in forearm blood flow during single and intermittent cold application. *Journal of Orthopaedic and Sports Physical Therapy*, *29*(3), 177–180.

Knight, C. A., Rutledge, C. R., Cox, M. E., Acosta, M., & Hall, S. J. (2001). Effect of superficial heat, deep heat, and active exercise warm-up on the extensibility of the plantar flexors. *Physical Therapy*, *81*(6), 1206–1214.

Laliberte, M. (2019). *Epsom salts are trendy, but do they actually work?* Retrieved from https://www.rd.com/health/wellness/does-epsom-salt-work/.

Laukkanen, J. A. (2018). *Some like it hot: The health benefits of saunas.* Retrieved from https://bottomlineinc.com/health/wellness/some-like-it-hot-the-health-benefits-of-saunas.

Lehmann, J. F., Masock, A. J., Warren, C. G., & Koblanski, J. N. (1970). Effect of therapeutic temperatures on tendon extensibility. *Archives of Physical Medicine and Rehabilitation, 51*(8), 481–487.

Lehmann, J. F., Warren, C. G., & Scham, S. M. (1974). Therapeutic heat and cold. *Clinical Orthopaedics and Related Research, 99,* 207–245.

Lentell, G., Hetherington, T., Eagan, J., & Morgan, M. (1992). The use of thermal agents to influence the effectiveness of a low-load prolonged stretch. *Journal of Orthopaedic and Sports Physical Therapy, 16*(5), 200–207.

Lewis, T. (1930). Observations upon the reactions of the vessels of the human skin to cold. *Heart, 15,* 177–208.

Magness, J., Garrett, T., & Erickson, D. (1970). Swelling of the upper extremity during whirlpool baths. *Archives of Physical Medicine and Rehabilitation, 51*(5), 297–299.

Malanga, G. A., Yan, N., & Stark, J. (2015). Mechanisms and efficacy of heat and cold therapies for musculoskeletal injury. *Postgraduate Medicine, 127*(1), 57–65.

Mayer, J. M., Ralph, L., Look, M., Erasala, G. N., Verna, J. L., Matheson, L. N., et al. (2005). Treating acute low back pain with continuous low-level heat wrap therapy and/or exercise: A randomized controlled trial. *The Spine Journal, 5*(4), 395–403.

Michlovitz, S., Hun, L., Erasala, G. N., Hengehold, D. A., & Weingand, K. W. (2004). Continuous low-level heat wrap therapy is effective for treating wrist pain. *Archives of Physical Medicine and Rehabilitation, 85*(9), 1409–1416.

Mirkin, G. (2021). *Why ice delays recovery.* Retrieved from http://drmirkin.com/fitness/why-ice-delays-recovery.html.

Mooventhan, A., & Nivethitha, L. (2014). Scientific evidence-based effects of hydrotherapy on various systems of the body. *North American Journal of Medical Sciences, 6*(5), 199–209.

Mun, J. H., Jeon, J. H., Jung, Y. J., Jang, K. U., Yang, H. T., Lim, H. J., et al. (2012). The factors associated with contact burns from therapeutic modalities. *Annals of Rehabilitation Medicine, 36*(5), 688–695.

Nakano, J., Yamabayashi, C., Scott, A., & Reid, W. D. (2012). The effect of heat applied with stretch to increase range of motion: A systematic review. *Physical Therapy in Sport, 13*(3), 180–188.

Park, K. N., Kwon, O. Y., Weon, J. H., Choung, S. D., & Kim, S. H. (2014). Comparison of the effects of local cryotherapy and passive cross-body stretch on extensibility in subjects with posterior shoulder tightness. *Journal of Sports Science & Medicine, 13*(1), 84–90.

Petrofsky, J., Bains, G., Prowse, M., Gunda, S., Berk, L., Raju, C., et al. (2009). Dry heat, moist heat and body fat: Are heating modalities really effective in people who are overweight? *Journal of Medical Engineering & Technology, 33*(5), 361–369.

Petrofsky, J. S., Laymon, M., & Lee, H. (2013). Effect of heat and cold on tendon flexibility and force to flex the human knee. *Medical Science Monitor, 19,* 661–667.

Prentice, W. E. (1982). An electromyographic analysis of the effectiveness of heat or cold and stretching for inducing relaxation in injured muscle. *Journal of Orthopaedic and Sports Physical Therapy, 3*(3), 133–140.

Quillen, W. S., & Rouillier, L. H. (1982). Initial management of acute ankle sprains with rapid pulsed pneumatic compression and cold. *Journal of Orthopaedic and Sports Physical Therapy, 4*(1), 39–43.

Ravanelli, N., Casasola, W., English, T., Edwards, K. M., & Jay, O. (2018). Heat stress and fetal risk. Environmental limits for exercise and passive heat stress during pregnancy: A systematic review with best evidence synthesis. *British Journal of Sports Medicine. 53*(13), 799–805.

Sapareto, S. A., & Dewey, W. C. (1984). Thermal dose determination in cancer therapy. *International Journal of Radiation Oncology, Biology, Physics, 10*(6), 787–800.

Schmidt, K. L., Ott, V. R., Röcher, G., & Schaller, H. (1979). Heat, cold, and inflammation. *Zeitschrift Fur Rheumatologie, 38*(11–12), 391–404.

Scialoia, D., & Swartzendruber, A. J. (2020). The R.I.C.E protocol is a myth: A review and recommendations. *The Sport Journal, 41*(2), 1–19.

Singh, H., Osbahr, D. C., Holovacs, T. F., Cawley, P. W., & Speer, K. P. (2001). The efficacy of continuous cryotherapy on the postoperative shoulder: A prospective, randomized investigation. *Journal of Shoulder and Elbow Surgery, 10*(6), 522–525.

Usuba, M., Miyanaga, Y., Miyakawa, S., Maeshima, T., & Shirasaki, Y. (2006). Effect of heat in increasing the range of knee motion after the development of a joint contracture: An experiment with an animal model. *Archives of Physical Medicine and Rehabilitation, 87*(2), 247–253.

Warren, C. G., Lehmann, J. F., & Koblanski, J. N. (1971). Elongation of rat tail tendon: Effect of load and temperature. *Archives of Physical Medicine and Rehabilitation, 52*(10), 465–474.

Warren, C. G., Lehmann, J. F., & Koblanski, J. N. (1976). Heat and stretch procedures: An evaluation using rat tail tendon. *Archives of Physical Medicine and Rehabilitation, 57*(3), 122–126.

Weston, M., Taber, C., Casagranda, L., & Cornwall, M. (1994). Changes in local blood volume during cold gel pack application to traumatized ankles. *Journal of Orthopaedic and Sports Physical Therapy, 19*(4), 197–199.

Wyper, D. J., & McNiven, D. R. (1976). Effects of some physiotherapeutic agents on skeletal muscle blood flow. *Physiotherapy, 62*(3), 83–85.

Yildirim, N., Ulusoy, M. F., & Bodur, H. (2010). The effect of heat application on pain, stiffness, physical function and quality of life in patients with knee osteoarthritis. *Journal of Clinical Nursing, 19*(7–8), 1113–1120.

Ylikahri, R., Heikkonen, E., & Soukas, A. (1988). The sauna and alcohol. *Annals of Clinical Research, 20*(4), 287–291.

Zankel, H. T. (1966). Effect of physical agents on motor conduction velocity of the ulnar nerve. *Archives of Physical Medicine and Rehabilitation, 47*(12), 787–792.

REVIEW AND APPLY YOUR KNOWLEDGE

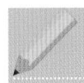 **MATCHING ONE: CONCEPT REVIEW**

Place the letter of the answer next to the number of the term or phrase that best describes it.

A. Conduction
B. Convection
C. Cryotherapy
D. Father Sebastian Kneipp
E. Friction
F. Conversion
G. Reduced edema
H. Hydrotherapy
 I. Cryokinetics
J. John Harvey Kellogg
K. Thermotherapy
L. Increased collagen extensibility

_____ 1. Massage technique used to administer ice massage.
_____ 2. Father of hydrotherapy.
_____ 3. Cold application combined with joint mobilizations.
_____ 4. An effect of heat application.
_____ 5. Transfer of a nonthermal form of energy (mechanical, electrical, chemical) into heat in the body.
_____ 6. Therapeutic use of cold.
_____ 7. Director of a sanitarium in Michigan where massage and water cures were part of the health regimen.
_____ 8. Therapeutic use of heat.
_____ 9. Transfer of heat by circulating currents of water or air between a warmer object/substance and a cooler object/substance.
_____ 10. An effect of cold application.
_____ 11. Transfer of heat between objects or substances that are in direct contact with each other.
_____ 12. Use of water in any of its forms for health promotion or treatment of various diseases and conditions.

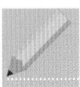 **MATCHING TWO: CONCEPT REVIEW**

Place the letter of the answer next to the number of the term or phrase that best describes it.

A. Contrast method
B. Swiss shower
C. Paraffin bath
D. Radiation
E. Steam bath
F. Whirlpool bath
G. Evaporation
H. Hydrostatic
 I. Vichy shower
J. Thalassotherapy
K. Sauna bath
L. Spa

_____ 1. Transfer of heat through heat rays.
_____ 2. Bath in a tub containing heated water that is continuously circulated.
_____ 3. External use of seawater.
_____ 4. Place where water treatments and other services are administered to encourage relaxation and rejuvenation of the mind and body.
_____ 5. Combines cold and heat in the same treatment.
_____ 6. Vapor bath taken in a ceramic-tiled room, cabinet, or canopy.
_____ 7. Dipping of a limb into heated wax and mineral oil.
_____ 8. Pressure exerted by fluids on an immersed object.
_____ 9. Warm water sprayed over a client lying on a shallow table. A horizontal water pipe is above the table and contains multiple downward-facing showerheads.
_____ 10. Dry heat bath received in a wood-lined room or cabinet.
_____ 11. Transfer or loss of heat when a liquid changes into a gas or vapor.
_____ 12. Warm water sprayed over a client sitting or standing in a shower containing multiple vertically wall-mounted and horizontally or ceiling-mounted showerheads.

MULTIPLE CHOICE: TEST YOUR KNOWLEDGE

Place the letter of the answer next to the number of the term or phrase that best describes it.

_____ 1. Who was the author of the book *My Water Cure*?
A. Father Sebastian Kneipp
B. Pehr Henrik Ling
C. George Henry Taylor
D. John Henry Kellogg

_____ 2. Which water-soluble agent made of magnesium sulfate was thought to reduce muscle aches and pains?
A. Baking soda
B. Epsom salt
C. Sea salt
D. Milk bath

_____ 3. Vapocoolant sprays use which method of heat transference?
A. Conduction
B. Convection
C. Radiation
D. Evaporation

_____ 4. Ultrasound uses which method of heat transference?
A. Conduction
B. Convection
C. Conversion
D. Radiation

_____ 5. Cold-induced vasodilation was first noted by Lewis and was called the:
A. inflammatory cascade.
B. hunting response.
C. gate control.
D. contrast method.

_____ 6. Which is the final sensation clients usually experience during cold application?
A. Numbness
B. Burning
C. Stinging
D. Aching

_____ 7. The application of heat creates what effect on blood flow?
A. Vasoconstriction
B. Vasodilation
C. Edema reduction
D. Compromised circulation

_____ 8. Which spa type offers treatments including Botox, laser, and skin resurfacing?
A. Day
B. Resort
C. Medical
D. Destination

_____ 9. The appropriate temperature range for tepid water is between _____ ° F.
A. 65–80
B. 80–95
C. 95–99
D. 99–104

_____ 10. Which hydrotherapy treatment often uses multiple downward-facing showerheads situated along a horizontal pipe running the length of the table?
A. Steam shower
B. Sauna shower
C. Swiss shower
D. Vichy shower

_____ 11. The spa technique that uses a fine, grainy exfoliant is a:
A. body scrub.
B. body polish.
C. body wash.
D. body wrap.

_____ 12. Which spa technique has a client laying in a foot or less of warm salt water within a dark soundproof tank?
A. Shirodhara
B. Turkish bath
C. Flotation therapy
D. Watsu

CRITICAL THINKING

But She's a Triathlete!

Chandra is 38 years old, a triathlete, and a regular receiver of massage. She has come to you to try a heat treatment for the first time. You explain how relaxing it can be, how it loosens muscles and collagen, and you will be better able to stretch her tissues afterward. You apply a hydrocollator pack to her back, and Chandra says the temperature is fine. You leave the pack on for 15 minutes, then massage and stretch the muscles in her back. As you are having her turn over, she says she feels dizzy and sees dark spots in front of her eyes. What is happening to Chandra? What is your best course of action?

Answers can include but are not limited to:

Chandra is in the beginning stages of fainting. Fainting is a sudden loss of consciousness associated with peripheral vasodilation, decreased blood pressure, and reduced heart rate and can occur during or immediately after thermotherapy. Because Chandra is very fit, it may be unexpected that Chandra would be starting to faint from the heat treatment. However, it can happen to anyone.

If a client feels faint during treatment, immediately stop the thermotherapy and lower the client's head and raise the client's feet. If a client feels faint getting up from treatment, ask the client to sit back down and remain in the seated position until the feeling of dizziness has subsided before standing and walking. To reduce the risk of fainting, keep the client's upper body elevated during treatment to reduce the degree of positional change.

In the future, Chandra would most likely benefit from another type of treatment with temperatures lower than the hydrocollator, or she may not be a good candidate for any type of thermotherapy.

PROFESSIONAL PRACTICE

At Your Service

The Transformation Station is a spa with a convention center. The average client is a one-time user of services, scheduling when there is free time during the convention. Brett has an appointment with practitioner Tara. During the intake, Brett says he scheduled the massage because he has been standing on his feet all day behind his vendor booth, selling items to convention participants. His feet and legs are killing him. He had heard another vendor talking about the great heat treatment she had received at the spa that relaxed her muscles. Brett requests a heat treatment on his calves. During the pretreatment interview, Tara discovers Brett has a history of DVT. He says he is fine now that he is taking an anticoagulant. Tara is concerned about Brett's health history. She is also conflicted because the management frowns upon turning clients away. What should Tara do?

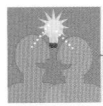

DISCUSSION

Massage and Cosmetology

Massage practitioners are allowed by law to perform spa treatments in some states, but in others there may be restrictions. Contact your state massage board and cosmetology board and ask what restrictions affect your practice. If available, post your findings on an Internet-based discussion board monitored by your instructor.

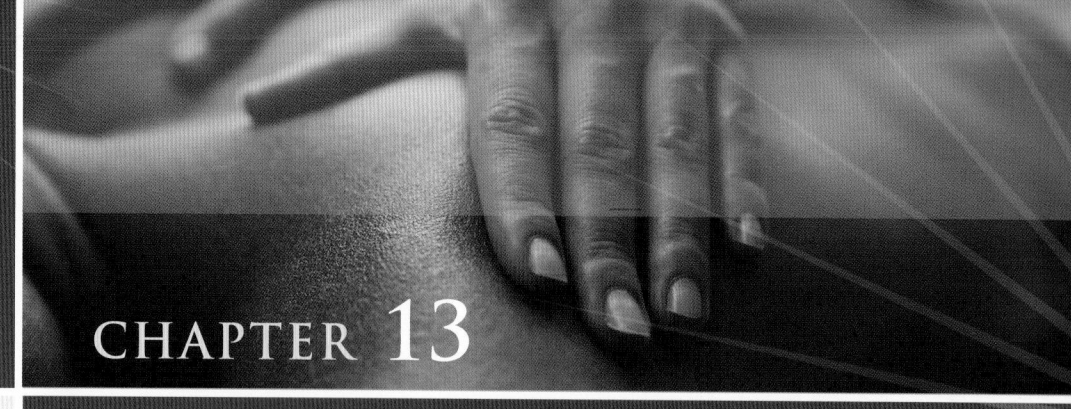

CHAPTER **13**

Foot Reflexology: Principles and Practice

LEARNING OBJECTIVES

After completing this chapter, the student should be able to:

1. Define reflexology and discuss how the body is mapped on the feet by zones, landmarks, and reflex points.
2. Describe basic techniques used in foot reflexology, list treatment guidelines, and perform a foot reflexology session.

INTRODUCTION

Reflexology, or *zone therapy*, is the application of pressure to specific points on the feet or hands; these points are believed to correspond with certain areas of the body (National Center for Complementary and Integrative Health [NCCIH], 2020). Reflexology is the fifth most widely used modality by massage practitioners (Federation of State Massage Therapy Boards [FSMTB], 2013) and studies indicate reflexology is safe for even fragile patients (NCCIH, 2020). Reflexology can be performed on other areas of the body such as the ears, but this chapter focuses on foot reflexology. Foot reflexology is different from nonspecific foot massage as pressure is not applied to specific points. Research is mixed regarding which is better for reducing symptoms in some populations (Gozuyesil & Baser, 2016; Williamson et al., 2002). Research related to foot reflexology is on Evolve.

Feet have been revered and considered sacred in many cultures. Jesus washed the feet of his disciples, and the practice of Pranāma in Indian culture traditionally includes touching the feet of elders as a signal of respect. Indigenous Americans believed the feet were sacred because they are in contact with the earth; therefore feet should be uncovered to receive the earth's life force.

Various forms of foot massage and reflexology have existed for over 5000 years with references found in many countries, including India, Egypt, China, and Japan. Early statues from India of the Hindu god Vishnu depict Sanskrit symbols placed on Vishnu's feet at the same location as points in reflexology. One of the earliest records depicting foot reflexology is a pictograph found in an Egyptian tomb dating to approximately 2500 BCE. It features a person giving a foot massage to another person. Underneath the pictograph is carved, "Do not hurt me." The carved response is, "I will act only to help you."

Reflexology developed out of zone therapy and the research and writings of American physicians William Fitzgerald and Joe Shelby Riley in the early 1900s. In 1911, German physician B. Barczewski published a paper on zone therapy and used the term "reflex massage." In 1955, German physician W. Kohlrausch published the book *Reflex Zone Massage*, stating the effects of pressure on specific points caused increased blood flow from reflexive action within arterial walls. Although reflexology does have many benefits, specific hemodynamic effects or blood flow to specific organs is not one of them (Jones et al., 2013). The term reflex massage became more widely used, and the term *zone therapy* was replaced with *reflexology*.

Reflexology was popularized in America by Eunice D. Ingham, a physiotherapist who is affectionately referred to as the mother of reflexology (Fig. 13.1). Ingham worked for Dr. Riley, and she began using reflexology on her patients. She spent most of her life mapping the location of reflex points on the feet. In 1938, she wrote and published *Stories the Feet Can Tell*, which contained case reports and foot maps she developed. These foot maps are still used today. Ingham spread her knowledge and love of reflexology

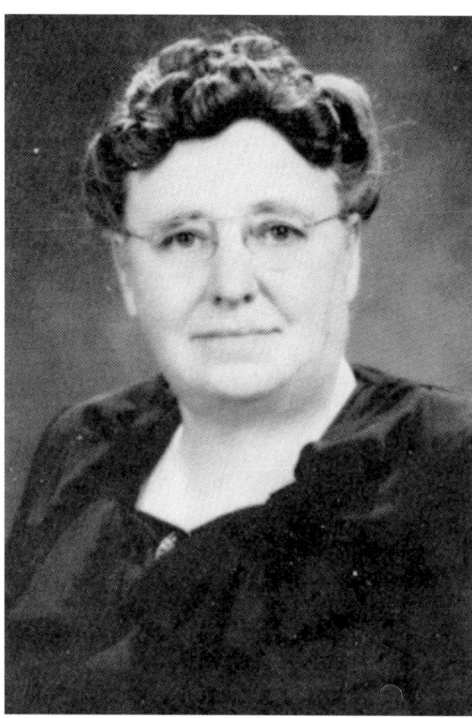

FIG. 13.1 Eunice D. Ingham (1889–1974). Ingham created the map used to locate reflex points still used today, and she is often referred to as the mother of reflexology. (Courtesy International Institute of Reflexology.)

through teaching, writing, and demonstrating reflexology from the 1930s through the early 1970s. Then, Ingham retired, and her nephew, Dwight Byers, took over the work. Byers established the International Institute of Reflexology (IIR), which still offers reflexology seminars worldwide.

Ancient Theories of Reflexology

According to ancient Eastern principles, all living things are surrounded by a life force. Life force has been called many things, including chi, qi, ki, and prana. Reflexology theory states life force flows through the body on 1 of 10 vertical pathways called zones, which give rise to reflexology's original name of zone therapy. When the body is in a state of health, energy flows freely along all the zones. Disease or pain impedes the flow of life force and represents an imbalance or obstruction. Imbalance of energy flow in any part of the zone will affect the entire zone.

> *Always do right. This will gratify some people and astonish the rest.*
>
> ~ **Mark Twain**

MAP OF THE BODY: ZONES, LANDMARKS, AND REFLEX POINTS

Maps of the feet help individuals locate reflex points within vertical zones and between horizontal landmarks. During a reflexology session, pressure is applied along zones, between landmarks, and on areas containing reflex points.

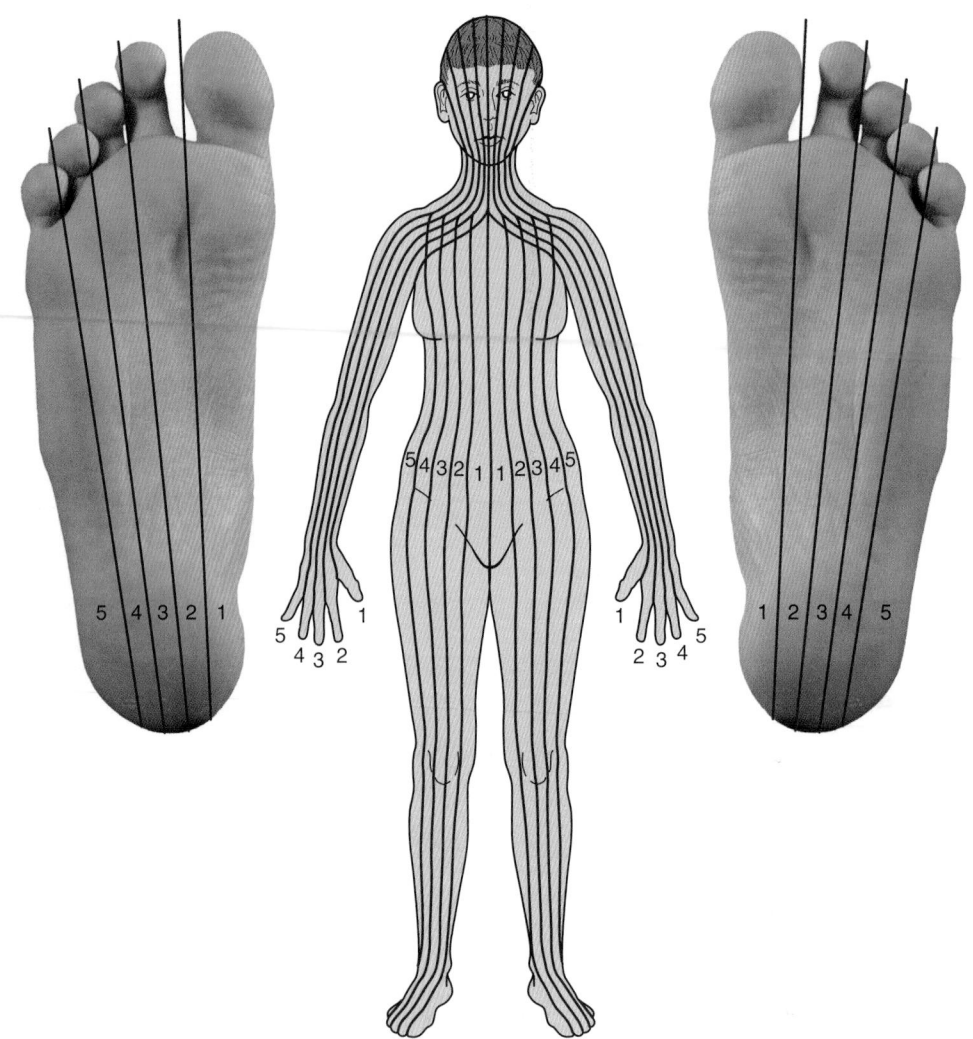

FIG. 13.2 Zones: 10 vertical pathways in the body *(central image)* and on the feet *(left* and *right images)* where life force flows.

Zones

The **zones** are 10 vertical pathways in the body where life force flows (Fig. 13.2). Five zones are in each foot and used to locate reflex points. Imagine a line passing from the area between each toe and then continuing straight up to the head. Zone 1 passes through the great toe or the first toe, zone 2 passes through the second toe, and so on, until you reach the smallest toe, which is zone 5. Every structure, including glands and organs, within a zone is connected energetically. Life force within the entire zone is stimulated when its corresponding areas on the foot are pressed, according to some theories of reflexology.

Landmarks: Lines and Areas

Landmarks are horizontal lines that cross the bottom or plantar surface of the foot and delineate areas containing reflex points (Fig. 13.3). The reproductive areas are on the sides of both feet, and the spinal areas are along the medial edge of both feet.

- **Neck/Shoulder Line**: The neck/shoulder line is between the base of the toes and the ball of the foot. The *head area* lies above the neck/shoulder line.

- **Diaphragm Line**: The diaphragm line is below the ball of the foot. The *chest area* lies between the neck/shoulder line and the diaphragm line.
- **Waistline**: The waistline is at the base of the fifth metatarsal. The *upper abdominal area* lies between the diaphragm line and the waistline. The *lower abdominal area* lies between the waistline and the pelvic line.
- **Pelvic Line**: The pelvic line is above the heel. The *pelvic area* lies below the pelvic line.

Reflex Points

Reflex points are points that correspond to body structures, including organs and glands. Reflex points and their positional relationships closely resemble the body (Fig. 13.4).

BASIC TECHNIQUES

Several basic techniques are used in foot reflexology. These include walking technique, point work, and relaxation techniques. Handheld tools can be used to apply pressure to reflex points.

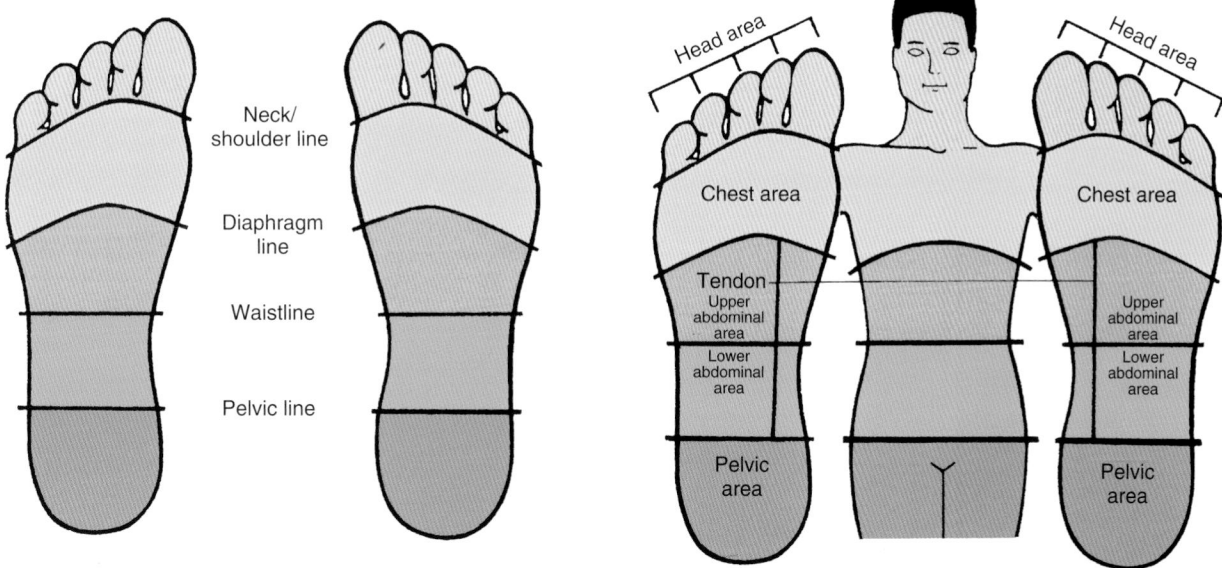

FIG. 13.3 Landmarks: Horizontal lines traverse the bottoms of the feet *(left image)*, delineate treatment areas *(right image)*. (From Norman, L. [1998]. *Feet first: A guide to foot reflexology*. New York: Simon & Schuster.)

Walking Technique

The walking technique is used to stimulate reflex points within an entire zone or areas between landmarks. Pressure is applied with the thumb on the bottom of the foot or with the fingers on the top of the foot. To perform the walking technique, bend and straighten the thumb (or finger) at the distal interphalangeal (DIP) joint; this creates the *walking* action. While the thumb of one hand is performing the walking technique, fingers on the same hand can support the foot receiving treatment. The nonworking hand can also support the treatment foot (Fig. 13.5).

Point Work Techniques

Point work is used when applying pressure to specific reflex points. There are two types of point work—direct pressure technique and hook-in and backup technique.
- **Direct Pressure Technique**. Locate a reflex point with your thumb or finger and apply direct pressure. To increase pressure, rotate, pivot, or flex the client's foot while your thumb (or finger) remains stationary.
- **Hook-In and Backup Technique**. Locate a reflex point with your finger or thumb and apply pressure. Next, flex or bend the DIP joint of the working finger or thumb while maintaining contact with the reflex point. Lastly, extend or straighten the DIP joint of the working finger or thumb while maintaining contact. These combined actions are similar to the walking technique but are essentially "walking in place." The alternating pressure is concentrated on one reflex point, and movement of the working finger or thumb pushes tissues aside; the client may experience increased pressure. This technique can be used on reflex points such as the pituitary, ileocecal valve, and sigmoid colon, just to name a few.

Relaxation Techniques

Manual relaxation techniques, sometimes called *desserts,* are used to relax the client before, during, and after a reflexology session. Techniques include the foot flop, the ankle flop (Fig. 13.6); and moving the foot and ankle into dorsiflexion, plantar flexion (Fig. 13.7), inversion, and eversion or wringing the foot (Fig. 13.8). The practitioner can also press and hold the base of the great toe, the base of the heel, or the solar plexus point. Press in during the client's inhalation and reduce pressure while maintaining contact during the client's exhalation. Do this for five breaths.

TREATMENT GUIDELINES

Reflexology can be practiced almost anywhere. The client's footwear is removed and they may be in the seated, prone, supine, or side-lying positions. Suggested guidelines for reflexology sessions include:
- Conduct a health assessment (see Chapter 10).
- Obtain consent for treatment (see Chapter 10).
- Rest the client's bare feet on a cushion covered by a clean drape.
- Wash your hands and disinfect any handheld tools before and after each reflexology session (see Chapter 9).
- Use efficient body mechanics during the session (see Chapter 7).
- Massage lubricants are not required. If used, apply only a small amount because your thumbs and fingers may slide off reflex points. Be sure the client is not allergic to lubricant ingredients prior to use.
- Begin the reflexology session with several relaxation techniques.

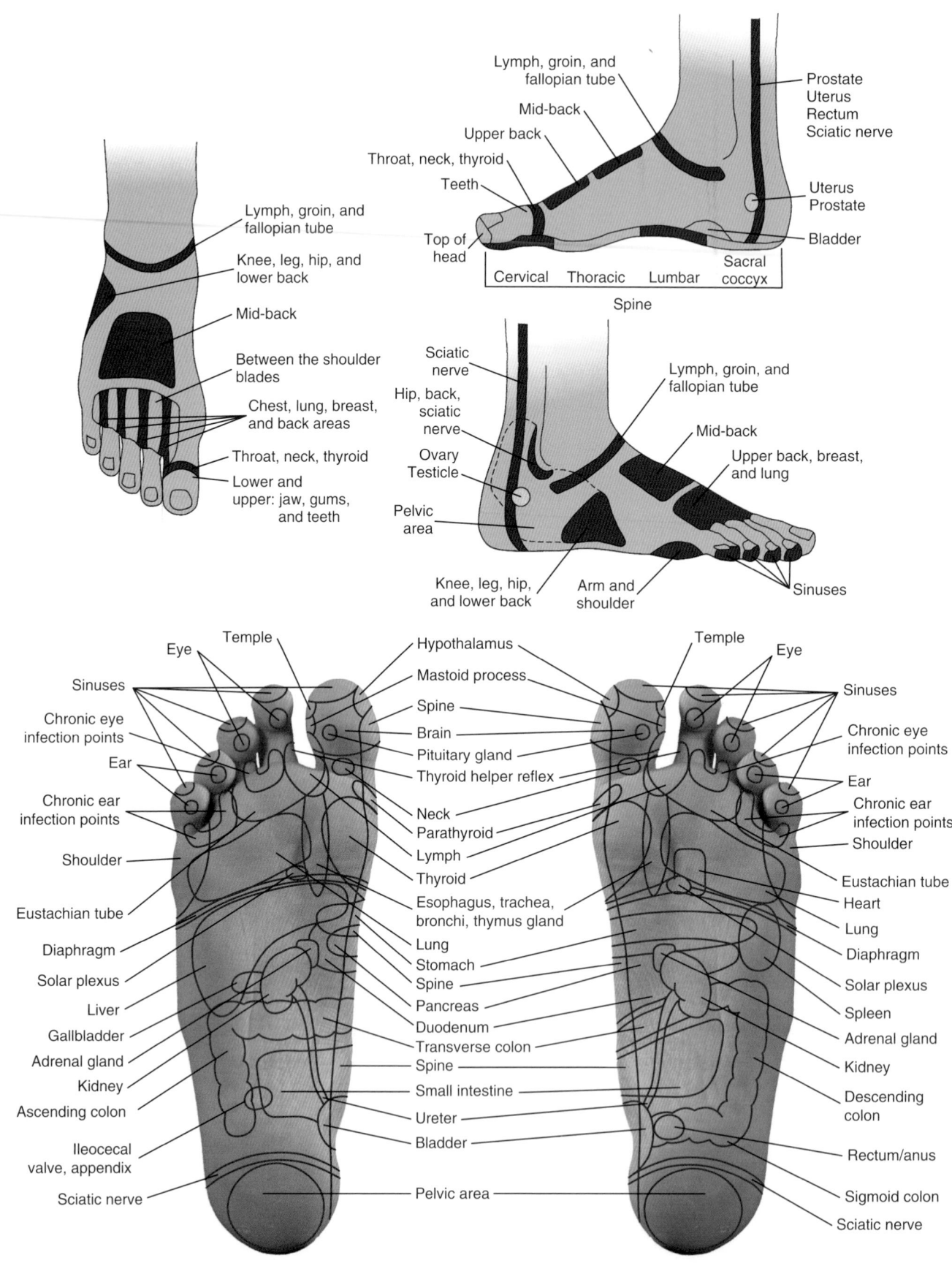

FIG. 13.4 Reflexology foot map.

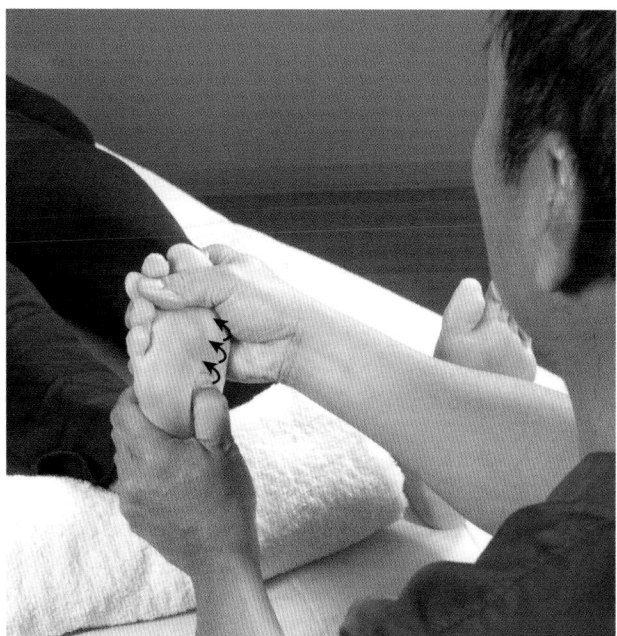

FIG. 13.5 The walking technique is used to apply pressure on points within an entire zone and areas between landmarks.

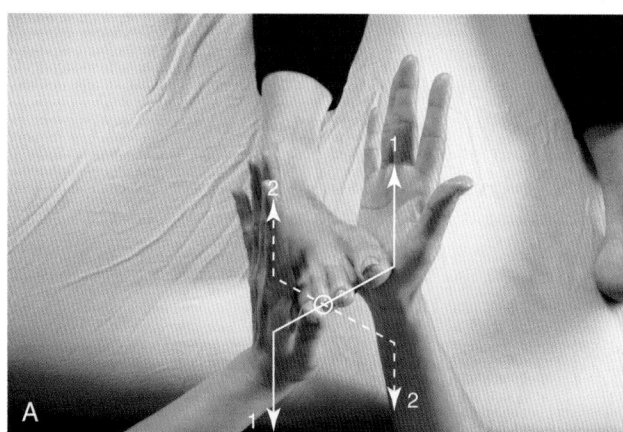

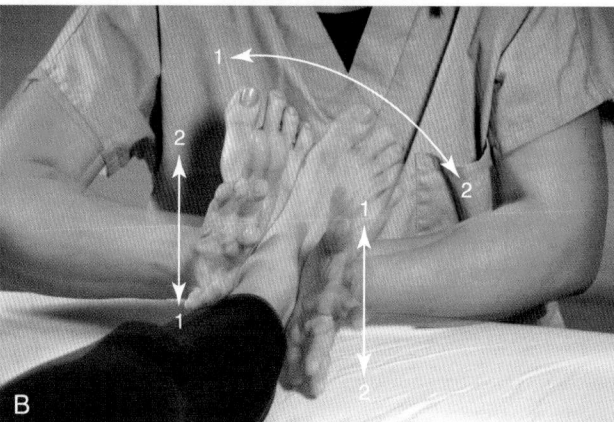

FIG. 13.6 Desserts include the foot flop (A) and the ankle flop (B).

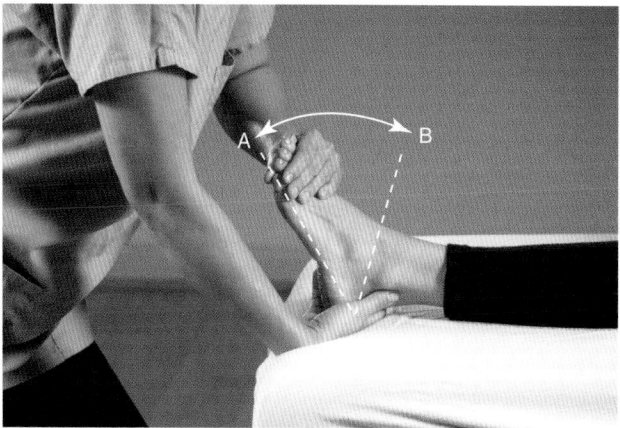

FIG. 13.7 Ankle plantar flexion (A) and dorsiflexion (B).

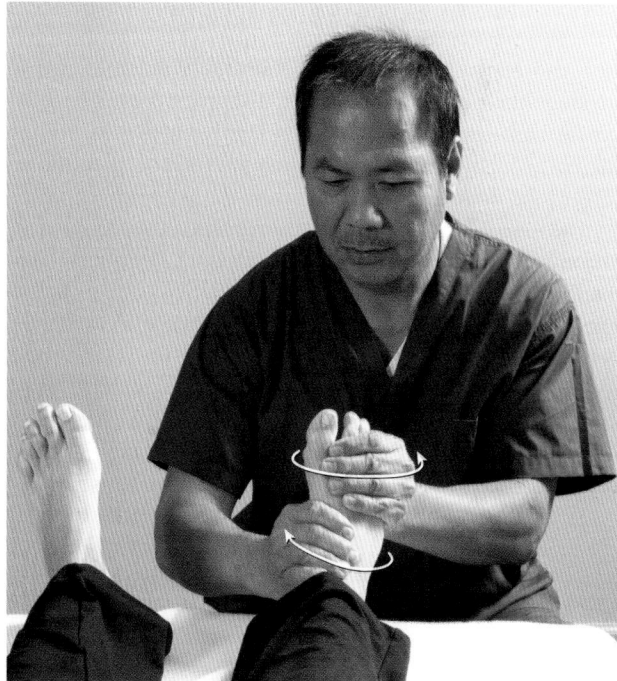

FIG. 13.8 Foot inversion and eversion or wringing.

- Use pressure according to the client's preference. Track the client's responses and make appropriate adjustments (see Chapter 8).
- Use fingertips rather than thumbs when applying pressure on the top of the foot because skin is thinner and there is less musculature.
- Thumbs may be more appropriate on the bottom of the foot. Knuckles can be used on the thick skin of the heels.
- If your hands begin to feel fatigued, use relaxation techniques.
- Remove excess lubricant after the session, assist with slipping socks and shoes onto the client's feet, and remove any bolsters before asking the client to stand.

Contraindications

Standard precautions, transmission-based precautions, and local contraindications applicable for massage may also be applicable for reflexology (see Chapter 9). Pregnancy, peripheral neuropathy, and client frailty are not contraindications for foot reflexology. *Local contraindications* include:

- Localized cysts
- Skin lesions such as ulcerations and fissures
- Viral skin infections such as warts
- Fungal infections such as athlete's foot
- Bacterial infections such as cellulitis
- Ingrown toenails if sensitive
- Gout
- Recent injury of the foot or ankle (avoid the affected foot for 72 to 96 hours while the area is locally inflamed).

FOOT REFLEXOLOGY SESSION

You can apply reflexology on yourself or teach clients to massage their own feet. You can also use a tennis ball, lacrosse ball, or racquetball to massage your feet by rolling the ball across the bottom of your foot as you press down toward the floor.

The foot can be divided into treatment areas: the head, chest, abdomen, pelvis, reproductive area, and spine. Horizontal landmarks mentioned previously (neck/shoulder, diaphragm, waistline, and pelvic lines) delineate five treatment areas on the bottom of the feet. Reproductive areas are on the sides of both feet. Spinal areas are along the medial edge of both feet from the base of the heel to the base of the top of the great toe. Use walking techniques to work treatment areas on the foot. Use point work techniques to massage specific reflex points.

Begin the foot reflexology session by establishing physical contact with the client. For example, place the thumbs on the client's solar plexus reflex points beneath the balls of the feet between the second and third toes. In reflexology, the solar plexus reflex point is referred to as the *key to relaxation*. Apply pressure to these points while the client inhales; release pressure while the client exhales. Follow the client's breath with your own. Repeat the press-and-release sequence five times. As the session progresses, you may return to the solar plexus reflex points to help your client relax, especially after point work over pressure-sensitive areas.

Head Area

The head area contains the toes. The great toe houses the reflex points for the pituitary gland. Locate the pituitary reflex point using your thumb. The point will often feel similar to a small pebble. The sinus reflex points are in the pads of each toe. Gently squeeze each pad to stimulate the sinus reflexes. Use the walking technique along the bottom and sides of each toe, pressing from the tip to the base to stimulate other reflex points.

Chest Area

The ball of the foot is the chest area, which contains the heart and lungs. In the body, the heart is two-thirds to the left of the midline and one-third to the right. This relationship is represented on the feet; the heart reflex is primarily on the left foot, with a small portion on the right foot.

Abdominal Area

The upper and lower abdominal areas are between the diaphragm line and the pelvic line. The spleen and stomach reflex points are on the left foot, and the liver and gallbladder reflex points are on the right foot. Another important area to stimulate is the pancreas reflex point on the left foot, just below the stomach reflex point.

Pelvic Area

The pelvic area is below the pelvic line. This area contains reflex points for the ascending colon and for portions of the transverse colon. The left foot contains reflex points for the rest of the transverse colon and for the descending colon. The reflex points for most of the urinary structures are in the pelvic area. The urinary bladder reflex point is where the pelvic line meets the arch of the foot.

Reproductive Area

The reproductive areas are on the heels and ankles. The uterus or prostate reflex points are on the medial or inside of the ankle, and the ovaries or testes reflex points are on the lateral or outside of the ankle. To locate the reflex points for the uterus or prostate, imagine a diagonal line drawn from the highest point of the medial ankle (medial malleolus) to the base of the heel; in the middle of the line are the uterus/prostate reflex points. Use the same measuring procedure to locate the ovaries or testes reflex points on the lateral ankle. The next area to work is the sciatic nerve reflex points. To locate these, imagine a stirrup running from beneath the heel, behind the ankle, and on both sides of the Achilles tendon.

Spinal Area

The spinal area is along the medial edge of both feet. As you look at the arch of the foot, notice how the medial edge possesses four distinct curves, similar to the vertebral column. The spinal area contains all the spinal reflex points. Use the walking technique along the spinal reflex points, pressing continuously from the base of the heel to the tip of the great toe.

E-RESOURCES

http://evolve.elsevier.com/Salvo/MassageTherapy

- Reflexology routine
- Chapter challenge
- Flash cards

DWIGHT BYERS

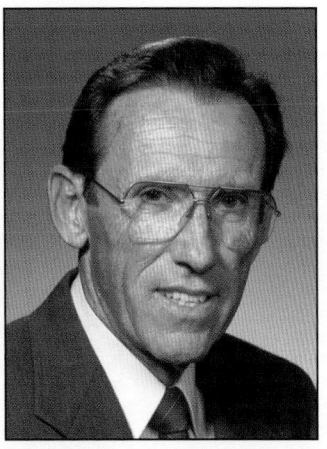

Whether it is curly hair, an outgoing personality, or a knack for music, there are some things that just seem to run in families. Nature versus nurture debates aside, it should be no surprise some of the important pioneers in the massage field caught the bodywork bug from their own family members. This was the case with Dwight Byers, one of the bright lights in the area of bodywork known as reflexology.

Byers's aunt, Eunice Ingham, was a physical therapist and the founder of reflexology. In the early 1930s, she worked with a physician who was interested in zone therapy, a method developed in the early 1900s that used pressure on different points of the feet to relieve pain. Ingham took this work a step further. After much experimentation and exhaustive notetaking, she developed what came to be known as *reflexology*.

Dwight Byers was not only Ingham's nephew, but also her early "guinea pig" as she developed her theories. Byers was skeptical at first, but as his hay fever and asthma disappeared, so did his doubt. Byers remembers those early days: "At first, we kind of laughed at her. I helped her carry her bags and set up. But soon I became fascinated, and eventually my sister and I began helping her teach."

Byers honed his anatomy skills as a medic in the US Army and later in mortuary science, and he began practicing reflexology part time. Following his aunt's death in 1974, Byers knew it would be up to him to safeguard the integrity of her work. He established the International Institute of Reflexology to preserve her method and share it with others. Byers also wrote the book, *Better Health with Foot Reflexology*, with these same aims in mind.

Byers is a strong believer that knowledge comes best through lots of experience. So, his advice to students? Practice. Then practice some more. "You've got to work on thousands of feet," he says. "My advice for beginning massage practitioners is to master your art. Don't be a jack-of-all-trades and master of none."

Byers's attitude toward assessments is equally pragmatic. After a student completes 200 hours of training in reflexology, he offers up his own feet for a session. He asks himself, "Would I pay to have this treatment done?" The answer determines whether the student is ready to call oneself a certified professional.

Dwight Byers still serves as the president of the International Institute of Reflexology and travels around the world to teach. Thanks to him, the legacy of his remarkable aunt will continue to spread and flourish, shared by reflexologists and massage practitioners across the globe.

REFERENCES

Federation of State Massage Therapy Boards (FSMTB). (2013). *Job task analysis*. Retrieved from https://www.fsmtb.org/media/1120/2012-jta.pdf.

Gozuyesil, E., & Baser, M. (2016). The effect of foot reflexology applied to women aged between 40 and 60 on vasomotor complaints and quality of life. *Complementary Therapies in Clinical Practice, 24*, 78–85.

Jones, J., Thomson, P., Irvine, K., & Leslie, S. J. (2013). Is there a specific hemodynamic effect in reflexology? A systematic review of randomized controlled trials. *Journal of Alternative and Complementary Medicine, 19*(4), 319–328.

National Center for Complementary and Integrative Health (NCCIH). (2020). *Reflexology*. Retrieved from https://nccih.nih.gov/health/reflexology.

Williamson, J., White, A., Hart, A., & Ernst, E. (2002). Randomised controlled trial of reflexology for menopausal symptoms. *BJOG, 109*(9), 1050–1055.

REVIEW AND APPLY YOUR KNOWLEDGE

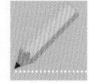 **MATCHING ONE: CONCEPT REVIEW**

Place the letter of the answer next to the term or phrase that best describes it.

A. Chi, qi, ki, prana
B. Desserts
C. Ingham
D. Landmarks
E. Massage lubricant
F. Mother of reflexology
G. Fifth
H. Reflexology
I. India
J. Ten
K. Fitzgerald and Riley
L. Zone therapy

_____ 1. Individuals whose research and writings helped develop reflexology.

_____ 2. Reflexology ranks number _____ in modalities most widely used by massage practitioners, according to the Federation of State Massage Therapy Boards.

_____ 3. The history of reflexology can be traced to countries, including Egypt, China, Japan, and _____.

_____ 4. Term originally used to describe reflexology.

_____ 5. Title by which Eunice Ingham is often referred.

_____ 6. Application of pressure to specific points on the feet or hands.

_____ 7. Total number of zones the feet possess.

_____ 8. Author of *Stories the Feet Can Tell*, published in 1938.

_____ 9. Horizontal lines on the bottom of each foot that delineate treatment areas and contain reflex points.

_____ 10. Manual relaxation techniques used before, during, and after a reflexology session.

_____ 11. Term to describe life force.

_____ 12. Product not required to perform reflexology treatments.

MATCHING TWO: CONCEPT REVIEW

Place the letter of the answer next to the term or phrase that best describes it.

A. Gout
B. Diaphragm line
C. Kohlrausch
D. Handheld tools
E. Peripheral neuropathy
F. Pelvic line
G. Point work techniques
H. Reflex points
I. Walking techniques
J. Zone 1
K. Zone 5
L. Zones

_____ 1. Term for the 10 vertical pathways through which life force flows.

_____ 2. Landmark below the ball of the foot.

_____ 3. Condition that is not a local contraindication for receiving reflexology.

_____ 4. Zone passing through the smallest toe.

_____ 5. Points that correspond to body structures, including organs and glands.

_____ 6. Technique used to work entire zones or areas between landmarks.

_____ 7. Landmark above the heel.

_____ 8. Can be used to apply pressure when doing point work.

_____ 9. Zone passing through the great toe.

_____ 10. Author of *Reflex Zone Massage*, published in 1955.

_____ 11. Local contraindication for foot reflexology.

_____ 12. Techniques used to stimulate specific reflex points.

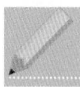

MULTIPLE CHOICE: TEST YOUR KNOWLEDGE

Place the letter of the answer next to the number of the term or phrase that best describes it.

_____ 1. The medial edge of the foot contains the:
   A. pelvic area.
   B. abdominal area.
   C. spinal area.
   D. reproductive area.

_____ 2. Reflexology foot maps still used today were primarily developed by:
   A. Fitzgerald.
   B. Riley.
   C. Ingham.
   D. Byers.

_____ 3. Who established the International Institute of Reflexology?
   A. Riley
   B. Byers
   C. Fitzgerald
   D. Ingham

_____ 4. Which area contains the pituitary reflex point?
   A. Spinal
   B. Abdominal
   C. Chest
   D. Head

_____ 5. Which of the following reflex points is on the medial or inside of the ankle?
   A. Prostate
   B. Ovaries
   C. Liver
   D. Lung

_____ 6. The "foot flop" is an example of what type of technique?
   A. Desserts
   B. Walking
   C. Point work
   D. Direct pressure

_____ 7. The "hook-in and backup technique" is an example of what type of technique?
   A. Desserts
   B. Walking
   C. Point work
   D. Relaxation work

_____ 8. Which of the following is a local contraindication for foot reflexology?
   A. Pregnancy
   B. Rosacea
   C. Athlete's foot
   D. Peripheral neuropathy

_____ 9. Which point is referred to as the "key to relaxation" in foot reflexology?
   A. Sciatic nerve
   B. Solar plexus
   C. Pituitary
   D. Heart

_____ 10. Which of the following reflex points is in the pads of each toe?
   A. Sinus
   B. Heart
   C. Colon
   D. Stomach

_____ 11. Which of the following reflex points is in the abdominal area of the right foot?
   A. Spleen
   B. Liver
   C. Stomach
   D. Pancreas

_____ 12. Which of the following reflex points is on the lateral or outside of the ankle?
   A. Colon
   B. Uterus
   C. Prostate
   D. Ovary

CRITICAL THINKING

May the Force Be With You

What are your thoughts about the concept of life force (ki, chi, qi, and prana)? What do think of reflexology alleviating symptoms and conditions in the body by balancing life force flow? Would you be willing to learn reflexology? Why or why not?

Answers can include, but are not limited to:

The answers to these questions are really going to depend on the reader's point of view about Eastern bodywork methods and traditional medicines. Every answer will be different. Some readers will have already studied reflexology or other Eastern bodywork methods and theory; some will not; some will be open to learning more about it; some will not and can be because of several things: personal interest, personal spiritual beliefs, previous education, personal experiences, and so forth.

PROFESSIONAL PRACTICE

Appearances Sometimes Make a Difference

Delores has been practicing massage for 10 years. Natalie, the wife of a prominent bank executive, contacted Delores late one afternoon and requested a massage for 9am the next day. Natalie arrives well dressed and has on beautiful makeup. During the pretreatment interview, she says she is attending an important fundraising event right after the massage, where she is being honored as the most generous donor. She says she gets nervous being in front of large groups of people and has booked the massage so she can be relaxed. Should Delores offer Natalie reflexology instead of a massage? Would this be a better option for Natalie and, if so, why? Would the effects be the same as for massage? How should she talk to Natalie about receiving reflexology instead of massage?

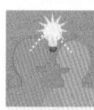

DISCUSSION

Should Reflexologists Obtain a Massage License?

There is a debate currently going on in the massage community. One side of the debate says reflexology is part of massage and if you want to practice reflexology, you must have a massage license (in states requiring a massage license). The other side of the debate says reflexology is not massage, and therefore, reflexologists are not required to obtain a massage license. What do you think and why? If available, post your reflections on an Internet-based discussion board monitored by your instructor.

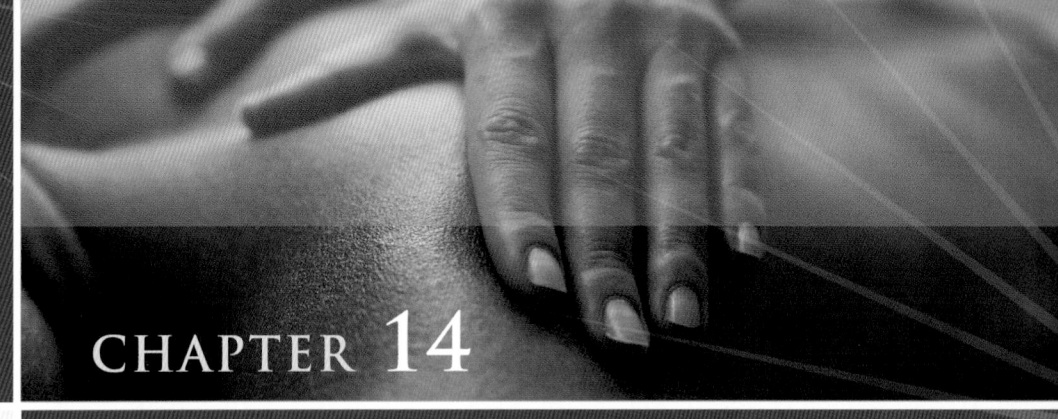

CHAPTER 14

Clinical Massage: Pain Theories and Pain Management, Clinical Assessments, and Clinical Application Methods

Michele J. Renee and Susan G. Salvo

The world as we have created it is a process of our thinking. It cannot be changed without changing our thinking.
—Albert Einstein

LEARNING OBJECTIVES

After completing this chapter, the student should be able to:

1. Define clinical massage and discuss past and present theories of pain, types of pain, pain perception, and pain management.
2. Discuss and perform clinical assessments, including range of motion, posture, gait observation, and tests for orthopedic conditions.
3. Outline types of sports massage, working with athletes, as well as soft tissue injuries, current protocols, massage modifications.
4. Identify application methods used in clinical massage, including trigger point therapy and myofascial release techniques.
5. Describe hospital-based massage, and discuss massage considerations for surgery, surgical scars, individuals in hospice care, and coping with death-related grief.

http://evolve.elsevier.com/Salvo/MassageTherapy

INTRODUCTION

Massage practitioners working in clinical settings are a growing trend. An estimated 250 hospitals in the United States offer massage services for inpatients, and competencies have been established (Academic Collaboration for Integrative Health [ACIH], 2017). Benefits of massage for hospitalized patients include reduced pain, increased relaxation and a sense of wellbeing, improved mood, enhanced mobility, increased participation in treatment, and faster recovery (Smith et al., 1999). Massage is the most recommended complementary approach by U.S. physicians to their patients, with psychiatrists leading the way in recommendations (Stussman et al., 2020). Physical and occupational therapists are hiring massage practitioners to work in their clinics. Chiropractors are taking advantage of the benefits of massage for their patients, employing practitioners, and billing insurance for massage services. In addition, massage practitioners are recognizing undiagnosed conditions and referring affected individuals to an appropriate healthcare provider (Mallory et al., 2018).

Clinical massage is massage used to rehabilitate injuries; manage medically diagnosed conditions, their treatments, or complications; and manage issues related to surgery. Examples of injuries are rotator cuff tears and plantar fasciitis; examples of medically diagnosed conditions are diabetes and asthma; examples of medical treatments are chemotherapy and dialysis; examples of disease complications are peripheral neuropathy and depression; examples of issues related to surgery are lymphedema and scar tissue.

Clinical massage may be prescribed by healthcare providers and include condition-related treatment goals. Prescriptions include CPT codes. The length of a session is often 15 minutes per code and treatment is applied to a specified area.

Clinical massage can also refer to the practice settings where massage services are provided, such as hospitals, physical therapy clinics, physical rehabilitation clinics, chiropractic clinics, sports clinics, medical facilities that provide services for military service members, oncology centers, and hospice care facilities. **Physical rehabilitation** is the restoration of an individual to a normal or near-normal function after a disabling disease or injury. Physical rehabilitation often begins soon after the causative event (in the case of injuries) and continues until the individual reaches *maximum medical improvement* (MMI). MMI is the point in the rehabilitative process when the condition is unlikely to improve, and no additional recovery is expected. MMI is usually determined by the patient's healthcare provider (*Mosby's Medical Dictionary*, 2021; *Stedman's Medical Dictionary*, 2005).

Clinical massage focuses on therapeutic or palliative goals. **Therapeutic** goals refer to curative measures used to treat diseases, disorders, or injuries. Examples of therapeutic goals are improved function, reduced recovery time, decreased scar tissue, and reduced edema. **Palliative** goals refer to noncurative measures used to improve a patient's quality of life. Examples of palliative goals are reduced pain, fatigue, nausea, insomnia, depression, and anxiety.

A **patient** is the recipient of medical/healthcare services. There are several types of patients. An **inpatient** is usually admitted to the hospital to receive medical/healthcare services and who stays in the hospital overnight. Inpatients may remain in the hospital for 1 day, or several days or weeks. An **outpatient** is not admitted to the hospital. Annual exams with a primary care physician or consultations with a cardiologist are examples of outpatient services, and care is usually provided in a medical office or outpatient center. In this chapter, the terms patients and clients are used interchangeably.

Massage can save money for patients, hospitals/clinics, and insurance companies. A cost analysis conducted at a pediatric pain clinic found that an interdisciplinary approach that included massage, acupuncture, biofeedback, and psychotherapy reduced inpatient and emergency department visits and saved the hospital a total of $36,228 per patient, per year, and saved the insurance company $11,482 per patient per year (Mahrer et al., 2018). Insurance companies may cover massage services for personal injury (PI), automobile and workers' compensation claims if these services are "medically necessary." Documentation of patient progress may be required to establish medical necessity. Prescriptions and insurance claim forms are discussed in Chapter 10.

This chapter aims to introduce students to clinical massage and to provide fundamental knowledge about pain and the management thereof, clinical assessments, working with sports and tactical athletes, soft tissue injuries, specialized application methods, working in hospital settings, postsurgical considerations, and in-hospice care settings. To accomplish these tasks, this chapter expands upon information covered in other chapters, including evidence-informed practice (see Chapter 5); massage techniques, mobilizations, and stretches (see Chapter 8); assessment, treatment planning, and documentation (see Chapter 10); fascia (see Chapter 18); joint movements (see Chapter 19); muscle contractions (see Chapter 20); and kinesiology (see Chapter 21). If practitioners want more information, they should pursue specialization through continuing education programs.

PAIN

Pain is an unpleasant sensory and emotional experience associated with, or resembling, actual or potential tissue damage (International Association for the Study of Pain [IASP], 2020). This widely accepted definition was introduced by the IASP and adopted by the American Pain Society and the World Health Organization. The definition of pain was updated in 2020 and included six key concepts.

- Pain is a personal subjective experience influenced by biologic, psychologic, and social factors.
- Pain and nociception are different. Pain is the experience whereas **nociception** is the encoding of the painful event (e.g., touching a hot stove, accidentally cutting yourself).

- People learn pain through life experiences.
- A person's subjective report of pain should be respected.
- Pain may have adverse effects related to physical functioning and psychosocial wellbeing.
- Verbal description is only one way in which pain is expressed. The inability to communicate does not negate the human or nonhuman/animal experience of pain.

Pain affects many people across a wide variety of demographics and is associated with a myriad of diseases and conditions. Pain affects more Americans than diabetes, cardiovascular disease, and cancer combined. It can limit a person's ability to work, sleep, care for their families, and engage in recreational activities. Poorly managed pain can lead to negative outcomes such as anxiety, depression, and financial hardship. Pain is cited as the main reason Americans seek healthcare services, is a major contributor to healthcare costs, and is a leading cause of disability (National Institutes of Health [NIH], 2015).

Massage can be effective in reducing pain, as reported by 92% of massage consumers. Twenty-nine percent of massage consumers use it to reduce or manage pain, and 33% receive massage for soreness, stiffness, or muscle spasm (American Massage Therapy Association [AMTA], 2021). The American College of Physicians published practice guidelines for adults with acute, subacute, and chronic lower back pain and recommended the use of nonpharmacologic treatments such as massage before prescribing pain-reducing medications (Qaseem et al., 2017).

Pain Theories: Past and Present

Pain represents a field of study that goes back several centuries. Pain theories include the intensity theory, Cartesian dualism theory, specificity theory, pattern theory, gate control theory, neuromatrix model, and the biopsychosocial model. Early theories considered pain to be a direct result of changes in tissues, but current research indicates that pain is more complex and involves the conversion of sensory signals into the perception of pain. How this conversion occurs is still not well understood. Let's explore pain theories, both past and present.

Intensity Theory

This theory dates back to Plato, who stated pain occurs when a stimulus is intense and lasts longer than usual.

Cartesian Dualistic Theory

Pain is a consequence of committing sin and akin to karma. Pain was connected to the soul and was how people who committed sin repented for their actions.

Specificity Theory

Pain is a specific sensation transmitted by specific receptors. Descartes expanded this theory, stating that pain resided in the pineal gland, making the brain the moderator of pain. Von Frey also contributed to this theory, postulating that there was a separate system in the body that perceived pain, cold, heat, and touch—much like hearing and vision (Fig. 14.1).

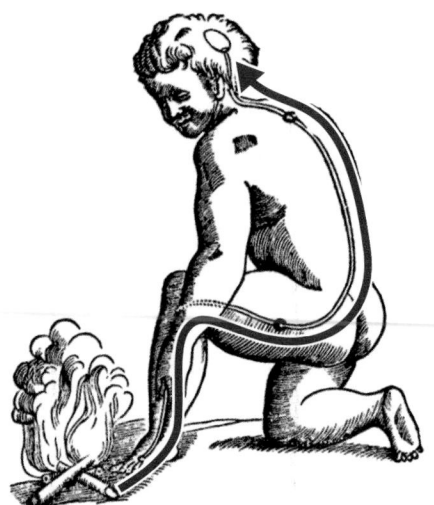

Specificity theory of pain
(16th Century)

FIG. 14.1 Specificity theory. This theory states that pain is a specific sensation transmitted by specific receptors.

Gate Control Theory

The gate control theory states that the spinal cord acts like a neurologic gate and controls whether or not pain signals enter the brain, which results in the experience of pain. When the gate is open, the brain receives the message, and when the gate is closed, the brain does not receive the message. Stimuli such as pressure (massage), motion, heat, and cold, travel on larger, more insulated (myelinated), and faster nerves compared with pain stimuli. The faster stimuli enter the spinal cord first, close the gate, and prevent pain messages from entering the brain (Melzack & Wall, 1965). However, the gate control theory did not explain chronic pain or painful conditions such as phantom limb pain.

Neuromatrix Theory

This theory states that pain is a multidimensional experience produced by a person's "neurosignature," or unique pattern of nerve impulses within a widely distributed network in the brain called the body-self neuromatrix. Pain is one possible output or expression of the neuromatrix after synthesizing various inputs (Fig. 14.2). The neurosignature is the soil on which seeds of incoming information or input fall. Any resultant plants can be thought of as output (Melzack, 2001). Let's look at types of input first.

- **Body sensations (somatosensory)**. This includes characteristics such as sensory location, distribution, frequency, duration, and intensity, as well as sensation qualities such as burning, tingling, and aching.
- **Emotions (affect)**. This is how we feel about incoming sensation.
- **Cognitive/mental processes**. This is what we think about the sensation, including memories of past experiences, personal beliefs and biases, cultural influences, and what the sensation might mean.

There are several types of outputs.

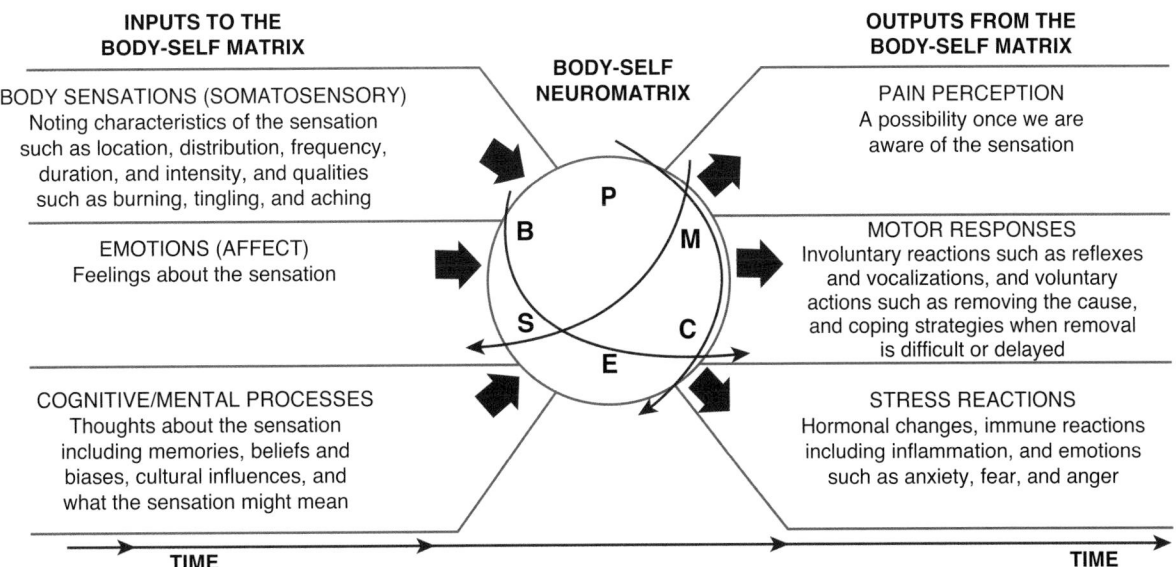

FIG. 14.2 Neuromatrix theory. This theory states that pain is a multidimensional experience produced by a person's unique pattern of nerve impulses within a widely distributed network in the brain called the body-self neuromatrix. (Modified from Melzack R. [2001]. Pain and the neuromatrix in the brain. *Journal of Dental Education*, 65[12], 1378–1382.)

- **Pain perception.** This is one possibility when we become aware of the sensation.
- **Motor responses.** This includes involuntary reactions such as reflexes and spontaneous vocalizations, as well as voluntary actions such as consciously removing the cause, and coping strategies when removal of the cause is difficult or delayed.
- **Stress reactions.** This includes hormonal reactions such as increases in cortisol, adrenaline, and endorphins; immune reactions such as inflammation; and emotional reactions such as anxiety, fear, and anger.

The neuromatrix model illustrates the concept of **neuroplasticity**, the brain's ability to form and reorganize synaptic connections, especially in response to experience. Repetition helps form new neural pathways. Neuroplasticity is one of the most important concepts in understanding pain and suggests neural networks are not fixed and can be modified.

Biopsychosocial Model

Pain, health, and disease are products of complex interactions between biologic factors (i.e., genetics, biochemical), psychologic factors (i.e., mood, behavior, personality), and social factors (i.e., culture, family relationships, socioeconomic status, community/social support). A multidimensional approach, rather than a unidimensional approach, is needed to address issues of health maintenance, disease prevention, and pain management (Engel, 1977). Ways to apply the biopsychosocial model in professional practice are listed in the section titled "Pain Management."

Types of Pain: Nociceptive and Neuropathic

Pain can be classified according to the type of nerve that is activated. **Nociceptive pain** is produced by nerves called nociceptors. This type of pain is caused by actual or potential tissue damage. **Neuropathic (neurogenic) pain**, also called neuropathy, is produced by non-nociceptive nerves. This type of pain is caused by damage to the nervous system itself. Examples of neuropathic pain is nerve compression or nerve entrapment (e.g., carpal tunnel syndrome, sciatica, nerve compression by tumors), neurologic infection (e.g., meningitis, shingles), neurologic diseases and conditions (e.g., Parkinson disease, multiple sclerosis, stroke), and nerve trauma (e.g., spinal cord or traumatic brain injuries). Other causes of neuropathic pain are radiation therapy, chemotherapy, and complications of surgical procedures such as amputations.

Types of neuropathies are central and peripheral. **Central neuropathy** originates in the central nervous system (CNS). **Peripheral neuropathy** originates in the peripheral nervous system (PNS). **Radiculopathy** is a type of neuropathy that originates in spinal nerve roots of the PNS. Radiculopathy originating in the cervical region is called *cervical radiculopathy*. Radiculopathy originating in the lumbar region is called *lumbar radiculopathy*. Neuropathies can cause pain and paresthesia—some cause motor dysfunction. **Paresthesia** includes abnormal sensations, such as burning, itching, numbness, tingling or pricking, often called "pins and needles," which may or may not include the sensation of pain.

Types of Pain: Acute and Chronic

Pain can be classified according to its duration. **Acute pain** lasts less than 30 days and is usually related to injuries, disease, or invasive procedures, such as surgery. The intensity, distribution, and characteristics of acute pain usually correspond with damaged tissues. Pain often dissipates as inflammatory responses diminish, damaged tissues heal, movement normalizes, and the affected individual resumes normal life. Acute pain is protective and predictable. **Subacute pain** may follow acute pain, and occur when inflammation subsides, but the person still experiences pain and impaired function.

Chronic pain persists past the normal healing times and reflects the state of the person's nervous system rather than the condition of the tissues (usually more than 3 to 6 months). Whereas acute pain is proportional, appropriate, and often coincides with inflammation, chronic pain is regarded as a problem in itself, and it is often difficult or impossible to determine when the pain started or its cause. Approximately 25.3 million U.S. adults (11.2%) have chronic pain every day, and nearly 40 million adults (17.6%) have severe pain (U.S. Department of Health and Human Services, 2018).

Types of Pain: Specific and Nonspecific

Pain can be classified by its underlying cause. **Specific pain** has a specific cause, such as tissue damage, deformity, disease, or a condition such as disc herniation. **Nonspecific pain** does not have an inflammatory, structural, or disease-related cause. Common locations of nonspecific pain are the lower back, neck, shoulders, hips, and knees. Most pain is nonspecific pain. In fact, 85% of lower back pain is classified as being nonspecific (Koch & Hänsel, 2019).

Pain Perception: Pain Threshold, Pain Tolerance, and Sensitization

Pain perception is the subjective reporting of a painful experience. Many factors influence pain perception, pain intensity, and duration, including gender, race and ethnicity, age, emotions including catastrophizing and ruminating, levels of physical activity, obesity, sleep deprivation, cold application, heat application, massage, and preexisting diseases including anxiety and depression (Adams et al., 2010; Cimpean & David, 2019; Daneau et al., 2019; Park et al., 2014; Park et al., 2016; Shankland, 2011; Shah et al., 2015; Thompson et al., 2016; Wandner et al., 2012; Yildirim et al., 2010; Zhang et al., 2013). The most important risk factor is the presence of pain in another area of the body (Mills et al., 2019). Pain perception is unique to each individual and can be experienced on a spectrum, from pain threshold on the low end to pain tolerance on the high end.

- **Pain threshold**. The *minimum* level of intensity perceived as painful. Some massage research studies use the term pressure pain threshold, which is the minimum amount of pressure that produces pain. Massage can reduce pressure pain threshold in persons who have painful conditions (Chatchawan et al., 2014; Kamali et al., 2019; Moraska et al., 2017).
- **Pain tolerance**. The *maximum* level of intensity perceived as painful, with any further pain being unbearable and intolerable.

Pain perception can be altered through a phenomenon called sensitization. **Sensitization** is a condition of a lower pain threshold and increased nervous system responsiveness, which results in pain hypersensitivity. During sensitization,

nerves detecting pain are more responsive and things typically not painful (e.g., handshake, hug), are now painful. Sensitization can be associated with chronic pain and conditions such as fibromyalgia, temporomandibular joint dysfunction, and migraine headaches. Types of sensitizations are central and peripheral.

- **Central sensitization**. Sensitization in the CNS (e.g., brain and spinal cord).
- **Peripheral sensitization**. Sensitization in the PNS (e.g., cranial and spinal nerves).

Sensitization may increase the size of a nerve's receptive field, or an area of the body where a single sensory nerve can detect sensations. It is unclear how sensitization occurs, but it may be related to physical or psychological trauma. However, just as the nervous system learns to "turn up" the volume on pain, it can learn ways to turn it down.

Pain Management

Pain management is a process of providing care that alleviates or reduces pain to a level of comfort that is acceptable to a client. In 2017, the Joint Commission began requiring hospitals to provide nonpharmacologic pain treatments, or to combine pharmacologic and nonpharmacologic approaches. Nonpharmacologic treatments include massage, chiropractic/osteopathic care, and acupuncture. This requirement is partially in response to the current opioid crisis (National University of Health Sciences [NUHS], 2017).

The misuse of and addiction to opioids, including prescription painkillers, constitutes a serious public health crisis. The Consortium Pain Task Force demands a call to action to increase access to effective, nonpharmacologic pain interventions, including massage. Furthermore, current guidelines now place massage and other nonpharmacologic approaches on the front line in treating acute, subacute, and chronic lower back pain. These guidelines suggest physicians should recommend participation in exercise such as walking and as many daily activities as possible, as this would likely reduce pain (Tick et al., 2018). Massage practitioners can encourage their clients to participate in these activities and explain to them that they are likely to increase function. This cognitive approach to pain management may also reduce anxiety, increase confidence, and give clients a sense of control over their recovery. The degree of pain experienced may be dependent on perceived levels of threat, real or imagined. Teaching clients the connection between thoughts and pain can assist them to understand this relationship better.

Management of pain is ideally a multidisciplinary approach, and pain management should include psychological and cognitive/behavioral interventions. Massage can be viewed as a psychological as well as a physical intervention. Walach et al. (2003) found that massage can be as effective as standard medical care in chronic pain conditions, and the effects thereof tended to last longer in the massage group, possibly because of its effect on the psychologic domain. To address the cognitive/behavioral aspects of pain, educate clients about pain and pain mechanisms, which have been found to reduce chronic pain, disability, and catastrophizing, as well as improve function (Louw et al., 2011). Furthermore, a client's beliefs about pain often predict if acute pain will become chronic (Ramond et al., 2011). Massage practitioners can positively influence clients' attitudes about their bodies and functional capacities and improve outcomes by being hopeful about prognosis, while minimizing verbal and nonverbal messages that may exacerbate fear and uncertainty. Other ways to improve client outcomes include:

1. Recognizing that relationships are central to providing quality care.
2. Using empathy, curiosity, self-awareness, and/or mindfulness when providing care.
3. Communicating evidence in ways that promote dialogue and trust.
4. Providing or encouraging multidisciplinary services.

CLINICAL ASSESSMENTS

Assessments are used to gather client information in order to make informed decisions about treatment. Some assessments indicate or contraindicate massage, or they may necessitate a referral to a medical specialist. However, all assessments begin with a client's health history. Pain was defined previously and pain assessments usually involve the use of visual, numeric, verbally descriptive, or pictorial scales. Clients' health history and pain scales are discussed in Chapter 10. Observational, palpatory, and movement assessments are conducted if warranted. If neurologic signs and symptoms or referred pain are involved, special orthopedic tests may be used. The goal is not to complete as many tests as possible, but to conduct only those assessments specific to the client's complaint or goal. **LEARNING TIP:** To help you remember the order in which assessments are conducted, use the acronym **HOPMNRS** for **H**istory, **O**bservation, **P**alpation, **M**ovement, **N**eurologic sign/symptoms, **R**eferred pain, and **S**pecial tests such as orthopedic assessments (Magee, 2020). As tests and their results are subject to error, no test is completely accurate, and some special tests have questionable clinical value (Hegedus et al., 2017; Lederman, 2011; Preece et al., 2008).

Obtain consent before beginning an assessment and explain briefly what you are planning to do, why you are doing it, how long it will take, what positioning will be required, and what equipment you will use, if any. Wash hands before and after the assessment, preferably in the client's presence. Warm your hands and any equipment before touching the client and be aware of the client's reactions.

Conduct assessments bilaterally and perform the test on the uninvolved side first. This side will be used as a baseline and serve as a treatment goal when conducting post-treatment assessments. Testing the uninvolved side first also helps give the client a sense of normal movement. Some assessments and observations may make clients feel uncomfortable or self-conscious, especially those related to posture or gait. This situation may prompt clients to adopt an unnatural stance or movement pattern, similar to smiling artificially when asked to pose for a picture. Acknowledge this possibility and conduct assessments in as relaxed a manner as possible to reduce the client's self-consciousness.

Range of Motion Assessment

Range of motion (ROM) is the amount of motion that occurs when one segment of the body moves in relationship to another segment of the body. Both active and passive ROM assessments can be performed on a client. ROM assessment is used to determine the absence or presence of pain, which structures might be limiting the movement, which soft tissues to address during the session, or if a referral is needed. Remember, ROM assessments are performed bilaterally, starting with the uninvolved side. Active resisted movements are part of several clinical massage applications, such as muscle energy techniques (METs) and proprioceptive neuromuscular facilitation (PNF), which are discussed later in this chapter. To review from Chapter 8, *passive range of motion* (PROM) is movement produced by external forces without voluntary contraction (e.g., client is passive while the practitioner performs the movement). *Active range of motion* (AROM) is movement produced by voluntary contraction (e.g., client actively moves the limb or body part). Active movements can be performed with assistance or against resistance.

ROM is limited by several barriers.

- **Physiologic barrier**. Limits in ROM caused by reaching the elastic limits of soft tissues that surround a joint (i.e., muscles, tendons, ligaments).
- **Anatomic barrier**. Limits in ROM caused by the shape of the bones at the joint. Do not move a client past their anatomic barrier as this may injure the client.
- **Restrictive (pathologic) barrier**. Limits in ROM caused by pathology or structural abnormality (i.e., contracture, osteophyte/bone spur) and prevents the person from reaching their normal physiologic barrier.

When performing PROM assessments, practitioners must be able to describe the feel of a joint when it reaches then end of its ROM. The term end-feel has evolved for this purpose. **End-feel** is the quality of resistance felt by the practitioner at the end of PROM. There are several types of end-feels.

- **Normal end-feel (physiologic)**. This occurs when normal anatomy stops the movement. Normal end-feel can be hard, soft, or firm and is determined by the structure stopping the motion.
  - **Hard end-feel**. This feels rigid or abrupt and occurs when bone-to-bone contact limits motion. For example, elbow extension is limited by contact with the olecranon process and bony floor of the olecranon fossa.
  - **Soft end-feel**. This feels mushy or spongy and occurs when motion is limited by increased resistance from muscles or skin. For example, elbow and knee flexion is limited by compression of muscles.

- **Firm end-feel**. This feels firm yet elastic with a slight give and occurs when motion is limited by joint capsules or ligaments. For example, finger extension is limited by tension in the metacarpophalangeal joint capsules.
- **Abnormal end-feel (pathologic)**. This occurs when motion stops before its normal end range because of an abnormal or pathologic condition, such as contracture, joint deformity, and swelling from edema or lymphedema.
- **Empty end-feel**. This occurs when no end-feel was noted because pain triggered protective muscle splinting.

Practitioners with an awareness of normal end-feel can better determine reasons for a joint's lack of motion or excessive motion and devise a more appropriate treatment plan.

Postural Assessment

A **postural assessment** is an observational evaluation of a client's relaxed, barefoot, standing posture and is used to determine postural abnormalities that may cause or contribute to a client's complaint (also called a *static postural assessment*). The practitioner observes specific landmarks after the client is asked to stand upright, look straight ahead, relax their shoulders, and let their arms hang naturally. Centrally located landmarks should be positioned along a vertical line—bilateral landmarks should be symmetric when comparing left to right. Palpation of these landmarks may be used if clothing obstructs their view.

Some practitioners use a plumb line or posture grid when conducting postural assessments. A plumb line determines the **line of gravity,** a vertical line through the center of an object to its base of support. The line of gravity is used as the midsagittal plane when assessing posture. A posture grid contains numbered horizontal and vertical lines, and provides rapid visual cues of an individual's posture. Ensure that the floor on which the client stands barefoot is level and, if a wall-mounted chart is used, it is mounted level with the floor.

Anterior Landmarks

Use a vertical line in the midsagittal plane to observe the following anterior landmarks (Fig. 14.3). This line should be equidistant between the knees and ankles and bisect the:
- Nasal septum
- Manubrium of the sternum
- Umbilicus
- Pubic symphysis
  Horizontal symmetry should be observed between the:
- Acromion processes
- Iliac crests
- Anterior superior iliac spines (ASIS)[a]
- Greater trochanters
- Tips of the fingers

---

[a]Anterior Superior Iliac Spine may be slightly lower in females due to natural elongation of this protuberance.

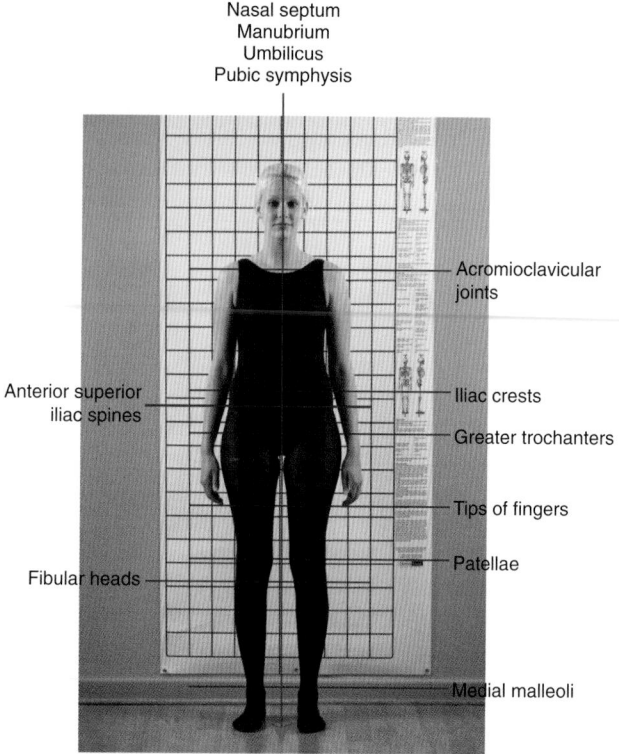

Nasal septum
Manubrium
Umbilicus
Pubic symphysis

Acromioclavicular joints

Anterior superior iliac spines

Iliac crests

Greater trochanters

Tips of fingers

Patellae

Fibular heads

Medial malleoli

FIG. 14.3 Postural assessment. Anterior landmarks, with the client standing in front of a posture grid.

- Bottom of the patellae
- Fibular heads
- Medial malleoli
  Also observe the following:
- Spaces between the trunk and the arms
- Knee alignment noting any positional abnormalities such as valgum (valgus position) or varum (varus position). **Valgum** occurs when the distal end of a bone or joint projects laterally. **Varum** occurs when the distal end of a bone or joint projects medially. In the knee, knock-kneed is called *genu valgum* and bowlegged is called *genu varum* (Fig. 14.4). **LEARNING TIP:** To help you remember the difference between val*gum* and va*rum* is "gum" keeps your knees together and "rum" keeps your knees apart.

Posterior Landmarks

Use a vertical line in the midsagittal plane (Fig. 14.5) to observe posterior landmarks. This line should bisect the:
- Occipital protuberance
- Vertebral spinous processes
- Sacral tubercles
- Coccyx
  Horizontal symmetry should be observed between the:
- Mastoid processes
- Base of the occiput
- Scapulae (acromion processes, scapular spines, inferior angles)
- Posterior superior iliac spines

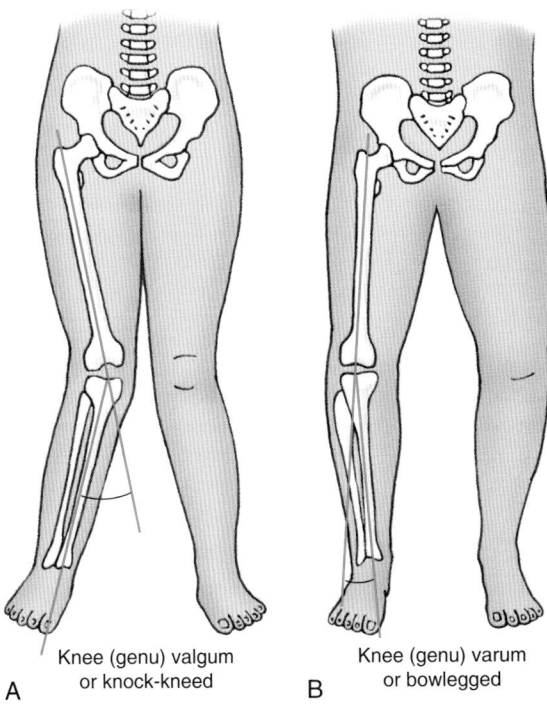

FIG. 14.4 Knee alignment abnormalities. (A) Knee valgum or knock-kneed; (B) knee varum or bowlegged. (From Muscolino, J. E. [2017]. *Kinesiology: The skeletal system and muscle function* [3rd ed.]. St. Louis: Mosby).

- Greater trochanters
- Medial malleoli
- Calcanei (singular, calcaneus)
  Also observe the following:
- Lateral positioning of the spine (scoliosis)
- Spaces between the medial borders of the scapulae and the spine
- Knee alignment noting any inward or valgus positioning (knock-knees) as well as any outward or varus positioning (bowlegged) observed anteriorly.

Lateral Landmarks

Use a vertical line in the frontal plane on the left and the right side of the body to observe lateral landmarks (Fig. 14.6). This line should bisect the:
- External auditory meatus
- Humeral head
- Greater trochanter
- Lateral epicondyle of the femur
- Lateral malleolus
  Also observe the following:
- Head positioned too far forward (anteriorly) or backward (posteriorly)
- Shoulders positioned too far forward (protracted) or backward (retracted)
- Spinal abnormalities in the upper back (hyperkyphosis) or lower back (hyperlordosis)
- Levels of the anterior and posterior iliac spines (excessive pelvic tilt)

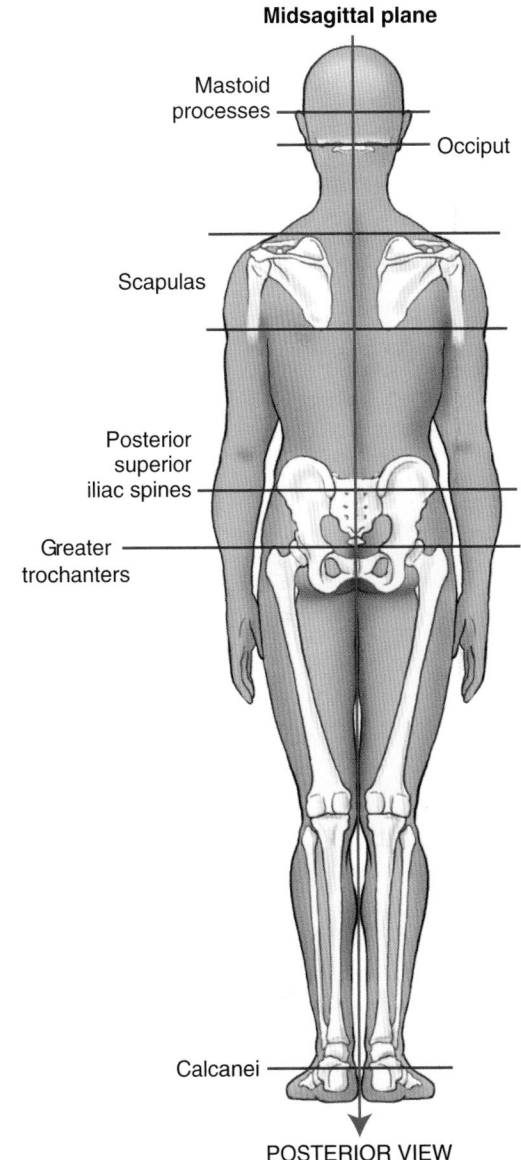

FIG. 14.5 Postural assessment. Posterior landmarks

- Knee hyperextension
  Along with the aforementioned landmarks, note symmetry in major muscle groups and between anterior and posterior musculature. Survey other signs of postural abnormalities such as:
- Differences in leg length
- Collapsed foot arches, which contribute to an unstable base of support
  Postural assessment is simply a snapshot of a client's posture at a particular moment in time, and some postural assessments were found ineffective and problematic (Borenstein et al., 2001; Lederman, 2011; Preece et al., 2008). Furthermore, Moriguchi et al. (2009) found significant differences among postural examiners when determining locations of particular landmarks, especially in overweight individuals. Additionally, avoid suggesting something is wrong if the client does not have a posture conforming to the "standard."

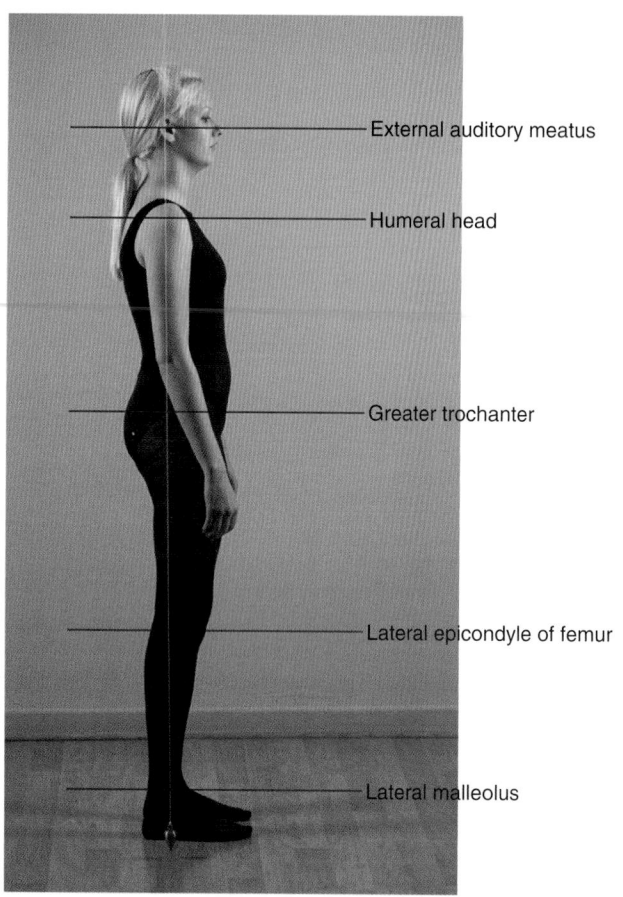

External auditory meatus

Humeral head

Greater trochanter

Lateral epicondyle of femur

Lateral malleolus

FIG. 14.6 Postural assessment. Lateral landmarks.

Many factors influence a client's posture, including their emotional state, proprioceptive and other types of neural input, diseases such as osteoporosis, spinal deviations such as scoliosis, and habitual movement patterns. If abnormalities are observed, they must be verified through an inquiry with the client or by the client's healthcare provider.

Gait Observation

Gait is a pattern of movement used while walking or running. The nervous and musculoskeletal systems work together to produce balance and coordination while the body is in motion. Gait patterns are influenced by health, disease, injury, age, personality, and sociocultural factors. Walking speed in older adults is an indicator of robust health or of frailty. Massage practitioners may choose to observe gait if walking difficulties were reported during the client intake. Ask a client to walk at their normal pace and observe gait from the front, the back, and the side.

The Gait Cycle

The **gait cycle** (or stride) is the sequence of events that begin when one foot contacts the ground and ends when the same foot contacts the ground again. Each gait cycle contains two steps (one step by each foot). The gait cycle, also called the *gait pattern*, occurs at varying speeds, on numerous terrains, and often while the person is carrying items (purses, luggage,

children, etc.), all of which can alter the body's center of gravity. **Cadence** is the number of steps taken per minute; also called *step rate*.

The gait cycle is divided into two phases (stance and swing phase) and eight events (Fig. 14.7). This highly orchestrated sequence involves movements of the hips, knees, and feet, as well as pelvic movements such as shifts and tilts. When the body is supported by only one leg, this is called **single-limb support**. When both feet are in contact with the ground at the same time, this is called **double-limb support**. When running, the double limb support is completely absent, a characteristic distinguishing running from walking. Phases and their associated events and periods are listed next.

- **Stance phase**. The timeframe between heel strike and heel off; occurs when the foot is in contact with the ground and bearing most of the bodyweight. The stance phase constitutes approximately 60% of the gait cycle.
  1. **Heel strike**. Begins when the heel strikes the ground and is the first part of double-limb support. Heel strike involves hip flexion, knee extension, and ankle dorsiflexion.
  2. **Flat foot (loading response)**. The body absorbs the impact of the foot on the ground while the hip extends and the knee slightly flexes.
  3. **Midstance**. The body is now supported by one leg and moves from impact absorption to forward propulsion. The hip extends further, the knee reaches maximal flexion, and then begins to extend.
  4. **Heel off (terminal stance)**. The heel leaves the ground and the hip extends, then flexes, while the knee flexes, and the ankle plantarflexes.
- **Swing phase**. The timeframe between pre-swing and terminal swing; occurs when the foot is not touching the ground, starts to advance forward, and bodyweight is on the other or contralateral foot. The swing phase constitutes approximately 40% of the gait cycle.
  5. **Toe off (pre-swing)**. The hip flexes, the knee flexes, the ankle plantarflexes, and the toes leave the ground.
  6. **Foot adjacent (initial swing)**. The hip extends, the knee flexes, the ankle dorsiflexes, and both feet are adjacent or near each other.
  7. **Leg vertical (mid-swing)**. The hip flexes, the knee flexes slightly, the ankle dorsiflexes slightly, and the leg is vertical.
  8. **Next heel strike (terminal swing)**. The hip flexes, the knee extends, the ankle moves to a neutral position, and the same heel strikes the ground again.

Gait can be observed more easily during the stance phase because of the greater length of time spent here. However, the swing phase can be demanding, as the body maintains balance while lifting and positioning the airborne limb. Gait observations may reveal **compensatory patterns**, or *compensatory movements*, which are conscious or unconscious movements used to correct imbalances and reduce discomfort. These patterns may occur from muscle weakness; structural asymmetry; a change in the body's center of gravity, such as in cases of advanced pregnancy; or gait disorders

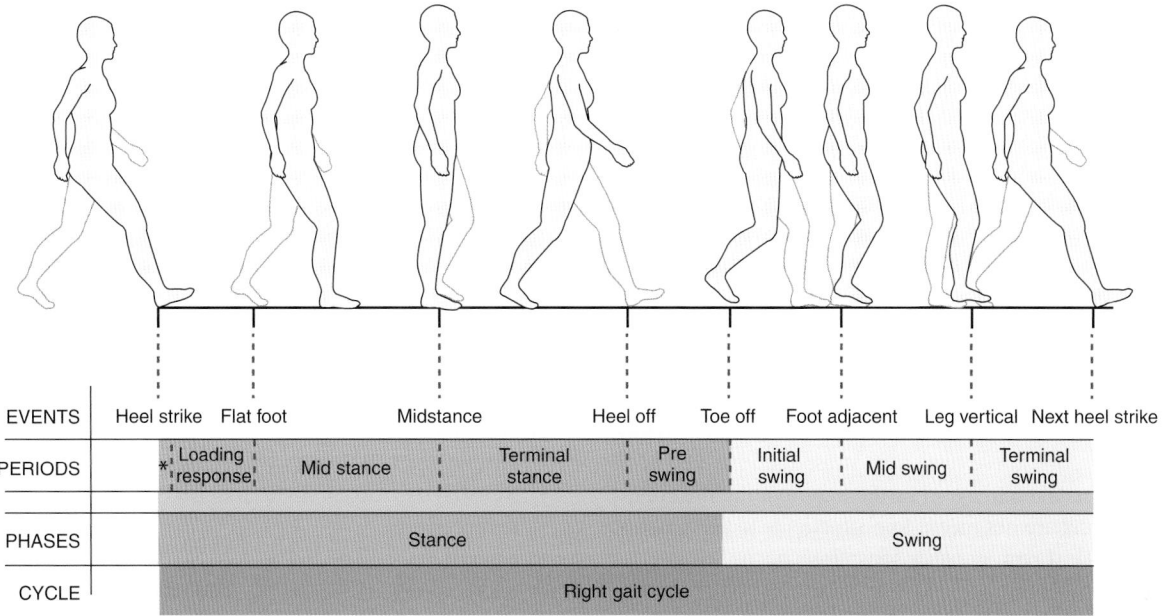

FIG. 14.7 Gait cycle on the right limb with associated stance or swing phases. (From Neumann, D. A. [2010]. *Kinesiology of the musculoskeletal system: Foundations for rehabilitation* [3rd ed.]. St. Louis: Mosby.)

from underlying conditions. Compensatory patterns may be caused by, or be a source of, muscle spasms and trigger points (TrPs). Compensation allows the body to function as close to optimal as possible. While massage practitioners may find some value observing gait, gait assessment or "analysis" is more effectively assessed by physical therapists and gait specialists (Harradine et al., 2018).

Gait Disorders

Gait disorders are altered gait patterns caused by deformities, amputations, muscle weakness or contracture, pain, or loss of motor control. Other factors include arthritic changes; diseases such as gout; surgeries that fuse joints; or foot problems such as bunions. Neurologic conditions, such as peripheral neuropathy, can also affect gait. Gait disorders can lead to loss of personal freedom, decreased quality of life, and increased risk of falls. Some gait disorders are so distinctive they have special names assigned to them.

- **Antalgic gait**. Limp adopted to avoid pain on weight-bearing structures. Antalgic gait is characterized by walking hesitancy and a short stance phase.
- **Ataxic gait**. Unsteady, uncoordinated, staggered gait with feet thrown out and irregular foot placement—the person often looks at the floor while walking due to a lack of proprioception. Ataxic gait is associated with cerebellar or sensory disturbances.
- **Hemiplegic gait**. Decreased walking speed, asymmetric step length, and decreased time spent in the stance phase. The hip flexes during walking, but not the knee. There is also a foot drop, and the lower extremity moves in a semicircle. Hemiplegic gait is associated with stroke.

- **Propulsive gait**. A stooped, rigid posture, with the head and neck bent forward. Steps are shorter and faster. Propulsive gait is associated with Parkinson disease.
- **Shuffling gait**. The person drags and shuffles their feet, and steps are shorter. Shuffling gait is also associated with Parkinson disease.
- **Scissor gait**. Knees and thighs cross in a scissor-like pattern and the person appears crouched over. Steps are slow and short. Scissor gait is associated with cerebral palsy.
- **Waddling gait**. Lateral movements of the trunk and hips are exaggerated, producing a waddling, duck-like walk. Waddling gait is associated with muscular dystrophy.

Orthopedic Assessments

Orthopedic assessments, or *special tests*, are used to determine the presence or absence of musculoskeletal or neurologic conditions. These assessments are not intended as diagnostic tools, as this is outside the scope of practice. A positive test suggests that the client has symptomology of the condition being tested and helps practitioners make professional judgments. For example, test results may guide treatment choices (i.e., carpal tunnel syndrome), while others indicate referral to the client's healthcare provider for medical evaluation (i.e., intervertebral disc pathology). The accuracy of the test depends on many factors, including interrater reliability, sensitivity, and specificity.

- **Interrater reliability**. Degree of agreement among two or more trained or expert raters. Zero percent to 15% is no to minimal agreement; 15% to 35% is weak agreement; 36% to 63% is moderate agreement; 64% to 81% is strong agreement, and 83% to 100% is almost perfect agreement (McHugh, 2012).

- **Sensitivity**. Ability of a test to detect a problem, or to measure a true positive.
- **Specificity**. Ability of a test to identify individuals who do *not* have a problem, or to measure a true negative.

Generally speaking, tests with low sensitivity and specificity did not perform well, and tests with a high sensitivity and specificity did perform well. Special tests with a sensitivity and specificity of around 90% performed well and have a good assessment value. Interrater reliability, sensitivity, and specificity are included with each test in this section when available.

Many tests listed are called "provocative tests" because they provoke the onset of symptoms. Because of this, inform clients that the test may cause pain and produce symptoms. Furthermore, these tests may stress the involved area, so care must be taken to avoid further aggravating the condition. These tests are not meant to push clients to the point of pain, but to see if pain or other sensations occur.

Before performing any tests, an area must be free from fracture or tumors (abnormal growths). Furthermore, any client with severe spasm or pain of unknown origin should not be evaluated with orthopedic assessments, and instead referred to their healthcare provider.

Full and Empty Can Tests (Rotator Cuff/Supraspinatus Lesions)

Ask the client to flex their shoulders 90 degrees. The thumb is up for the full can test and thumb is down for the empty can test (Fig. 14.8A and B). The practitioner places one hand on the client's forearm and applies downward pressure while the client resists. A positive test produces shoulder weakness and/or pain.
- **Interrater reliability**: Unavailable

- **Sensitivity**: 70%; 89% for full can and empty can, respectively
- **Specificity**: 81%; 59% for full can and empty can, respectively

Speed Test (Bicep Tendinopathy/Shoulder Labrum Tear)

This test assesses long head biceps tendinopathy (LHBT) and superior labral tear from anterior to posterior (SLAP) lesions. Ask the client to flex their shoulder 90 degrees, elbow extended, and palm facing up or supinated. The practitioner places one hand above the wrist and applies downward pressure while the client resists. A positive test produces shoulder pain.
- **Interrater reliability**: Unavailable
- **Sensitivity**: 56%; 44% for LHBT and SLAP lesion, respectively
- **Specificity**: 57%; 64% for LHBT and SLAP lesion, respectively

Apley Scratch Test (Shoulder Dysfunction)

Ask the client to bring their hands together on their back—one hand from above and the other from below with both hands arriving somewhere between the shoulders, possibly grasping hands (Fig. 14.9). Essentially, the client is using shoulder flexion, extension, adduction, abduction, and medial and lateral rotation to "scratch" between their scapulae. This action is repeated on the other side while the practitioner notes any differences. A positive test is decreased mobility on one side when comparing both sides. However, the client's dominant side is often more limited, and a positive test does not always indicate dysfunction.
- **Interrater reliability**: Unavailable

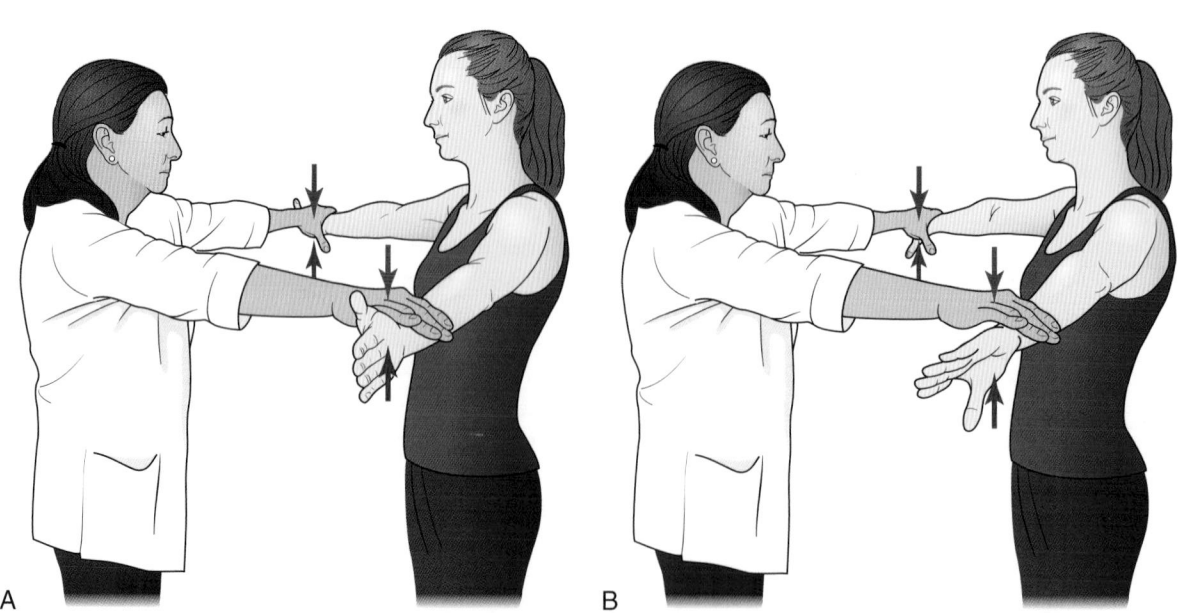

A   B

FIG. 14.8 The full can test (A) and the empty can test (B) can be used to assess problems with the rotator cuff including supraspinatus lesions. (From Swartz, M. [2021]. *Textbook of physical diagnosis* [8th ed.]. Philadelphia, PA: Elsevier.)

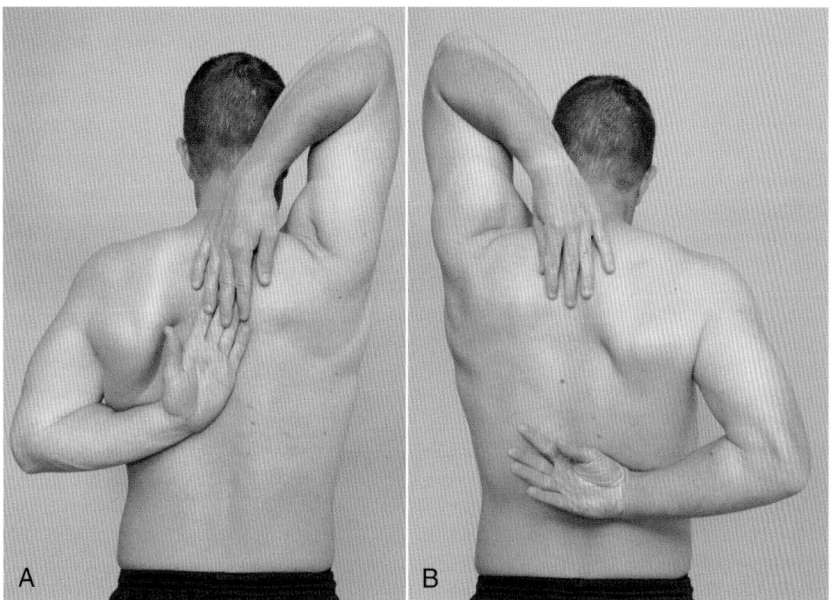

FIG. 14.9 The Apley's scratch test can be used to assess shoulder dysfunctions on the right (A) and left (B) sides of the body. The dominant side is often more limited, so a positive test result does not always indicate shoulder dysfunction. (From Magee, D. [2014]. *Orthopedic physical assessment* [6th ed.]. St. Louis: Saunders.)

- **Sensitivity**: Unavailable
- **Specificity**: Unavailable

Adson Test (Thoracic Outlet Syndrome)

Ask the client to externally rotate, abduct, and extend their shoulder—the practitioner palpates the radial pulse on the same side (Fig. 14.10). The client is asked to inhale and hold their breath while extending the neck and rotating the head toward the tested shoulder. The test is positive if the client reports paresthesia during this action or if the pulse fades, indicating hypertonicity of the scalenes and vascular/neurologic compromise.

- **Interrater reliability**: Low evidence
- **Sensitivity**: 94%
- **Specificity**: 53%

Roos Test (Thoracic Outlet Syndrome)

The client stands or sits with shoulders externally rotated and abducted 90 degrees, and elbows flexed 90 degrees (as if to "surrender"). The elbows should be pushed back slightly (Fig. 14.11). Next, ask the client to slowly clench and open the hands (every 2 to 3 seconds) for up to 3 minutes or until they can no longer continue because of pain. This position stretches the neurovascular bundle and can exacerbate symptoms of thoracic outlet syndrome. A positive test produces heaviness or weakness in the arms, or numbness, tingling, or paresthesia in the hands. Also, look for discoloration in the hands, which is another positive sign. Minor fatigue is not a positive sign.

- **Interrater reliability**: Unavailable
- **Sensitivity**: 84%
- **Specificity**: 30%

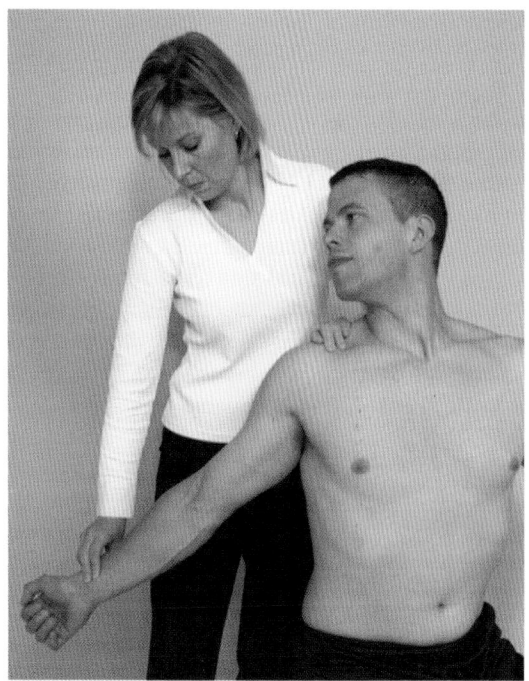

FIG. 14.10 The Adson test can be used to assess thoracic outlet syndrome.

Phalen Test (Carpal Tunnel Syndrome)

Ask the client to maximally flex both wrists and press the backs of the hands together so the forearms form a straight line with elbows pointing laterally—this position is maintained for up to 1 minute (Fig. 14.12). This position stretches the median nerve and can exacerbate symptoms of carpal tunnel syndrome. A positive test produces pain, numbness,

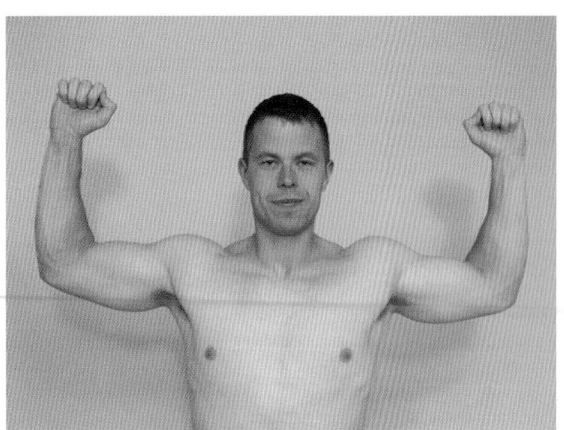

FIG. 14.11 The Roos test can be used to assess thoracic outlet syndrome.

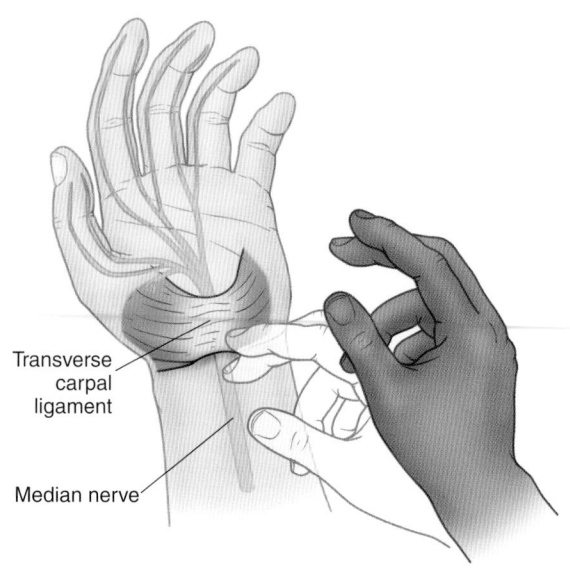

FIG. 14.13 The Tinel sign test can be used to assess carpal tunnel syndrome.

tingling, or paresthesia that occurs in the area of median nerve distribution (thumb, index, middle, and lateral half of ring fingers). A reverse Phalen is the same procedure applied in wrist extension and has similar clinical value.

- **Interrater reliability**: 54%
- **Sensitivity**: 66%
- **Specificity**: 72%

Tinel Sign Test (Carpal Tunnel Syndrome)

Ask the client to flex the elbow on the affected side, and supinate the forearm so the palm faces up, and slightly extend the wrist. Lightly tap the anterior middle wrist above the transverse carpal ligament four to six times using one or two fingertips (Fig. 14.13). The test is positive if pain, numbness, tingling, or paresthesia occurs in the area of median nerve distribution (thumb, index, middle, and lateral half of ring fingers). The Tinel sign test can be used on other areas of the body, such as the medial elbow (ulnar nerve), the lateral neck (brachial plexus), and the medial ankle (tibial nerve).

- **Interrater reliability**: Unavailable

- **Sensitivity**: 50%
- **Specificity**: 80%

Shoulder Abduction Test/Bakody Sign (Cervical Disc Symptomology)

Ask the client to elevate the arm and rest the forearm on top of their head; this position is maintained for approximately 30 seconds (Fig. 14.14). Test the asymptomatic side first to establish a baseline, followed by the symptomatic side. The test is positive if symptoms decrease, as this position reduces tension on the nerve root.

- **Interrater reliability**: 20%
- **Sensitivity**: 43%
- **Specificity**: 90%

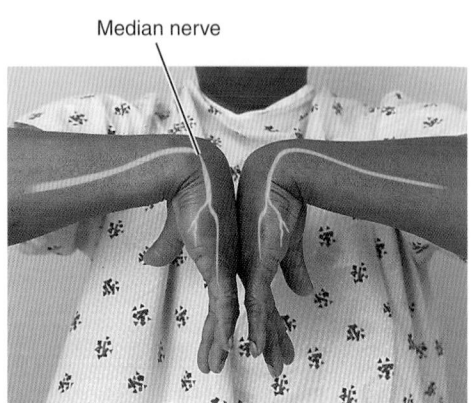

FIG. 14.12 The Phalen test can be used to assess carpal tunnel syndrome. (From Wall, R. M., Hockberger, R. S., & Gaushe-Hill, M. [2018]. *Rosen's emergency medicine: Concepts and clinical practice* [9th ed.]. St. Louis: Elsevier.)

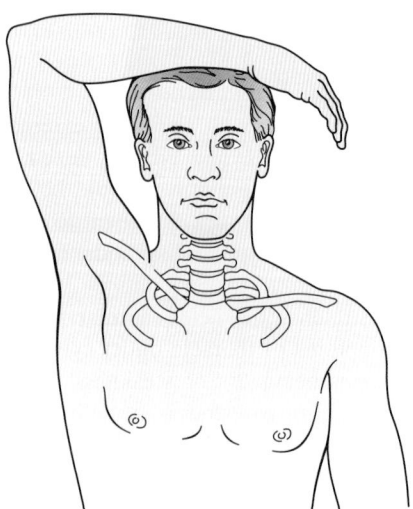

FIG. 14.14 The shoulder abduction test (Bakody sign) can be used to assess cervical disc symptomology.

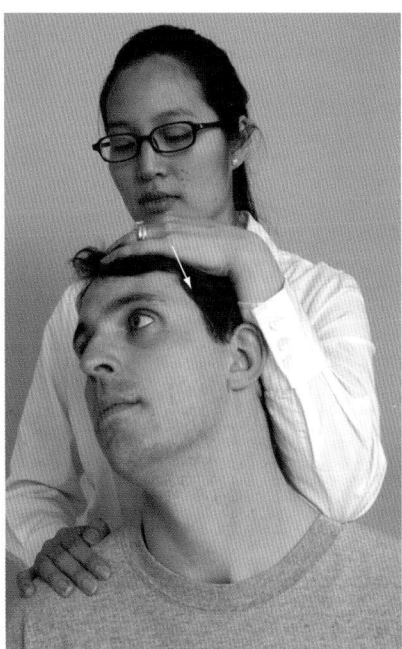

FIG. 14.15 The cervical compression test (Spurling test) can be used to assess cervical disc symptomology. (From Magee, D. [2021]. *Orthopedic physical assessment* [7th ed.]. St. Louis: Elsevier.)

Cervical Compression Test/Spurling Test (Cervical Disc Symptomology)

The client sits while the practitioner places one hand on top of the client's head and applies gentle downward pressure (Fig. 14.15). The test is positive if pain or paresthesia occurs, possibly radiating down the adjacent upper extremity.

- **Interrater Reliability**: 46%
- **Sensitivity**: 55%
- **Specificity**: 92%

Straight Leg Raise Test (Lumbar Disc Symptomology)

This test may identify lumbar disc pathology and the radiculopathy of sciatica. Assess the unaffected side first. Ask the client to lie supine, while the practitioner passively flexes the hip by lifting the leg off the table (Fig. 14.16). A positive test occurs when pain and paresthesia occurs down the opposite leg, as this action causes the pathologic disc to compress the spinal nerve root. Symptoms are more likely to occur when hip flexion reaches 35% to 70%. Be sure and discontinue the leg raise when symptoms occur or when full ROM is achieved.

- **Interrater reliability**: 68%
- **Sensitivity**: 68%
- **Specificity**: 56%

FABER Test/Patrick Test (Hip/Sacroiliac Symptomology)

FABER stands for **F**lexion, **AB**duction, and **E**xternal **R**otation. Ask the client to lie supine with one hip externally rotated, knee flexed, and leg resting on the opposite thigh (figure-4 position) (Fig. 14.17). Ensure that the ankle is unrestricted and not on the opposite thigh. Stabilize the opposite ilium at the ASIS, and place the other hand on the medial flexed knee. Apply downward pressure on the knee until you reach the end of PROM. The test is positive if pain is produced in the hips (buttock or groin) or in the Sacroiliac region.

- **Interrater reliability**: 60%
- **Sensitivity**: 60%
- **Specificity**: 29%

Varus Stress Test (Lateral Collateral Ligament Integrity)

Ask the client to lay supine with knees extended. Place one hand on the medial thigh above the knee and the other hand on the ankle (Fig. 14.18). Externally rotate the tibia slightly and apply lateral pressure above the knee while stabilizing the ankle. This action will stress the lateral collateral ligament. Repeat the test, but with knees flexed 20 to 30 degrees (a bolster can be used). A positive test produces pain and excessive gaping on the lateral side of the knee.

- **Interrater reliability**: 43%
- **Sensitivity**: 91%
- **Specificity**: 17%

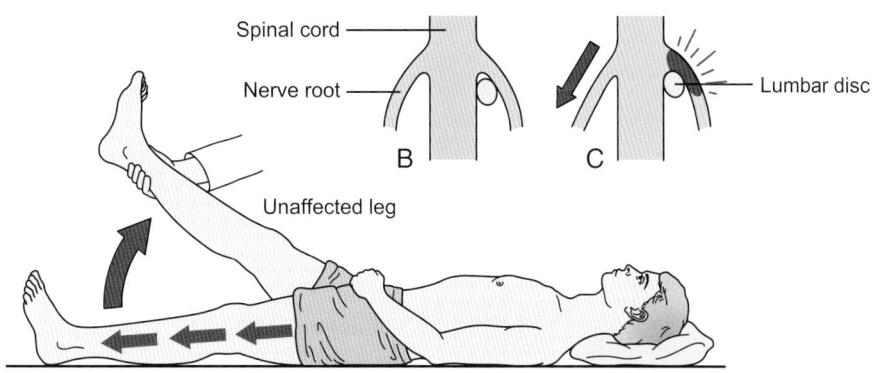

FIG. 14.16 The straight leg raise test can be used to assess lumbar disc symptomology. Passive flexion of the hip (A). Spinal cord and nerve root before the test (B). Compression of the spinal nerve root by the pathologic lumbar disc during the test (C).

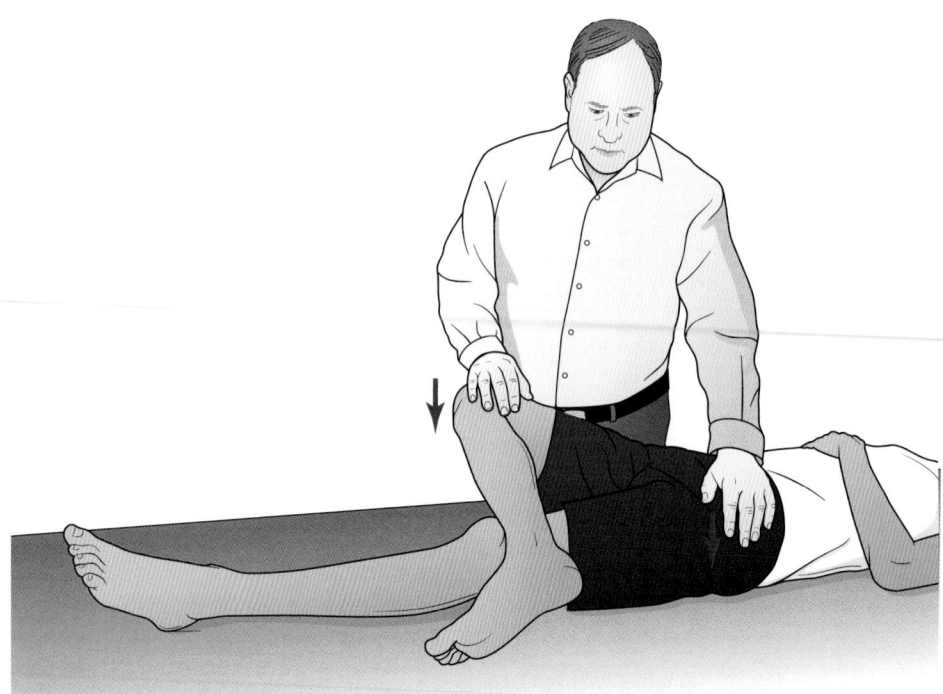

FIG. 14.17 The FABER (Patrick) test can be used to assess hip or sacroiliac symptomology. (From Swartz, M. [2021]. *Textbook of physical diagnosis* [8th ed.]. Philadelphia: Elsevier.)

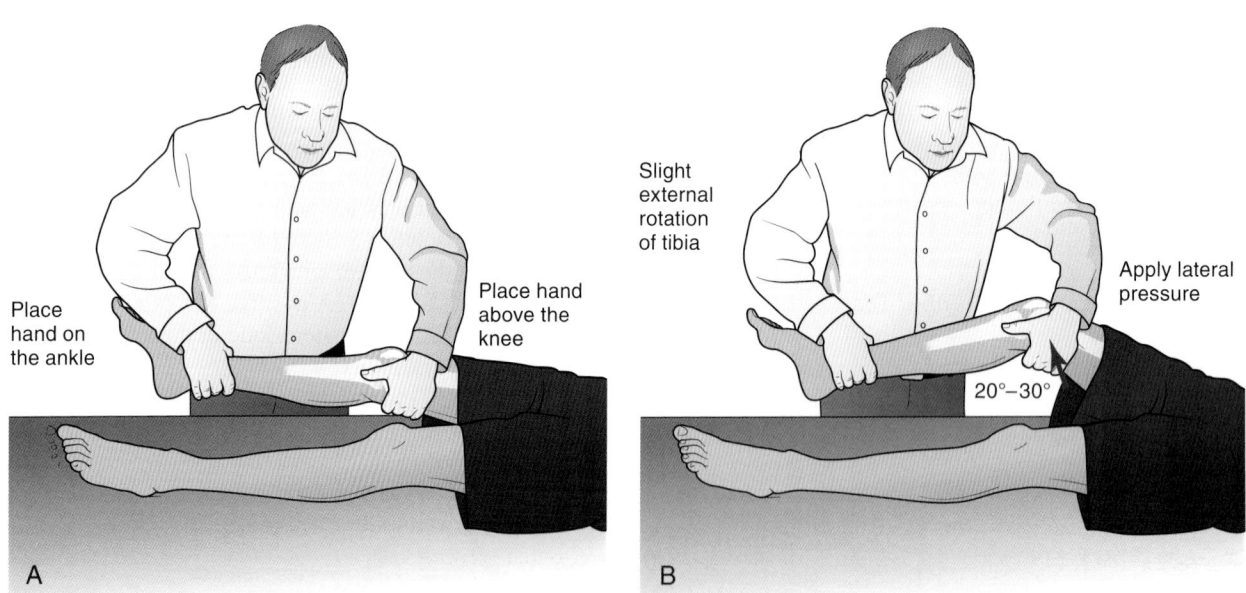

Place hand on the ankle

Place hand above the knee

Slight external rotation of tibia

Apply lateral pressure

20°–30°

A

B

FIG. 14.18 The varus stress test can be used to assess the integrity of the lateral collateral ligament. Position of the limb before the test (A). External rotation of the tibia and application of lateral pressure during the test (B). (From Swartz, M. [2021]. *Textbook of physical diagnosis* [8th ed.]. Philadelphia: Elsevier.)

Valgus Stress Test (Medial Collateral Ligament Integrity)

Ask the client to lay supine with knees extended. Place one hand on the lateral thigh above the knee and the other hand on the ankle (Fig. 14.19). Externally rotate the tibia slightly and apply medial pressure above the knee while stabilizing the ankle. This action will stress the medial collateral ligament. Repeat the test, but with knees flexed 20 to 30 degrees (a bolster can be used). A positive test produces pain and excessive gaping on the medial side of the knee.

- **Interrater reliability**: 43%

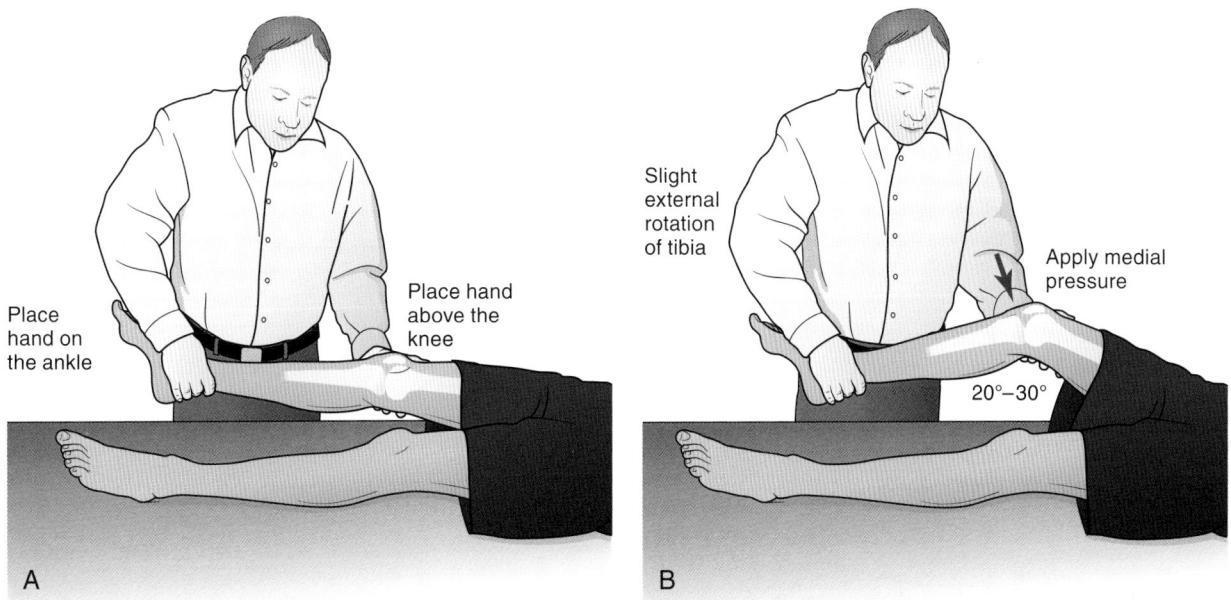

FIG. 14.19 The valgus stress test can be used to assess the integrity of the medial collateral ligament. Position of the limb before the test (A). External rotation of the tibia and application of medial pressure during the test (B). (From Swartz, M. [2021]. *Textbook of physical diagnosis* [8th ed.]. Philadelphia: Elsevier).

- **Sensitivity**: 50%
- **Specificity**: 98%

Anterior Drawer Test (Anterior Talofibular/Anterior Cruciate Ligament Integrity)

Ask the client to lie supine. To test for anterior talofibular ligament integrity, the practitioner places one hand above the ankle to stabilize the leg and the other hand over the

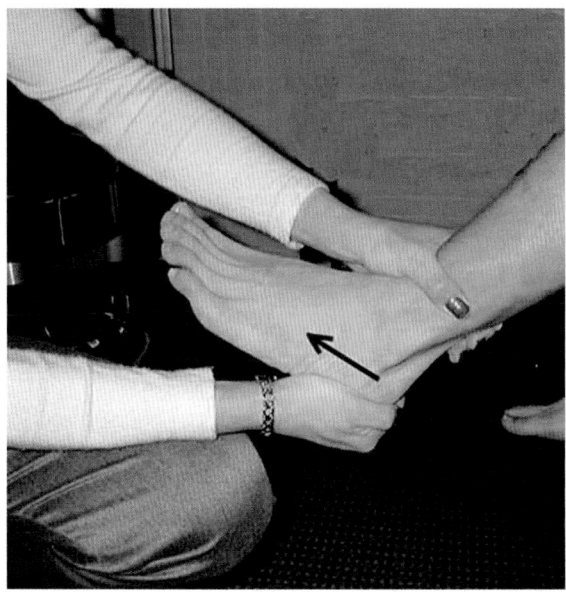

FIG. 14.20 The anterior drawer test performed on the ankle can be used to assess the integrity of the anterior talofibular ligament. (From Brinker, M. R., & Miller, M. D. [1999]. *Fundamentals of orthopaedics*. Philadelphia: Saunders).

heel (Fig. 14.20). Next, pull the foot anteriorly—this action is similar to opening a drawer. The test is positive when the foot slides forward, possibly with a clunk. The client may experience pain during this action. The practitioner can test for anterior cruciate ligament (ACL) integrity by applying the anterior pull below the knee while it is flexed (Fig. 14.21).

- **Interrater reliability**: 82%
- **Sensitivity**: 78% (laxity); 96% (rupture)
- **Specificity**: 39% (laxity); 83% (rupture)

Calf Squeeze Test/Thompson Test (Achilles Tendon Integrity)

The client lies prone with both feet off the edge of the table. The practitioner squeezes the client's calf several times while observing passive plantarflexion. A positive test occurs when the foot does not plantarflex during the calf squeeze.

- **Interrater reliability**: Unavailable
- **Sensitivity**: 96%
- **Specificity**: 93%

SPORTS MASSAGE AND WORKING WITH ATHLETES

As stated in the introduction, Clinical massage includes sports massage and working with athletes. **Sports massage** is the application of massage techniques to address the needs of athletes in competitive and recreational settings. In sports massage—before, between, or shortly after an event—techniques are usually applied through clothing and without lubricant. Lubricants may interfere with the athlete's ability to sweat (leading to possible overheating) and may interfere

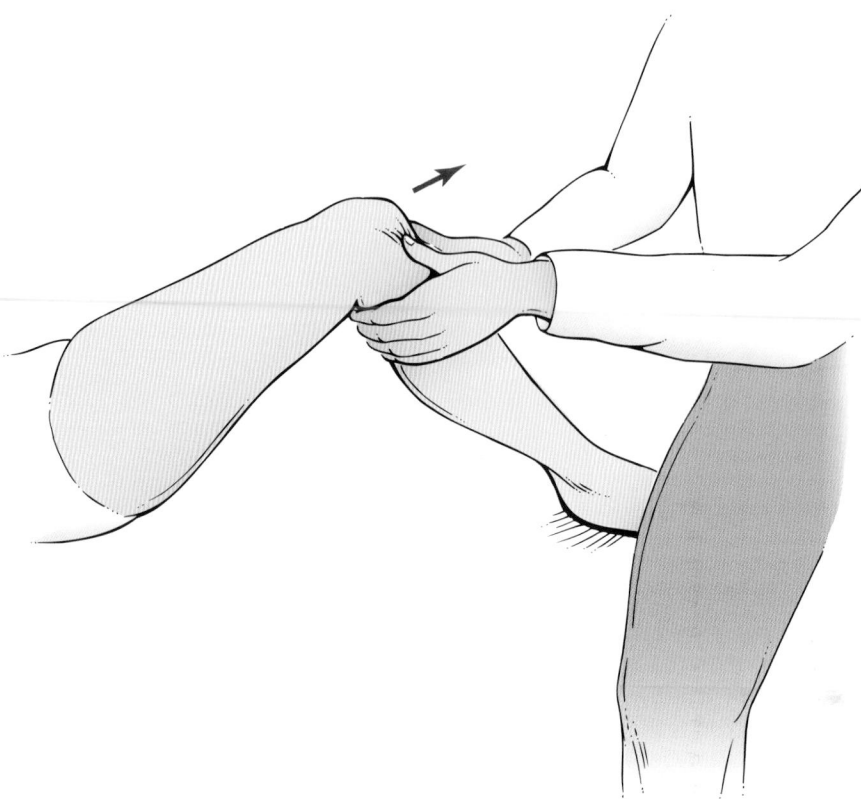

FIG. 14.21 The anterior drawer test performed on the knee can be used to assess the integrity of the anterior cruciate ligament. (From Swartz, M. [2021]. *Textbook of physical diagnosis* [8th ed.]. Philadelphia: Elsevier.)

with performance. For example, lubricants on the hands of gymnasts may cause them to lose grip on parallel bars.

Elite, professional, amateur, and tactical athletes may seek services from massage practitioners. An **athlete** is someone who possesses a natural or acquired ability needed to participate in a sport. Examples of sports in which athletes participate include baseball, football, basketball, tennis, golf, rodeo, and running. Some stage performers and musicians consider themselves athletes, a *tactical athlete* is someone in a service profession who has physical fitness and performance requirements associated with their job. Examples of tactical athletes are people in military service members; law enforcement, such as police officers; and first responders, such as firefighters and paramedics. This section discusses sports massage types and specific massage considerations when working with military personnel.

Types of Sports Massage

There are several types of sports massage, which include pre-event, inter-event, post-event, maintenance, and rehabilitative. Pre-, inter-, and post-event sports massages are often provided for a group of athletes (after a triathlon, tennis match, or rodeo tournament, for example) (Fig. 14.22). These events are generally part of a fun, high-energy atmosphere, and may sometimes serve as fundraisers. In some communities, groups of licensed

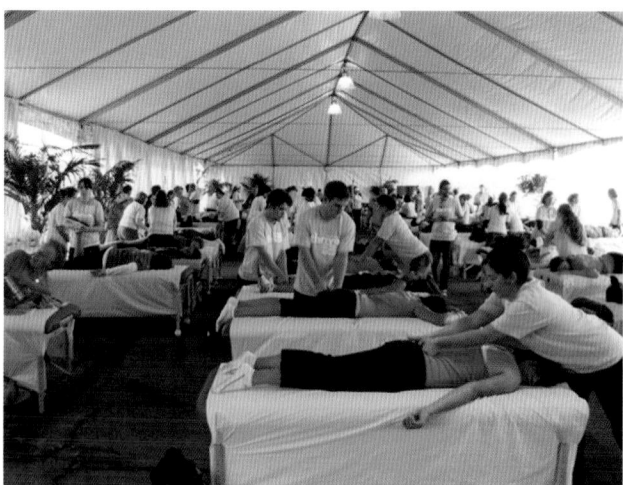

FIG. 14.22 Post-event sports massage after an athletic event. (Courtesy Gina Fong Seidler, National Holistic Institute.)

practitioners form a sports massage team and provide massages for free or for a small fee.

Pre-Event Massage

Pre-event sports massage is given 2 or fewer hours before the event. Techniques are more general than specific and usually consist of brisk movements applied using moderate pressure—they should leave the athlete ready for action. Sessions are brief, 15 or fewer minutes, and bolsters and headrests are not used (to save time).

Inter-Event Massage

Inter-event sports massage occurs between events or within 1 or 2 days before the next event. If applied immediately after the event, ensure that the athlete has cooled down before the massage (i.e., is no longer sweating). The cooling down phase can last 3 to 10 minutes and allows heart and respiration rates to return to normal. Maintain a general focus and avoid deep or specific work on athletes who will compete in ≥24 hours.

Post-Event Massage

Post-event sports massage occurs 30 minutes to 6 hours after the event. Sessions are 10 to 20 minutes in duration. Ensure that the athlete has cooled down thoroughly before massage (i.e., is no longer sweating and cardiorespiratory rates are within normal range). Swedish massage techniques such as effleurage and petrissage are used to reduce delayed-onset muscle soreness and promote rest and recovery. Avoid tapotement or deep, specific techniques, as the athlete's muscles may spasm easily in their hypersensitive state. **Delayed-onset muscle soreness** (DOMS), or *post-exercise muscle soreness*, is pain or discomfort in skeletal muscles following unaccustomed or strenuous physical activity. DOMS occurs several hours after the activity, and soreness is felt most strongly 24 to 72 hours afterward. DOMS is thought to be caused by eccentric (lengthening) contractions, which create microtrauma in muscle fibers. DOMS is sometimes mistakenly believed to be caused by a build-up of lactic acid, but lactic acid is involved in muscle fatigue, not muscle soreness. Massage is effective in reducing or preventing DOMS and is more effective than hot/cold treatments and static stretching (Choroszewicz et al., 2020; Nekouei et al., 2020; Guo et al., 2017).

Maintenance Massage

Maintenance sports massage occurs between training sessions or events and usually lasts 30 to 60 minutes. These sessions can be planned in advance to align with the 'athlete's training and events schedule, with the most important sessions scheduled first (e.g., several days before or after the event depending on travel time, during recovery weeks, after hard or long workouts). The goal of maintenance massage is to address any soreness, work on sports-specific muscles that are tight, improve performance, and prevent injury. Maintenance massage is a blend of general massage techniques, myofascial techniques, TrP approaches, and deep tissue applications, and others. The intensity of the massage is determined by the athlete's training schedule—the closer to a sports event, the less intrusive the massage technique should be.

Rehabilitative Massage and Soft Tissue Injuries

Rehabilitative sports massage addresses the injury rehabilitation needs of athletes. Most sports injuries are **soft tissue injuries**, which is trauma to muscles, their tendons, and to ligaments. Common soft tissue injuries include tennis or golfer's elbow, rotator cuff strain, shin splints, plantar fasciitis, and muscle sprains and strains (i.e., hamstrings, Achilles tendon, groin, lower back). Specific massage considerations for these conditions are detailed in Chapters 19 and 20.

The initial response to soft tissue injury is **acute inflammation**, an immediate response to tissue damage characterized by localized swelling, heat, redness, pain, and a loss of

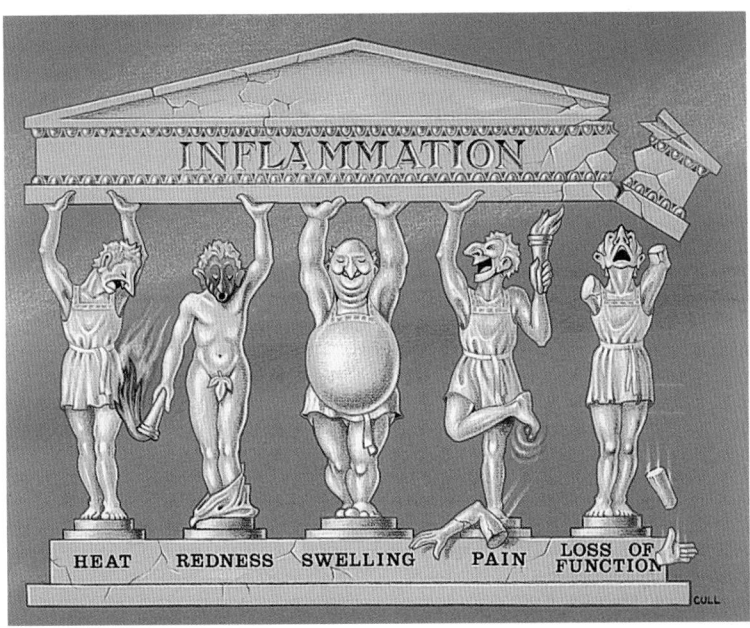

FIG. 14.23 Inflammation. Signs and symptoms. (Reprinted by permission of Professor Peter Cull, London University.)

function. **LEARNING TIP**: To help you remember these characteristics, use the acronym **S-H-A-R-P** for **S**welling, **H**eat, **A** loss of function, **R**edness, and **P**ain (Fig. 14.23). Acute inflammation is usually protective, beneficial and serves to eliminate pathogens and foreign agents. It also removes damaged tissues and creates an environment that maximizes tissue repair. Acute inflammation occurs regardless of how soft tissue trauma occurred (sports injury, slips and falls, vehicle accidents), and is usually of short duration, lasting approximately 72 hours (3 days) after initial onset, but can last up to 5 days. **Subacute inflammation** is the period after the acute inflammation. It is characterized by swelling and pain but lacks heat and redness. Subacute inflammation usually begins on day 4 and may last 2 to 6 weeks.

Several factors affect how fast tissues heal. Nutrition is important because the healing process requires increased amounts of nutrients. For example, dietary protein is important because most of the structural components of tissues are proteins. Vitamin C is needed for the normal production and maintenance of tissue components, especially collagen. Vitamin C also strengthens and promotes the formation of new capillary beds. Good blood circulation is essential, so that oxygen, nutrients, white blood cells, and platelets are transported to the injured site. Blood and lymph flow promotes healing, because it removes excess tissue fluid, bacteria, foreign bodies, and debris.

Different tissue types heal at varying rates. Epithelial cells divide rapidly and regenerate quickly. Cartilage heals slowly, or not at all, because it lacks blood supply. Muscle has an extensive blood supply and can heal relatively quickly, whereas bone tissue takes longer to heal, and tendons and ligaments take even longer because they have reduced blood supply.

Tissues heal faster in people who are younger. The younger body is generally in a better nutritional state, provides better blood supply to tissues, and has a higher metabolic rate. This means tissues in a younger person's body can synthesize needed materials and divide more quickly.

Protocols During the Acute Inflammation Phase
Recommended protocols used during the acute phase of inflammation are M-C-E and M-E-A-T. **M-C-E** stands for **Move–Compress–Elevate**. Instruct clients to move safely when they can (and often), using pain as a boundary. Soft tissues can be compressed with bandages or cloth and the injured area can be elevated whenever possible. **M-E-A-T** stands for **Movement–Exercise–Analgesics–Treatment**. Again, instruct clients to move safely when they can and often, using pain as their boundary. They can also exercise as pain decreases and use topical or oral analgesics for pain, but not antiinflammatories. Treatment depends on the injury and ranges from massage, acupuncture, laser therapy, ultrasound, steroid injections, to surgery.

Ice is no longer recommended during the acute phase because it interrupts or delays the inflammatory cascade, which reduces the delivery of oxygen and decreases some aspects of revascularization needed for healing and recovery. Ice can be used to reduce pain and swelling during the subacute phase after acute inflammation has resolved. Consider limiting ice application to 10 or fewer minutes and for no more than a total of 6 hours. After the initial swelling has decreased, a heat application may be used as pain relief. Compression and elevation can help control swelling and do not appear to interfere with the inflammatory process.

Massage and Soft Tissue Injuries
For massage practitioners in nonclinical settings, such as private practice and spa/wellness facilities, avoid the recently injured area until acute inflammation has subsided and the area has entered the subacute phase, which is usually 4 to 6 days after the initial injury. The transition from acute to subacute occurs once the area is no longer warm and red but may still be swollen and painful. Elevate the injured area during this time, which may help reduce swelling.

If signs and symptoms of acute inflammation exceed day 6, they may be related to something more serious, such as infection rather than inflammation. In these cases, a referral should be made to the client's healthcare provider for evaluation and possible treatment before proceeding with massage.

For massage practitioners in clinical settings, such as hospitals, physical therapy, and chiropractic clinics, the attending healthcare provider is responsible for the initial screening and diagnosing of clients who have been in a recent injury-producing event. They will determine when massage services are appropriate. **NOTE**: Scar tissue massage is discussed in the section on surgery.

Tactical Athletes
As stated in the introduction, **tactical athletes** are people in service professions who have physical fitness and performance requirements associated with their job (military, police officers, firefighters, paramedics). They often face stressful situations under life-threatening conditions, while carrying heavy gear and equipment. Helmets and night vision goggles can strain neck and shoulder muscles. Standard military helmets weigh 4 lb, night vision goggles on helmets weigh 2 lb, and flight helmets weigh 2 to 4 lb. As reference, the average football helmet weights 2 to 3 lb. Individuals with extended daily exposure to heavy headgear are at increased risk of neck pain, muscle fatigue, and headaches. Moreover, when headgear weight is combined with vibration and shock movements in vehicles and aircrafts, it increases the risk for neck pain.

Carrying rucksacks, fire hoses, body armor, weapons, and other heavy equipment and supplies takes a physical toll on the body. The average load is 60 to 120 lb. Years of running on hard surfaces, extended periods of wearing heavy boots, being in confined spaces, falling from military vehicles, or accidents and exposure to improvised explosive devices (IEDs) can also cause pain and/or contribute to injury.

Because these tasks are physically challenging, tactical athletes are at high risk for soft tissue injuries. Not surprisingly, training injuries are the number-one noncombat-related reason for lost duty time or removal from deployment in military service members. Injuries to the neck, shoulders, feet, ankles, knees, and lower back are common. Careful consideration of the client's specific job, combined with a comprehensive health history, will direct treatment goals. Furthermore, the work involved can take an enormous emotional toll. Posttraumatic stress disorder (PTSD) may surface during service or later in life. PTSD manifests in several ways and ranges from unnoticeable to serious. Loud noises, bright lights, or unexpected events (sudden opening of a door) may generate a startle response. For new clients, the response may be unexpected for them also.

Another common issue is hearing loss resulting from regular exposure to noisy vehicles and equipment, as well as weapon fire and blasts. In fact, 80% of military service members have hearing loss in one or both ears (Sefton & Burkhardt, 2016). During the intake, consider asking if the client has hearing issues. If confirmed, ask if the client has a preferred side for hearing when communicating, and keep this in mind during conversations. More information regarding how to modify treatment for clients with hearing impairments is detailed in Chapter 11. Research related to massage for military personnel, veterans, and their families is on Evolve.

CLINICAL MASSAGE: APPLICATION METHODS

Practitioners of clinical massage may employ focused massage and stretching techniques and/or use of handheld tools, some of which are briefly discussed in this section. These sections are summaries of entire systems of treatment and proficiency of these methods come from their study and practice. Keep in mind that, over time, these systems have been updated and may be practiced differently today compared with how they were originally intended.

Furthermore, keep in mind that using these methods does not necessarily give practitioners of clinical massage an advantage over techniques used by practitioners of wellness massage, especially for reducing pain or improving function. Indeed, research has found no significant or meaningful differences between general techniques of effleurage, petrissage, friction, tapotement, and vibration and focused techniques of myofascial release (MFR) and TrP therapy for producing these outcomes (Cherkin et al, 2011; Romanowski et al, 2012).

Apply scope of practice guidelines and standards of care such as avoiding treatment over endangerment sites, unless the application of pressure is light (i.e., manual lymphatic drainage [MLD]). Avoid treating the area during the acute phase of inflammation, which is usually 72 hours (3 days). Use the acronym S-H-A-R-P (Swelling, Heat, A loss of function, Redness, and Pain) to recall the signs and symptoms of acute inflammation. The following steps are recommended for all application methods in this section.

1. Assess the client and determine if the selected method is safe and appropriate.

2. Explain the method, reasons why it was selected, and sensations the client is expected to feel (e.g., pulling, pressure, stinging), potential side effects (i.e., irritation from tape, petechial rash from scraping tools, cupping marks, soreness, etc.), and adverse events. Because the client may not fully comprehend what a petechial rash or cupping marks look like, provide images so that consent will be valid.
3. Obtain consent.
4. Apply the method.
5. Document. Include treatment details such as the type of method and tools used; why it was administered; the application area and duration of application; position of the client; and the client's response or treatment outcome.

Muscle Energy Techniques/Proprioceptive Neuromuscular Facilitation

Muscle energy techniques (MET) and **proprioceptive neuromuscular facilitation** (PNF) are methods that combine isometric contraction and stretching to improve treatment outcomes. The isometric contraction and stretching accomplish several things. First, the tension generated by muscle contraction activates Golgi tendon organs, which temporarily inhibit contraction. The isometric contraction also causes mild muscle fatigue, which temporarily reduces the muscle's ability to contract. METs and PNF take advantage of this brief vulnerability and passively stretch the muscle, which resets the stretch receptors to a new increased resting length.

METs and PNF were developed about the same time in history (1940s), but by different professionals. METs were developed by osteopaths (Mitchell Jr. and Sr.) and used to correct bone positions. PNF was developed by physical therapists (Kabat and Knott) and used to strengthen weak muscles. The term "muscle energy" refers to the energy of muscle contraction (Chaitow & DeLany, 2008; Wright & Drysdale, 2008). The term "PNF" refers to activation of proprioceptors, or stretch receptors within the muscle, to facilitate neuromuscular function (Page, 2012). PNF recommends a stronger contraction and longer stretch period compared to METs. Both METs and PNF use muscle contraction and stretching and are based on neurologic laws outlined by Sherrington (see Chapter 23). Additionally, both METs and PNF are equally effective in decreasing pain, increasing ROM, and improving function (Kumari et al., 2016).

Because both MET and PNF are stretching techniques, follow all cautions and contraindications related to stretching listed in Chapter 8.

1. Stretch the target muscle(s) to a barrier, which is either at the pain threshold or where resistance is first noted.
2. Ask the client to contract the stretched muscle against a resistance provided by the practitioner. For METs, the client uses about 25% of their strength; for PNF, the client uses 50% of their strength. An elastic band, strap, or immobile object can be used to provide resistance.
3. Maintain the contraction for 3 to 10 seconds for METs; For PNF, the contraction is maintained for 10 to 30 seconds. Some practitioners use pulsed contractions.

4. Next, the client relaxes while the practitioner re-stretches the muscle, locates a new barrier (ROM likely increased), and repeats the stretch/contract/stretch sequence two to four more times.

There are several techniques of METs.

- **Post-isometric relaxation (PIR)**. Stretch/contract/stretch of the target muscle.
- **Reciprocal inhibition (RI)**. Stretch/contract/stretch of the target muscle's antagonist.
- There are several techniques of PNF.
- **Contract relax (CR)**. Stretch/contract/stretch of the target muscle. CR is basically PIR. CR is also called *hold relax*.
- **Antagonist contract (AC)**. Stretch/contract of the target muscle's antagonist. AC is basically RI.
- **Contract relax antagonist contract (CRAC)**. Combines CR and AC and involves stretch/contract/stretch of the target muscle and its antagonist.

Positional Release Therapy/Strain-Counterstrain

Positional release therapy (PRT) or **strain-counterstrain** (SCS) is the placement of a target muscle into a shortened, comfortable position. This location is called the *position of ease,* or place where pain is relieved. Essentially, PRT is the opposite of stretching because the muscle attachments are brought closer together instead of farther apart. The theory behind how PRT/SCS works is that, when tissues are pushed together, compressed, twisted, or unkinked, pain signal activity decreases (Bethers et al., 2021). PRT/SCS were developed by Lawrence Jones, D.O. in the 1950s. PRT/SCS is also called *passive positioning* or *ortho-bionomy*; the latter term was coined by Arthur Pauls, D.O. PRT/SCS can be applied as follows:

1. Locate a tender point in a muscle.
2. Without reducing applied pressure, ask the client to relax while the practitioner shortens the muscle. The action ceases when the client reports a pain reduction and only the experience of pressure.
3. Reduce pressure and maintain only light contact over the point for 60 to 90 seconds.
4. Return the body to an anatomically neutral position while the client remains relaxed.
5. Recheck the tender point—expect a 50% to 100% reduction in pain. The area can be retreated until the desired effect is achieved.

Manual Lymph Drainage

Manual lymphatic drainage (MLD) is gentle, superficial skin stretching applied along lymphatic pathways combined with diaphragmatic breathing to promote lymph flow and reduce or prevent swelling. Skin stretching techniques include circling, scooping, pumping, and rotating. MLD is used as a preventive measure; as a postoperative measure for surgeries such as mastectomy, liposuction, and joint replacement surgery; or for palliative care. In cases of lymphedema, MLD reroutes lymph flow around areas where lymphatic vessels have been surgically removed or damaged.

MLD is more effective when combined with other methods such as PNF, elastic therapeutic tape (ETT), or *complete decongestive therapy* (practitioner-applied MLD with compressive garments/bandaging, skin care, gentle active movements, self-applied MLD). MLD contraindications include congestive heart failure, kidney failure, and lymphedema from active cancer. MLD was developed by the Danish physicians Emil and Estrid Vodder in the 1930s. Along with the Vodder method, practitioners interested in MLD can become certified in the Földi, Leduc, and Casley-Smith methods. All methods have several common elements.

- Sessions begin and end with diaphragmatic breathing to stimulate lymph flow in lymphatic ducts.
- Techniques are applied slowly and rhythmically, using light pressure, and without lubricant.
- Movements include a resting phase, which allows the skin to return to its original position.
- Techniques are applied to proximal unaffected areas first, usually in cervical, axillary, and inguinal areas (areas of superficial lymph nodes). Distal affected areas are treated last. This approach allows lymph to move more efficiently.

Elastic Therapeutic Tape

Elastic therapeutic tape (ETT) is thin, stretchy, elastic tape applied to the skin. ETT can stretch 120% to 140% of its original length after applied and then recoils to its original unstretched length—this action creates a pulling force. Several brands of ETT are available, including KinesioTape and RockTape. ETT was developed by Kenzo Kase in the 1970s. Theories suggest ETT increases interstitial spaces and decompresses activated pain receptors. ETT improves ROM, decreases pain, and reduces swelling (Chen et al., 2018; Mostafavifar et al., 2012; Pop et al., 2014; Thelen et al., 2008; Williams et al., 2012).

ETT is waterproof and breathable. However, it needs to be patted dry with a towel when it becomes wet from swimming, bathing, or sweating. ETT should not be applied over skin lesions, skin rashes, or sunburn. The main, but rare, side effect is skin irritation. ETT can be applied as follows:

1. Select the area of tape application.
2. Cut the length of tape needed, which is approximately 2″ longer than the treatment area. Additionally, cut and shape the tape to fit the width and contours of the treatment area (Y-shaped, fan-shaped, donut-shaped). Cut the tape ends in a crescent or semicircle to prevent premature peeling.
3. Skin should be clean, dry, and free of lubricants. Alcohol wipes can be used to prepare the area. If body hair is limiting tape adhesion, hair in the treatment area may need to be trimmed or shaved.
4. Apply the tape by removing the backing, stretching it about 50% without pulling the tape ends, and placing it over the treatment area. The treatment area itself can be elongated by stretching prior to tape application. Avoid touching the adhesive side of the tape after removing the backing, as this may decrease the adhesive strength.

5. Rub the surface of the tape to activate the heat-sensitive adhesive.

Wait at least 1 hour after tape application before swimming, bathing, or engaging in activities that cause sweating. When applied properly, ETT can last 3 to 5 days. To remove ETT, peel it off slowly in the direction of body hair. Baby or cooking oil can be applied before removal, as it helps to break down the tape adhesive—allow it to soak in for a few minutes before slowly removing the tape.

Instrument-Assisted Soft Tissue Mobilization

Instrument-assisted soft tissue mobilization (IASTM) uses handheld tools with round edges to scrape the skin in multiple directions. This action breaks down fibrosis and adhesions, and facilitates remodeling so tissues are restructured in ways that promote movement—the same principle applies to transverse/cross-fiber friction. In fact, some studies refer to IASTM as instrument-assisted cross-fiber massage. The use of handheld tools allows deeper penetration into tissues while reducing stress on the practitioner's hands.

IASTM is most commonly used for tendonitis, carpal tunnel syndrome, plantar fasciitis, rotator cuff injuries, and scar tissue. IASTM evolved from Gua Sha, which is a component of traditional Chinese medicine. However, Gua Sha is used to stimulate the body's energy, called qi or chi, and not for musculoskeletal conditions. IASTM often produces a reddish/purple rash called petechiae caused by friction-induced broken capillaries. Other side effects include soreness and bruising (Kim et al., 2017). While evidence supports its use to reduce pain and improve ROM, there is currently no consensus on best practices, such as the best type of instrument or how much pressure to apply to achieve optimal results (Cheatham et al., 2019; Seffrin et al., 2019).

Cupping Therapy

Cupping therapy uses plastic, silicone, or glass cups placed on the skin to create suction and lift the tissues. Negative pressure is generated by withdrawing trapped air from the cup, either mechanically by pumping it out, or thermally by cooling heated air (the latter is called *fire cupping*). Negative pressure causes the skin and fascia beneath the cup to lift, which causes skin reddening from increased perfusion (movement of fluids through capillaries into interstitial spaces). Cupping therapy is also called *fascial cupping*. Cupping therapy, like IASTM, originated from traditional Chinese medicine. Cups come in various sizes. Larger cups create stronger suction and are used for large muscular areas such as the back and legs. Smaller cups create a weaker suction and are used for smaller areas such as the forearms and face. There are two types of cupping therapy.

- **Dry cupping**. Use of suction only.
- **Wet cupping**. Use of suction and bloodletting. The skin is pricked with a needle. This type of cupping is invasive and outside a massage practitioner's scope of practice. There are several types of cupping therapy techniques.
- **Static cupping**. The cup remains on the skin for the duration of treatment (i.e., called parking).

- **Shaking/rotational cupping**. The cup is shaken or rotated while in a stationary position.
- **Flash cupping**. The cup is repeatedly released and replaced on the skin for the duration of treatment.
- **Glide cupping**. The cup is moved across lubricated skin for the duration of treatment.

Cupping therapy can reduce pain, increase function, and reduce cellulite (Arslan et al., 2015; Saha et al., 2017; Wang et al., 2017). Cupping often leaves temporary marks on the skin, which disappears in 3 to 4 days but can linger for up to 10 days (Moura et al., 2018). In fact, clients may elect not to receive cupping therapy because of this side effect (Hong et al., 2020). In addition to contraindications related to all massage methods (i.e., skin lesions, infectious disease), cupping is not recommended for people taking anticoagulant medications or who have blood disorders. Dry cupping therapy can be applied as follows:

1. Place a clean cup over the treatment area and mechanically remove the air by squeezing it or by using a pumping device. This action causes the skin to rise into the cup.
2. Apply the cupping technique of your choice (static, shaking/rotational, flash, gliding). If the cup pops off the skin before treatment is complete, re-apply the cup and continue.
3. Treatment duration ranges 3 to 5 minutes.

Cupping therapy and cupping tapotement are different. Cupping tapotement is part of postural drainage and percussion (PD&P), an airway clearance technique used on the back and chest to loosen mucus in the lungs so it can be removed by coughing. PD&P is used as part of treatment in respiratory conditions such as pneumonia and is discussed in *Mosby's Pathology for Massage Professionals*.

Trigger Points Therapy

Trigger points (TrPs) are hyperirritable tender spots in taut palpable bands within skeletal muscle and associated fascia. As a result of this, TrPs are also called *myofascial trigger points*. TrPs cause pain and/or motor dysfunction and autonomic phenomena. Examples of motor dysfunction are muscle stiffness, weakness, or limited movement. Examples of autonomic phenomena are pallor, sweating, and watering eyes. Palpation of TrPs can also cause referred pain, jump signs, and/or local twitch responses (Lavelle et al., 2007; Travell & Simons, 1983). Not all trigger points should be palpated, such as within endangerment sites.

- **Referred pain**. Pain perceived at a location other than the site of painful stimulus or origin. Referred pain patterns are proximal or distal to the TrP in about 73% of cases. Distal pain patterns are more common than proximal pain patterns. Referred pain occurs in or around the point the other 27% of cases. TrPs and their pain referral patterns are fairly consistent from one person to another (Fig. 14.24). Sharp, stabbing, shooting, numbing, or electric-type pain may occur from pressure over nerves rather than TrPs and should be avoided.

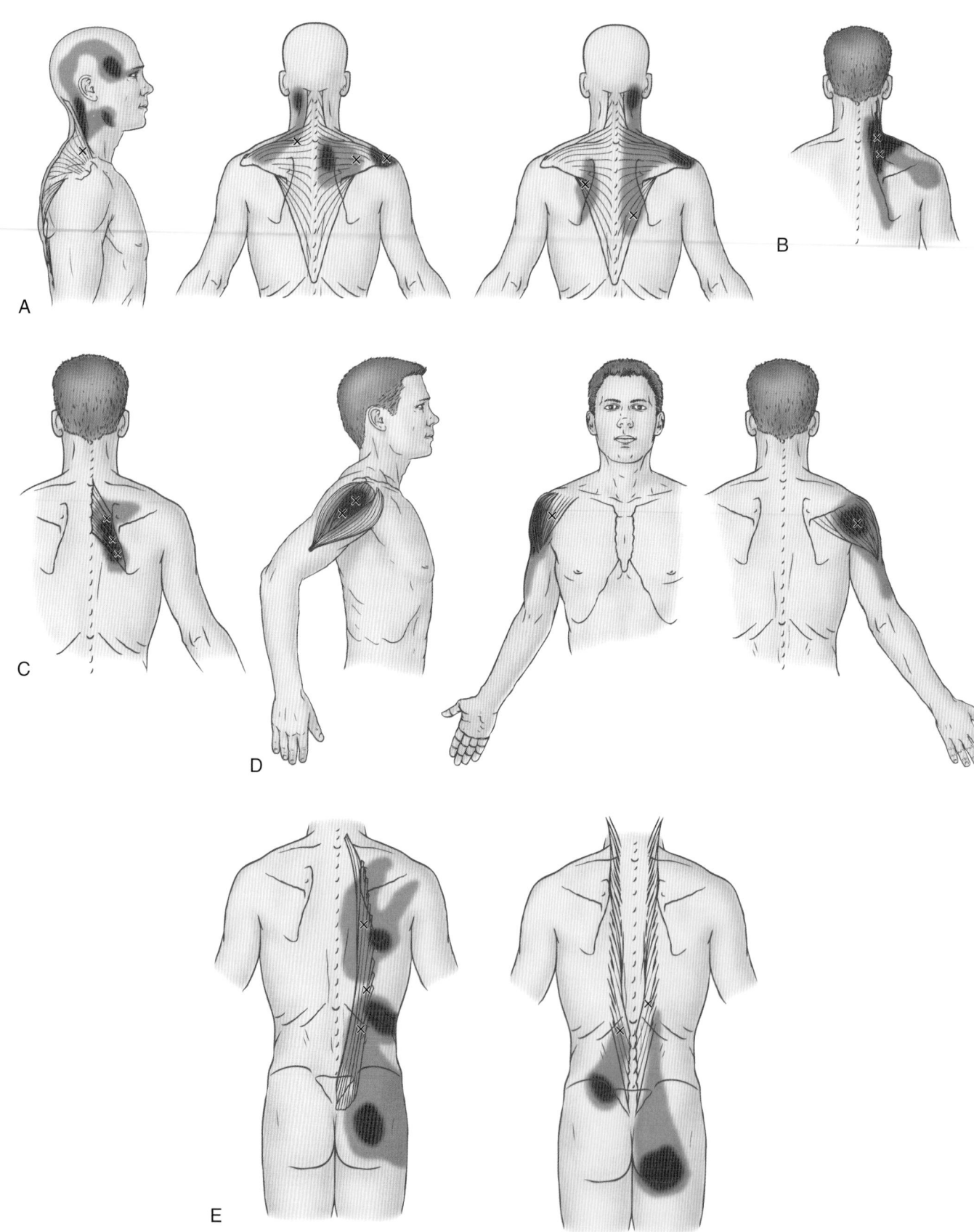

FIG. 14.24 Commonly treated muscles with their associated trigger points (indicated by Xs) referral patterns (indicated by red shading). (A) Trapezius. (B) Levator scapula. (C) Rhomboids. (D) Deltoids. (E) Erector spinae (iliocostalis, longissimus).

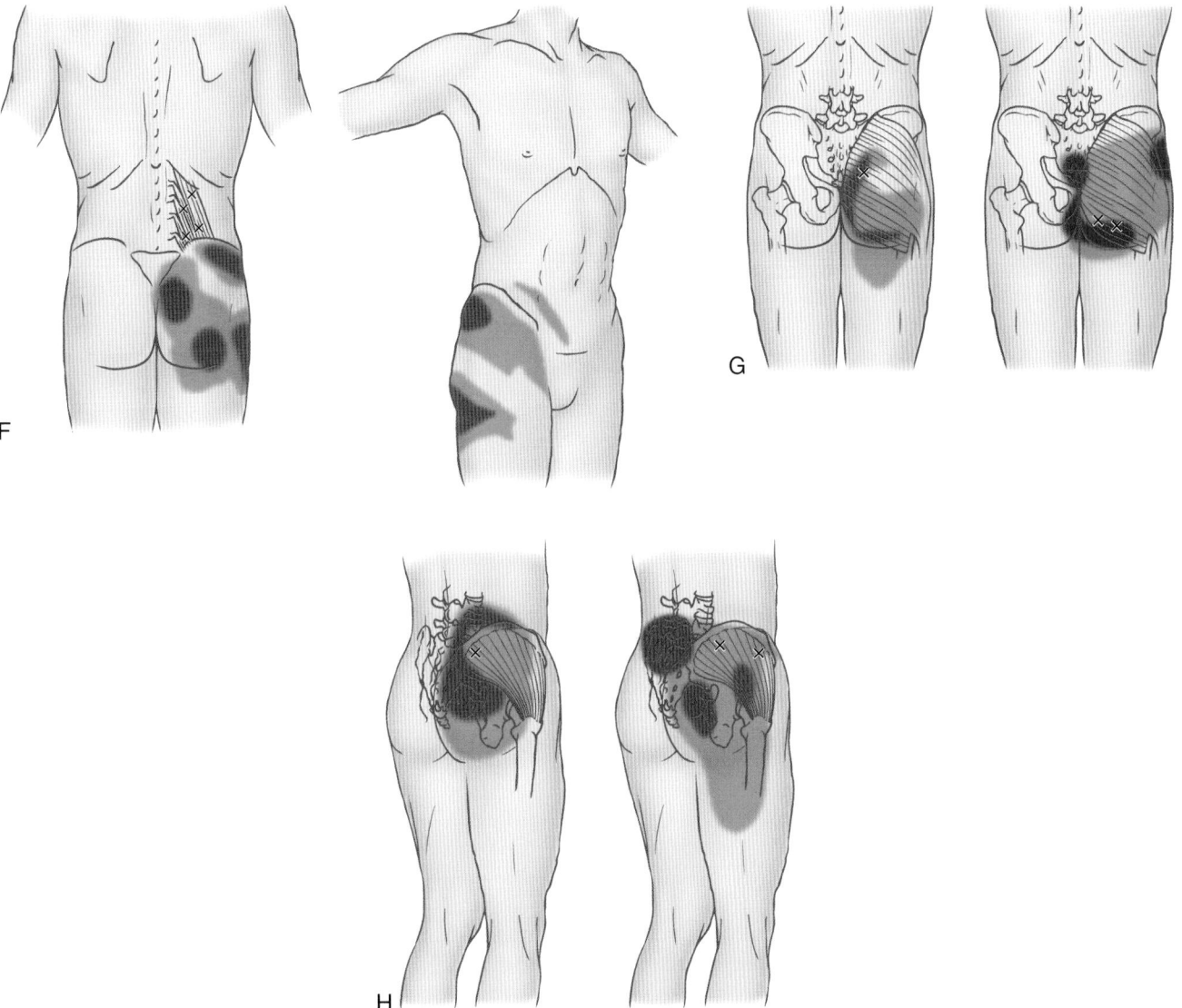

FIG. 14.24, cont'd (F) Quadratus lumborum. (G) Gluteus maximus. (H) Gluteus medius. (From Muscolino, J. E. [2009]. *The muscle and bone palpation manual*. St. Louis: Mosby.)

- **Jump sign**. A grimace, wince, or vocalized response that seems out of proportion to the amount of applied pressure. The person may also move or "jump" involuntarily or jerk the arm or other body area.
- **Local twitch response**. A transient visible or palpable contraction as tense muscle fibers of the TrP contract during pressure application.

  Trigger points can be classified as active, latent, or satellite.
- **Active trigger points**. These may be painful all the time or elicit pain when pressed and the person recognizes them as being familiar.
- **Latent trigger points**. Same characteristics as active TrPs but cause no pain until pressed and the person does not recognize them as being familiar. When latent TrPs are pressed, the client may comment, "I didn't even realize it hurt there."

- **Satellite trigger points**. These form within pain referral zones of active or latent TrPs.

  Several hypotheses attempt to explain TrP development. The most widely accepted hypothesis is the *integrated hypothesis*, which states TrPs develop by excessive release of acetylcholine by presynaptic neurons. Muscle strain, overuse, or direct trauma "trigger" sustained contraction and form taut bands in the muscle. Sustained contraction causes local ischemia and reduced availability of oxygen, nutrients, and adenosine triphosphate (ATP). ATP is needed to stop the contraction by release of the myosin heads from actin. Local ischemia also causes the release of bradykinins, norepinephrine, catecholamines, cytokines and other inflammatory mediators, and substance P (the latter increases pain perception). Other factors contributing to TrP development are myofascial dysfunctions, arthritis, and temporomandibular joint dysfunction, nutritional deficiencies (vitamins B, C, D, iron, and magnesium), structural asymmetry (leg length discrepancy, scoliosis), lack of flexibility, stress, and emotional trauma (Gerwin et al., 2004; Shah et al., 2015). Quintner and Cohen (1994) suggested TrPs may be caused by nerve compression within the nervi nervorum. The nervi nervorum is the nervous system's own nervous system, and it innervates the sheaths surrounding nerves. Cathie (1974) noted that many common TrPs coincide with areas where nerves pass through fascial sheaths. This helps explain why TrPs can be found in noncontractile tissue such as fascia and the existence of latent and satellite TrPs.

Trigger point therapy is the use of manual pressure over TrPs. Pressure is usually applied with the fingertips or the hands, but forearms, elbows, feet, or handheld tools can be used. TrP therapy is also called *myotherapy* and *neuromuscular therapy*. Commonly used manual techniques are transverse friction and sustained compression and are equally effective (Fernandez-de-las-Penas et al., 2006). Sustained compression was once called *ischemic compression*—Travell and Simons (1998) coined the term because the skin initially blanches pale or becomes ischemic on release of pressure before becoming hyperemic and pinkish red.

Travell and Simons, authors of the most credible and scholarly source on TrPs and TrP therapy (*Myofascial Pain and Dysfunction: The Trigger Point Manual*), do not recommend manual pressure on all TrPs, such as within endangerment sites. In these areas, non-manual techniques such as METs or PNF are more appropriate for inactivating myofascial TrPs. TrP therapy in non-endangerment sites can be applied as follows.

1. Locate a TrP using manual pressure. The pressure can be applied over bare skin, through the drape, or through clothing. When applied to bare skin, it should be lubricant free or lightly lubricated.
   - Some practitioners use the **T-A-R-T** method for locating TrPs, which stands for **T**issue changes, **A**symmetry, **R**ange of motion (ROM) variations, and **T**enderness. *Tissue changes* include variations in texture or thickness and the formation of taut bands, as well as changes in temperature. *Asymmetry* is noted when comparing one side of the client's body to its equivalent on the other side. Note asymmetric movement patterns, end-feel, and pain during *ROM assessments*. Also note *tenderness* or pain when the point is pressed.
2. Press or massage the point for 10 to 20 seconds. Pressure of 6 to 7 on a 10-point pressure scale is recommended—ask for client feedback and adjust the level of pressure accordingly. Heat or superficial warming friction can be used before or between pressure/massage applications.
3. After the TrP is treated, passively stretch the muscle to help increase its resting length. Repeat sequence if needed.

Myofascial Release

Myofascial release (MFR) is low-load, long-duration skin stretching. Myofascial refers to muscles and related fascia.

Fascia may hold memories due to a *neurofascial connection,* wherein higher centers of the brain activate autonomic and endocrine pathways, and manual therapies may aid in their improved function (Tozzi, 2014). Robert Ward, D.O., a student of Ida Rolf, the originator of Structural Integration, or Rolfing, first coined the term "MFR" in the 1960s. However, John Barnes, P.T. popularized the method in the 1970s. Fascia is discussed in Chapter 18.

Superficial fascia contains an enzyme called *hyaluronidase*, which allows it to change temporarily to a watery gelatinous consistency (called sol-gel conversion) when subjected to mechanical pressure or heat. This property is called *thixotropy* (Juhan, 1987). While thixotropy is interesting, it is clinically irrelevant, as superficial fascia reverts back to its prior state when pressure or heat stops. MFR can reduce pain and muscle soreness, increase ROM, improve relaxation, and enhance recovery after athletic performance (Chen et al., 2021; Kerautret et al., 2021). MFR can be applied in the following ways, as listed below. Several techniques address myofascial tissues (skin rolling, deep effleurage, IASTM, and cupping therapy), not just the MFR technique mentioned below.

1. Gently move and stretch unlubricated skin until a tissue barrier or point of slight resistance is noted (Fig. 14.25A). One hand can anchor the tissue while the other hand moves and stretches the skin (see Fig. 14.25B).
2. Maintain this position for 90 to 120 seconds. During this time, the tissue barrier will increase as tissues soften and lengthen. Do not glide across the skin. Two hands/thumbs can be used to move the skin in the same or opposite direction; the latter resembles an S-shape (Fig. 14.26).
3. Repeat sequence in several planes of movement (e.g., vertically, horizontally, obliquely).

HOSPITAL-BASED MASSAGE THERAPY

Hospital-based massage therapy (HBMT) includes massage services provided in hospital or medical settings. HBMT is used in military hospitals, cancer treatment centers, infusion centers (i.e., chemotherapy, dialysis); maternity centers for labor and delivery; intensive care units including neonatal units; postacute rehabilitation centers; medical-postsurgical; therapy clinics; and behavioral health facilities (Fig. 14.27). The type of care offered in hospital and healthcare settings can be defined by the level of care, duration of stay, and projected patient outcomes including acute care, long-term care, and home healthcare, and are discussed next. Hospice care is also a type of care given in these settings and is discussed in a later section.

- **Acute care**. Time-sensitive care administered both rapidly and frequently to improve patient outcomes. Acute care includes preventive, curative, rehabilitative, and palliative interventions. The duration of acute care is usually 30 or fewer days, with 4 days being the average length of stay.

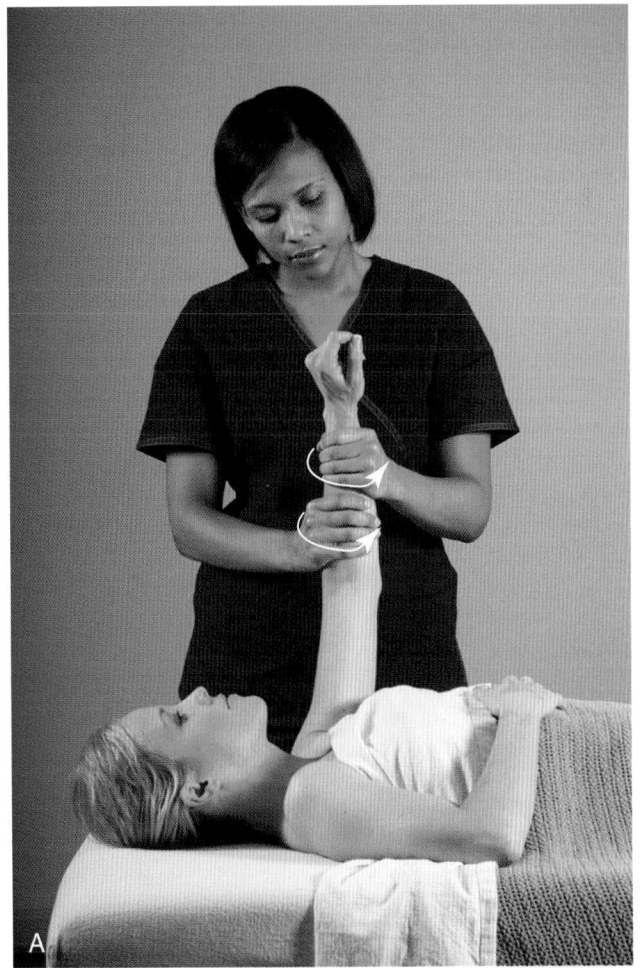

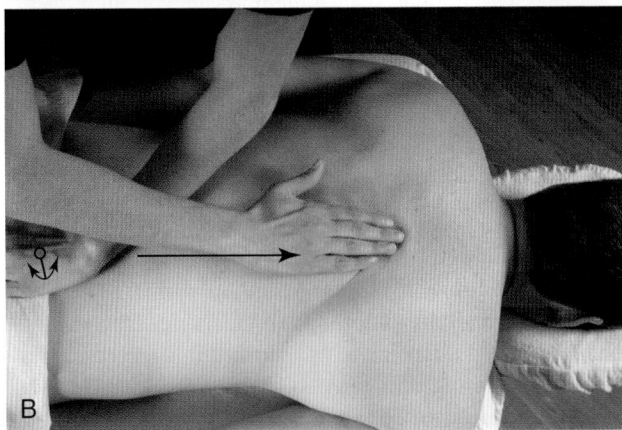

FIG. 14.25 Myofascial release. Two hands can stretch the tissue in the same direction (A), or one hand can anchor the tissue while the other hand stretches the tissue (B).

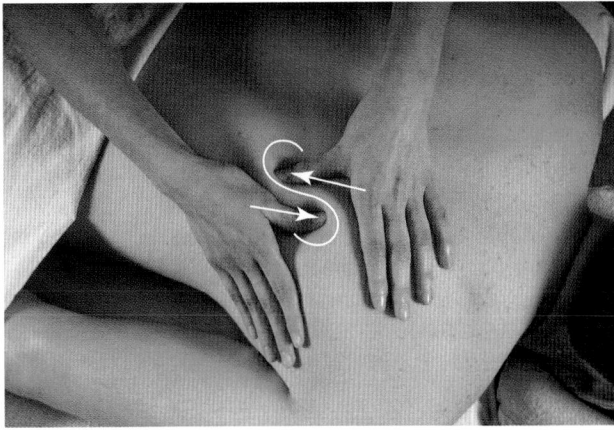

FIG. 14.26 Myofascial release techniques. Both hands/thumbs can stretch the tissue in opposite directions, which can resemble an S-shape.

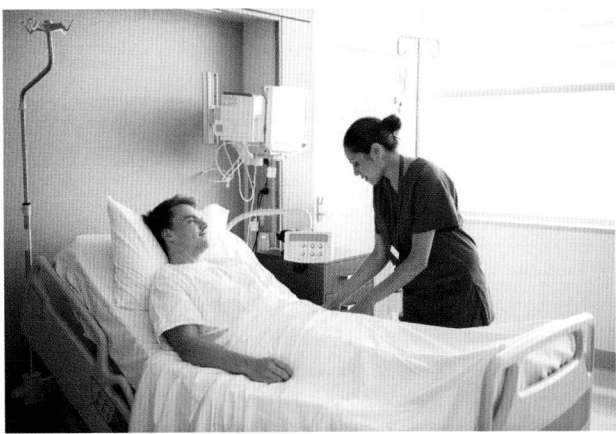

FIG. 14.27 Hospital-based massage therapy. This is found in a variety of medical environments, including military hospitals, cancer treatment centers, nonprofit and for-profit hospitals, therapy clinics, and behavioral health facilities. (Copyright © istock.com.)

- **Long-term care**. Medical and nonmedical care to patients with chronic illnesses, disabilities, or who are medically fragile and unable to care for themselves. The length of stay is usually 30 or more days. Nonmedical care includes help with activities such as dressing, bathing, and using the toilet. Long-term care may be provided in extended-stay, subacute rehabilitation, skilled nursing, and assisted living facilities. Long-term care can also be provided at home.
- **Home healthcare**. Medical and nonmedical care provided in the patient's home or residence. Medical care includes skilled nursing care, physical, occupation, respiratory, or speech therapy, and nonmedical care, as mentioned previously. Home healthcare is usually less expensive, more convenient, and as effective as care received in medical settings. Moreover, patients report increased satisfaction with home healthcare compared to other settings.

Surgery

Surgery is a medical specialty that uses operative instruments and procedures to correct deformities or defects, investigate or treat diseases, repair injuries, and help improve body function or appearance. Surgery can also be used to remove a baby from the uterus (i.e., cesarean section—see Chapter 11). Approximately 48 million surgeries are performed in the U.S. annually. The most common surgeries are for cardiovascular conditions, followed by digestive system surgeries and musculoskeletal surgeries. Surgeries can either be minor or major.

- **Minor surgery**. Involves local anesthesia and is minimally invasive. Most surgical procedures are superficial, only affecting the outermost portions of the body. The risk of infection is reduced, recovery time is shorter, and there is less scarring compared with major surgery. Examples include removing skin lesions such as warts or moles, breast biopsies, cataract surgery, and dental extractions. Minor surgery is also called *day surgery* or *outpatient surgery*.
- **Major surgery**. Involves general anesthesia, respiratory assistance, and entering a body cavity so the surgeon has access to the work area. Major surgery has a higher risk of infection and longer recovery period, and usually leaves a larger scar. Examples of major surgeries are open-heart surgery, gastric bypass surgery, joint replacement surgery, and Cesarean section. Major surgery is also called *inpatient surgery*.

After surgery, the surgical wound begins to heal and likely produces a scar. Wound healing and scar formation happen in four sequential and overlapping stages, often referred to as the "cascade of healing." While wound healing is discussed in the context of surgical wounds, it applies to any wound, including those from injuries.

- **Stage 1: Hemostasis**. This stage involves mechanisms to stop the bleeding from broken blood vessels (see Chapter 26).
- **Stage 2: Inflammation**. This stage focuses on destroying bacteria and removing debris in preparation for the growth of new tissue. The scar is swollen, warm, red, and often painful. This stage lasts for approximately 2 weeks.
- **Stage 3: Proliferation (regeneration)**. The body begins to fill and cover the wound site by depositing collagen. Scars in this stage are characterized by 3 Rs: red, raised, and rigid. This stage lasts up to 8 weeks.
- **Stage 4: Remodeling (maturation)**. The new tissue in the wound matures, collagen fibers reorganize, and excess collagen dissipates. The scar becomes both strong and flexible, but not as much as normal skin. Mature scars also lack pigment, glands, and hair follicles found in normal skin. The remodeling stage can last from 12 to 18 months.

Massage and Surgery

For major surgery, massage can begin once the client is medically stable. *Medical stability* occurs when vital signs, such as pulse, temperature, and blood pressure are within normal limits; the client is conscious and comfortable; and the prognosis is good to excellent. Communicate with the patient care coordinator if the client is still under medical supervision and follow their directives. Position the client for comfort. A side-lying position may be needed to avoid pressure on areas containing incisions, drain tubes, or medical devices, such as catheters or pacemakers. The

incision, or cut, produced by surgical instruments during the operation and areas near the incision are avoided until sutures or staples are removed and the incision is dry (not moist or open) and into the remodeling (maturation) phase. This may take up to 8 weeks after surgery or longer. In addition, the area around the incision should not be manipulated in a way that places stress on it while it is healing. Avoid vigorous massage techniques on the lower extremities (thighs and legs) for 12 weeks after surgery because of increased risk of blood clots or venous thromboembolism (Kuznar, 2010; Sweetland et al., 2009).

For minor surgery, the same general guidelines apply, with one exception. If it appears that blood clot risk after minor surgery is low and brief, light pressure on the lower extremities may not be warranted. Instead, screen for blood clots by looking for signs and symptoms such as unilateral leg swelling, heat, redness or noticeable discoloration, pain, and tenderness. If present, avoid massage to the affected lower extremity.

Massage and Scars

The wound scar is a local contraindication until the area is dry and in the remodeling (maturation) phase. This timeframe is 8 weeks or longer. Use deep friction and skin-rolling near and directly over the scar with or without lubricant. Massage tissues in several directions (superior, inferior, medial, lateral, clockwise, counterclockwise) because scar tissue is arranged haphazardly. Begin with light pressure and progress to deeper pressure. Inquire about pressure sensitivity and adjust it below the client's pain tolerance. Discontinue scar tissue massage and refer clients to their healthcare provider if the scar is redder, warmer, or more painful upon subsequent sessions (Moffitt Cancer Center [MCC], 2008). Teach clients how to massage their own scars if the tissues are in accessible areas.

Hospice Care

Hospice care is a type of medical care that provides palliative services to patients and their families who are facing a life-limiting illness. Common palliative services include medications and nonpharmacologic interventions, such as massage, music therapy, guided imagery, breathing techniques, gentle movements, such as yoga and tai chi, acupuncture, and pet therapy. Cancer was the most common diagnosis among Medicare hospice patients, followed by heart disease and dementia. Patients with a principal diagnosis of dementia spent the most time in hospice care (National Hospice and Palliative Care Organization [NHPCO], 2020).

Massage and Hospice Patients

Massage for patients in hospice care is provided in several settings, including a private residence; nursing home, or other institutionalized care facility; a dedicated hospice center; or in an acute care hospital. Massage practitioners may be required to participate in an orientation and follow guidelines set forth by the hospice agency. If you enter the room and other people are present such as visitors or team members, introduce yourself and state why you are there. Be willing to massage the patient in a busy room or wait until team members are finished with their tasks.

Space is often limited in hospice settings, so portable massage tables are usually not appropriate. In many instances, individuals will be massaged where they are positioned, which may include lying in a bed or sitting in a recliner. If massaging the patient in a bed, the practitioner can raise, lower, or tilt the bed to help preserve good body mechanics and accommodate the patient's comfort. The bedrails can be adjusted, and the footboard and headboard removed if needed, except if the patient is at risk of falling.

Assist with untying and retying garments such as hospital gowns. Drape clean linens over anything touching the patient's body during the massage. When undraping, fold linens back instead of tucking them beneath the patient, which may require lifting the patient. Patients may wear their own clothing. In these cases, work through clothing, as undressing and redressing may be difficult.

Use an unscented massage lubricant, creme or lotion provided by the facility, or the patient's own product (used with permission). Use techniques of light pressure and slow speed. Touch-based techniques such Healing Touch, M-technique, and Reiki are also appropriate. When the massage begins, ask patients to inform you if they experience any discomfort, and tell them if it occurs, modifications will be made immediately to reduce the discomfort. Keep in mind patients may choose to not give feedback, so be keenly aware of their responses. The length of the session may be 30 to 60 minutes but actual "hands-on" time may be shorter, and more time may be needed for comfort measures such as arranging pillows and blankets.

Coping With Dying, Death, and Grief

Massage practitioners working in hospice care will experience loss of patients and death-related grief. It is vital that they have supportive measures in place. These may include opportunities to debrief with staff, group therapy, and the ability to take time off, as needed, to cope.

On receiving the news of dying, the patient and the patient's family and friends may experience a wide range of diverse emotional responses. These responses can have a direct impact on the palliative aspects of hospice care. One of the common models of the psychologic processes involved with loss was introduced by Kübler-Ross et al. (1972), a Swiss psychiatrist, as the five stages of grief. The amount of time each stage takes, and its overall process,

varies per patient. The stages of grief are denial, anger, bargaining, depression, and acceptance. In each one of these stages, healthcare providers should respect the patient's responses and allow the patient the autonomy to make the transition throughout each phase. A patient may neither experience the stages in order, nor experience all of the stages.

- **Stage 1: Denial**. The denial stage serves as a protective coping mechanism. It is normal for the patient to behave in a manner suggesting nothing has changed and support a positive outcome.
- **Stage 2: Anger**. When denial ends, anger reveals itself by blaming or angered behavior. It is quite possible for the patient to exhibit signs of resentment, rage, and envy. This is often the most difficult stage for caregivers. The patient wants to be recognized and allowed to express emotions.
- **Stage 3: Bargaining**. In this stage the person makes statements toward religious figureheads or caregivers as bargaining favors for extension of life. This is the stage in which the patient realizes their looming absence in milestones of those around them. An example of this may be a father who wants to see his daughter graduate.
- **Stage 4: Depression**. This stage is the beginning of withdrawal in which the person needs space to internalize and self-assess feelings of death and the process of leaving the people and places to whom the patient has bonded. Heightened spirituality is often a part of this phase.
- **Stage 5: Acceptance**. In this final stage, the patient comes to terms with death and experiences peace about dying. Not every patient will make it to acceptance.

Dying is a natural process in which the body begin to systematically shut down. There are emotional, physical, and spiritual aspects to dying. The process will be unique for each patient and may be impacted by the patient's cultural foundation, belief system, and support system. It is important for the massage practitioner to partner with the patient and family, supporting them without judgment or criticism. It is a great honor to be present during end-of-life care.

I would like to thank Judith DeLany, Alice Sanvito, Monica Reno, and Michael Breaux for their past contributions on this chapter.

E-RESOURCES

http://evolve.elsevier.com/Salvo/MassageTherapy

- Chapter challenge
- Flash cards
- Additional information

RONALD MELZACK

Imagine losing a limb to amputation and then experiencing years of chronic pain in the missing limb. You know it's not there. You can see it's not there. It's been years since the amputation. Yet, you experience excruciating pain daily. Doctors were perplexed by this phenomenon for years, struggling to find a way to provide relief for this frustrating problem.

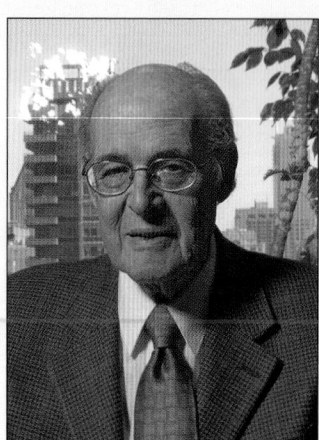

Ronald Melzack spent his career helping us understand how the brain gathers information about pain and processes it. Ronald Melzack was born on July 19, 1929, in Montreal, Canada. He was from a working-class family, and was the only sibling in his family to attend a university. After a rocky start in college, he found success in the psychology program at McGill University. He received his MSc from McGill in 1951 and his PhD in 1954.

After receiving his PhD, Melzack chose to further his research at the University of Oregon. His work in William Livingston's physiology laboratory exposed him to the puzzle of phantom limb pain. A woman whose leg had been amputated complained of terrible pain in the same leg that had been removed. He took note of this and would research phantom limb pain in depth later in his career.

Melzack eventually became a faculty member at the Massachusetts Institute of Technology. This is where he met Patrick Wall, whose research centered on the nature of pain. At the time, pain was understood as something simple: the greater the tissue damage, the greater the pain felt. Melzack and Wall challenged this way of thinking in 1965 when they published a paper about their gate control theory of pain, which proposed that pain messages encounter nerve gates in the spinal cord that control whether these signals are allowed to pass through to the brain.

By 1975, Melzack had gathered over 100 words to describe pain. With the help of a statistician, he was able to quantify each descriptor. This led to the creation of the McGill Pain Questionnaire, a leading, global method of measuring pain in research.

Melzack's later research into phantom limb pain also helped him develop the concept of a neuromatrix; he published a paper about this in 1989. This concept proposed that the brain and spinal cord, and not tissue damage, were responsible for the production of pain, and that various parts of the CNS work together to produce pain. It also proposed that we are born with a genetically determined neural network that generates our perception of the body and is responsible for generating chronic pain, even when no limbs are present. For example, a substantial number of children who are born without a limb feel a phantom pain in the missing limb, suggesting that there is a sort of neuromatrix subserving body sensation. Because chronic pain doesn't function as a warning, the neuromatrix concept offers an explanation for the mechanisms that may underlie some kinds of chronic pain and outlines new forms of treatment.

Melzack is also the author of several textbooks about pain, as well as a book of Inuit stories. In 1994, he received the Prix du Québec for research in pure and applied science, recognizing him as a Laureate of the highest honor. His work represents a substantial volume of our understanding of pain today. Melzack passed away on December 22, 2019.

What Einstein did for physics, he (Melzack) has done for pain research and management.

—**The Canadian Medical Hall of Fame**

REFERENCES

Academic Collaboration for Integrative Health (ACIH). (2017). *Hospital-based massage therapy: Competencies for optimal practice in integrated environments*. Retrieved from https://static1.squarespace.com/static/55861f1ae4b01ea9a58583a7/t/5b365b12352f537eda523d69/1530288918205/HBMT_Competencies_2018.pdf.

Adams, R., White, B., & Beckett, C. (2010). The effects of massage therapy on pain management in the acute care setting. *International Journal of Therapeutic Massage & Bodywork, 3*(1), 4–11.

American Massage Therapy Association (AMTA). (2021). *Massage profession research report*. Retrieved from https://www.amtamassage.org/publications/massage-profession-research-report/.

Arslan, M., Kutlu, N., Tepe, M., Yilmaz, N. S., Özdemir, L., & Dane, S. (2015). Dry cupping therapy decreases cellulite in women: A pilot study. *Indian Journal of Traditional Knowledge, 4*(3), 359–364.

Bethers, A. H., Swanson, D. C., Sponbeck, J. K., Mitchell, U. H., Draper, D. O., Feland, J. B., et al. (2021). Positional release therapy and therapeutic massage reduce muscle trigger and tender points. *Journal of Bodywork and Movement Therapies, 28*, 264–270.

Borenstein, D. G., O'Mara, J. W., Jr., Boden, S. D., Lauerman, W. C., Jacobson, A., Platenberg, C., et al. (2001). The value of magnetic resonance imaging of the lumbar spine to predict low-back pain in asymptomatic subjects: A seven-year follow-up study. *The Journal of Bone and Joint Surgery*, *83*(9), 1306–1311.

Cathie, A. G. (1974). *Papers and selected writings and lectures of Angus G. Cathie.* Colorado Springs: American Academy of Osteopathy.

Chaitow, L., & DeLany, J. (2008). *Clinical Application of Neuromuscular Techniques* (2nd ed., Vol. I). Edinburgh: Churchill Livingstone.

Chatchawan, U., Eungpinichpong, W., Sooktho, S., Tiamkao, S., & Yamauchi, J. (2014). Effects of Thai traditional massage on pressure pain threshold and headache intensity in patients with chronic tension-type and migraine headaches. *Journal of Alternative and Complementary Medicine*, *20*(6), 486–492.

Cheatham, S. W., Baker, R., & Kreiswirth, E. (2019). Instrument assisted soft-tissue mobilization: A commentary on clinical practice guidelines for rehabilitation professionals. *International Journal of Sports Physical Therapy*, *14*(4), 670–682.

Chen, S. M., Lo, S. K., & Cook, J. (2018). The effect of rigid taping with tension on mechanical displacement of the skin and change in pain perception. *Journal of Science and Medicine in Sport*, *21*(4), 342–346.

Chen, Z., Wu, J., Wang, X., Wu, J., & Ren, Z. (2021). The effects of myofascial release technique for patients with low back pain: A systematic review and meta-analysis. *Complementary Therapies in Medicine*, *59*, 102737.

Cherkin, D. C., Sherman, K. J., Kahn, J., Wellman, R., Cook, A. J., Johnson, E., et al. (2011). A comparison of the effects of 2 types of massage and usual care on chronic low back pain: A randomized, controlled trial. *Annals of Internal Medicine*, *155*(1), 1–9.

Choroszewicz, P., Dobosiewicz, A. M., & Badiuk, N. (2020). Sports massage as a method of preventing delayed onest muscle soreness. *Pedagogy and Psychology of Sport*, *6*(2), 104–112.

Cimpean, A., & David, D. (2019). The mechanisms of pain tolerance and pain-related anxiety in acute pain. *Health Psychology Open*, *6*(2), 2055102919865161.

Daneau, C., Cantin, V., & Descarreaux, M. (2019). Effect of massage on clinical and physiological variables during muscle fatigue task in participants with chronic low back pain: A crossover study. *Journal of Manipulative and Physiological Therapeutics*, *42*(1), 55–65.

Engel, G. L. (1977). The need for a new medical model: A challenge for biomedicine. *Science*, *196*(4286), 129–136.

Fernandez-de-las-Penas, C., Alonso-Blanco, C., Fernandez-Carnero, J., & Miangolarra-Page, J. C. (2006). The immediate effect of ischemic compression technique and transverse friction massage on tenderness of active and latent myofascial trigger points: A pilot study. *Journal of Bodywork and Movement Therapies*, *10*(1), 3–9.

Gerwin, R. D., Dommerholt, J., & Shah, J. P. (2004). An expansion of Simons' integrated hypothesis of trigger point formation. *Current Pain and Headache Reports*, *8*(6), 468–475.

Guo, J., Li, L., Gong, Y., Zhu, R., Xu, J., Zou, J., et al. (2017). Massage alleviates delayed onset muscle soreness after strenuous exercise: A systematic review and meta-analysis. *Frontiers in Physiology*, *8*, 747.

Harradine, P., Gates, L., & Bowen, C. (2018). Real time non-instrumented clinical gait analysis as part of a clinical musculoskeletal assessment in the treatment of lower limb symptoms in adults: A systematic review. *Gait Posture*, *62*, 135–139.

Hegedus, E. J., Wright, A. A., & Cook, C. (2017). Orthopaedic special tests and diagnostic accuracy studies: House wine served in very cheap containers. *British Journal of Sports Medicine*, *51*(22), 1578–1579.

Hong, M., Lee, I. S., Choi, D. H., & Chae, Y. (2020). Attentional bias toward cupping therapy marks: An eye-tracking study. *Journal of Pain Research*, *13*, 1041–1047.

International Association for the Study of Pain. (2020). *IASP announces revised definition of pain*. Retrieved from https://www.iasp-pain.org/publications/iasp-news/iasp-announces-revised-definition-of-pain/.

Juhan, D. (1987). *Job's body: A handbook for bodywork*. Barrington, NY: Station Hill Press.

Kamali, F., Mohamadi, M., Fakheri, L., & Mohammadnejad, F. (2019). Dry needling versus friction massage to treat tension type headache: A randomized clinical trial. *Journal of Bodywork and Movement Therapies*, *23*(1), 89–93.

Kerautret, Y., Guillot, A., Eyssautier, C., Gibert, G., & Di Rienzo, F. (2021). Effects of self-myofascial release interventions with or without sliding pressures on skin temperature, range of motion and perceived well-being: A randomized control pilot trial. *BMC Sports Science, Medicine & Rehabilitation*, *13*(1), 43.

Kim, J., Sung, D. J., & Lee, J. (2017). Therapeutic effectiveness of instrument-assisted soft tissue mobilization for soft tissue injury: Mechanisms and practical application. *Journal of Exercise Rehabilitation*, *13*(1), 12–22.

Koch, C., & Hänsel, F. (2019). Non-specific low back pain and postural control during quiet standing-a systematic review. *Frontiers in Psychology*, *10*, 586.

Kübler-Ross, E., Wessler, S., & Avioli, L. V. (1972). On death and dying. *JAMA*, *221*(2), 174–179.

Kumari, C., Sarkar, B., Banerjee, D., Alam, S., Sharma, R., & Biswas, A. (2016). Efficacy of muscle energy technique as compared to proprioceptive neuromuscular facilitation technique in chronic mechanical neck pain: A randomized controlled trial. *International Journal of Health Sciences and Research*, *6*(11), 152–161.

Kuznar, W. (2010). Increased risk of thromboembolism 12 weeks after surgery. *American Journal of Nursing*, *110*(3), 17.

Lavelle, E. D., Lavelle, W., & Smith, H. S. (2007). Myofascial trigger points. *Anesthesiology Clinics*, *25*(4), 841–851.

Lederman, E. (2011). The fall of the postural-structural-biomechanical model in manual and physical therapies: Exemplified by lower back pain. *Journal of Bodywork and Movement Therapies*, *15*(2), 131–138.

Louw, A., Diener, I., Butler, D. S., & Puentedura, E. J. (2011). The effect of neuroscience education on pain, disability, anxiety, and stress in chronic musculoskeletal pain. *Archives of Physical Medicine and Rehabilitation*, *92*(12), 2041–2056.

Magee, D. J. (2020). *Orthopedic Physical Assessment* (7th ed.). St Louis: Elsevier.

Mahrer, N. E., Gold, J. I., Luu, M., & Herman, P. M. (2018). A cost-analysis of an interdisciplinary pediatric chronic pain clinic. *The Journal of Pain*, *19*(2), 158–165.

Mallory, M. J., Hauschulz, J. L., Do, A., Dreyer, N. E., & Bauer, B. A. (2018). Case reports of acupuncturists and massage therapists at Mayo clinic: New allies in expediting patient diagnoses. *Explore (NY)*, *14*(2), 149–151.

McHugh, M. L. (2012). Interrater reliability: The kappa statistic. *Biochemia Medica (Zagreb)*, *22*(3), 276–282.

Melzack, R. (2001). Pain and the neuromatrix in the brain. *Journal of Dental Education*, *65*(12), 1378–1382.

Melzack, R., & Wall, P. D. (1965). Pain mechanisms: A new theory. *Science*, *150*(3699), 971–979.

Mills, S. E. E., Nicolson, K. P., & Smith, B. H. (2019). Chronic pain: A review of its epidemiology and associated factors in population-based studies. *British Journal of Anaesthesia*, *123*(2), 273–283.

Moffitt Cancer Center. (2008). *Managing your scar*. Retrieved from https://moffitt.org/media/1086/managing_your_scar.pdf.

Moraska, A. F., Schmiege, S. J., Mann, J. D., Butryn, N., & Krutsch, J. P. (2017). Responsiveness of myofascial trigger points to single and multiple trigger point release massages: A randomized, placebo controlled trial. *American Journal of Physical Medicine & Rehabilitation*, *96*(9), 639–645.

Moriguchi, C. S., Carnaz, L., Silva, L. C., Salasar, L. E., Carregaro, R. L., Sato, T., et al. (2009). Reliability of intra- and interrater palpation discrepancy and estimation of its effects on joint angle measurements. *Manual Therapy*, *14*(3), 299–305.

Mosby's Medical Dictionary. (2021). (11th ed.). St. Louis: Mosby Elsevier.

Mostafavifar, M., Wertz, J., & Borchers, J. (2012). A systematic review of the effectiveness of kinesio taping for musculoskeletal injury. *The Physician and Sportsmedicine, 40*(4), 33–40.

Moura, C. C., Chaves, É. C. L., Cardoso, A. C. L. R., Nogueira, D. A., Corrêa, H. P., & Chianca, T. C. M. (2018). Cupping therapy and chronic back pain: Systematic review and meta-analysis. *Revista Latino-Americana de Enfermagem, 26*, e3094.

National Hospice and Palliative Care Organization (NHPCO). (2020). *NHPCO releases new facts and figures report on hospice care in America.* Retrieved from https://www.nhpco.org/hospice-facts-figures/.

National Institutes of Health (NIH). (2015). *NIH analysis shows Americans are in pain.* Retrieved from https://nccih.nih.gov/news/press/08112015.

National University of Health Sciences (NUHS). (2017). *Joint Commission calls for hospitals to provide complementary and alternative medicine for pain.* Retrieved from https://www.nuhs.edu/joint-commission-calls-for-hospitals-to-provide-complementary-and-alternative-medicine-for-pain/.

Nekouei, P., Majlesi, S., Nekooei, P., Ghasemabad, K. H., & Alemi, B. (2020). Comparison between the impact of vibration and static stretching as two massaging methods on the prevention of delayed onset muscle soreness in healthy non-athlete males. *Archives of Physical Medicine and Rehabilitation, 101*(12), e134.

Page, P. (2012). Current concepts in muscle stretching for exercise and rehabilitation. *International Journal of Sports Physical Therapy, 7*(1), 109–119.

Park, K. N., Kwon, O. Y., Weon, J. H., Choung, S. D., & Kim, S. H. (2014). Comparison of the effects of local cryotherapy and passive cross-body stretch on extensibility in subjects with posterior shoulder tightness. *Journal of Sports Science & Medicine, 13*(1), 84–90.

Park, S. J., Yoon, D. M., Yoon, K. B., Moon, J. A., & Kim, S. H. (2016). Factors associated with higher reported pain levels in patients with chronic musculoskeletal pain: A cross-sectional, correlational analysis. *PLoS One, 11*(9), e0163132.

Pop, T. B., Karczmarek-Borowska, B., Tymczak, M., Hałas, I., & Banaś, J. (2014). The influence of kinesiology taping on the reduction of lymphoedema among women after mastectomy—preliminary study. *Contemporary Oncology, 18*(2), 124–129.

Preece, S. J., Willan, P., Nester, C. J., Graham-Smith, P., Herrington, L., & Bowker, P. (2008). Variation in pelvic morphology may prevent the identification of anterior pelvic tilt. *The Journal of Manual & Manipulative Therapy, 16*(2), 113–117.

Qaseem, A., Wilt, T. J., McLean, R. M., Forciea, M. A., Clinical Guidelines Committee of the American College of Physicians, & Denberg, T. D. (2017). Noninvasive treatments for acute, subacute, and chronic low back pain: A clinical practice guideline from the American college of physicians. *Annals of Internal Medicine, 166*(7), 514–530.

Quintner, J. L., & Cohen, M. L. (1994). Referred pain of peripheral nerve origin: An alternative to the "myofascial pain" construct. *The Clinical Journal of Pain, 10*(3), 243–251.

Ramond, A., Bouton, C., Richard, I., Roquelaure, Y., Baufreton, C., Legrand, E., et al. (2011). Psychosocial risk factors for chronic low back pain in primary care—a systematic review. *Family Practice, 28*(1), 12–21.

Romanowski, M., Romanowska, J., Grześkowiak, M. (2012). A comparison of the effects of deep tissue massage and therapeutic massage on chronic low back pain. *Stud Health Technol Inform, 176*, 411–414.

Saha, F. J., Schumann, S., Cramer, H., Hohmann, C., Choi, K. E., Rolke, R., et al. (2017). The effects of cupping massage in patients with chronic neck pain—a randomised controlled trial. *Complementary Medicine Research, 24*(1), 26–32.

Seffrin, C. B., Cattano, N. M., Reed, M. A., & Gardiner-Shires, A. M. (2019). Instrument-assisted soft tissue mobilization: A systematic review and effect-size analysis. *Journal of Athletic Training, 54*(7), 808–821.

Sefton, J. M., & Burkhardt, T. A. (2016). Introduction to the tactical athlete special issue. *Journal of Athletic Training, 51*(11), 845.

Shah, J. P., Thaker, N., Heimur, J., Aredo, J. V., Sikdar, S., & Gerber, L. (2015). Myofascial trigger points then and now: A historical and scientific perspective. *PMR, 7*(7), 746–761.

Shankland, W. E., II. (2011). Factors that affect pain behavior. *Cranio: The Journal of Craniomandibular Practice, 29*(2), 144–154.

Smith, M. C., Stallings, M. A., Mariner, S., & Burrall, M. (1999). Benefits of massage therapy for hospitalized patients: A descriptive and qualitative evaluation. *Alternative Therapies in Health and Medicine, 5*(4), 64–71.

Stedman's medical dictionary (28th ed.). (2005). Philadelphia, PA: Lippincott Williams & Wilkins.

Stussman, B. J., Nahin, R. R., Barnes, P. M., & Ward, B. W. (2020). U.S. physician recommendations to their patients about the use of complementary health approaches. *Journal of Alternative and Complementary Medicine, 26*(1), 25–33.

Sweetland, S., Green, J., Liu, B., Berrington de González, A., Canonico, M., & Reeves, G., et al. (2009). Duration and magnitude of the postoperative risk of venous thromboembolism in middle aged women: Prospective cohort study. *BMJ (Clinical Research Ed.), 339*, b4583.

Thelen, M. D., Dauber, J. A., & Stoneman, P. D. (2008). The clinical efficacy of kinesio tape for shoulder pain: A randomized, double-blinded, clinical trial. *The Journal of Orthopaedic and Sports Physical Therapy, 38*(7), 389–395.

Thompson, T., Correll, C. U., Gallop, K., Vancampfort, D., & Stubbs, B. (2016). Is pain perception altered in people with depression? A systematic review and meta-analysis of experimental pain research. *The Journal of Pain, 17*(12), 1257–1272.

Tick, H., Nielsen, A., Pelletier, K. R., Bonakdar, R., Simmons, S., Glick, R., et al. (2018). Evidence-based nonpharmacologic strategies for comprehensive pain care: The consortium pain task force white paper. *Explore (New York), 14*(3), 177–211.

Tozzi, P. (2014). Does fascia hold memories? *Journal of Bodywork and Movement Therapies, 18*(2), 259–265.

Travell, J. G., & Simons, D. G. (1983). *Myofascial pain and dysfunction: Trigger point manual of the upper extremities.* Baltimore, MD: Williams & Wilkins.

Travell, J. G., & Simons, D. (1998). *Myofascial pain and dysfunction, the trigger point manual* (2nd ed.). Baltimore, MD: Lippincott Williams and Wilkins.

U.S. Department of Health and Human Services, National Center for Complementary and Integrative Health. (2018). *Chronic pain: In depth.* Retrieved from https://www.nccih.nih.gov/health/chronic-pain-in-depth.

Walach, H., Güthlin, C., & König, M. (2003). Efficacy of massage therapy in chronic pain: A pragmatic randomized trial. *Journal of Alternative and Complementary Medicine, 9*(6), 837–846.

Wandner, L. D., Scipio, C. D., Hirsh, A. T., Torres, C. A., & Robinson, M. E. (2012). The perception of pain in others: How gender, race, and age influence pain expectations. *The Journal of Pain, 13*(3), 220–227.

Wang, Y. T., Qi, Y., Tang, F. Y., Li, F. M., Li, Q. H., & Xu, C. (2017). The effect of cupping therapy for low back pain: A meta-analysis based on existing randomized controlled trials. *Journal of Back and Musculoskeletal Rehabilitation, 30*(6), 1187–1195.

Williams, S., Whatman, C., Hume, P. A., & Sheerin, K. (2012). Kinesio taping in treatment and prevention of sports injuries: A meta-analysis of the evidence for its effectiveness. *Sports Medicine, 42*(2), 153–164.

Wright, P., & Drysdale, I. (2008). A comparison of post-isometric relaxation (PIR) and reciprocal inhibition (RI) muscle energy techniques applied to piriformis. *International Journal of Osteopathic Medicine, 11*(4), 158–159.

Yildirim, N., Filiz Ulusoy, M., & Bodur, H. (2010). The effect of heat application on pain, stiffness, physical function and quality of life in patients with knee osteoarthritis. *Journal of Clinical Nursing, 19*(7–8), 1113–1120.

Zhang, Y., Zhang, S., Gao, Y., Tan, A., Yang, X., & Zhang, H. (2013). Factors associated with the pressure pain threshold in healthy Chinese men. *Pain Medicine, 14*(9), 1291–1300.

REVIEW AND APPLY YOUR KNOWLEDGE

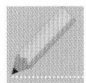 **MATCHING ONE: CONCEPT REVIEW**

Place the letter of the answer next to the number of the term or phrase that best describes it.

A. Acute pain
B. Chronic pain
C. Clinical massage
D. Gate control theory
E. Neuromatrix theory
F. Neuroplasticity
G. Palliative methods
H. Pain
 I. Sensitization
J. Pain tolerance
K. Pain threshold
L. Therapeutic methods

_____ 1. Pain lasting less than 30 days and usually related to injuries, disease, or invasive procedures, such as surgery.

_____ 2. The brain's ability to form and reorganize synaptic connections, especially in response to experience.

_____ 3. Unpleasant sensory and emotional experience associated with, or resembling, actual or potential tissue damage.

_____ 4. Curative measures used to treat diseases, disorders, or injuries.

_____ 5. The *maximum* level of intensity perceived as painful and any more would be unbearable.

_____ 6. Noncurative measures used to improve a patient's quality of life.

_____ 7. Theory stating pain is a multidimensional experience produced by a person's "neurosignature" or unique pattern of nerve impulses within the brain.

_____ 8. Theory that states the spinal cord acts like a neurologic gate and controls if pain signals enter the brain.

_____ 9. Condition of lowering the pain threshold and increased nervous system responsiveness, resulting in pain hypersensitivity.

_____ 10. The *minimum* level of intensity perceived as painful.

_____ 11. Pain that persists past normal healing times and reflects the state of the person's nervous system rather than the condition of the tissues.

_____ 12. Massage used to rehabilitate injuries, manage medically diagnosed conditions, their treatments or complications, and manage issues related to surgery.

MATCHING TWO: CONCEPT REVIEW

Place the letter of the answer next to the number of the term or phrase that best describes it.

A. Maximum medical improvement
B. Pain management
C. Compensatory patterns
D. Local twitch response
E. Hospice care
F. Gait cycle
G. Delayed-onset muscle soreness
H. Myofascial release
 I. Sports massage
J. Antalgic gait
K. Tactical athlete
L. Trigger points

_____ 1. Process of providing care that alleviates or reduces pain to a level of comfort acceptable to a client.

_____ 2. Sequence of events which begins when one foot contacts the ground and ends when the same foot contacts the ground again.

_____ 3. Point in the rehabilitative process when the condition is unlikely to improve and no additional recovery is expected.

_____ 4. Limp adopted to avoid pain on weight-bearing structures and is characterized by walking hesitancy.

_____ 5. Someone in a service profession who has physical fitness and performance requirements associated with their job.

_____ 6. Application of massage techniques to address the needs of athletes in competitive and recreational settings.

_____ 7. Pain or discomfort in skeletal muscles following unaccustomed or strenuous physical activity.

_____ 8. Type of medical service that provides palliative care to patients and their families who are facing a life-limiting illness.

_____ 9. Transient visible or palpable contraction as tense muscle fibers of the TrP contract during pressure application.

_____ 10. Massage technique that uses low-load, long-duration skin stretching.

_____ 11. Hyperirritable tender spots in taut palpable bands within skeletal muscle or its associated fascia and, when pressed, cause pain and/or motor dysfunction and autonomic phenomena.

_____ 12. Conscious or unconscious movements used to correct imbalances and reduce discomfort.

MULTIPLE CHOICE: TEST YOUR KNOWLEDGE

Place the letter of the answer next to the number of the term or phrase that best describes it.

_____ 1. A common location of nonspecific pain is the:
A. elbow
B. ankle
C. wrist
D. lower back

_____ 2. Which is the amount of motion that occurs when one segment of the body moves in relationship to another segment of the body?
A. Range of motion
B. Gait cycle
C. Postural analysis
D. Proprioception

_____ 3. The encoding of a painful event is called:
A. neuromatrix
B. nociception
C. neuroplasticity
D. neurogenic

_____ 4. Which term refers to pain caused by damage to the nervous system?
A. Nociceptive pain
B. Neuropathic pain
C. Nonspecific pain
D. Subacute pain

_____ 5. Which clinical assessment might a practitioner utilize as a plumb line?
A. Range of motion assessment
B. Postural assessment
C. Gait assessment
D. Orthopedic assessment

_____ 6. Which gait disorder is characterized by decreased walking speed, asymmetric step length, and is associated with a stroke?
A. Antalgic
B. Ataxic
C. Hemiplegic
D. Propulsive

_____ 7. Which orthopedic assessment could be used to test for carpal tunnel syndrome?
A. Adson test
B. Roos test
C. Phalen test
D. Spurling test

_____ 8. Which orthopedic assessment could be used to test for anterior cruciate ligament instability?
A. Varus stress test
B. Valgus stress test
C. Anterior drawer test
D. Calf squeeze test

_____ 9. An example of a tactical athlete is a:
A. golfer
B. runner
C. skydiver
D. paramedic

_____ 10. Which type of sports massage occurs between training sessions and usually lasts 30 to 60 minutes?
A. Pre-event
B. Post-event
C. Maintenance
D. Rehabilitation

_____ 11. Which describes a trigger point that does not cause pain until pressed and the client does not recognize it as familiar?
A. Active
B. Latent
C. Satellite
D. Referred

_____ 12. Massage on scars is a local contraindication until the wound has reached the _____ healing stage.
A. hemostasis
B. inflammation
C. proliferation
D. remodeling

CRITICAL THINKING

Lighten Up!

Clients experience pressure from massage subjectively. This means even though the massage practitioner may use exactly the same pressure on two different clients, one client may think it is too light, whereas the other may feel it as painful. Why is this?

Answers can include but are not limited to:

Pain is complex; multifaceted; and includes sensory, emotional, cognitive, and sociocultural components, all of which can influence pain perception. Pain perception is the subjective interpretation of an unpleasant experience. Many factors influence pain perception, including gender; race and ethnicity; age; emotions, including catastrophizing and ruminating; levels of physical activity; obesity; sleep deprivation; cold application; heat application; massage; and preexisting diseases, which include anxiety and depression. The most important risk factor for pain is the presence of another site of pain within the body. Terms frequently used in discussions of pain perception are pain thresholds and pain tolerance levels. Pain threshold is the point at which pain from a stimulus is perceived. Pain tolerance is the point at which any more intensity would be unbearable.

Pain perception can be altered through a phenomenon called sensitization. Sensitization is a condition of a lower pain threshold and increased nervous system responsiveness, which results in pain hypersensitivity. During sensitization, nerves detecting pain are more responsive to stimuli from things that are typically not painful, including a handshake or a hug. Sensitization can be associated with chronic pain and conditions such as fibromyalgia, temporomandibular joint dysfunction, and migraine headaches. The types of sensitization include central and peripheral. Central sensitization is sensitization in the CNS. Peripheral sensitization is sensitization in the PNS. Sensitization may increase the size of a nerve's receptive field, or the area of the body wherein nerves can detect sensations. It is unclear how sensitization occurs, but it may be related to physical or psychological trauma. However, just as the nervous system learns to "turn up" the volume on pain, it can learn ways to turn it down.

PROFESSIONAL PRACTICE

What's Pain Got to Do With It?

Garrett was in a bicycle accident about 10 days ago. He was wearing his helmet. As he fell, the left side of his head struck the side of a mailbox, which stretched the left side of his neck. He did not feel any pain right after the accident, but the next day his head, neck, and right shoulder were in pain. Garrett saw his doctor, who recommended rest and pain medication. This helped, but each morning Garrett felt the pain as intensely as he had the day after the accident.

Audrey, one of Garrett's colleagues, referred him to Baila, a massage practitioner who had helped her. Garrett made an appointment for that day. He told Baila that he felt pain in his right shoulder and neck most of the time and that, 2 days ago, he began to feel tingling in his right arm and hand.

During postural assessments, Baila noticed right lateral flexion of the neck and an elevated right shoulder. When she asked Garrett to flex his neck laterally to the left, he felt sharp pain in the left side of his neck. During palpation, Baila felt dense, hypertonic tissues on the right side of the neck and overstretched weak muscles on the left. She suspected tingling in his right arm may be from hypertonic tissues compressing a nerve, but sharp pain on the left made her wonder about the possibility vertebrae may also have suffered trauma.

At the time Garrett visited Baila, was his pain acute, subacute, or chronic? Should Baila discuss her findings and concerns with Garrett's doctor before initiating massage? Should Baila recommend Garrett return to his doctor for a more thorough medical examination before initiating massage treatments? If she does believe further medical testing is necessary to determine whether any vertebral damage is present, is it acceptable for Baila to rely on her training and experience to treat the spasms and overstretched tissues today? If Baila performs a massage today, should she treat trigger points if she finds them?

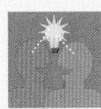

DISCUSSION
Chronic Pain

New studies about chronic pain suggest it may not always be the result of tissue damage. Explain how a person who was in a motor vehicle accident 6 months ago is still experiencing back pain. Which techniques would you use for this client and why? Cite studies in your answer if possible.

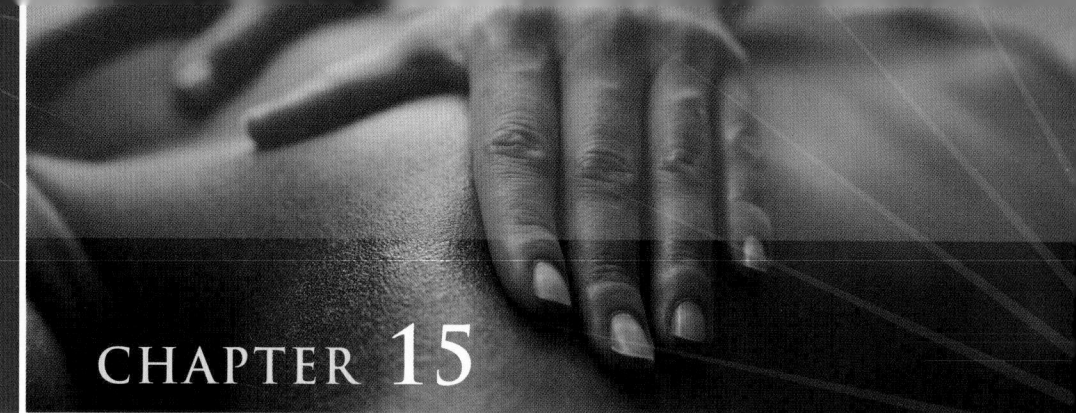

CHAPTER 15

Seated Massage: Principles and Practice

LEARNING OBJECTIVES

After completing this chapter, the student should be able to:

1. Define seated massage and list things to consider when buying a massage chair.
2. Perform preseated massage procedures, a basic seated massage routine, and postseated massage procedures.

INTRODUCTION

Seated massage is performed on a seated, clothed individual usually in an open, public space (Palmer, 2012). Seated massage, or *chair massage,* came to prominence through the efforts of David Palmer, whose vision was to make massage convenient and affordable for anyone, anywhere, and anytime. Palmer introduced seated massage to the corporate world in the early 1980s. Working at large corporations such as Apple, Inc. and Pacific Bell, Palmer developed a unique chair for the client to sit on during the massage. Techniques used during seated massage were derived from an Eastern-style massage called *amma* or *tuina* and a European-style massage, which includes compression, stretching, joint mobilizations, and tapotement or percussion. In 1986, Palmer coined the term *"onsite massage"* and began teaching this method and selling the newly developed massage chair.

Today, seated massage may be done exclusively or incorporated into other methods. Most seated massage is performed while the client sits in a specially designed massage chair mentioned previously, but it may also be performed while the client sits in a regular chair, a stool, or on the ground. Seated massage techniques are also used for clients in wheelchairs or clients in institutional care facilities.

Seated massage techniques do not require massage lubricants, and sessions are typically brief (15 minutes) but can last 30 minutes or longer. The practitioner focuses on the client's areas of complaint, which are typically the back, neck, and shoulders. The cost of seated massage is usually $10 to $20 per session, with the average cost $1 to $2 per minute. Massage practitioners can use seated massage as their primary modality and source of income or as a secondary modality to supplement their income. Enterprising practitioners have brought seated massage to every venue imaginable, including airports, beauty salons, large and small businesses, concerts (public and backstage), chiropractic offices, day spas, numerous events such as fairs and festivals, golf courses, health food stores, hospitals, locker rooms, offices, private practices, retail stores, schools, shopping malls, sporting events, car washes, and even street corners. Massage emergency response teams (MERTs) often use seated massage as their primary treatment protocol. Sponsored by the American Massage Therapy Association, MERTs were deployed during the rescue efforts after the September 11, 2001, terror attack on the World Trade Center and the Pentagon. MERTs were also used on rescue workers and others at the disaster sites including hurricanes Andrew and Katrina.

Performing onsite massage requires planning and knowledge of logistics. For example, parking may be quite a distance away from the location where the onsite massage will occur, requiring a lengthy transportation of the massage chair and supplies. Depending on the location, the massage practitioner may find themself setting up the chair in a tiny space, in the middle of a lobby, or outside, at the mercy of weather. The massage practitioner usually needs to provide

---

BOX 15.1

Onsite Massage Events: What to Bring

- Massage chair (or other seated system)
- Clean reusable or disposable face rest covers, pillowcases, and modesty towel/cloth (for clients who wear skirts)
- Cleaning supplies such as hand sanitizer and disinfectant for chair fabric
- Paper towels, facial tissue, and trash bags
- Clipboard, signup sheets, consent forms, and pens
- Music or white noise source such as mobile device app
- Clock or stopwatch
- Name tags, business cards, and appointment calendar (paper or digital)
- Bank bag and small bills for change, receipt book, and tip jar
- Drinking water and snack foods
- Stool for sitting and pad for kneeling on the floor
- Sunscreen, sunglasses, cap, or hat (if working outdoors)
- Extra set of work clothes
- First aid kit

---

all the supplies for onsite massage and needs to pack them efficiently. A list of items to bring to onsite massage events can be found in Box 15.1.

BUYING A MASSAGE CHAIR

Massage chairs can be purchased through massage table manufacturers. Primary features of a massage chair include the seat, knee, and chest pads, the arm shelf, and the face rest (Fig. 15.1). Purchase a massage chair from reputable, well-established manufacturers because they tend to provide superior customer service and offer a trial period so the chair can be returned for a full refund if the buyer is not satisfied. They also sell accessories to accompany their chairs. The

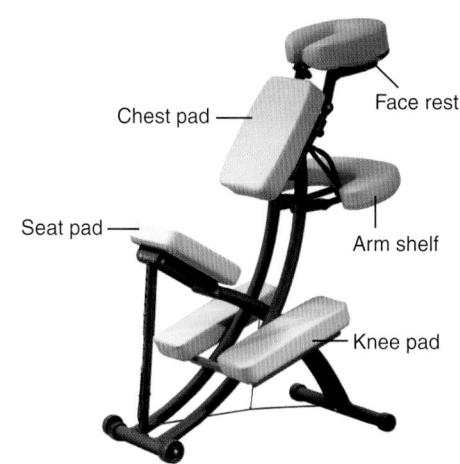

FIG. 15.1 A massage chair with features labeled. (Courtesy Oakworks Massage Tables.)

following factors should be kept in mind when selecting a massage chair:

- **Stability**. A creaky or wobbly chair may make clients feel anxious and unsafe. The arm shelf should be strong enough to withstand deep pressure techniques performed on a client's forearms.
- **Transportability**. The chair should be lightweight and easy to transport because it will be moved to different locations.
- **Operability**. The chair should be set up and taken down quickly and easily.
- **Adjustability**. The chair should be adjustable to fit a variety of body shapes and sizes but not so many that time is spent making unnecessary adjustments. For example, the position of the arm shelf should be high enough off the floor so the client is comfortable, and the practitioner can maintain efficient body mechanics when massaging the client's forearms and hands. However, only one or two quick adjustments, not three or four, should be needed to put the arm shelf in place.

New premium massage chairs cost $500 and up. Economically priced massage chairs range from $150 to $250. If seated massage is performed only occasionally (a few times a year), an economical chair may suffice so long as it is well constructed and structurally sound. Some manufacturers offer desktop face support, which can be clamped to or balanced on the edge of a counter, table, or desk with a chest pad hanging vertically over the edge (see Fig. 11.21).

PRESEATED MASSAGE PROCEDURES

Conduct a client health assessment and establish a treatment plan to address your client's treatment goals (see Chapter 10). As a precautionary measure, do not use deep or vigorously applied massage techniques on individuals who are frail or who have bone or joint pathologies, including osteoporosis, spondylolysis, spinal stenosis, and bone cancer (Guo et al., 2013; Wang et al., 2014; Wu et al., 2010).

Ensure the area where the seated massage will take place is wide enough to allow the practitioner to move completely around the chair. If the chair was transported in a carrying case, place it away from the massage area to reduce fall risks for you and the client. Be prepared to cover and/or disinfect all components that directly contact the client's skin. Cover the face rest cushion with a clean fabric or disposable face rest cover, or a paper towel. Cover the arm shelf with a clean fabric or disposable cover or wipe the shelf with disinfecting agent.

Instruct the client on how to sit in the chair properly by demonstration and verbal explanation using specific directions such as, "Sit on the seat and place your knees and legs on these cushions while resting your forearms on the arm shelf and your face in the crescent-shaped pillow."

Make any adjustments to the chair before the massage begins. Primary adjustments are (1) the seat height, (2) chest pad height, (3) face rest height and angle, and (4) arm shelf height (Fig. 15.2). Clients will typically arch their backs or

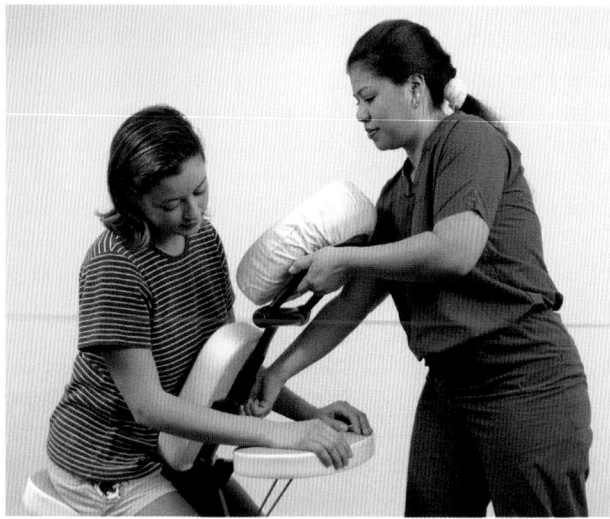

FIG. 15.2 The massage practitioner makes adjustments to the height of the face rest and chest pad before the massage begins. Chair adjustments are tailored to the individual client.

slump over if the chair is not adjusted properly for their height. The client's back should be straight with the shoulders relaxed and not elevated. The face rest frame should be positioned with the neck slightly flexed. Once chair adjustments are complete, ask clients if additional adjustments are needed to provide maximum comfort. Wash and dry your hands before the massage begins (see Chapter 9).

If massaging seated clients using a regular chair and not a massage chair, use a *tripod position*.

This position helps ensure the client's body is supported during seated massage and promotes ease of breathing. An unsupported seated position is not recommended, as clients would tire easily from providing counterbalance. The three parts of the tripod in the seated position are:

1. Feet on the floor;
2. Buttocks on the chair seat or bed; and
3. Hands or elbows on the thighs, or a table (see Fig. 7.15).

The area of the seated massage may be noisy. Establish a nonverbal communication method such as hand gestures before the massage begins. For example, ask clients to raise a hand if they are experiencing discomfort from massage pressure, which will be responded to immediately. A 5-point pressure scale can be used and indicated by the number of fingers extended on a raised hand. In this situation, one extended finger represents light pressure, three fingers represent moderate pressure, and five fingers represent deep or uncomfortable pressure. In most cases, pressure should be maintained between three and four (Turkeltaub et al., 2014) (Fig. 15.3).

Be culturally sensitive when using hand gestures during a seated massage, as what is meant by someone from the United States may be interpreted differently by someone from different regions of the globe. For example, the "thumbs-up" symbol in the United States is a sign of approval, but in the Middle East, it means to "stick it where the sun does not shine." The "okay" sign means satisfactory

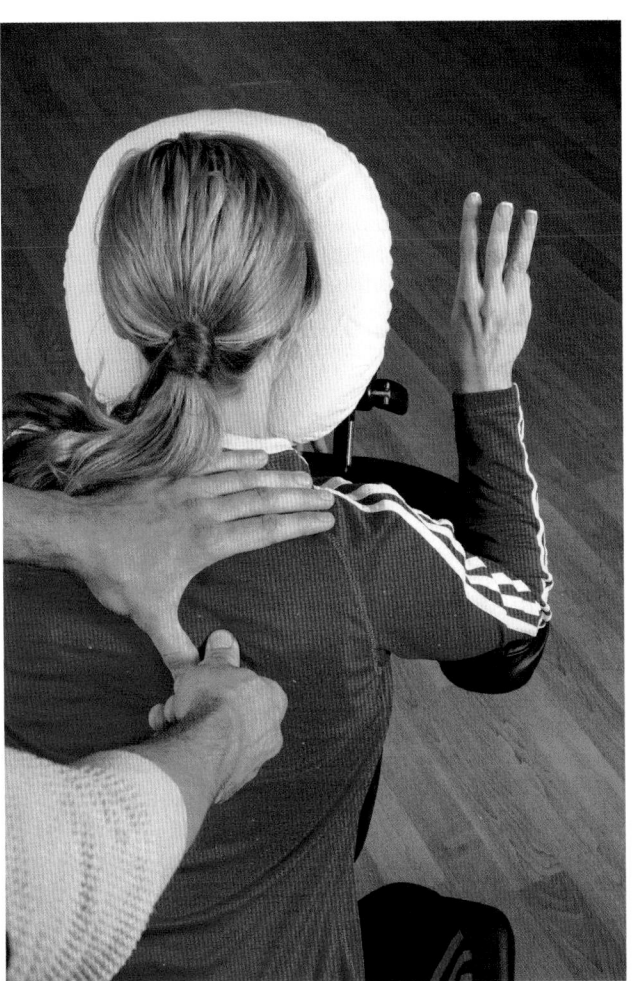

FIG. 15.3 Client raising three fingers to indicate the level of pressure sensitivity.

in the United States but signifies money in Japan, zero/worthless in France, and the equivalent of sticking up your middle finger in Brazil.

Ultimately, your only source of funding is satisfied clients.

—Tim Mullen

SEATED MASSAGE ROUTINE

The following routine can be completed in approximately 15 minutes. Spend more time on the client's areas of complaint. Gentle stretches or passive range of motion (PROM) can also be incorporated into the seated massage routine. Stretches for the forearm, wrist, and hand can be done while clients lean forward in the massage chair. Neck and shoulder stretches can be done while clients sit up straight in the chair.

Upper Back and Neck

Begin with massage techniques such as compression so clients will be familiar with your touch and establish their individual pain threshold while receiving massage pressure. With pressure preferences noted, apply compression to the paraspinal muscles using the heels of the hands or loosely clenched fists. Next, move inferiorly a hand width at a time starting between the scapulas and ending just above the ilium of the pelvis. Then move back superiorly a hand width at a time until you return to the starting point. Repeat on the other side.

Next, stand directly behind the client at the center of their back. With your arms outstretched, a slight bend in the elbows, apply compression to both sides of the paraspinals simultaneously using the heels of both hands. If this movement is uncomfortable to your wrists, change to a loosely clenched fist. Repeat this pattern but apply deep circular friction using loosely clenched fists. Make four to eight circles with each hand, working up and down the paraspinals. Periodically ask clients how they are feeling. Adjust pressure as needed.

Move to the client's side and petrissage (knead) the muscles within the cervical laminar groove moving from the occipital bone to the shoulders using lighter pressure—the thumb and second finger can be used for this technique (Fig. 15.4). Then reverse direction. **NOTE**: When the client's face is in the face rest, the neck is unsupported. The cervical region is the most mobile region of the spine (Neumann, 2010), which makes this area vulnerable to injury from external forces, especially deep perpendicular pressure. Therefore, the posterior neck is massaged using lighter pressure while the client is in the chair using the face rest.

Use deep circular frictions with the heel of your hand or fingertips on the trapezius and rhomboids between the spinous processes and medial border of the scapulae. Use one hand to support the anterior aspect of the shoulder while using the other hand to massage the area. If this area is one of the client's areas of complaint, spend more time here. You can use your thumb or guided elbow for additional pressure. For broader, less specific pressure, use the blade of the ulna. Apply more precise pressure by flexing the elbow so only the olecranon process is in contact with the tissue. Use your other hand to guide and stabilize the elbow (Fig. 15.5). When massage to this area is complete, move lateral to the shoulder and apply circular frictions to the tendons of the rotator cuff muscles.

Apply circular friction to the area below the scapulae using the heels of the hands, working both sides of the spine. This action addresses the latissimus dorsi and paraspinals.

Lower Back

Palpate the client's waistline, being careful not to elicit a tickle response. After locating the lateral end of the 12th rib, apply deep friction with your thumbs or the heel of your hand along its inferior surface. Using circular friction, massage the edges of the lumbar spine in the transverse processes. Use deep circular friction in thumb width increments from L1 to the iliac crest. Change direction of pressure and massage the superior surface of the iliac crest laterally to the

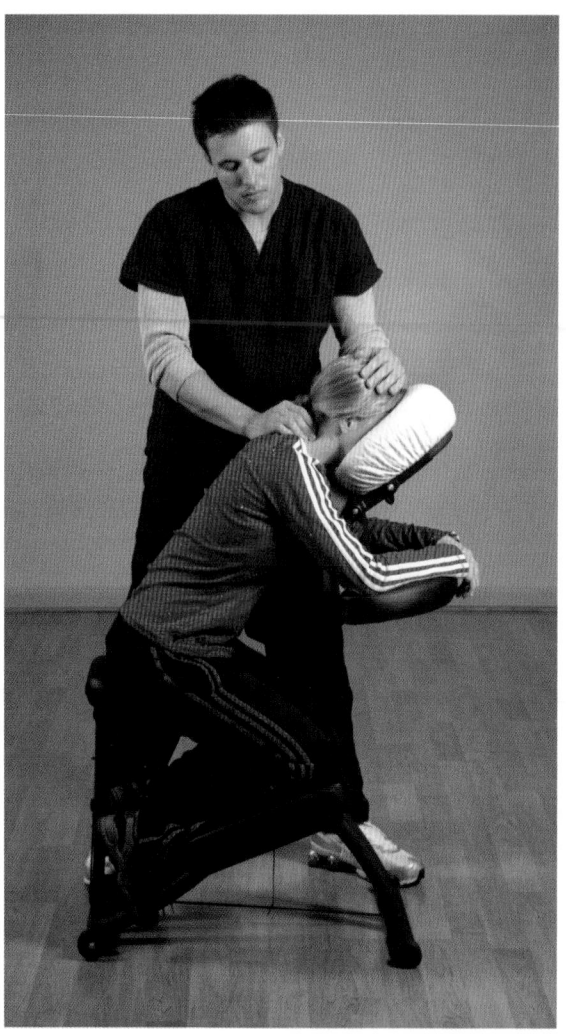

FIG. 15.4 Massage practitioner massaging muscles in the cervical laminar groove.

midline of the body. This action addresses the quadratus lumborum in the lower back.

The lower portion of the paraspinals can now be massaged more thoroughly using fingertips, thumbs, or guided elbows. Treat one side at a time with deep circular or cross-fiber friction, using sustained pressure on tender areas. Apply friction from medial to lateral, allowing the client to rock slightly in the chair. If clients do not like the rocking motion for any reason, discontinue it immediately and use a different technique.

Upper Extremity

Use petrissage, rolling, jostling, nerve strokes, or compressions to massage arm muscles such as biceps and triceps. Facing the front of the chair and slightly to one side, place the client's forearm with the palm down on the arm shelf to massage the posterior forearm muscles. Apply compression to the extensor group with the heel of your hand, working from wrist to elbow (Fig. 15.6). Repeat this sequence three times, then rotate the palm up and apply three sets of compression to the flexor group. Reposition the palm down and use circular friction applied with the heel of your hand. Work from wrist to elbow in 1- to 2-inch intervals, using 5 to 10 circles on each spot. Repeat this sequence three times. Turn the client's palm up again and repeat the circular friction sequence on the flexor group.

Apply circular friction to all sides of the wrist using your thumbs. Grasp the client's hand, shake out the upper extremity, and return it to the arm shelf. Repeat the entire sequence on the other upper extremity.

Face and Scalp

Using the tips or pads of the fingers, apply circular friction to the temples, jaw, face, and forehead (Fig. 15.7). During

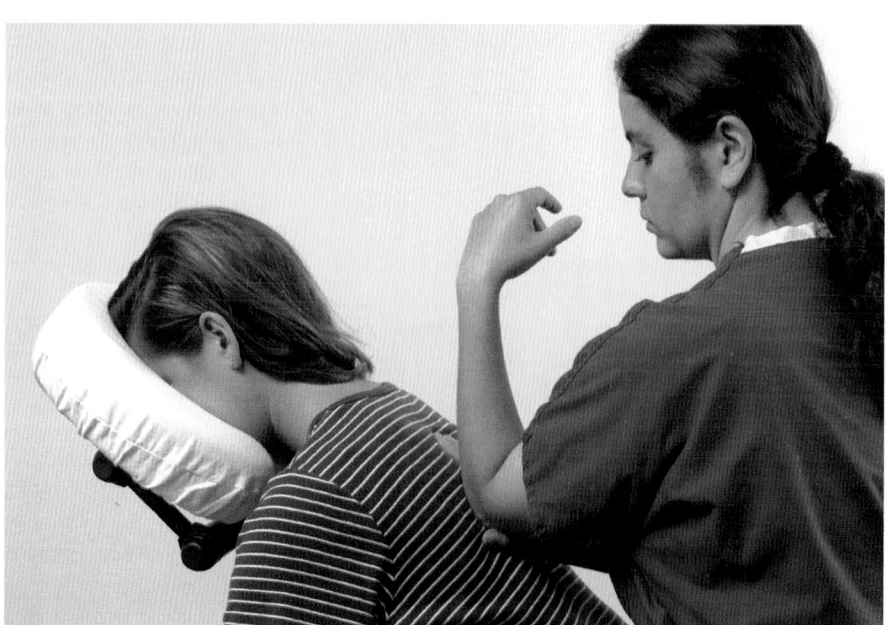

FIG. 15.5 Guided elbow technique. Pressure can become deeper and more specific by flexing the elbow. Notice how the practitioner uses the opposite hand to guide and stabilize the elbow.

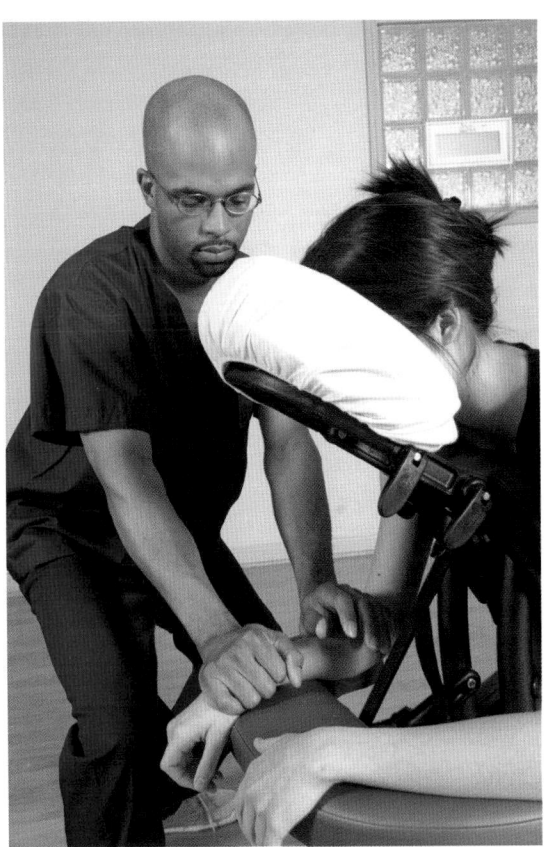

FIG. 15.6 Massage practitioner applying compression to the extensor group on the client's posterior forearm.

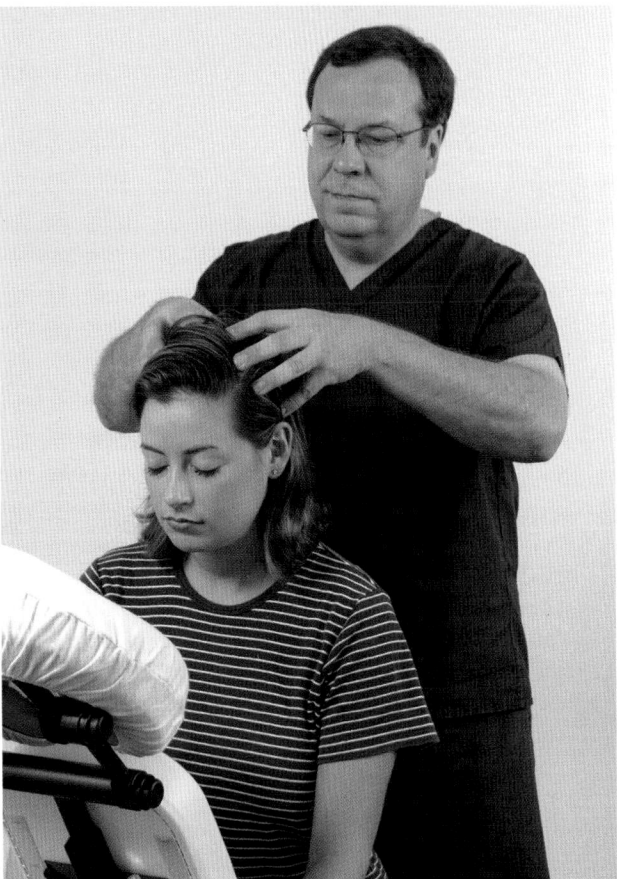

FIG. 15.7 The massage practitioner can use the fingertips to apply circular friction to the scalp.

scalp massage, the tissue can be shifted back and forth across the skull using friction in any direction. Gentle tapping or pincement is appropriate on the scalp, especially as part of your closing techniques. Although facial and scalp massage can feel great while in a chair, some clients do not want their hair or makeup disturbed, so obtain consent first.

Closing Techniques

As the seated massage session concludes, return to more generalized massage techniques such as compression. If the goal is to leave the client relaxed, finish with some general effleurage (gliding) and slowly applied nerve strokes on the back and shoulders. If the client is returning to work and needs to be more alert, finish with tapotement, superficial friction, and briskly applied nerve strokes. Tapping tapotement on the head and hacking or loose fist beating on the shoulders and back, and over the hips and lateral thighs, are stimulating ways to finish the massage.

POSTSEATED MASSAGE PROCEDURES

Tell the client the massage is over and ask them to get off the chair slowly and carefully. Be sure your client has all their personal items such as eyeglasses, keys, or mobile devices. After you collect your fees and thank the client for their time, state you hope the massage was beneficial and to consider recommending seated massage to others. Have business cards available and schedule another appointment if requested by the client. Wash and dry your hands, disinfect the chair fabric, complete documentation notes, take a few deep breaths, and get ready for the next client.

E-RESOURCES

http://evolve.elsevier.com/Salvo/MassageTherapy

- Chapter challenge
- Flash cards
- Video 15-1: Seated Massage

DAVID PALMER

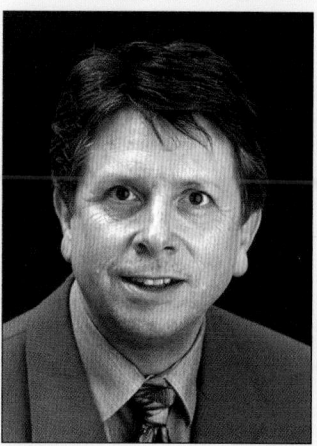

Touch is for everyone. For the rich and the poor. The busy and the bored. The shy and the outgoing. But what we think of as a standard massage session (let us say an hour long), Swedish massage in a private office business setting is not always accessible—to people who cannot get away from work for an entire hour; to people who cannot afford it; to people without transportation; or to people who, for personal or religious reasons, are not okay with being unclothed, even with impeccable draping.

Enter chair massage. It is quick, it is inexpensive, and it can take place anywhere. Chair massage is quickly becoming ubiquitous. You can find it in airports, at the mall, at staff appreciation events, even at the farmers' market. This was not an accident. It is due entirely to the personal mission of one man: David Palmer.

Palmer was born in 1947, and his massage career began in 1980. He ended up as the director of a massage institute specializing in Eastern-style massage. He quickly realized there was a disconnect between what the massage professionals wanted to provide and what kind of massage people were interested in receiving. It was difficult to convince people that paying quite a bit of money to enter a private room, remove all their clothing, and be rubbed with oils by a relative stranger was not a creepy activity, much less a worthwhile endeavor. The lack of touch in American culture led to people being frightened of such a thing. Palmer states: "They were selling a graduate-level understanding of the field of touch to a population who had not even begun kindergarten regarding touch." It might have been just what the public needed, but it was extremely difficult to sell.

The solution? Make it quick, public, and affordable. How frightening would massage be if performed on a fully clothed client, seated in a chair, right out in the open? In 1983, Palmer decided to design a special chair just for this purpose. He took the idea of a slanted chair with leg rests he had seen and added a head rest

and chest support. He enlisted a French cabinetmaker as his partner, and in 1986, the first massage chair was available for sale.

Not content with simply providing the tools, Palmer began teaching chair massage techniques. He founded Touch-Pro International, which teaches a specific form of chair massage, inspired by acupressure, which is not only beneficial to clients, but also protects the practitioner by promoting excellent body mechanics. Former AMTA President Scott Lamp said of Palmer: "David may not have been the first to discover chair massage, but, like Columbus, there is no doubt he was the first to put it on the map."

Palmer's work, like many people with a strong vision, has not been without controversy in the massage field. Some feel the availability of an inexpensive chair massage will lower the amount of money people are willing to pay massage practitioners. His opinion that a simple chair massage does not require the practitioner to receive as much education as a clinical massage practitioner providing table work has sparked many debates. Still, Palmer has stayed true to his principles. He confesses, "I'm one of those unreformed 1960s brats who thinks it's still possible to change the world."

Palmer's vision for the future? "To make touch a positive social value in our culture." He says, "Parents are afraid to touch their kids; teachers cannot touch their students; it's crazy out there. My feeling is we need to shift that around, and massage is a vehicle for doing that because it provides structured touch."

And the world seems to agree. Chair massage is a quickly growing field. Most massage schools now include chair massage in their curricula. David Palmer teaches, speaks, and writes extensively, and he is universally known as "the father of chair massage." Whether you dream of owning a soothing spa or working in a medical clinic, do not for a second underestimate the power of chair massage. Because it is true the world can always use a little bit more touch.

REFERENCES

Guo, Z., Chen, W., Su, Y., Yuan, J., & Zhang, Y. (2013). Isolated unilateral vertebral pedicle fracture caused by a back massage in an elderly patient: A case report and literature review. *European Journal of Orthopaedic Surgery & Traumatology, 23*(Suppl. 2), S149–S153.

Neumann, D. A. (2010). *Kinesiology of the musculoskeletal system: Foundations for rehabilitation* (2nd ed.). St. Louis: Elsevier.

Palmer, D. (2012). *On the side of angels.* Retrieved from https://touchpro.com/821/.

Turkeltaub, P. C., Yearwood, E. L., Friedmann, E. (2014). Effect of a brief seated massage on nursing student attitudes toward touch for comfort care. *Journal of Alternative and Complementary Medicine, 20*(10), 792–729.

Wang, J. Y., Wu, P. K., Chen, P., Yen, C. C., Hung, G. Y., Chen, C. F., et al. (2014). Manipulation therapy prior to diagnosis

induced primary osteosarcoma metastasis: From clinical to basic research. *PLoS One, 9*(5), e96571.

Wu, P. K., Chen, W. M., Lee, O. K., Chen, C. F., Huang, C. K., & Chen, T. H. (2010). The prognosis for patients with osteosarcoma who have received prior manipulative therapy. *The Journal of Bone and Joint Surgery, 92*(11), 1580–1585.

REVIEW AND APPLY YOUR KNOWLEDGE

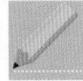

MATCHING: CONCEPT REVIEW

Place the letter of the answer next to the number of the term or phrase that best describes it.

A. Hand gestures
B. Amma or tuina
C. Primary massage chair adjustments
D. Convenient and affordable
E. Palmer
F. Demonstrate and explain how to sit in the chair properly
G. Factors to consider when selecting a massage chair
H. Massage lubricant
I. Osteoporosis
J. Seated or chair massage
K. Tripod position
L. 15 to 30 minutes

_____ 1. Massage techniques performed on a seated, clothed individual usually in an open, public space.

_____ 2. Stability, transportability, operability, and adjustability.

_____ 3. Product not required for seated massage techniques.

_____ 4. What practitioners should do before clients sit in their massage chairs.

_____ 5. Typical length of a seated massage treatment.

_____ 6. Position that supports seated clients when the practitioner is using a regular chair and not a massage chair.

_____ 7. Reasons why seated massage may appeal to clients, according to Palmer.

_____ 8. Can be used in noisy environments to indicate sensitivity to pressure.

_____ 9. Eastern-style massage from which many chair massage techniques were derived.

_____ 10. Persons with this condition should not receive deep or vigorously applied massage techniques during seated massage.

_____ 11. Individual who introduced seated massage in the workplace in the early 1980s.

_____ 12. Seat height, chest pad height, face rest height and angle, and arm shelf height.

MULTIPLE CHOICE: TEST YOUR KNOWLEDGE

Place the letter of the answer next to the number of the term or phrase that best describes it.

_____ 1. David Palmer coined which term?
  A. Seated massage
  B. Preseated massage
  C. Onsite massage
  D. Chair massage

_____ 2. Most seated massage is performed while the client sits:
  A. in a massage chair.
  B. in a regular chair.
  C. on a stool.
  D. on the ground.

_____ 3. Which of the following is true of seated massage?
  A. Lubricant is required
  B. Clients fully disrobe
  C. Sessions are typically brief
  D. Sessions are typically in private

_____ 4. The average cost of a seated massage is:
  A. $1 to 2 per minute
  B. $5 per minute
  C. $7 per minute
  D. $10 per minute

_____ 5. Which describes a massage chair's ability to be set up and taken down quickly and easily?
  A. Stability
  B. Sustainability
  C. Operability
  D. Adjustability

_____ 6. Which describes a massage chair's ability to fit a variety of body shapes and sizes?
  A. Stability
  B. Sustainability
  C. Operability
  D. Adjustability

_____ 7. Which factor may require the establishment of a nonverbal communication before the massage begins?
  A. The noise level of the environment.
  B. The need for ample setup time.
  C. The lack of privacy.
  D. The difficulty of the techniques.

_____ 8. If a client is sitting in a regular chair and not a massage chair, which of the following is recommended?
   A. tripod
   B. prone
   C. supine
   D. fowler

_____ 9. Seated massage routines are well-suited to address which of the following areas?
   A. Lower legs
   B. Upper back
   C. Abdominals
   D. Pectorals

_____ 10. A typical seated massage begins with work in which region?
   A. Hips
   B. Scalp
   C. Hands
   D. Shoulders

_____ 11. A closing technique on the scalp might include:
   A. effleurage.
   B. petrissage.
   C. gentle tapping.
   D. decompression.

_____ 12. How frequently should the massage chair be disinfected?
   A. Once a day
   B. Once an hour
   C. Between each client
   D. Between each location

CRITICAL THINKING

Chair Massage to the Rescue

Clara is working as an independent contractor for a local massage office. Because she is the newest massage practitioner there, she does not have as many clients as the other practitioners yet and wants to work on building her client base. She has been considering buying a massage chair and doing onsite massage to complement her practice at the local massage office. What are the realities of this approach for Clara?

Answers can include but are not limited to:

A massage chair may be less expensive than a massage table, so it is a lower cost of equipment investment. Clara may also be able to borrow or rent a massage chair instead. There are many different settings in which a chair massage can be performed, so Clara has a variety from which to choose. Because clients are fully clothed, they may be more receptive to chair massage than table massage, and the cost for the treatment is less. However, Clara could use the treatment as an opportunity to ask clients to consider seeing her for a table massage at her massage office.

Clara will need to purchase a massage chair and the supplies needed to perform onsite massage. She will need to do research for events at which to perform chair massage, and she may need to pay a fee to attend the event. Clara will also need to market chair massage to various types of companies who may or may not be receptive to it. She needs to be fully aware of all the logistics of setting up and performing chair massage onsite.

PROFESSIONAL PRACTICE

Seated Massage During Pregnancy

Cyndi saw her obstetrician a few days ago because she has been feeling fatigued. She's 40 years old and going to give birth to her first child in 3 months. During her visit, Dr. Grayson noticed her patient fidgeting, clenching her fists, and having a stressed look on her face. She took her blood pressure for a second time and, as she suspected, Cyndi's blood pressure was slightly higher than at the beginning of the visit. Cyndi's obstetrician referred her to a massage practitioner with training in pregnancy massage. She suggested a weekly massage could help relax her nerves and keep her blood pressure in a healthy range.

Cyndi's employer recently began a wellness program allowing each employee to have two 10-minute chair massages each month at the employer's expense. Cyndi learns the practitioner hired by her employer is not certified in prenatal massage. Should Cyndi opt for chair massage? If so, how often and of what duration? What considerations need to be made for positioning Cyndi on the chair? Does the practitioner need clearance from Dr. Grayson?

DISCUSSION

Table Versus Chair

When would a seated massage be more advantageous over table massage? Be sure your discussion includes types of conditions, life stages, and clinical settings. If available, post your reflections on an Internet-based discussion board monitored by your instructor.

I would like to thank Ralph Stephens for his prior contributions on this chapter.

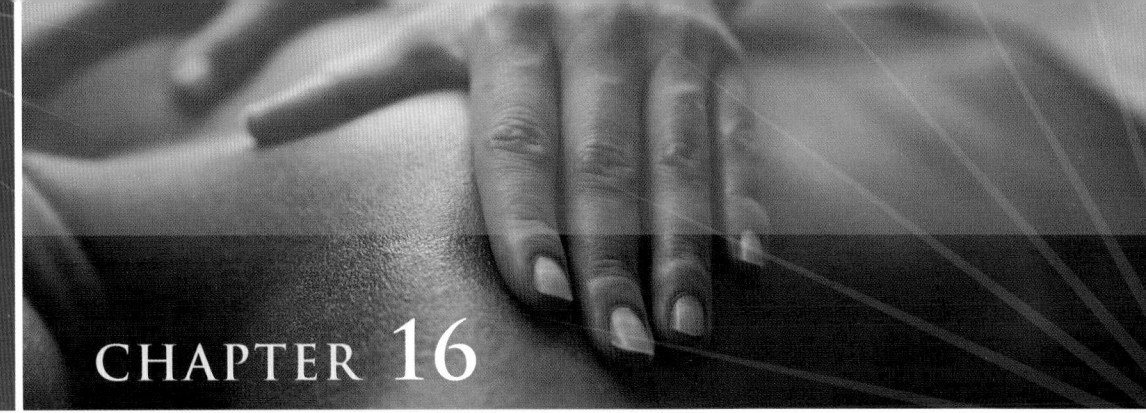

CHAPTER 16

Asian Bodywork Therapy: Shiatsu, Thai Massage, and Ayurvedic Principles

Experience is the hardest kind of teacher. It gives you the test first and the lesson afterward.

—Anonymous

LEARNING OBJECTIVES

After completing this chapter, the student should be able to:

1. Define Asian bodywork therapy and describe the five phases or elements, the channels, and ways to assess energetic imbalances.
2. Discuss shiatsu, Zen shiatsu, Thai massage, Ayurvedic principles, and the chakras and their characteristics.

INTRODUCTION

Many massage methods originated in various regions of Asia (e.g., China, Japan, India, Thailand) and have developed under the influences of many great teachers. Asian bodywork therapy (ABT) is a profession with nationally recognized standards of education. Although many ABT methods exist (Jin Shin Do, tuina, etc.), this chapter provides an overview of ABT, with a focus on shiatsu, Thai massage, Ayurvedic principles, and chakras. These methods can be easily incorporated into a massage practice. However, an exclusive practice of ABT requires training and guidance from experienced instructors. Should the material presented in this chapter stimulate your curiosity, seek further training to expand your knowledge.

ASIAN BODYWORK THERAPY

ABT is the use of pressure and/or soft tissue manipulation to treat the body, mind, and spirit, including the electromagnetic or energetic fields in and surrounding the body. ABT is based upon traditional Chinese medical principles for assessing the body's energetic system and uses traditional Asian techniques to balance this energetic system for the promotion, maintenance, and restoration of health (American Organization for Bodywork Therapies of Asia [AOBTA], n.d.). Traditional Chinese medicine (TCM) may include the use of acupuncture, herbs, essential oils, exercise (e.g., tai chi, qi gong), dietary principles, moxibustion (use of heat from burning an herb called mugwort or moxa placed over or on the skin to stimulate acupoints), gua sha (a skin-scraping technique), and cupping therapy (plastic, silicone, or glass cups placed on the skin to create a suction and lift the tissue). In addition, liniments, compresses, and herbal baths can be used. *Consult your state laws to be sure you are within your scope of practice before using any of these methods on your clients.*

Vital Energy (Ki, Chi, Qi, and Prana)

Vital energy, or life force, creates and connects all things and all phenomena existing in the universe. This includes everything that manifests physically in nature and in the human body, including emotions, thoughts, and spirit. This energy, also called **ki** (Japanese [pronounced "chee"]), **chi** or **qi** (Chinese [also pronounced "chee"]), **prana**, and sometimes *ojas* (Sanskrit [pronounced "o-juss"]). Ki demonstrates itself as movement and vibration. Solid material and inanimate objects have a vibration observed at a microscopic level in the vibration and movement of atoms. Electrons spin around protons, and they constantly collide against each other and other atoms, releasing energy. The force of attraction and repulsion between the protons and electrons and the spaces between them are also manifestations of energy in the form of magnetic fields. The human body also generates a magnetic field that can be measured.

Studies done on particles of light have shown any given particle can be observed as a particle of matter or a wave of energy at the same time. This interchangeability between matter and wave (nonmatter) introduces the concept of relativity, which is further expanded in the field of quantum physics. This concept provides a model for the theories of Asian medicine and ABT.

Pauline Sasaki, a disciple of the renowned teacher Shizuto Masunaga and the creator of quantum shiatsu, describes the observable energetic phenomena as variations in the speed of vibration in which material aspects have the slowest speed of vibration (and therefore are easier to see with the naked eye) and spiritual aspects have the fastest. The faster the vibration is, the harder it is to observe its manifestations, although by increasing the development of our sensory system, we may be able to sense them. We can observe the effects of these faster vibrations in electricity; although we cannot see electricity itself, we can feel a current running through our bodies when we experience an electrical shock.

Yin and Yang

The text *Yellow Emperor's Classic of Internal Medicine* is highly regarded in Chinese medicine. It dates from 300 to 100 BCE. It is here theories of yin and yang are first mentioned and the model for the creation of ki is provided. The **Tai Ji** symbol represents yin and yang formed by a complete circle divided into two sides symbolizing duality, or the dynamic struggle between opposites. Tai Ji means "supreme ultimate" or "grand terminus." One side of the circle is black, and one side is white, each containing a smaller circle of the opposite color, symbolizing the nonabsolute quality of all things (Fig. 16.1). The four main aspects of yin and yang are (1) opposite yet relative, (2) interdependent, (3) mutually consuming, and (4) intertransforming.

The two sides of the Tai Ji move toward each other in a circular motion, which is a representation of all life processes. During the day (yang), the light of the sun decreases to make way for the darkness of night (yin), and night comes to end by bringing light (yang) into the darkness (yin). The constant movement of one thing into its opposite is what generates ki. In this example, a moment of the day exists, after sunset or before sunrise, called *twilight,* when it is difficult to tell whether it is day or night. Day and night are relative to each other and also relative to where the observer is placed. Another example is how one season transforms

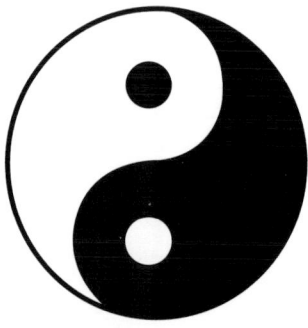

FIG. 16.1 Tai Ji symbol of yin and yang formed by a complete circle divided into two sides.

into the next—winter into spring, spring into summer, and so forth. Even in the utmost yin of winter, there is a seed of yang, as shown by dormant seeds within the earth waiting for spring. Even in the utmost yang of summer, there is a seed of yin, as shown by the stillness creatures tend to have on the hottest days of summer.

In Chinese, yin and yang literally mean "the dark or shadow side of the hill" and "the light or sunny side of the hill," respectively. The Tai Ji poetically and graphically represents a dynamic observed in the duality of the day-night or lightness–darkness cycle and in all aspects of nature. The **yang**, or sunny side of the hill, has more light, warmth, and activity, and so movement exists. Plants grow easily and have foliage and seeds attracting insects and birds. The **yin**, or shadowy side of the hill, is darker, the temperature is cooler, plants grow more slowly, more dampness can be found, and less overall activity exists compared with the sunny side. Male and female, up and down, inside and outside, slow and fast, matter and energy, passive and active, contraction and expansion are just some of the yin and yang pairs. When comparing yin and yang qualities, remember one is not better than the other and one is not necessarily right and the other wrong. They are simply different aspects of the same oneness or ki manifestation (Table 16.1). They mutually create and balance each

other; thus, one is necessary for the other to exist. They have equal value relative to one another and are essentially two sides of the same coin. In this way, health is a dynamic equilibrium between yin and yang.

In ABT, a symptom such as pain can be assessed energetically as either predominantly yin or predominantly yang and treated accordingly. Pain as a manifestation of a *yang* imbalance is a feeling of heat, agitation, and restlessness; the area appears red, is warm to the touch, and feels hard and inflamed. The pain is often sharp, can move around, and is frequently found in the upper part of the body. The person may feel additional pain if the affected area is touched. Pain as a manifestation of a *yin* imbalance is a feeling of cold, weakness, weight, and lethargy; the pain is dull rather than sharp and feels deep. The skin is discolored or dark, and it feels good to the client if the area is touched directly. Yang type of pain can be observed in acute phases of injury; yin type of pain can be observed in chronic and prolonged phases of a disease.

If a person is living with persistent physical pain, over time they will become emotional, impatient, angry, or depressed, which are emotional aspects. Also affected are the client's self-perception, ability to succeed in life's pursuits, and outlook on life, which are mental aspects. Even the person's relationships with others and with the universe, which are social and spiritual aspects, will be affected.

A yang imbalance would be addressed with soothing (yin) techniques to help disperse excess energy. For a yin imbalance, it is desirable to bring in more movement (yang) to break up the stagnation of energy or tone up or strengthen the deficiency or weaknesses. Using some of the opposite qualities helps restore the movement between yin and yang. This method will help the client regain balance.

All of me, why not take all of me.

—**Billie Holiday**

The Five Phases or Five Elements

The **five phases**, or *five elements*, refer to wood, fire, earth, metal, and water, and are used to describe nature and individuals. Each phase, or element, has particular characteristics and interacts with other phases in important ways. The term *phases* is preferred because it describes dynamic rather than static states of energy.

The five phases are correlated with different stages of the biologic cycle, including birth, growth, climax, decay, and death. Other correlations are seasons of the year (with the fifth season being late summer, or the transition between summer and fall); bodily organs; sense organs; bodily secretions; colors; flavors; smells; and sounds; times of the day; emotions; and body–mind–spirit function. The five phases also illustrate how energy behaves at different stages. Each phase influences and is influenced by the other phases. Health is an expression in which all five phases are in harmony with each other.

It is important to note everyone has all five phases within them. Although one phase tends to be more dominant, paying

TABLE 16.1 Relative Correspondences of Yin and Yang	
YIN	**YANG**
Feminine	Masculine
Dark	Light
Cold (numb)	Hot (inflamed)
Moist	Dry
Interior	Exterior
Chronic	Acute
Anterior	Posterior
Medial	Lateral
Inferior	Superior
Community	Competition
Earth	Heaven
Water	Fire
Moon	Sun
Slow (still, lethargic)	Fast (restless, energetic)
Static, storing, conserving	Transforming, changing
Substantial	Nonsubstantial
Matter	Energy
Soft, mushy tissue	Hard, congested tissue
Concave	Convex
Passive (inhibited)	Active (excited)
Pale tongue	Red tongue
Thin pulse	Full pulse
Contraction	Expansion
Deficiency	Excess
Pain is dull, achy, stiff	Pain is sharp or moving
Deep	Shallow (on the surface)
Client says "Mm-mm-mm."	Client says "Ouch!"

TABLE 16.2 Five Phases (Elements) Correspondences

ELEMENT	ORGAN SYSTEMS	SEASON	COLOR	SENSE ORGAN	FUNCTION	EMOTION
Fire	HT/SI	Summer	Red	Tongue	Emotional stability	Joy
	HP/TH				Assimilation Circulation Protection	
Earth	SP/ST	Late summer	Yellow	Mouth	Digestion Nourishment Support	Pensiveness
Metal	LU/LI	Autumn	White	Nose	Respiration Intake of ki Letting go (LI)	Grief
Water	KID/BL	Winter	Black/dark blue	Ears	Store essence Impetus	Fear
Wood	LIV/GB	Spring	Green	Eyes	Gather ki for decisive action	Anger Frustration

HT/SI, Heart, Small Intestine; *HP/TH,* Heart Protector, Triple Heater; *KID/BL,* Kidney, Bladder; *LIV/GB,* Liver, Gallbladder; *LU/LI,* Lung, Large Intestine; *SP/ST,* Spleen-Pancreas, Stomach.

attention to the other phases is equally important to maintain balance in life. See Table 16.2 for a list of associations and correspondences of the five phases.

Wood

The wood phase is associated with exuberance and fast growth observed in the spring as seeds sprout, new shoots appear on branches of trees, and activity that decreases during the winter suddenly picks up. Green, the color of foliage at its peak, is the color associated with the wood phase. People also react to the influence of the spring; the wood phase is observed in the renewed hope and bursts of energy often experienced with the first sunny days after a long winter. Strong winds are common in spring, and so wind is associated with the wood phase and is recognized as an element of its influence. In a person, this dynamism can be observed as the emotional irritation developing when exposed to a draft of air for a long time. In addition, a burst of anger has similar behavior to a burst of wind. It pushes and may break things for a few moments then suddenly disappear—the same as when anger calms down once it has been vented (from Latin *ventus,* meaning "wind").

The wood organ systems are (1) Liver—stockpile or store ki for decisive action and to distribute ki where it is needed, and (2) Gallbladder—govern decision making and store and excrete bile. People who have a lot of wood element in their makeup tend to be athletic and in charge. For example, an Olympic triathlete most likely has a lot of the wood element, as do chief executives of Fortune 500 companies. Sour flavor and the craving for oils and fats can also be related to wood.

Frustration, which can be repressed anger, is also associated with the wood phase. Anger and frustration are emotions closely associated with the Liver, whereas courage, or lack thereof, is associated with the Gallbladder. By working Liver or Gallbladder channels or their corresponding points on the surface of the skin, you can help someone with chronic anger to change or moderate their behavior.

Fire

Fire provides light, warmth, and spark, a lively and colorful dynamic. The fire phase is associated with the color red, summer, heat, bitter flavor, the tongue, the cardiovascular system, the emotion of joy, speech, sweat, insight, and inspiration. The main functions of fire's organ systems are (1) Heart—emotional stability, (2) Small Intestine—assimilation, (3) Heart Protector—circulation, and (4) Triple Heater—protection. Together, they are interpreters of experience.

People who have a lot of fire tend to be the life of the party. They are engaging and charismatic and like to connect with people. Most entertainers have a lot of fire in their bodily makeup. On the other hand, a person with weak fire can appear shy or dull. Fire can manifest in the face. A full red complexion shows strong or excess fire, whereas pale cheeks can indicate deficient fire.

TCM views too much of any emotion as problematic, and this is no exception for joy; just as an intense fire can be damaging, constant joy and excitement can cause or be a result of emotional unrest. Regular meditation practice is useful for a fire imbalance.

Earth

Being "down to earth" is an expression summing up the centering, stable quality of the earth phase. Between all the other phases, a moment of transition exists ruled by the earth. All foods come from the soil and therefore are associated with earth. Mother Earth in her bountiful generosity, receptivity, and patience provides everything we need. The act of eating has a calming, satisfying, and comforting effect. People eat "comfort foods" when sick or depressed. Comfort foods remind us of home, with their warmth, safety, and sweet smells. This phase is associated with moisture, singing, sweet flavor, the lips, and saliva.

People who show love for their home and family tend to have a lot of earth in their makeup. They tend to be the ones who have everyone home for the holidays and make big holiday dinners. They are concerned that everyone's needs are being met.

The yellow color associated with earth comes from the color of the soil in the region of northern China, where the theory of five phases supposedly originated (Huang He, Yellow River). Carefully observing a person's face can sometimes reveal a yellow hue or coloring pointing to an earth phase imbalance, probably affecting the Spleen or Stomach. Foggy thinking, heaviness of the body, and craving for sugar are all signs of an earth imbalance.

Metal

From the soil deep in the earth, minerals are extracted to make strong and valuable metals. During our history as human beings, the metal blade of swords and of other weapons has shaped much of our civilization. The borders of countries have been determined by wars fought with metal weapons or by the influence of commerce based on precious metals. Gold is the agreed-upon measure of material worth in many societies. *Value, worth, structure, shape,* and *border* are some of the words associated with the metal phase. The border of our body, the skin, and keeping healthy psychologic boundaries are necessary to protect ourselves from unwanted, outside influences. A sense of self-worth (metal), for example, is gained and supported from the grounded (earth) knowledge of ourselves. The Lungs and Large Intestine organ systems are also associated with metal. In TCM, Lung gathers ki from the air and creates wei (protective) ki, which circulates along the surface of the body as a defense. Our first breath and last breath mark the beginning and end boundaries of our life in physical form. The Large Intestine's function of elimination or letting go is what helps rid the body of waste. It also applies to unwanted emotional or mental structures we no longer need. The nose, the color white, autumn, grief, mucus, dry climate, and craving for pungent and spicy flavors are also associated with the metal phase. The main functions of the metal organ systems are (1) Lungs—intake of ki, and (2) Large Intestine—elimination.

Those who have a lot of metal in their makeup like to sort, organize, and eliminate what is not necessary. They crave an orderly existence. As children, they most likely insisted on coloring inside the lines and tend to gravitate toward occupations such as accounting.

Water

Water takes the shape of whichever vessel contains it, be it a glass or channel carved into rock, but water keeps its unique characteristics, such as fluidity and adaptability, and is always flowing downward. These characteristics are what give water its power and energy, as with a stream coming down the mountain. If the mountain slopes are gentle, then water will move smoothly and easily in a continuous flow.

If rocks and branches interrupt the stream, then water will go around, jump over, or carve into the obstacles until it finds its way through. Willpower is a trait associated with the water phase. Water rules the functioning of the Kidney and Bladder organ systems, whose task is to provide the impetus (the "get up and go" energy) for life. The Kidney and Bladder are in charge of the purification process and the balance of water in the body. The bones, bone marrow, teeth, central nervous system, ears, hearing, the emotion of fear, winter, black or dark blue color, urine, groaning sounds, and craving for salty foods are all correspondences to the water phase. The main functions of these organ systems are (1) Kidney—stores life essence, and (2) Bladder—stores and excretes urine.

People who have a lot of water in their makeup like to spend time alone, preferably doing something creative such as writing poetry or doing art; most artists have a great deal of water in their makeup.

Water is a precious and essential element for survival because our bodies are mostly water. The water element is sensitive to the pressure of stress in modern life. The adrenal glands produce adrenaline for the fight-or-flight response when we are frightened and is also part of this organ system.

Creative/Promoting and Control Cycles

The five phases have underlying cycles contributing to balance or imbalance (Fig. 16.2).
- **Creative/Promoting Cycle.** This describes how a phase feeds, nourishes, or generates the next phase in line. This cycle is often described as the mother-child relationship. In the example of water nourishing wood, water is the mother and wood is the child.

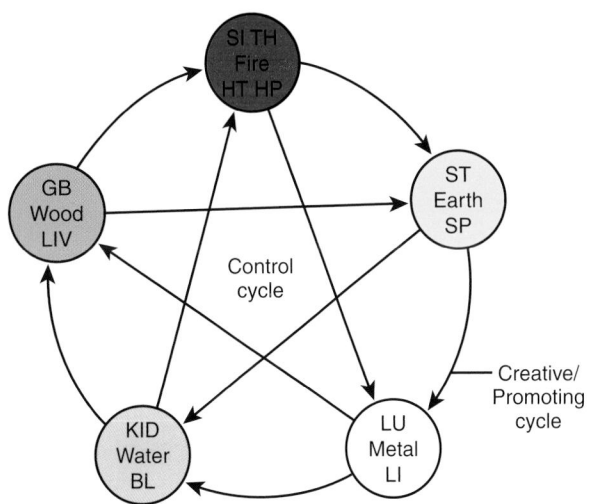

FIG. 16.2 Five phases with cycles and associated channels. The creative/promoting cycle feeds, nourishes, or generates the next phase in line. The control cycle is a system of checks and balances, which keeps any one phase from overacting. *BL,* Bladder; *GB,* Gallbladder; *HP,* Heart Protector; *HT,* Heart; *KID,* Kidney; *LI,* Large Intestine; *LIV,* Liver; *LU,* Lung; *SI,* Small Intestine; *SP,* Spleen-Pancreas; *ST,* Stomach; *TH,* Triple Heater.

- **Control Cycle.** This is a system of checks and balances, which keeps any one phase from overacting. For example, when a tree (wood) gets too tall, an axe (metal) is used to control its height.
  - **Overacting (Insulting) Cycle.** This is a pathologic version of the control cycle where there is excessive control weakening or suppressing the phase being controlled. This counteractive cycle inverts or goes in the opposite order of the creative/promoting cycle.

The following examples illustrate use of the cycles in client assessment.

Wood creates fire – In a client who has a lot of fire-associated symptoms, such as redness on the face, agitation, and inappropriate emotional responses, the practitioner checks the fire channels and the wood channels. In this case, wood is the mother creating or generating fire, which is described as the child. Too much wood can generate too much fire. The fire phase might be tamed by controlling the amount of fuel (wood) stoking the flame. The reverse situation might also happen. A client without "sparkle" and who has a pale face and is constantly feeling cold and showing other signs of lack of fire might be treated by strengthening the mother phase, which is wood.

Earth controls water – Since the beginning of time, farmers along riverbanks know when the river rises and floods its banks, it may have dire consequences for their crops and livelihood. A strong earth element will keep water under control, just as a dam or riverbank does. If the water phase (ruling the Kidney, Bladder, and water balance in the body) overacts, then it can swamp the earth-ruled function of the Spleen and Stomach, dampening the Spleen's function. This action can slow down digestion and increase bloating, tiredness, and edema, under which conditions fluids become backed up in the interstitial space between the cells. A strong earth phase helps keep everything in its place (one of the Spleen's functions). A person with an Earth imbalance would do well to exercise; eat cooked foods such as stews, grains, and soups; and receive treatments to strengthen the Spleen and Stomach organ systems.

The Channels and the Hara

Channels, or meridians, are pathways in the body through which energy circulates. They are bilateral and contain acupoints (discussed later in the chapter). These channels move the vital substances—ki, essence, blood, body fluids, and spirit—to the zang-fu organs (discussed in a later section). Channels are the connections of the material body to the nonmaterial body (e.g., energy field surrounding the body). Channels distribute, balance, and connect the ki of the interior organs with the surface body. Channels help "move the ki and blood, regulate the yin and the yang, moisten the tendons and the bones, and benefit the joints" (Huang's *Yellow Emperor's Classic of Internal Medicine,* 1966). Ki circulates through the channels in a fixed direction, with one channel ending where the next channel begins, making one continuous interconnected channel. Yin channels connect with yang channels on the extremities, yang channels connect with

yang channels on the head, and yin channels connect with yin channels on the torso. The flow of ki follows the Chinese clock—a time system based on circadian or biologic cycles in which each organ system has a time of the day when ki activity peaks, starting with the lungs channel and ending with the liver channel (Fig. 16.3). The Chinese clock is also called the "noon-to-midnight law."

There are 12 regular channels located bilaterally and symmetrically. These channels are named after their associated organ systems. Names of the channels use capital or upper-case letters to differentiate them from anatomic organs (i.e., Heart is the channel, whereas the heart is the anatomic organ). If you find a client has a Heart channel imbalance, this does not necessarily mean there is an illness or disease of the anatomic heart, so avoid making statements such as, "You have a problem with your heart." Hearing this statement may cause anxiety in the client about a possible medical condition affecting the heart, and it clearly falls outside your scope of practice.

The channels occur in yin and yang pairs and each channel has a specific location in the hara where its ki is easily accessed (see Fig. 16.18). The **hara** is the body's center of focused power and energy. Within the hara is the **tanden** (dan t'ian, dan tien), the sea of ki, 1 to 2 inches below and behind the navel. In Japan, a person is said to "have good hara" when they enjoy good health, stability, and strength. Several qi gong and tai chi exercises and meditations can be used to develop the tanden because it is the center of power for the practice of martial arts. It is the point at which the

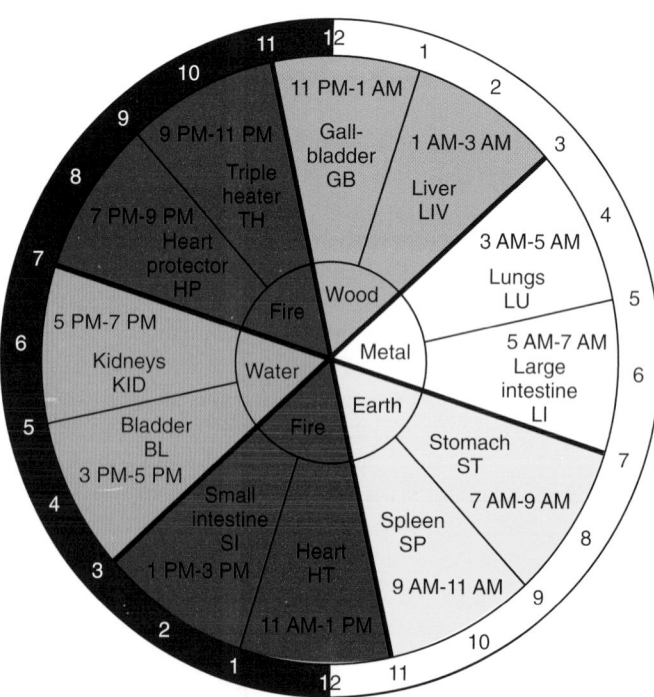

FIG. 16.3 Chinese clock or noon-to-midnight law. This time system is based on circadian or biologic cycles in which each organ system has a time of the day when its ki is at its peak of activity.

person physically embodies the ki of the earth as their own state of being, allowing ki to permeate every action they do.

In addition, each channel has a time of day when ki flow is at its peak (see Figs. 16.3). When an imbalance occurs in a channel, symptoms may flare up at the time of the day corresponding with a particular channel. For example, if someone wakes up every night between 1 am and 3 am, then it may point to a Liver imbalance.

1. **Lung Channel (LU)**. Yin organ, metal energy, and rules 3 to 5 am (Fig. 16.4)
2. **Large Intestine (LI)**. Yang organ, metal energy, and rules 5 to 7 am (Fig. 16.5)
3. **Stomach (ST)**. Yang organ, earth energy, and rules 7 to 9 am (Fig. 16.6)
4. **Spleen (SP)**. Yang organ, earth energy, and rules 9 to 11 am (Fig. 16.7)
5. **Heart (HT)**. Yin organ, fire energy, and rules 11 am to 1 pm (Fig. 16.8)
6. **Small Intestine (SI)**. Yang organ, fire energy, and rules 1 to 3 pm (Fig. 16.9)
7. **Bladder (BL)**. Yang organ, water energy, and rules 3 to 5 pm (Fig. 16.10)
8. **Kidney (KID)**. Yin organ, water energy, and rules 5 to 7 pm (Fig. 16.11)
9. **Heart Protector (HP)/Pericardium (P)**. Yin organ, fire energy, and rules 7 to 9 pm (Fig. 16.12)
10. **Triple Heater (TH)**. Yang organ, fire energy, and rules 9 to 11 pm (Fig. 16.13)
11. **Gallbladder (GB)**. Yang organ, wood energy, and rules 11 pm to 1 am (Fig. 16.14)
12. **Liver (LIV)**. Yin organ, wood energy, and rules 1 to 3 am (Fig. 16.15)

Triple Heater (Triple Warmer, Triple Burner) refers to three "heaters," "warmers," or "burners" in the body.

- **Upper Heater**. This is above the diaphragm and regulates intake. It includes the head, heart, pericardium, throat, and lungs.
- **Middle Heater**. This extends from the diaphragm to the navel and controls transformation. It includes the stomach, spleen, liver, and gallbladder.
- **Lower Heater**. This is below the navel and regulates the separation of nutrients and wastes and the elimination of wastes. It includes the kidneys, bladder, intestines, and sex organs.

The eight extraordinary vessels work as reservoirs for the 12 regular channels, supplementing their function and pooling and storing ki as needed to preserve balance in the whole system. The Governing and Conception vessels are the only extraordinary vessels with their own exclusive points, and the 12 regular channels provide points to access the other extraordinary vessels. The Conception (Ren), Governing (Du), Penetrating (Chong), and Belt (Dai) vessels are particularly important in the formation and support of the embryo.

Tsubos (Acupoints)

Tsubos, or **acupoints**, are points along channels where energy concentrates and surfaces. Tsubo is Japanese for "container" or "vase." There are 361 points in the body. Tsubos have specific actions when stimulated by pressure, needle insertion (acupuncture), heat application (moxibustion), essential oils, or application of vibration via a tuning fork. Tsubos are identified by the name of the channel plus a number that increases in sequential order from the beginning of the channel to the end (SP1, SP2, SP3, and so forth). Some tsubos have a Chinese name suggesting geologic features, such as KID1 (bubbling spring), LI4 (union valley), and HP7 (great mound).

Cun

A **cun** (pronounced "soon") is a body measurement used to find tsubos. Each cun is measured by the width of the client's own thumb knuckle. For example, ST36 (leg three miles) is 3 cun below the lower edge of the patella, and 1 cun lateral to the crest of the tibia (Fig. 16.16).

Kyo and Jitsu

Kyo and jitsu are Japanese terms describing quantities of energy or the activity in a tsubo. **Kyo** means "empty, yin, depleted, or not enough ki." **Jitsu** means "full, yang, excessive, or too much ki." Kyo and jitsu also refer to the unique quality of ki, such as responsive or sluggish, soft or hard, and expansive or contractive.

Pressure is applied into the channel perpendicular to kyo and jitsu tsubo. In a kyo tsubo, the pressure will be applied longer as the ki gathers. In a jitsu tsubo, the pressure will be applied just long enough to disperse excess ki. In most instances, when you press on a kyo tsubo, it feels as though you can go deep. It can feel soft, cool, nonresponsive, or sluggish; energy in the tsubo is lacking. The ki projected in the form of pressure is welcoming. While pressing on the point, visualize you are calling ki to the tsubo, helping to draw energy toward it. This technique is called *tonification*. The ki pouring into the kyo tsubo comes from other places in the client where it is not needed or has an excess amount, as well as from the universe. When you feel something start to stir or move in the tsubo, move to another point. By bringing the attention to the kyo tsubo, your own ki initiates a process of transformation. This does not mean you are pouring your own ki into the tsubo, as in a gasoline filling pump. By respecting the Zen shiatsu principles of touch (see later discussion), your own energy field will be expanded. Because of this expansion, you should not feel drained at the end of a session.

A jitsu tsubo feels full of energy. The point may feel hard, warm, and superficial. Your pressure feels pushed out or resisted and it feels as if you cannot stay on the point long. The intention is to disperse excess ki in the jitsu tsubo. This technique is called *sedation*. The main difference between tonification and sedation techniques is the practitioner's objective.

This entire system is designed to be self-regulating. As with yin and yang, kyo and jitsu are relative to each other. Every jitsu tsubo has a corresponding kyo tsubo somewhere down the channel; its depletion is supplying the excess of the other point, and every kyo point has a jitsu point that needs to overwork to balance the deficiency. You sometimes

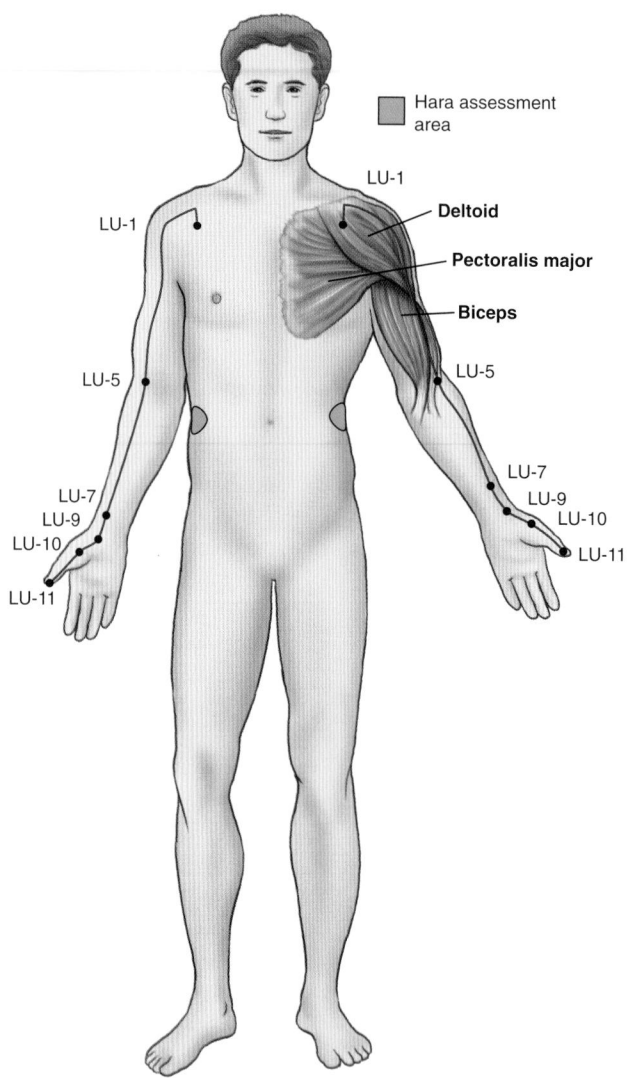

FIG. 16.4 Lung *(LU)* channel and associated hara assessment area; anterior view.

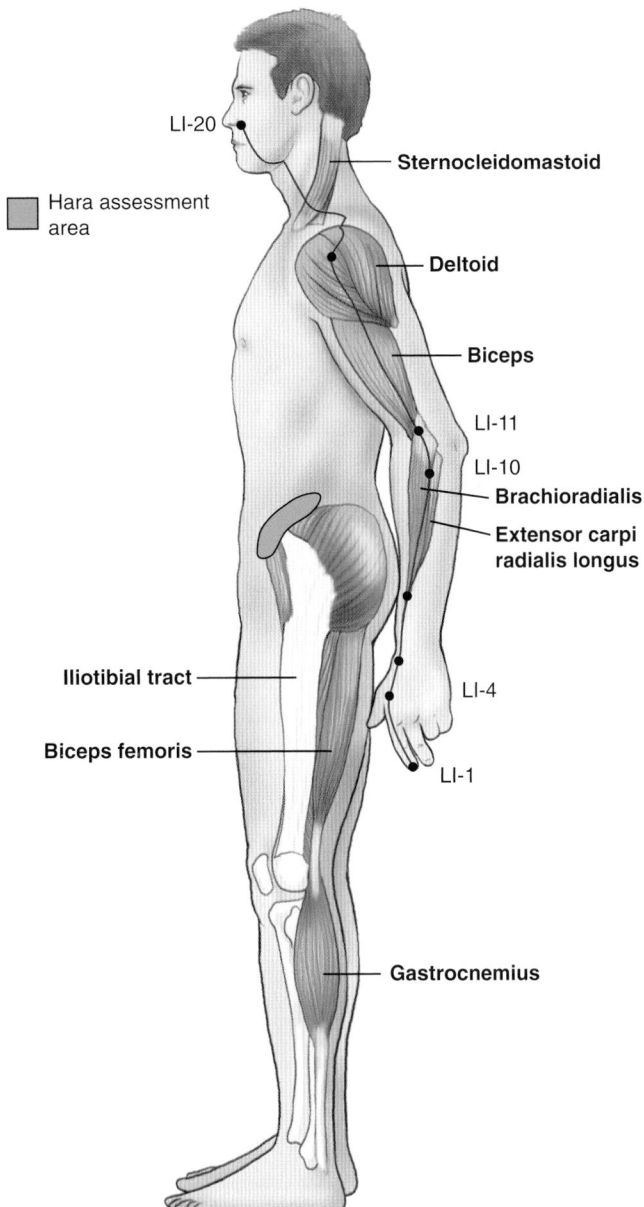

FIG. 16.5 Large Intestine *(LI)* channel and associated hara assessment area; lateral view.

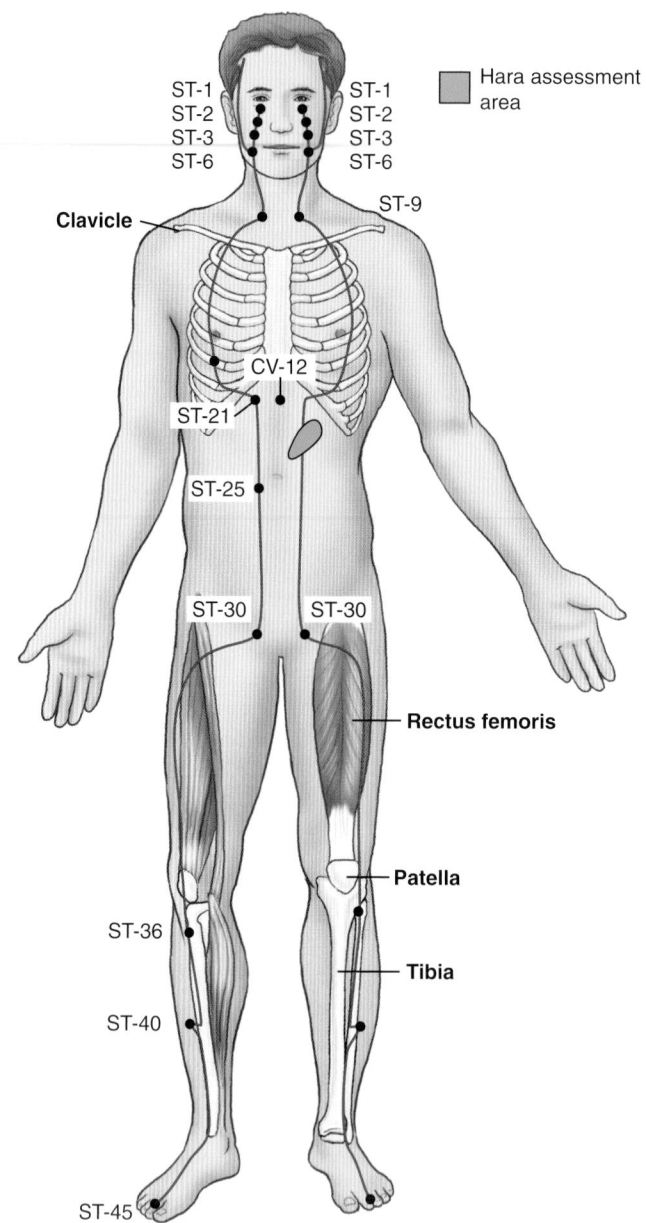

FIG. 16.6 Stomach *(ST)* channel and associated hara assessment area. *CV*, Conception vessel; anterior view.

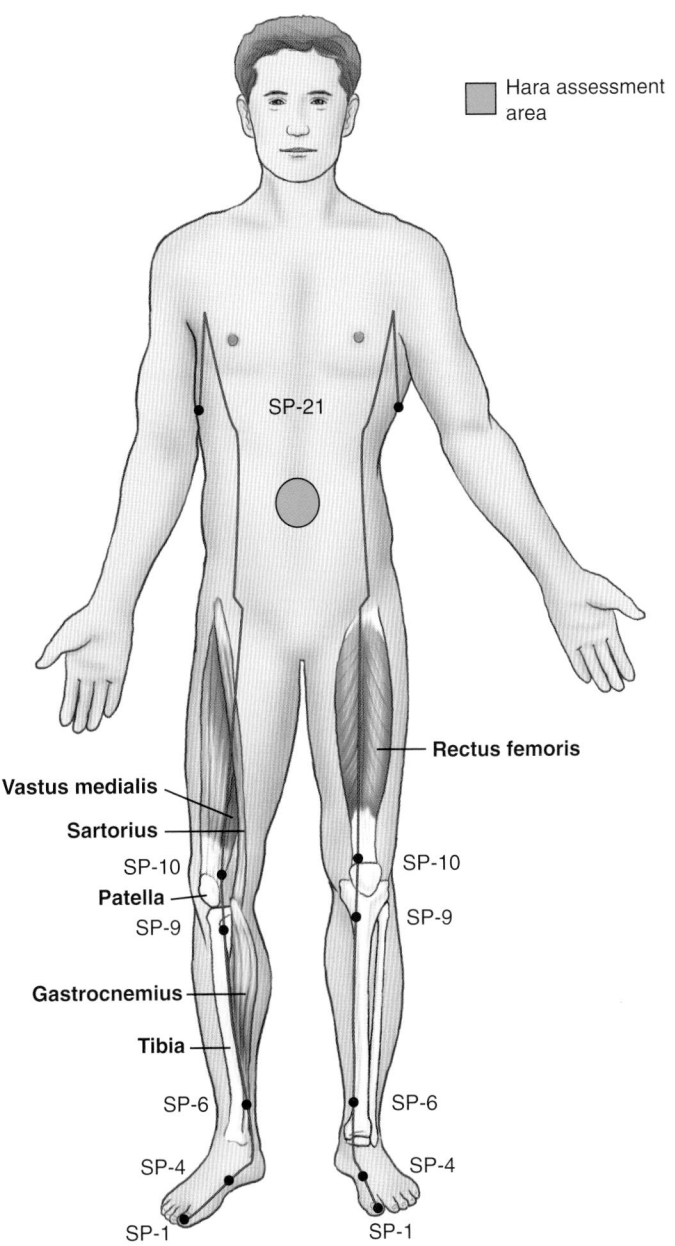

Hara assessment area

SP-21

Rectus femoris

Vastus medialis

Sartorius

SP-10

Patella

SP-9

Gastrocnemius

Tibia

SP-6

SP-4

SP-1

SP-10

SP-9

SP-6

SP-4

SP-1

FIG. 16.7 Spleen *(SP)* channel and associated hara assessment area; anterior view.

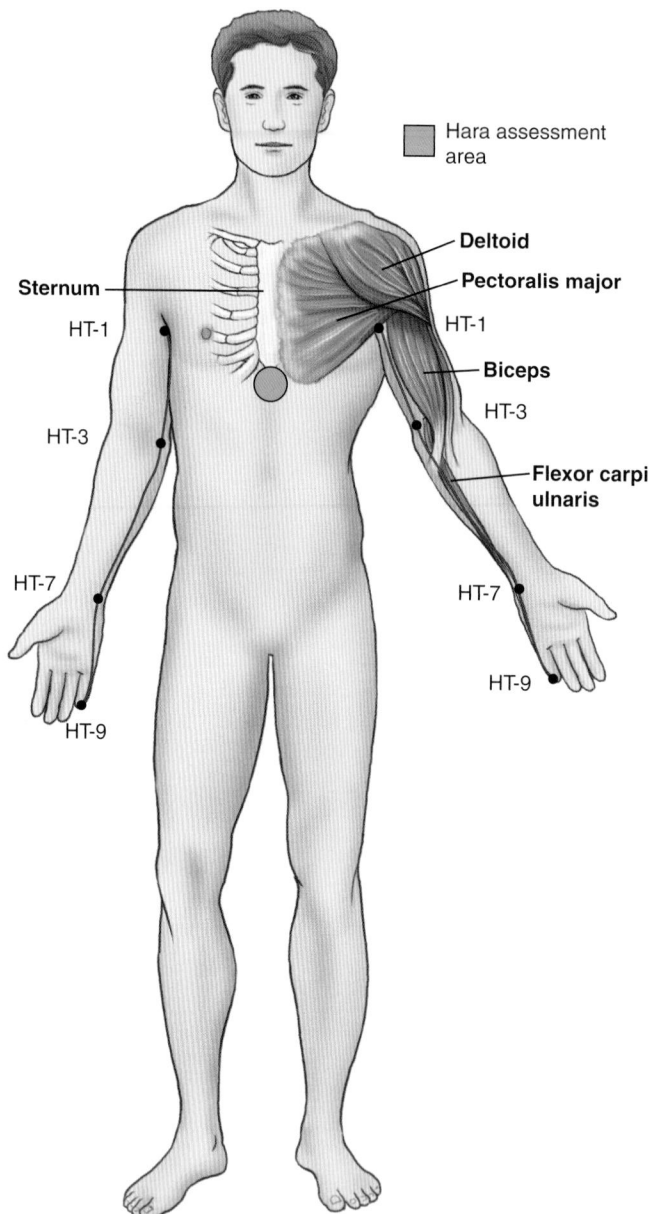

FIG. 16.8 Heart *(HT)* channel and associated hara assessment area; anterior view.

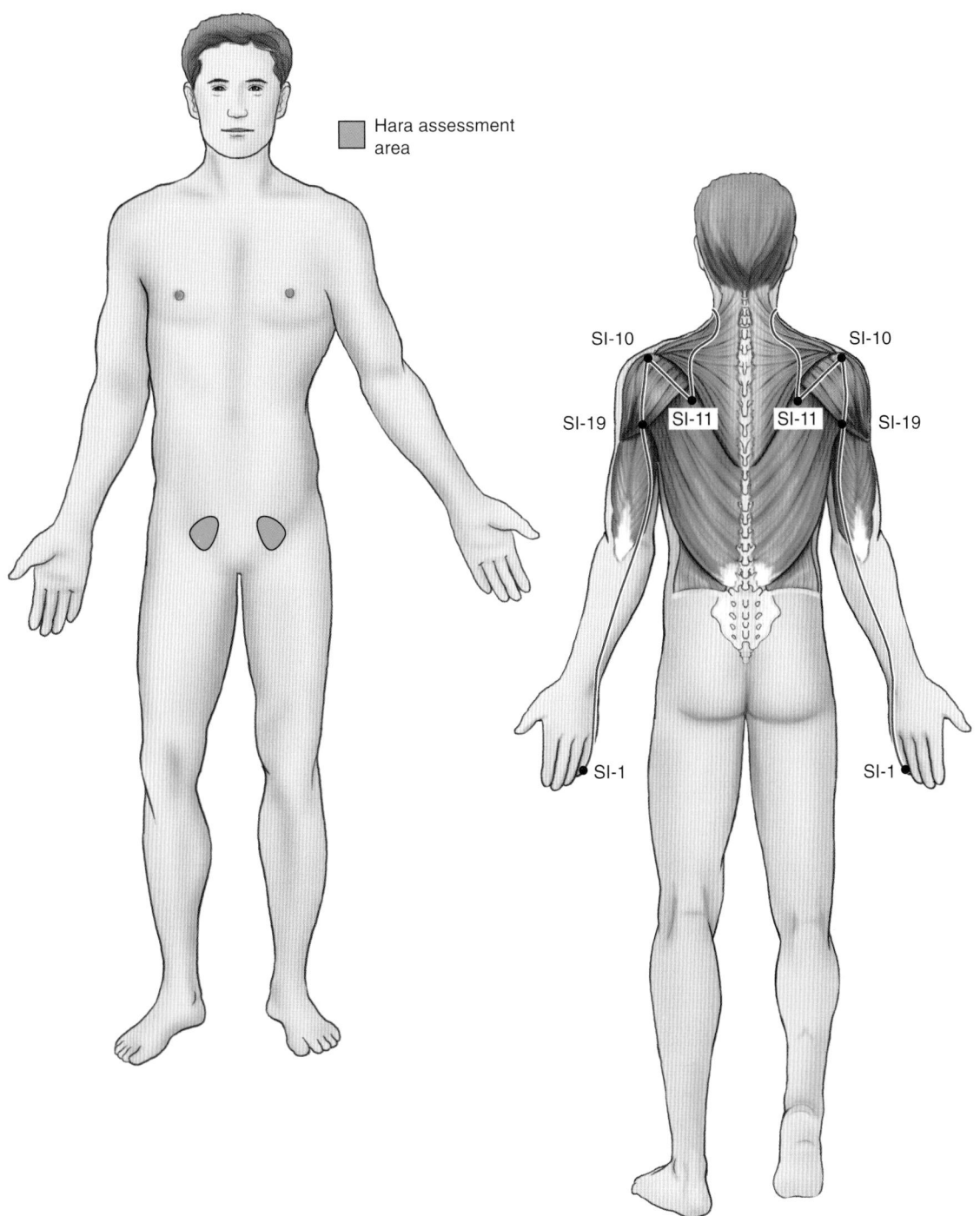

FIG. 16.9 Small Intestine *(SI)* channel (posterior and lateral views) and associated hara assessment area (anterior view).

Continued

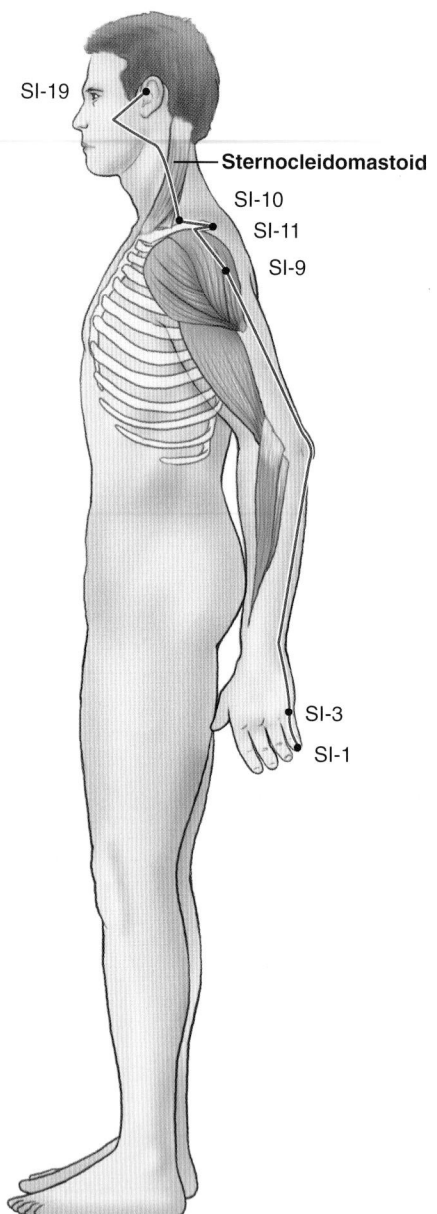

FIG. 16.9, CONT'D

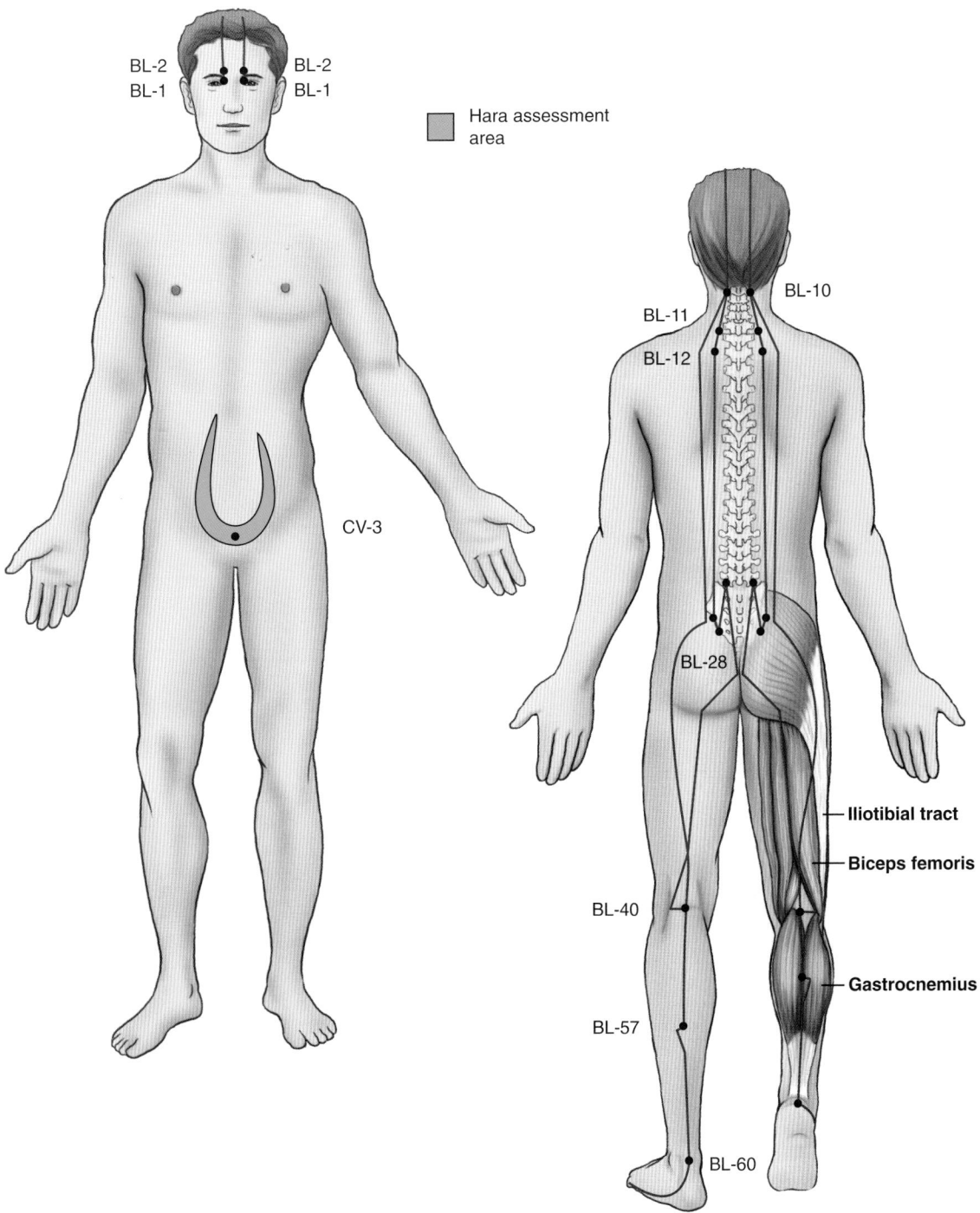

FIG. 16.10 Bladder *(BL)* channel and associated hara assessment area. *CV,* Conception vessel; anterior and posterior views.

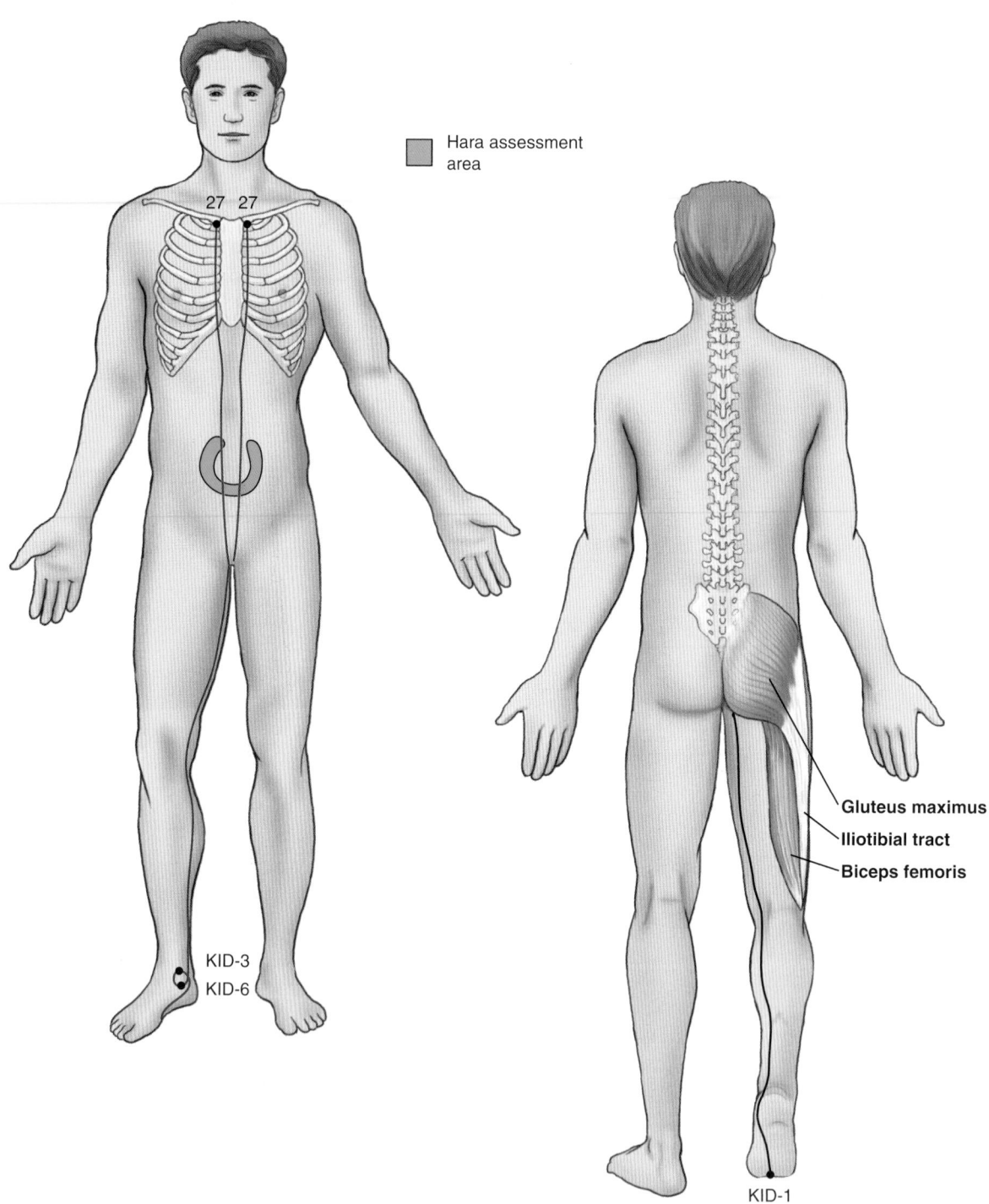

FIG. 16.11 Kidney *(KID)* channel and associated hara assessment area; anterior and posterior views.

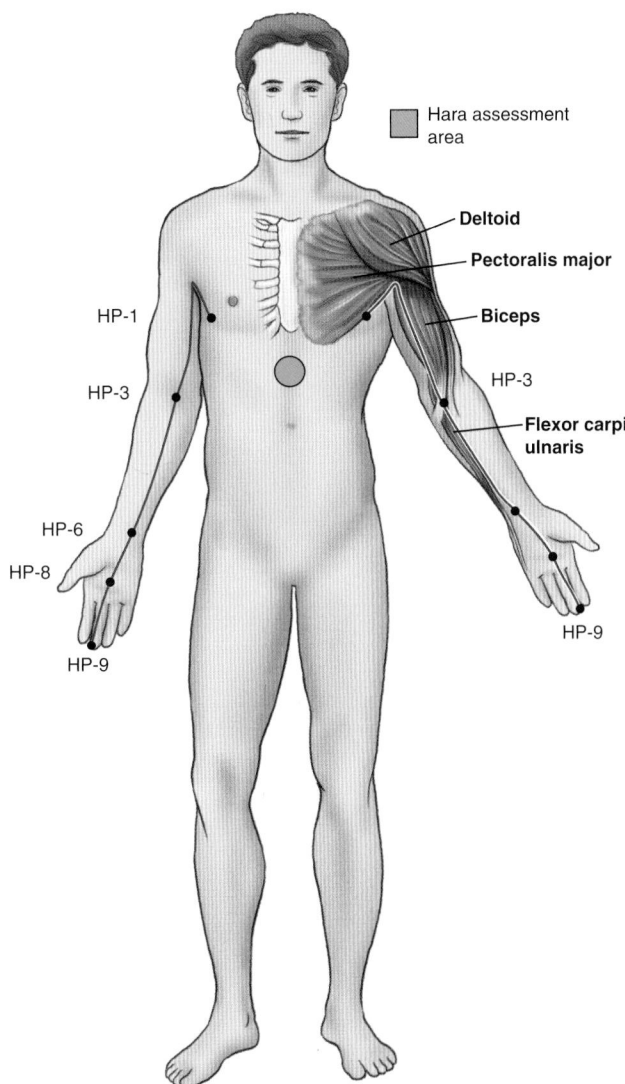

FIG. 16.12 Heart Protector *(HP)* channel and associated hara assessment area; anterior view.

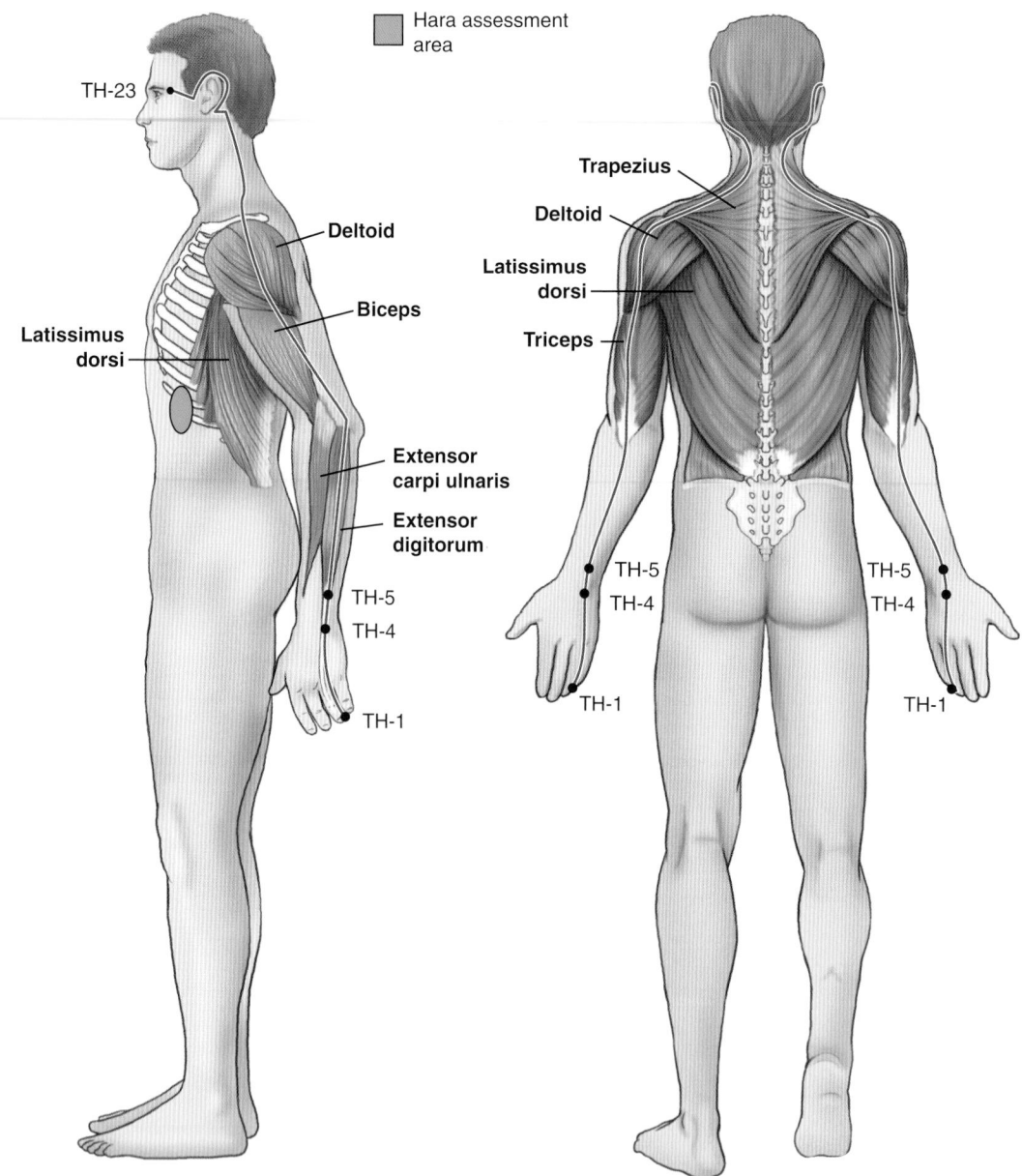

FIG. 16.13 Triple Heater *(TH)* channel and associated hara assessment area; lateral and posterior views.

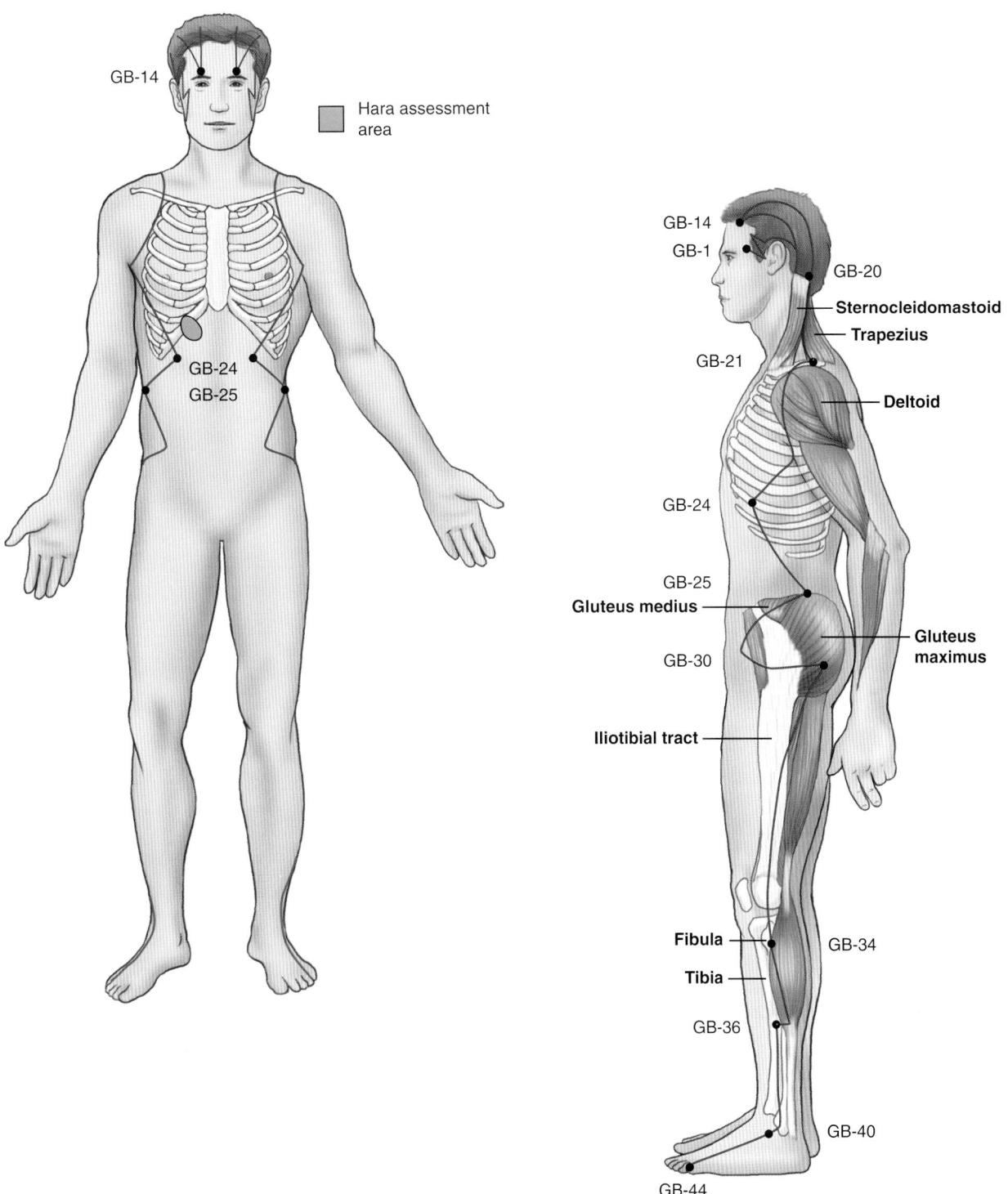

FIG. 16.14 Gallbladder *(GB)* channel and associated hara assessment area; anterior and lateral views.

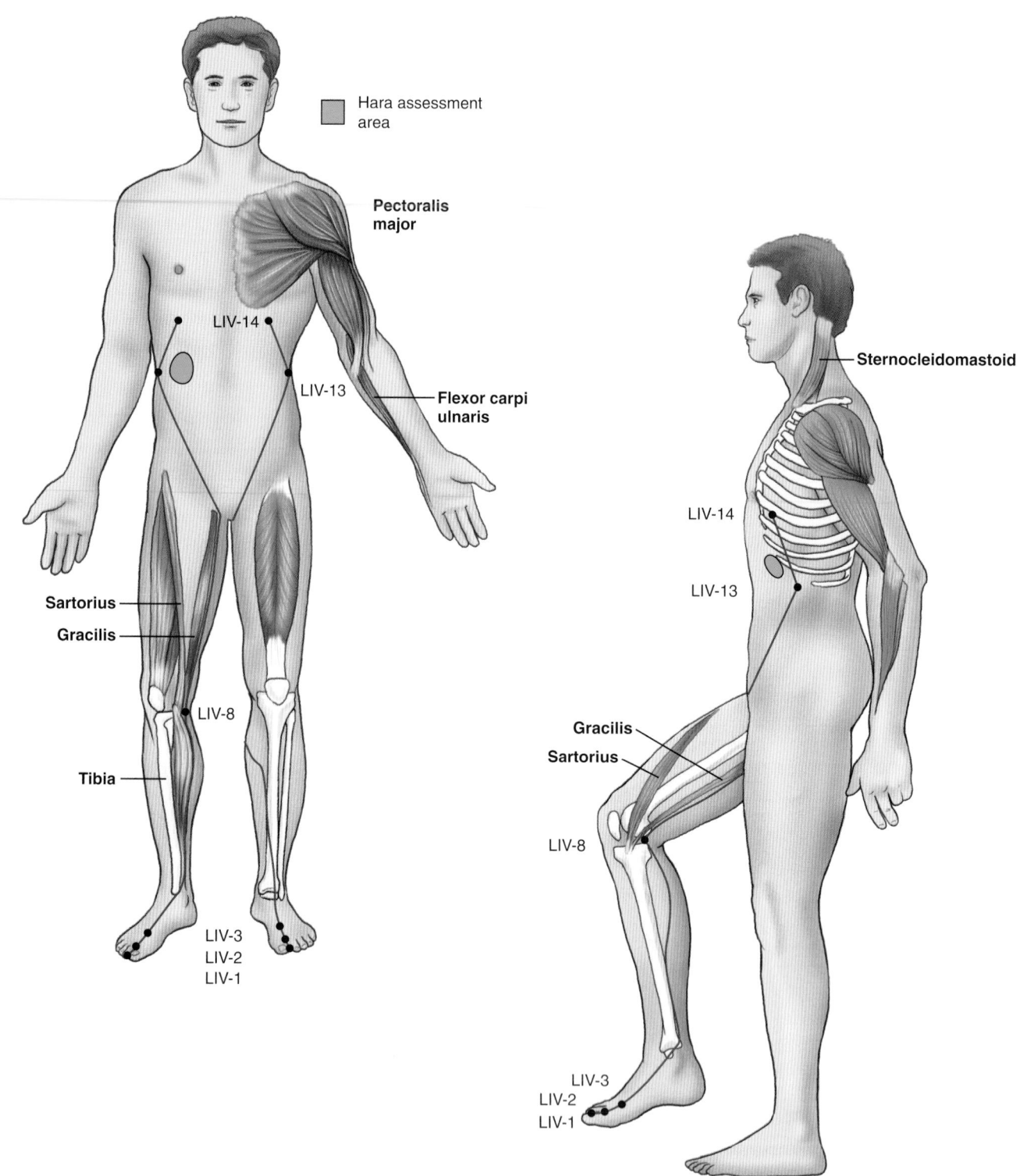

FIG. 16.15 Liver *(LIV)* channel and associated hara assessment area; anterior and lateral views.

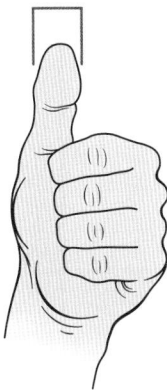

FIG. 16.16 Cun. The length of a cun is determined by the client's own thumb knuckle and is used to find tsubos.

find kyo and jitsu points next to each other on the same channel. You may also find channels predominantly kyo or predominantly jitsu. These determinations can be made during hara assessment (discussed later). Although other channels may be addressed during treatment, the focus will be on balancing out the most kyo channel and the most jitsu channel. Through tonification and sedation, the goal is to even out or harmonize ki in the entire channel. This process will balance ki throughout all the channels.

The practitioner should first find and address the kyo channel because this will initiate balance in the whole system. If you push ki away from a jitsu tsubo without first identifying and tonifying the kyo tsubo, it may feel temporarily better but the results will not last long. In fact, by the time you go back to the first identified jitsu tsubo, it will already start to change before it is touched again. Therefore the treatment strategy is to:

1. Identify kyo and jitsu tsubos.
2. Tonify the kyo tsubos.
3. If necessary, disperse or sedate the jitsu tsubos.
4. Check for changes until ki evens out throughout the whole channel or system.

Zang-Fu Organs

The zang-fu organs are two organ systems which contain their associated channels; they are divided into yin and yang pairs. The functions of the organ systems are the physical, emotional, mental, and spiritual aspects of human existence. Emotional nourishment is as important for full development as food is. Mental stimulation and nourishment, such as learning, is vital for the development of intellectual capabilities. It is the same as nourishing your relationships with yourself, others, and the universe to help you have a spiritually rich life. A good flow of energy through the channels and vessels to the whole system keeps the zang-fu organs, and the body nourished, which is the foundation for health. An imbalance anywhere in the system—or an interruption, blockage, or depletion of the flow of energy—will affect not only the area but also the system as a whole.

- **Zang Organs (Yin)**. These are the Heart, Liver, Lungs, Kidney, Heart Protector, and Spleen. They tend to be

solid organs. Their main functions are to manufacture and store essential substances, including ki, blood, and body fluids.
- **Fu Organs (Yang)**. These are the Small Intestine, Gallbladder, Large Intestine, Bladder, Triple Heater, and Stomach. They tend to be hollow organs. Their main functions are to receive and digest food, and to transmit and excrete wastes.

Zang-fu organs correspond with other organs; elemental forces in nature (discussed under the theory of the 5 phases); climatic conditions such as dampness, heat, cold, and dryness; colors, sounds, flavors, smells, times of the day, and seasons; and other characteristics. ABT can be used as a preventive measure by identifying imbalances and restoring the flow of energy before symptoms manifest. The ABT practitioner must remember the aim is not just to fix a particular problem or symptom but to restore the flow of energy overall. This action will help ensure zang-fu organs are functioning properly.

Fish will be the last one to discover water.

—Einstein

ASSESSING ENERGETIC IMBALANCES

Practitioners of ABT use various methods to assess energetic imbalances. Clients might be experiencing physical or emotional aspects of one of the five phases, or have an affinity or aversion pointing to a particular phase. They might have a more yin or a more yang condition. They may have weakness or excess in a particular channel. All these ideas put together, plus the valuable addition of the practitioner's experience, can help the practitioner tailor the session to the specific needs of the client. The main assessment methods used to assess energetic imbalances are looking, listening and smelling, palpating, and asking.

Looking

The practitioner can tell a lot about the client's state of health and personality by observing how the client looks and behaves, their physical constitution, body proportions, posture, gait, mannerisms, level of activity, and strength in movement. You can check the face color (hue), circles under the eyes, condition of hair and nails, redness or discoloration of the skin, and "sparkle," or lack of, in the eyes. Looking at the tongue, or tongue assessment, is regularly used by ABT practitioners to determine internal conditions of the body. Redness on the tip of the tongue, for example, can point to heat in the Heart. A thick white coating or fur at the back of the tongue might point to coldness in the Kidney or Bladder. An enlarged tongue with scalloped edges may point to a deficiency of the Spleen. Deep cracks at the center might point to a deficiency of the Stomach. When looking at the client, keep your gaze relaxed. This increases your peripheral vision. This way, you can have a one-shot look and impression of the whole person, instead of parts or specific details. The details will later fit into the big picture. Another way is to look at the space larger than just the physical body of the client. This space contains the physical body and the energy field around the client.

Listening and Smelling

Listening refers not only to what the person is saying but also to how it is being said, what is not being said, and tone of voice. Is a complaining, angry, or sad tone heard? Is the client talking in a hushed voice, growling, or shouting? Does it sound as though the person is holding their breath? Do they have a dry mouth? You can sometimes distinguish a particular smell associated with the person such as sweet (relating to earth), burnt (relating to fire), damp (relating to earth and water), rancid (relating to wood), rotten (relating to metal), or putrid (relating to water).

Palpating

You can check specific reflex areas in the abdomen, or hara, and compare energetic states of different organ systems (see the "Hara assessment" section). Many ABT practitioners rely on feeling the pulses at three different places on each of the client's wrists. This skill gives information on the ki, zang-fu organs, and channels. As the practitioner works, they check the skin texture and firmness, temperature changes, and areas of pain in the client's body. Areas of pain are called *Ah shi points*. Ah shi, which means "that's it," elicits a reaction from a client when touched. Other points palpated for assessment are Shu and Yu (transporting) points on the back and Bo or Mu (alarm) points on the front of the body.

Asking

The practitioner can inquire specifically about the client's symptoms, sleep patterns, elimination, digestion, appetite, diet, exercise, menstruation patterns, and health history, as well as climatic likes or dislikes. For example, a person might strongly dislike cold, heat, or drafts of air, or a symptom might worsen on damp or rainy days. These can point to imbalances in specific elements.

In the beginner's mind there are many possibilities, but in the expert's mind there are only a few.
—Shunryu Suzuki

SHIATSU AND ZEN SHIATSU

Shiatsu is a Japanese ABT method using applied pressure along energy channels to restore, maintain, or balance the flow of ki. The term shiatsu literally means "finger (shi) pressure (atsu)," but hands, elbows, knees, and feet are also used and, when appropriate, joint mobilizations and stretches. As discussed previously, tsubos are found along the channels and are places ki is easily accessed.

Based on TCM, shiatsu had been used in Japan for centuries until it was banned, alongside other folk medicine methods, during the U.S. occupation of Japan after World War II. In the 1950s, Tokujiro Namikoshi created a style of shiatsu using Western anatomic references instead of traditional Chinese–Japanese nomenclature. Thanks to his efforts, the Ministry of Health in Japan approved his style of shiatsu as medical treatment. The Namikoshi Shiatsu School, which he created, is still open today; and this style of shiatsu is very popular in Japan.

Shiatsu is traditionally done on an individual lying on a floor mat while the client is fully clothed, and no lubricants are used (Fig. 16.17). Shiatsu is adaptable to almost any environment and situation. It is popular not just for relaxation and wellbeing but also in pregnancy; during labor; in

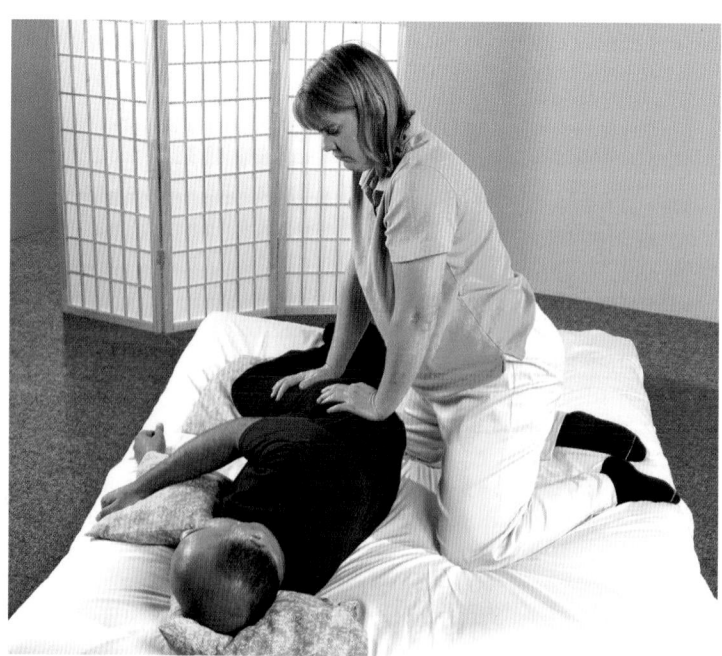

FIG. 16.17 Practitioner administering shiatsu on a fully clothed client lying on a floor mat. (From Anderson, S. [2008]. *The practice of shiatsu.* St. Louis: Mosby.)

critical care of patients in hospitals; for emergency relief support; and in corporate, military, and other settings.

There have been several types of shiatsu taught in recent years. In the late 1990s, Ruthie Piper developed **ashiatsu**, a form of shiatsu performed with the practitioners' feet while holding onto a stabilizing tool for balance (e.g., wooden bars or ropes suspended from the ceiling, parallel gymnastics bars, a stool, chair, or bench). In most cases, the client is unclothed, draped with linens, and lies on a table instead of a matt. Right about the same time, Harold Dull developed **watsu**, performed on a floating client while the practitioner stands in about 3 feet of water and helps them float while applying shiatsu techniques.

Another type of shiatsu is **Zen shiatsu**, which is a bodywork style that is heavily dependent on the mental state of the practitioner. The Zen part of Zen shiatsu does not have a religious connotation, as in Zen Buddhism. Instead, the Zen in Zen shiatsu is the meditative or contemplative state of mind in which the Zen shiatsu practitioner must be to perceive and connect with the ki of both the client and the self.

Shizuto Masunaga, the creator of Zen shiatsu, graduated from the Japan Shiatsu College in 1959 and later studied with Namikoshi, but he took a different approach. Masunaga trained at the university as a psychologist but also studied ancient Chinese medicine in which mind–spirit references to clinical practice were commonplace. After meticulous research, Masunaga came up with an expanded model of health in which emotional and mental aspects of the person were taken into consideration and blended into the physical touch technique of shiatsu. He created a new chart of channels extending the classical channels and contributed hara assessments of the channels. Widely used in shiatsu schools throughout the world today, hara assessment provides a focus for treatment.

The emphasis of Zen shiatsu techniques is to have an in-the-moment understanding of the quality and movement of ki. Although the functions and actions of individual tsubos are essential to learn and use in practice, it is more important to be in touch with the entire channel, for it is what guides the practitioner during the session.

Principles

Principles of Zen shiatsu provide a way for the practitioner to be relaxed and aware throughout the session while maintaining a clear mind. One of the ways to help the practitioner and the client stay centered is to be present and pay attention to the process as it unfolds from moment to moment. The practitioner's hands receive feedback and reactions from the client as they work. The practitioner should be able to interpret this information so they can adapt, creating a technique appropriate for the client. Although the practitioner follows a routine, especially at the beginning of training, no two sessions will be the same because the practitioner will tailor Zen shiatsu treatments to each client. The principles of Zen shiatsu are:

- Be relaxed.
- Use body weight, not force.

- Move from the hara.
- Use a two-handed connection.
- Use stationary, perpendicular pressure.
- Project ki.
- Work one channel before moving to another channel.

Be Relaxed
Some ABT methods emphasize the practitioner's muscular strength when applying techniques and therefore are quite physical, using strength through muscular contraction. Of course, once muscular contraction reaches a threshold, it cannot be sustained for prolonged periods. The practitioner can push the threshold to sustain the contraction with practice, just like weight lifters, but there is a point at which the muscles need to rest before they can contract again. It is difficult for a practitioner to keep high levels of contraction throughout the hour or more of a typical session, never mind doing many sessions in a day. In addition, if the practitioner's effectiveness is tied to muscular strength, then much stress is continually placed on muscles to remain in a contracted state.

Zen shiatsu is based on the opposite principle—namely, the practitioner must be relaxed to be effective. Being relaxed does not mean the practitioner's touch will be light or ineffective. They can perform any task that demands physical power while keeping a sense of openness and relaxation. Think of the grace of a top-class dancer or skater, whose muscular effort is guided by a prevailing sense of calmness and fixed attention even in the midst of a challenging performance.

Being aware of your body, consciously releasing areas of tension, breathing fully, having a comfortable posture, and adjusting it to keep relaxed and open during the session are some of the ways to ensure you do not use muscular force in a purely contractive way. Besides, helping clients relax is almost impossible if the practitioner is not relaxed. As the practitioner relaxes and expands their energy field, awareness of their surrounding space increases. The perception of the client increases, as does what is needed during the session. The expansion of their field happens in all directions at the same time. As the practitioner's energy field expands downward, the connection to the earth increases. As the practitioner's field expands forward, the connection with the client increases. As the practitioner expands upward, a connection is made with cosmic ki to help inspire and guide the session. When the practitioner relaxes and expands their ki, coming in contact with the client's ki in the channels is relatively easy and more effective.

Use Body Weight, Not Force
Using the weight of the practitioner's body to apply pressure is the most effective way to ensure a supportive and effective touch and will help them better perceive the client's reaction. Effective body mechanics include having an aligned spine; a good connection of the legs, knees, and feet to the floor; and arms extended with elbows slightly flexed

or unlocked. Good alignment also protects the practitioner from injury.

Move From the Hara

Moving from the hara means the practitioner's body is connected to the earth and they work from a grounded sense of self. Simple exercises, such as bringing your breathing down to the hara, can help you center yourself and feel grounded very quickly. Zen shiatsu practitioners relax their hara and face it toward the area on the client's body on which they are working.

Use Two-Handed Connection

Having both hands in contact with the client as you work contributes to stability, support, and continuous connection. Throughout the session, the practitioner's hands become more yin (receptive, feeling, slower, supportive) or more yang (active, faster, directive). The practitioner's more yin "mother hand" stays in one place, supporting and feeling the reaction of the work. The "child hand," or working hand, is more yang and active, moving along the channel. Ideally, both practitioner's hands are on the same channel. Feeling the reaction underneath the mother hand is relatively easy if the practitioner's hand and wrist are relaxed. The practitioner's hands connect through the client's channel, forming a closed circuit that includes hara, mother hand, child hand, and the client's channel or area worked. The practitioner's awareness of the client's subtle reactions is increased by visualizing a sphere of ki within this closed circuit. As the practitioner moves around the client, at least one hand remains on the client to provide a sense of connection.

Use Stationary, Perpendicular Pressure

Approach the area of work using stationary perpendicular pressure. This allows the energetic connection with ki in the channels. Touch that approaches the surface of the skin nonperpendicular creates tissue resistance, bringing up dense, slow vibrations of ki. This approach restricts the practitioner's work to only the physical range of ki. It can be effective, but it is "hit or miss," and the effect will be localized. When leaning with the body weight perpendicularly into the channel to apply pressure, the practitioner reaches the full range of vibrations of the channel—emotional, mental, spiritual, and physical, thus stimulating the whole channel at once. The practitioner adjusts the angle of pressure, adapting to the different curvatures of the body to ensure perpendicularity, then leans into the channel until the ki is contacted. Pressure is released before proceeding to the next area. Circling, rubbing, or moving the thumb or palm on the area restricts the practitioner's work to the physical and local aspects of the area.

Project Ki

By relaxing the body weight perpendicularly into a channel, the practitioner allows their ki to project itself beyond the point of contact with the surface of the client's skin, allowing better contact with the client's ki. The practitioner can visualize the area as a sphere and project ki toward the center of the sphere.

Work One Channel before Moving to Another Channel

As a rule, the practitioner follows along the same channel instead of jumping back and forth from different channels or areas of the body. The practitioner continues along the entire channel, moving around the client in a consistent, fluid manner.

Techniques: Palming and Thumbing

The two main techniques used in Zen shiatsu are palming and thumbing.

Palming

Palming is done with relaxed hands placed on the client's body. The practitioner extends the arms and brings the body weight forward until they feel the pressure under their palms. Palming is a good way to assess the quality of ki in the channel and compare different sensations on each area being worked.

Thumbing

Thumbing is done with thumbs extended and relaxed fingers. The practitioner's elbows are slightly flexed or unlocked, and the shoulders are relaxed or dropped. The thumb should be aligned with the wrist, elbow, and shoulders. The practitioner should be mindful of not flexing the distal interphalangeal joint but keeping it extended instead. The point of contact of the thumb with the channel should be midway between the pad and the nail of the thumb, taking care not to be too close to the nail. Thumbing can be done effectively only if the practitioner's nails are clipped short.

Both palming and thumbing are done rhythmically while following the direction of the flow of ki in the client's channels. The direction of work is different when the client is supine and when the client is prone.
- Client Supine
  - From the hara down the legs to the feet along the yang channels on the lateral aspect of the legs
  - From the chest out to the arms along the yin channels
  - From the chest up to the head
- Client Prone
  - From the base of the neck, laterally to shoulders and arms
  - From the base of the neck down along the back toward the sacrum
  - From the sacrum toward the feet

Hara Assessment

Hara assessment is palpating the client's hara to assess reflex areas of the channels. The aim of hara assessment is to find the most kyo channel and the most jitsu channel. The hara assessment areas for these channels will react reflexively to each other, indicating the focus of the client's treatment. Working the kyo–jitsu pair of channels is the fastest and most direct way to balance the client's whole system.

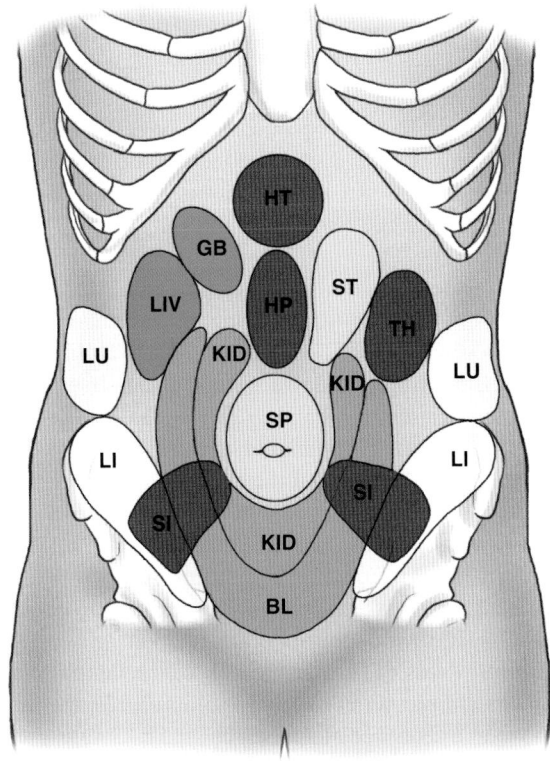

FIG. 16.18 Hara and channel reflex areas. Locate the most kyo or jitsu channel helps determine the focus of the client's treatment.

Each channel has a specific location in the hara in which its ki is most easily accessed (Fig. 16.18).

The practitioner compares the overall energetic state of the client and gains a clearer picture of where imbalances may be found, then checks each channel location in a specific order. The following is how a Zen shiatsu practitioner performs a hara assessment:

- Sit in a comfortable position by the client's hara so all the channel assessment areas are easily reached.
- Align your spine and center yourself by bringing attention to the connection of the legs to the earth and breathing from your hara.
- Place your mother hand on the side of the client's trunk.
- With the child hand, gently and perpendicularly palpate each of the client's hara assessment areas with relaxed fingertips. The pressure should be light and comfortable for the client but still deep enough to be present and make contact with the ki.
- Feel for the client's most kyo area, comparing all areas with even pressure and for an equal amount of time.
- Feel for the client's most jitsu area, comparing all the areas with even pressure and for an equal amount of time. To find the kyo and jitsu reaction, the practitioner:
- Place the mother hand on the client's most kyo area, contacting the ki.
- Place the child hand on the client's most jitsu area and feel for a reaction in the most kyo area, underneath their

mother hand. There may be a feeling of subtle movement or change under the fingertips.

If the practitioner does not get a reaction of any kind with the most jitsu area, the mother hand is left on the client's most kyo area, and with the child hand, make another round of the remaining assessment areas, this time pressing a bit more deeply than before until the area that reacts is found. This will be the jitsu channel used during the client's treatment. Some guidelines for hara assessment:

- Channels such as Kidney, Bladder, Large Intestine, Small Intestine, and Lung have either broad or bilateral diagnostic areas in the hara. They need to be palpated evenly. If one side feels jitsu and the other side of the same channel assessment area feels kyo, then the practitioner should discard them and look for an alternative one with a consistent kyo or jitsu feeling throughout the whole area to be assessed.
- One channel of a yin and yang pair (LV/GB, LU/LI, HT/SI, and so forth) cannot be the most kyo and the other the most jitsu.

THAI MASSAGE

Thai massage consists of stretching and compression on points along energy channels to balance energy and restore health. In Thailand, Thai massage is called *partner yoga* and **Nuad Bo'Rarn** (pronounced new-odd bo-rahrn). Nuad is Thai for "to touch with the intention of imparting healing." Bo'Rarn is Sanskrit for "something ancient and revered." Thai massage practitioners work very slowly and in a quiet, meditative state, like Zen shiatsu. Clients remain clothed and lie on a padded mat resting on the floor or on a raised platform.

Thai massage is a key component of traditional Thai medicine. The origins of Thai medicine date back 5000 years and are rooted in the traditions of Ayurvedic medicine of ancient India. When the Buddhist culture moved from India to Thailand approximately 2200 years ago, Ayurvedic medicine came as well. Over time, Ayurvedic medicine mingled with the healing traditions of the indigenous people of Thailand. This led to a new and distinct system of Thai medicine. For the people of Thailand, this healing method is held in high regard and recognized as an important part of their cultural heritage. There are several branches of Thai medicine: herbal medicines, nutrition and food cures; spiritual/psychologic practices; and Nuad Bo'Rarn, or hands-on healing work. Many stretching techniques are derived from yogic tradition. As with yoga and all practices of massage and bodywork, proper body mechanics are essential for the health and longevity of the practitioner and for the safety and benefit of the client.

Principles

To better understand traditional Thai medicine, you must also have a basic understanding of Ayurveda. Please refer to the Ayurvedic section later. According to Thai medical theory, human beings are composed of a synergistic blend of three distinct essences in a continuous interplay between and with each other. These are the (1) human body, (2) energy, and (3) citta. The human body is a combination of all physical attributes, including the material aspects of a person. Energy is the organizing force bringing together all aspects of a human being into a unified functioning whole. Like the healing traditions of China and Japan, the Thai massage system postulates the body possesses energy channels called **Sen**. These channels are not identical to the channels of traditional Chinese medicine or shiatsu, although there are some similarities. Sen channels originate near the navel, deep in the abdominal cavity, and flow to the sensory orifices, to the excretory orifices, and along the extremities to the hands and feet. For more information on Sen, please refer to the books listed in the bibliography.

Citta encompasses all the aspects of the nonphysical body, including thoughts, emotions, will, and spiritual aspirations. Citta is invoked by our creativity, imagination, intentionality, dreams, and wonderment. Citta is unique to human beings and separates humans from all other living creatures on earth.

The application of Thai massage is seen as an expression of spiritual practice. Thai massage practitioners seek to work in a concentrated and meditative state and, through touch and intention, impart these qualities to the client. Practitioners are encouraged to bring these qualities along with their highest aspirations and spiritual philosophy into their everyday life. This is expressed succinctly in the Four Divine States of Mind of Buddhist philosophy, which are:

1. Loving kindness
2. Compassion
3. Mental equanimity (i.e., evenness of mind even under stress)
4. Vicarious joy and happiness (i.e., empathy)

Techniques

Thai massage is divided into two very different styles: the northern style developed in North Thailand, and the southern style developed in South Thailand. The southern style is performed rapidly and sometimes abruptly. The northern style is performed more slowly, but not too slow. This section focuses on northern-style Thai massage. This slowness serves two purposes:

- Supports, enhances, and encourages a meditative state in both the practitioner and the client. Thai massage requires great balance and sensitivity from the practitioner.
- Protects the client and practitioner from injury. The client is guided into yoga postures (asanas). Some of these postures can be demanding. Because the technique is performed very slowly and with acute awareness, all techniques can be stopped or adjusted for maximum safety and effectiveness.

Thai massage is done with the client in all four positions: supine, prone, side lying, and seated. The client remains clothed. Lubricants are rarely used. Some styles of Thai massage use herbal compresses as compression tools. Stretching techniques are an important part of Thai massage.

Central to Thai massage is the practitioner's intent to affect vata, or wind. The wind element in the Thai language is referred to as *pen lom*. Rhythmic compressions can be used to facilitate the correct movement of wind in the body and to relieve wind if it has become stuck or stagnant. In addition to the thumb, finger, and hand techniques, the practitioner must learn to use their forearms, elbows, feet, legs, knees, and entire body weight to skillfully apply Thai massage techniques. The practitioner's body weight stabilizes a region of the client's body with compression while stretching techniques are applied. Working the Sen energy channel in a particular direction is not emphasized. Techniques are performed both up and down energy channels without regard to tonification or sedation strategies as seen in shiatsu. The techniques used in Thai massage are:

1. **Palm Press (PP)**. Use of the entire palm to apply downward compression. The practitioner works with a straight elbow while shifting body weight (Fig. 16.19).
2. **Palm Circle (PC)**. Use of the entire palm as well as hand and fingers to make circular movements. Palm circles are used most often on the abdominal region.
3. **Thumb Press (TP)**. Use the ball of the thumb to apply downward pressure to specific points. Often, the thumbs move in a sequence along Sen channels. Care is given to not hyperextend the joints of the thumb.
4. **Finger Circles (FC)**. Use the tips of the fingers moving in a circular or rotational direction. Finger circles are

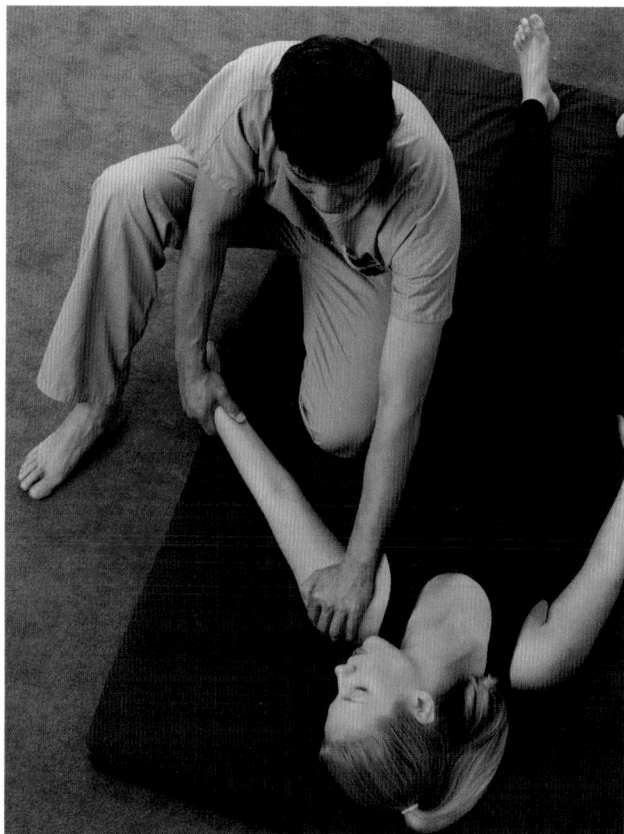

FIG. 16.19 Thai massage. Practitioner uses their entire palm during the palm press.

most often used along the sternum, in the intercostal spaces, and on the face.

5. **Thumb Circle (TC).** Use of the thumb moving in a circular or rotational direction. While the thumbs are moving, the wrist and fingers remain relaxed. This technique is used most often on the face and head and over bony areas.

6. **Elbow Press (EP).** Use of the tip of the elbow to create a deep, penetrating compression. The elbow is placed on the body and the practitioner exerts a slow downward pressure. The elbow press is most often used on the hips, upper trapezius, and soles of the feet.

7. **Forearm Rolling Pin (FRP).** This involves a moving downward pressure. The entire length of the ulna is placed on the body and then the radius is rotated over the ulna back and forth. This procedure is applied along the iliotibial band and upper trapezius.

8. **Foot Press (FP).** Use of the entire sole of the foot to deliver compression. The foot press is often paired with a pulling action to create a force/counterforce. For example, the practitioner presses with their foot into the client's medial thigh (adductors) of a bent knee while simultaneously pulling the client's ankle. The counterforce deepens the foot compression.

9. **Knee Press (KP).** This is performed with the practitioner in a kneeling position while placing their knees on the client's body. This technique is especially suited for the bottom of the client's foot or the gluteal region.

10. **Stretching Techniques (ST).** This is accomplished by creating a force/counterforce in various locations of the body. Stretching is done with the client in any of the four positions. Stretching creates elongation and expansion and helps open up joint spaces.

1-2-3-2-1 Pattern

Most techniques are performed in a 1-2-3-2-1 pattern. For example, two-handed palm presses applied to the medial thigh with one leg flexed in the yoga tree position. The first palm press is applied just superior to the knee joint (position #1). The second palm press is done proximal to the first, a little higher up the thigh (position #2). The next palm press is even more proximal, closer to the inguinal groove (position #3). The next palm press is now distal to position #3, back at position #2, and finally, the last palm press of the sequence is back at position #1, just superior to the knee joint. This pattern is very rhythmic and soothing and is repeated at various locations on the body during a Thai massage session.

AYURVEDA

Ayurveda is the traditional Hindu system of medicine that maintains or improves health through diet, massage, yoga, yogic breathing, and the use of herbal preparations. Ayurveda is one of the world's oldest healing systems and closely adheres to the principle of a fundamental connection between microcosm and macrocosm. Humans are the microcosm, or tiny representations of the universe, which is the macrocosm.

Contained within each person is everything making up the surrounding world. The interconnectedness of humans and their world makes it impossible to understand one completely without the other. This section discusses the fundamental principles and practices of traditional Ayurveda as understood from their original Sanskrit sources and traditional practitioners.

The Doshas

According to Ayurveda, there are five great elements present in everything in the universe. These elements are earth, air, fire, water, and space (or ether). These elements manifest in the human body as three basic principles or energies known as the **doshas** (pronounced *doe-shuh*). Doshas and the seven dhatus (tissues) and three malas (waste products) all make up the human body. The Sanskrit word *dosha* means a "fault" or "defect." When these elements are not balanced, they disrupt the normal functioning and cause bodily malfunctions. The three active doshas, or *tri-doshas*, are vata, pitta, and kapha. Everyone has vata, pitta, and kapha, but usually, one is primary, one is secondary, and the third is least prominent. When an imbalance occurs, they disrupt the normal functioning of the body, which may lead to disease manifestation. An imbalance indicates an increase or decrease in one, two, or all three of the doshas. Because the qualities of each dosha help determine the individual's makeup, they provide the basis for ascertaining which dosha or combination of doshas may be causing the imbalance.

Vata

Vata means "wind" and is the combined elements of air and space. Vata governs movement and nervous system functions. Vata is below the navel and in the bladder, large intestines, pelvic region, thighs, bone marrow, and legs; its principal seat is the colon. When disrupted, its primary manifestation is gas and muscular or nervous energy, which may lead to pain. The qualities of vata are dryness, cold, light, irregularity, mobility, roughness, and abundance. Dryness occurs when vata is disturbed and is a side effect of motion. Too much dryness produces irregularity in the body and mind.

Pitta

Pitta means "bile," which is the combined elements of fire and water. Pitta governs digestion, metabolism, hunger, thirst, sight, courage, and mental activity. Pitta is between the navel and the chest and in the stomach, small intestines, liver, spleen, skin, and blood; its principal seat is the stomach. When disrupted, its primary manifestation is acid and bile, which can lead to inflammation. Pitta is hot, light, intense, fluid, liquid, putrid, pungent, and sour. Heat appears when pitta is disturbed. The intensity of excessive heat produces irritability in the body and mind.

Kapha

Kapha means "phlegm" and is the combined elements of earth and water. Kapha governs lubrication and structure and maintains the body's solid nature, tissues, sexual power, and strength. It also controls patience. The normal locations of kapha are the upper part of the body, the thorax, head, neck, upper portion of the stomach, pleural cavity, fat tissues, and areas between joints; its principal seat is the lungs. When it is disrupted, its primary manifestation is fluids and mucus, which can lead to swelling, with or without discharge. Kapha is heavy, cold, stable, dense, soft, and smooth. Heaviness occurs when kapha is disturbed and results from firmness caused by kapha. The viscosity of excessive kapha produces slowness in the body and mind.

The Dhatus

The seven **dhatus** are the tissues that support the body functions. Each dhatu is responsible for and nourish the dhatus that come next in the following order. The first dhatu is formed by consumed food and beverage. The end product of all dhatus is *ojas*, or immunity.

- **Rasa**. Plasma and lymph
- **Rakta**. Blood
- **Mamsa**. Muscle or flesh
- **Meda**. Fat
- **Asthi**. Bone, ligaments, and tendons
- **Majja**. Nervous tissue
- **Shukra and Arthava**. Male and female reproductive tissues of semen and ova

The Malas

The **malas** are waste products and include sweat, urine, and feces. A fourth category of other waste products includes fatty excretions from the skin and intestines, ear wax, mucus of the nose, saliva, tears, hair, and nails. It is important to flush out these waste products regularly and excesses could lead to ill health and disease.

Prakriti

Prakriti is our body type or basic constitution. Prakriti is determined at conception and remains until death. The four factors influencing a person's constitutional type are (1) the father, (2) the mother (particularly her food intake), (3) the womb, and (4) the season of the year they were born. A large imbalance of the doshas in the mother will affect the growth of the embryo and fetus, and a moderate excess of one or two of the doshas will affect the constitution of the child. Seven normal body constitutions exist and are based on the three doshas: vata, pitta, kapha, vata-pitta, pitta-kapha, vata-kapha, and sama. The last is a state in which all three occur in equal proportions. It is the best condition but is extremely rare.

Most people are a combination of doshas, in which one dosha predominates. In general, vata types tend to be anxious and fearful, exhibit light and "airy" characteristics, and are prone to vata diseases. Pitta types are aggressive and impatient, exhibit fiery and hotheaded characteristics, and are prone to pitta diseases. Kapha types are stable and entrenched, if not sluggish at times; they exhibit heavy, wet, and earthy characteristics and are prone to kapha diseases.

These concepts are the principal factors helping the Ayurvedic practitioner determine the correct course of treatment to be administered to a client for a particular ailment.

Nadis

Similar to the traditional channels of TCM, the **nadis** are channels in the body where prana energy flows. Although the concept of the bodily winds or pranas occurs in Ayurveda, the development of the notion of the nadis is restricted to the system of yoga in India. Nadis are sometimes viewed as extending only to the skin of the body but are often thought to extend to the boundary of the aura. The three main nadis include sushumna, ida, and pingala, but a total of 72,000 nadis are said to exist in the body. Nadis start from the central channel along which they are found and radiate from the chakras (see discussion in next section) to the periphery, then the nadis gradually become thinner. Prana flow is stimulated through the practice of **pranayama**, or breath control, and by manual pressure on **marma points**, which are located along the nadis.

Chakras

Chakras are the energy centers in the body along the central channel, or sushumna. In the Ayurvedic tradition, the word *chakra* comes from a Sanskrit word meaning "wheel" or "circle." The functions of the chakras are to receive, process, and distribute energy and to keep the spiritual, mental, emotional, and physical health of the body in balance. The earliest mention of chakra, found in Rigveda, dating from about 1500 BCE, refers to the wheel of a carriage or of the Sun's chariot. An early reference to an energy center in the body is found in Yoga Upanishads (circa 600), one of the oldest texts of the Vedas. The chakra system came to be an integral part of the Tantric yoga philosophy and practice in India. The main text about chakras came to the West in a translation by the Englishman Sir John Woodroffe, alias Arthur Avalon, in the book *The Serpent Power*, published in 1919. The book lists seven basic chakras, and they all exist within the subtle body, present along with the physical body.

Chakras are described in ascending order from the base of the spine to above the head (Fig. 16.20), even though they may express themselves externally at points along the front of the body (navel, heart, throat, and so forth). All chakras are associated with a color, an element, a sound, a symbol (a different number of lotus petals in each chakra), and many other distinguishing characteristics. Although some discrepancies exist, here are the more traditional chakra characteristics.

Root Chakra (First Chakra)

Location: Base of the spine in the perineum
Sanskrit name: Muladhara
Gland: Adrenal medulla
Symbol: Four-petaled lotus
Color: Blood-red
Element: Earth

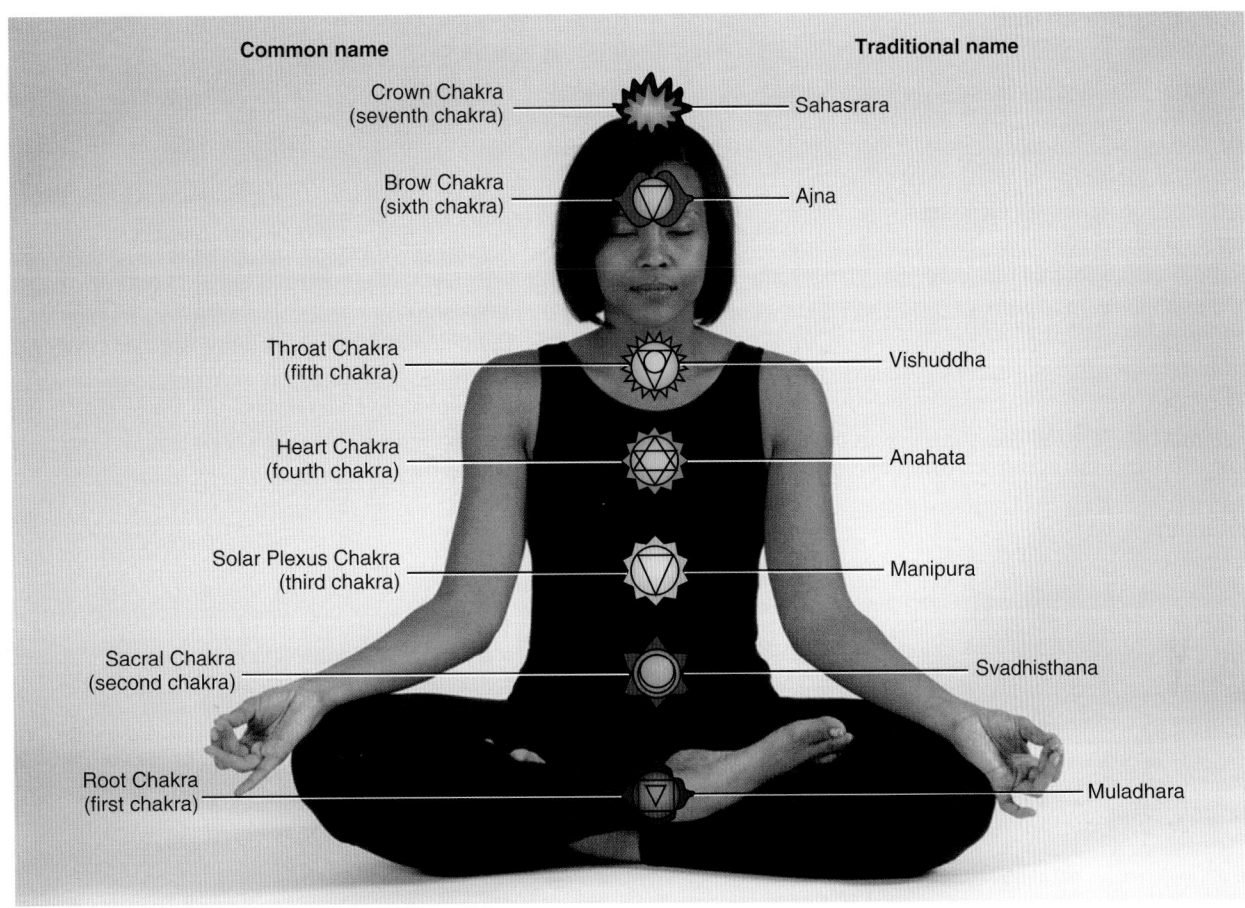

FIG. 16.20 The seven chakras. Traditional names, common names, and their locations.

Qualities: Grounding, patience, structure, stability, security, survival
Essential oils: Cinnamon, garlic, sandalwood
Gem: Ruby
Herb: Mugwort
Musical note: C

Sacral Chakra (Second Chakra)
Location: Sacrum, 2 inches below the navel and 2 inches into the pelvis
Sanskrit name: Svadhisthana
Gland: Gonads
Symbol: Six-petaled lotus
Color: Orange
Element: Water
Qualities: Wellbeing, sexuality, sensuality, pleasure, abundance, seat of the emotions
Essential oils: Jasmine, neroli, orange blossom
Gem: Moonstone
Herb: Cedar
Musical note: D

Solar Plexus Chakra (Third Chakra)
Location: Below the sternum and just above the navel

Sanskrit name: Manipura
Gland: Pancreas
Symbol: Ten-petaled lotus
Color: Yellow
Element: Fire
Qualities: Self-worth, self-esteem, confidence, personal power, mentality
Essential oils: Lemon, grapefruit, juniper
Gem: Yellow sapphire, topaz, citrine
Herb: Rosemary
Musical note: E

Heart Chakra (Fourth Chakra)
Location: Midchest
Sanskrit name: Anahata
Gland: Thymus
Symbol: Twelve-petaled lotus
Color: Green
Element: Air
Qualities: Unity, love, peace, purity, and innocence
Essential oils: Rose, carnation, lily of the valley
Gem: Emerald, rose quartz
Herb: Lavender
Musical note: F

Throat Chakra (Fifth Chakra)
Location: Throat
Sanskrit name: Vishuddha
Gland: Thyroid
Symbol: Sixteen-petaled lotus, circle
Color: Blue or turquoise
Element: Ether (contains all elements)
Qualities: Communication, will, creativity, truthfulness, integrity
Essential oils: Blue chamomile, gardenia, ylang-ylang
Gem: Blue sapphire, blue pearl
Herb: Wintergreen
Musical note: G

Brow Chakra (Sixth Chakra)
Location: Between the eyebrows (third eye or eye of psychic vision)
Sanskrit name: Ajna
Gland: Pineal
Symbol: Two-petaled lotus
Color: Indigo
Element: The cosmos
Qualities: Intuition, discernment, wisdom, imagination, knowledge
Essential oils: Camphor, sweet pea
Gem: Amethyst

Herb: Sage
Musical note: A

Crown Chakra (Seventh Chakra)
Location: Top of skull or just above the skull
Sanskrit name: Sahasrara
Gland: Pituitary
Symbol: 1000-petaled lotus
Color: White (sometimes purple) or white streaked with purple
Element: The cosmos
Qualities: Enlightenment, grace, beauty, serenity, oneness with all that is
Essential oils: Violet, lavender, lotus
Gem: Alexandrite
Herbs: Frankincense and myrrh
Musical note: B

E-RESOURCES

http://evolve.elsevier.com/Salvo/MassageTherapy

- Chapter challenge
- Flash cards
- Additional information

SHIZUKO YAMAMOTO

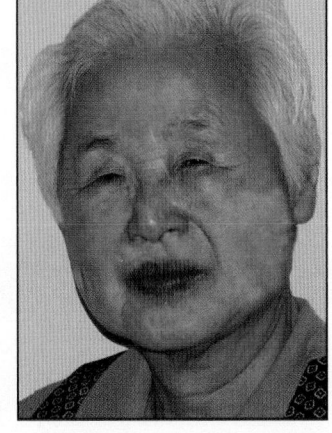

In the 21st century, the notion of preventive care and wellness as a solution to the healthcare crisis is not revolutionary. But Shizuko Yamamoto has been practicing and teaching these ideals since the 1940s, saying, "If society is to continue without extreme financial and emotional burdens, significant change must occur. The numbers of people afflicted with serious illnesses are ever-increasing. A fundamental and rapid change to preventive healthcare and holistic techniques is essential to turn around humankind's race toward degeneration."

Shizuko Yamamoto was born in Tokyo in 1924, the youngest of five children. Although she was in her early twenties, Yamamoto developed eye problems. Doctors suspected she had leukemia, and in her own words, she "just didn't feel well." She endured 10 unsuccessful operations to treat her eyes, spent 3 years in and out of hospitals, and several more years hiding out at home, attempting to recover from the surgeries and subsequent depression. With her trust in Western medicine eroded, she agreed to her parent's request to receive treatment from their shiatsu practitioner, and her interest in Eastern healing arts was born.

Yamamoto began with yoga, which led her to change her diet and begin a macrobiotic lifestyle. (Not a diet, she is quick to point out, a lifestyle.) Macrobiotics is based on a regimen of eating whole grains, local fruits and vegetables, and avoiding most animal products. In addition to the types of food included in macrobiotics, there are several guidelines regarding how and when to eat.

Meanwhile, she completed beginner training at the Namikoshi and Nishizawa schools of shiatsu, learning the modality, which involves applying pressure to certain points on the body to balance ki, or life force.

She began teaching yoga, and when students struggled in their progress, she provided shiatsu treatments to help them along. To compensate for her small stature, barely 5 feet 3 inches, she created a barefoot shiatsu technique, saving her hands from overuse and extending her career exponentially. As she expanded into martial arts training, Yamamoto learned more about the universal principles of how nature functions. This motivated a change in her shiatsu style, teaching styles, and her own macrobiotic lifestyle, as she integrated meditation and corrective exercises into each.

Yamamoto says, "We are nature's creation. Our bodies should be organic. We need clean water and a good environment. We are not just existing as ourselves; we are part of the planet, otherwise we cannot survive." Yamamoto's teachings are the embodiment of this idea. She founded a holistic beauty school in Japan, where students learned about macrobiotic foods, healthful cooking, yoga, and exercise, alongside facial treatments and cosmetics.

At the urging of a colleague, Yamamoto moved to the United States to concentrate on promoting and teaching macrobiotic activities. At the time she settled in New York, the state was struggling with the legality of macrobiotic practitioners. Yamamoto obtained a job helping to cook a macrobiotic menu for a film star, which led to her employment in a macrobiotic restaurant. As her co-workers complained about various aches and pains, she gave quick shiatsu treatments. Word spread, and in a short time, Yamamoto was making a living as a shiatsu practitioner.

As Yamamoto integrated all of her knowledge into full treatment plans for clients and friends, she also began to travel, providing bodywork and teaching throughout the United States and abroad. In 1986 she founded the International Macrobiotic Shiatsu Society, an organization dedicated to spreading natural complementary and alternative healing techniques to maintain and regain health. She pioneered the blending of bodywork with the macrobiotic lifestyle to create macrobiotic shiatsu, based on the idea that health is the natural condition of human beings and illness can be treated and avoided through natural means.

Yamamoto is the author of several books, including *Barefoot Shiatsu, The Shiatsu Handbook*, and *Whole Health Shiatsu*, and still lives in New York City. Her work, life, and teachings form a coherent whole, each part complementing and supporting the others. In a world where many massage practitioners struggle to balance work and life, this is a lesson we can all learn from Shizuko Yamamoto.

I would like to thank Richard Gold, Diego Sanchez, Georgia Tetlow, and Kenneth Zysk for past contributions to this chapter.

REFERENCES

American Organization for Bodywork Therapies of Asia. (n.d.). *About Asian bodywork therapy*. Retrieved from https://www.aobta.org/page/Def_Scope_Profession.

Huang, D. (1966). *The yellow emperor's classic of internal medicine*. Chapters 1–34 translated from the Chinese with an introductory study by Ilza Veith. Berkeley: University of California Press.

BIBLIOGRAPHY

Anderson, S. K. (2008). *The practice of shiatsu*. St Louis: Mosby.

Apfelbaum, A. (2003). *Thai massage: Sacred body work*. New York: Penguin Group.

Balaskas, K. (2002). *Thai yoga massage: How to use traditional Thai massage, yoga, and breathwork for healing and spiritual harmony*. Dallas: Element Books Ltd.

Beinfeld, H., & Korngold, E. (1992). *Between heaven and earth: A guide to Chinese medicine*. New York: Random House.

Beresford-Cooke, C. (2003). *Shiatsu theory and practice: A comprehensive text for the student and professional* (2nd ed.). St Louis: Elsevier.

Brennan, B. A. (1993). *Light emerging: The journey of personal healing*. New York: Random House.

Chow, K. T. (2004). *Thai yoga massage: A dynamic therapy for physical wellbeing and spiritual energy*. Rochester: Inner Traditions/Bear & Company.

Chow, K. T., & Moody, E. (2006). *Thai yoga therapy for your body type: An ayurvedic tradition*. Rochester: Inner Traditions/Bear & Company.

Connelly, D. (1994). *Traditional acupuncture: The law of the five elements*. Laurel, MD: Tai Sophia Institute.

Dash, B., & Lalitesh, K. (1980). *Basic principles of ayurveda*. New Delhi: Asia Book Corp of America, Concept Publishing.

Dash, V. B. (1990). *Fundamentals of ayurvedic medicine*. Twin Lakes, WI: Lotus Press.

Dubitsky, C. (1997). *Bodywork shiatsu: Bringing the art of finger pressure to the massage table*. Rochester, VT: Inner Traditions International.

Ellis, A. (1994). *Fundamentals of Chinese acupuncture*. Brookline, MA: Paradigm Publications.

Ferguson, P. (2000). *Take five: The five elements guide to health and harmony*. Dublin: Gill & MacMillan.

Gold, R. (2006). *Thai massage: A traditional medical technique* (2nd ed.). St. Louis: Elsevier.

Holland, A. (1999). *Voices of qi: An introductory guide to traditional Chinese medicine* (2nd ed.). Berkeley, CA: North Atlantic Books.

Judith, A., & Ravenwolf, S. (1999). *Wheels of life: A journey through the chakras*. Woodbury, MN: Llewellyn Worldwide.

Kaptchuk, T. J. (2010). *The web that has no weaver: Understanding Chinese medicine*. Lincolnwood, IL: RosettaBooks.

Krishan, S. (2003). *Essential ayurveda: What it is and what it can do for you*. Novato, CA: New World Library.

Lad, V. (1993). *Ayurveda: The science of self-healing*. Twin Lakes, WI: Lotus Press.

Lad, V. (2007). *Textbook of ayurveda: A complete guide to clinical assessment*. Albuquerque, NM: Ayurvedic Press.

Leggett, D. (1999). *Recipes for self-healing*. London: Meridian Press.

Leslie, C. M., & Young, A. H. (1992). *Paths to Asian medical knowledge*. Berkeley, CA: University of California Press.

Lundberg, P. (2009). *The book of shiatsu: A complete guide to using hand pressure and gentle manipulation to improve your health, vitality, and stamina*. New York: Simon & Schuster.

Maciocia, G. (1995). *Tongue diagnosis in Chinese medicine*. Vista, CA: Eastland Press.

Maciocia, G. (2005). *Foundations of Chinese medicine: A comprehensive text*. St Louis: Elsevier.

Masunaga, S., & Ohashi, W. (1997). *Zen shiatsu: How to harmonize yin and yang for better health*. Tokyo: Japan Publications.

Matsumoto, K. (1983). *Extraordinary vessels*. Brookline, MA: Paradigm.

Meulenbeld, G., Wujastyk, J. M., & Wujastyk, D. (2001). *Studies on Indian medical history*. Amsterdam: Egbert Forsten.

Nadkarni, A. K. (1989). *Indian materia medica*. New Delhi: Popular Prakashan.

Namikoshi, T. (1997). *Complete book of shiatsu therapy: Health and vitality at your fingertips*. Tokyo: Japan Publications.

Pitman, V. (2004). *On the nature of the whole, Indian medical tradition series* (Vol. 7). New Delhi: Motilal Banarsidass.

Salguero, C. P., & Roylance, D. (2011). *Encyclopedia of Thai massage*. Findhorn Press.

Sharma, H. M., & Clark, C. (2002). *Contemporary ayurveda: Medicine and research in maharishi ayurveda*. St Louis: Elsevier.

Sharma, P. V. (1999). *Essentials of ayurveda*. New Delhi: Motilal Banarsidass.

Svoboda, R. E. (1998). *Prakriti: Your ayurvedic constitution*. Twin Lakes, WI: Lotus Press.

Svoboda, R. E., & Lade, A. (1996). *Tao and dharma: Chinese medicine and ayurveda*. Twin Lakes, WI: Lotus Press.

Tsu, L. (2009). *Tao te ching*. Translated by G Fu Feng and J English. New York: Vintage Books.

Upadhyay, S. D. (1986). *Nadivijana*. Delhi, India: Chaukhamba Sanskrit Pratisthan.

Xinnong, C. (2010). *Chinese acupuncture and moxibustion*. Beijing: Beijing Foreign Languages Press.

Zimmermann, F. (1999). *Jungle and the aroma of meats: An ecological theme in hindu medicine*. New Delhi: Motilal Banarsidass.

Zysk, K. G. (1993). The science of respiration and the doctrine of the vital winds in ancient India. *Journal of the American Oriental Society, 113*(2), 198–213.

Zysk, K. G. (1997, 2000). *Asceticism and healing in ancient India.* Medicine in the buddhist monastery. Revised edition. New Delhi: Motilal Banarsidass. Vol 2 of Indian Medical Tradition.

Zysk, K. G. (2001). New age ayurveda or what happens to Indian medicine when it comes to America. *Traditional South Asian Medicine, 6*(6), 10–26.

Zysk, K. G. (2007). The bodily winds in ancient India revisited. *Journal of the Royal Anthropological Institute, 13*, 105–115.

Zysk, K. G. (2008). *Siddha medicine in Tamil Nadu*. Copenhagen: National museet.

Zysk, K. G. (2010). Traditional medicine in India: Ayurveda and siddha. In M. Micozzi (Ed.), *Fundamentals of complementary and alternative medicine* (4th ed.). St. Louis: Elsevier.

REVIEW AND APPLY YOUR KNOWLEDGE

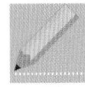

MATCHING ONE: CONCEPT REVIEW

Place the letter of the answer next to the number of the term or phrase that best describes it.

A. Asian bodywork therapy
B. Channels
C. Gua sha
D. Five phases or elements
E. Hara
F. Jitsu
G. Ki
H. Kyo
I. Looking, listening and smelling, palpating, and asking
J. Chi or qi
K. Shiatsu
L. Tsubos

_____ 1. Examples are earth, wood, fire, metal, and water.
_____ 2. Methods used by Asian bodywork practitioners to assess energetic imbalances in their clients.
_____ 3. Japanese Asian bodywork method using applied pressure along energy channels to restore, maintain, or balance the flow of ki.
_____ 4. Term used to describe a quality of energy that is full, yang, excessive, or too much ki.
_____ 5. Term used to describe a quality of energy that is empty, yin, depleted, or not enough ki.
_____ 6. Use of pressure and/or manipulation to treat the body, mind, and spirit, including the electromagnetic or energetic fields in and surrounding the body.
_____ 7. Chinese term for vital energy or life force.
_____ 8. Japanese term for vital energy or life force.
_____ 9. Pathways in the body through which energy circulates.
_____ 10. Points along channels where energy concentrates and surfaces.
_____ 11. The body's center of focused power and energy.
_____ 12. A skin-scraping technique used in traditional Chinese medicine.

MATCHING TWO: CONCEPT REVIEW

Place the letter of the answer next to the number of the term or phrase that best describes it.

A. Ayurveda
B. Chakras
C. Dosha
D. Kapha
E. Moxibustion
F. Nadis
G. Pitta
H. Prakriti
I. Solar plexus
J. Cupping therapy
K. Thai massage
L. Zang-Fu organs

_____ 1. Technique in which heat from burning an herb called mugwort is placed over or on the skin to stimulate acupoints.
_____ 2. Technique in which plastic, silicone, or glass cups are placed on the skin to create a suction and lift the tissue.
_____ 3. In Ayurveda, a person's unique natural constitution.
_____ 4. Term used to describe yin and yang organ systems and their associated channels.
_____ 5. A form of partner yoga consisting of stretching and compression; also called Nuad Bo'Rarn.
_____ 6. In Ayurveda, the combination of all five elements (earth, air, fire, water, and space or ether) making up the human body.
_____ 7. Another term for the third chakra.
_____ 8. In Ayurveda, the body's energy centers along a central channel.
_____ 9. In Ayurveda, the dosha made up of the elements of earth and water.
_____ 10. In Ayurveda, channels in the body where prana energy flows.
_____ 11. In Ayurveda, the dosha made up of the elements of fire and water.
_____ 12. Traditional Hindu system of medicine that maintains or improves health through diet, massage, yoga, yogic breathing, and herbal preparations.

MULTIPLE CHOICE: TEST YOUR KNOWLEDGE

Place the letter of the answer next to the number of the term or phrase that best describes it.

_____ 1. What is the symbol that represents yin and yang?
   A. Ojas
   B. Ventus
   C. Tai Ji
   D. Kyo Jitsu

_____ 2. Which element is associated with spring, the color green, and the liver?
   A. Wood
   B. Fire
   C. Earth
   D. Metal

_____ 3. Which element is associated with autumn, the color white, and the lungs?
   A. Wood
   B. Fire
   C. Earth
   D. Metal

_____ 4. Ki follows the Chinese clock, which is a system of time based on:
   A. nature's seasons.
   B. biologic cycles.
   C. spiritual balance.
   D. moon phases.

_____ 5. The flow of ki is at its peak in which channel from 11 am to 1 pm?
   A. Stomach
   B. Liver
   C. Kidney
   D. Heart

_____ 6. The width of a client's thumb knuckle determines which of the following?
   A. Tsubo
   B. Cun
   C. Kyo
   D. Jitsu

_____ 7. Which of the following is classified as a Yin organ?
   A. Liver
   B. Gallbladder
   C. Stomach
   D. Bladder

_____ 8. Which form of Asian bodywork involves floating the client in water?
   A. Shiatsu
   B. Ashiatsu
   C. Watsu
   D. Zen shiatsu

_____ 9. In Thai medical theory, what is the term that encompasses all the aspects of the nonphysical body, including thoughts, emotions, will, and spiritual aspirations?
   A. Sen
   B. Cun
   C. Pitta
   D. Citta

_____ 10. In Ayurveda, which is the term for the waste products of the body and include sweat, urine, and feces?
   A. Dosha
   B. Dhatus
   C. Vata
   D. Malas

_____ 11. Which of the seven dhatus refers to blood?
   A. Rasa
   B. Rakta
   C. Meda
   D. Majja

_____ 12. Which chakra is associated with intuition, psychic vision, and the color indigo?
   A. Crown
   B. Brow
   C. Throat
   D. Heart

CRITICAL THINKING

Thai Massage and Pregnancy

Do you think Thai massage is safe to perform on a pregnant client? What considerations is your answer based on?

Answers can include but are not limited to:

Thai massage can be performed on many different types of clients. The positioning and techniques can be modified according to the client's comfort, vitality, and existing conditions and need. Traditional Thai massage is performed on a futon on the floor, but if a client is unwilling or unable to get down on the futon, some of the techniques can be adapted to working on a massage table. If the client is 4 or more months pregnant, she would need to be propped in a semireclining position for supine work, whether she is on a futon or massage table. To perform Thai massage techniques on her back and posterior legs, she would need to be propped in side-lying or lateral recumbent position. Because clients remain fully clothed for Thai massage, draping is not a concern when positioning the client.

Stretching techniques are an important part of Thai massage. These techniques stimulate stretch receptors and convey a variety of signals to the brain. Stretching increases flexibility, improves range of motion and posture, restores balance within and between muscle groups, and relieves pain and suffering. However, because of the release of the hormone relaxin, caution is warranted for Thai massage stretching and joint mobilization techniques. In addition, the application of pressure may need to be adjusted, especially over any varicosities.

An area of concern for newly pregnant clients is the possibility of a miscarriage. For this reason, Thai massage, just like Western massage, could be considered a contraindication during the first trimester.

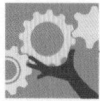

PROFESSIONAL PRACTICE

Synergy

Marcia has pain in her medial ankle accompanied by paresthesia. She also has pain in her back and shoulders. Marcia's doctor recommended massage or shiatsu. She was given the contact information for Jerry, a massage practitioner, and Sarah, a shiatsu practitioner. Marcia decided to schedule appointments with both.

Jerry focused on reducing scar tissue from the sprains and deactivating trigger points in her legs, shoulders, and back. For

2 days after treatment, Marcia found it easier to stand and walk. She felt minor relief in her back, but the ankle pain persisted. Sarah focused on the Kidney and Bladder channels, where she found stagnation. For the next 2 days, Marcia's back pain was reduced and she felt a surge in energy she had not experienced in years.

Marcia wants to continue seeing both practitioners but wants to be sure their treatments are complementary. What can Marcia do to ensure treatments are synergistic?

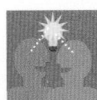

DISCUSSION

Cultural Differences

Western medicine and Eastern medicine have both been evolving for centuries but within different cultures. Contrast and compare each approach to health and disease. If available, post your reflections on an Internet-based discussion board monitored by your instructor.

Work is love made visible
—Kahlil Gibran

CHAPTER 17

Business Practices: Getting Started, Marketing, Professional Development, Accounting, and Planning

LEARNING OBJECTIVES

After completing this chapter, the student should be able to:

1. Discuss licensing, types of insurance, employment opportunities, business entities, zoning, startup costs, and taxes.
2. Outline business practices, including how to determine fees for services and discuss bartering, tipping, and various business policies.
3. Describe marketing strategies, including mission statements, business cards, professional profiles, websites, blogs, social media, gift cards, value-added services, and retail products.
4. Discuss professional development and business resources, such as continuing education, board certification, mentors, preceptors, business coaches, business contracts, and proposals.
5. Define accounting and delineate types of financial statements.
6. Write a business plan.

http://evolve.elsevier.com/Salvo/MassageTherapy

INTRODUCTION

There are many reasons why individuals choose a career in massage. For some, it is the fulfillment experienced by helping others who have a diminished quality of life because of stress, pain, or injury. For others, it is the flexible work hours, financial rewards, or the opportunity of owning or running a business. In fact, 72% of massage practitioners describe themselves as sole practitioners at least part of the time (American Massage Therapy Association [AMTA], 2022).

When looking at characteristics of individual massage practitioners, this is what we find: 82% enter the massage profession as their second career, and 86% of practitioners are female (AMTA, 2022). Comparing gender gaps of the massage profession to the nursing profession, we find a similar trend in that 76% to 90% of healthcare workers are female (Day & Christnacht, 2019).

What does a work week look like? Massage practitioners spend an average of 24 hours a week giving massages and see an average of 44 clients a month. Seventy percent of a workday is spent giving massages, and the other 30% of the time is spent on business-related tasks such as bookkeeping, managing supplies, maintaining equipment, marketing, and client scheduling.

What does the financial picture look like in various practice settings? Massage practitioners are making an average of $85 for 1 hour of massage services when working in a client's home, and practitioners working in a massage franchise or chain are making an average of $25 for 1 hour of massage services; these amounts include tips (AMTA, 2022).

Massage businesses are thriving. Companies holding the largest market share in the massage industry are Massage Envy, Hand and Stone Massage, and Elements (IBISWorld, 2020). Health and service businesses are among the industries with the best track record of operational longevity. So, what factors contribute to business failure? A study conducted by the University of Tennessee found that 46% of business failures are due to incompetence, and 30% are due to unbalanced experience or lack of managerial experience (Statistic Brain Research Institute, 2018). Business incompetence includes emotional pricing or no knowledge of pricing, cost of living higher than the business income, nonpayment of taxes, lack of business planning, and lack of finance knowledge or record keeping knowledge. Other reasons for business failure identified by Mason (2021) were not expending enough effort; having unrealistic expectations; unwillingness to take responsibility; choosing a business that is not profitable; failing to clearly define and understand the consumer market, consumers, and consumer buying habits; failure to anticipate or react to the competition or to changes in technology; overdependence on a single consumer; and believing they can do everything alone without outside assistance.

Don't assume a door is closed. Push on it.
—**Marian Wright Edelman**

GETTING STARTED

This section discusses activities most massage school graduates must complete to enter the profession such as getting a state license, professional insurance, and other requirements. This section also features information regarding employment opportunities, types of employment, various business entities, zoning, startup costs, and taxes.

Professional License

A **license** is official permission granted to an individual by a legal authority to do, to use, or to own something. The term license also refers to the document issued to the licensee. A **professional license** restricts the practice of an occupation to those who hold a license. In contrast, certification restricts the use of a title, but not the practice, to those who are certified. Professional licensure seeks to protect the public by enforcing standards that restrict practice to qualified individuals who have met certain educational requirements and earned a passing score in a competency examination—such as the Massage and Bodywork Licensing Examination, or MBLEx. Licensing criteria vary from state to state, but most states require a minimum of 500 classroom hours and participation in a student practicum or public clinic. Individuals who do not have a professional license in licensed states are not permitted to perform the same procedures that licensed individuals can. Currently, the Council of State Governments is developing an interstate compact so practitioners who have an unencumbered state license in their home state have the privilege to practice in a remote state that is a member of the interstate compact. As of 2021, only three states do not regulate the practice of massage.

Insurance

Insurance is an agreement by a company or governmental agency to provide compensation for specified losses, damages, illness, or death in return for payments called *premiums* given to the insurance provider. Most people pay their premiums monthly. The document containing the terms and conditions of the insurance agreement is called the *insurance policy*. Some policies have an *insurance deductible*, which is a set amount the policyholder must pay every year before the insurance company starts paying. This amount varies by policy, and some policies have no deductible. There are several types of insurances such as liability, disability, workers' compensation, and health insurance.

Professional Liability Insurance

Massage practitioners are liable or responsible for any negative outcomes related to the care they provide to the public. Substandard or negligent care may result in a lawsuit filed against the practitioner to remedy the damages they caused.

Professional liability insurance helps protect the service provider from bearing the full cost of a legal defense and helps pay for damages awarded by the courts if the provider is found negligent. Professional liability insurance is also called *malpractice insurance* and *errors and omissions (E&O) insurance.* Most lawsuits claim the practitioner owed the client a duty of care; the practitioner through the massage breached that duty; the breach caused an injury; and the injury caused the client physical, psychological, and/or financial damages (Coble, 2016). Many states require licensees to have professional liability insurance. Most professional associations offer this type of insurance to their members. Professional liability insurance can be obtained by massage students while they are enrolled in a training program.

Commercial General Liability Insurance

Commercial general liability insurance (CGL) is a type of liability insurance that helps protect businesses from bearing the full cost of defending against claims for damages resulting from negligence associated with property and day-to-day business operations. Examples of claims include bodily injuries from slips and falls while a client is in the office, or property damage when a tree limb falls and damages a client's car. CGL insurance is also called *premises liability insurance.*

Disability and Workers Compensation Insurance

Disability insurance provides income protection if a person is unable to work because of disease or injury. The Social Security Administration (2021) projects one quarter of today's 20-year-olds will become disabled before reaching the age of 67. Thus, disability is a major economic risk—especially when the reduced ability to earn income is combined with growing health-related costs. **Workers' compensation insurance** provides income to employees who are unable to work because of a job-related injury. Workers' compensation insurance may include reimbursement or payments of medical expenses. Employers are often required to have workers' compensation to cover their employees in the event of job-related injuries.

Health Insurance

Health insurance covers part or all of the medical expenses for diseases, conditions, and injuries. The policy is administered and managed by a central organization such as a governmental agency or a private entity. Some policies include a *copayment,* or copay, which is the flat fee paid during each medical appointment or when filling a prescription. The insurance copay is usually a relatively small amount and may or may not count toward your deductible.

Employment Opportunities and Types of Employment

A career in massage offers many employment opportunities in healthcare; fitness and wellness; beauty and spa industries; and the travel, recreational, and hospitality industries.

An alphabetical list of employment opportunity examples includes:
- Acupuncture clinics
- Airports
- Athletic teams and dance companies
- Casinos
- Chiropractic clinics
- Corporate wellness programs
- Cruise lines
- Day spas
- Dentist offices
- Facial, nail, and beauty salons
- Golf, tennis, and country clubs
- Gyms and health clubs
- Hospitals
- Hotels
- Massage franchises
- Nursing homes
- Onsite massage in offices
- Pain management clinics
- Physical therapy, rehab, and sports medicine clinics
- Private practice
- Psychiatric treatment centers
- Resorts
- Rodeos
- Shopping malls
- Upscale grocery stores
- Veterinarians and racetracks (animal massage)

There are several types of employment, and practitioners can work full time or part time. What constitutes full time can vary by culture and by employer. In any type of employment, the employer often determines the hours of the day and days of the week of employment (U.S. Bureau of Labor Statistics, 2021).
- **Full time employment**. Usually works ≥35 hours a week.
- **Part time employment**. Usually works ≤35 hours a week.
- **Casual employment**. Works when needed and does not have a fixed schedule.
- **Contract employment**. Works on a fixed-term or contractual basis for an agreed-upon length of time.
- **Commissioned employment**. Works and receives commission payments rather than an hourly or weekly pay rate.

Employers generally provide the place where massage services are administered, the tools and materials needed to administer the services, and exercise some control over the service such as time of service, length of time spent providing the service, and fees clients pay for services rendered. In addition, employers are responsible for collecting taxes and providing compensation to employees.

Self-employed individuals may be **independent contractors**—individuals who have specialized skills, training, or licensure that allows them to work without supervision. Independent contractors often provide their own tools and equipment, work in more than one location, and are not required to sign a noncompete agreement. A self-assessment quiz is on Evolve to see if self-employment is a good choice for you.

Self-employed individuals receive a fee based on completion of a task, and the fee is usually determined by the independent contractor—not the individual who is receiving the service or the business who utilizes independent contractors.

Contracting businesses occasionally mischaracterize employees as independent contractors. This may arise from businesses wanting to avoid employers' responsibilities such as withholding income taxes, contributing to Social Security, paying unemployment insurance, and obtaining workers' compensation insurance. This mischaracterization can expose an employer to penalties and interest for missing tax payments. Employees treated as independent contractors may take legal action for gaps in Social Security and unemployment compensation coverage. If an employee fails to pay income tax due, the employer may have to pay the employee's taxes to the extent of the tax-withholding shortfall. Massage practitioners considering an independent contractor relationship should obtain advice from a lawyer or accountant to confirm if a proper characterization of the relationship exists.

Developing a Resume and Curriculum Vitae

Resumes and curricula vitae are important documents to help job applicants present themselves as the best candidate to prospective employers. A **resume** is a summary of an individual's education, experiences, and accomplishments related to a particular skill set. Resumes are typically one page in length and organized in reverse-chronological order, with the most current events listed first. A **curriculum vitae** (CV) is an in-depth overview of a person's education, experiences, and accomplishments and is also organized in reverse-chronological order. CVs are longer in length compared with resumes.

A well-prepared resume or CV gives prospective employers an insight into your professional career potential. Resumes and CVs are essentially forms of advertisement, and the person applying for the position is the product advertised. As such, resumes and CVs are vehicles to help individuals get to the next step of potential employment—the job interview. These are the sections of a resume or CV.

- **Contact Information**: Include your name, mailing address, contact numbers, email address, and a link to an online professional profile that includes a professional portrait photograph.
- **Qualifications Summary**: A bulleted list of four to six points outlining outstanding career achievements. This section is omitted if the individual is just starting their career.
- **Professional Work Experience**: This contains only the experiences relevant to the job for which you are applying. As a rule, each experience should have a list of three to five bullet points of main duties and achievements associated with the job experience.

- **Education**: Include names of universities, community colleges, or technical schools; location of the schools (city, state); dates attended; and degrees awarded.
- **Additional Sections**: Sections such as publications, awards and honors, and additional skills can be added to highlight special skills you possess. For example, are you fluent in a second language or do you possess computer software skills such as Photoshop?

When creating your resume or CV, choose easy-to-read fonts and follow the 24, 12, 10 format: your name is in 24-pt font, all headers are in 12-pt font, and all bullet points are in 10-pt font. This divides the resume or CV into easy-to-read sections.

Job Interviews

A job interview is a formal meeting between a candidate and a representative of a company who is seeking to hire workers. The main objectives of the interview are for both sides to identify benefits the candidate can add to and get from the company. There are several kinds of interviews such as screening, electronic or phone, sequential, and panel interviews. *Screening interviews* are used by companies to narrow the applicant pool. *Electronic* or *phone interviews* may be used when the applicants and companies are in different geographic regions. Treat electronic or phone interviews as if they were face to face and have important documents on hand. *Sequential interviews* occur when applicants are interviewed by different individuals within the company, sometimes within the same day. During a *panel interview*, applicants are interviewed by a panel or group. Multiple applicants can be interviewed at the same time.

Know enough about the company to speak authoritatively during the interview. Topics may include the company's recent stock price if publicly traded, its mission statement, names of the chief executive officers, and any current relevant news that could affect the business (Hansen, n.d).

A list of common interview questions is on Evolve. Use them to prepare and practice your responses. What most employers are looking for is evidence of problem-solving skills, the ability to work in a team, and a strong work ethic. Other abilities and attributes important to employers and recruiters are analytical skills, written and verbal communication skills, leadership skills, tact, a friendly/outgoing personality, and computer skills (National Association of Colleges and Employers, 2020).

Research suggests wearing formal business attire rather than casual attire has a positive impact on business interactions such as job interviews (Fig. 17.1) (Menafn, 2020). Find out their policies on tattoos, body art, and body piercings and use these policies to inform your appearance for the interview. Arrive at least 15 minutes before the interview and bring extra copies of your resume or CV. Shut off all portable electronic devices.

When responding to questions, showcase skills and experiences that fit the job and emphasize critical thinking, but keep responses short and to the point. Never badmouth a previous employer, boss, or co-worker. Ask questions

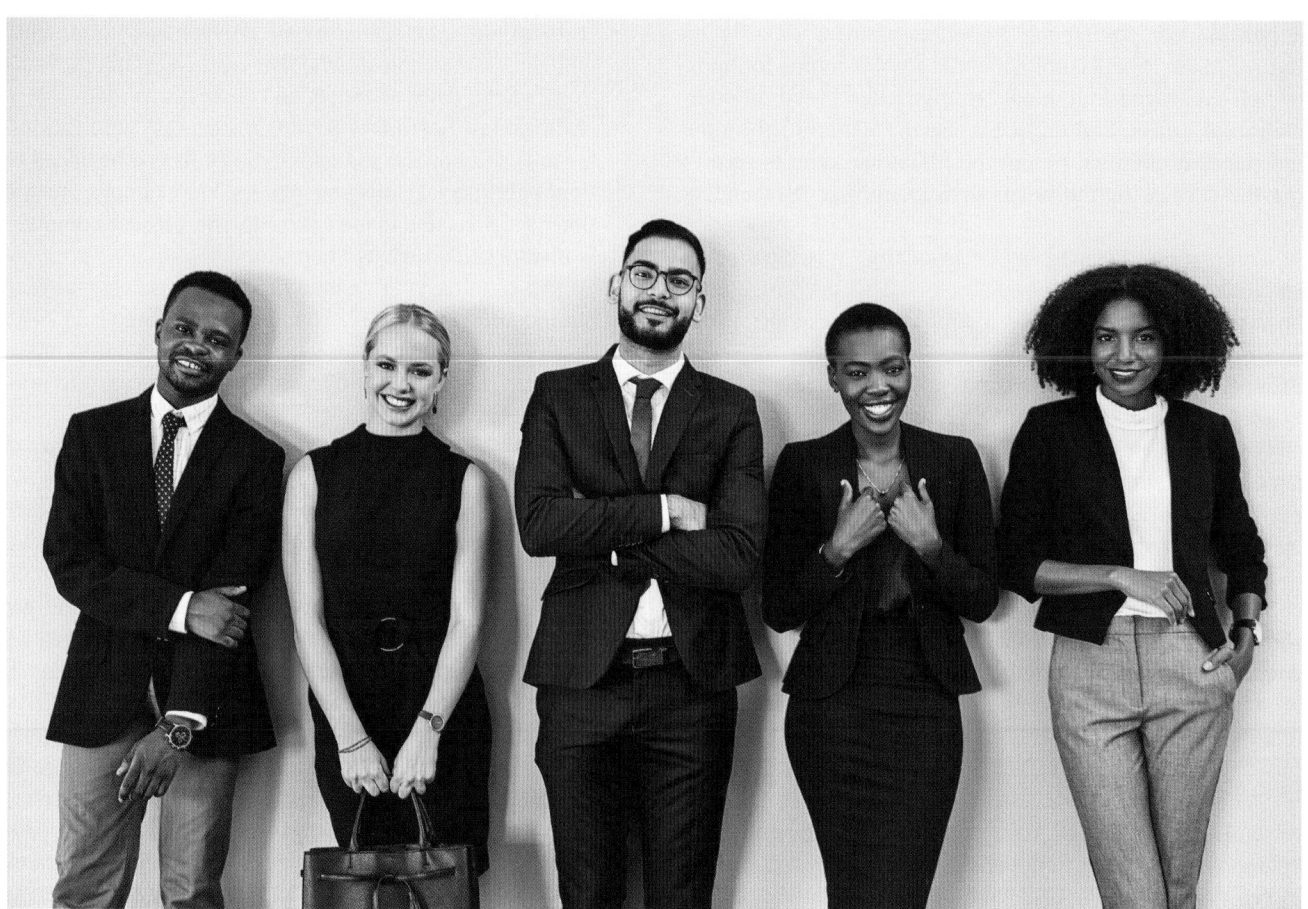

FIG. 17.1 Dress for success for job interviews. (Copyright © istock.com/LumiNola.)

displaying interest in the job such as job expectations, the work environment, management style, promotions and performance reviews, and compensation. Use body postures that convey empathy such as eye contact, facial expressions depicting warmth, an open body posture, and tone of voice that conveys confidence and compassion. Negative forms of body language include slouching, looking off in the distance, being distracted by electronic devices, chewing gum, and mumbling.

As the interview winds down, ask about the next steps in the process and the timetable the employer expects to use to decide about the position. Lastly, thank the interviewer before leaving and write a thank-you note sent via email or postal mail shortly after the interview.

Business Entities

Self-employed practitioners or independent contractors must choose a business entity or legal business structure. Common choices among for-profit businesses include sole proprietorships, partnerships, and corporations. Each entity has tax and liability consequences. Consult a lawyer, accountant, and other business experts before starting your business to establish the proper structure that meets both short-term and long-term goals, and savings, investment,

tax consequences, and health insurance responsibilities. In addition, avoid using a business account for personal transactions. If you share expenses with other practitioners, maintain separate business entities by not commingling funds.

Sole Proprietor

A **sole proprietorship** is a business of a single owner. Legally, no distinction exists between the business and the owner. Business profits and debts are the owner's, and the business terminates upon the owner's death. The owner assumes any business risks to the extent of their personal assets, whether the assets are used in the business or are personally owned. Although a sole proprietorship is not a separate legal entity from its owner, it is a separate entity for accounting purposes. Any business financial activities (deposits of massage fees) are maintained separately from the owner's personal financial activities (i.e., mortgage payments). The advantages of a sole proprietorship are that they are easy to start and the least expensive type of business entity to operate. Profits and losses are reported on Schedule C of an individual Form 1040 tax return. The disadvantage is the owner is personally liable and any court judgments may involve personal assets.

Partnerships: General and Limited

Business partnerships are owned by two or more entities. The main types of business partnerships are general and limited. **General partnerships** are an agreement between two or more individuals who conduct the business for profit, and each partner contributes money, property, labor, or skill, and they share the business's profits and losses. Partners have unlimited personal liability for the business's debts. **Limited partnerships** limit the personal liability of partners according to the amount that partner invested into the company. Partners must file a certificate of limited partnership with the proper state authorities. Tax Form 1065 is used by partnerships to file federal tax returns annually with the Internal Revenue Service (IRS). Partnerships must also submit a completed Schedule K-1. The K-1 is a partner's share of income and deductions reported on their individual tax return (Form 1040).

Limited Liability Company

Limited liability companies (LLCs) are a blend of partnerships and corporations. Members of an LLC have flexible involvement in the company and receive financial rewards similar to a partnership but have less exposure to risks similar to a corporation (discussed next).

Corporations: C- and S-Corporations

Corporations are legal business entities who are granted a charter by the state in which they operate. Articles of incorporation must be filed with the state to establish a corporate entity. Some states require filing of certain documents such as the minutes to shareholder meetings and some require annual payments. Corporations have privileges and liabilities distinct from its board of directors or the shareholders. A **shareholder**, also called a stockholder, is a person or business (e.g., partnership, corporation) that owns at least one share of a stock. **Shares** are units of equity and ownership in a corporation. Profits may be distributed in the form of dividends (capital gains), and share value may increase as the value of the corporation grows.

- **C-Corporation**: C-corporation's earnings are taxed by the Internal Revenue Service at the corporate level and again at the shareholder level (called *double taxation*). C-corporations cannot pass losses through to shareholders.
- **S-Corporation**: Subchapter S-corporations are corporations of a certain size and structure that file specific paperwork with the Internal Revenue Service requesting Subchapter S status. S-corporations operate the same as C-corporations but earnings are not taxed on a corporate level but "flow through" to the shareholder's tax returns.

Zoning

Zoning is the dividing of geographic areas into zones so a city or municipality can restrict the number and types of buildings within the zone as well as how these buildings are used. Approximately 36% of massage practitioners provide massages in their homes (AMTA, 2022). If planning to conduct a massage business in a residential zone, compliance with zoning ordinances or restrictive covenants is required. Zoning ordinances for home or residential offices might include restricting the number of employees, limiting the number of parked vehicles, disability access, the number of client visits per day, lawn/home signage, retail sale restrictions, and limits on the percentage of the home dedicated to business operations.

Startup Costs

Startup costs are expenses incurred before a business opens. Most startup costs for massage businesses include equipment such as massage tables, a music system, massage linens and lubricants, furniture and fixtures, office supplies, office rental deposits and utility deposits, phones and phone service plans, legal and professional services, insurance premiums, licenses and permits, advertising, printing costs, personnel, cash in a business account, and a petty cash account. The Internet is a good source for business startup cost calculators. Some startup costs become regular operating expenses such as replacing linens, lubricants, and office supplies.

Taxes and Tax Deductions

Taxes are sums of money levied upon income or revenue, property, and sales, which is then given to a government to carry out its functions, such as expenditures on war, law enforcement, protection of property, public transportation, and the operation of government itself. Taxes are also used to fund public services, such as welfare, education, healthcare, and pensions for disabled and elderly persons.

Gross income is the total amount of income earned over a period of time by an individual/household or a company. Gross income is also called *gross earnings*. **Net income** is the amount an individual, household, or a company makes after deducting allowable expenses and taxes. Net income is also called *net earnings*. **Income taxes** are taxes owed on personal and business income and on unearned income such as dividends and rental property. In many countries such as the United States, the income tax rate is progressive—higher income earners pay a higher tax rate compared with lower income earners.

Employers deduct a percentage of employee wages (currently 7.65%) for Social Security and Medicare tax. The employer "matches" the amount deducted from the employee's salary and remits the approximately 15.3% to the IRS as Employee Taxes. These taxes fund the Social Security payments employees can draw during retirement. The employer issues a W-2 form annually. This form contains the employee's wages, tips, and compensations, as well as withholdings. This and other forms are used to determine whether additional taxes are owed or if a refund is expected. Individuals and businesses file federal and state income tax returns annually, or once a year. Taxable income is total income minus allowable deductions. Individuals use Form 1040 to file their annual income tax return with the IRS.

Self-employment taxes are taxes levied on small business owners who derive income directly from consumers as opposed to individuals who are employees (see the earlier section on income tax). Self-employed individuals are required to pay both the employer's and employee's portion of Social Security and Medicare taxes, which is currently 15.3%.

Tax deductions are expenses that reduce taxable income and usually result from expenses incurred to produce the income. Other factors affecting the amount of income tax owed are exemptions and tax credits. A main difference between tax deductions, tax exemptions, and tax credits is that deductions and exemptions reduce taxable income, and tax credits reduce the amount of tax owed. Obtain a list of deductions, exemptions, and credits from authoritative sources such as tax professionals and governmental agencies. Examples of potential tax deductions include:

- Accounting and bookkeeping fees
- Advertising and promotional fees
- Books and periodicals
- Business-related insurance payments
- Continuing education (CE) and continuous professional development (CPD) expenses
- Conventions and conferences of business and trade organizations
- Gifts to and the entertaining of current or prospective clients (limits apply)
- Internet and hosting service charges
- Laundry and cleaning services
- Legal, consulting, and professional services
- License, certification, and permit fees
- Office and massage supplies
- Postage and shipping fees
- Printing and duplication fees
- Rent
- Repairs to office or equipment
- Service charges related to financial transactions and merchant fees
- Uniforms and personal protective equipment (PPE)
- Utilities and telephone services

The Length of Time Business Records Are Kept

Business records include business expense receipts, bank and financial institution records, and tax returns. Generally, business records that support an item of income, deduction, or credit shown on your tax return must be kept until the period of limitations for the tax return expires. *Period of limitations* is the time tax returns can be amended to claim a credit or refund or time period in which the IRS can assess additional tax (Internal Revenue Service [IRS], 2020). Unless otherwise stated, the years specified refer to the period after the tax return was filed. Returns filed before the due date are treated as if they were filed on the due date.

1. Keep records for 3 years if situations (4), (5), and (6) below do not apply to you.

2. Keep records for 3 years from the date you filed your original return or 2 years from the date you paid the tax, whichever is later, if you file a claim for credit or refund after you file your return.
3. Keep records for 7 years if you file a claim for a loss from worthless securities or bad debt deduction.
4. Keep records for 6 years if you do not report income that you should report, and it is more than 25% of the gross income shown on your return.
5. Keep records indefinitely if you do not file a return.
6. Keep records indefinitely if you file a fraudulent return.
7. Keep employment tax records for at least 4 years after the date that the tax becomes due or is paid, whichever is later.

Writing a novel is like driving a car at night. You can see only as far as your headlights, but you can make the whole trip that way.

—E. L. Doctorow

BUSINESS PRACTICES

This section discusses business practices, including setting fees (if self-employed), bartering, tips from clients, policies for clients who cancel or fail to show up for their scheduled appointments, and managing conflict.

Determining Fees for Services

If the massage practitioner is self-employed or an independent contractor, the business or service provider usually determines the fees clients are expected to pay for massage services. Most business and service providers set a fee based on time intervals such as 30-, 50-, 60-, 80-, or 90-minute sessions. Some businesses and service providers charge one fee for self-care, relaxation, or wellness massage and a higher fee for healthcare or therapeutic massage, deep pressure massage, or for specialized methods such as manual lymphatic or neuromuscular techniques of equivalent times.

To determine an hourly rate, add all costs (labor/salary and overhead) and profits, then divide this amount by the number of billable hours. The calculation may look like this: if you work 40 hours per week and take 2 weeks of vacation per year—40 (hours per week) times 50 (weeks worked per year) equals 2000 hours per year. Next, deduct nonbillable hours. These are hours spent doing tasks such as cleaning/disinfecting, scheduling, and marketing. This number is about 30% (AMTA, 2022). This adjustment reduces 2000 hours per year to 1400 billable hours per year. Then calculate costs, determine an annual salary, add in annual overhead expenses, and include a profit margin (Fishman, n.d.).

Let's look at salary first. The AMTA (2022) states annual earnings for massage practitioners average $29,439. The U.S. Bureau of Labor Statistics (2022) found the median annual salary for massage practitioners is $46,900. For calculations, take the average of these two amounts, which is an annual salary of about $38,170.

Next, calculate overhead costs and include advertising, insurance premiums, and taxes. Then add a profit—most businesses calculate between 10% and 20% (Fishman, n.d.). Again, use the average, which is 15%. Your calculations and resultant hourly rate may look something like this:

$$\$38,170 + \$20,000 = \$58,170 \text{ (salary and overhead)}$$

$$\$58,170 \times 15\% = \$8726 \text{ (15\% profit)}$$

$$\$58,170 + \$8726 = \$66,896 \text{ (annual costs and 15\% profit)}$$

$$\$66,896/1400 = \$47.78 \text{ (hourly rate)}$$

Lastly, examine what other providers are charging to see if this fee should be adjusted up or down. Make note of what recent graduates are charging versus what experienced practitioners are charging for similar services and consider the location of the business when making comparisons. Depending on market conditions, the business or provider may be able to charge more or might have to accept less.

Rescheduling Clients

Massage is a client-retention business, so a marketing strategy is client rescheduling. Asking clients to make another appointment is the best way to fill your schedule. Statistically speaking, current clients will likely reschedule when asked because the probability of selling to existing customers is between 60% and 70%. Those are good odds. These appointments can be scheduled on a weekly basis, every other week, monthly, or another regular interval.

If clients do not want to reschedule at this time, give them a smile and say an equivalent of, "Okay, you know how to reach me when you are ready to get back on the massage table."

Bartering

Bartering is the nonmonetary exchange of goods or services. An example of bartering is plumbers exchanging plumbing services for massage services from a massage practitioner. You must include in gross income in the year of receipt the fair market value of goods or services received from bartering. Generally, you report this income on Schedule C, Form 1040 (IRS, 2021a).

Tips

Tips, or *gratuities,* are discretionary money given to service providers by their consumer. Tips include:
- Cash received directly from customers.
- Tips from customers who give it through electronic settlements or payments. This includes credit cards, debit cards, gift cards, or other electronic payment methods.
- Tips received through tip pools, tip splitting, or other tip sharing arrangements.

The amount of the tip varies and is usually based on the total cost of services provided and the perceived quality of service given. Tips are common in massage industries that provide wellness or self-care massages such as spas and franchises/chains and in some private practices. Individuals who own the business or who are self-employed and receive the full price of the massage may or may not be tipped—consumers may only tip those who receive only a portion of the fee. Tips are also less common in clinics, hospitals, and institutionalized care facilities providing massages.

Tips should not be solicited by the business or the practitioner, and every client should receive the same level of care. Good tippers should not receive preferential treatment. Cash and noncash tips are considered income and are subject to federal income taxes. Cash tips received by an employee in any calendar month are subject to Social Security and Medicare taxes and must be reported to the employer. If the total tips received by the employee during a single calendar month from a single employer are less than $20, then these tips are usually not required to be reported (IRS, 2021b). Tips and their amounts are considered social customs and vary between countries. For example, tipping is common in the United States and Canada and less common in parts of Asia and Europe.

Cancellation and No-Show Policies

Self-employed massage practitioners must determine how cancellations and no-shows of previously scheduled appointments are handled. For cancellation policies, decide how far in advance clients can cancel with or without penalties. Examples of penalties are full or partial collection of the fee associated with the canceled appointment or a set fee such as $25.00. Also, determine how and when this fee will be collected. For no-show policies, also determine any associated penalties, including how and when a no-show fee will be collected. Consider having a policy that penalizes the practitioner if they cancel an appointment; this policy should be equivalent to the cancellation policy expected of clients. These policies should be clearly stated during the informed consent procedure. Chapter 10 discusses informed consent. Consider waiving penalties for scheduling changes in certain circumstances such as sudden illness.

Managing Conflict

Conflict is a fact of business life. Individuals have differing values and priorities, opinions will vary, and miscommunication and misunderstandings occur—all of which may create conflict.

Massage practitioners must use empathetic approaches to manage conflict. This can make the difference between positive and negative outcomes. These strategies are discussed under Making Professional Decisions in Chapter 2.

MARKETING

Marketing is defined as activities used to create, communicate, deliver, and exchange products and services that have value for consumers, clients, and the society at large.

Marketing promotes public awareness of a business. Examples of marketing activities include developing a mission statement and professional profile, launching and updating a website and social media campaigns, having a blog, and offering retail sales. Marketing is everything you do to get clients in the door and on the massage table. The next step to marketing is to get them to come back, then for clients to refer their friends and family.

Within the massage industry, marketing usually involves educating potential clients about what massage can do for them and about the massage business and/or the massage practitioner(s). If consumers do not perceive a need or benefit for your products and services, they are not likely to become regular clients. Massage offers many benefits from stress and pain reduction to improved function (see Chapter 6).

Marketing connects consumers to businesses through information, which may involve the use of advertising and publicity. **Advertising** is the use of persuasive messages to influence consumer buying habits, usually by paid announcements. Examples of advertising include print advertising (newspaper, magazines, brochures), broadcast advertising (television, radio), outdoor advertising (signs, banners, billboards), and digital advertising (social media, search engines). In contrast, **publicity** is free media exposure. Examples of publicity include writing an article on a blog or website, being interviewed on a podcast or webinar, giving public lectures at local civic groups, or offering complimentary chair massages at local events.

The goal of advertising is to attract new customers by defining a target market and reaching out to them with effective selling messages. A **target market** is a group of consumers that is more likely to want or need your products or services—a subset of the total business market. This process involves looking at characteristics or qualities of the group you believe your products or services will appeal to. Examples of a target market are high-stress executives, people committed to wellness, people with chronic pain, people with specific healthcare conditions (e.g., temporomandibular dysfunction), pregnant females, athletes, and seniors. Once the target market is identified, businesses can make better decisions about how to market their services and what the selling message should entail.

Businesses may consult with professional advertising agencies to develop advertising strategies. These agencies can provide clients a *media kit,* which includes population statistics by groups (females, males, age groups) and demographics about household incomes, education levels, and occupations. The kit also includes a price sheet, a history of the company, its mission statement, biographical data on the owners, and any advantages regarding buying their particular medium over competing media.

As access to technology expands, many business owners and practitioners are developing their own advertising through digital means. The use of social media and text message advertising has become ubiquitous. However, when texting to market yourself to others, be mindful of the Telephone Consumer Protection Act (TCPA). This requires businesses and/or organizations to receive written consent from individuals before sending SMS/text messages to them. Obtaining an individual's phone number—whether it belongs to a potential client, existing client, or former client—is not receiving consent or permission to contact them. Exceptions to the TCPA may include appointment reminders and delivery notifications (Griffith, 2018).

Marketing and Massage Client Demographics

What are common characteristics of massage clients? Most clients were had a college degree, were in higher income bracket, and had children. Clients between the ages of 45 and 54 received more massages than any other age group. Why do consumers use massage? Massage is mainly used for general health/wellness, relaxation, and stress reduction. Massage is also used for musculoskeletal soreness, stiffness, and pain (AMTA, 2022; Sundberg et al, 2017).

Where are clients receiving massages? Most massages are performed at a spa, a massage practitioner's office, or a massage franchise or chain. Clients are also receiving massages at beauty salons, hotels, resorts, health clubs, physical therapy, and chiropractic clinics, or in their homes. The least-used locations for massage service delivery are massage school clinics, physician/medical offices, and hospitals (AMTA, 2022).

How are these clients locating practitioners? Massage clients stated referrals are their primary method of locating massage practitioners (77%), followed by internet websites (48%) and social media (38%). Approximately 30% of massage clients found practitioners through local community events or locator services (AMTA, 2022),

Mission Statement

A **mission statement** is a single statement of a business's purpose—what it does, how it does it, and why it does it. It can also describe the business's culture, core values, ethics, and goals—what it wants to accomplish on a larger scale. A mission statement acts like a compass and represents a business's path. A mission statement directs business decisions, and it should be evident in what direction a business is moving after reading its mission statement. This contrasts with a vision statement, which represents the end point rather than the path it took to get there.

Mission-driven businesses are more successful compared with businesses without a mission. Mission statements can also drive consumer loyalty, foster engagement among colleagues and consumers, and focus strategic planning (Groscurth, 2014). A good mission statement should be short, memorable, inspiring, and consumer-oriented (Kerin & Peterson, 2012). Examples of mission statements are featured next.

- Google: To organize the world's information and make it universally accessible and useful.
- Starbucks: To inspire and nurture the human spirit—one person, one cup, one neighborhood at a time.
- Twitter: To give everyone the power to create and share ideas and information, instantly, without barriers.
- Coca-Cola: To refresh the world. To inspire moments of optimism and happiness. To create value and make a difference.
- REI: To inspire, educate, and outfit for a lifetime of adventure and stewardship.

There are several ways to write a mission statement. One way is to use the following steps:

1. Write down key words or phrases. Perhaps gather ideas from others.
2. Write down your defining characteristics. Your mission statement should reflect your style and your personality. How do you want your clients to remember you? What makes you different? If you want to be known for something, reflect it in your mission statement. Ask yourself: Why do I do what I do? What inspires me to do this work? What do I believe about it?
3. Narrow these down into the best, most interesting, and tangible ideas. Instead of saying you "make the world a better place," state how you plan to do it, such as delivering quality service. It is recommended to leave out jargon and buzzwords such as cutting edge, paradigm, and synergy.
4. Once your first draft is written, put it away for a few days, then reread it. How does it make you feel now? If it does not excite you, start over. If you are excited, great! Share it with others and ask for feedback. Finally, does it pass the t-shirt test? In other words, does it fit on a t-shirt? Would you wear it?

Business Cards

Business cards are small cards containing a professional name, business name, occupation, email address, physical address, website, and other contact information. Business cards are one of the most potent—yet often ignored—marketing tools. Business cards are often the first item prospective clients receive, so they are the first opportunity you have to make a good impression. Consider using a professional designer unless you have requisite skills in card design. Why? It is easy to spot a poorly designed card, which may not give prospective clients a good impression.

Keep your card design simple and graphics symbolic to the products and services you offer. Consider putting a photo of yourself on the card so people can continue to "put your face" to the name on the card long after the initial contact. Information should be well-spaced. Avoid card designs that are cluttered. Use easy-to-read fonts and compare both letters and numbers. In some font styles, 5 looks like 3, and 6 looks like 8. Proofread all information before it goes to print. Be creative, have fun, and remember—this is your business face.

SUSAN G. SALVO
123.455.6868

SUSAN G. SALVO
123.455.6868

SUSAN G. SALVO
123.455.6868

SUSAN G. SALVO
123.455.6868

The physical act of handing someone a business card may be more important than the card itself. Use a card as part of a conversation once you have a better understanding of the other person's needs or interests. As you hand someone the card, look the person in the eye, smile, and state clearly what you do and why it is valuable. People will often remember what you do easier than they remember your name—which is another reason why business cards are so important. You want people to remember when they come across your card in a pocket or billfold later. Hand out cards often; consider giving out two or three at a time and say they may know someone who needs massage services.

Professional Profile

A **professional profile** is a written summary of professional skills, strengths, and key experiences. Also called a *professional summary,* a professional profile lists what you have to offer consumers. A professional profile can serve as an "About Me" page on a website or a blog, a "Bio" on Twitter or a "Summary" on LinkedIn professional networking services. Like business cards, your professional profile may be the first point of contact between you and potential clients, so make a good impression. Getting a massage is a personal experience and a good professional profile helps clients connect with you.

A professional profile should be well thought out and carefully written; it takes planning and reflection. What accomplishments are you proud of? What has brought you joy? Your accomplishments may include working at a local theater or writing a travel blog. Writing about yourself may be difficult, and it may be worthwhile soliciting help from others as they may mention characteristics and traits you had not considered.

Ideally, have three profiles of different lengths: a micro, a short, and a long profile. Each profile will serve slightly different purposes.

- **Micro Profile**. These are usually one sentence using ≤30 words. It functions like a sales pitch; something you might use on Twitter.
- **Short Profile**. These are approximately one paragraph of ≤100 words. It covers all essential information; something you might use on LinkedIn.
- **Long Profile**. These can be an entire page or approximately 500 words; something you would use on your website or blog.

Write the long profile first and edit it down to create the short and micro profiles. When using the short or micro profile, consider adding a hyperlink to the long profile for those who want to read more about you. Most professional profiles follow a similar format. Honeysett (2020) recommends this template.

[Name] is a [title] who works with [who you help] to [how you help them].

[First name] [knows/believes] [what you know/believe about the work you do].

[First name] has [landed/secured/garnered/worked at/ supported] [insert your most compelling experiences and wins]. [First name] is a [trained/certified/ awarded] [insert relevant trainings, awards, honors, etc.]. [First name] holds a [insert degree] in [insert area of study] from [insert university].

NOTE: The second sentence is the most important as it tells people "why" you do what you do. You can add some flavor to the profile by including something completely unexpected that lets readers know your other interests. This can run the gamut from you are also a wine sommelier to you frequently play Pokémon with your kids. These are great conversation starters.

End your profile with contact information and perhaps hyperlinks to your email, your website, a Skype account, or social sharing sites. After it is written and edited, check and double-check spelling and grammar. Get your friends to proofread it and ask them to be brutally honest. Also remember your profile should be reviewed and updated often, perhaps on a quarterly basis.

In the end, we will conserve only what we love, we will love only what we understand, we will understand only what we are taught.
—**Baba Dioum (Senegalese conservationist)**

Websites

Websites are places on the internet where one or more pages of information are found. Websites are vital to businesses, and for good reason. We live in a digital world; a website is the center of a business's digital or online presence. Consumers use the internet to locate products and services, and a website increases the likelihood your business will be found. Indeed, the Internet has a wider reach than any other form of advertising.

Even if consumers do not contact you or make an appointment, they can learn about your products and services as well as your qualifications by reading your professional profile. A website helps you establish credibility, and consumers may choose your business over others because of your website. Consumers can contact you, make appointments, purchase gift cards, download forms, and access informative videos, your blog, or social networking sites on your website.

When selecting a domain name, choose one easy to remember and spell and ends in ".com," as most consumers assume that Uniform Resource Locators, or URLs, end in .com. Many massage organizations and associations offer a free webpage or website as part of membership benefits or may provide discounts for design and hosting services.

You can hire someone to design your website, or you can design one yourself. Choose a color scheme that fits your business message. Females generally like blue, purple, and green and do not like gray, orange, and brown. Males generally like blue, green, and black and do not like purple, orange, and brown. Blue represents trust. Black adds a sense of luxury and value. Bright colors such as red, orange, and yellow are best for your call-to-action page. Use white to create space (Patel, n.d.).

Design elements that increase user engagement include navigation, graphical representation, organization, content utility, purpose, simplicity, and readability (Garett et al, 2016). Recommended tabs for a massage website include (1) Benefits of Massage, (2) Services and Prices, (3) First Visit, (4) Location, (5) About Me, and (6) Contact. If you have a blog or use social media such as Facebook to promote your business, be sure links are on your home page as well.

Your profile page, commonly called "About Me" or "About Us," is the second most visited page on a website (Patel, 2021). Always include a professional photograph of yourself. Best practices for a profile picture include (1) smiling with teeth showing, (2) wearing a dark-colored suit or light-colored button-down shirt, (3) jawline showing that includes its shadow, (4) head-and-shoulders or head-to-waist photo, (5) asymmetric composition, (6) unobstructed eyes, and (7) no squinting (Lee, n.d.).

Blogs

A **blog** is a discussion or informational website often written using diary-style entries called *posts*. The term *blog* is a shortened or truncation of the phrase weblog (web log). As a marketing tool, a blog can engage your target market, attract or retain clients, drive traffic to your website, gain the attention of search engines, and establish yourself as an authority in your field through educating readers. Blog visitors can read about new products and services, ways to improve health or quality of life, have their questions about massage answered, or gain a broader perspective about topics. Consumers enjoy getting a glimpse of the more personal side of a business, and they may feel more connected to you after reading your blog post or personal page. Readers can also participate in discussions by posting comments. Think of a blog as a more relaxed website in which you can share your perspective on relevant topics. Keep in mind professional boundaries regarding self-disclosure as outlined in Chapter 2.

Keep blog posts between 350 and 1000 words. Readers tend to skim blogs, so keep them brief. If you need a longer post, consider writing two blogs. The most important thing is to provide useful and meaningful content. Examples of blog posts are "Five Stretches You Can Do at Home to Reduce Lower Back Pain" and "Massage Reduces Symptoms of Fibromyalgia." Use images that help you convey information. Most bloggers post regularly—weekly or monthly at a minimum. Be sure your blog links to your website and social media sites (Pringle, 2013).

Social Media

Social media is a website where members of virtual communities can interact with each other. Examples of social media include Facebook, Instagram, Twitter, YouTube, Snapchat, LinkedIn, Google+, and Pinterest. Originally, social media was used to share life events. Now, it is also used to network with colleagues, create career and educational opportunities, collaborate on projects, fundraising, play virtual games, and promote businesses.

According to the Pew Research Center (2021), 7 in 10 Americans use social media to connect with one another, engage with news content, share information, and for entertainment. YouTube and Facebook are the most widely used platforms, and their users are the most broadly represented of the population as a whole. Smaller percentages of Americans use sites such as Twitter, Pinterest, Instagram, and LinkedIn. Among adults under the age of 30, Instagram, Snapchat, and TikTok were commonly used social media platforms. Approximately 7 in 10 Facebook users and 6 in 10 Instagram and Snapchat users visit these sites at least once a day.

Because of their popularity and widespread use, social network sites are an important marketing tool and can be used for many of the same reasons blogs are used: to engage your target market, attract or retain clients, and drive traffic to your website. If you are using social media as a marketing tool and work for a business, be sure to comply with Health Insurance Portability and Accountability Act (HIPAA) laws and business policies related to use of social media, which may include posting restrictions. Common social media HIPAA violations include posting pictures or videos of clients without written consent, posting information that could allow clients to be identified, posting gossip about clients, and sharing pictures or videos taken inside a facility in which clients or client records are visible. Posting restrictions include private groups within social media platforms.

Digital citizenship is the responsible and ethical use of technology by anyone who uses computers, the Internet, and digital devices. As stated in Chapter 2, soliciting or accepting friend requests from clients creates dual relationships, and clients may have access to private information from the practitioner's personal page. Before posting or responding to a post, take time to think about the impact and possible consequences it may have on others and on yourself before "sharing." Self-reflect before you self-reveal. Ask yourself three essential questions:

1. Where is this coming from? Posts should come from a place of kindness, fairness, or inquiry. Avoid posting anything when you are angry, hurt, or offended. This includes responding to comments.
2. If my parent, partner, children, clients, or colleagues saw this, what would they think? Be sure your posts or comments do not negatively affect other people. This may include avoiding discussions of religion or politics or posting comments that might be taken as offensive, insulting, or controversial.
3. Can this come back to haunt me? Once you post something—whether a comment, a picture, or a video—it can be viewed, copied, pasted, shared, and distributed in ways you did not intend. Inflammatory remarks or images of you intoxicated or insufficiently dressed can be viewed by clients and prospective business contacts. If a post prevents a client from making an appointment, hinders future business opportunities, or attracts the wrong kind of client, the risks far outweigh the benefits. In addition, prospective employers often view your social networking sites as part of the vetting process.

Gift Cards, Value-Added Services, and Retail

Gift cards, or **gift certificates**, are vouchers given as a "gift" to pay for services and/or products. Gift cards are great marketing tools, and they often bring new clients into a business. Most often, people who purchase and give gift cards are clients, and because they enjoy the service they want to share it with others. This is *word-of-mouth* advertising. People tend to trust services and products recommended by friends, family, and co-workers. Furthermore, gift cards can be used to spread goodwill as donations for charitable causes. Building public relations within the community is one way to grow your business.

The federal Credit Card Accountability Responsibility and Disclosure (CARD) Act of 2009 and some state laws regulate gift certificates and cards. Currently, gift certificates and gift cards cannot expire within 5 years from the date purchase or activation. Gift certificates and gift cards used as a promotion, reward, or part of a loyalty program are often exempt from this rule, provided they meet certain requirements such as gift cards donated to charities (Morton, 2016).

Other marketing strategies include offering additional services and retail. **Value-added services** are those offered to consumers for little or no cost. Businesses can use value-added services to market less popular services such as reflexology or increase earnings for popular services such as adding essential oils to lubricant and up-charging the client for an aromatherapy massage. **Retail**, selling good for use rather than for resale, is another way to market services, especially if the items are designed to support reasons why clients are receiving massage services. For example, if clients are receiving a massage to relax, retail items such as stress-reducing aromatherapy products, candles, or bath salts. If clients are receiving a massage to manage pain, retail items such as massage tools, liniments, and neck pillows. Be sure some retail items are easily affordable. Retail what you use yourself or what you recommend.

> *The greatest discovery of my generation is that a human being can alter his life by altering his attitudes.*
> —**William James**

PROFESSIONAL DEVELOPMENT AND BUSINESS RESOURCES

Massage practitioners will continue to grow and develop professionally after graduation and obtaining their first job (Box 17.1). Professional resources and supportive networks

---

BOX 17.1

Qualities of a Professional Massage Practitioner

Massage practitioners should have knowledge of techniques and principles that include an understanding of legal and ethical issues. They must also acquire a working knowledge of and acceptance for human nature and individual characteristics. Daily contact with a wide variety of people with a host of problems and concerns is a significant part of their work. Courtesy, compassion, and common sense are often cited as the *three Cs* most vital to the success of a massage practitioner.

In fact, the first responsibility of a massage practitioner is always to provide safe, competent, courteous, and compassionate care to clients. Other characteristics of a professional massage practitioner include:

- Has an aptitude for working with their hands
- Is computer literate
- Has good communication skills that include writing, speaking, and listening
- Maintains professional boundaries and integrity
- Avoids dual relationships
- Is trustworthy and exhibits a sense of responsibility
- Prepares and maintains client records
- Keeps client information confidential
- Leaves private concerns at home
- Has patience in dealing with others and the ability to work as a member of a team
- Practices with competence and within the scope of practice determined by state law
- Projects a favorable image
- Possesses expertise that comes through three main sources: technical competence, social validation (through a formal recognition of training and status), and reputation
- Exhibits a relaxed attitude when meeting new people
- Starts and ends each session on time and lets nothing interrupt a session
- Has an understanding of and empathy for others
- Uses appropriate guidelines when releasing information
- Uses empathy and tact when managing conflict
- Has a willingness to learn new skills and techniques

---

are vital for the health and longevity of any career or business. This section discusses continuing education, board certification, mentors, preceptors, business coaching, contacts, and proposals.

Continuing Education and Board Certification

Continuing education is education to ensure ongoing competence relevant to professional practice after leaving a system of formal education such as a college, university, or vocational/trade school. Continuing education is usually required for license renewal with the licensee providing evidence of participation in and/or completion of educational and professional activities. CE courses can be taken as seminars, presentations, webinars, distance learning, or other similar types of programs. CE, also called *continuous professional development*, is used to increase skills in a particular line of work. In some states, CE is optional.

Board certification is the examination of a person's professional qualifications by a group of peers, often in a specialty of practice (e.g., pregnancy massage, oncology massage, lymphatic massage) and granting the person a title if qualifications are met. The process is voluntary and different from the process of licensure, the latter of which sets the minimum competency requirement to practice massage. Board certification in the massage profession can be obtained by the National Certification Board for Therapeutic Massage and Bodywork (NCBTMB). As mentioned previously, certification restricts the use of the title but not the practice. Practice restrictions are achieved through state licensure and legally defined scope of practice.

Mentors, Preceptors, Coaches, and Business Resources

A **mentor** is an experienced and trusted advisor who provides counsel, guidance, support, and encouragement. Mentoring relationships support mentees—or protégés—in developing their self-confidence and professional competencies. Critical to the success of mentoring are creating a relationship of trust, clearly defining roles and responsibilities, establishing short-term and long-term goals, and having open and supportive communication and collaborative problem solving. Mentoring relationships are rewarding to both parties, and some relationships become lifelong. Associations such as the American Massage and Therapy Association and the Alliance for Massage Education have mentoring programs. Some practitioners have more than one mentor.

A **preceptor** is an experienced individual within a healthcare facility who is paired with a newly hired individual during the orientation period. A preceptor teaches the new practitioner about the company's policies and procedures and helps with the acquisition of skills related to the position. Preceptors are often responsible for the new practitioner's professional activities for just the orientation period or may be extended for several weeks or months.

A mentor-type relationship often develops once the formal preceptor–practitioner relationship ends.

A **business coach** is an individual who has business experience and oversees, assists, and guides a novice businessperson in developing, starting, or growing a business. Business coaches can offer a unique coaching experience that is focused on specific challenges massage practitioners face. New practitioners can benefit from the guidance and encouragement from a coach while starting and growing a business. Business coaches can help empower practitioners during the evolution of a long-term career. Coaches can clarify goals and objectives to empower practitioners to pursue and create massage therapy-related projects that are aligned with their vision. Whereas mentors and preceptors are often individuals within your field, business coaches may not be, which can promote much-needed objectivity. Business coaches may be chiropractors, physical therapy practitioners, small business owners, bankers, or consultants.

Additional business resources include the Small Business Administration and the Service Corps of Retired Executives. Colleges and universities that have business and/or marketing departments often have advanced students or graduates that can assist practitioners in preparing business proposals or locating business resources.

Don't overlook business resources within professional massage organizations. Becoming a member of one or more massage organizations helps keep you current with developing trends. Professional membership also provides a forum for the exchange of ideas with people who truly understand your professional issues while actively supporting the industry. Attend massage conferences and conventions often. Nothing is quite as inspiring as hundreds of people gathered together who share a common experience.

"Two heads are better than one," and one person cannot possibly know everything about managing a business. It is important to reach out to others and ask for their advice. Learning from the experience and mistakes of others can save you time and money. Find professionals you admire, who are successful, and who are willing and able to support you with advice. Give something back to the support person. Money may not be appropriate in some circumstances, but find a service the mentor or coach needs such as cooking or babysitting, or give gifts such as books or even massages. Show the person you appreciate their time and expertise. Remember, regardless of what advice is offered, decisions are ultimately your own.

Business Contracts and Proposals

Contracts are written agreements that outline expectations, duties, and responsibilities in business relationships—these can be legally binding and enforceable by law. Contracts help delineate expectations, duties, and responsibilities. Ensure the contract (1) clarifies the business relationship of each party (e.g., lessor or lessee, employer or employee, partner or independent contractor), (2) contains the duration of the agreement such as 6 months or 1 year, and (3) predetermines on what grounds the contract can be terminated if before the agreed-upon time. Have an attorney review the contract before dated signatures are collected. Everything is negotiable, but negotiate before signing.

Proposals are simply plans or suggestions put forward for consideration and discussion in business relationships. For example, massage practitioners may write proposals to recommend inclusion of massage services in a gym or onsite massage services in a business complex. Most proposals undergo a vetting period by all involved parties before being adopted. When submitting a proposal, include your resume or CV (discussed previously) and list the objectives, anticipated outcomes, methods of evaluating outcomes, and logistics—the what, when, and where section of the proposal. If you are familiar with the facility, recommend a specific location where services will be provided. Briefly discuss physical arrangements, such as room dimensions, bathroom locations, lighting, equipment, and supplies. Are you proposing full-time or part-time work? Will services be available during the day, evenings, or on weekends and holidays? Consider proposing part-time availability and increased hours of operation as demand for services increases. What hours of the day will services be offered, and who will pay for them?

A proposal should also list who should be contacted as ideas are developed and problems arise and a mutually agreed-on mediator (third party) to help settle disputes. Include sections on proposed budgets and amounts you are contributing, if any; the names and amounts of funds received from other participants; and the amount you are requesting from the agency or corporation, if any. Suggest plans for additional fundraising, if needed. The budget should include expenses for the proposed project. If income is generated, who will benefit financially? This section should also include payment schedules and payment methods.

Both contracts and proposals outline ideas, help avoid communication problems, state specifically how problems will be handled and who will handle them when they do arise, and help keep both parties focused on the business venture.

I am indeed rich, since my income is superior to my expense, and my expense is equal to my wishes.
—Edward Gibson

ACCOUNTING

Accounting is the process of measuring, processing, and communicating financial and nonfinancial information. This information is summarized in financial statements and shared with external entities such as bankers, investors, and regulators. Accounting is known as the *language of business.*

The recording of financial transactions is called **bookkeeping**. Massage practitioners can hire an accountant or bookkeeper to assist with accounting and tax reporting needs. Some practitioners use professional accounting software packages such as FreshBooks, Intuit Quickbooks Pro, Sage, and Wave. This section discusses basic accounting terms and financial statements. Review the section titled "Length of Time Business Records Are Kept" for the period of time a business must keep financial records.

Petty Cash Accounting

Petty cash is a small amount of cash a business keeps on hand to pay for inexpensive items such as office supplies and postage. A common accounting method used to set up a petty cash account is to withdraw the desired amount of cash (e.g., $100) and keep it in an envelope or small lock box. As the cash is used to pay for inexpensive items, the receipts are placed in the envelope or box. When the cash is all used up, it is replenished by another cash withdrawal. At any given time, the total in the petty cash account should equal the amount of cash remaining plus the business receipts.

Financial Statements

Financial statements are written records that convey financial information and financial performance of individuals, businesses, and corporations. Key financial statements include a (1) balance sheet, (2) cash flow statement, and (3) profit and loss statement (P&L). Financial statements are standardized with relevant information and may be audited by governmental and regulatory agencies to ensure accuracy and for licensing, tax, financing, or investing purposes.

Balance Sheet

A **balance sheet** is an overview of a business's assets, liabilities, and shareholder's equity on a specific date—it is a snapshot in time. The date at the top of the balance sheet tells you when the snapshot was taken, which is generally at the end of a fiscal year. The balance sheet formula is (assets = liabilities + equity). Let's look at some definitions.

- **Assets.** Valuable economic resources to which an individual or business has a legal claim. Examples of assets are property, equipment, inventory, money in the bank, and monies owed to the company (i.e., accounts receivable). Assets include trademarks and patents.
  - A **trademark** is an image or phrase that identifies your goods or services. The owner of the trademark has the right to prevent others from using a similar image or phrase.
  - A **patent** is an invention or title owned by a legal entity and, for a set period, gives that entity the sole right to exclude others from making, using, or selling it.
- **Liabilities.** Debts or obligations an individual or business (debtor) owes to another individual or business (creditor) and is payable in money, goods, or services. Examples of liabilities include money owed to suppliers, vendors, or creditors (i.e., accounts payable), operating expenses such as rent, utilities, wages, and taxation authorities.
- **Equity.** An individual's or business's net worth. Equity is determined by deducting liabilities for the assets (assets − liabilities = equity). Equity is also referred to as capital.

This financial statement is called a "balance sheet" because equity must equal, or be in balance with, assets minus liabilities. A balance sheet is also called a *statement of financial condition*.

Cash Flow Statement

A **cash flow statement** reports the movement of cash provided to the company (moving *into* the company) and the movement of cash used by the company (moving *out of* the company) during a period of time such as a month, quarterly (every 3 months), or annually (every 12 months). If more money moves into the business than is distributed, the cash balance increases, and the business is said to have a *positive cash flow*. Conversely, if more money moves from the company than is provided, the business has a *negative cash flow*. Because cash flow is regarded as the life-giving blood of a business, keeping track of these amounts and having the opportunity to regulate these amounts may make the difference between whether your business thrives or not.

Profit and Loss (Income) Statement

Profit and loss statements report an individual's or business's financial performance (both profits or income and losses or expenses) during a particular period of time. The main purpose of the P&L statement is to convey if an individual or business is making a profit or a loss. However, it can be very effective in showing whether income is increasing when compared with other time periods. One important thing to remember about income statements is they represent a period of time (as do cash flow statements). This contrasts with the balance sheet, which represents a single moment in time.

BUSINESS PLAN

A **business plan** is a document that describes a business's organization, services and products, marketing strategy, management style, financial projections, future plans, and strategies for achieving them. Although this chapter provides much of the market research, you will spend twice as much time, if not more, researching and analyzing business data as you spend actually writing a business plan. It is vital you are as objective as possible so you can write and carry out a realistic business plan. Seek advice from mentors and coaches when needed to gain objectivity.

A business plan outline can help individuals organize their thoughts rather than staring at a blank page waiting for inspiration to strike. The following sections are frequently seen in a business plan (Stockton, 2019). However, not all categories will fit your situation. For example, a business plan for a person who is self-funding and not trying to attract investors will likely not have a section requesting funds. Write your business plan to include a combination of sections that makes the most sense for your business and your needs.

Executive Summary

Briefly state the background of the company, where it is today, where it is headed, and why it will be successful or more successful in the future. Include a mission statement, brief description of products/services, basic information about the company's organization, and location. Include financial information and growth plans if you are asking for financing. Although this is the first section, it is usually the last section written as it is a summary of the entire plan and includes a little information from all sections.

Company Description

Describe the company, the clients or consumers it plans to serve, and how your products and services will meet their needs. Be specific about the types of problems your business plans to solve. Explain any competitive advantage you have that will make your business successful. This section is where you boast about your strengths.

Market Analysis

Describe your industry, its current conditions and outlook, and its target market. Include discussions on competition, how well the competition is doing, and their strengths and weaknesses. Look for trends and themes suggesting why they are successful. Include what competitors are charging for their services and products.

Organization and Management

Discuss the company's legal structure (business entity) and who will manage it. Include an organizational chart, if applicable. Also provide a professional profile of key members that includes their qualifications, experience, and education relevant to their role in the company.

Services or Products

Describe the services and products you offer or plan to offer. Outline the hours of the day and days of the week the business will operate. Include information regarding service or product costs, suppliers, and services or products that may be added in the future. Include what your fee schedule looks like and how these fees were determined.

Marketing and Sales

Describe how you plan to attract and retain clients. Include a description of how sales occur. Discuss strategies for penetrating the market and promoting sales.

Funding Request

If asking for funding, this is the section where you make the request. Include the current amount requested, how funding will be used, and projections about future funding needs and how those funds will be used. Specify if funds are needed to buy equipment or supplies, pay salaries or insurance premiums, or cover specific bills until the business is making a profit.

Financial Analysis and Projections

Include financial analyses to support the idea the business will be successful. If the business is established, include balance sheets, cash flow statements, and P&L statements for the past 3 to 5 years. Also include a financial projection for the next 5 years. Explain the projections and make sure they match your funding requests.

Appendix

Use your appendix to provide supporting documents or other materials where specifically requested. Common items included are personal and business credit histories, images of products, references, copies of licenses and certifications, legal documents, insurance policies, and contracts and contact information for consultants.

E-RESOURCES

http://evolve.elsevier.com/Salvo/MassageTherapy

- Chapter challenge
- Flash cards
- Additional information
- Business plan

BENNY VAUGHN

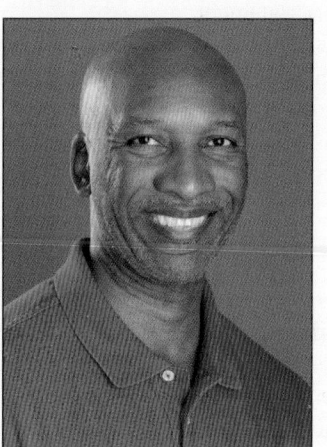

The classic old schoolyard retort is, "It takes one to know one!" Although the saying generally does not do too well at impressing playground bullies, it can be true in the world of massage. Anyone, given the skills, education, and passion, can work with any kind of client, but having "been one" yourself can give you extra insight. People who have been pregnant may be drawn to pregnancy massage. Many massage practitioners who have experienced injuries find they can relate to clients in a rehabilitation setting. For Benny Vaughn, being an athlete led him to the field of sports massage.

Vaughn was born in 1951 in Georgia. Being a Black child in that time and place was not easy; schools, buses, movie theaters, and most public areas were segregated, and there were few clear opportunities for success. But his world changed in 1960 when his father, an Army cook, was transferred to Germany. For the first time in his life, Vaughn lived in an integrated community at a time when people back in the United States were dying for that right. It gave him a global perspective and changed his view of what was possible in the world.

An athletic youth, Vaughn's track and field skills allowed him to attend the University of Florida in 1969 on a full athletic scholarship. Always looking for ways to improve athletic performance, he read about how some European athletes were using massage to speed recovery from training, competition, and injury. Vaughn was intrigued. After graduating with a degree in Health Education, he decided to attend massage therapy school and learn this skill for himself.

After graduating from the American Institute of Massage Therapy, Vaughn landed his first massage job at the Gainesville Executive Health Club. His teacher, Bruce Simer, continued to mentor him. Simer taught Vaughn the importance of customer satisfaction and encouraged him to educate his clients about the benefits of massage in addition to simply providing excellent massages.

Vaughn knew he had extra barriers to break through to have a successful massage career. A Black male massage practitioner in the American South needed to be more professional, more patient, and more attuned to clients' needs to overcome prejudices against people of color. As a result, Vaughn pushed himself to excel, and he eventually became known as one of the foremost experts on sports massage of the time.

Now, Vaughn is a certified athletic trainer and a certified strength and conditioning specialist on top of his massage license and other certifications. He has been a member of the sports medicine staff for the U.S. track and field teams at multiple Olympic Games as well as multiple track and field World Championships. He owns and operates the Benny Vaughn Athletic Therapy Center in Fort Worth, Texas, and worked with athletes at the 2004 Olympics in Athens, the 2008 Olympics in Beijing, the 2012 Olympics in London, and the 2021 Olympics in Japan. Although he teaches regularly, he still sees himself as a massage practitioner first and a teacher second, treating a full schedule of clients.

You may notice there is no Benny Vaughn Method of sports massage. This is by design. Vaughn understands great massage is not about this or that technique—it is about skills and developing a useful treatment plan, whatever sources the techniques come from. He says, "In the end, the names we use for massage techniques really indicate belief systems and philosophies. Simply calling it something other than touch or massage does not make the outcome better for that individual client. It is the combination of skill, experience, and compassion of the massage practitioner that carries powerful results for the client."

Skill, experience, and compassion: These are three areas in which Benny Vaughn excels. Whatever clients you choose to work with and whatever modalities you use, keep these three prerequisites in mind. Without them, no special training or fancy certificates will get you anywhere. But with them, you can overcome anything.

REFERENCES

American Massage Therapy Association (AMTA). (2022). *Massage profession research report*. Evanston, IL: ATMA.

Coble, C. (2016). *Massage injuries: can you sue?* Retrieved from https://blogs.findlaw.com/injured/2015/08/massage-injuries-can-i-sue.html.

Day, J. C., & Christnacht, C. (2019). *Women hold 76% of all health care jobs, gaining in higher-paying occupations*. Retrieved from https://www.census.gov/library/stories/2019/08/your-health-care-in-womens-hands.html.

Fishman, S. (n.d.). *How much should you charge for your services? How to price your services to attract business and make a profit*. Retrieved from https://www.nolo.com/legal-encyclopedia/business-services-charge-how-much-30158.html.

Garett, R., Chiu, J., Zhang, L., & Young, S. D. (2016). A literature review: website design and user engagement. *Online Journal of Communication and Media Technologies, 6*(3), 1–14.

Griffith, S. (2018). *Telephone Consumer Protection Act Compliance (TCPA)*. Retrieved from https://help.simpletexting.com/compliance-consent-and-legal-stuff/compliance-and-consent/tcpa-compliance.

Groscurth, C. (2014). *Why your company must be mission-driven*. Retrieved from http://www.gallup.com/businessjournal/167633/why-company-mission-driven.aspx.

Hansen, R. S. (n.d.). *10 best job interview tips for job seekers*. Retrieved at https://www.livecareer.com/career/advice/interview/job-interview-tips.

Honeysett, A. (2020). *The professional bio template that makes everyone sound accomplished*. Retrieved from https://www.themuse.com/advice/the-professional-bio-template-that-makes-everyone-sound-accomplished

Interactive Biodiversity Information System [IBIS] World. (2020). *Massage franchises industry in the United States: market research report*. Retrieved from https://www.ibisworld.com/united-states/market-research-reports/massage-franchises-industry/.

Internal Revenue Service. (2020). *How long should I keep records*? Retrieved from https://www.irs.gov/businesses/small-businesses-self-employed/how-long-should-i-keep-records.

Internal Revenue Service. (2021a). *Bartering income: topic no. 420*. Retrieved from https://www.irs.gov/taxtopics/tc420

Internal Revenue Service. (2021b). *Tip recordkeeping and reporting*. Retrieved from https://www.irs.gov/businesses/small-businesses-self-employed/tip-recordkeeping-and-reporting

Kerin, R. A., & Peterson, R. A. (2012). *Strategic marketing problems: cases and comments* (13rd ed.). Upper Saddle River, NJ: Prentice Hall, Inc.

Lee, K. (n.d.). *The research and science behind finding your best profile picture*. Retrieved from https://buffer.com/library/best-profile-picture-science-research-psychology/

Mason, M. K. (2021). *What causes small businesses to fail?* Retrieved from http://www.moyak.com/papers/small-business-failure.html.

Menafn, G. (2020). Dress for success: how clothes influence our performance. Retrieved from https://menafn.com/1100974172/Dress-for-success-How-clothes-influence-our-performance.

National Association of Colleges and Employers. (2020). *Key attributes employers want to see on students' resumes*. Retrieved at https://www.naceweb.org/talent-acquisition/candidate-selection/key-attributes-employers-want-to-see-on-students-resumes/

Morton, G. (2016). *National conference of state legislatures: gift cards and gift certificates statues and legislation*. Retrieved from http://www.ncsl.org/research/financial-services-and-commerce/gift-cards-and-certificates-statutes-and-legis.aspx.

Patel, N. (n.d.). *How to use the psychology of color to increase website conversions*. Retrieved from https://neilpatel.com/blog/psychology-of-color-and-conversions/

Patel, N. (2021). *The 4 most important pages on tour website (and how to optimize them)*. Retrieved from https://blog.hubspot.com/marketing/optimize-important-website-pages

Pew Research Center. (2018). *Social media fact sheet*. Retrieved from https://www.pewresearch.org/internet/fact-sheet/social-media/

Pringle, S. (2013). *Blogging best practices: the ideal length for the perfect blog post*. https://www.business2community.com/blogging/blogging-best-practices-the-ideal-length-for-the-perfect-blog-post-0577303.

Social Security Administration. (2021). *Fact sheet: social security*. Retrieved from https://www.ssa.gov/news/press/factsheets/basicfact-alt.pdf.

Statistic Brain Research Institute. (2018). *Startup business failure rate by industry*. Retrieved from http://www.statisticbrain.com/startup-failure-by-industry/.

Stockton, B. (2019). *How to write a business plan in 9 steps*. Retrieved from https://fitsmallbusiness.com/business-plan/

Sundberg, T., Cramer, H., Sibbritt, D., Adams, J., & Lauche, R. (2017). Prevalence, patterns, and predictors of massage practitioner utilization: results of a US nationally representative survey. *Musculoskeletal Science and Practice, 32,* 31–7.

United States Department of Labor Statistics. (2021). *Concepts and definitions*. https://www.bls.gov/cps/definitions.htm

United States Department of Labor Statistics. (2022). *Occupational employment statistics: massage therapists*. https://www.bls.gov/ooh/healthcare/massage-therapists.htm.

REVIEW AND APPLY YOUR KNOWLEDGE

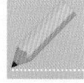

MATCHING ONE: CONCEPT REVIEW

Place the letter of the answer next to the number of the term or phrase that best describes it.

A. Advertising
B. Blog
C. Curriculum vitae
D. Board certification
E. Marketing
F. Mentor
G. Professional liability
H. Mission statement
I. Professional license
J. Corporation
K. Social media
L. Sole proprietorship

_____ 1. An experienced and trusted advisor who provides counsel, guidance, support, and encouragement.

_____ 2. Informational website using diary-style entries called posts.

_____ 3. Term used to describe a business of a single owner.

_____ 4. Websites where members of virtual communities can interact with each other.

_____ 5. Insurance that helps protect a service provider from bearing the full cost of legal defense and helps pay for damages awarded by the courts if the provider was found negligent.

_____ 6. Describes why a business exists and its core objectives.

_____ 7. Official permission granted by a legal authority to an individual to practice in an occupation.

_____ 8. In-depth overview of a person's education, experiences, and accomplishments.

_____ 9. Legal business entity that has its own privileges and liabilities distinct from its board of directors or shareholders.

_____ 10. Examination of a person's professional qualifications by a group of peers, often in a specialty of practice, and granting the person a title if qualifications are met.

_____ 11. Activities used to create, communicate, deliver, and exchange offerings that have value for customers, clients, and the society at large.

_____ 12. The use of persuasive messages to influence consumer's buying habits, usually by paid announcements.

MATCHING TWO: CONCEPT REVIEW

Place the letter of the answer next to the number of the term or phrase that best describes it.

A. Accounting
B. Assets
C. Barter
D. Business plan
E. Taxes
F. Contracts
G. Equity
H. Independent contractors
I. Tips
J. Liabilities
K. Deductions
L. Zoning

_____ 1. Debts or obligations an individual or business owes to another individual or business.

_____ 2. Dividing geographic areas so a city or municipality can restrict the number of and types of buildings within the area, as well as how the buildings are used.

_____ 3. Measuring, processing, and communicating financial and nonfinancial information.

_____ 4. Valuable economic resources to which an individual or business has legal claim.

_____ 5. Document that describes a business's organization, services and products, marketing strategy, management style, and financial projections, future plans, and strategies for achieving them.

_____ 6. A business's net worth determined by deducting liabilities from assets.

_____ 7. Nonmonetary exchange of goods or services.

_____ 8. Discretionary money given to service providers by their consumers.

_____ 9. Written agreements that outline expectations, duties, and responsibilities and can be legally binding and enforceable by law.

_____ 10. Individuals who have special skills, training, or licensure that allows them to work without supervision.

_____ 11. Money paid on income, property, and sales of goods or services, which is given to a governmental agency to carry out its many functions.

_____ 12. Expenses that reduce taxable income.

MULTIPLE CHOICE: TEST YOUR KNOWLEDGE

Place the letter of the answer next to the number of the term or phrase that best describes it.

_____ 1. What is the set amount a policyholder must pay every year before an insurance company starts paying?
   A. Insurance claim
   B. Insurance deductible
   C. Insurance policy
   D. Insurance reinstatement

_____ 2. Which type of insurance provides income protection if a person is unable to work because of disease or injury?
   A. Professional liability
   B. Disability
   C. Premises liability
   D. Health

_____ 3. A business entity that is owned by two or more entities that share in the profits and losses is a:
   A. C-corporation
   B. S-corporation
   C. Sole proprietorship
   D. Business partnership

_____ 4. What is an agreement by a company or governmental agency to provide compensation for specified losses, damages, illness, or death in return for payments called premiums?
   A. Share
   B. Gratuity
   C. Insurance
   D. Installment

_____ 5. What is a unit of equity and ownership in a corporation called?
   A. Bitcoin
   B. Share
   C. Tax deduction
   D. Installment

_____ 6. What is an average profit percentage to use when calculating hourly fees for services?
   A. 1%
   B. 5%
   C. 15%
   D. 25%

_____ 7. The fair market value of bartered goods or services must be included in one's _____ when filing taxes.
   A. Gross income
   B. Net income
   C. Gratuities
   D. Deductions

_____ 8. What is the term used to describe the amount an individual/household or a company makes after deducting allowable expenses and taxes?
   A. Equity
   B. Petty cash
   C. Gross income
   D. Net income

_____ 9. What is the primary method clients use to locate massage practitioners?
   A. Referrals
   B. Websites
   C. Social media
   D. Locator services

_____ 10. Which of the following best describes free media exposure?
   A. Vision statement
   B. Publicity
   C. Advertisement
   D. Billboards

_____ 11. What is a group of consumers more likely to want or need your products or services?
   A. Target market
   B. Social media
   C. Population sample
   D. Cultural cohort

_____ 12. What is the responsible and ethical use of technology by anyone who uses computers, the Internet, and digital devices?
   A. Location boundary
   B. Standard of care
   C. Digital citizenship
   D. Value-added service

CRITICAL THINKING

How You Do Anything Is How You Do Everything

Meredith and Tony were in the same class at their massage school. They have remained friends now that they have graduated, but Tony had noticed some behaviors on Meredith's part that concerned him a little. For example, in the student breakroom she would talk about the clients she worked on in the student clinic, sometimes making fun of their bodies; or she would find a particular male client "hot." Often, she would not have her homework done on time and would have many reasons why it wasn't complete. Although she seemed to learn massage techniques easily, she would get impatient if the instructor needed to spend more time with other students. Once, Tony came up to her outside the school building, and he accidentally heard Meredith on her cell phone making a date with one of the teaching assistants.

Meredith and Tony recently met for lunch. After catching up for a few minutes, Meredith told Tony she was let go from a local massage business after working there 2 weeks. She didn't understand why—she had gone out of her way to suck up to the manager, and she always got extra-large tips from her male clients. She thought the problem was that the other massage practitioners were jealous of her and her skills, and she had let another practitioner know she hadn't been hired to fold linens in between clients. That was someone else's job. Now Meredith needed to find another place to work and was wondering if Tony had any suggestions for her.

Answers can include but are not limited to:

As the old saying goes, "How you do anything is how you do everything." Meredith displayed behaviors as a massage student she most likely carried into her professional massage setting. She does not see these behaviors related to her lack of success as a professional massage practitioner and is blaming others for being fired.

Tony can point out to her the attributes of an ethical and professional massage practitioner, and that those same attributes she had as a student carried into her professional massage practice. Meredith needs to do some serious self-evaluation and make sincere changes if she is to be successful as a massage practitioner.

Massage practitioners should have knowledge of techniques and principles that include an understanding of legal and ethical issues. They must also acquire a working knowledge of and acceptance for human nature and individual characteristics. Daily contact with a wide variety of people with a host of problems and concerns is a significant part of their work. Courtesy, compassion, and common sense are often cited as the *three Cs* most vital to the success of a massage practitioner.

In fact, the first responsibility of a massage practitioner is always to provide competent, courteous, and compassionate care to clients. Other characteristics of a professional massage practitioner are in Box 17.1.

PROFESSIONAL PRACTICE

Which Way to Go?

Spend time thinking about and researching which market sector you want to go into after graduation. Examples of market sectors are relaxation and spa settings, rehabilitation and clinical settings, corporate settings, and mobile massage. Factor in your unique personality, skill sets, values, reasons for becoming a massage practitioner, and what you need from your business. Write this down and share it with your teachers and classmates.

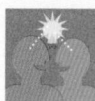

DISCUSSION

Break or Burden

Becky is a newly licensed massage practitioner who landed a job as an independent contractor at a local chiropractic office. She has just entered her third month at the clinic. Tom, the office manager, expects Becky to be on the premises Monday through Friday from 10 am to 6 pm. When Becky is not taking care of massage clients, she is expected to answer the phone and fold newly laundered linens.

Today, Tom gave Becky a list of clients who have not been in the clinic for over 6 months. Becky is expected to call each client and introduce herself as the new massage practitioner and suggest they schedule an appointment. Becky is upset.

Why do you think Becky is upset? If available, post your reflections on an Internet-based discussion board monitored by your instructor.

CHAPTER 18

Not all who wander are lost.
—J.R.R. Tolkien

Introduction to the Human Body: Medical Terminology, Cells, Tissues, and Body Compass

LEARNING OBJECTIVES

After completing this chapter, the student should be able to:

1. Define anatomy, physiology, homeostasis, and allostasis, and discuss medical terminology.
2. Discuss cells and cell processes.
3. Outline tissues and tissue types.
4. State types of membranes, and give examples.
5. Describe the body compass, including anatomic position and planes.
6. Detail directional terms, body cavities, and body regions.

http://evolve.elsevier.com/Salvo/MassageTherapy

INTRODUCTION

You are about to embark on an unforgettable journey—a new path of self-discovery—into your own self. To begin, you have to learn a new language—a language of science and medicine. Most of these terms have their roots in Latin and Greek. Learning this language is crucial to your studies that follow because your skill and effectiveness in performing massage, especially designing client-centered treatment plans, depend on your understanding of anatomy, physiology, and pathology. These terms and concepts will be reinforced many times in the remaining chapters. Remember, the key to retaining information is repetition.

A clear visual picture of the many arrangements of cells and tissues will help you feel what is beneath your hands as you apply massage techniques. As massage practitioners, you will be evaluating, comparing, and then reevaluating all of the numerous tissue types you are palpating and manipulating. You will be gliding across the epidermis (largely epithelial and nervous tissues); compressing and stretching fascia (connective tissue); kneading deltoids and trapezius (muscle tissue); and chucking between metacarpals (connective tissue).

Nearly everyone has some basic understanding of anatomy and physiology, if not from prior education classes, then from practical experience of one's own body. Our bodies are physiologic masterpieces. As you read this textbook, your heart is pumping blood, your lungs are moving air, your pupils are adjusting to reading conditions, and your nerves are monitoring both internal and external environments. These processes are dynamic and occur within us every second we are alive. During this study of anatomy and physiology, many wonders will be revealed. The philosopher Plato once noted the "acquiring of knowledge is just a form of recollection." Learning anatomy and physiology is simply becoming aware of who you already are. Next, let's look at several important concepts.

Anatomy is the study of the structures of the human body and their positional relationships to one another. The study of anatomy can be approached in several ways. *Gross anatomy* is the study of larger body structures, such as bones, muscles, and organs. *Microscopic anatomy* is the study of smaller structures such as cells and tissues, which are seen through a microscope. Cells and tissues make up larger structures such as organs found in gross anatomy. *Comparative anatomy* studies commonalities and differences between structures of all life forms. *Surface anatomy* studies relationships of structures found on the surface of the body and how they relate to internal structures.

Physiology is the study of how the body and its individual parts function in normal body processes. As with anatomy, there are different approaches to the study of physiology. *Comparative physiology* is the study of similarities and differences in vital body processes. *Developmental physiology* is the study of embryonic development. *Pathophysiology* and *pathology* are the studies of disease.

To better understand the relationship between anatomy and physiology, a theater metaphor may be helpful. The cast of characters are the "structures" of the play (anatomy). The plot, or how characters interact, is the "function" of the play (physiology).

Homeostasis is the constant and stable internal environment within a narrow range despite changes that occur in the external environment. For example, normal body temperature is approximately 98.6°F irrespective of room temperature. Other examples of homeostasis are normal blood sugar levels, blood pressure, and heart/respiration rates. **Allostasis** is the process of achieving homeostasis through physiologic and behavioral changes. For example, the body responds to changes in internal temperature by increasing heat production or releasing excess heat—this process will continue until homeostasis or normal body temperature is achieved. Homeostasis and allostasis are regulated primarily by the nervous and endocrine systems, which are featured in Chapters 23 and 24.

As we begin our study, definitions of anatomic terms are important, so everyone speaks and understands a common language.

MEDICAL TERMINOLOGY

Many students enter science-based courses knowing they have to learn and remember extensive lists of terminology. Although each discipline has its own set of relevant terms, there are some common principles that apply to scientific and medical terminology. When the Romans conquered Greece, the knowledge and languages of both cultures merged. The legendary doctors Hippocrates of Cos and Galen of Pergamon are credited for many of the Greek and Latin medical terms used today.

Medical words are often made up of several components or parts, and knowing these will help you to remember them or help you decipher their meaning. These parts are a *root*, a *prefix*, and a *suffix*.

The **root** or stem is the main or most basic part of a word. Some words combine two roots with the connecting vowel *o*. For example, combining the root *cardi-*, Greek for "heart," and the root *vascular*, Latin for "vessel," becomes a new word *cardi-o-vascular* or *cardiovascular*, which means pertaining to the heart and its vessels. See Vocabulary Builder: Common Root Words and Their Meanings for more word roots.

A **prefix** is letters added at the beginning of a root word to change its meaning. It can elaborate or qualify the word. For example, *pre-* is a prefix meaning "before" or "front." Add *pre-* before the root *cancer* and it becomes *precancerous*, denoting a stage of disease that may lead to cancer but cancer has not yet developed. See the Vocabulary Builder: Common Prefixes, Their Meanings, and Examples table for more prefix information.

A **suffix** is letters added at the end of a word to change its meaning. It can also denote the type of word, such as an adjective or a noun. Suffixes can also indicate value, quality, action, or relation such as gender, size, number, or type. For example, *-ectomy* is a suffix meaning "to cut out," as in surgery. Add *-ectomy* behind the word *appendix,* and the new term is *appendectomy*, or surgical removal of the appendix. See Vocabulary Builder: Common Suffixes, Their Meanings, and Examples and Vocabulary Builder: Commonly Used Plural Endings tables for more information.

As you study anatomy and physiology, it is helpful to become familiar with prefixes, suffixes, and root words. Think of them as building blocks put together in many different ways to form words. This way, if you know what the building blocks mean, you do not have to memorize every new term you encounter. Instead, you can figure out its meaning. An example is *cardiomyopathy. Cardi-* means heart; *myo-* means muscle; and *-pathy* means disease. Therefore *cardiomyopathy* means heart muscle disease. Another example is *myalgia.* You already know *myo-* means muscle, so you know this term has something to do with muscles. Understanding that *-algia* means pain means you now know *myalgia* means muscle pain. Another example is *neuralgia.* You already know *-algia* means pain, so you know this term has something to do with a type of pain. Understanding that *neuro-* means nerves means you know *neuralgia* means nerve pain.

To assist in learning pronunciations, echo back terms (either mentally or subvocally) your instructor says aloud. Or use a web-based program with audio features. Along with correct pronunciation, correct spelling is crucial because some medical terms look or sound similar. For example, *ileum* is a section of the small intestine and *ilium* is a bone in the pelvis. When in doubt, use a medical dictionary or electronic medical spell-checker.

Vocabulary Builder: Common Prefixes, Their Meanings, and Examples

PREFIX	MEANING	EXAMPLE
a-, an-	Lacking, without, not	Asymptomatic, anaerobic
ab-	Away from, absent	Abduction, abnormal
ad-	Toward, near to, increase	Adduction, adjust
adeno-	Gland	Adenoma, adenitis
allo-	Other, different	Allostasis, allopathic
angio-	Vessel	Angiogram, angioma
ante-	Front, before, toward	Anterior, ante mortem
anti-	Against, opposed	Antifungal, antibody
auto-	Self	Autoimmune, autonomic
bi-, di-	Twice, double, two	Biceps, diencephalon
bio-	Life	Biology, biohazard
cephal-	Head	Cephalitis, cephalalgia
circum-	Around	Circumduction, circumcision
contra-	Opposite, against	Contraindication, contralateral
cryo-	Extreme cold	Cryotherapy, cryoablation
cyto-	Cell	Cytoplasm, cytomegaly
de-	Separate, away from, down	Decapitate, decompose
dia-	Through	Diaphragm, diarrhea
dis-	Apart, away	Dislocation, dissection
dors-	Back	Dorsal, dorsiflexion
dys-	Difficult, bad, labored	Dysfunction, dysplasia
ecto-, exo-, ex-	On the outer side	Ectoderm, exocrine, excise
endo-	Within, inside	Endometrium, endocardium
epi-	Upon, over, in addition to	Epicondyle, epicardium
extend-	Straighten	Extension, extensor
flex-	Bend	Flexion, flexibility
glu-, gly-	Sugar, sweet	Glucose, glycosuria
histo-	Tissue	Histology, histamine
hetero-	Dissimilar	Heterocellular, heterogeneous
homeo-, homo-	Like, same	Homeopathy, homogenous
hydro-	Water or hydrogen	Hydromassage, hydrophobia
hyper-	Over, above, excessive	Hyperextension, hypertension
hypo-	Under, below, deficient	Hypodermic, hypovolemia
hyster-	Uterus, womb	Hysterectomy, hysteroscopy
infra-	Under, below, beneath	Infraspinatus, infrahyoid
inter-	Between, together	Intercostal, interarticular
intra-	Within	Intravenous, intravascular
lipo-	Lipid, fat	Lipoma, liposuction
meso-	Middle	Mesentery, mesoderm
meta-	Beyond, after, change	Metabolism, metacarpals
micro-	Small	Microvilli, microscope
mono-	One, single	Mononuclear, monoaxial
multi-	Many	Multifidus, multipennate
narco-	Sleep, numbness, stupor	Narcolepsy, narcotic
necro-	Death	Necrosis, necropsy
ophthalmo-	Eye	Ophthalmic, ophthalmologist
ot-	Ear	Otitis, otologist
para-	Alongside, beside	Parasympathetic, paranormal
patho-	Disease	Pathology, pathogen
peri-	Around, surrounding	Periosteum, periodontal
post-	Rear, after, behind	Posterior, postmortem
pre-, pro-	Before, front	Prenatal, protuberance
quad-	Four	Quadriceps, quadratus
re-	Again, back	Realign, retract
recto-	Straight	Rectum, rectus
retro-	Backward	Retroperitoneal, retrovert
sub-	Under, beneath, below	Subscapular, subcutaneous
super-, supra-	Above, over	Superficial, supraspinatus
syn-, sym-	Together, with, joined	Synarthrotic, symbiotic
therm-	Heat	Thermal, thermotherapy
trans-	Across, over, beyond, through	Transverse, transfusion
tri-	Three	Triceps, triaxial
uni-	One	Unilateral, uniaxial

Vocabulary Builder: Common Root Words and Their Meanings

ROOT	MEANING	ROOT	MEANING	ROOT	MEANING
Abdomin(o)-	Abdomen	Hepat(o)-	Liver	Rect(o)-	Rectum
Aden(o)-	Gland	Hydr(o)-	Water	Rhin(o)-	Nose
Adren(o)-	Adrenal gland	Hyster(o)-	Uterus	Splen(o)-	Spleen
Angi(o)-	Vessel	Ile(o)-, ili(o)-	Ileum	Sten(o)-	Narrow, constriction
Arteri(o)-	Artery	Laryng(o)-	Larynx	Stern(o)-	Sternum
Arthr(o)-	Joint	Mamm(o)-	Breast, mammary gland	Stomat(o)-	Mouth
Bronch(o)-	Bronchus, bronchi	Mast(o)-	Mammary gland, breast	Therm(o)-	Heat
Card-, cardi(o)-	Heart	Men(o)-	Menstruation	Thorac(o)-	Chest
Cephal(o)-	Head	My(o)-	Muscle	Thromb(o)-	Clot, thrombus
Chondr(o)-	Cartilage	Myel(o)-	Spinal cord, bone marrow	Thyr(o)-	Thyroid
Col(o)-	Colon	Nephr(o)-	Kidney	Tox(o)-	Poison
Cost(o)-	Rib	Neur(o)-	Nerve	Toxic(o)-	Poison, poisonous
Crani(o)-	Skull	Ocul(o)-	Eye	Trache(o)-	Trachea
Cyan(o)-	Blue	Ophthalm(o)-	Eye	Ur(o)-	Urine, urinary tract, urination
Cyst(o)-	Bladder, cyst	Orth(o)-	Straight, normal, correct	Urethr(o)-	Urethra
Cyt(o)-	Cell	Oste(o)-	Bone	Urin(o)-	Urine
Derma-	Skin	Ot(o)-	Ear	Uter(o)-	Uterus
Duoden(o)-	Duodenum	Ped(o)-	Child, foot	Vas(o)-	Blood vessel, vas deferens
Encephal(o)-	Brain	Pharyng(o)-	Pharynx	Ven(o)-	Vein
Enter(o)-	Intestines	Phleb(o)-	Vein	Vertebr(o)-	Spine, vertebrae
Fibr(o)-	Fiber, fibrous	Pnea-	Breathing, respiration		
Gastr(o)-	Stomach	Pneum(o)-	Lung, air, gas		
Gloss(o)-	Tongue	Proct(o)-	Rectum		
Gyn-, gyne-, gynec(o)-	Woman	Psych(o)-	Mind		
Hem-, hema-, hem(o)-	Blood	Pulm(o)-	Lung		
Hemat(o)-	Blood	Py(o)-	Pus		

Adapted from Fritz, S. (2016). *Essential sciences for therapeutic massage* (5th ed., table 3.2). St Louis, MO: Elsevier.

Vocabulary Builder: Common Suffixes, Their Meanings, and Examples

SUFFIX	MEANING	EXAMPLE
-algia	Pain	Fibromyalgia, neuralgia
-blast	Bud or sprout, developing	Osteoblast, collagenoblast
-cele	Tumor, herniation, pouch	Meningocele, rectocele
-clast	Destroy or break down	Angioclast, osteoclast
-cyte	Cell	Hemocyte, osteocyte
-ectomy	Excision or to cut out	Tonsillectomy, appendectomy
-emia	Blood condition	Hyperemia, lipidemia
-er	Agent, person	Trainer, dispatcher
-gen	Produce, create	Carcinogen, fibrinogen
-gram	To record	Electrocardiogram, angiogram
-ia, -osis, -ism	State or condition	Anemia, cyanosis, embolism
-iatry	Healing	Psychiatry, podiatry
-itis	Inflammation	Arthritis, dermatitis
-megaly	Great, large	Cardiomegaly, splenomegaly
-oid	Shaped	Rhomboid, cuboid
-ologist	Specialist in a particular study	Biologist, histologist
-ology	Study of	Urology, biology
-oma	Tumor	Neuroma, lipoma
-osis	Condition	Lordosis, sclerosis
-pathy	Disease	Neuropathy, retinopathy
-otomy	Incision or to cut into	Colostomy, lumpectomy
-penia	Poverty	Osteopenia, thrombocytopenia
-plasia	To form	Hyperplasia, dysplasia
-rrhage, -rrhea	Abnormal or excessive flow	Hemorrhage, diarrhea
-scopy	To view or examine	Arthroscopy, cystoscopy
-stasis	Control, stopping	Homeostasis, hemostasis
-trophy	Nourish, grow, develop	Hypertrophy, dystrophy
-tropy	Turning, changing	Thixotropy

Vocabulary Builder: Commonly Used Plural Endings

SINGULAR	PLURAL	EXAMPLES
-a	-ae	scapula/scapulae
-en	-ina	foramen/foramina
-is	-es	testis/testes
-is	-ides	iris/irides
-nx	-ges	larynx/larynges
-on	-a	mitochondrion/mitochondria
-um	-a	bacterium/bacteria
-us	-i	nucleus/nuclei
-x	-ces	thorax/thoraces
-y	-ies	cavity/cavities

LEVELS OF ORGANIZATION

The human body can be thought of as a universe made up of small components organized as a functional unit. This organization follows a hierarchy or is ordered from the most simple to the most complex and is *chemical, cellular, tissue, organ, organ system,* and *organism* (Fig. 18.1).

The **chemical level** encompasses chemical elements or biochemistry of the body. Examples of chemicals are atoms, compounds, gases such as oxygen, minerals such as iron, and molecules such as deoxyribonucleic acid (DNA). The **cellular level** is cells and provides functions vital for life such as muscle and nerve cells. The **tissue level** is groups of cells, all of which possess similar structure and perform specific functions such as epithelial and connective tissues.

The **organ level** is composed of structures containing two or more tissue types such as the kidneys and the bladder. Terms are used to indicate regions of organs and spaces with hollow structures.

- **Cortex.** Outer region of an organ (e.g., cerebral cortex).
- **Medulla.** Inner region of an organ (e.g., adrenal medulla).
- **Lumen.** Space within a hollow tube (e.g., intestines and blood vessels).

The **organ system level** is a group of related organs with complementary functions arranged into systems performing physiologic processes. Examples are the respiratory system and the digestive system. Each organ system is discussed in a separate chapter. The highest and most complex organizational level is the **organism level** and represents a living entity. Each organism is composed of several organ systems to promote life. Examples of organisms are *Homo sapiens,* fish, frogs, and butterflies.

CELLS AND CELLULAR PROCESSES

The **cell** is the smallest structural and functional unit existing as a self-sustaining entity. Cells are the building blocks of the human body. Scientists estimate between 75 and 100 trillion cells are present in the body at any given moment. Most cells are microscopic in size and cannot be seen with the naked eye. Some of the smallest cells are red blood cells, which are so tiny several million red blood cells would fit on the tip of a ballpoint pen. One of the largest body cells is the female sex cell or ovum (egg), which is approximately the size of the period at the end of this sentence.

Cells are made up of chemical building blocks called *elements.* The main elements are carbon, oxygen, hydrogen, and nitrogen. *Trace elements,* or minerals, are also present in cells. Examples of trace elements are calcium, iron, iodine, sodium, and potassium. Trace elements are important for cellular functions. Calcium is needed for blood clotting; iron is necessary to make hemoglobin, which transports oxygen in blood; and iodine is needed to make thyroid hormones, which influence metabolism. **Metabolism** is the biochemical processes that occur within a living organism to maintain life. Besides elements and trace elements, water makes up approximately 60% to 80% of all cells. The study of cells is called *cytology.*

To gain a better understanding of cells, we will study the anatomy and physiology of a typical or *composite* cell. Bear in mind there is no such thing as a typical cell—this model was created for study purposes. To accomplish its many functions, cells move substances where they are needed. Some of these processes require energy, and others do not.

Parts of a Cell

The following section discusses the parts of a cell (Fig. 18.2). These parts include the cell membrane, cytoplasm, and organelles (Table 18.1).

Cell Membrane

Each cell is surrounded by a **cell membrane** or *plasma membrane*. This membrane separates intracellular fluid from extracellular fluid. The cell membrane is responsive to changes

TABLE 18.1 Cell Structures and Functions

CELL STRUCTURES	FUNCTIONS
Cell membrane	Facilitates exchange of nutrients and wastes
Cytoplasm	Most cellular activities occur here
Endoplasmic reticulum	Transport materials. The cell's "roadways."
Golgi body	Synthesizes proteins and fats/lipids, then packs and stores them. The cell's "packing and shipping plants."
Mitochondrion	Takes in nutrients, breaks them down, creates ATP, and site of cellular respiration. The cell's "power plant."
Lysosome	Break down unneeded proteins, destroy pathogens, and remove cellular debris. The cell's janitors or "garbage disposals."
Nucleus	Directs most metabolic activities such as growth and reproduction. Contains DNA and RNA. The cell's "control center."

ATP, Adenosine triphosphate; *DNA,* deoxyribonucleic acid; *RNA,* ribonucleic acid.

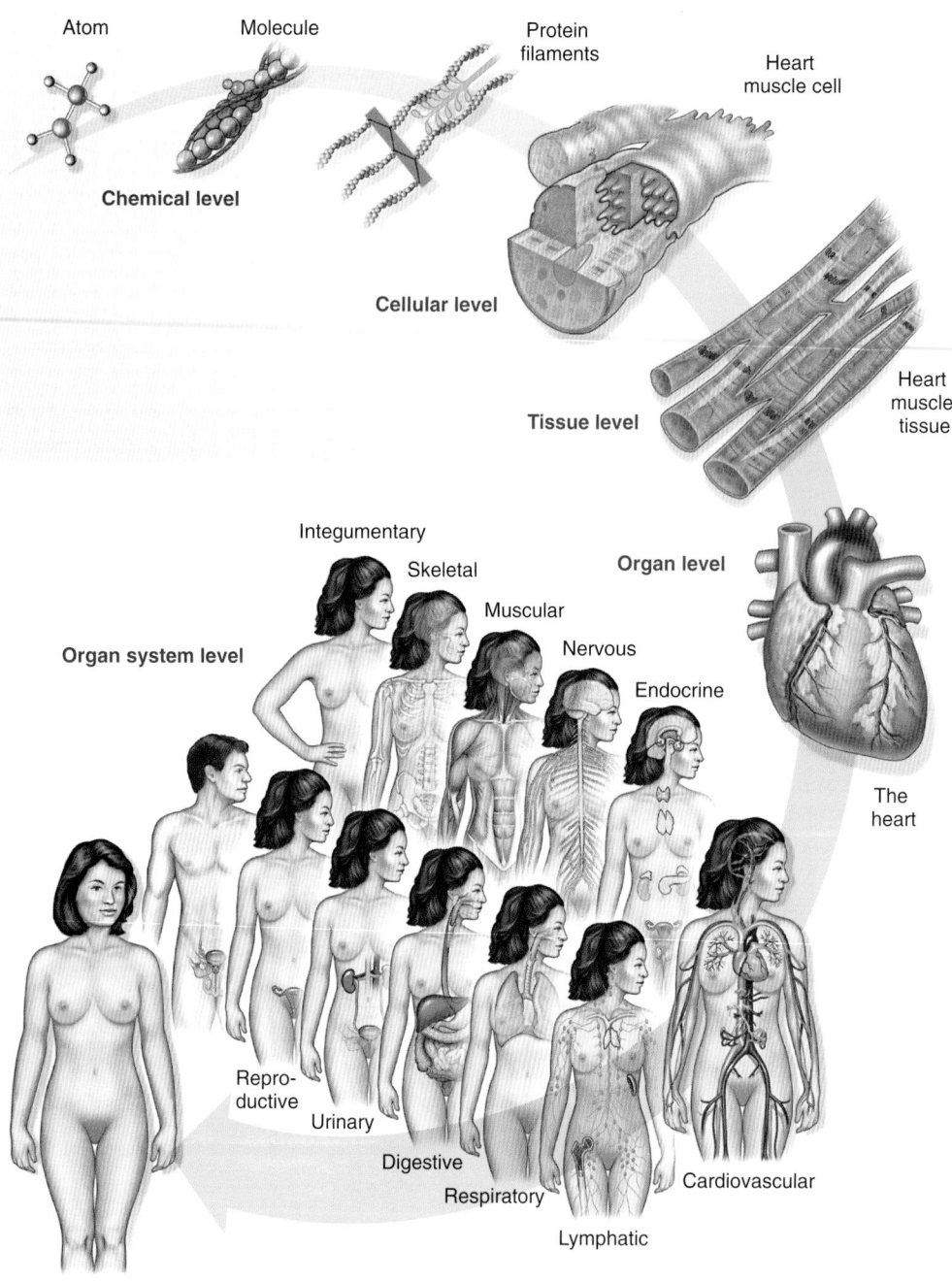

Atom　　Molecule

Protein filaments

Heart muscle cell

Chemical level

Cellular level

Tissue level

Heart muscle tissue

Integumentary

Skeletal

Muscular

Nervous

Endocrine

Organ level

Organ system level

The heart

Repro-ductive

Urinary

Digestive

Respiratory

Lymphatic

Cardiovascular

Organism level

FIG. 18.1 Levels of organization from the least complex *(chemical level)* to the most complex *(organism level).* (From Patton, K. T., & Thibodeau, G. A. [2010]. *Anatomy & physiology* [7th ed.]. St. Louis, MO: Mosby.)

inside and outside the cell. The membrane is semipermeable, which functions like gates in a fence, allowing some materials to pass and limiting or blocking the passage of others. This action facilitates the exchange of nutrients and wastes. Some cell membranes contain receptors for hormones or other regulatory chemicals, which can alter cell metabolism. These processes can be passive or active, which are discussed later. Think of the cell membrane as the "gatekeeper" of the cell.

Cytoplasm

Cells contain a gel-like intracellular fluid called **cytoplasm** or *protoplasm.* Floating in cytoplasm are structures called organelles, discussed next. Most cellular activities, such as metabolism and cell division, occur in cytoplasm. The portion of cytoplasm not contained within organelles is called *cytosol.* The portion of cytoplasm within organelles is called *endoplasm.*

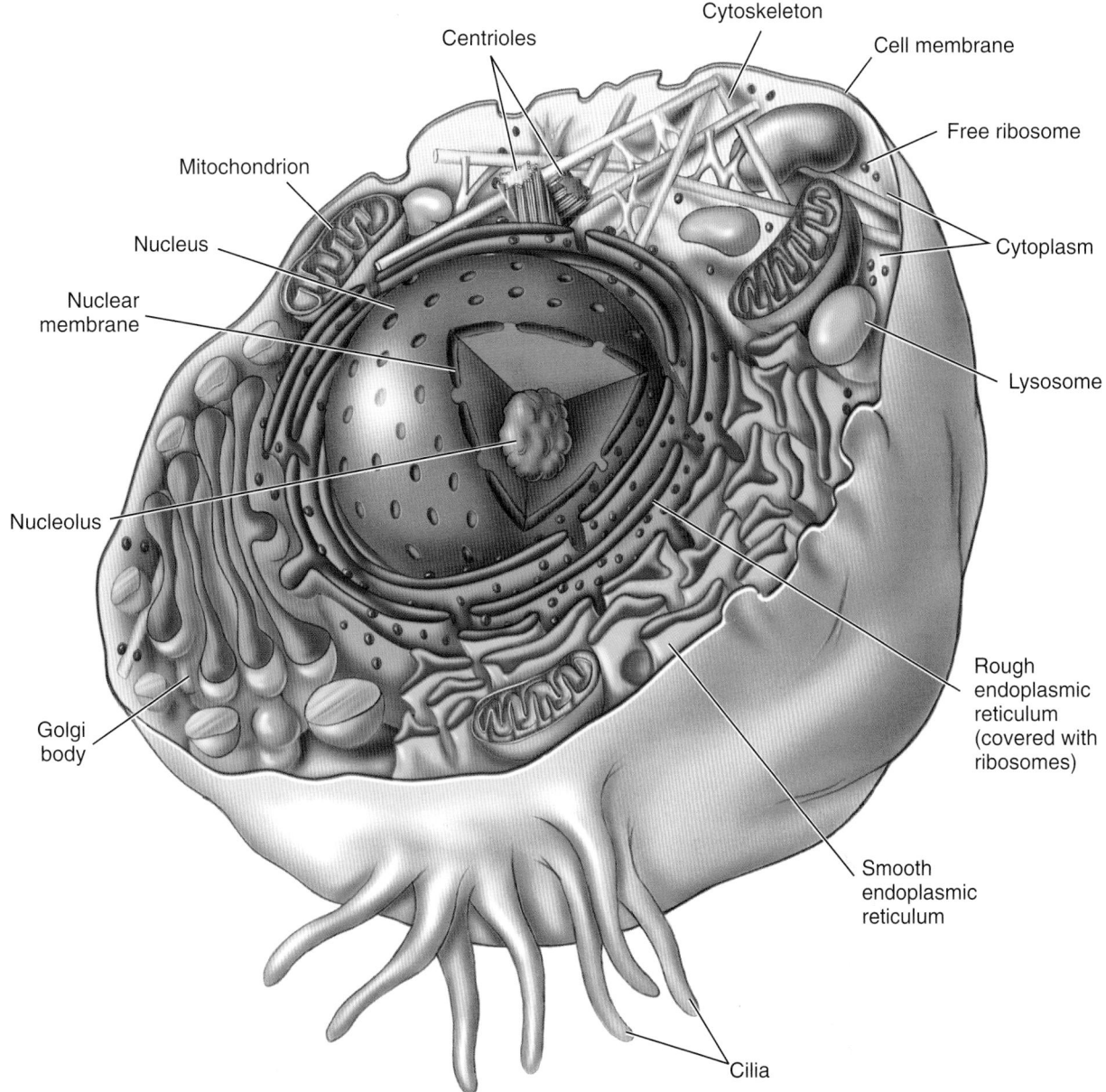

FIG. 18.2 A typical or composite cell. This cell possesses hairlike projections called cilia. (From Herlihy, B. [2011]. *The human body in health and illness* [4th ed.]. St. Louis, MO: Mosby.)

Organelles

Within the cell are structures called **organelles.** Each organelle possesses distinct structures and functions. Some organelles function in reproduction, some store materials, and some metabolize nutrients.

The **endoplasmic reticulum** (ER) is a network of curved sacs arranged in parallel rows. Pieces of the ER can break off and become parts of other organelles or even parts of the cell membrane. This allows the ER to transport materials. Think of the ER as the cell's "roadways." ER can be classified as rough or smooth. Rough ER is spotted with ribosomes. **Ribosomes** are small granules of ribonucleic acid (RNA) and are the "protein factories." Some ribosomes float freely (called *free ribosomes*). Some ribosomes attach to the ER, which gives it a rough appearance and is called *rough ER. Smooth ER* does not contain ribosomes.

Golgi bodies, or *Golgi complexes,* are a series of separate horizontal membranous sacs stacked on top of each other. They synthesize proteins and fats or lipids, then pack and store them. Think of the Golgi bodies as the post office or the "packing and shipping plants." When needed, proteins and fats are wrapped in a piece of Golgi body membrane and are moved within the cell or outside the cell to be used elsewhere in the body.

Mitochondria are oval organelles that look like partitioned sausages. The mitochondria's interior contains numerous chambers called *cristae*—these increase the surface area for improved productivity. These organelles take in nutrients, break them down, and create **adenosine triphosphate** (ATP), the cell's energy molecule. Think of mitochondria as the cell's "power plant." The biochemical process is called cellular respiration. Some cells have several thousand mitochondria, and others have none. Muscle cells need a lot of energy for muscle contraction so they have a lot of mitochondria. Red blood cells lack mitochondria. If a cell feels it is not getting enough energy, more mitochondria can be created. Sometimes mitochondria can grow larger or combine with other mitochondria, depending on the needs of the cell.

Lysosomes are membranous organelles that have broken off from Golgi bodies. The size of lysosomes changes with their activity level. They are small during inactive periods and large during active periods. Lysosomes break down unneeded proteins and destroy pathogens with enzymes. Lysosomes also release enzymes at injury sites to help remove cellular debris. Think of lysosomes are the cell's janitors or "garbage disposals." Lysosomes can trigger self-digestion to decrease the number of cells, such as shrinking the size of the uterus after childbirth.

Centrioles are paired, tubular structures that assist cell division by organizing chromosomes. These organelles are usually found near the nucleus. Cells without centrioles are incapable of cell division (e.g., red blood cells).

Nucleus is the spherical shaped and often largest organelle. Each nucleus contains clusters of proteins, DNA, and RNA, which help form chromosomes, or our genetic code. Humans possess 23 pairs of chromosomes. A discussion of chromosomes is found in Chapter 25. A porous nuclear membrane surrounds the nucleus. Smaller structures within the nucleus called *nucleolus* help to synthesize proteins. Think of the nucleus as the cell's "control center" because it directs most metabolic activities, including growth and reproduction. All cells have at least one nucleus at some time in their existence. Red blood cells lose their nuclei as they mature, and skeletal muscle cells possess many nuclei.

Cytoskeleton

Many cells contain a network of microfilaments and microtubules called **cytoskeleton.** This network serves as scaffolding material to provide an internal structure to the cell. The cytoskeleton helps to move substances across the membrane. The cytoskeleton may organize itself as cellular extensions, such as *microvilli, cilia,* and *flagella.*

- **Microvilli**. Fingerlike projections found in the lining of the lower gastrointestinal tract and in the proximal tubule within the kidneys. Microvilli helps increase the surface area, which improves absorption (see Fig. 29.5).
- **Cilia**. Hairlike projections on the lining of the upper respiratory tract. Cilia help sweep mucus toward the throat so it can be swallowed. Cilia are also found in the lining of the female reproductive tract to help move the ova toward the uterus.
- **Flagellum**. Whiplike solitary projection providing cellular locomotion. Flagella are found on sperm cells and on some bacteria such as protozoa.

Cellular Processes: Passive

Passive processes, or *passive transport,* do not require energy or activity of the cell membrane. Molecules move because of differences in concentration, pressure, or temperature. These differences are called *gradients,* and they are the driving forces behind the movement of molecules down a gradient. For example, molecules move from an area of high concentration to low concentration, from an area of high pressure to low pressure, and from an area of high temperature to low temperature. Movement will continue until differences in concentration, pressure, or temperature are equal. Passive processes do not require energy, but they are dynamic—molecules continue to move even after equilibrium has occurred. Passive processes include *diffusion*, *osmosis*, and *filtration*.

Diffusion

Diffusion is the movement of molecules from an area of high concentration to an area of low concentration to equalize concentrations. During diffusion, molecules simply spread out, or diffuse, in a given space or across a cell membrane. For example, when a lump of sugar is dropped into a glass of water, the concentration of sugar is highest where the cube first lands. Over time, the cube dissolves and sugar moves throughout the liquid until the concentration of sugar is distributed equally (Fig. 18.3). Time needed for diffusion to occur can be reduced by stirring or heating the liquid. Some respiratory, cardiovascular, and digestive organs perform their functions through diffusion.

Osmosis

Osmosis is the movement of water across a cell membrane from an area of low concentration to high concentration to equalize concentration on both sides of the membrane. Water moves instead of molecules to create equilibrium. Osmosis is a type of diffusion and is used when the membrane is selectively permeable; it allows water to move but not one or more molecules. Movement of water continues until concentrations equalize (Fig. 18.4). The kidneys filter blood and manufacture urine using osmosis.

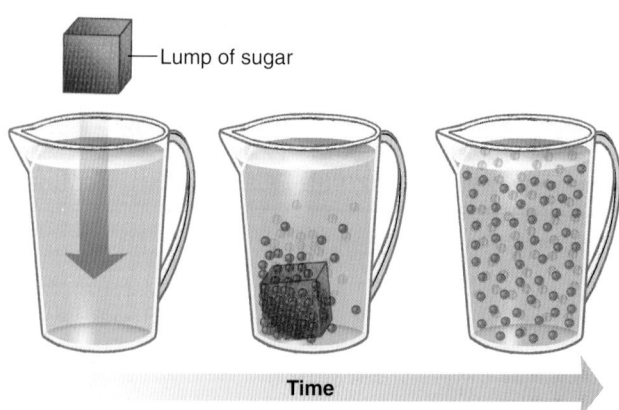

FIG. 18.3 Diffusion is a passive cell process in which molecules move from an area of high concentration to an area of low concentration to equalize concentrations.

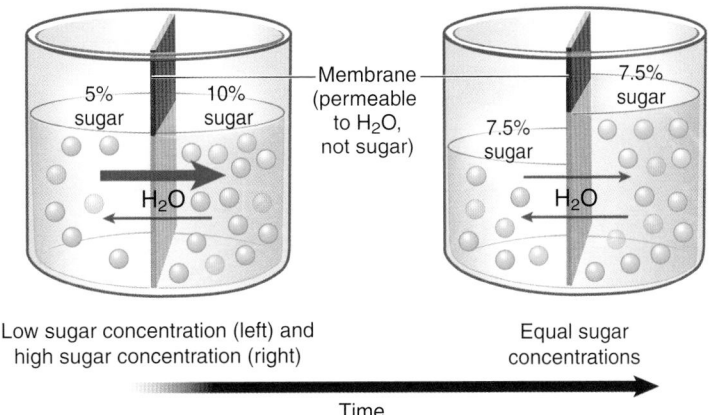

FIG. 18.4 Osmosis is a passive cell process in which water moves across a membrane from an area of low concentration to high concentration to equalize concentrations on both sides of the membrane. (From Patton, K., & Thibodeau, G. [2014]. *The human body in health and disease* [6th ed.]. St. Louis, MO: Mosby.)

Filtration

Filtration is the movement of water and molecules across a cell membrane because of pressure. Blood pressure pushes nutrients and wastes out of blood capillaries into cells within tissues. The sizes of pores within cell membranes determine which molecules pass and which do not. For example, pores in the kidney's filtration membrane are small and only allow the passage of tiny molecules such as water and wastes; larger molecules such as proteins and blood cells remain in blood. Pores in the filtration membrane in the liver are large, allowing the passage of both large and small molecules.

Cellular Processes: Active

Active processes, or *active transport,* require cells to expend energy to help move molecules across its membrane. These molecules must move against their concentration gradients, or uphill instead of down, as seen in passive processes. In other words, molecules move from an area of low concentration to an area of high concentration. These molecules will travel in the opposite direction only when forced by pumping mechanisms or by vesicles powered by the cell's energy.

Transport by Pumps

Pump mechanisms use carrier molecules within cell membranes. Because of their location, carrier molecules are also called *membrane pumps.* They function like a clamshell. When a certain ion binds to a carrier molecule, the shell closes on one side and reopens on the other side, essentially moving the ion across the cell membrane.

Two examples of transport by pumps are muscle and nerve cells. Muscle cells use pumps to move calcium ions, which help muscles contract and relax. Nerve cells use pumps to move sodium and potassium ions, which help nerves conduct impulses. Pump mechanisms require ATP produced by the cell's mitochondria. Energy released during the breakdown of ATP is used to fuel the pump.

Transport by Vesicles

Vesicles are small spherical sacs that import and export various substances. The main processes of transport by vesicles are *endocytosis* and *exocytosis.*

- **Endocytosis.** Process of moving substances inside the cell. To accomplish this, the cell's cytoskeleton pulls apart and draws inward to form an indentation. The target molecule is then surrounded and pulled inside the cell. Types of endocytosis are *phagocytosis* and *pinocytosis,* which are vital to immune responses.
  - **Phagocytosis** *(cell eating).* The molecule drawn inside the cell fuses with lysosome, which coats it with enzymes and digests it. This essentially kills the molecule, which is often a pathogen, such as bacteria. The digested products are released by exocytosis.
  - **Pinocytosis** *(cell drinking).* This is almost identical to phagocytosis except the targeted substance is liquid and not solid. Pinocytic cells are more common than phagocytic cells.
- **Exocytosis.** Process of moving substances outside the cell. A membrane-enclosed vesicle inside the cell joins the cell membrane, which moves it outside the cell. Exocytosis is used by cells secreting digestive enzymes, hormones, and mucus, as well as nerve cells secreting chemicals called neurotransmitters.

TISSUES

Tissues are groups of similar cells acting together to perform specific functions. Tissues organize themselves into organs. *Organs* are groups of two or more tissue types performing specialized functions. Tissues have a wide variety of shapes, sizes, and arrangements, which varies from a thin sheet of single cells to thick walls containing millions of cells. The study of tissues is called *histology.* All tissues are surrounded by an extracellular *matrix* or *ground substance.*

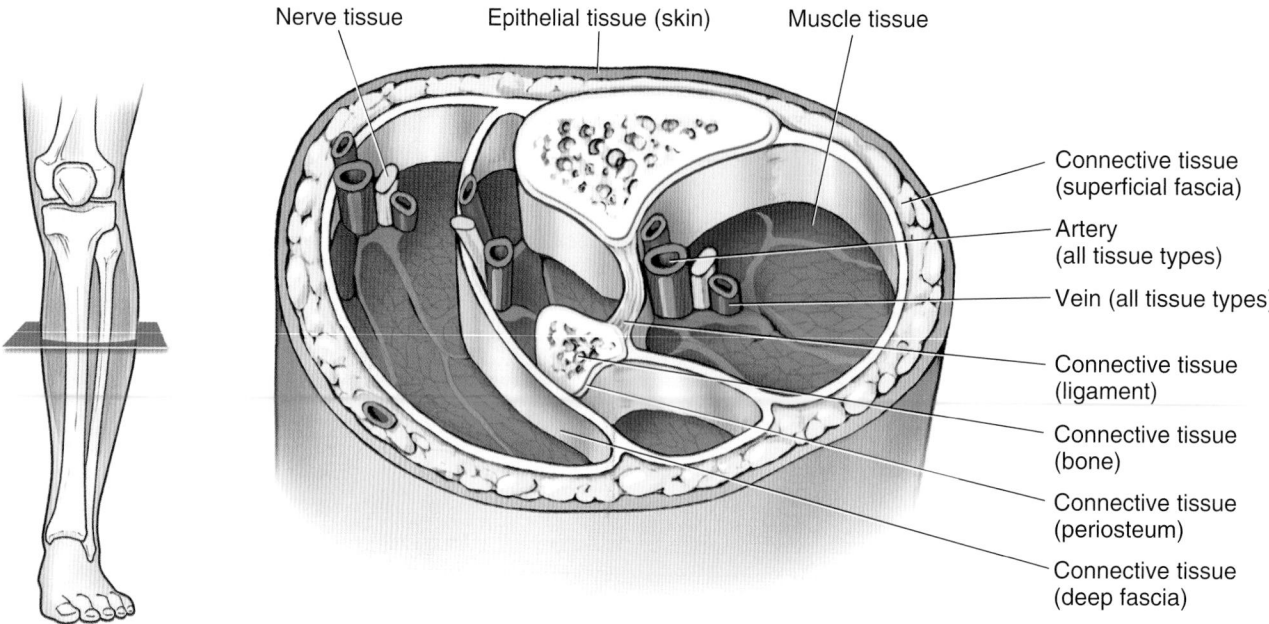

Nerve tissue   Epithelial tissue (skin)   Muscle tissue

Connective tissue (superficial fascia)
Artery (all tissue types)
Vein (all tissue types)
Connective tissue (ligament)
Connective tissue (bone)
Connective tissue (periosteum)
Connective tissue (deep fascia)

FIG. 18.5 Cross-section view of the leg with principal tissue types identified (*white*, connective tissue; *red*, muscle tissue).

Principal types of tissue are *epithelial tissue, connective tissue, muscular tissue, and nervous tissue* (Fig. 18.5).

- **Epithelial Tissue.** Covers external and internal structures, such as the external surface of the skin and the internal lining of the heart and blood vessels, and lines open and closed body cavities. Epithelial tissue provides protection, absorption, secretion, excretion, and sensation.
- **Connective Tissue.** Forms the framework for organs and glands and for the body as a whole. Connective tissue provides transportation and defense and connects and supports other tissues.
- **Muscle Tissue.** Found in hollow organs and tubes; some are attached to bones. Muscle tissue produces movement and heat and helps maintain body posture.
- **Nervous Tissue.** Found in the brain, spinal cord, and nerves. Nervous tissue detects sensory input, provides interpretative functions, coordinates motor output, and facilitates higher mental functioning and emotional responsiveness.

Interstitial fluid is found in the extracellular spaces between the tissues. This fluid is primarily water and contains substances, such as salts, sugars, fatty acids, amino acids, hormones, and neurotransmitters. Interstitial fluid bathes cells and provides a transport medium for nutrients, gases, and wastes. Interstitial fluid, blood plasma, and lymph are chemically similar. Interstitial fluid is more plentiful than plasma or lymph.

Tissues develop early in the embryo. By day 16, three embryonic tissue layers are beginning to differentiate. From superficial to deep, these layers are *ectoderm, mesoderm,* and *endoderm* (Fig. 18.6). These layers will later develop into all tissues and organs of the body.

- **Ectoderm.** Outermost layer and gives rise to structures of the nervous system, including special senses (vision, hearing/balance, smell, taste), and epidermis of the skin (touch).
- **Mesoderm.** Middle layer and develops into muscles, bones, and other connective tissues.
- **Endoderm.** Innermost layer and becomes epithelial tissue lining body's cavities, passages, and internal organs.

Epithelial Tissue

Epithelial tissue, or *epithelium,* lines or covers external and internal body structures and lines open body cavities (e.g., the digestive, respiratory, urinary, and reproductive tracts) and closed body cavities (e.g., the dorsal and ventral cavities). A type of epithelium called *endothelium* covers internal surfaces of blood and lymphatic vessels. *Glandular epithelium* is found in endocrine and exocrine glands and contains secretory cells.

Epithelial tissue is made up of closely packed cells and arranged in one or more layers. This tissue has a high rate of cell division and regenerates quickly. Epithelium is bound to underlying tissues by a thin permeable layer called a *basement membrane*. Permeability of the basement membrane is important because epithelium does not contain blood vessels and receives oxygen and nutrients by diffusion from capillaries in underlying tissues.

As mentioned previously, epithelial tissue provides protection, absorption, secretion, excretion, and sensation. It offers *limited protection* from mechanical injury, harmful chemicals, invading pathogens, and excessive water loss. It can *absorb* nutrients and gas exchange through epithelium of the digestive and respiratory tracts. It can *secrete* hormones, enzymes, mucus, and other lubricating fluids. It can *excrete* wastes, such as urine and sweat. It also detects

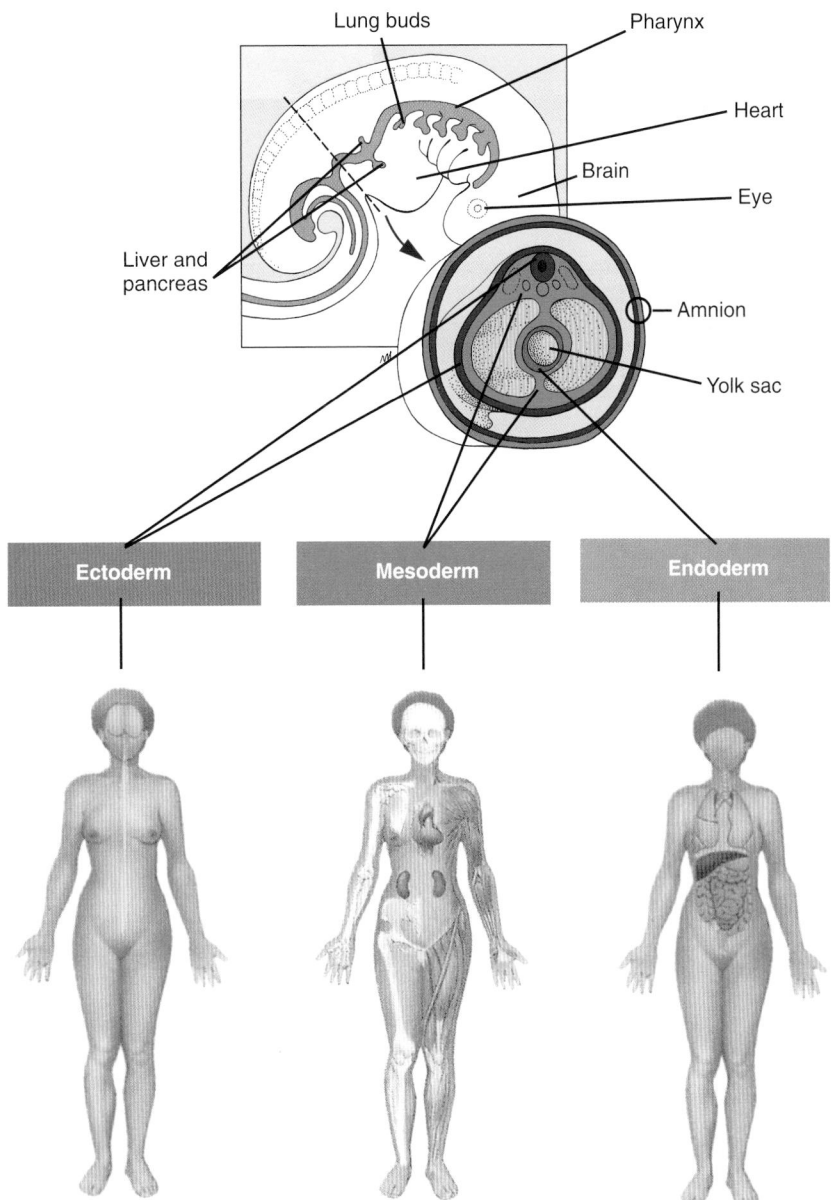

FIG. 18.6 Embryologic tissue layers of ectoderm *(nervous tissue),* mesoderm *(muscle and connective tissues),* and endoderm *(epithelial tissue and internal organs).* (From Thibodeau, G. A., & Patton, K. T. [2007]. *Anatomy & physiology* [6th ed.]. St. Louis, MO: Mosby.)

sensations by using receptors embedded in the skin, tongue, nose, eyes, and the ears.

Epithelial tissue can be classified by its number of layers as simple or stratified. *Simple epithelium* is one cell thick, and *stratified epithelium* is two or more cells thick. Epithelial tissue can also be classified by its shape as squamous, cuboidal, or columnar. *Squamous* is flat shaped, *cuboidal* is cube shaped, and *columnar* is column shaped. In some cases, these classifications are combined to describe epithelium, such as *simple squamous* found in the lungs and *stratified squamous* found in the mouth and skin. *Pseudostratified epithelium* has the appearance of multiple layers but is actually a single layer of cells with nuclei at different levels. *Transitional epithelium* combines all shapes and

permits stretching of structures such as the urinary bladder (Fig. 18.7).

Connective Tissue

Connective tissues connect, support, transport, and defend, as mentioned previously. It *connects* tissues to each other (e.g., muscles to muscles, muscles to bones, bones to bones). It *supports* organs and glands via a mesh framework and supports the body as a whole. It *transports* nutrients and wastes and *defends* the body through processes such as blood clotting and immune responses. Connective tissue is the most abundant tissue type (Table 18.2). Types of connective tissue are
- Fibrous
- Bone

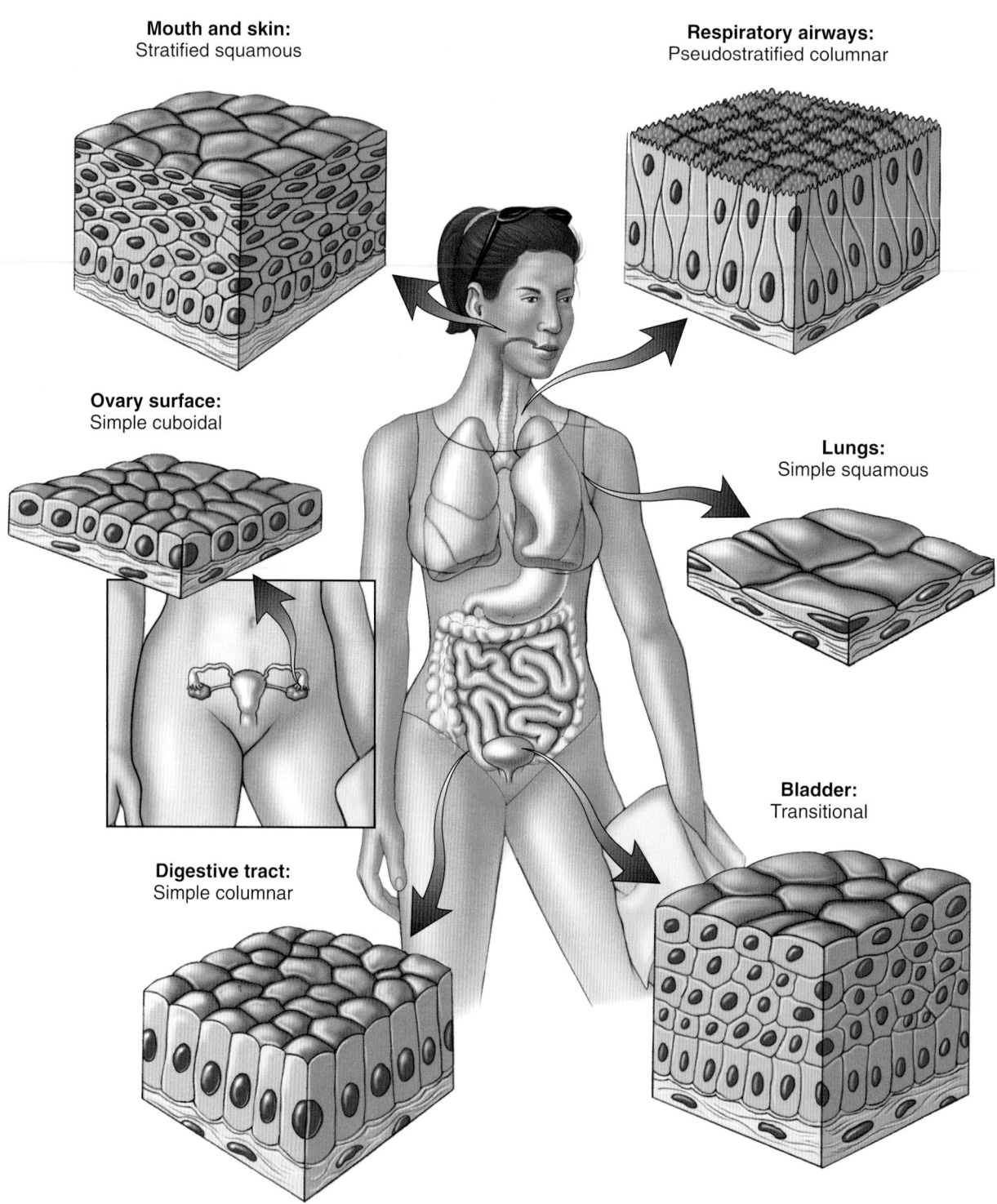

Epithelial Tissue

Mouth and skin:
Stratified squamous

Respiratory airways:
Pseudostratified columnar

Ovary surface:
Simple cuboidal

Lungs:
Simple squamous

Bladder:
Transitional

Digestive tract:
Simple columnar

FIG. 18.7 Epithelial tissue: Types and locations anterior view. (From Herlihy, B. [2011]. *The human body in health and illness* [4th ed.]. St. Louis, MO: Mosby.)

- Cartilage
- Blood

Connective tissue consists of protein fibers distributed in an extracellular matrix. Precursor cells called **fibroblasts** produce the protein fibers found in connective tissues.

Fibroblasts also contribute to wound healing and tissue repair. Types of protein fibers are *elastin, reticulin,* and *collagen.* Elastin fibers are flexible and elastic; reticular fibers are thin, delicately woven strands. Collagen is the most abundant type, is tough and durable, and makes up approximately 25%

TABLE 18.2 Connective Tissue Types

TYPE	CHARACTERISTICS
Areolar (loose)	Most widely distributed connective tissue. Elastic glue and connects structures to each other and permits movement between them. Found largely in the hypodermis layer (superficial fascia).
Adipose (loose)	Fat cells called adipocytes and stores surplus food, insulates and conserve heat, and cushions structures.
Reticular (loose)	Supportive framework in bone marrow, lymph nodes, liver, and spleen. Traps harmful substances.
Regular (dense)	Connects muscle to bone and bone to bone. Examples are tendons, and ligaments.
Irregular (dense)	Same as regular dense tissue, but fibers are stronger and thicker and arranged irregularly. Examples are deep fascia, periosteum surrounding bone, and outer capsules of organs.
Elastic (dense)	Elastic and recoils after stretching. Found in walls of blood vessels and the bronchi.
Bone	Provides support, protection, and muscle attachment sites. Types are compact and spongy.
Cartilage	Strong and protective and capable of withstanding repeated stress. Types are hyaline, fibrocartilage, and elastic.
Blood	Transports respiratory gases, nutrients, and waste products. Includes erythrocytes, leukocytes, thrombocytes, and plasma.

of all protein in the body. Degenerative changes in collagen's molecular structure contribute to aging.

Types and amounts of protein fibers and characteristics of matrix distinguish one connective tissue type from another (Fig. 18.8). For example, cartilage contains few protein fibers and a type of matrix that traps water to form a firm gel. Bone contains fewer protein fibers in a hard mineralized matrix, so it is denser. Blood lacks protein fibers in its liquid matrix, unless a clot needs to form. Then fibroblasts help to produce fibrin strands to form and stabilize a blood clot. The ratio of fibers and matrix for ligaments and fascia is somewhere between blood and bone.

Connective tissue has a wide variety of vascularity or blood vessel supply. Some tissues, such as those found in the skin's dermis, are highly vascularized. Tendons and ligaments have few blood vessels. Cartilage has very little to no blood vessels. Vascularity influences healing rates. Injured tendons and ligaments heal very slowly. Cartilage may not heal at all.

Fibrous Connective Tissue

Fibrous connective tissue is the packing material of the body. It supports structures, attaches them to each other, fills in spaces between structures, and helps keep them in their proper places. Fibrous connective tissue has two subclasses which are loose and dense connective tissue. Loose connective tissue is divided into (1) areolar, (2) adipose, and (3) reticular. Dense connective tissue is divided into (1) regular, (2) irregular, and (3) elastic.

- **Areolar Tissue.** This is the most widely distributed connective tissue and functions like elastic glue. It connects structures to each other and permits movement between them. Along with adipose tissue, loose fibrous connective tissue forms the hypodermis layer (superficial fascia). Areolar tissue contains an enzyme called *hyaluronidase*, allowing it to change temporarily to a watery consistency when subjected to heat or mechanical pressure. This property is called *thixotropy* and is discussed in Chapter 14. Research suggest that hormones such as estrogens may play a role in fascial stiffness and sensitization (Fede et al, 2016).
- **Adipose Tissue (Body Fat).** This consists mainly of fat cells called adipocytes and serves as storage for surplus food. It also insulates the body to conserve heat and cushions structures such as the heart, kidneys, and some joints.
- **Reticular Tissue.** This resembles areolar tissue, but its matrix contains only reticular fibers. This provides the supportive framework within bone marrow, lymph nodes, liver, and spleen. Reticular fibers trap harmful substances as they travel in blood and lymph and provide defensive functions.
- **Dense *Regular* Tissue.** Connects muscle to bone (tendons, aponeurosis) and bone to bone (ligaments). Protein fibers are arranged in parallel rows and are slightly wavy, which gives them elasticity and tensile strength and the ability to resist pulling forces in one or two directions.
- **Dense *Irregular* Tissue.** This has the same structural elements as dense regular tissue, but fibers are stronger and thicker and arranged irregularly. This tissue is found in areas where tension is exerted from multiple directions. This is found in deep fascia, periosteum surrounding bone, and outer capsules of the kidneys and spleen.
- **Elastic Connective Tissue.** These are found in the walls of the blood vessels and the bronchi and recoil after being stretched by blood as the heart beats or by air during exhalation.

More about fascia – **Fascia** is sheets of connective tissue enveloping the body beneath the skin, enclosing muscle and nerve cells, and compartmentalizing muscles into muscle groups; it provides for their attachment to bone and other structures. Fascia encompasses both loose and dense connective tissues mentioned previously. Fascia helps to stabilize structures and allows tissues to slide over each other during movement. Fascia plays a unifying role within the soft tissue system. In fact, Gerlach and Lierse (1990) referred to the phenomenon as the *bone-fascia-tendon system* because it was difficult to identify where one tissue type ended and another began. Fascia is divided into two types according to its location in the body.

- **Superficial Fascia.** Located under skin, is continuous with the dermis, and is composed of loose areolar connective tissue. Superficial fascia can even contain nerve receptors, and blood vessels and skeletal muscle if they are located superficially (i.e., muscles of fascial expression).

Connective Tissue

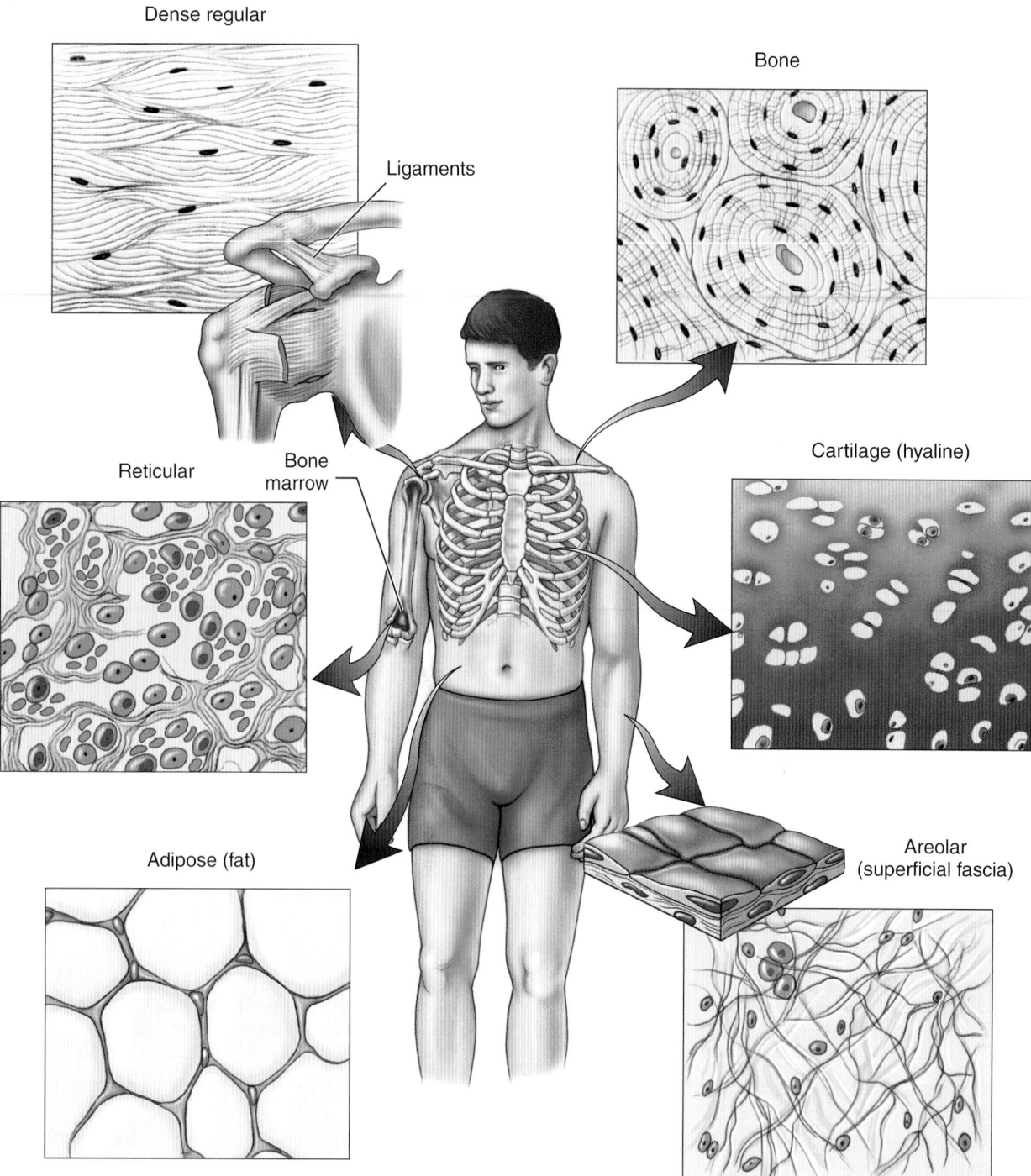

FIG. 18.8 Connective tissues: select types and locations, anterior view. (From Herlihy, B. [2011]. *The human body in health and illness* [4th ed.]. St. Louis, MO: Mosby.)

- **Deep Fascia.** Extends from superficial fascia, surrounds deeper structures, and is composed of dense irregular connective tissue. Deep fascia is tight-fitting and maintains the contour of the associated anatomic structures. Deep fascia may be given unique names that define their location (thoracolumbar fascia, plantar fascia) or their unique characteristics (fascia lata).

Bone

Bone is the hardest connective tissue. Mature bone cells called *osteocytes* become embedded in collagen and mineral salt crystals. These crystals make up more than 50% of the bone matrix, giving bone its characteristic firmness. Bones are part of the skeletal system, provide support and protection, and serve as muscle attachment sites. Bones also store minerals and fats and produce blood cells. Types of bone are *compact* and *spongy* (see Fig. 19.1). Bones are discussed in more detail in Chapter 19.

- **Compact Bone.** These form the hard outer shell of bone.
- **Spongy Bone.** Thin latticework beams inside the bone, giving it a spongy appearance.

Cartilage

Cartilage is strong and protective and capable of withstanding repeated stress and has a tough, rubbery matrix. Temporary cartilage, found in the early fetal skeleton, is later replaced by bone. Permanent cartilage retains its tough rubbery quality, except during certain disease processes and in advanced age. Cartilage is avascular (lacking blood supply), and nutrients reach the cells by diffusion from the surrounding environment—this movement is very slow. As previously mentioned, injuries to cartilage heal slowly, if at all. Cartilage can be divided into *hyaline, fibrocartilage,* and *elastic.*

- **Hyaline Cartilage.** Firm and smooth composed of cells in a translucent, pearly-blue matrix. Hyaline is the most prevalent type of cartilage; it covers the articulating surfaces of bones, connects ribs to the sternum, and is found in the nose, ears, trachea, and smaller respiratory tubes.
- **Fibrocartilage.** The strongest and most durable cartilage type and serves as shock absorbers. It is found between vertebrae (intervertebral discs) and in the knee (meniscus).
- **Elastic Cartilage.** The softest and most pliable cartilage type and gives shape to the external nose and ears. It is also found in internal structures (e.g., larynx [voice box]).

Blood

Blood is liquid connective tissue and transports respiratory gases, nutrients, and waste products. Components of blood include blood cells called *erythrocytes, leukocytes,* and *thrombocytes* and fluid called *plasma.* Plasma makes up approximately 55% of whole blood, and blood cells compose approximately 45%. See Chapter 26 for more information.

- **Erythrocytes.** Transports oxygen and carbon dioxide to and from cells.
- **Leukocytes.** The body's mobile army and serves as part of the body's defense mechanism by destroying or inactivating pathogens and foreign agents.
- **Thrombocytes.** Helps blood to clot, reducing or stopping blood loss from small breaks in vessels.
- **Plasma.** Straw-colored liquid in which blood cells are suspended.

Muscle Tissue

Muscle tissue is regarded as the movement specialist of the body. Muscle tissue can respond to a stimulus, contract or shorten, extend or stretch and lengthen, and returns to its original shape after movement. Types of muscle tissue are *skeletal, cardiac, and smooth* (Fig. 18.9). Their names often suggest their locations (Table 18.3).

- **Skeletal Muscle.** Attaches to skeletal bones and is the most abundant muscle tissue type. Skeletal muscle cells, or muscle fibers, are long, cylindrical, and threadlike. Muscle cells

contain many small, elongated nuclei located peripherally. They also contain dark and light bands, giving them a striated or striped appearance when viewed microscopically. Skeletal muscle is under voluntary control, meaning their movement can be consciously willed. Skeletal muscles are featured in Chapters 20 and 21.

- **Cardiac Muscle.** Located in the heart wall and helps the heart to contract repeatedly to pump blood. Cardiac muscle is involuntary. Like skeletal muscle, cardiac muscle contains striations or stripes. Cardiac muscle cells are Y or H shaped. These shapes allow cells to fit together like clasped fingers and create the heart's spherical shape. Between these cells are intercalated discs which assist in nerve transmission so heart contractions are synchronized. Cardiac muscle cells are mononucleated but can be multinucleated, and nuclei are oval shaped and centrally located. More information on cardiac muscle can be found in Chapter 26.
- **Smooth Muscle.** Found in hollow visceral organs such as the stomach, bladder, and uterus, and within tubes such as the intestines and blood vessels. Smooth muscle is also called *visceral muscle.* Smooth muscle cells are long, narrow, and spindle shaped (pointed at both ends). They contain one oval-shaped centrally located nucleus and have a smooth appearance because they do not possess striations or stripes. Smooth muscle is primarily involuntary and cannot be controlled by will. Consuming

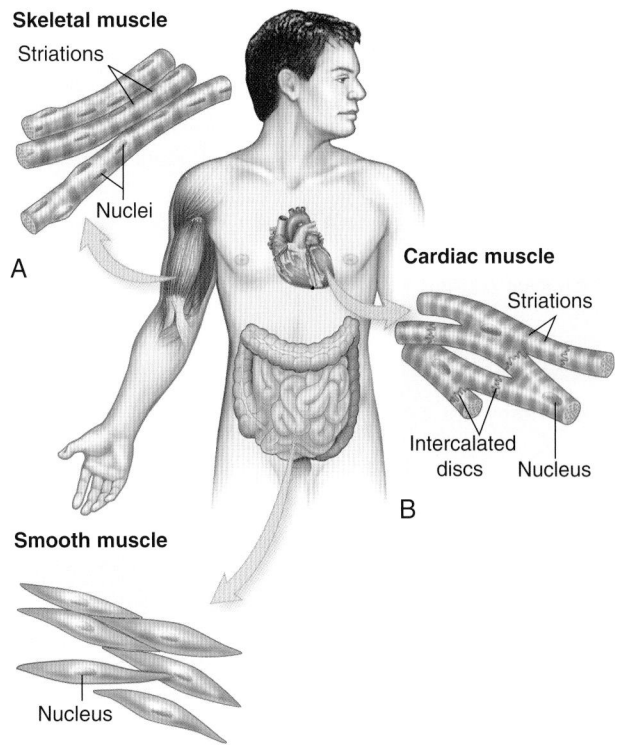

FIG. 18.9 Muscle tissue: types and locations which include (A) skeletal muscle, (B) cardiac muscle, and (C) smooth muscle (anterior view). (From Patton, K., & Thibodeau, G. [2014]. *The human body in health and disease* [6th ed.]. St. Louis, MO: Mosby.)

TABLE 18.3 Muscle Tissue Characteristics: A Comparison			
TYPES	**SKELETAL**	**CARDIAC**	**SMOOTH**
Synonyms	Voluntary	Heart	Visceral
Striations	Yes	Yes	No
Number of nuclei	Multinucleate	Mononucleate (can be multinu-cleated)	Mononucleate
Location of nuclei	Peripherally located	Centrally located	Centrally located
Shape of nuclei	Small, elongated	Oval-shaped	Oval-shaped
Shape of cells	Long, cylindrical, and threadlike	Y- or H-shaped	Spindle-shaped
Voluntary or involuntary	Voluntary	Involuntary	Involuntary
Distinguishing characteristics	Striped and multinucleated	Intercalated discs	Shape of cells
Discussion	Attaches to bones and most abundant muscle tissue type	In the heart wall and helps heart to contract repeatedly to pump blood	In hollow visceral organs or tubes, such as stomach, bladder, and uterus, and in tubes such as intestines and blood vessels

little energy, these cells are adapted for long, sustained contractions.

Nervous Tissue

Nervous tissue is in the brain and spinal cord and within nerves. Nerve cells, or *neurons,* transmit nerve impulses. As mentioned previously, nervous tissue detects sensory input, provides interpretative functions, coordinates motor output, and facilitates higher mental functioning and emotional responsiveness. Nerve tissue also secretes chemical messengers called *neurotransmitters,* which assist impulse conduction. Nervous tissue is discussed in more detail in Chapter 23. Nerve cells have three principal parts (Fig. 18.10).

- **Dendrites**. Transmit impulses to the cell body.
- **Cell Body**. Contains the nucleus and other organelles.
- **Axon**. Transmits impulses away from the cell body. Nerve cells can possess several axonal extensions. Some axons are surrounded by a myelin sheath, a white fatty material that insulates axons and prevents impulse "leakage" to adjacent neurons.

MEMBRANES

Membranes are thin, soft, pliable sheets of tissue that cover the body, line body cavities, and cover organs within body cavities. Membranes help protect internal and external surfaces and anchor structures to each other. Most membranes also secrete lubricating fluids. Some membranes are named by their predominant tissue type (e.g., epithelial and connective tissue membranes). Some membranes are named by the substances they secrete (e.g., mucous, serous, synovial).

Epithelial Membranes

Epithelial membranes are composed of epithelial tissue and the connective tissue to which it attaches. Types of epithelial membranes are *cutaneous, mucous, and serous membranes.*

- **Cutaneous Membranes.** Cover external body surfaces and includes the skin. Skin is both tough and supple and contains

numerous oil and sweat glands. The integumentary system, which includes the skin, is discussed in Chapter 22.

- **Mucous Membranes.** Line body cavities that open to the outside. Examples of mucous membranes are linings of the digestive, respiratory, urinary, and reproductive tracts. Mucous membranes, or *mucosae,* secrete a viscous fluid called *mucus,* which coats, lubricates, and protects associated structures.
- **Serous Membranes.** Line closed body cavities that do not open directly to the outside and cover organs inside those cavities. Serous membranes consist of two layers—a parietal layer and a visceral layer. The *parietal layer* covers the walls of body cavities like wallpaper and often adheres to it. The *visceral layer* covers the visceral organs within the body cavity. Serous membranes secrete thin, watery *serous fluid,* which is found between the parietal and visceral layers. Serous fluid lubricates the membrane and reduces friction when organs in the thoracic or abdominopelvic cavity move against each other or the cavity wall. Serous membranes are named by their location. For example, serous membranes are the pericardium, which surrounds the heart; the pleura, which surrounds the lungs; and the peritoneum, which surrounds the organs in the abdominopelvic cavity.

Connective Tissue Membranes

Connective tissue membranes are composed solely of connective tissues. Types of connective tissue membranes are *synovial and meningeal membranes* (Fig. 18.11). Like serous membranes, connective tissue membranes line cavities that do not open to the outside.

- **Synovial Membranes.** Lines cavities of freely movable joints such as the shoulder, hip, elbow, and knee. These membranes secrete a thick, clear fluid into the joint cavity called *synovial fluid* or *synovium.* Synovial fluid provides nutrition and lubrication of the articular cartilage so they can move freely without friction. Synovial membranes also line flattened saclike structures called *bursae.* Bursae are found near select joints. See Chapter 19 for more information.

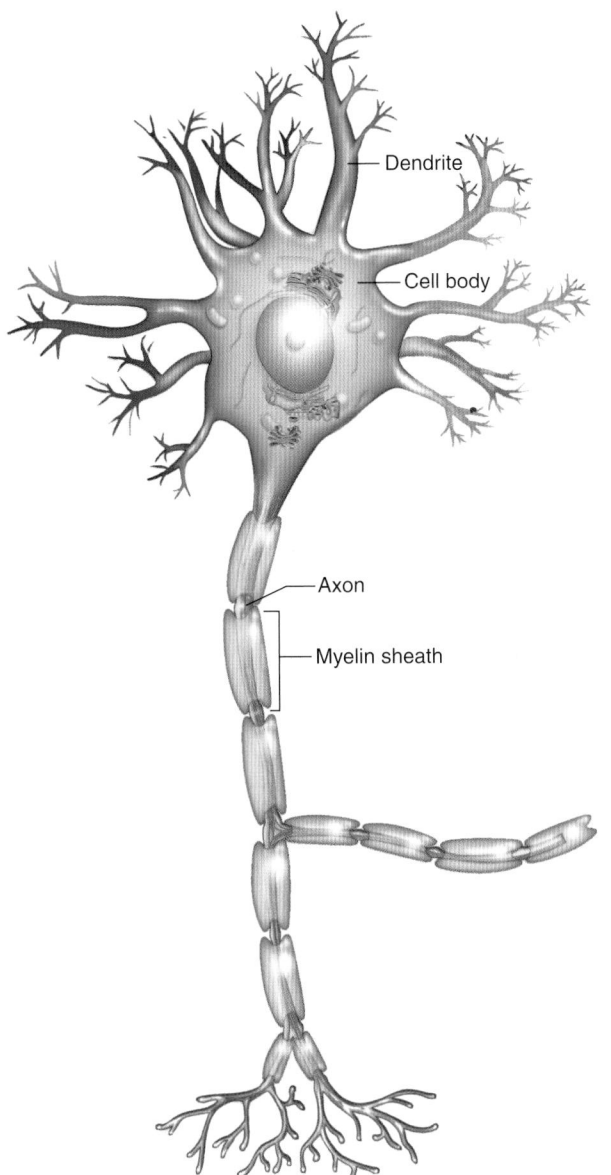

FIG. 18.10 Nerve tissue is composed of nerve cells. Nerve cells have three principal parts: a cell body, which contains the nucleus and other organelles; dendrites, and an axon. Some axons are surrounded by a myelin sheath. (From Patton, K., & Thibodeau, G. [2014]. *The human body in health and disease* [6th ed.]. St. Louis, MO: Mosby.)

- **Meningeal Membranes.** Lines spaces within the dorsal cavity, which contain the brain and spinal cord. Meningeal membranes, or *meninges*, provide protection for these vital structures. Cerebrospinal fluid fills the spaces between the inner and middle meningeal layers; serous fluid fills the spaces between the middle and the outer meningeal layers (see Fig. 23.6).

A mind, once stretched by a new idea, never regains its original dimension.

—**Oliver Wendell Holmes**

BODY COMPASS: ANATOMIC POSITION, PLANES, DIRECTIONAL TERMS, BODY CAVITIES, AND BODY REGIONS

The body compass is the tool used to locate or describe directions, positions, and locations of body structures. Every good map has a compass indicating north, south, east, and west. The map also has references, such as scales to indicate distance (e.g., miles) or grids to indicate location. Without references, maps would be of little or no use. Imagine trying to read a map if you cannot understand terms or phrases such as *south, 5 miles, 1 block,* or *by the lake.* The body compass helps students to navigate the body including planes, quadrants, cavities, and regions.

Anatomic Position

When describing locations of body structures, a standard posture known as the **anatomic position** is used (Fig. 18.12). In this position, the body is standing upright and facing forward, the arms are at the sides, palms are facing forward with the thumbs to the side, and feet are hip-distance apart with toes pointing forward.

Body Planes

Planes are transparent flat surfaces dividing the body into three dimensions of left/right, front/back, and top/bottom. Planes lie at right angles and provide references for height, depth, and width (Fig. 18.13). The three cardinal planes are *sagittal, frontal,* and *transverse.* Movements take place in planes and are discussed in Chapter 19.

Sagittal Plane

The **sagittal plane** bisects or cuts the body front to back and divides it into right and left sections. The **midsagittal plane,** or *median plane,* is used to describe the sagittal plane that runs through the midline marked by the navel, dividing it into equal right and left halves. Sagittal planes run parallel to the left and to the right of the midsagittal plane. Forward and backward movements occur in the sagittal plane.

Frontal Plane

The **frontal plane,** or *coronal plane,* bisects the body side to side and divides it into front (anterior) and back (posterior) sections. Side-to-side movement occurs in the frontal plane.

Transverse Plane

The **transverse plane,** or *horizontal plane,* bisects the body horizontally and divides the body into top (superior) and bottom (inferior) sections. Twisting or rotational movements occur in the transverse plane.

Directional Terms

Directional terms describe location and direction of particular body structures when the person is standing in the anatomic position (Fig. 18.14).

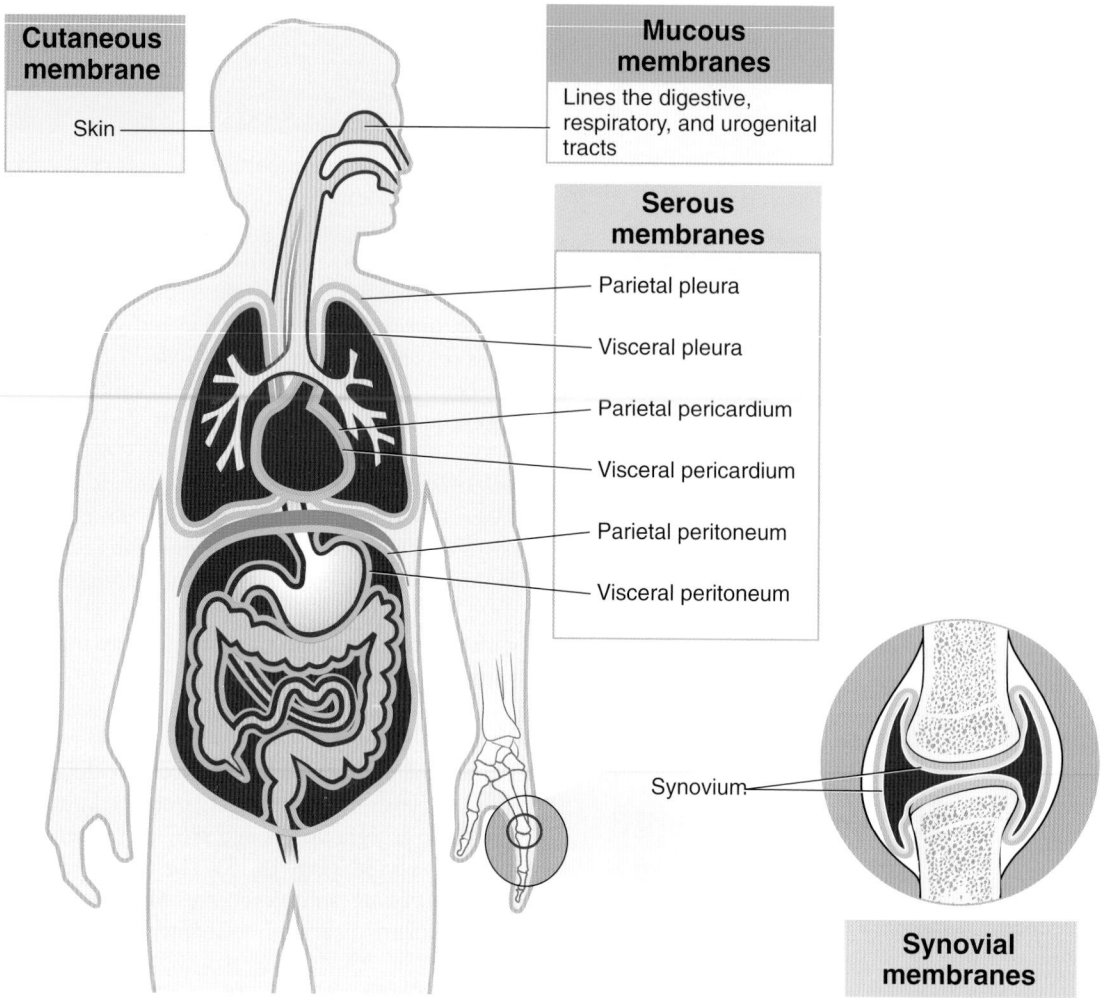

FIG. 18.11 Membranes: types and locations, anterior view. Meningeal membranes are not featured.

Left
To the left of the body or a structure—the subject's left, not your left. *Example: The heart is primarily on the left side of the body.*

Right
To the right of the body or a structure—the subject's right, not your right. *Example: The liver is primarily on the right side of the body.*

Superior
Situated above or toward the head end. *Example: The jaw is superior to the neck.*

Inferior
Situated below or toward the tail end. *Example: The sacrum is inferior to the skull.*

Anterior
On the front side of a structure. Anterior is also known as ventral. *Example: The heart is anterior to the vertebral column.*

Posterior
On the back of a structure. Posterior is also known as dorsal. *Example: The vertebral column is posterior to the sternum.*

Medial
Oriented toward or near the midline of the body. *Example: The nose is medial to the ears.*

Lateral
Oriented farther away from the midline of the body. *Example: The ribs are lateral to the vertebral column.*
   NOTE: Medial and lateral refers to centrally located areas, such as the trunk.

Ipsilateral (Homolateral)
Related to the same side of the body. *Example: The right hand is ipsilateral to the right elbow.*

Contralateral
Related to opposite sides of the body. *Example: The right foot is contralateral to the left foot.*

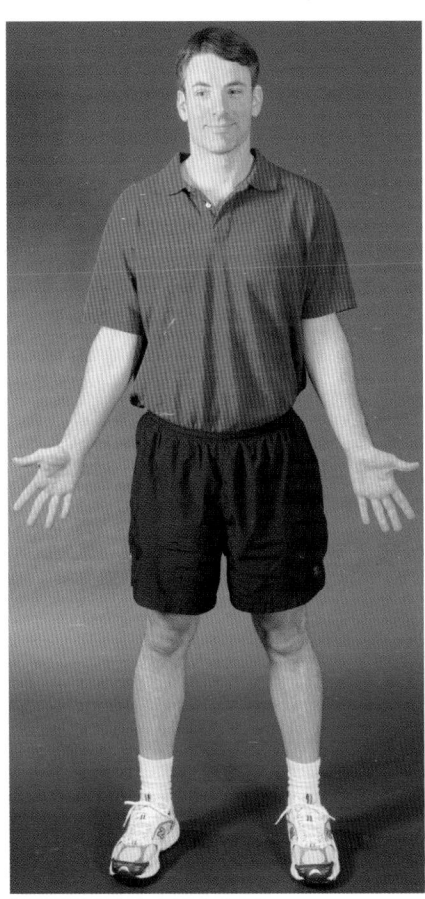

FIG. 18.12 Anatomic position is used when describing the locations of body structures (anterior view).

Proximal

Nearer to the point of reference, usually toward the trunk of the body. *Example: The hip is proximal to the knee.*

Distal

Farther from the point of reference, usually away from the trunk of the body. *Example: The foot is distal to the knee.*

NOTE: Proximal and distal refer mainly to structures in the upper and lower extremities.

Superficial

Relative to the outside or external surface of a structure. *Example: The skin is superficial to the muscles.*

Deep

Relative to or situated within the body. *Example: The heart is deep to the skin.*

Body Cavities

A **body cavity** is a hollow space and often contains organs and other structures and is often filled with fluid. The two main body cavities are the *dorsal cavity* and the *ventral cavity* (Fig. 18.15).

Dorsal Cavity

The **dorsal cavity** is on the backside or posterior aspect of the body. The dorsal cavity is further divided into the *cranial* and *spinal cavity.*

- **Cranial Cavity.** In the skull and contains the brain.
- **Spinal (Vertebral) Cavity.** In the vertebrae of the spinal column and contains the spinal cord.

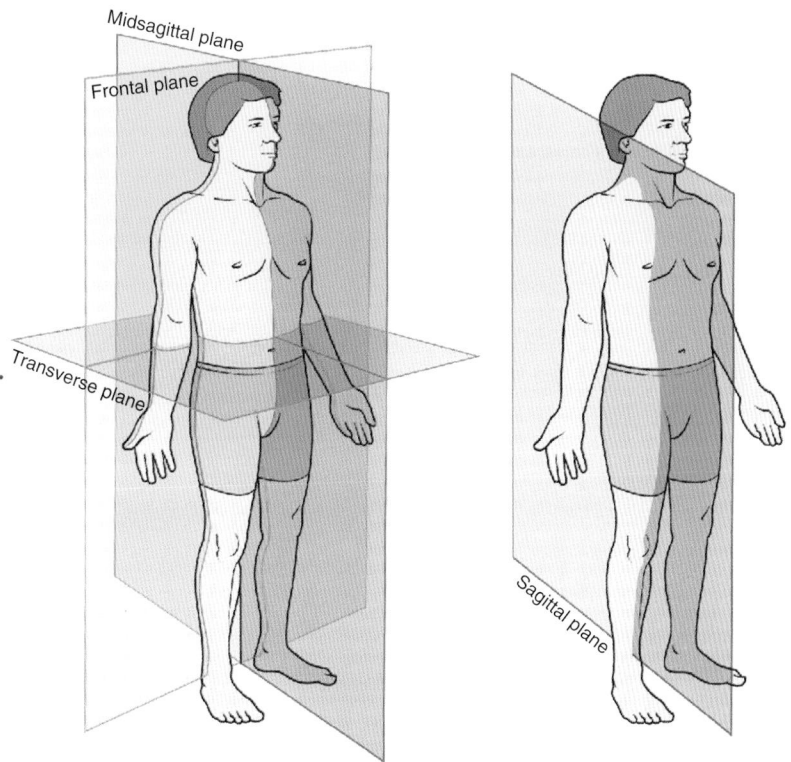

FIG. 18.13 Planes of the body, anterior view *(left image).* Sagittal planes run parallel to the left or to the right of the midsagittal plane *(right image).*

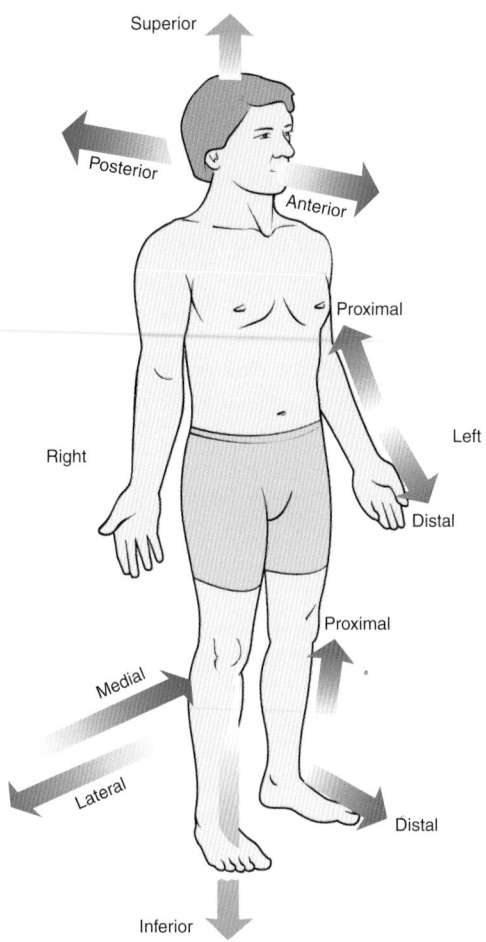

FIG. 18.14 Directional terms, anterior view.

Ventral Cavity

The larger **ventral cavity** is on the front side or anterior aspect of the body. The ventral cavity is divided by the diaphragm into the *thoracic* and *abdominopelvic cavity.*

- **Thoracic Cavity.** Contains the *pleural cavities,* which surround the lungs, and the *mediastinum,* which is the space between the lungs. The mediastinum houses the *pericardial cavity*, which contains the heart and great vessels (aorta, superior and inferior venae cavae), esophagus, and trachea.
- **Abdominopelvic Cavity.** Contains the abdominal and pelvic cavities. The *abdominal cavity* contains the digestive organs. The *pelvic cavity* contains the reproductive and some urinary organs.

Abdominal Quadrants and Regions

There are several ways to divide the abdomen into sections. One way uses four sections or quadrants. The other way uses nine regions (Fig. 18.16). Both assist in locating abdominal organs or signs and symptoms related to illness or disease. As a reminder, left and right refer to left and right of the body being viewed, not left and right of the viewer.

Abdominal Quadrants

To divide the abdomen into quadrants, one line is drawn horizontally and another one is drawn vertically, intersecting at the umbilicus. From right to left and from top to bottom, they are the (1) right upper quadrant, (2) left upper quadrant, (3) right lower quadrant, and (4) left lower quadrant.

Abdominal Regions

To divide the abdomen into nine regions, two horizontal lines and two vertical lines are used to create a tic-tac-toe–like design. From right to left and from top to bottom, they are the

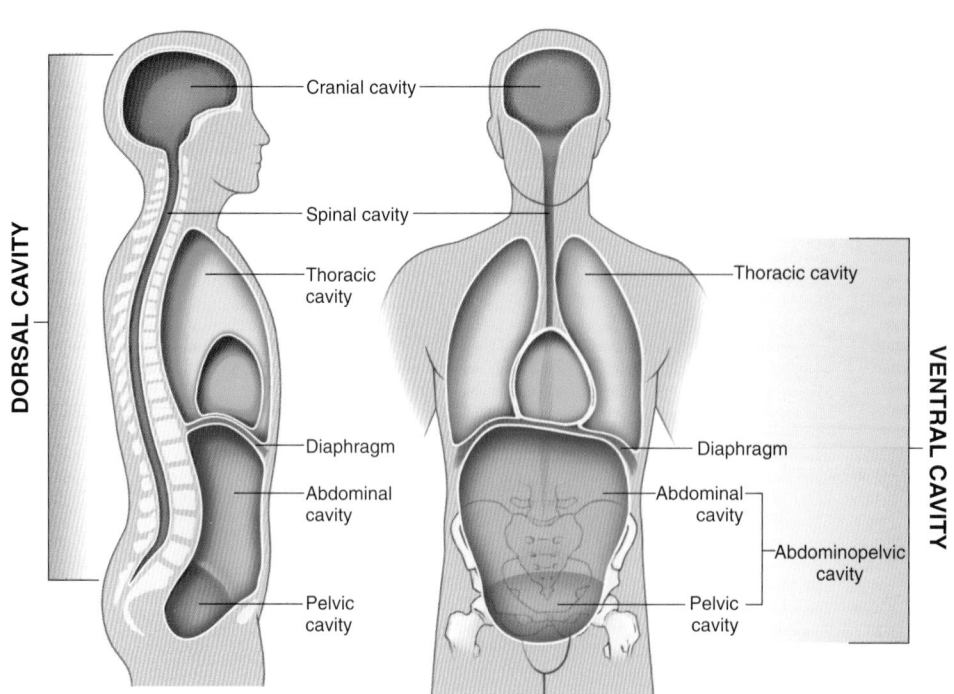

FIG. 18.15 Body cavities: types and locations viewed laterally *(left image)* and anteriorly *(right image).*

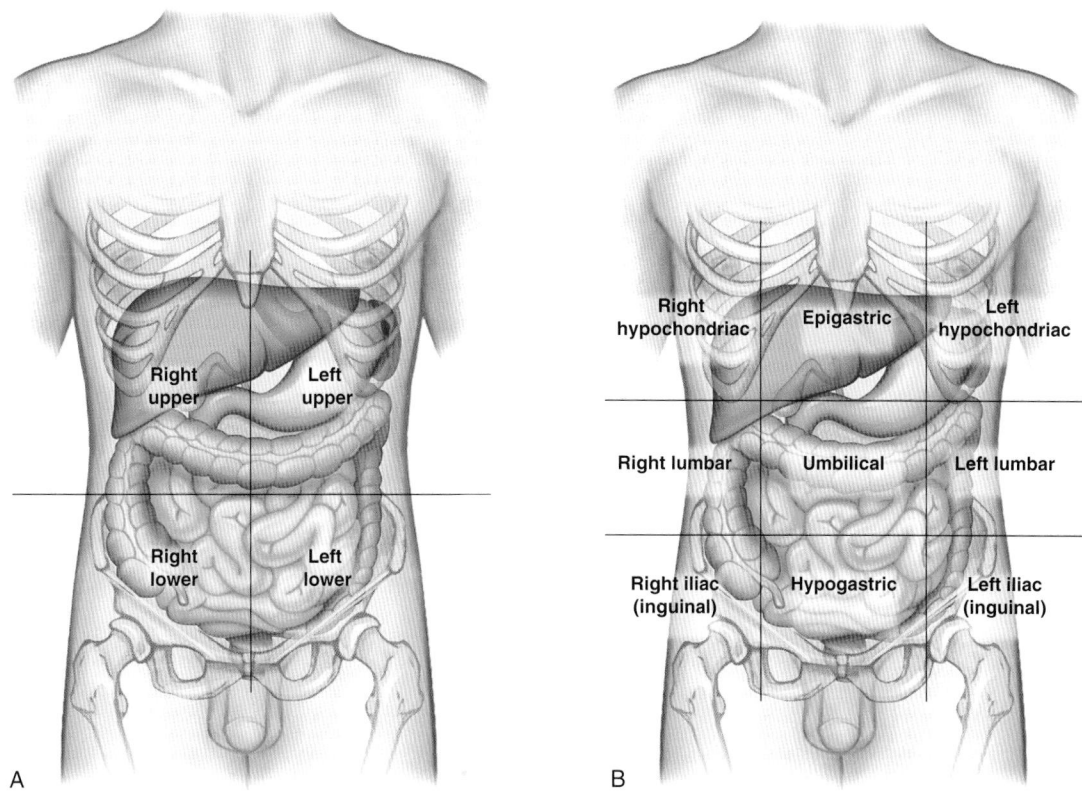

FIG. 18.16 Abdominal quadrants (A) and regions (B), anterior views. (From Patton, K., & Thibodeau, G. [2014]. *The human body in health and disease* [6th ed.]. St. Louis, MO: Mosby.)

(1) right hypochondriac region, (2) epigastric region, (3) left hypochondriac region, (4) right lumbar region, (5) umbilical region, (6) left lumbar region, (7) right iliac or inguinal region, (8) hypogastric region, and the (9) left iliac or inguinal region.

Body Regions

The body can be divided into the axial region and the appendicular regions of the upper and lower extremities (Fig. 18.17). These are presented next.

Axial Region

The axial region contains the head, neck, and torso or trunk.

1. **Cephalic:** Head
2. **Cranial:** Upper skull
3. **Temporal:** Side of skull
4. **Facial:** Face
5. **Frontal:** Forehead
6. **Orbital:** Eye; *ophthalmic* means "pertaining to the eye"
7. **Zygomatic:** Upper cheek
8. **Nasal:** Nose
9. **Buccal:** Cheek wall within the mouth
10. **Oral:** Mouth
11. **Otic:** Ear; *auricular* means "pertaining to the ear"
12. **Mandibular:** Lower jaw
13. **Occipital:** Lower back skull
14. **Cervical:** Neck; *nuchal* means "pertaining to the nape or back of the neck"
15. **Thoracic:** Chest, area between the neck and diaphragm
16. **Abdominal:** Abdomen; superior region of the abdominopelvic cavity
17. **Pelvic:** Pelvis; inferior region of the abdominopelvic cavity
18. **Pectoral:** Breast area or upper anterior thorax; *mammary* means "pertaining to the breast"
19. **Sternal:** Middle of the chest; breastbone
20. **Costal:** Ribs
21. **Umbilical:** Navel or central abdomen; pertaining to the umbilical cord
22. **Vertebral:** Spinal column
23. **Sacral:** Sacrum of the spinal column
24. **Coccygeal:** Bottom of the spinal column or coccyx area; upper region of the gluteal cleft
25. **Lumbar:** Lower back or loin area between the ribs and hips; *flank* means "pertaining to the side region(s) of the lumbar area"
26. **Gluteal:** Buttocks formed by the gluteal muscles
27. **Sacroiliac:** Between the sacrum and pelvic bones
28. **Perineal:** Between the anus and the genitals

Upper Extremity

The upper extremity, or upper limb, contains the arms, forearms, hands, and connections to the axial regions via the shoulders.

1. **Clavicular:** Collar bone
2. **Acromial:** Top of shoulder
3. **Scapular:** Shoulder blade

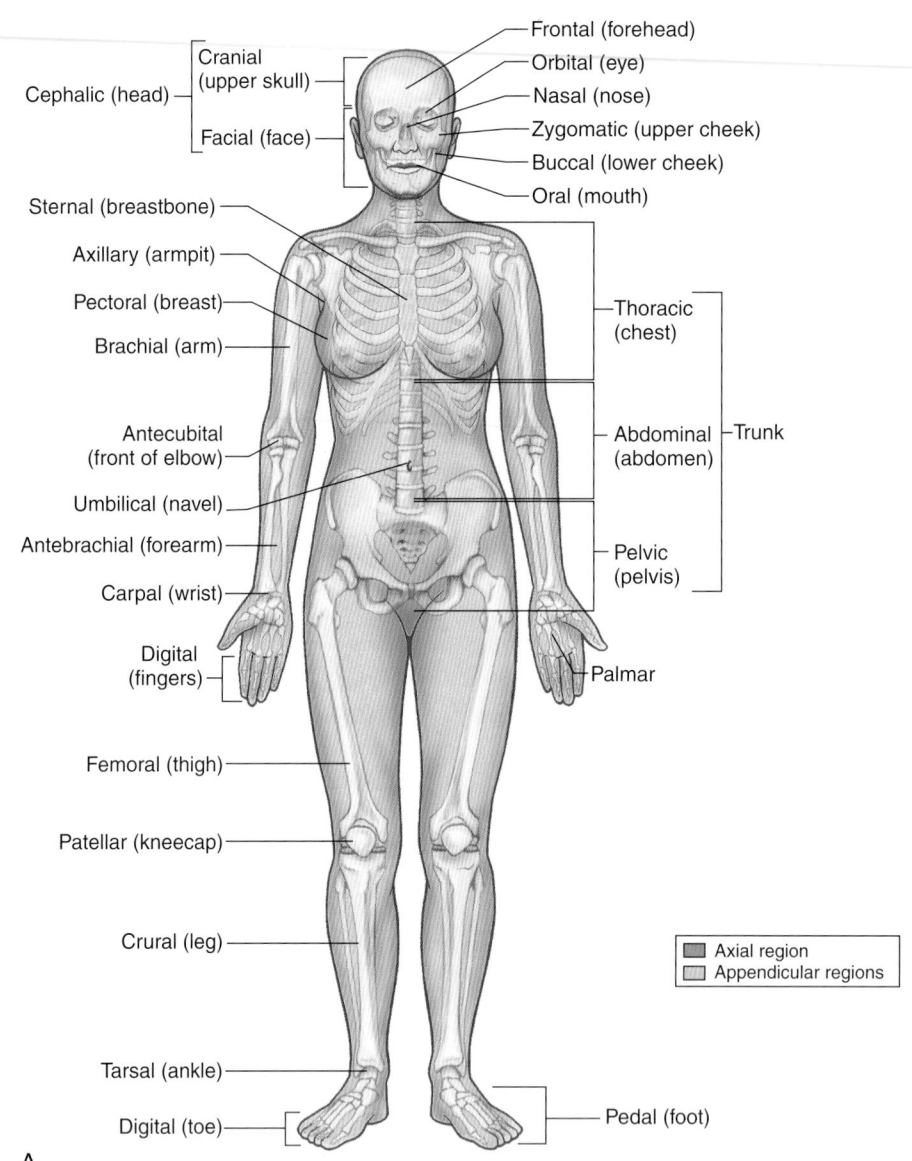

Frontal (forehead)
Orbital (eye)
Nasal (nose)
Zygomatic (upper cheek)
Buccal (lower cheek)
Oral (mouth)

Cranial (upper skull)
Cephalic (head)
Facial (face)

Sternal (breastbone)
Axillary (armpit)
Pectoral (breast)
Brachial (arm)

Antecubital (front of elbow)
Umbilical (navel)
Antebrachial (forearm)
Carpal (wrist)

Digital (fingers)

Femoral (thigh)

Patellar (kneecap)

Crural (leg)

Tarsal (ankle)
Digital (toe)

Thoracic (chest)

Abdominal (abdomen)   Trunk

Pelvic (pelvis)

Palmar

Axial region
Appendicular regions

Pedal (foot)

A

FIG. 18.17 Body regional terms in the axial and appendicular skeleton. (A) Anterior view.

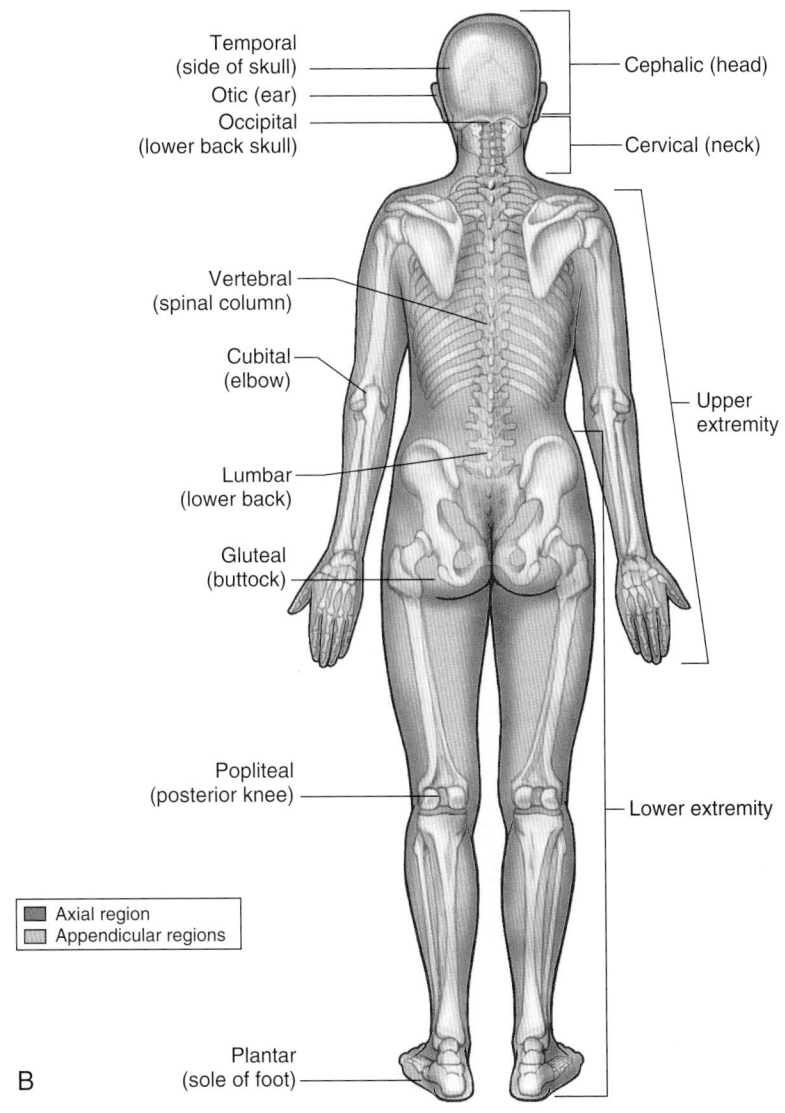

FIG. 18.17—CONT'D (B) Posterior view. (From Patton, K., & Thibodeau, G. [2014]. *The human body in health and disease* [6th ed.]. St. Louis, MO: Mosby.)

4. **Deltoid:** Curve of the shoulder formed by the deltoid muscle
5. **Axillary:** Armpit
6. **Brachial:** Arm; between the shoulder and elbow
7. **Antebrachial:** Forearm; between the wrist and elbow
8. **Cubital:** Elbow
9. **Antecubital:** Front of the elbow; bend of the elbow
10. **Carpal:** Wrist
11. **Palmar:** Anterior surface or palm of the hand; *volar* means "pertaining to the palm"
12. **Dorsum:** Posterior surface of the hand
13. **Pollex:** Thumb
14. **Digital:** Fingers or toes; *phalangeal* means "pertaining to the finger or toes"

Lower Extremity

The lower extremity, or lower limb, contains the thighs, legs, and feet and connections to the axial regions via the hips.

1. **Coxal:** Hip
2. **Pubic:** Genital area over the pubic symphysis
3. **Groin:** Area between thigh and abdomen; *inguinal* means "pertaining to the groin"
4. **Femoral:** Thigh; between the hip and knee
5. **Patellar:** Kneecap
6. **Popliteal:** Posterior knee
7. **Crural:** Leg; between the knee and ankle
8. **Calf:** Posterior leg; *sural* means "pertaining to the calf"
9. **Tarsal:** Ankle
10. **Pedal:** Foot or feet

DEANE JUHAN

Deane Juhan is a bodyworker, one of the first Trager-trained instructors, an anatomy teacher and lecturer for the Trager Institute, and author of *Job's Body: A Handbook for Bodyworkers*. As the title suggests, the book offers an answer to the age-old question of "why?" regarding the Old Testament book of Job... but that is just for starters. The book explores "the various ways through which intuitive and informed touch can positively affect a wide variety of symptoms and help to change people's lives for the better." The book was 9 years in the making, which is surprising, considering the manner in which Juhan's words easily flow during casual conversation.

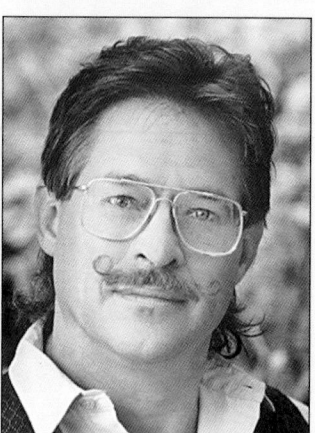

Copyright © Karen Kurlinden Photography.

Born to a woman who had poor taste in men and a soldier who did not hang around to become a father, Juhan was later adopted, growing up as an only child in Glenwood Springs, Colorado. His father worked for the state and never drew a large salary, but his parents were wise about using resources and were determined their only child's education would receive top priority in their lives.

Juhan describes himself as an underachiever in high school. The University of Colorado introduced him to a whole new way of living, and he admits to being caught up in the novelty of its hip, liberal atmosphere until his junior year, when "his rudder finally bit the water," he says. At this point in his life, he became interested in the aspects of art, science, and civilization.

Juhan learned about Esalen, a workshop and meeting place for developing human potential in Big Sur, California, while working on his dissertation in literature. He actually managed to sneak in and start doing massage. He was so good at it. Juhan's first experience in anatomy was developing slides and lectures for *Structural Integration* for *Rolfing* lectures, but when he witnessed Milton Trager, he was hooked and abandoned all other methods to learn the Trager Approach.

"It was love at first sight," says Juhan. "I was attracted to his quality of being. It was his rich avuncular benevolence without all the preliminary folderol made me want to learn to do what he did, so I threw myself into it and gave it my all."

The goal in a Trager session is to connect with the client's sensory information, process what the practitioner helps the client discover or rediscover, then help the client wake up to the possibility for long-term change through movement. The practitioner lays down new patterns by repeating a movement message again and again. The feeling finally becomes etched on the client's awareness, creating an experience of length, relaxation, and pain-free movement.

Juhan reminds us the only thing we truly know about the world is the way the body responds to it, and no one can know how our bodies are responding to stimuli the way we each individually can. In short, we are, to a very great degree, responsible for our own wellbeing.

Juhan writes in *Job's Body: A Handbook for Bodyworkers*, "For Job this was revelation—the perception that God was in his very flesh, in the throbbing of his heart, in the singing of his nerves, in the coiling of his muscles, to be touched and felt more intimately than an embrace."

As a beginning massage practitioner, you are probably not seeking a revelation so much as you are a direction. You can probably guess Juhan's advice is to look within. Choose the modality that will, according to Juhan, "flower in your psyche or experience. Look for what turns you on, look for what you love, not what the market says is hot."

11. **Calcaneal:** Heel
12. **Dorsum:** Top of foot
13. **Plantar:** Bottom or sole of foot; *volar* means "pertaining to the sole of the foot"
14. **Hallux:** Large or big toe
15. **Digital:** Toes or fingers; *phalangeal* means "pertaining to the toes or fingers"

E-RESOURCES

http://evolve.elsevier.com/Salvo/MassageTherapy

- Chapter challenge
- Flash cards

BIBLIOGRAPHY

Abrahams, P. H., Spratt, J. D., Loukas, M., & van Schoor, A. N. (2003). *Abrahams' and McMinn's clinical atlas of human anatomy* (8th ed.). St Louis: Elsevier.

Applegate, E. (2010). *The anatomy and physiology learning system* (4th ed.). Philadelphia: Saunders.

Como, D. (Ed.). (2016). *Mosby's dictionary of medicine, nursing, and health professions* (10th ed.). St Louis: Elsevier.

Fede, C., Albertin, G., Petrelli, L., Sfriso, M., Biz, C., De Caro, R., Stecco, C. (2016). Hormone receptor expression in human fascial tissue. *European Journal of Histochemistry, 60*(4), 2710.

Frazier, M. S., & Drzymkowski, J. W. (2015). *Essentials of human diseases and conditions* (6th ed.). St Louis: Elsevier.

Gerlach, U. J., & Lierse, W. (1990). Functional construction of the superficial and deep fascia system of the lower limb in man. *Acta Anatomica (Basel), 139*(1), 11–25.

Haubrich, W. S. (2003). *Medical meanings: a glossary of word origins* (2nd ed.). New York: American College of Physicians.

Herlihy, B. (2017). *The human body in health and illness* (6th ed.). St Louis: Saunders.

Hubert, R. J., & VanMeter, K. C. (2018). *Gould's pathophysiology for the health professions* (6th ed.). Philadelphia: Saunders.

Huether, S. E., McCance, K. L., & Brashers, V. L. (2019). *Understanding pathophysiology* (7th ed.). St Louis: Mosby.

Kalat, J. W. (2013). *Biological psychology* (11th ed.). Belmont, Calif: Cengage Learning.

Kapit, W., & Elson, L. M. (2013). *The anatomy coloring book* (4th ed.). New York: Benjamin Cummings.

Kumar, V., Abbas, A. K., & Aster, J. C. (2015). *Robbins & Cotran pathologic basis of disease* (9th ed.). St Louis: Mosby.

Lauderstein, D. (2012). *The deep massage book: How to combine structure and energy in bodywork*. Taos: Redwing Book Company.

Marieb, E. N., & Keller, S. M. (2018). *Essentials of human anatomy and physiology* (12th ed.). New York: Benjamin Cummings.

McCance, K. L., & Huether, S. E. (2019). *Pathophysiology: The biological basis for disease in adults and children* (8th ed.). St Louis: Mosby.

Myers, T. W. (2014). *Anatomy trains: Myofascial meridians for manual and movement therapists* (3rd ed.). Churchill Livingstone: Elsevier.

Netter, F. H. (2018). *Atlas of human anatomy* (7th ed.). St Louis: Mosby.

Patton, K. T. (2019). *Anatomy and physiology* (10th ed.). St Louis: Elsevier.

Patton, K. T., Thibodeau, G. A., & Douglas, M. M. (2012). *Essentials of anatomy and physiology* (4th ed.). New York: Pearson.

REVIEW AND APPLY YOUR KNOWLEDGE

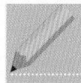

MATCHING ONE: CONCEPT REVIEW

Place the letter of the answer next to the number of the term or phrase that best describes it.

A. Adipose
B. Anatomy
C. Cytoplasm
D. Fibrocartilage
E. Diffusion
F. Epithelium
G. Hyaline
H. Mitochondria
I. Interstitial
J. Nervous
K. Nucleus
L. Pathology

_____ 1. Cell's "control center" because it directs most metabolic activities, including growth and reproduction.

_____ 2. Connective tissue type serving as storage for surplus food and insulation to conserve body heat.

_____ 3. Cell's "power plant" because it creates adenosine triphosphate (ATP), the cell's energy molecule.

_____ 4. Study of disease.

_____ 5. Connective tissue found between vertebrae and in the knee.

_____ 6. Tissue covering external and internal body structures and provides protection, absorption, secretion, excretion, and sensation.

_____ 7. Gel-like intracellular fluid.

_____ 8. Study of body structures and their positional relationships to one another.

_____ 9. Fluid found in the extracellular spaces between the tissues.

_____ 10. Connective tissue covering the articulating surfaces of bone.

_____ 11. Tissue that detects sensory input, provides interpretative functions, and coordinates motor output.

_____ 12. Movement of molecules from an area of high concentration to an area of low concentration to equalize concentrations.

MATCHING TWO: CONCEPT REVIEW

Place the letter of the answer next to the number of the term or phrase that best describes it.

A. Anatomic position
B. Allostasis
C. Costal
D. Serous
E. Frontal
F. Homeostasis
G. Contralateral
H. Popliteal
I. Proximal
J. Synovial
K. Antebrachial
L. Ventral

_____ 1. Membrane that lines closed body cavities and covers organs inside those cavities.

_____ 2. Plane bisecting the body side to side and dividing it into anterior and posterior sections.

_____ 3. Membrane lining cavities of freely movable joints such as the shoulder, hip, elbow, and knee.

_____ 4. Body cavity containing thoracic and abdominopelvic subdivisions.

_____ 5. Term synonymous with ribs.

_____ 6. Term synonymous with posterior knee.

_____ 7. Standard posture used when describing locations of body structures.

_____ 8. The process of achieving homeostasis through physiologic and behavioral changes.

_____ 9. Term synonymous with forearm.

_____ 10. Directional term meaning nearer to the point of reference, usually toward the trunk of the body.

_____ 11. Directional term meaning the opposite side of the body.

_____ 12. Maintenance of a constant and stable internal environment within a narrow range despite changes that occur in the external environment.

MULTIPLE CHOICE: TEST YOUR KNOWLEDGE

Place the letter of the answer next to the number of the term or phrase that best describes it.

_____ 1. The highest and most complex organizational level is the:
    A. cellular.
    B. organ.
    C. organism.
    D. chemical.

_____ 2. Which term describes the outer region of an organ?
    A. Inferior
    B. Medulla
    C. Lateral
    D. Cortex

_____ 3. The organelles that assist cell division by organizing chromosomes are the:
    A. Mitochondria.
    B. Centrioles.
    C. Nuclei.
    D. Lysosomes.

_____ 4. The movement of water across a cell membrane from an area of low concentration to high concentration to equalize concentration on both sides of the membrane is:
    A. filtration.
    B. osmosis.
    C. diffusion.
    D. pressure.

_____ 5. What is the process of moving substances outside the cell?
    A. Endocytosis
    B. Phagocytosis
    C. Pinocytosis
    D. Exocytosis

_____ 6. The internal lining of the heart and blood vessels are made of which a type of tissue?
    A. Epithelial
    B. Connective
    C. Muscular
    D. Nervous

_____ 7. Smooth muscle fibers are shaped like a:
    A. cylinder.
    B. rectangle.
    C. spindle.
    D. square.

_____ 8. Which describes the anatomic position?
    A. Palms to the side with thumbs facing forward
    B. Palms facing forward with thumbs to the side
    C. Palms facing backward with thumbs drawn in
    D. Palms to the side with thumbs drawn in

_____ 9. Which plane bisects the body into equal right and left halves?
    A. Frontal
    B. Transverse
    C. Coronal
    D. Midsagittal

_____ 10. Which is found in the axial region?
    A. Axillary
    B. Clavicular
    C. Mandibular
    D. Cubital

_____ 11. Which term refers to space within a hollow tube?
    A. Cortex
    B. Medial
    C. Lumen
    D. Distal

_____ 12. Which term means leg or between the knee and the ankle?
    A. Popliteal
    B. Plantar
    C. Carpal
    D. Crural

CRITICAL THINKING

What Is All This Nonsense?

You have a classmate who is overwhelmed by all the new terms in anatomy and physiology. He does not understand how to break down the words and says they all just seem like a jumble of letters. How can you help your classmate understand and learn the information needed in massage education?

Answers may include but are not limited to:

Many scientific and medical terms possess one or more parts: a *root, a prefix,* and a *suffix.* Once you have become familiar with parts of words, it will be easier to determine the meaning of terms you will encounter during your studies.

A root is the main part of a word, or its foundation. Some words combine two roots, such as *cardi-,* Greek for "heart," and *vascular,* Latin for "vessel." A vowel is often used to combine two roots to aid in pronunciation. The most common combining vowel is the letter *o.* When combining *cardi-* and *vascular,* the new word is *cardi-o-vascular* or *cardiovascular.*

A prefix is placed before a root word to alter its meaning. For example, *pre-* is a prefix meaning "before" or "front." Add *pre-* before the root *cancer* and it becomes *precancerous,* denoting a stage of disease that may lead to cancer, but cancer has not yet developed.

A suffix is placed after a root word to alter its meaning. For example, *-ectomy* is a suffix meaning "to cut out," as in surgery. Add *-ectomy* behind the word *appendix,* and the new term is *appendectomy,* or surgical removal of the appendix.

Learning medical terms can be daunting initially, but with time and practice, you will reap many rewards, including better marks on examinations. You will soon discover medical terminology makes sense and is easy to understand once you are familiar with the basics.

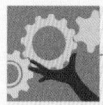

PROFESSIONAL PRACTICE

The Knee Bone Is Connected to the Thigh Bone...

Callista has just graduated from massage school and has started working at a local massage franchise. Her first client this morning is a chiropractor, who tells her his left sacroiliac joint is painful, leading to ipsilateral tightness in the muscles of his gluteal, femoral, popliteal, and calf regions. This has led to contralateral compensation in the muscles of his right vertebral, costal, and pectoral regions, and he is experiencing some tightness there as well. What areas of the body is the chiropractor describing? How should Callista focus on these areas during the treatment?

DISCUSSION

Childhood Cancer

Neuroblastoma is one of the most common cancers in children. Research what type of cancer this is, how it develops, how it is treated, and what massage considerations apply. If available, post your reflections on an Internet-based discussion board monitored by your instructor.

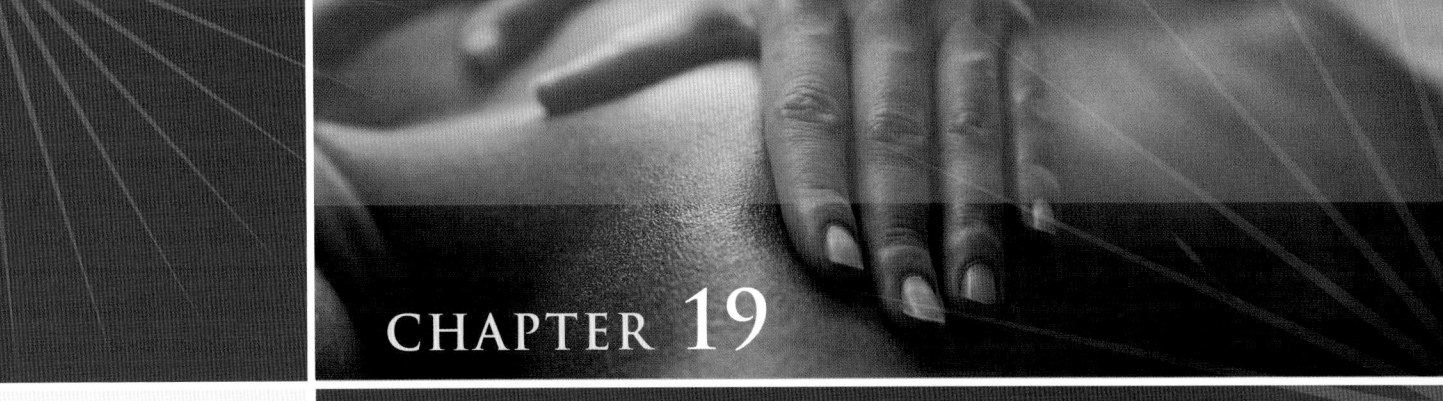

CHAPTER 19

Skeletal System, Pathologies, Disorders, and Injuries

LEARNING OBJECTIVES

After completing this chapter, the student should be able to:

1. List anatomic structures and physiologic processes related to the skeletal system and discuss bone tissue, bone cells, ossification, bone growth, and bone remodeling.
2. Classify bones by their size and shape, and discuss long bone anatomy and divisions of the skeleton.
3. Classify joints by their structure and function, and discuss synovial joint anatomy, types of synovial joints, and synovial joint movements.
4. Describe skeletal pathologies, disorders, and injuries and state their massage modifications.

http://evolve.elsevier.com/Salvo/MassageTherapy

INTRODUCTION

The skeletal system consists of individual and fused bones, joints, and their associated connective tissues, such as ligaments and cartilage. Bones themselves are living tissue and have an extensive blood supply. The skeletons we see in anatomy classes, laboratories, and museums are actually the mineral salts that remain after death.

Bones are the hard connective tissues that make up the skeletal system. The adult human body contains 206 named bones. This number does not include additional sesamoid bones in the hands and feet or sutural bones in the skull. The numbers of these bones vary from person to person, and the actual number may change over a person's lifetime. For example, if an individual has a sedentary lifestyle, then changes to one that involves consistent manual labor, they can develop additional sesamoid bones in their hands.

Bones are steel girders of the body, forming its internal framework. Second only to tooth enamel, bones are the hardest tissue in the body, yet they are relatively light, somewhat flexible, and able to resist certain amounts of tension and external forces. Massage practitioners need an in-depth understanding of the skeletal system to locate bony landmarks for muscle attachments and to identify endangerment sites.

Osteology is the study of bones. Use Table 19.1 to help you understand terms of the skeletal system.

ANATOMY

Basic anatomy of the skeletal system includes:
- Bones—including associated structures, such as cartilage
- Joints—including associated structures, such as ligaments

TABLE 19.1 Word Meanings

WORD	MEANING
Amphi	Gr. on both sides
Arthr, arthro	Gr. joint
Blast	Gr. germ cell or bud
Bursa	Gr. a leather sac
Chondr	Gr. cartilage
Clast	Gr. to break
Crepitus	L. crackling or rattling (sound)
Diarthrotic	Gr. two; joint
Epiphysis	Gr. upon, over; to grow
Haversian	Havers, British physician and anatomist (1650–1702)
Ligament	L. to bind or a band
Ossicle	L. little bone
Os, ossi	Gr. bone
Osteo, osseo	L. bone
Periosteum	Gr. around, about; L. bone
Sesamoid	Gr. sesame seedlike; shaped
Skeleton	Gr. dried up
Symphysis	Gr. together with, joined; to grow
Synarthrotic	Gr. together, joint
Volkmann	German physician (1800–1877)

Gr., Greek; *L.,* Latin.

PHYSIOLOGY

Functions of the skeletal system are:
- Support—The skeletal system provides support for the body through a bony framework.
- Protection—Bones help protect internal organs.
- Movement—Bones are attachment sites for tendons of skeletal muscles. Movements occur as muscles pull on, and reposition, bones during muscle contraction. Therefore, bones function as levers to provide movement (see Chapter 20 for information on levers).
- Blood cell production—Blood cells are produced in the red marrow of bones, especially long bones, through a process called *hematopoiesis.*
- Fat storage—Fats are stored in yellow bone marrow and are released when needed.
- Mineral storage—Minerals, such as phosphorus, magnesium, and sodium, and mineral compounds, such as calcium phosphate and calcium carbonate, are stored in bone and are released when needed.

BONE CELLS, BONE TISSUE, OSSIFICATION, BONE GROWTH, AND BONE REMODELING

Bones contain several types of cells. Bone, or *osseous tissue,* is a type of connective tissue. Bones change, or remodel, throughout life. These structures and processes are discussed next.

Bone Cells: Osteoblasts, Osteocytes, and Osteoclasts

Bone tissue contains three main cells. **Osteoblasts** or bone-forming cells, **osteocytes** or mature bone cells, and **osteoclasts** or bone-destroying cells. Osteoblasts secrete a substance that mineralizes bone tissue. Some osteoblasts become trapped in this material, which leads to their maturation and transformation to become osteocytes.

Osteoclasts secrete a substance that dissolves minerals left by osteoblasts, leaving behind small cavities which will be refilled later by minerals produced by osteoblasts. *LEARNING TIP:* To help you remember the difference between the osteoblasts and osteoclasts: Osteo**B**lasts **B**uild bone and osteo**C**lasts **C**rush bone.

Bone Tissue: Compact Bone and Spongy Bone

Types of bone tissue include compact bone and spongy bone; they are named by their relative density or how tightly tissues are packed together (Fig. 19.1). **Compact bone** forms the hard outer shell of bone and constitutes approximately 80% of the total adult bone mass. Compact bone contains many cylindrical-shaped units that run lengthwise and are called *osteons* or *Haversian systems.* Each osteon surrounds a *central (Haversian) canal* that contains blood vessels, lymphatic vessels, and nerves. Central canals are interconnected by *transverse (Volkmann) canals.* These

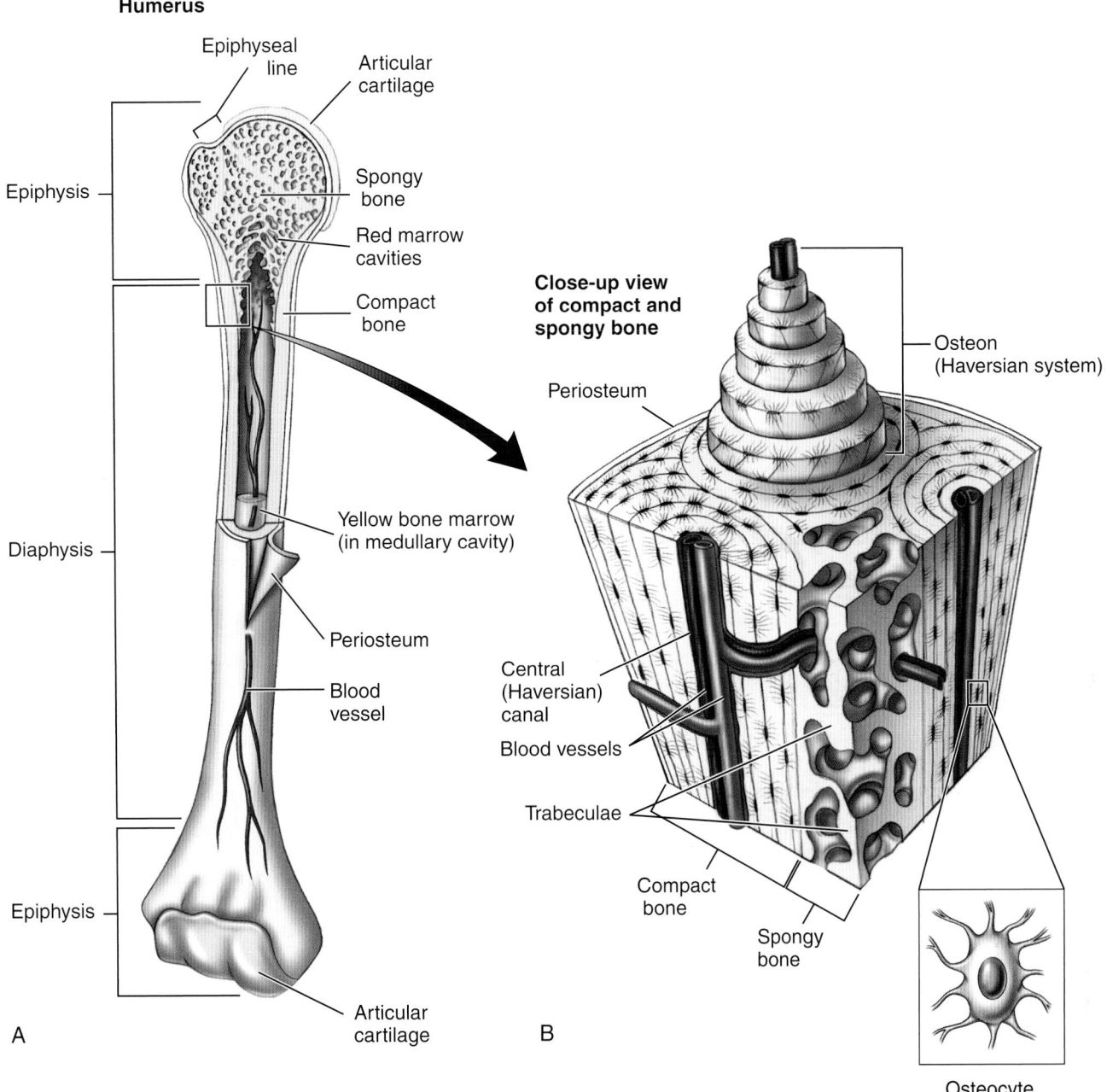

Humerus

FIG. 19.1 Bone anatomy. (A) Structures of a long bone. (B) Compact and spongy bone, close-up view. The transverse (Volkmann) canal extending from the central (Haversian) is not labeled. (From Herlihy, B. [2011]. *The human body in health and illness* [4th ed.]. St. Louis, MO: Mosby.)

canals also contain blood vessels, lymphatic vessels, and nerves.

Spongy bone, or *cancellous bone,* is lighter and less dense than compact bone and constitutes approximately 20% of the total bone mass. Spongy bone contains thin strips called *trabeculae,* giving it a spongy appearance. Trabeculae are arranged to provide maximum strength, similar to braces that support a building. In fact, trabeculae can rearrange themselves if the direction of stress changes. Small, irregular cavities created by the trabeculae contain red bone marrow, which houses blood-forming cells.

Ossification and Bone Growth

Ossification, or *osteogenesis,* is the process of bone tissue development by osteoblasts. This process begins during fetal development and continues throughout adulthood. Even after full adult stature is achieved, bones continue to remodel, the latter of which is discussed in the next section.

Types of ossification are intramembranous and endochondral. Both types are essential for fetal growth and development. **Intramembranous ossification** is bone development from membranes, such as those found in the flat bones of the skull. Intramembranous ossification also occurs

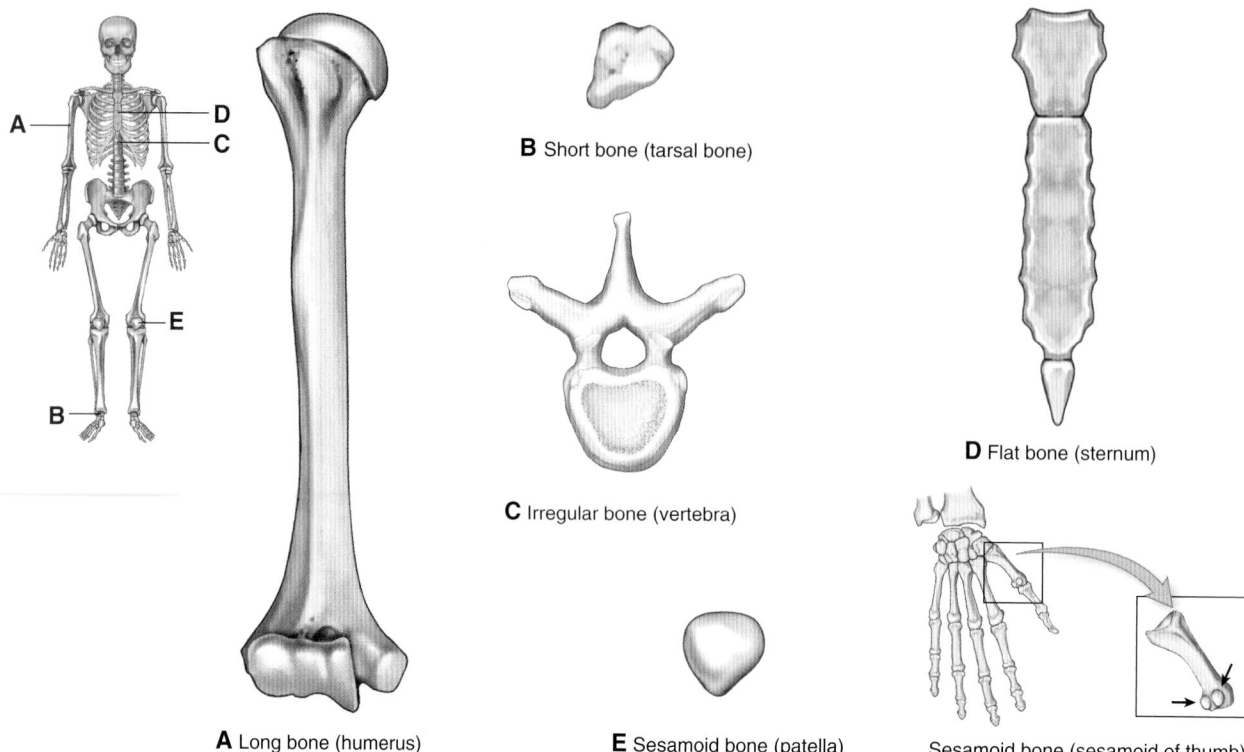

FIG. 19.2 Classification of bones by shape and size. Long bone (A), short bone (B), irregular bone (C), flat bone (D), and sesamoid bone (E). (From Patton, K. T., & Thibodeau, G. A. [2013]. *Anatomy & physiology* [8th ed.]. St. Louis, MO: Mosby.)

after birth and during the healing phase of bone fractures. **Endochondral ossification** is bone development from cartilage. The fetal skeleton is mainly cartilage. Osteoblasts in cartilage secrete minerals that transform some of the cartilage into bone. As the baby develops further, most of the cartilaginous skeleton is replaced with bone, except for articular surfaces within joints and parts of the nose and ribs.

Bone growth continues throughout childhood until the early part of the second decade of life. At this time, bone growth ceases. Sites where bone growth occurs are found in the section titled "Epiphyses, Articular Cartilage, Epiphyseal Plate, and Epiphyseal Line."

Bone Remodeling

Bone remodeling is the process of bone destruction by osteoclasts and bone formation by osteoblasts. Bone remodeling begins after bone growth is complete and continues throughout life. Both bone formation and destruction (or resorption) occur at approximately the same rate, so bone density in healthy bone is relatively constant. Many factors affect bone remodeling including age, gender, levels of physical activity, nutrition, and medication use. The body can detect increases in workload and respond by increasing bone mass or density. This phenomenon is called **Wolff law** (German anatomist and surgeon Julius Wolff [1836–1902]), and it states that bone is laid down in areas of high stress and reabsorbed in areas of low stress. If the loading on a bone increases, the bone can remodel to become stronger. The

inverse is also true—if the loading on a bone decreases, the bone will become less dense and weaker.

Hormones play a role in bone remodeling. When blood calcium levels are low, parathyroids secrete parathyroid hormone, which raises blood calcium levels by stimulating osteoclasts and inhibiting osteoblasts. When blood calcium levels are high, the thyroid secretes calcitonin, which lowers blood calcium levels by stimulating osteoblasts and inhibiting osteoclasts. In addition, growth hormone secreted by the anterior pituitary promotes bone growth, and bone growth is influenced by gonadal hormones, such as estrogens and testosterone.

CLASSIFICATION OF BONES BY SHAPE AND SIZE

Bones can be classified by their shape and size (Fig. 19.2). These classifications include long, short, flat, irregular, and sesamoid.

Long

Long bones are longer than they are wide. Long bones are those of the arm (humerus), forearm (ulna and radius), thigh (femur), and leg (tibia and fibula).

Short

Short bones are generally small, cube-shaped, and contain multiple articulating surfaces. Short bones are those of the wrists (carpals) and the ankles (tarsals).

Flat

Flat bones possess a broad, flat surface. Flat bones are those of the chest (sternum), upper back (scapula), ribcage, pelvis, and the skull.

Irregular

Irregular bones are oddly shaped and do not fit well in other shape/size categories. Irregular bones are found in the skull and spine (vertebrae).

Sesamoid

Sesamoid bones are small bones embedded in tendons and ligaments. Sesamoid bones are round and found in the knee (patella), hands, feet, and throat (hyoid).

LONG BONE ANATOMY

A long bone contains several essential structures (see Fig. 19.1A).

Diaphysis, Periosteum, and Medullary Cavity

The **diaphysis** is the cylindrical shaft of the long bone. Blood vessels enter the diaphysis through a small opening called the *nutrient foramen* (foramina, *plural*). The **periosteum** surrounds the diaphysis and is a dense, fibrous sheath containing blood and lymphatic vessels, nerves, and osteoblasts for growth and fracture healing. The periosteum is like the bone's life support system. Periosteum attaches to the underlying bone via perforating fibers called *Sharpey fibers*. Bones in the forearms and legs are connected by extensions of the periosteum called the *interosseous membrane* or *interosseous ligament* (see Fig. 21.8). This structure provides additional muscle attachment sites and divides muscles into compartments.

The **medullary cavity** is the hollow space within the diaphysis. The medullary cavity is filled with red and yellow bone marrow. In infancy, red bone marrow fills the medullary cavity and provides blood-forming cells. Red bone marrow in later life is found just in cavities between trabeculae in spongy bone. In adulthood, the medullary cavity is filled with yellow marrow, which functions as fat storage. The surface of the medullary cavity is lined with a thin connective membrane called *endosteum,* which contains osteoclasts.

Epiphyses, Articular Cartilage, Epiphyseal Plate, and Epiphyseal Line

The two ends of a long bone are the **epiphyses** (epiphysis, *sing.*). **Articular cartilage** covers the surfaces of the epiphyses. The type of cartilage is hyaline and provides smooth surfaces for movement within joints. Periosteum does not extend over the articular cartilage.

An **epiphyseal plate** of hyaline cartilage is found near the ends of growing bone, allowing them to increase in length. Cartilage within the epiphyseal plate (also called *growth plate*) continues to grow throughout childhood until the early part of the second decade of life.

At this time, cartilage growth in the epiphyseal plate ceases and completely ossifies and leaves behind an **epiphyseal line**.

DIVISIONS OF THE SKELETON

The skeletal system is divided into distinct regions. They are the (1) axial skeleton and the (2) appendicular skeleton (Fig. 19.3). Specific bony markings and their significance are discussed in Chapter 21.

Axial Skeleton

The **axial skeleton** consists of 80 named bones along the skeleton's central axis and includes the skull, vertebral column, sternum, and the ribs.

Skull

The skull consists of 29 bones: *8 cranial bones* (1 frontal, 2 parietal, 2 temporal, 1 occipital, 1 sphenoid, 1 ethmoid); *14 facial bones* (2 maxilla, 2 zygomatic, 2 palatine, 1 mandible, 2 lacrimal, 2 nasal, 2 inferior conch, 1 vomer); *6 ear ossicles* in the ear canal (2 malleus, 2 incus, 2 stapes), and *1 hyoid bone*. The skull may contain small bones with the sutures called *sutural,* or *Wormian,* bones.

Vertebral Column

There are 26 bones in the vertebral or spinal column: *7 cervical* vertebrae, *12 thoracic* vertebrae, *5 lumbar* vertebrae, *1 sacrum,* and *1 coccyx.*

Sternum

There is one sternal bone.

Ribs

There are 24 individual or 12 pairs of ribs.

Appendicular Skeleton

The **appendicular skeleton** consists of bones of the shoulder and pelvic girdles and bones of the upper and lower extremities. There are 126 named bones in the appendicular skeleton.

Shoulder Girdle

There are four bones in the shoulder (pectoral) girdle: *two scapulae* and *two clavicles.*

Upper Extremities

There are 60 bones in the upper extremity, 30 bones on each side. There are *2 humeri, 2 ulna, 2 radii, 16 carpals, 10 metacarpals,* and *28 phalanges.* The hands contain small sesamoid bones.

Pelvic Girdle

There are two bones in the pelvic girdle or pelvis. Each of these two pelvic bones are made up of three fused bones—*ilium, ischium,* and *pubis.*

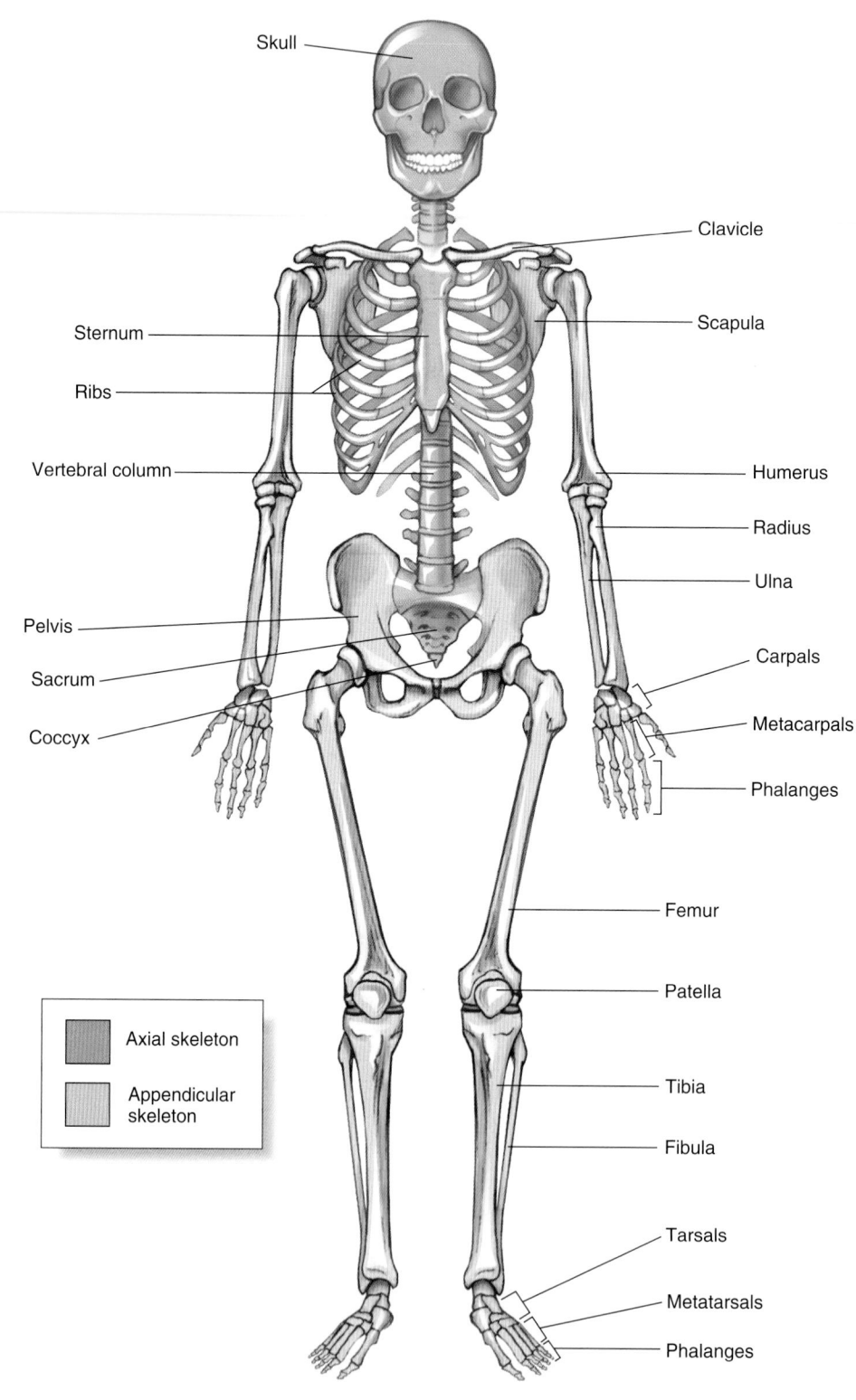

A   ANTERIOR VIEW

FIG. 19.3 Axial and appendicular divisions of the skeleton. (A) Anterior view.

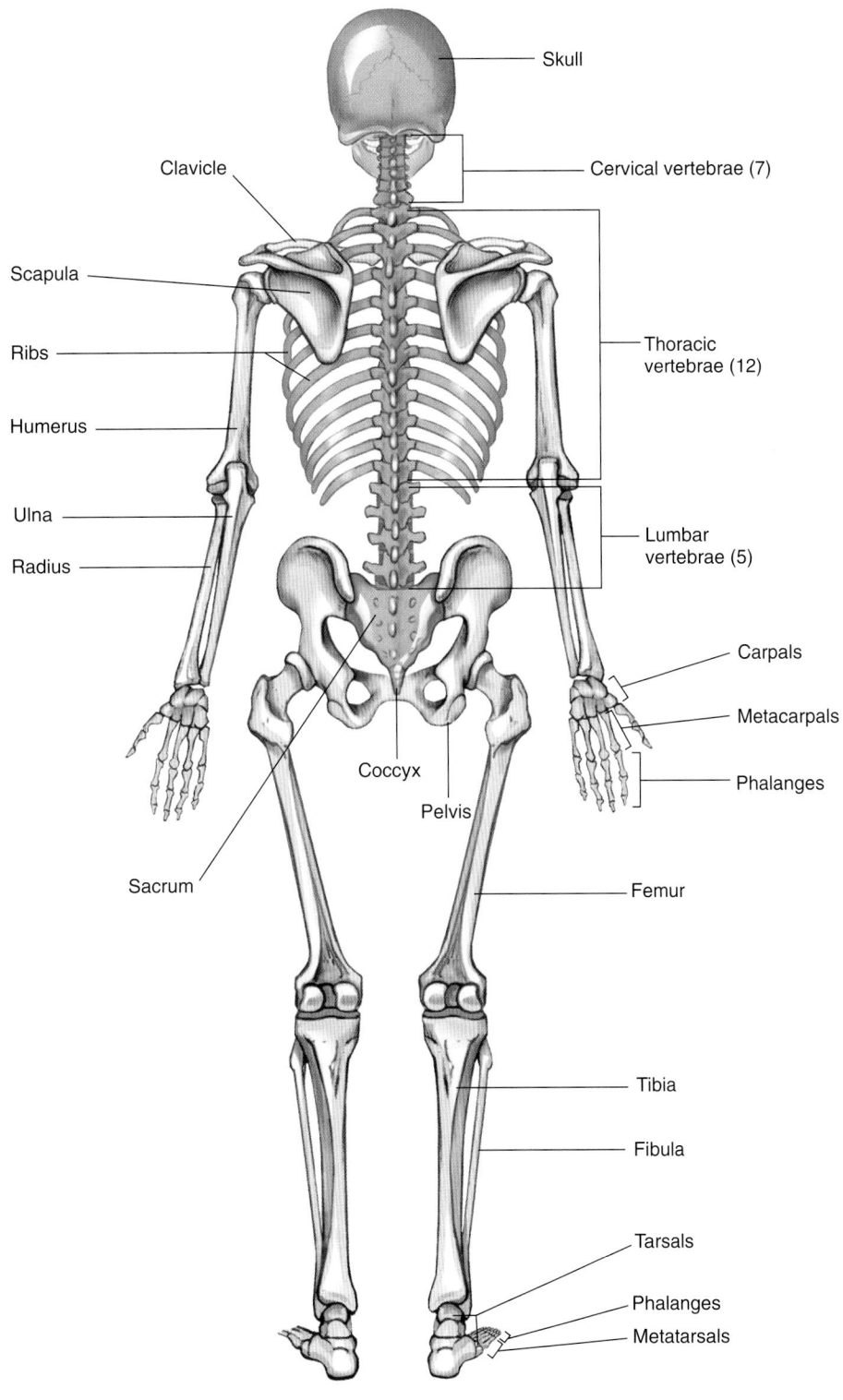

Skull

Clavicle

Cervical vertebrae (7)

Scapula

Ribs

Thoracic
vertebrae (12)

Humerus

Ulna

Radius

Lumbar
vertebrae (5)

Carpals

Metacarpals

Coccyx

Phalanges

Pelvis

Sacrum

Femur

Tibia

Fibula

Tarsals

Phalanges

Metatarsals

B   POSTERIOR VIEW

FIG. 19.3—CONT'D (B) Posterior view. (From Patton, K., & Thibodeau, G. [2014]. *The human body in health and disease* [6th ed.]. St. Louis, MO: Mosby.)

Lower Extremities

There are 60 bones in the lower extremity, 30 bones on each side. There are *2 femurs*, *2 patellae*, *2 tibias*, *2 fibulas*, *14 tarsals*, *10 metatarsals*, and *28 phalanges*. The feet contain small sesamoid bones.

> *It always seems impossible until it's done.*
> ~ **Nelson Mandela**

JOINTS

Joints are where two or more bones come together or join. Other terms for joints are *articulation* and *arthrosis* (*arthro-* means "joint"). Most joints allow the body to move in response to muscular forces or external forces. This movement may be small, as seen between the bones in the spine, or quite mobile, as seen between the bones of the shoulder. Joints also help bear the weight of the body and provide stability. Every bone in the skeleton articulates with at least one other bone, except the hyoid bone in the throat. Joints can be classified according to their structure or tissues within the joint and by their function or amount of movement permitted by the joint.

Structural Classification of Joints

Structural classifications divide joints into fibrous, cartilaginous, or synovial, depending on the anatomic structures within the joint and the absence or presence of a joint capsule (Fig. 19.4). Corresponding functional classifications are listed in *italics*.

Fibrous Joints

Bones in fibrous joints are joined by dense fibrous connective tissue, and fibrous joints do not have a joint capsule. The skull contains fibrous joints called *sutures*. Fibrous joints resemble *synarthrotic joints*.

Cartilaginous Joints

Bones in cartilaginous joints are joined by cartilage (fibrocartilage and occasionally hyaline) and cartilaginous joints do not have a joint capsule. Cartilaginous joints allow more movement than fibrous joints but less than synovial joints. The pelvis contains a cartilaginous joint called the pubic symphysis. Cartilaginous joints resemble *amphiarthrotic joints*.

Synovial Joints

Bones in synovial joints have synovial membranes and are enclosed by a joint capsule which contains a joint cavity

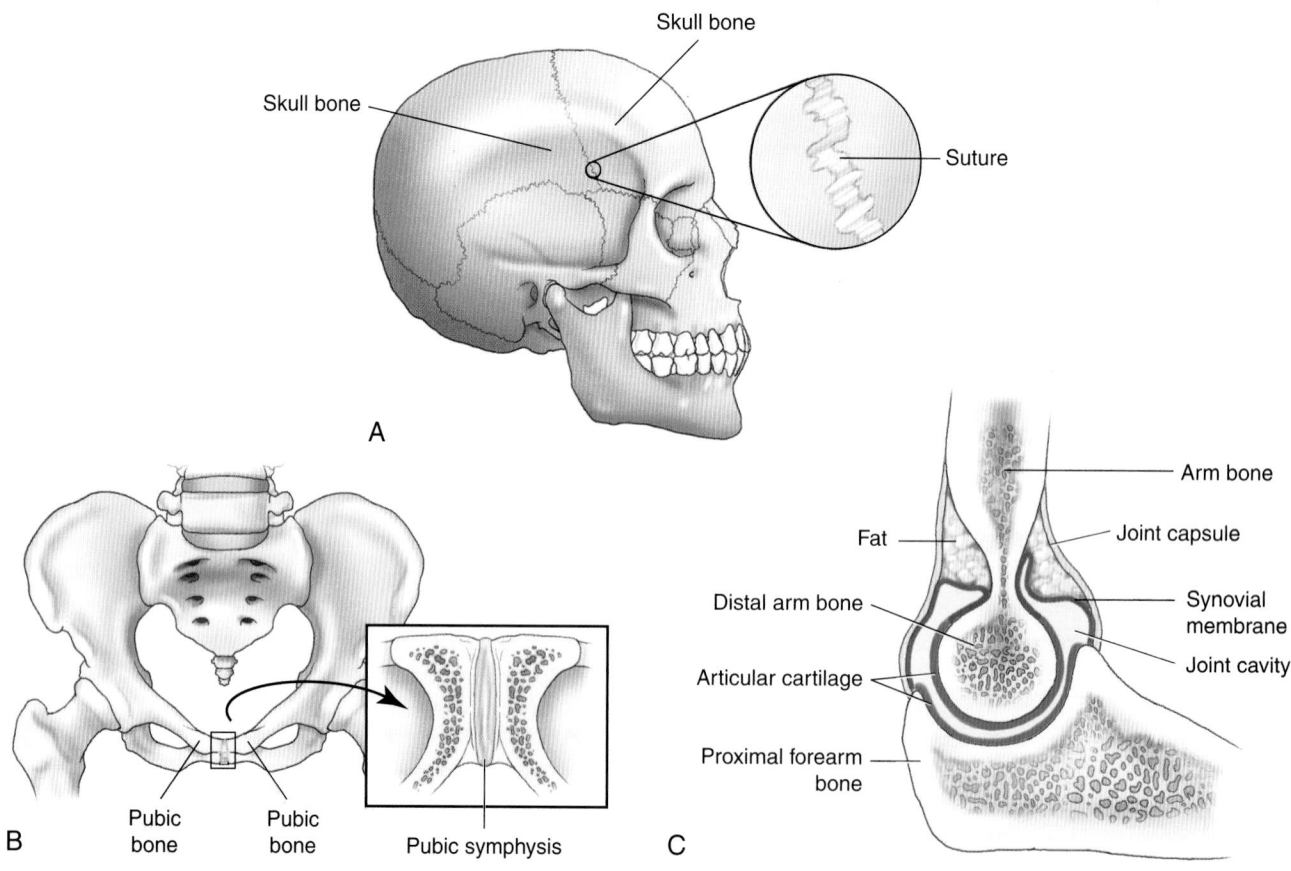

FIG. 19.4 Structural classification of joints. (A) Fibrous joints have dense fibrous connective tissue. The skull contains fibrous joints called sutures. (B) Cartilaginous joints have cartilage. Between the two pelvic bones is a cartilaginous joint called the pubic symphysis. (C) Synovial joints have synovial membranes enclosed by a joint capsule which contains a joint cavity filled with synovial fluid. The elbow is a synovial joint. (From Muscolino, J. E. [2011]. *Know the body*. St. Louis, MO: Mosby.)

filled with synovial fluid. Surfaces of articulating bones possess cartilage. Other structures associated with synovial joints are featured in the next major section. Synovial joints are the most movable and most common joints in the body. Synovial joints resemble *diarthrotic joints*.

Functional Classification of Joints

Functional classifications divide joints into synarthrotic, amphiarthrotic, or diarthrotic, depending on the joint's movement capacity. Corresponding structural classifications are listed in *italics*. ***LEARNING TIP**:* To help you remember the functional classification of joints, use the word **S-A-D** for **S**ynarthroses—**A**mphiarthroses—**D**iarthroses.

Synarthrotic Joints

Movement in synarthrotic joints, or synarthroses, is not permitted or extremely limited under normal conditions. Synarthrotic joints are common in the axial skeleton and include most joints in the skull (sutures) and joints holding teeth in their sockets (gomphoses). Synarthrotic joints resemble *fibrous joints*.

Amphiarthrotic Joints

Amphiarthrotic joints, or amphiarthroses, are slightly movable joints. Amphiarthrotic joints are common in the axial skeleton and include joints between the vertebrae (intervertebral joints) and the joint between the pubic bones (symphysis pubis). Amphiarthrotic joints resemble *cartilaginous joints*.

Diarthrotic Joints

Diarthrotic joints, or diarthroses, are freely movable joints. Diarthrotic joints are common in the appendicular skeleton and include joints in the shoulders (glenohumeral joints) and hips (acetabulofemoral joints). Diarthrotic joints resemble *synovial joints*.

SYNOVIAL JOINT ANATOMY

Synovial joints, or diarthrotic joints, are freely movable, and contain several distinguishing characteristics. These joints have a double-layered structure called a **joint capsule** or articular capsule. The joint capsule is highly innervated and has a rich blood supply. The outer layer of the capsule is fibrous and surrounds the joint like a sleeve. The space between the two layers is called the **joint cavity**. The inner layer of the joint capsule is lined with a **synovial membrane** that secretes a thick clear liquid called **synovial fluid**. This fluid, also called *synovium*, provides nutrition and lubrication of the articular cartilage so the joint can move easily and without friction. The amount of synovial fluid production depends on the level of joint activity. **Ligaments** help unite articulating bones, which strengthens the joint. **Articular cartilage**

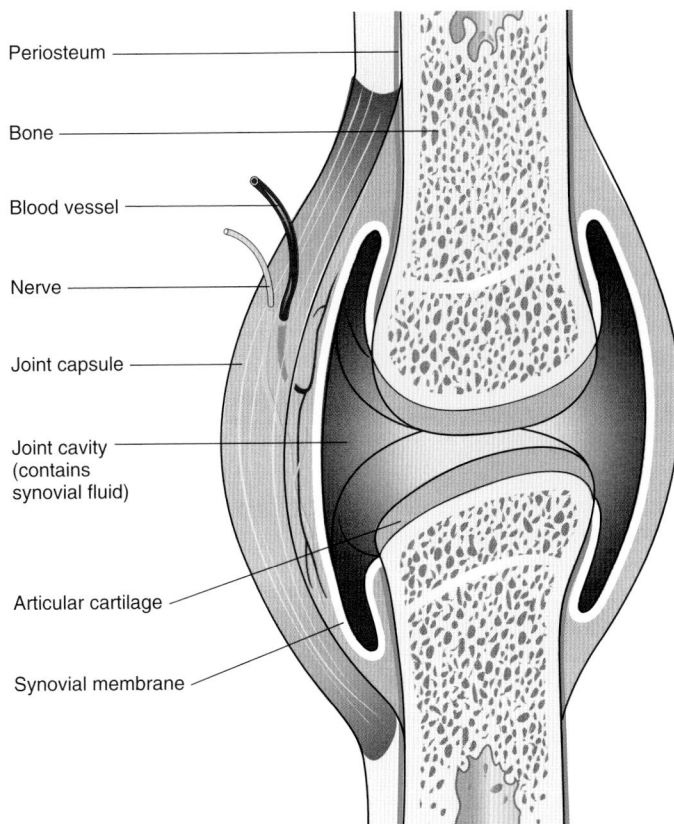

Periosteum

Bone

Blood vessel

Nerve

Joint capsule

Joint cavity (contains synovial fluid)

Articular cartilage

Synovial membrane

FIG. 19.5 Synovial joint structures. Synovial joints are enclosed by a joint capsule. Cartilage covers the articulating bone surfaces. The joint cavity is lined with a synovial membrane that secretes synovial fluid.

covers the articulating surfaces of bone (Fig. 19.5). This type of cartilage is hyaline, which has a firm and smooth consistency and is pearly or bluish white in color. Articular cartilage decreases friction during movement and increases shock absorption. Some joints, such as the shoulder and the hip, also have a **labrum**, a ring of fibrocartilage around the edge of the articular cartilage to increase its surface area.

Accessory Structures: Fat Pads, Bursae, Synovial Sheaths, and Menisci

Some synovial joints, such as the knee, contain **fat pads**, which protect articular cartilages and fill spaces within the joint as they change shape during movement. Many synovial joints contain **bursae**, flattened saclike structures between ligaments or tendons and bones to reduce friction (Fig. 19.6). Some joints contain **synovial sheaths** or *tendon sheaths,* which are elongated bursae surrounding tendons to increase their gliding capacity. Bursae and synovial sheaths are lined with synovial membranes that secrete synovial fluid. Areas in the body where synovial sheaths are found include the forearms and wrist and the legs and ankles. Crescent-shaped fibrocartilaginous pads called **menisci** are found in the knees and the jaw (see Fig. 21.16). Menisci act as shims to make irregular bone shapes fit together, help the joints move smoothly, and serve as shock absorbers.

TYPES OF SYNOVIAL JOINTS

Most body movements, such as getting out of a chair, running, or throwing a ball are the action of several joints working together and providing actions around various axes. Joints can be classified based on the number of axes they move around. Each group contains two types of joints named by their shape (Fig. 19.7). Table 19.2 compares types of joints, their movements, and examples of each.

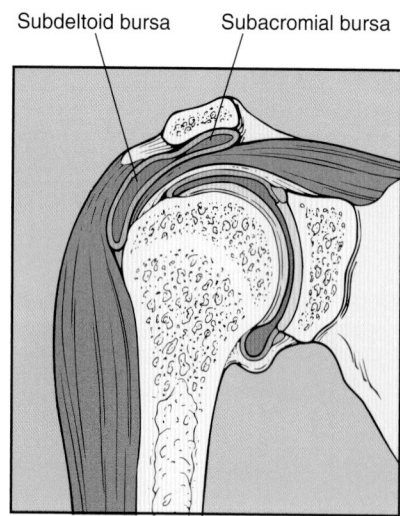

Subdeltoid bursa   Subacromial bursa

FIG. 19.6 Bursae of the shoulder joint. Bursae are flattened saclike structures between ligaments or tendons and bones to reduce friction. (From Frazier, M. S. [2013]. *Essentials of human diseases and conditions* [5th ed.]. St. Louis, MO: Saunders.)

Uniaxial Joints

Uniaxial joints move around only one axis and in one plane. Types of uniaxial joints are hinge and pivot.

Hinge Joints

Hinge joints possess a convex surface on one bone that fits into a concave surface of another bone. Movements in hinge joints are similar to that of two boards hinged together, allowing the angle of the joint to decrease, causing flexion, or to increase, causing extension. Examples of hinge joints are the elbow between the arm bone and the forearm bones (humeroulnar and humeroradial joints) and the ankle between the leg bones and a tarsal bone (talocrural joint).

Pivot Joints

Pivot joints possess a ringed or notched surface of one bone that fits into a projection of another bone. Movements in pivot joints are limited to rotation. Examples of pivot joints are between a projection of the second cervical vertebra and a ring-shaped portion of the first vertebra (atlantoaxial joint), and between a projection of a forearm bone and a notch of the other forearm bone (proximal and distal radioulnar joints).

Biaxial Joints

Biaxial joints permit movements around two perpendicular axes and in two perpendicular planes. Types of biaxial joints are saddle and condyloid or ellipsoidal.

Saddle Joints

Saddle joints possess a concave surface of one bone that fits into a convex surface of another. This positional relationship resembles a rider in a "saddle." Saddle joints are found in the thumb and the shape of the bones at the joint makes it possible for the thumb to swing in an arc and touch the tips of the fingers and grip objects. Specific movements are flexion, extension, abduction, adduction, opposition, reposition, and circumduction. There are two saddle joints in the body: between the thumb's metacarpal and the wrist's trapezium bone (first carpometacarpal joint).

Condyloid (Ellipsoidal) Joints

Condyloid joints possess an oval-shaped surface or condyle of one bone(s) that fits into a depression or socket of another bone(s). This position allows one bone to travel back and forth (flexion and extension) and side to side (abduction and adduction). Examples are the joint between the oval-shaped projections in the skull and depressions on the first cervical vertebra (atlantooccipital joint) and between the distal ends of the lateral forearm bone and the depressions of several carpal bones (radiocarpal joints).

Multiaxial Joints

Multiaxial joints permit movement around three axes and in three planes. Types of multiaxial joints are ball and socket and gliding.

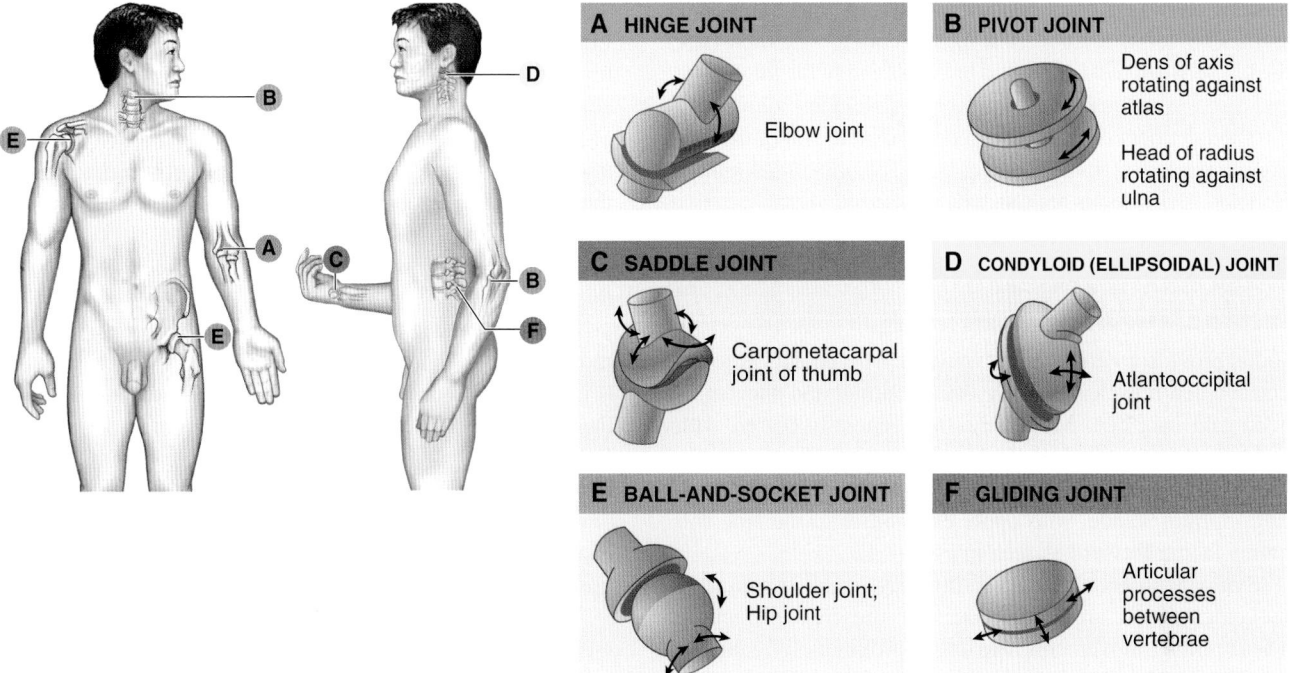

FIG. 19.7 Types of synovial joints and their locations. (A) Hinge. (B) Pivot. (C) Saddle. (D) Condyloid (Ellipsoidal). (E) Ball and Socket. (F) Gliding. Hinge and pivot are uniaxial joints. Saddle and condyloid are biaxial joints. Ball and socket and gliding joints are multiaxial joints.

TABLE 19.2 Synovial Joints, Movements, and Examples

NAME OF JOINT	MOVEMENT	EXAMPLE
Hinge	Uniaxial: allows flexion and extension	Elbow joint between the arm bone and the two forearm bones (humeroulnar and humeroradial joints) and ankle joint between the medial leg bone and a tarsal bone (talocrural joint)
Pivot	Uniaxial: allows rotation	Joint between a projection of the second cervical vertebra and a ring-shaped portion of the first vertebra (atlantoaxial joint) and joint between a projection of one forearm bone and a notch of the other forearm bone (distal radioulnar joint)
Saddle	Biaxial: allows flexion/extension, abduction/ adduction, opposition/ reposition, and circumduction	Joint between the thumb's metacarpal and trapezium carpal bone (first carpometacarpal joint)
Condyloid/Ellipsoidal	Biaxial: allows flexion/extension, abduction/ adduction	Joint between the two oval-shaped projections on the skull and two depressions on the first cervical vertebra (atlantooccipital joint) and joint between the distal end of the lateral forearm bone and the depressions of several carpal bones (radiocarpal joints)
Gliding	Multiaxial: allows flexion/extension, inversion/ eversion, and lateral flexion and rotation of the vertebral column	Joint between bones in the wrist (intercarpal joints), joint between bones in the feet (intertarsal joints), and joint between bones of the vertebral column (facet joints)
Ball and socket	Multiaxial: allows flexion/extension, abduction/ adduction, circumduction, and rotation	Joint between the ball-shaped proximal end of the thigh bone and a socket of the pelvic bone (acetabulofemoral joints) and joint between the ball-shaped proximal end of the arm bone and a socket in the shoulder blade (glenohumeral joints)

Gliding Joints

Gliding joints are interactions of relatively flat surfaces of articulating bones. This position allows limited but complex movement along all axes. As a group, gliding joints are the least mobile of all synovial joints. Examples of gliding joints are between bones in the wrist (intercarpal joints) and between bones in the feet (intertarsal joints). Gliding joints are also called *planar joints*.

Ball and Socket Joints

Ball and socket joints consist of the ball-shaped end of one bone and a socket-shaped surface of another bone. This position allows the first bone to move in many directions. Ball and socket joints are our most movable joints. Examples are the hip between the ball-shaped proximal end of the thigh bone and a socket in the pelvic bone (acetabulofemoral joints), and the shoulder between the ball-shaped proximal end of the arm bone and a socket in the shoulder blade (glenohumeral joints). Ball and socket joints are also called *spheroid joints*.

TYPES OF SYNOVIAL JOINT MOVEMENT

Joints provide a variety of movements. Movements at joints occur when muscles crossing them contract and shorten or relax and lengthen. Movements are generally paired with their opposite, such as flexion and extension. Human body movements are described in relation to the anatomic position: upright stance, with upper extremities to the side and palms facing forward as seen in Fig. 18.12.

Synovial joints also have **joint play**, small involuntary movements that are independent of muscle contraction. These gliding movements measure approximately ⅛ inch in any plane and occur along the contours of the joint surfaces. Joint capsule laxity allows for joint play.

Some joint movements cause painless noises, or **crepitus**, which may be described as creaking, cracking, grating, crunching, or popping sounds. Synovial fluid, which lubricates joints, can accumulate gas while the joint is not being used. Crepitant sounds are thought to be caused by tiny bubbles of nitrogen forming in synovial fluid, which sometimes burst when the joint is stretched (Brakke, 2016; Nelsen, 2015). These sounds are both common and normal during joint movement. Crepitus may occur in joints affected by diseases, such as osteoarthritis (OA) or rheumatoid arthritis (RA). Crepitus is also used to describe any noise originating in the body, including flatulence released by the digestive tract, and lungs crackling from respiratory disease.

Flexion and Extension

Flexion is bending a joint so that the angle between the bones decreases (Fig. 19.8). Examples of joints permitting flexion are the fingers, toes, elbows, hips, knees, neck, shoulders, spine, and wrists.

Extension is straightening a joint so that the angle between the bones increases (see Fig. 19.8). Examples of joints permitting extension are the fingers, toes, elbows, hips, knees, neck, shoulders, spine, and wrists. **Hyperextension** is overextending the joint beyond its normally straightened position, as in moving the head back to look upward. Some joints that permit extension also permit hyperextension. Flexion and extension occur in the sagittal plane.

Abduction and Adduction

Abduction is movement away from the midline (Fig. 19.9). Examples of joints permitting abduction are the hips and shoulders. Abduction of the fingers or toes spreads the fingers or toes apart; the midline of the hand is the middle finger, and the midline of the foot is the second toe.

Adduction is movement toward the midline (see Fig. 19.9). Examples of joints permitting adduction are the hips and shoulders. Adduction also brings the extremity across the midline of the body. Adduction of the fingers or toes moves them together. As mentioned above, the midline of the hand is the middle finger, and the midline of the foot is the second toe. Abduction and adduction occur in the frontal plane. *LEARNING TIP:* To distinguish adduction from abduction, remember **add**uction **add**s to the midline.

Radial deviation (wrist abduction) occurs as the hand moves toward the radius and away from the midline (Fig. 19.10). **Ulnar deviation** (wrist adduction) occurs as the hand moves toward the ulna and midline (Fig. 19.11). Radial and ulnar deviations occur in the frontal plane. *LEARNING TIP:* To distinguish the difference between radial and ulnar deviation, remember the letter **L** is in both u**L**nar and **L**ittle finger. During u**L**nar deviation, the **L**ittle finger moves toward the u**L**na.

Horizontal adduction occurs as the shoulder or hip moves the extremity toward the midline or anteriorly in the horizontal plane. **Horizontal abduction** occurs as the shoulder or hip moves the extremity away from the midline or posteriorly in the horizontal plane (see Fig. 19.11).

Adduction of the thumb, or **opposition**, moves it toward the other fingers or in contact with the pad of any finger on the same hand (Fig. 19.12). Abduction of the thumb, also called **reposition**, returns the thumb to its anatomic position next to the index finger.

Circumduction

Circumduction is conical movement in which one end of the body is relatively fixed and the other end moves in a circle. The fixed end is usually proximal, and the moving end distal. Circumduction is a combination of several movements including flexion, adduction, extension, and abduction (Fig. 19.13). Joints permitting circumduction include the shoulder and hip. Circumduction occurs in the sagittal and the frontal planes.

Rotation

Rotation occurs when a bone pivots or rotates around its own central axis (Fig. 19.14). **Left/right rotation** refer to the direction of rotation and are used to describe joint movement in the central axis, such as the neck and spine. Rotation occurs in the horizontal plane.

Lateral (external) rotation and **medial (internal) rotation** refer to the direction of rotation. Lateral rotation is rotation away from the midline and medial rotation is rotation toward the midline. These terms are used for joints of the appendicular skeleton, such as the shoulder, hip, and knee (the knee can be rotated slightly when flexed). Lateral and medial rotations occur in the horizontal plane.

Upward and downward rotations are movements of the scapula and are defined by movements of the shoulder socket or glenoid cavity. **Upward (superior) rotation**

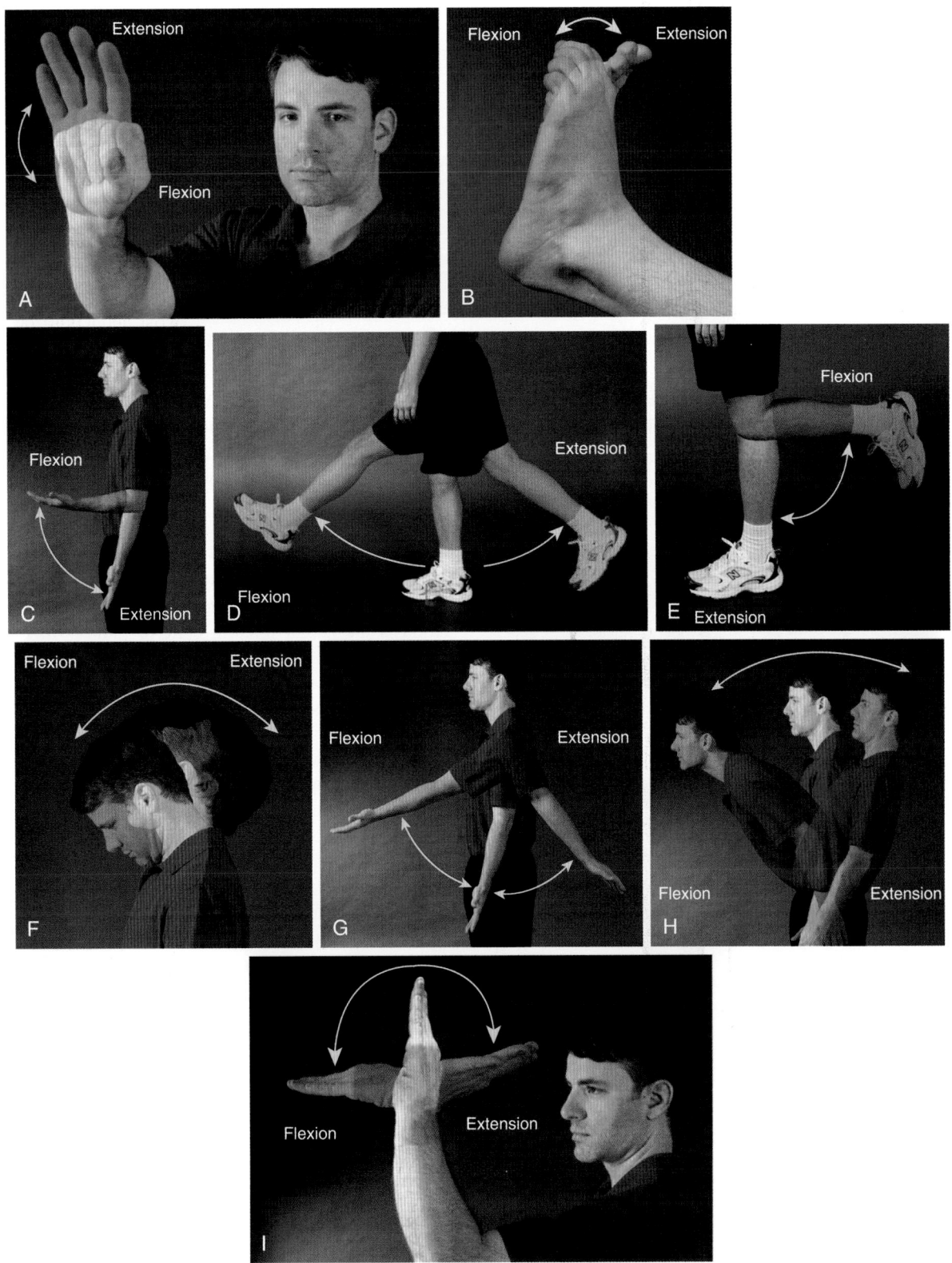

FIG. 19.8 Flexion and extension. (A) Fingers. (B) Toes. (C) Elbow. (D) Hip. (E) Knee. (F) Neck. (G) Shoulder. (H) Spine. (I) Wrist.

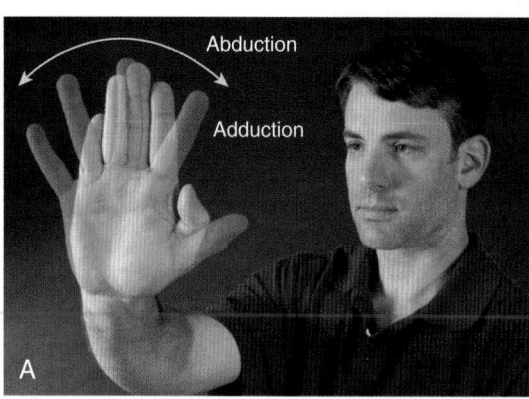
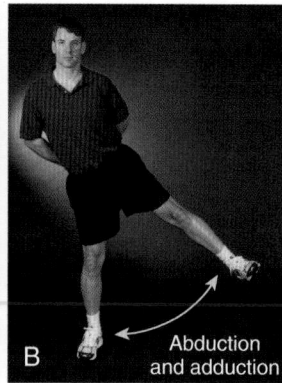
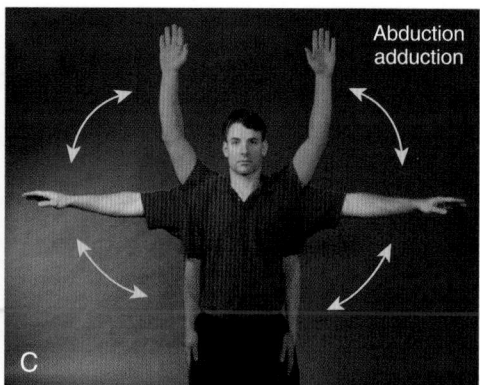

FIG. 19.9 Abduction and adduction. (A) Fingers. (B) Hip. (C) Shoulders.

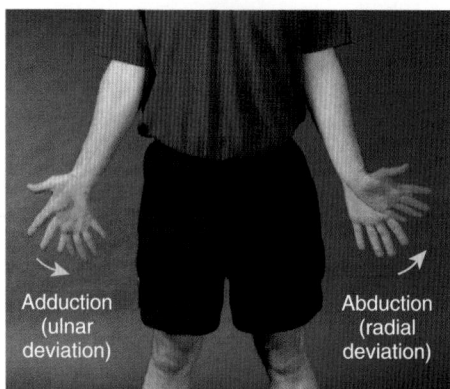

FIG. 19.10 Adduction (ulnar deviation) and abduction (radial deviation) of the wrists.

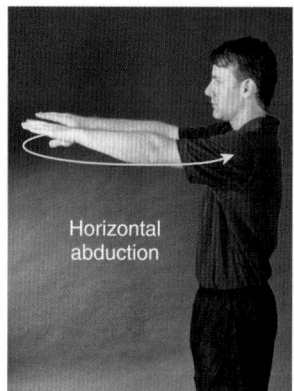

FIG. 19.11 Horizontal abduction of the shoulder.

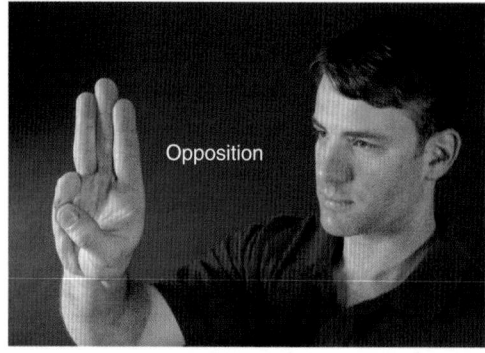

FIG. 19.12 Opposition of the thumb (adduction).

occurs when the glenoid cavity moves upward or superiorly (Fig. 19.15). **Downward (inferior) rotation** occurs when the glenoid cavity moves downward or inferiorly (see Fig. 19.15). Upward and downward rotation occur in the frontal plane.

Supination and Pronation

Supination and pronation are rotational movements of the forearm. The only bone moving during supination and pronation is the lateral forearm bone or radius. *LEARNING TIP:* To remember which bone moves during supination and pronation, the **R**adius does the **R**otating.

Supination is lateral rotation in which the bones of the forearm are in a parallel position and the palms face anteriorly. If the elbows are flexed, supination turns the palms so that they face up or superiorly (Fig. 19.16). *LEARNING TIP:* s**UP**ination contains the word **UP** and is needed to hold a c**UP** of so**UP**.

Pronation is medial rotation in which the bones of the forearm cross to form an X and the palms face posteriorly. If the elbows are flexed, pronation turns the palms so that they face down or inferiorly (see Fig. 19.16). *LEARNING TIP:* **Pron**ation is the palm turned downward, so you are **Pron**e to spill a cup of soup. Supination and pronation occur in the horizontal plane.

Plantar Flexion and Dorsiflexion

Plantar flexion is movement of the ankle so that the foot moves inferiorly—the toes are pointing down toward the ground (Fig. 19.17). Plantar flexion is also written as plantarflexion and both terms are used interchangeably. *LEARNING TIP:* To distinguish between plantar flexion and dorsiflexion, remember **Plant**ar flexion **Plant**s the toes in the earth.

Dorsiflexion is movement of the ankle so that the foot moves superiorly—the toes are pointing up (see Fig. 19.17). Plantar flexion and dorsiflexion occur in the sagittal plane.

Inversion and Eversion

Inversion occurs when the foot rotates medially and the plantar surface of the foot faces the midline. When both feet are inverted, the soles face each other (Fig. 19.18). The foot

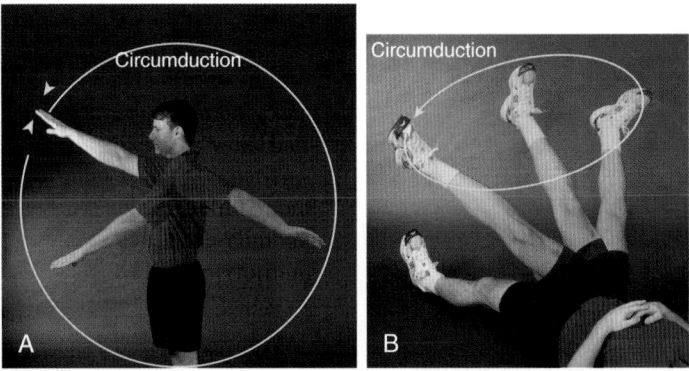

FIG. 19.13 Circumduction. (A) Shoulder. (B) Hip.

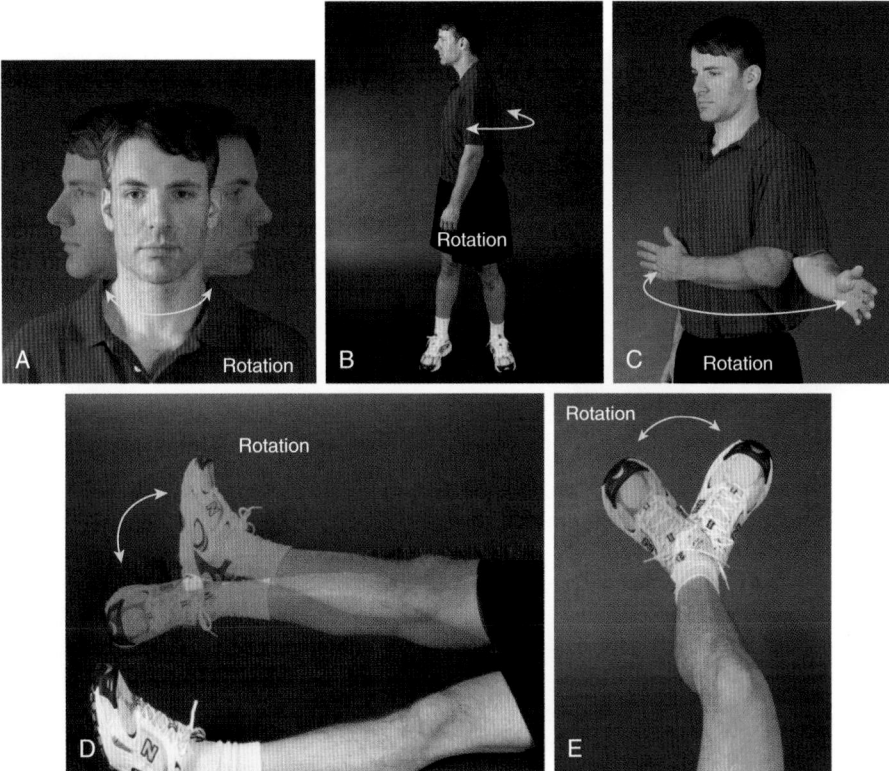

FIG. 19.14 Rotation. (A) Neck. (B) Spine. (C) Shoulder (with elbow flexed). (D) Hip. (E) Knee (with knee flexed).

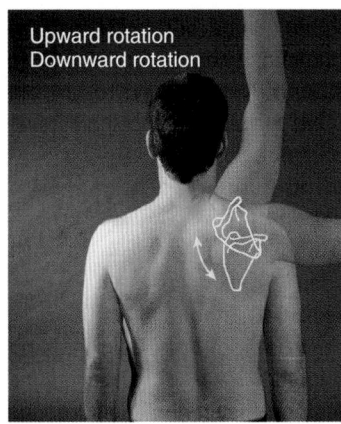

FIG. 19.15 Upward (superior) and downward (inferior) rotation of the scapula.

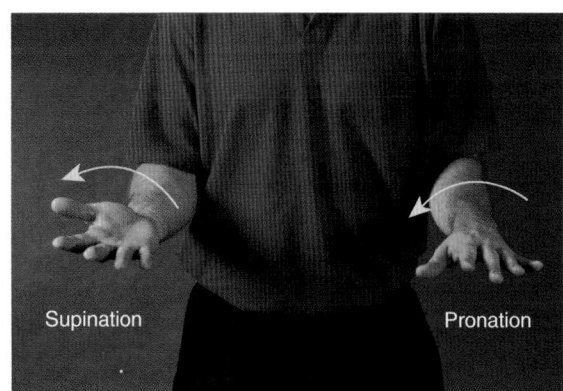

FIG. 19.16 Supination and pronation of the forearm (with elbows flexed).

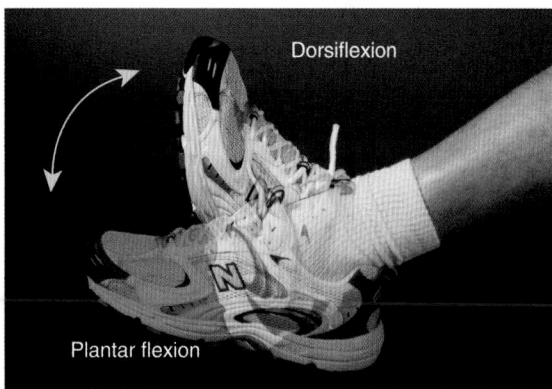

FIG. 19.17 Plantar flexion and dorsiflexion of the ankle.

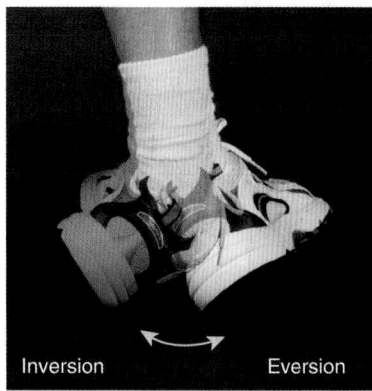

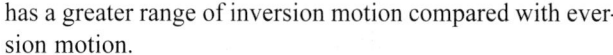

FIG. 19.18 Inversion and eversion of the foot.

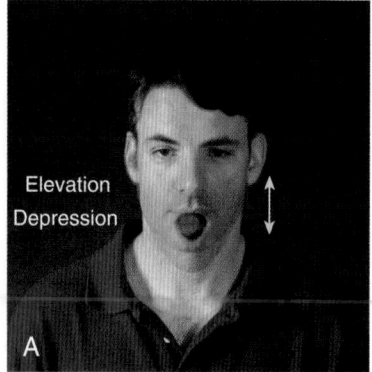

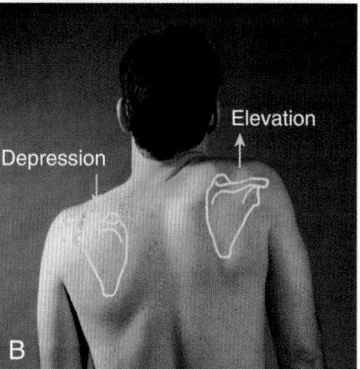

FIG. 19.19 Elevation and depression. (A) Jaw. (B) Shoulder blade.

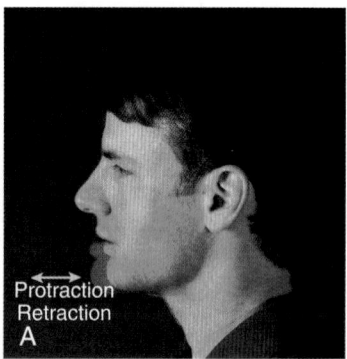

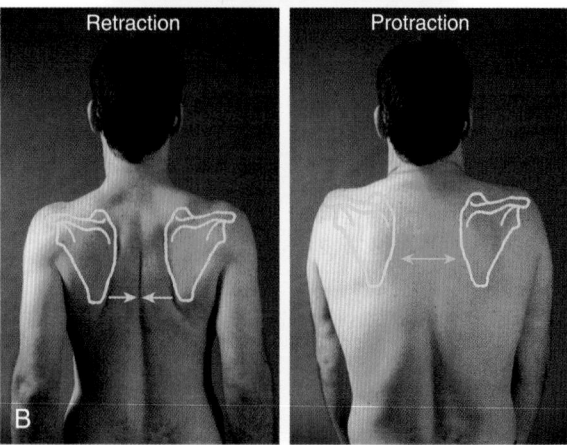

FIG. 19.20 Protraction (protrusion) and retraction (retrusion). (A) Jaw. (B) Shoulder blade.

has a greater range of inversion motion compared with eversion motion.

Eversion occurs when the foot rotates laterally and the plantar surface of the foot faces away from the midline. When both feet are everted, the soles do not face each other (see Fig. 19.18). Inversion and eversion occur in the frontal plane.

Elevation and Depression

Depression and elevation are downward and upward movements. **Elevation** is superior or upward movement, essentially raising or lifting the shoulder blade (scapula) or jaw (mandible) (Fig. 19.19).

Depression is inferior or downward movement, essentially lowering or dropping the shoulder or jaw (see Fig. 19.19). Elevation and depression occur in the frontal plane.

Protraction and Retraction

Protraction and retraction are anterior and posterior movements of the shoulder blade (scapula) or jaw (mandible). **Protraction** (protrusion) is movement in an anterior or forward direction (Fig. 19.20).

Retraction (retrusion) is movement in a posterior or backward direction (see Fig. 19.20). Protraction and retraction occur in the horizontal plane.

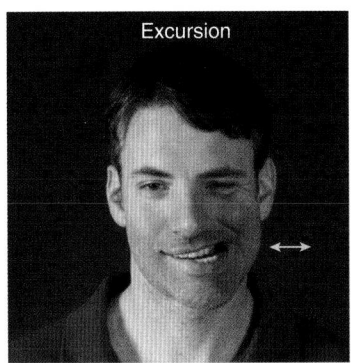

FIG. 19.21 Excursion (lateral deviation) of the jaw.

Excursion

Excursion (lateral deviation) is side-to-side movements of the jaw or mandible. **Lateral excursion** moves the jaw away from the midline, toward the right or left sides. **Medial excursion** returns the jaw to the midline position (Fig. 19.21). Excursion occurs in the horizontal plane.

SKELETAL PATHOLOGIES, DISORDERS, AND INJURIES

Featured next are common pathologies, disorders, and injuries of the skeletal system listed alphabetically. Each item includes a brief description and massage-related modifications. Many injuries in this section undergo stages of inflammation; this topic is discussed in Chapter 14. A more extensive list and related research is found in the current edition of *Mosby's Pathology for Massage Professionals* (2022).

Adhesive Capsulitis (Frozen Shoulder)

Adhesive capsulitis occurs when the shoulder joint capsule becomes thick and chronically inflamed, causing pain and limited range of motion. As the condition progresses, adhesions develop, making active movement even more difficult. The condition is called "frozen" shoulder because the more pain is felt, the less likely the shoulder is moved, which causes more stiffness, and leads to more pain and less movement—a continuous cycle causing the shoulder to be frozen in one position. Adhesive capsulitis affects up to 5% of the population and is more common in females between 40 and 60 years of age. However, males with adhesive capsulitis are at greater risk for a longer period of recovery and greater disability. Typically, only one shoulder is affected. Some people develop adhesive capsulitis in the opposite shoulder. Signs and symptoms of adhesive capsulitis are divided into three stages.

- **Freezing stage**. In this stage, there is a gradual onset of a dull shoulder ache and stiffness that slowly develops into pain, which occurs both at rest and during movement. The shoulder stiffness increases, reducing range of motion. This stage lasts between 6 weeks and 9 months.
- **Frozen stage**. During this stage, shoulder pain may lessen, but remains stiff and movement is difficult. This

makes it harder to complete daily activities. This stage lasts from 2 to 6 months.
- **Thawing (recovery) stage**. In this stage, shoulder pain lessens, and range of motion slowly improves.

Massage and Adhesive Capsulitis

Massage can be applied to the area at any stage because the inflammatory process associated with adhesive capsulitis is chronic in nature and not acute. Inquire about pressure sensitivity over affected areas and adjust it according to the client's preference. Massage, especially deep friction massage, over shoulder muscles may reduce pain and improve mobility. Consider incorporating gentle shoulder passive range of motion (PROM) and traction using the pendulum method.

Shoulder PROM/traction (pendulum method). Asking the client to lay prone near the edge of the table and allow the affected arm to hang over the table's edge. The client's shoulder should be close to the table edge to allow maximum traction. The client's hanging hand should not touch the floor; adjust the table height higher if needed. Gently move the client's arm, swinging it back and forth like a pendulum for approximately 30 seconds. Afterward, allow the client to rest in this position for up to 5 minutes. During this time, the client may gently swing their arm back and forth or in a circle. Recommend this passive activity be done at home while standing or lying down on a bed or table, allowing gravity to gently traction the shoulder joint. As the client's condition improves, the client can add a 3-pound dumbbell during the homecare activity.

Baker Cyst

A **Baker cyst** is a fluid-filled pouch that forms in the popliteal space behind the knee. Baker cysts are more common in older adults. As many as one in five people with knee problems develop a Baker cyst. A Baker cyst is also called a *popliteal cyst*. It is commonly caused by inflammation of the knee, such as seen in various types of arthritis or from a knee injury, especially a meniscal tear. These situations cause the knee to produce excess synovial fluid that leaks out and forms a pouch-like structure in the popliteal space. Thrombophlebitis deep vein thrombosis [DVT] and accompanying blood clots below the cyst may occur as a rare complication.

Massage and Baker Cyst

Screen the client for DVT by looking for signs and symptoms: unilateral leg swelling, heat, redness or noticeable discoloration, and pain. If present, avoid massage to the affected lower extremity and recommend medical testing by their healthcare provider. Massage has been found safe with precautions taken, such as screening for DVT and avoiding the affected limb (Ng et al., 2018). If signs and symptoms of DVT are not present, avoid the affected popliteal area. Use a soft bolster behind the knees while the client is supine. Coexisting medical conditions (osteoarthritis, knee injury) should be factored into the treatment plan.

Bursitis

Bursitis is inflammation of a bursa, a flattened saclike structure between ligaments or tendons and bones that acts as a cushion to reduce friction. The body contains more than 150 bursae found between tendons, bony prominences, and some muscles. The most common locations of bursitis are the shoulder (subacromial, subcoracoid, and subscapular bursitis); elbow (olecranon bursitis [student's elbow]); hip (trochanteric, and ischial bursitis [weaver's bottom]); knee (prepatellar [housemaid's knee], infrapatellar bursitis [clergyman's knee]); the heel (calcaneal bursitis); and the base of the great toe (metatarsophalangeal bursitis). Bursitis can also occur in or near surgically replaced joints. Bursitis may be either acute or chronic. Acute bursitis has a sudden onset. Chronic bursitis results from long-standing bursitis and may lead to changes in tissues, such as calcification and adhesion formation.

Massage and Bursitis

For acute cases, treat the affected area as a local contraindication. Elevate the affected area during the massage, which may help reduce swelling. Once inflammation has resolved, local massage can begin.

For chronic cases, position the client for comfort. For example, avoid the side-lying position in cases of hip or trochanteric bursitis. In cases of metatarsophalangeal bursitis, use a higher-than-normal (8 inches) bolster in front of the ankles to prevent the affected toe from touching the massage table while the client is prone; undrape the foot to prevent uncomfortable pressure on the affected toe while the client is supine. Massage muscles that cross affected joints. Adjust the pressure according to the client's preference.

Dislocations and Subluxations

A **dislocation** is the temporary displacement of bones within a joint, with complete loss of contact between articulating surfaces. Usually, one bone is forced out of place while another remains in a normal position. A **subluxation** is a partial dislocation, with some contact remaining between articulating surfaces. Dislocations are most often seen in people younger than 20 years. The most commonly dislocated joints are the shoulders and fingers. The jaw and shoulder joints are susceptible to recurrent dislocations.

Massage and Dislocations/Subluxations

During the acute inflammation phase, treat the affected area as a local contraindication. If possible, elevate the affected limb during the massage, which may help reduce swelling. If the client is wearing a cast or splint, do not apply heat to distal areas to prevent swelling.

Once acute inflammation has resolved or entered the subacute phase, local massage can begin. Inquire about sensitivity over affected areas and adjust pressure accordingly. For chronically dislocated joints, avoid traction and PROM, as they have varying degrees of permanent ligament laxity, and may dislocate easily from the externally applied forces.

Fractures

Any crack or break in a bone is called a **fracture**. The highest incidence rates occur in males between the ages of 15 and 24 years and in adults 65 years and older. The number of hip fractures is expected to rise sharply from 1.66 million in 1990 to 6.3 million by the year 2050, mainly due to an increase in the aging population. Pathologic fractures may result in people with osteoporosis from lack of bone density. In fact, if a person with osteoporosis sustains a hip fracture related to a fall, medical experts now believe a spontaneous pathologic fracture was more likely to have caused the fall, rather than vice versa.

Fractures are broadly classified as complete or incomplete and as open or closed. *Complete fractures* occur when the bone breaks all the way through; *incomplete fractures* occur when the bone is damaged but is still in one piece. *Open fractures*, formerly known as compound fractures, describe fractures in which the skin is broken. In *closed fractures*, formerly called simple fractures, the skin over the broken bone is intact.

Massage and Fractures

While the bone is immobilized, treat the affected area as a local contraindication. If on a limb, elevate the affected area to help reduce swelling. Massage proximal to the area to help reduce any edema. If the client is wearing a cast or splint, do not apply heat to distal areas to prevent swelling.

Once healing is complete and bone union has occurred (determined by the healthcare provider), massage of the affected area can begin. Inquire about pressure sensitivity over affected areas and adjust it according to the client's preference. Coexisting medical conditions, such as osteoporosis or cancer, should be factored into the treatment plan.

Ganglion Cyst

A **ganglion cyst** is a fluid-filled pouch that forms on tendons or joints, usually the wrists or hands (90% of cases). Cysts can also develop near other joints, such as the knees, ankles, and feet. The cyst can be single or multiple growths. Ganglion cysts can be small, the size of a pea, or up to an inch (2.5 cm) in diameter. With rest, ganglia tend to decrease in size slightly. Females are more likely to be affected than males (3:1). Ganglia tend to recur after they spontaneously disappear or are treated. A ganglion cyst was previously known as a "Bible bump" because of the once-common treatment of hitting the cyst with a Bible or other large book.

Massage and Ganglion Cyst

Avoid the affected area because pressure may cause the cyst to rupture or cause radial nerve damage (Jin, 2011).

Gout

Gout is arthritis caused by accumulation of uric acid crystals, usually the base of the great toe (first metatarsophalangeal joint). Gout can also occur in other joints, such as the ankles, knees, fingers, wrists, and elbows. Gout typically develops after many years (15 to 30 years) of asymptomatic hyperuricemia. Prevalence rates are 15 to 35 people per 1000. Increased incidence of gout occurs in males, in people with a high body mass index, and in people who consume alcohol regularly. Gout is also called *gouty arthritis* and *metabolic arthritis*. Gout occurs in three stages: (1) asymptomatic hyperuricemia, (2) acute gout, and (3) chronic tophaceous gout. During the acute stage, pain develops suddenly, and the person has difficulty walking. Initial bouts may last a few days and subside spontaneously. Acute episodes may start to occur more frequently, with bouts lasting several weeks, which may signal the transition into chronic gout. During this stage, pain is not as severe, but affected joints become deformed and movement becomes limited. Painless nodules called *tophi* may form in subcutaneous tissues over the ear, extensor surfaces of the arms and feet, and over the Achilles' tendon and patella.

Massage and Gout

Massage is postponed if the client has fever. The client may receive the massage after being fever-free for 24 hours without the use of fever-reducing drugs, such as ibuprofen or acetaminophen (Centers for Disease Control and Prevention [CDC], 2018).

Afterward, the massage can be performed while avoiding affected areas, which is usually the great toe. Avoid traction and PROM on these areas. While the client is prone, use a higher-than-normal (8 inches) bolster in front of the ankles to prevent the affected toe from touching the massage table. While the client is supine, undrape the foot to prevent uncomfortable pressure on the affected toe. Avoid massage over nodules, which can be present in chronic cases. Coexisting conditions (kidney dysfunction) should be factored into the treatment plan.

Hyperkyphosis (Kyphosis)

Hyperkyphosis is an exaggeration of the normal posterior kyphotic curvature in the thoracic spine. A kyphotic curvature is normal (20 to 40 degrees), but hyperkyphosis refers to an excessive rounding of more than 45 to 50 degrees. Hyperkyphosis and hyperlordosis may co-exist. Rounded shoulders and a dowager's hump are sometimes classified as mild forms of hyperkyphosis, the latter being related to osteoporosis.

Hyperkyphosis can cause back pain when lying down, difficulties in breathing, and a reduction of function during activities of daily living, such as getting out of chairs or difficulty looking up while walking and driving. Hyperkyphosis is also called hunchback.

Massage and Hyperkyphosis

Position the client for comfort, which may include the use of a neck pillow while the client is supine or side-lying. While the client is prone, consider placing a pillow or other supportive cushion under the clavicles or upper chest to reduce discomfort in the thoracic spine.

Avoid traction and PROM on the thoracic spine and affected nearby joints. If pain management is a treatment goal, some relief can be gained by massage of the involved muscles, such as pectoralis major and minor, serratus anterior, and rhomboids major and minor. Coexisting medical conditions (osteoporosis, arthritis) should be factored into the treatment plan.

Hyperlordosis (Lordosis)

Hyperlordosis is an exaggeration of the normal anterior lumbar curvature and increased anterior pelvic tilt. A lordotic curvature is normal, but hyperlordosis refers to an excessive curvature. Untreated progressive hyperlordosis can lead to degenerative disc disease or herniated lumbar discs. Hyperlordosis and hyperkyphosis may coexist. Hyperlordosis is also called *swayback* or *saddleback*.

The most common cause of hyperlordosis is postural compensation for increased abdominal mass or girth, such as is seen in advanced pregnancy or obesity. Compensation occurs by unconsciously tightening lower back muscles to maintain balance when standing because the body's center of gravity is altered. Hyperlordosis may accompany spinal injury or diseases such as osteoporosis, or spondylolisthesis. Sometimes the cause is not identified.

Massage and Hyperlordosis

Position the client for comfort, which may include a higher-than-normal (8 inches) bolster behind the knees while the client is supine. This positional modification may reduce an anterior pelvic tilt. While the client is lying prone, consider placing a pillow or other supportive cushion under the abdomen to reduce discomfort in the lumbar spine. Avoid traction and PROM of the lumbar spine and affected nearby joints. If pain management is a treatment goal, some relief can be gained by massage of the involved muscles, such as quadratus lumborum, paraspinals, and gluteals. If the lower extremities are involved, massage the quadriceps, hamstrings, and calf muscles. Coexisting conditions (pregnancy, osteoporosis, spondylolisthesis) should be factored into the treatment plan.

Lyme Disease

Lyme disease is arthritis caused by bacteria and affects joints such as the hip and knee, as well as the skin, the heart, and the nervous system. Lyme disease was first detected in 1975 in Lyme, Connecticut, and has since been reported throughout North America and in other countries. Incidence is currently on the rise. Lyme disease is also called *Lyme arthritis*.

Lyme disease is caused by four species of bacteria. *Borrelia burgdorferi* and *Borrelia mayonii* are the leading causes Lyme disease in the United States. *Borrelia afzelii* and *Borrelia garinii* are the leading causes of Lyme disease in Europe and Asia. The causative bacterium is introduced into the body by a bite of an infected black-legged tick, commonly called a deer tick. The bacteria enter through the skin and then into the bloodstream, then migrate to the joints, lymph nodes, and other parts of the body. The tick is carried by animals, such as deer or mice and in their habitat, which are low bushes and tall grass in wooded areas. These ticks are most active in the summer months. In most cases, transmission occurs only after the tick is attached for long periods of time, from 36 to 48 hours. There is emerging evidence suggesting the causative bacteria may also be transmitted between humans during sexual activity with an infected person.

Massage and Lyme Disease

Massage is postponed if the client is experiencing systemic inflammation indicated by fever. The client may receive the massage after being fever-free for 24 hours without the use of fever-reducing drugs, such as ibuprofen or acetaminophen.

During massage, treat skin lesions and rashes as local contraindications. Avoid traction and PROM on affected joints. Because a person with Lyme disease tends to have recurrent episodes, inquire about symptoms before each massage.

Osgood-Schlatter Disease

Osgood-Schlatter disease is patellar tendinitis at the tibial tuberosity occurring in immature bone. The tibial tuberosity is below the knee. This condition usually occurs in just one knee, but both knees can be affected. It is seen more often in young athletes aged 11 to 14 years who participate in sports involving running, jumping and sudden changes of direction, such as soccer, basketball, volleyball, tennis, and gymnastics. Incidence rates were once higher in males than in females (3:1), but rates are near equal as more females become involved in sports.

Massage and Osgood-Schlatter Disease

If acute inflammation is present, treat the knee area as a local contraindication. Massage can be applied to the thigh area, especially the quadriceps. Massage both the affected and nonaffected side because thigh muscles on the nonaffected side may be tight and sore from overcompensation. Inquire about pressure sensitivity over affected areas and adjust pressure according to the client's preference. Massage the quads with knees flexed as well as extended (use a bolster behind the knees when the client is supine and in front of the ankles when the client is prone). These positions will ensure the quads are massaged in at least two positions (shortened and lengthened). Avoid overstretching the quads on the affected side.

Osteoarthritis and Spondylosis

Osteoarthritis (OA) is age-related arthritis characterized by inflammation of the joint capsule and progressive joint damage, and eventual loss of articular cartilage. OA is the most common form of arthritis and is seen among older adults; OA is almost universal in people older than 75 years. OA most often affects joints of the spine, hands, feet, hips, and knees. OA is also called *degenerative joint disease, degenerative arthritis*, and *wear and tear arthritis*.

Spondylosis is osteoarthritis of the spine, which affects the intervertebral discs and facet joints. Cervical spondylosis affects the neck (the most common type of spondylosis), and lumbar spondylosis affects the lower back.

Both osteoarthritis and spondylosis can lead to the formation of bony projections or bone spurs called *osteophytes* at joint margins. Osteophytes can project into neighboring tissues. If osteophytes press against spinal nerves, the person may experience radicular pain. Osteophytes can cause *spinal stenosis*, the abnormal narrowing of vertebral spaces, such as the central canal and intervertebral foramen. While bone overgrowth from osteophytes is the most common cause of spinal stenosis, it can also be caused by herniated discs, tumors, or spinal injuries.

Massage and Osteoarthritis/Spondylosis

Position the client for comfort. If the client has a contracture of the hand, consider placing a rolled-up washcloth in the palm during the massage to reduce pain and discomfort. Inquire about sensitivity over joints affected by OA and adjust pressure accordingly. Cold or moist heat applications may be used on affected areas to manage pain. The Arthritis Foundation (n.d.) recommends massage therapy to reduce pain and improve function in joints affected by arthritis. Avoid traction and PROM on the spine, hip, and other affected joints.

Osteoporosis

Osteoporosis is loss of normal bone density and increased bone porosity. Bones become brittle and weak, and can be described as compressible, like a sponge rather than dense like a brick; this increases the risk of fractures. A simple task such as bending over and picking up a book can cause a pathologic fracture in people with severe osteoporosis. A *pathologic fracture* is a broken bone caused by disease rather than an injury. Osteoporosis often progresses silently for decades and may not be diagnosed until a fracture occurs. The most common sites of osteoporosis-related fractures are the spine, the proximal femur, and the wrists.

Osteoporosis is the most common bone disease and women account for 80% of osteoporosis cases. A hip fracture is the most debilitating complication of osteoporosis, given that more than half of adults hospitalized for hip fractures do not return to their former level of functioning.

Massage and Osteoporosis

Position the client for comfort, especially in cases of spinal deviations, such as hyperkyphosis. This may include the use of a neck pillow while the client is supine or side-lying. While the client is prone, consider placing a small pillow or other supportive cushion under the clavicles or upper chest to reduce discomfort in the thoracic spine. Research suggests massage using light pressure is best for clients with osteoporosis as they are susceptible to fracture from low-weight external forces (Guo et al., 2013; Jeon et al., 2019). Only gentle PROM, such as mild rocking should be applied to affected areas (i.e., spine, hips, wrists).

Patellofemoral Pain Syndrome and Chondromalacia Patellae

Patellofemoral pain syndrome is pain and stiffness in front or around the patella, or kneecap. It is most commonly seen in young athletes, but it is seen in nonathletes as well. Estimates indicate that 1% to 3% of young athletes experience knee pain, with the most common cause being patellofemoral pain syndrome. Knee pain and stiffness can make climbing stairs, kneeling down, sitting cross-legged, and performing other everyday activities difficult. Patellofemoral pain syndrome is also called *patellofemoral syndrome, jumper's knee,* or *runner's knee.*

Chondromalacia patellae (CMP) is the softening and degeneration of articular cartilage on the posterior patella. Athletes and people who have arthritis or who are obese are at increased risk of CMP. The terms patellofemoral syndrome and chondromalacia patellae are often used interchangeably.

Massage and Patellofemoral Pain Syndrome/ Chondromalacia Patellae

If acute inflammation is present, treat the knee as a local contraindication. Massage can be applied to the thigh area, especially the hamstrings and quadriceps; the latter has the patella embedded in its tendons. Adjust the pressure according to the client's preference. Consider massaging these muscles in both shortened and lengthened positions. Using a bolster behind the knees when the client is supine and in front of the ankles when the client is prone will shorten the hamstrings and lengthen the quads. However, avoid overstretching the quads on the affected side.

Rheumatoid Arthritis and Juvenile Rheumatoid Arthritis

Rheumatoid arthritis (RA) is arthritis caused by an autoimmune response in which the body attacks, inflames, and destroys synovial joint membranes. Over time, joint inflammation spreads throughout the joint capsule, to articular cartilages and surrounding ligaments, then to underlying bone. RA often affects small joints of the fingers first, such as the metacarpophalangeal joints, and then progresses to joints of the wrists and elbows. However, the reverse is also seen. RA may also affect the spine, temporomandibular joints, and hips. RA usually displays bilateral involvement, with a high incidence of crippling deformity. RA also affects structures such as the skin, lungs, heart, and blood vessels. Between 1% and 2% of adults have RA, mostly women (3:1), and it usually strikes in the third or fourth decade of life. However, the incidence increases with age, affecting 5% of adults 70 years and older. The course of disease is marked by exacerbations and remissions. During each period of exacerbation, joint structures are damaged further. Some people experience a single episode and recover spontaneously, but most will have recurrent and persistent bouts.

RA that develops in children and adolescents is called **juvenile rheumatoid arthritis** (JRA). As in adult RA, JRA is marked by periods of exacerbation and remission. When comparing adult RA with JRA, several important differences emerge. Clinical manifestations unique to JRA include large joints being most affected; fusion or ankylosing of cervical spine is common if the disease progresses; joint pain is less severe; and subcutaneous nodules are absent. JRA affects an estimated 250,000 children in the United States, mainly females (4:1). Approximately 75% of cases experience complete remission and only a small number develop severe joint deformity.

Massage and Rheumatoid Arthritis/Juvenile Rheumatoid Arthritis

Avoid areas containing subcutaneous nodules. Vigorous massage is contraindicated during periods of exacerbation. During this time, massage using light pressure can be used. Superficial heat applications (e.g., moist heat packs, paraffin baths) can be used to reduce pain and joint stiffness and should not exceed 15 minutes. Cold applications can be safely used, but most individuals with RA prefer heat. Prolonged deep heat, such as from spa tubs and immersion baths, is contraindicated as these may increase the temperature in joint capsules and possibly contribute to joint damage (Goodman & Fuller, 2017).

Scoliosis

Scoliosis is an abnormal lateral curvature in the normally straight vertical line of the spine, usually in the thoracic region. The lumbar and cervical regions also may be involved. It occurs more frequently in females than in males (5:1). Most cases begin during the growth and development of puberty. The degree of curvature ranges from mild to severe, with some mild cases becoming more severe as the child grows. Severe cases reduce the size of the ribcage and may cause reduced lung capacity. Early detection and intervention are important; screenings are provided in elementary and secondary schools. Part of the screening involves the child leaning forward in front of a healthcare provider. If shoulder elevation is uneven and a hump appears on one side of the back, the child may have scoliosis. Other indicators include an uneven waistline and one scapula more prominent compared with the other. The hip and shoulder alignment is also uneven, with one shoulder and one hip higher than the other (usually on the opposite side). The person may lean to one side and clothes may not fit or hang properly.

Massage and Scoliosis

Experiment with several positional variations using pillows, bolsters, and other supportive cushions to find the position most comfortable for the client. Depending on the severity of the condition, lying prone or supine may be uncomfortable for the client. Clients with scoliosis may prefer a side-lying position with a small pillow placed at the waist. It may be helpful to ask the client about sleeping positions, making appropriate positional modifications when needed. Address tension in back muscles. Avoid traction and PROM of the thoracic spine and affected nearby joints. Coexisting medical conditions (osteoporosis, osteoarthritis) should be factored into the treatment plan.

Spondylolisthesis and Spondylolysis

Spondylolisthesis is an anterior displaced vertebra, usually L4 or L5. Varying degrees of severity have been seen. Spondylolisthesis is classified by the percentage of anterior displacement using the Meyerding system, which ranges from grade I to IV. Grade I is 1% to 25%; Grade II is 26% to 50%; Grade III is 51% to 75%; and Grade IV is 76% to 100%.

Severe cases can result in spinal deformities, such as hyperlordosis or hyperkyphosis (see prior entries). However, most cases of spondylolisthesis are low grade, stable, and asymptomatic. The two most common forms of spondylolisthesis are isthmic and degenerative.

- **Isthmic (spondylolytic) spondylolisthesis**. The most common cause of isthmic spondylolisthesis is **spondylolysis**, a fracture in the pars interarticularis. This thin portion of the lamina is between the superior and inferior articular facets. In many cases, the fracture goes unnoticed into adulthood, and then is found during diagnostic tests for other conditions. Some cases are caused by traumatic injury. This is the most common form in people younger than 65 years.
- **Degenerative spondylolisthesis**. This type of spondylolisthesis is caused by OA in the lumbar spine. Changes within intervertebral discs and spinal ligaments reduce the stability of the lumbar spine, causing the vertebrae to slip forward. Degenerative forms are more likely to occur in females compared to males (3:1). This is more common in adults over age 65 years.

Massage and Spondylolisthesis/Spondylolysis

Position the client for comfort, which may include using a higher-than-normal (8 inches) bolster under the knees while supine or a cushion under the lower abdomen while prone. Use only light pressure over the lumbosacral region. In addition, avoid traction and PROM on the lumbar spine. Coexisting medical conditions (arthritis) should be factored into the treatment plan.

Sprain

A **sprain** is an injury caused by an overstretched or torn ligament. This can happen when a joint is forced into an unnatural or unstable position, such as twisting the ankle or knee. It can also be the result of trauma, such as a motor vehicle accident. Common locations for sprains are the ankle, wrist, elbow, and knee. Sprains can be classified into three grades or degrees of severity: first, second, and third.

- **Grade 1 (1st degree)**. Affected ligaments are overstretched and damaged microscopically but are not torn. The joint is stable, and the person is usually able to move or continue with an activity, but with slight discomfort.
- **Grade 2 (2nd degree)**. Affected ligaments are torn. Swelling is noted, and the surrounding muscles splint to restrict movement. Joint instability is moderate, and the area is painful without movement.
- **Grade 3 (3rd degree)**. Affected ligaments are completely ruptured and swelling is significant. A snapping sound is often heard at the time of injury and there is a palpable depression in the area of the rupture. Joints

are unstable and a piece of the bone may be torn away (avulsion fracture). The person is unable to move or continue with an activity.

Massage and Sprains

While acute inflammation is present, treat the area as a local contraindication. If on a limb, elevate the affected area to help reduce swelling during the massage. If the client is wearing a cast or splint, do not apply heat to distal areas to prevent swelling.

Once acute inflammation has resolved or is in the subacute phase, local massage can begin. Massage, especially friction massage, may promote healing of tendons and ligaments. Inquire about pressure sensitivity over affected areas and adjust it below the client's pain tolerance. Avoid overstretching the injured area.

Temporomandibular Disorders

Temporomandibular disorder (TMD) is a term used to describe a group of conditions that cause pain and dysfunction of the temporomandibular joint (TMJ) and muscles controlling joint movement. Approximately 10 million Americans have some form of TMD. This condition is more common in females than in males. In most cases, TMD is unilateral. Many terms are used to describe TMD, including TMJ syndrome and TMJ disease. However, the term TMD is preferred and recommended by the American Academy of Orofacial Pain (AAOP) and other professionals. The AAOP classifies TMD into two types, myogenic and articular. Occasionally, both types are present simultaneously.

- **Myogenic TMD**. This is the most common form and only involves the masticatory muscles (i.e., masseter, temporalis, medial and lateral pterygoids). Myogenic TMD may be seen in individuals who have myofascial disorders or injuries, such as whiplash-associated disorder.
- **Articular TMD**. This is joint-related and described as an abnormal relationship between the articular discs and the coronoid processes of the mandible.

Massage and Temporomandibular Disorders

Avoid the prone position if it causes the client facial or jaw pain. For myogenic cases of TMD, apply friction massage to the temporalis and masseter muscles, sustained compression on trigger points in the masseter, and skin rolling on the masseter (Miernik et al., 2012). Intraoral friction of the masseter requires the donning and doffing of disposable gloves. Massage to the posterior neck and shoulders may be performed before or after specific TMD massage techniques. Because some cases of TMD are associated with psychosocial stress, massage using techniques that promote relaxation is indicated during the end of the session.

E-RESOURCES

http://evolve.elsevier.com/Salvo/MassageTherapy

- Chapter challenge
- Flash cards

IDA PAULINE ROLF

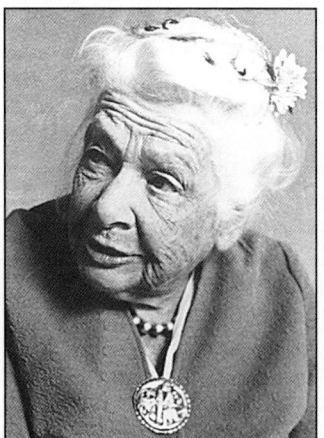

As a well-off woman born in 1896, there were a limited number of appropriate life paths Ida Rolf could reasonably be expected to take. There was getting married. There was... not getting married. There was the possibility of getting some education as well. What could not have been planned for was Rolf came of age in the midst of the First World War, when women began to fill many roles vacated by the young men who left for the battlefields abroad. And so it was that she became a researcher of biochemistry at the Rockefeller Institute, despite opposition from her own family.

Rolf's research led to her earning a PhD in biochemistry from Columbia's College of Physicians and Surgeons in 1920. She continued her research at the Rockefeller Institute after graduating and became an associate there. Always an independent thinker, she investigated fields ranging from mathematics and physics (which she studied at the Swiss Technical Institute) to osteopathy and yoga.

Through her varied studies, Rolf came to believe that bodies in their ideal state were balanced by gravity, but postural dysfunction caused by trauma, poor posture, or imbalanced work caused the body, and particularly the fascia, to work against gravity, expending needless energy and causing ever-increasing structural problems in the various body tissues as the body compensated.

In response to this understanding, Rolf developed a system for manually realigning the connective tissue of the body, gradually going from one section of the body to another and from superficial to deep over a series of sessions. She called this process *structural integration*. Today, structural integration is an umbrella term for a variety of methods sharing the same philosophy, whereas the technique specifically taught by Ida Rolf is called *Rolfing*.

Rolf did not keep this method to herself, but taught it to those who were willing to put in the effort required to learn. She maintained high standards for her students, encouraging them to gain experience and wait until they were extremely competent before considering themselves Rolfers. Although she expected much from her students, she was also committed to making the educational process accessible to them, developing a series of 10 sessions applied by practitioners for a wide variety of physiologic dysfunctions.

Over time, the world began to take more notice of her work, with research on its effectiveness being published in reputable medical journals. Although Ida Rolf passed away in 1979 at the age of 83, her work lives on through the Rolf Institute of Structural Integration, in Boulder, Colorado. The institute not only certifies new Rolfers but also promotes research. There are currently more than 1500 practicing Rolfers, and many more people practicing variations of structural integration have branched off in form but maintain the same basic philosophy about the functioning of the human body.

Rolf's lifelong commitment to independent thought served her well, and today her eponymous technique is used by people ranging from competitive athletes to people who are faced with severe physiologic dysfunction and chronic pain. Although not many know the story of this strong-minded woman, her name lives on in the practitioners who make use of her knowledge and the many clients they serve.

REFERENCES

Arthritis Foundation. (n.d.). *Benefits of massage*. Retrieved from http://www.arthritis.org/living-with-arthritis/treatments/natural/other-therapies/massage/massage-benefits.php.

Brakke, R. (2016). *What is crepitus*? Retrieved from https://www.arthritis-health.com/types/general/what-crepitus.

Centers for Disease Control and Prevention. (2018). *Guidance for school administrators to help reduce the spread of infection*. Retrieved from https://www.cdc.gov/flu/school/guidance.htm

Goodman, C. C., & Fuller, K. S. (2017). *Pathology for the physical therapist assistant* (2nd ed.).. St Louis: Elsevier.

Guo, Z., Chen, W., Su, Y., Yuan, J., & Zhang, Y. (2013). Isolated unilateral vertebral pedicle fracture caused by a back massage in an elderly patient: a case report and literature review. *European Journal of Orthopaedic Surgery and Traumatology,* (Suppl. 2), S149–S153.

Jeon, C. H., Chung, N. S., Lee, H. D., & Won, S. H. (2019). Case report: electrical automated massage chair use can induce osteoporotic vertebral compression fracture. *Osteoporosis International 30*(7), 1533–1536.

Jin, P. L. (2011). Case of radial nerve damage caused by improper massage for ganglion cyst. *Zhongguo Zhen Jiu, 31*(7), 630.

Miernik, M., Wieckiewicz, M., Paradowska, A., Wieckiewicz, W. (2012). Massage therapy in myofascial TMD pain management. *Advances in Clinical and Experimental Medicine, 21*(5), 681–685.

Nelsen, E. (2015). *Why do your knuckles pop*? Retrieved from https://www.youtube.com/watch?v=IjiKUmfaZr4

Ng, A. H., Francis, G. J., Sumler, S. S., Liu, D., & Bruera, E. (2018). The efficacy and safety of massage therapy for cancer inpatients with venous thromboembolism. *Journal of Cancer Research and Clinical Oncology, 7*, 203.

Salvo, S.G. (2022). *Mosby's pathology for massage professionals* (5th ed.). St Louis: Mosby.

BIBLIOGRAPHY

Abrahams, P. H., Spratt, J. D., Loukas, M., & van Schoor, A. N. (2003). *Abrahams' and McMinn's clinical atlas of human anatomy* (8th ed.). St Louis: Elsevier.

Applegate, E. (2010). *The anatomy and physiology learning system* (4th ed.). Philadelphia: Saunders.

Como, D. (Ed.). (2016). *Mosby's dictionary of medicine, nursing, and health professions* (10th ed.). St Louis: Elsevier.

Frazier, M. S., & Drzymkowski, J. W. (2015). *Essentials of human diseases and conditions* (6th ed.). St Louis: Elsevier.

Goodman, C. C., & Fuller, K. S. (2015). *Pathology: Implications for the physical therapist* (4th ed.). St Louis: Elsevier.

Hubert, R. J., & VanMeter, K. C. (2018). *Gould's pathophysiology for the health professions* (6th ed.). Philadelphia: Saunders.

Haubrich, W. S. (2003). *Medical meanings: A glossary of word origins* (2nd ed.). New York: American College of Physicians.

Herlihy, B. (2017). *The human body in health and illness* (6th ed.). St Louis: Saunders.

Huether, S. E., McCance, K. L., & Brashers, V.L. (2019). *Understanding pathophysiology* (7th ed.). St Louis: Mosby.

Marieb, E. N., & Keller, S. M. (2018). *Essentials of human anatomy and physiology* (12th ed.). New York: Benjamin Cummings.

McCance, K. L., & Huether, S. E. (2019). *Pathophysiology: The biological basis for disease in adults and children* (8th ed.). St Louis: Mosby.

Netter, F. H. (2018). *Atlas of human anatomy* (7th ed.). St Louis: Mosby.

Patton, K. T (2019). *Anatomy and physiology* (10th ed.). St Louis: Elsevier.

Patton, K. T., Thibodeau, G. A., & Douglas, M. M. (2012). *Essentials of anatomy and physiology* (4th ed.). New York: Pearson.

Porter, R. S. (2011). *The Merck manual of diagnosis and therapy* (19th ed). Whitehouse Station, NJ: Merck Sharp and Dohme Corp.

Taber, C. W. (2021). *Taber's cyclopedic medical dictionary* (24th ed.). Philadelphia: FA Davis.

REVIEW AND APPLY YOUR KNOWLEDGE

MATCHING ONE: CONCEPT REVIEW

Place the letter of the answer next to the number of the term or phrase that best describes it.

A. Arthrosis
B. Labrum
C. Diaphysis
D. Epiphyses
E. Hyaline
F. Menisci
G. Osteoblasts
H. Osteoclasts
I. Periosteum
J. Red bone marrow
K. Sesamoid
L. Synovial

_____ 1. Cylindrical shaft of a long bone.
_____ 2. Where blood cells are produced, especially in long bones.
_____ 3. Small bones embedded in tendons and ligaments.
_____ 4. Term synonymous with joint.
_____ 5. Joint type containing an external dense fibrous capsule and an internal cavity lined with a fluid-secreting membrane.
_____ 6. Bone-destroying cells.
_____ 7. Type of cartilage covering articular surfaces of bone.
_____ 8. Dense, fibrous sheath surrounding the diaphysis.
_____ 9. Ends of a long bone.
_____ 10. Crescent-shaped fibrocartilage pads in select joints to help irregular bones fit together and move smoothly.
_____ 11. Ring of fibrocartilage around the edge of articular cartilage to increase its surface area.
_____ 12. Bone-forming cells.

MATCHING TWO: CONCEPT REVIEW

Place the letter of the answer next to the number of the term or phrase that best describes it.

A. Adduction
B. Appendicular
C. Axial
D. Ball and socket
E. Bursae
F. Diarthroses
G. Extension
H. Plantar flexion
I. Medullary cavity
J. Saddle
K. Synarthroses
L. Hinge

_____ 1. Flattened saclike structures between ligaments or tendons and bones.
_____ 2. Movement in these joints is not permitted or is extremely limited.
_____ 3. Hollow space within the diaphysis of a long bone.
_____ 4. Skeletal region that includes the skull, vertebral column, sternum, and ribs.
_____ 5. Movement of the ankle so the foot moves inferiorly—toes pointing down.
_____ 6. Uniaxial joints allowing flexion and extension.
_____ 7. Movement toward the midline.
_____ 8. Biaxial joint in the thumb.
_____ 9. Skeletal region that includes bones of the upper and lower extremities and bones of the shoulder and pelvic girdles.
_____ 10. Straightening a joint so the angle between the bones increase.
_____ 11. Joint type resembling synovial joints.
_____ 12. Multiaxial joints in the shoulder and hip.

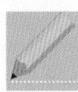

MULTIPLE CHOICE: TEST YOUR KNOWLEDGE

Place the letter of the answer next to the number of the term or phrase that best describes it.

_____ 1. Which of the following is a function of the skeletal system?
A. Temperature regulation
B. Exchange of gases
C. Mineral storage
D. Interpretive functions

_____ 2. What type of cell is responsible for dissolving minerals in bones?
A. Osteoblast
B. Osteoclast
C. Osteocyte
D. Osteophyte

_____ 3. The sternum and scapula are which type of bone?
A. Flat
B. Long
C. Short
D. Sesamoid

_____ 4. Which ankle movement occurs when the foot moves superiorly, and the toes point up?
A. Inversion
B. Pronation
C. Dorsiflexion
D. Supination

_____ 5. Which is a uniaxial joint?
A. Gliding
B. Ball-and-socket
C. Saddle
D. Pivot

_____ 6. What is the process of bone destruction by osteoclasts and bone reformation by osteoblasts?
A. Bone remodeling
B. Crepitus
C. Bone deviation
D. Ossification

_____ 7. A conical movement in which one end of the body is relatively fixed and the other end moves in a circle is:
A. rotation
B. circumduction
C. pronation
D. supination

_____ 8. Which is movement away from the midline?
A. Adduction
B. Abduction
C. Protraction
D. Opposition

_____ 9. Adhesive capsulitis is a condition also known as:
A. frozen shoulder
B. Bible bump
C. swayback
D. Still disease

_____ 10. A temporary displacement of the bones within a joint with complete loss of contact between articulating surfaces is a:
A. sprain
B. dislocation
C. strain
D. contracture

_____ 11. Abnormal lateral curvature in the vertical line of the spine is:
A. hyperkyphosis
B. hyperlordosis
C. spondylolysis
D. scoliosis

_____ 12. An injury caused by an overstretched or torn ligament is a:
A. fracture
B. sprain
C. strain
D. contracture

CRITICALTHINKING

What Do You Really Know?

All you know about your next massage client is that she is female and 76 years old. What ways do you think you might need to modify the massage for her? What is the best source of information for you to design a client-centered treatment?

Answers can include but are not limited to:

There is a possibility because the client is female and in her 70s she has osteoporosis and/or osteoarthritis. Osteoporosis requires modification in the application of pressure. Osteoarthritis requires modifications for joint mobilizations, or they may be contraindicated all together. However, it is important not to assume that the client is frail because of her age. She may be very active, she could lift weights, or she could run marathons. The best source of information to design a client-centered treatment is the client herself. Having access to a thorough health history is important, as well as asking the client about her levels of activity, medications she may be taking, and how she is feeling. These are the foundations of an individualized massage treatment.

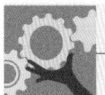

PROFESSIONAL PRACTICE

Rheumatoid Arthritis

Betty is a 52-year-old woman who was diagnosed with rheumatoid arthritis 10 years ago. Her hands are deformed, and she experiences periods in which joints in her hands are warm, swollen, and tender to the touch. During this time, hand movements are painful. Because of inactivity during these times, she has lost overall muscle strength; her leg muscles show evidence of sarcopenia. To help slow disease progression, Betty began taking corticosteroids. Betty has scheduled a massage appointment with you on Tuesday. How should you proceed? What are appropriate modifications you might implement for her? What home self-care would you suggest, if any?

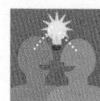

DISCUSSION

Hip Replacement Surgery

Many clients with osteoarthritis will undergo surgery to replace damaged joints. The most common joint replaced is the hip joint. Use an online search engine to locate a video on the surgical procedure (an animated video is recommended). After viewing, list at least two considerations you would apply to a client who had surgery (1) 1 month ago and (2) 1 year ago. List your rationale for each consideration. If available, post your list on an Internet-based discussion board monitored by your instructor. Allow your list to be vetted by classmates. After it is fully vetted, post your revised list.

CHAPTER 20

Muscular System, Pathologies, Disorders, and Injuries

If there is one door in the castle you have been told not to go through, you must. Otherwise, you'll just be rearranging furniture in rooms you've already been in.

—Anne Lamott

LEARNING OBJECTIVES

After completing this chapter, the student should be able to:

1. List anatomic structures and physiologic processes related to the muscular system and describe muscle fibers, connective tissues, and muscles.
2. Explain mechanisms involved in muscle contraction.
3. Classify muscles by their lever system, their shape, their actions, and how many joints they cross.
4. Describe muscular pathologies, disorders, and injuries and state their massage modifications.

INTRODUCTION

The thought of being alive brings to the forefront ideas of movement—heartbeat, facial expressions, and rise and fall of the chest with each breath. These visible signs of life are produced by muscle contractions. Years ago, physiologists believed skeletal muscles contracted by folding, similar to an accordion, or by changes in the diameter of each cell. Some researchers hypothesized muscles grew or perhaps moved the way springs move. In 1969, Hugh Huxley, a British biologist, discovered that muscle contraction does not occur by folding or springing. Shortening or lengthening of a muscle occurs from changes in the relative positions of one small part of a muscle cell to another.

This chapter examines one of the largest systems of the body—the muscular system, which provides body movement. We will explore muscle cells and how they contract. We will discuss types of muscles and how they arrange themselves to perform specific functions. Attributes of individual muscles, such as origins and insertions, as well as their specific actions, are discussed in Chapter 21. *Myology* is the study of the muscular system. The muscular system is important for massage practitioners to understand, and this system is key to learning kinesiology; practitioners will likely see clients with muscular pathologies, disorders, and injuries.

ANATOMY

Basic anatomy of the muscular system includes:
* Skeletal muscles—including associated structures such as tendons and aponeuroses
* Related deep fascial structures

PHYSIOLOGY

Important functions of skeletal muscles are:
* Movement—Skeletal muscles contract to pull on bones, producing movement. There are approximately 640 skeletal muscles in the body. Contraction of skeletal muscles also facilitates the movement of blood and lymph.
* Posture maintenance—**Posture** refers to positions of the body, such as standing and sitting, over a base of support. These positions are maintained by a skeletal framework and muscle tone. **Muscle tone**, or *tonus,* is continuous and partial muscle contraction even while muscles are at rest. For instance, muscles can maintain a stationary position while standing by, contracting continuously. Muscle tone is mediated by receptors called muscle spindles (see Chapter 23). Although we can exert conscious control over our posture, many postural changes are unconscious. *Stance* is a deliberate or particular way of standing (e.g., foot stance).
* Heat production—Muscle contractions produce heat. Skeletal muscles are the most metabolically active structures in the body and produce a significant amount of heat. This mechanism is called **thermogenesis** and is important for maintaining body temperature. In addition, when the body becomes chilled, skeletal muscles contract rapidly (i.e., shivering) to produce additional heat.

MUSCLE FIBERS, CONNECTIVE TISSUES, AND SKELETAL MUSCLES

Skeletal muscles are groups of contractile tissue surrounded by connective tissue, attached to bones, and can produce movement at joints. Skeletal muscles are the organs of the muscular system. Each organ consists of skeletal muscle tissue, connective tissue, nerve tissue, and vascular tissue. See Table 20.1 to help you understand terms of the muscular system. Many parts of a muscle contain the word stem *sarco-*, which means "flesh," to indicate their association with muscle cells. For example, *sarcolemma* is the cell membrane, *sarcoplasm* is the cytoplasm, and *sarcoplasmic reticulum* is the endoplasmic reticulum.

Muscle Fibers

Muscle tissue is composed of muscle cells called **muscle fibers.** They are called muscle fibers because of their threadlike shape, which often runs the length of the entire muscle. Muscle fibers possess unique characteristics compared with other cells, such as numerous mitochondria and nuclei (the latter is on the periphery). Furthermore, muscle fibers possess properties of excitability, contractility, extensibility, and elasticity.
* **Excitability.** The ability to respond to a stimulus, usually a motor neuron.
* **Contractility.** The ability to shorten. For example, to flex the elbow, the biceps muscle must contract.

TABLE 20.1 Word Meanings

WORD	MEANING
antagonist	*Gr.* to struggle against
aponeurosis	*Gr.* to become; sinew
atrophy	*Gr.* lacking, without, not; to grow
concentric	*L.* toward the middle
eccentric	*Gr.* away from the middle
fatigue	*L.* to tire
fascia	*L.* strong central structural unit or band
fascicle	*L.* little bundle
flaccid	*L.* flabby
Golgi tendon organs	Golgi, Italian histologist (1844–1926)
hypertrophy	*Gr.* over, above, excessive; to grow
isometric	*Gr.* same or equal measure
isotonic	*Gr.* same or equal tension
myo	*Gr.* muscle
pennate	*L.* feather
retinaculum	*L.* to retain
sarco	*Gr.* flesh
spasm	*Gr.* a convulsion
synergist	*Gr.* together, work
tendon	*L.* to stretch

Gr., Greek; *L.,* Latin

- **Extensibility.** The ability to lengthen or stretch. For example, as the triceps muscle must extend for the bicep muscle to contract and flex the elbow. Lack of muscle extensibility is called *spasticity*.
- **Elasticity.** The ability to return to a precontraction after lengthening or stretching.

Groups of muscle fibers bundled together within a muscle are called **fasciculi** (fascicle, *singular*). Parts of a muscle fiber are presented next.

Sarcolemma

Sarcolemma is the cell membrane. Folds in the sarcolemma, called **motor end plates,** contain receptors for **acetylcholine** (ACH), the neurotransmitter involved in muscle contraction. This process is discussed in the section titled "Muscle Contraction."

Sarcoplasm

Sarcoplasm is intracellular fluid and is equivalent to cytoplasm in typical cells.

Myofibrils, Sarcomeres, and Filaments

Myofibrils are the slender fibers that contain repeating compartments called sarcomeres. **Sarcomeres** are the structural units of muscle contraction. The end of a sarcomere is called a *Z line* or *Z disc*. Z lines are named because of their jagged appearance (from the German "Zwischenscheibe").

Sarcomeres contain thin and thick strands called **filaments** (myofilaments). There are two types of filaments arranged in alternating parallel rows. This arrangement gives skeletal muscles a striped or striated appearance. Hence, skeletal muscle is also called *striated muscle*. A cross-section view of a sarcomere with its thick and thin filaments looks like a honeycomb (Fig. 20.1). ***LEARNING TIP:*** To help remember the names of the filaments, myosin, the thick filament, is the "thicker" or longer word, and actin, the thin filament, is a "thinner" or shorter word.

- **Thin Filaments.** These are made of three proteins: *actin, tropomyosin,* and *troponin.* Actin is strung together like a twisted double-strand of beads. Thin filaments are

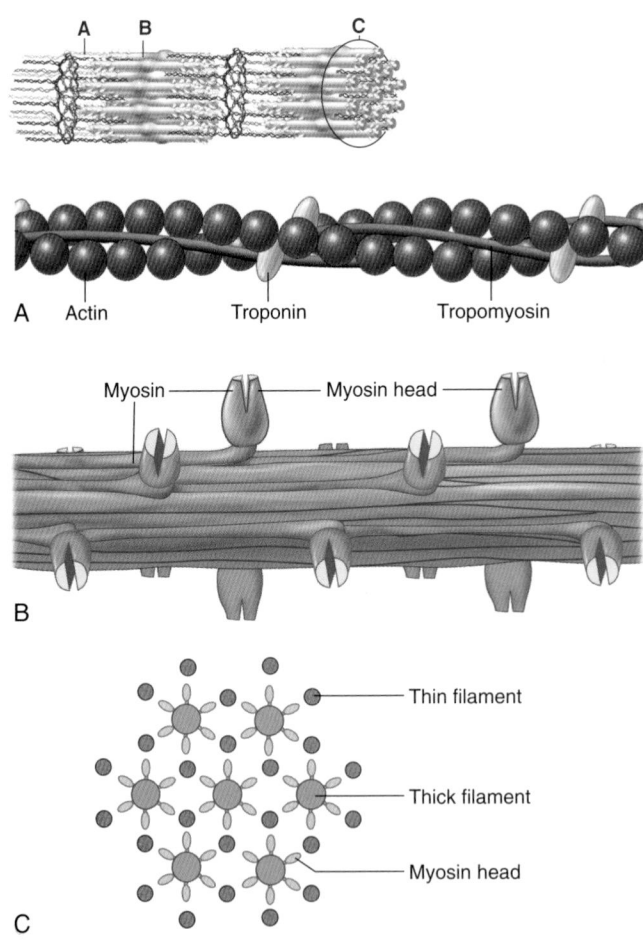

FIG. 20.1 Filaments within the sarcomere. (A) Thin filaments made up of three proteins: actin, tropomyosin, and troponin. (B) Thick filaments are entirely myosin. Myosin heads stick out from bundles and angle toward the thin filaments. (C) Cross-section view of a sarcomere to show relative positions of thin and thick filaments and the myosin heads. Sarcomeres are stacked in a honeycomb arrangement. (From Patton, K. T., & Thibodeau, G. A. [2010]. *Anatomy & physiology* [7th ed.]. St. Louis, MO: Mosby.)

attached to Z lines and extend toward the center of the sarcomere.

- **Thick Filaments.** These contain proteins called *myosin,* which "motors" the contraction of muscle fibers. Myosin is in the center of the sarcomere and is not attached to the Z lines. Myosin is shaped like golf clubs with shafts of the clubs bundled together. Myosin heads stick out from the bundles and angle toward thin filaments (see Fig. 20.1B).

Bands, Lines, and Zones in Sarcomeres

Sarcomeres contain bands, lines, and zones. **I bands** are the combined thin filaments and Z lines. **Z lines** are the borders of each sarcomere, mentioned previously. **H zone** is the center of a sarcomere containing only thick filaments. **A bands** run the entire length of thick filaments and includes the H zone (see Fig. 20.5).

Sarcoplasmic Reticulum

The **sarcoplasmic reticulum** (SR) is a system of interconnected hollow tubes surrounding myofibrils. The SR stores and releases calcium (Ca) and plays a role in muscle contraction. The SR contains extensions called **transverse tubules,** or "T tubules," which branch out to all parts of the muscle fiber. They are called *transverse* because they are positioned transversely across the SR (Fig. 20.2). This arrangement allows for synchronous contraction of the entire muscle fiber despite that the signal to contract is transmitted along the muscle fibers' exterior or sarcolemma.

Connective Tissues

Connective tissues surround muscle fibers, muscles, anchor muscles to bones, and stabilize their tendons (Fig. 20.3). The connective tissue layers that help define parts of a muscle (e.g., muscle, fascicle, fiber) are presented next.

- **Epimysium.** This thick outer layer of connective tissue surrounds the entire muscle or muscle group (i.e., quadriceps), which allows it to contract while maintaining structural integrity. Epimysium is also called *deep fascia* and is continuous with superficial fascia found under the skin.
- **Perimysium.** The middle connective tissue layer surrounds each fascicle. This arrangement allows the nervous system to produce specific movements by activating only part of a muscle. Perimysium also provides both vascularization and innervation of the muscle.
- **Endomysium.** The thin inner layer of connective tissue surrounds individual muscle fibers within the fascicle and lies against the sarcolemma. The endomysium is the first link in the transference of force or pull on tendons, and ultimately bone, to produce movement.

Tendons are dense bands of connective tissue that attach muscles and muscle groups to bones. The function of tendons is to move the attached bone. **Aponeurosis** is a broad, flat tendon that attaches muscles to bone, muscles to other muscles, or muscles to superficial fascia under the skin. Tendons and aponeuroses serve the same function and differ only in shape—tendons are cord-like, and aponeuroses are flat. Tendons in the wrists and ankles are surrounded by synovial sheaths to increase their gliding capacity during contraction.

Retinaculum is a band of connective tissue surrounding tendons to help keep them in place. It is not part of muscle. The function of retinaculum is to stabilize tendons; they may also function as pulleys. Retinacula are found primarily around the elbows, knees, ankles, and wrists.

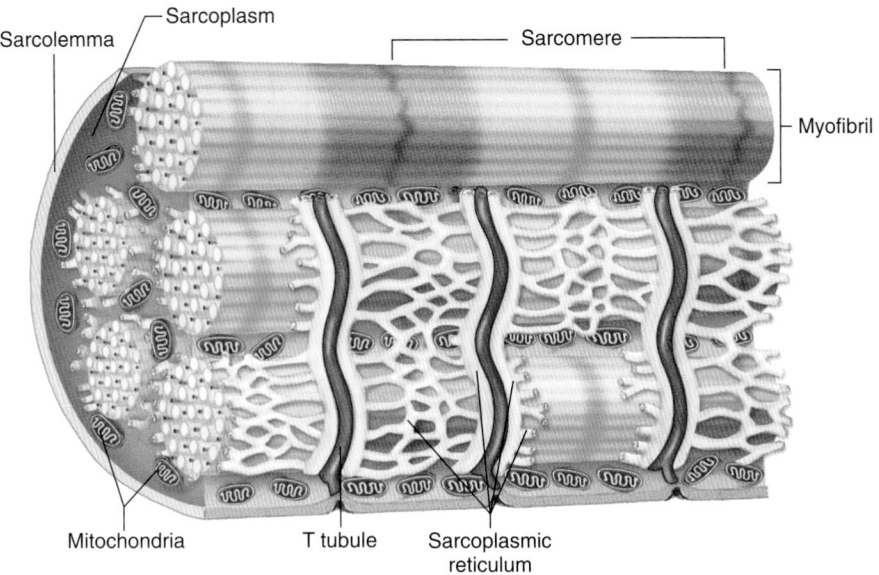

FIG. 20.2 Muscle fiber. Muscle fibers are encased by the sarcolemma (*cross-section view*). The sarcoplasmic reticulum and their transverse or T tubules surround the myofibrils and helps transport the nerve impulse into the muscle fiber. (From Patton, K., & Thibodeau, G. [2014]. *The human body in health and disease* [6th ed.]. St. Louis, MO: Mosby.)

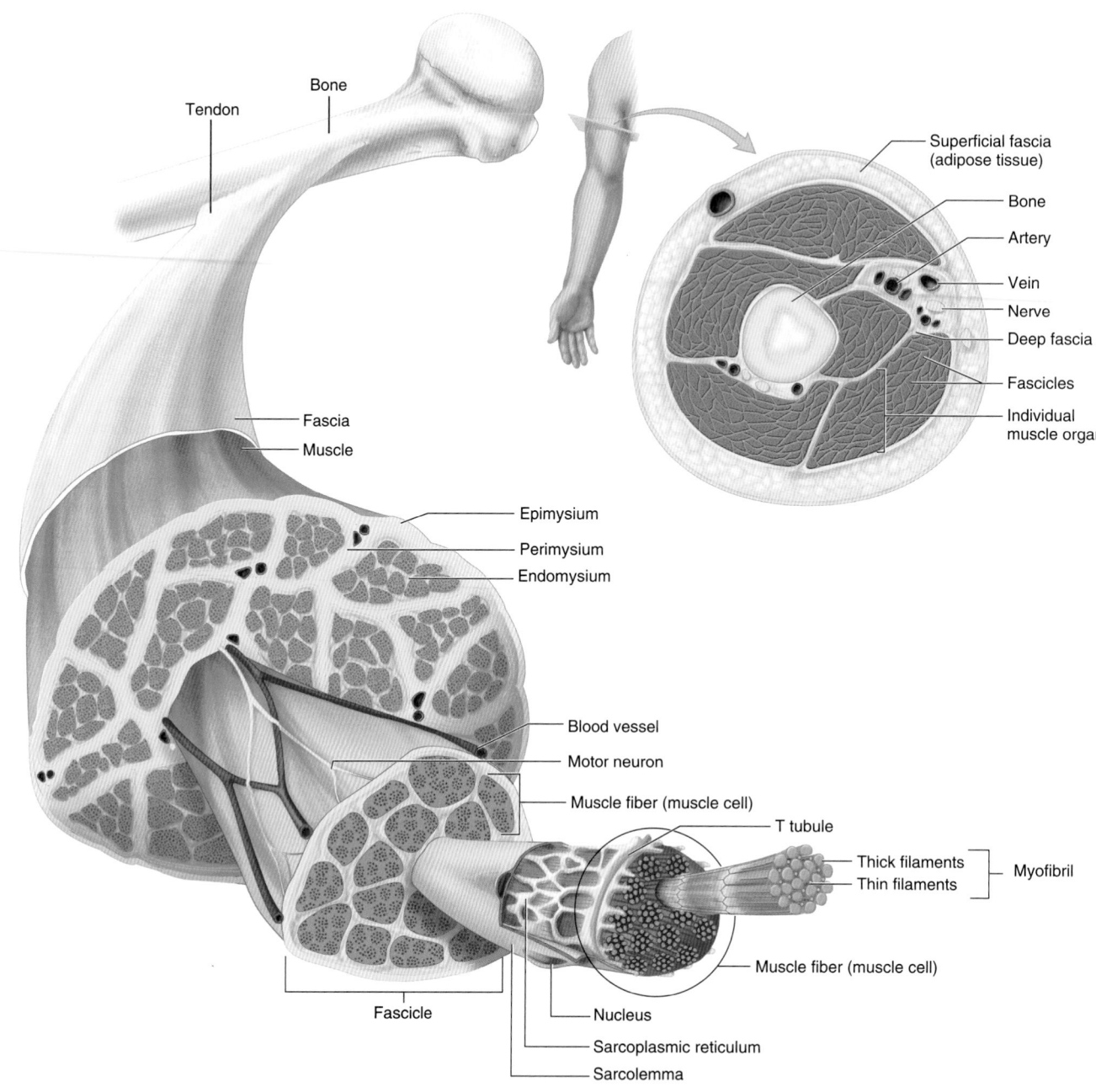

FIG. 20.3 Skeletal muscle anatomy, from muscle organs, to fascicles, to muscle fibers, to myofibrils (*left image*). Cross-section view of the midarm with structures labeled (*right image*). (From Patton, K., & Thibodeau, G. [2014]. *The human body in health and disease* [6th ed.]. St. Louis, MO: Mosby.)

Parts of a Skeletal Muscle

Skeletal muscles cross at least one joint and attach to at least two adjacent bones or other structures. To generate movement, sarcomeres in the wide central portion of the muscle, or muscle **belly,** change the length of the muscle, and cause tendons to move bones at their associated joints (Fig. 20.4).

Muscle attachments are classified functionally by what the bone is doing, or not doing, during movement. **Origins** are the attachments on the less movable bone or bone that remains inactive during contraction. Origins are usually more medially or proximally compared with insertions. For these reasons, origins are sometimes referred to as *proximal attachments*. Origins also tend to be larger, more extensive, and are red when featured on skeletons in classrooms and textbooks.

Insertions are the attachments on the bone that move during contraction. Insertions are usually more laterally or distally compared with origins. For these reasons, insertions are sometimes referred to as *distal attachments*. Insertions also tend to be smaller and are blue when featured on skeletons in

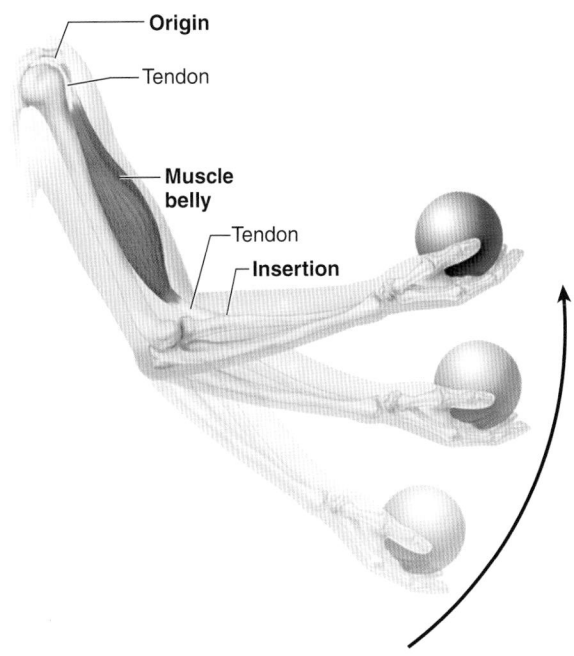

FIG. 20.4 Parts of a skeletal muscle. Origin, belly, and insertion. The insertion moves toward the origin as the biceps brachii shortens to flex the elbow (*posterior view*). (From Patton, K., & Thibodeau, G. [2014]. *The human body in health and disease* [6th ed.]. St. Louis, MO: Mosby.)

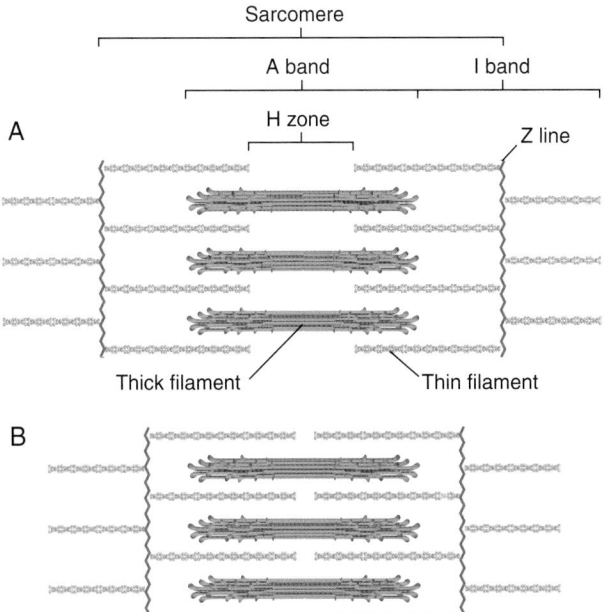

FIG. 20.5 The sliding filament model. (A) The I band and H zone are relatively wide when the muscle is not shortened. (B) Contracting muscle fiber. Actin and myosin filaments slide past one another; the filaments themselves do not become shorter. The Z lines are pulled closer to the center of the sarcomere, which shortens it. (Modified from Kirov, E. [2022]. *Herlihy's the human body in health and illness* [1st ANZ ed.]. Sydney, Australia: Elsevier.)

classrooms and textbooks. Insertions usually move toward origins (see Fig. 20.4). However, the opposite can occur.

Functional reversibility occurs when muscles reverse their relationship between attachment sites—origins move toward their insertions. For example, trapezius has its origins on the spine and the skull, and its insertions are on the scapula. Actions of trapezius include movements of both the skull and the scapula. Thus, the terms origin and insertion are helpful, but they do not always provide the information needed to ascertain a muscle's action. Specific actions of skeletal muscles are in Chapter 21.

To review, the progression from macroscopic structures to microscopic structures are:

Muscle → fascicle → musclefiber → myofibril
→ sarcomere → filaments

MUSCLE CONTRACTION

As stated previously, muscle fibers have properties of excitation, contraction, extensibility, and elasticity. These properties allow muscles to shorten and lengthen and move the body. **Muscle contraction** is the development of tension in muscle fibers through cross bridging. **Cross bridging** is the cycle that begins with excitation by a motor neuron, which causes the thick filaments to cross and bridge the gap between them and the thin filaments. Once this occurs, thick filaments attach and slide the thin filaments toward the center of the sarcomere, shortening the I bands and the H zones, and pulling the Z lines closer together; the filaments themselves

do not become shorter (Fig. 20.5). This sliding causes the muscle to move and later return to their original length. The schema used to describe this process is the *sliding filament model*. The neuromuscular junction facilities excitation and is discussed next.

Neuromuscular Junction

The **neuromuscular junction** is the synaptic connection between a motor neuron and a muscle fiber. This is where the nervous system transmits signals to the muscular system. The neuromuscular junction has three main parts (Fig. 20.6).

- **Motor Neuron.** This presynaptic structure transmits impulses from the nervous system to muscle fibers. Synaptic vesicles at terminal ends of the motor neuron are filled with ACH, the neurotransmitter involved in muscle contraction.
- **Synaptic Gap (Synapse).** The space between the motor neuron and the motor end plate. When activated, ACH is released from the motor neuron's synaptic vesicles, crosses the synaptic gap, and attaches to receptor sites on the motor end plate.
- **Motor End Plate.** This postsynaptic structure involves folded sections of the sarcolemma. The motor end plate contains receptor sites for ACH released by the motor neuron.

Excitation of the Motor End Plate

The binding of ACH to receptor sites on the motor end plate causes excitation of the muscle fiber. The impulse travels

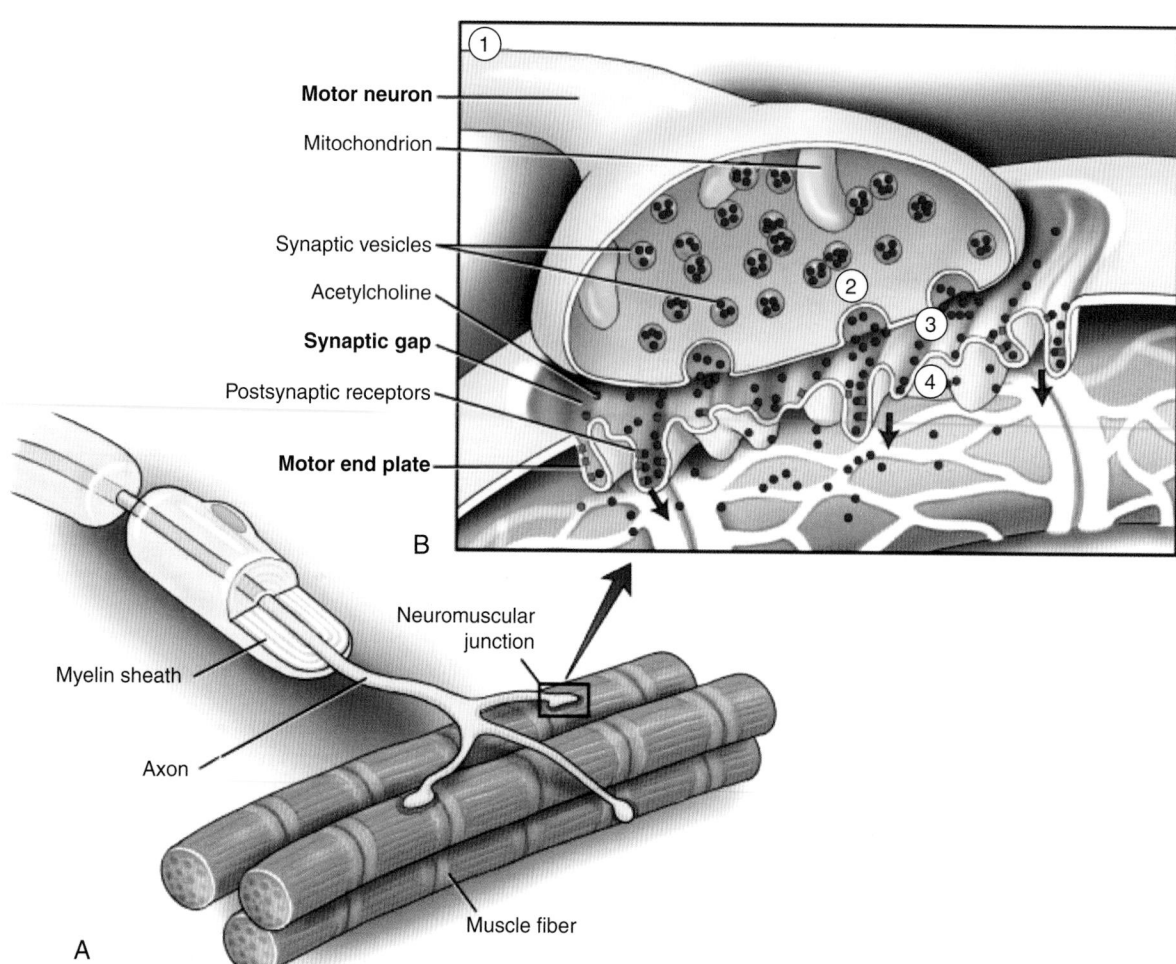

FIG. 20.6 Neuromuscular junction and motor unit. (A) The motor unit which is a single motor neuron and all the muscle fibers it innervates. (B) The neuromuscular junction (motor neuron, synaptic gap, motor end plate) and steps involved in the transfer of information at the neuromuscular junction. (1) The impulse travels down the motor neuron, causing the release of acetylcholine by the synaptic vesicles (2). Acetylcholine crosses the synaptic gap (3) and attaches to receptor sites on the motor end plate (4). (Modified from Kirov, E. [2022]. *Herlihy's the human body in health and illness* [1st ANZ ed.]. Sydney, Australia: Elsevier.)

through the T tubules into the SR, which causes Ca to be released into the sarcoplasm containing sarcomeres (see Fig. 20.6).

Contraction

Muscle contraction occurs when myosin heads bind to actin, causing the thin filaments to slide past the thick filaments. This sliding only happens in the presence of calcium. Myosin is chemically attracted to actin. Troponin and tropomyosin are regulatory proteins, which cover actin's binding sites and prevent myosin from attaching. When Ca enters the sarcomere, troponin and tropomyosin become displaced and expose the binding sites on actin and allow cross bridging. Myosin heads are hinged at their base and, once the binding sites are exposed, myosin attached to actin and slides it toward the center of the sarcomere, or H zone. This action is called the *power stroke* (Fig. 20.7). If adenosine triphosphate

(ATP) is present, myosin heads detach from actin, toggle back to their original position, then attach to the next exposed binding site on actin and repeat the power stroke. As a reminder, ATP is made by the cell's mitochondria and is the cell's energy molecule that prepares myosin for the next power stroke. Power strokes will continue if Ca is present. Events involved in contraction take just a few thousandths of a second. Excitation of the motor end plate and contraction are often called *excitation-contraction coupling*.

Relaxation

Almost immediately after the SR releases Ca into the sarcoplasm, it is actively pumped back into the SR. Within a few milliseconds, much of the Ca is recovered. Freed from its Ca bonds, troponin and tropomyosin slide back and cover the actin's binding sites. This action causes myosin heads to return to their precontraction state. The muscle is now at rest.

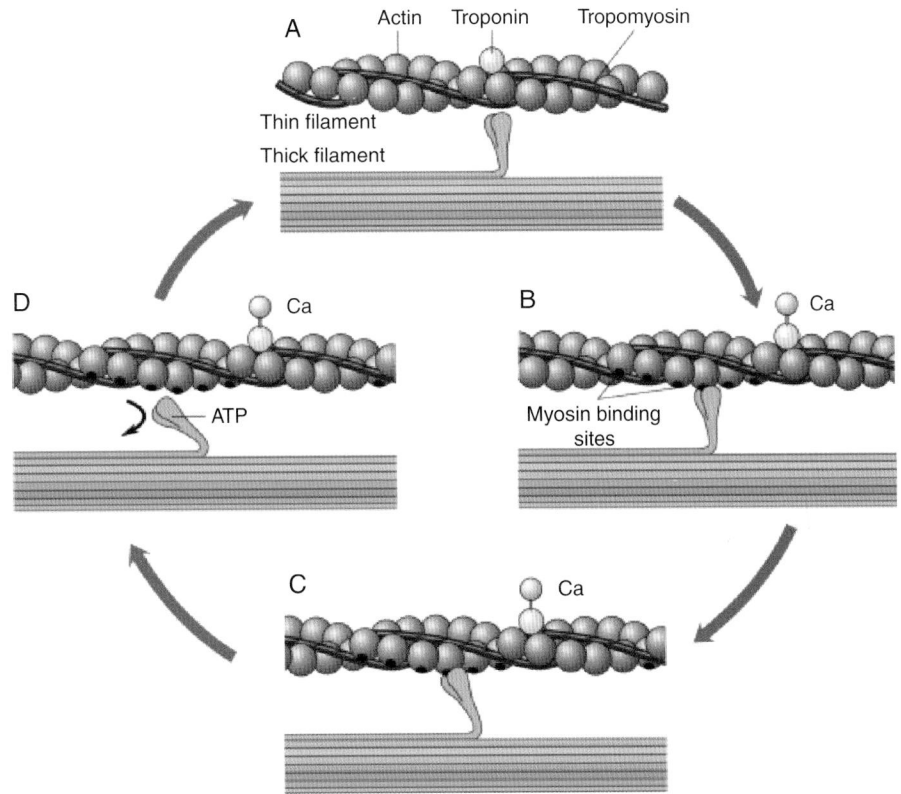

FIG. 20.7 Muscle contraction. (A) The muscle is resting, and actin's binding sites are covered by tropomyosin. (B) During contraction, Ca is released from the sarcoplasmic reticulum, causing tropomyosin to move and expose the binding sites on actin. Myosin can now bind to actin, forming a cross-bridge. (C) Myosin's power stroke causes the thin filament to slide and the sarcomere to shorten. (D) If adenosine triphosphate is present, myosin detaches, toggles back, and can reattach to the next binding site along actin if Ca is present. (Modified from Kirov, E. [2022]. *Herlihy's the human body in health and illness* [1st ANZ ed.]. Sydney, Australia: Elsevier.)

Motor Units, All-or-None Law, and Recruitment

Muscles can contain thousands of muscle fibers and are innervated by many motor neurons. These structures form functional groups called *motor units.* A **motor unit** is a single motor neuron and all muscle fibers it innervates (see Fig. 20.6A). A motor neuron may branch off and connect to anywhere between 2 and 2000 individual muscle fibers.

When a motor neuron transmits a nerve impulse, all muscle fibers within the motor unit receive the impulse to contract. The muscle fiber will contract to its fullest ability, or it will not contract at all—there are no partial contractions. Conversely, if a muscle fiber fails to receive a stimulus, it will not contract, and the muscle fiber will remain at its resting length. This principle is known as the **all-or-none law** or the *all-or-none response.*

The all-or-none law is true only for motor units, not the entire muscle. There are many motor units linked to a single skeletal muscle. The nervous system regulates the amount of muscular contraction by activating only the motor units needed to perform a given action. If more force is required, additional motor units are recruited. For example, more motor units are needed to pick up a book compared with a pencil. The process of motor unit activation based on need is known as **recruitment.**

> *All of us invent ourselves. Some of us have more imagination than others.*
>
> ~ **Cher**

Energy Sources for Muscle Contraction

The main sources of energy for muscle contraction are ATP, glucose, and oxygen. ATP is the cell's energy molecule and is produced by mitochondria. The more mitochondria a muscle fiber has, the more ATP it can produce and the more performance it can provide. Muscle fibers can even produce more mitochondria when needed to facilitate periods of physical activity. This partly explains how some people who initially can barely run a quarter of a mile can train to run marathons.

Besides ATP, contractions require glucose and oxygen. During rest, oxygen is stored in myoglobin within the sarcoplasm. **Myoglobin** is a red respiratory pigment similar to hemoglobin in red blood cells—they both store oxygen. When oxygen decreases rapidly, as it does during prolonged physical activity, oxygen is quickly replenished by myoglobin.

Concentration of ATP in muscle is typically low because the ATP produced during contraction is used up rapidly. To produce more ATP, the body breaks down glucose. If there is plenty of glucose in the blood, muscles have a readily available supply. Excess glucose is stored as glycogen predominantly in liver and muscle cells. When blood glucose levels are low and ATP is still needed, muscles can convert glycogen to glucose. The breakdown of glucose, or *glycolysis,* occurs in two stages.

The first stage is *anaerobic glycolysis* because oxygen is not used. It begins when muscles start contracting. Anaerobic glycolysis does not contribute a large amount of energy (the equivalent of two ATP molecules), and its contribution is brief (30 to 60 seconds). Lactic acid forms as a byproduct of anaerobic glycolysis. Some lactic acid diffuses into the blood, returns to the liver, and is converted back to glycogen. This process is one reason why a person may continue to breathe heavily after physical activity. We must repay the *oxygen debt* by using oxygen gained by heavy breathing to process the lactic acid.

The next stage is *aerobic glycolysis* because oxygen is used to produce energy. This process creates the equivalent of 36 ATP molecules. Oxygen is delivered and carbon dioxide is expelled by muscle fibers through mitochondrial cellular respiration (see Chapter 18). Aerobic glycolysis continues as long as oxygen is available.

Muscle fatigue is the decline in muscle's ability to generate force. This occurs when nerve impulses are no longer generated, or when muscles run out of ATP, glucose, or oxygen. In comparison, **delayed-onset muscle soreness** (DOMS) is caused by temporary muscle damage and inflammation, usually starting on the day following the physical activity. It usually peaks within 48 hours.

Types of Skeletal Muscle Contractions

Muscle contractions can be classified by whether muscle length changes or remains unchanged and if they shorten or lengthen during contractions (Fig. 20.8).

- **Isotonic Contractions.** During isotonic contractions, muscle length changes. Because isotonic contractions

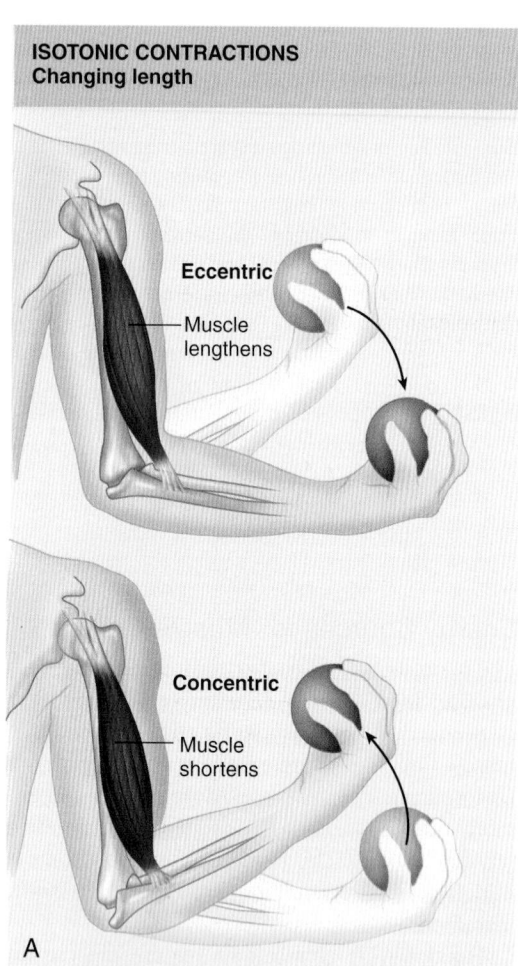

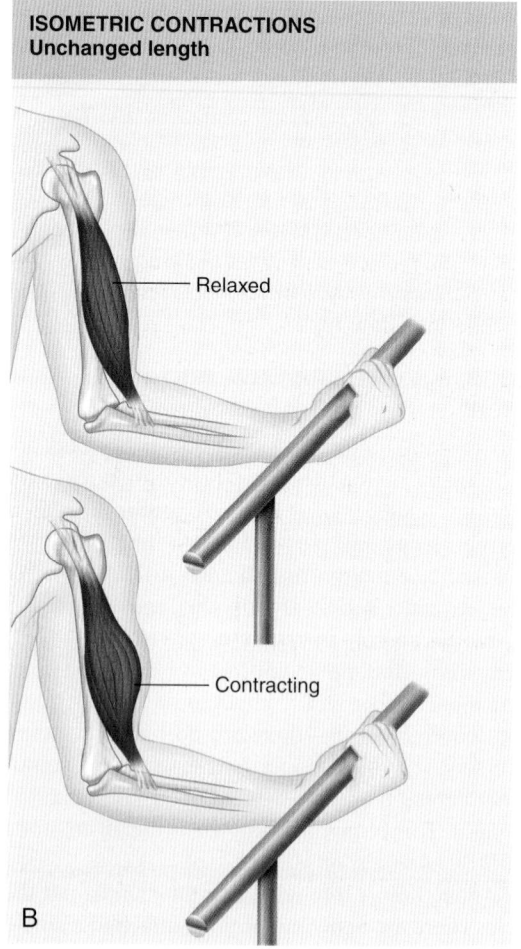

FIG. 20.8 Isotonic and isometric muscle contractions. (A) Isotonic contraction of eccentric (muscle lengthens) and concentric (muscles shortens) contractions. (B) Isometric contraction is where muscle length remains unchanged, and movement does not occur after contraction (*anterior views*). (From Patton, K., & Thibodeau, G. [2014]. *The human body in health and disease* [6th ed.]. St. Louis, MO: Mosby.)

involve movement, they are also called *dynamic contractions*. Isotonic contractions can be subclassified as concentric or eccentric contractions.

- **Concentric Contractions.** Muscles shorten during concentric contractions. Examples of concentric contractions are shortening of biceps brachii during elbow flexion or shortening of quadriceps femoris during knee extension.
- **Eccentric Contractions.** Muscles lengthen during eccentric contractions. Eccentric contractions oppose concentric contractions and serve to control movements and protect joints. Examples of eccentric contractions are the lengthening of biceps brachii during the lowering phase of biceps curls or the lengthening of quadriceps femoris during the lowering phase of knee extension. DOMS is thought to be caused by eccentric (lengthening) contractions, which create microtrauma in muscle fibers.

Isometric Contractions. During isometric contractions, muscle length remains the same and movement does not occur (see Fig. 20.8B). Isometric contractions are those that hold some yoga poses in stationary positions. Isometric contractions often occur in fixators or stabilizers because they stabilize joints so primary muscles (called *agonists and synergists*) can perform the desired action. Because isometric contractions do not involve movement, they are also called *static contractions*.

Types of Muscle Fibers

Muscle fibers were initially classified as fast twitch or slow twitch based on their speed of contraction. This division also corresponds to their structural differences, with fast twitch appearing white and slow twitch appearing red. These discoveries led to the current typing of muscle fibers; type 1 and type 2 are described next.

- **Type 1 (Red or Slow Twitch).** Type 1 contains large amounts of myoglobin and mitochondria, and many blood capillaries. Because of these characteristics, they have a redder color. They also have a greater capacity for slow or sustained contraction and take longer to fatigue (Table 20.2). Most *postural* or *core muscles* are type 1. Marathon runners tend to have more slow twitch muscles in their lower extremities compared to other athletes.

- **Type 2 (White or Fast Twitch).** Type 2 contains fewer myoglobin, mitochondria, and blood capillaries compared with Type 1. Because of these characteristics, they are lighter in color. They are also more suited for movement, contract faster, for shorter periods of time, and they fatigue more quickly. Most *phasic* or dynamic muscles are type 2. Sprinters and tennis players tend to have more fast twitch muscles in their lower extremities compared to other athletes.

Postural and Phasic Muscles

The terms postural and phasic describes muscles by their function and was first used by Janda (1983). **Postural muscles** are involved in maintaining an upright posture (e.g. spinal and calf muscles), while **phasic muscles** are responsible for movement (e.g. glutes and shoulder muscles). Postural muscles tend to shorten and tighten in response to overuse, underuse or trauma, whereas phasic muscles tend to lengthen and weaken in response to these types of stimuli.

CLASSIFYING MUSCLES BY LEVERS, SHAPES, ACTIONS, AND JOINTS

Muscles can be classified by the lever system they use to produce movement, by their shape, the actions they provide, or the number of joints they cross.

Classifying Muscles by Lever

Skeletal muscle movements usually involve leverage, or using a lever to move an object. A lever is a rigid bar that moves on a fixed point called the *fulcrum* when force is applied. Muscles, bones, and joints work together to create movement by acting as lever systems. A lever has three parts.

- **Load.** This is the weight of the body or object to be moved.
- **Pull.** This is the effort or muscle contraction needed to move the bone or lever.
- **Fulcrum.** This is the joint.

Lever systems are organized into classes according to how the **Load**, **Pull**, and **Fulcrum** are arranged (Fig. 20.9).

Class 1 Lever

In **class 1 levers,** the fulcrum or joint is positioned between the load and the pull or muscle, or L−F−P. This arrangement resembles a seesaw or pair of scissors. The skull sitting on top of the vertebral column is an example of a class 1 lever. In this example, the *pull* or **P** is produced by posterior neck muscles, the *fulcrum* or **F** is the joint between the first vertebra and the skull, and the *load* or **L** is the weight of the skull.

Class 2 Lever

Class 2 levers have the pull at one end, the load in the middle, and the fulcrum at the other end, or P−L−F. This arrangement resembles a wheelbarrow. An example of a class 2 lever is rising on the toes. The calf muscles provide the *pull* or **P**, the *load* or **L** is the weight of the body, and the *fulcrum* or **F** is at the joints between the foot and the toes.

TABLE 20.2 Type 1 and Type 2 Muscle Fiber Comparison		
CHARACTERISTIC	**TYPE 1**	**TYPE 2**
Color	Red	White
Contraction Rate	Slow twitch	Fast twitch
Duration	Long	Short
Resistance to Fatigue	Fatigue resistant	Fatigue easily
Capillary Density	High	Low
Mitochondrial Density	High	Low

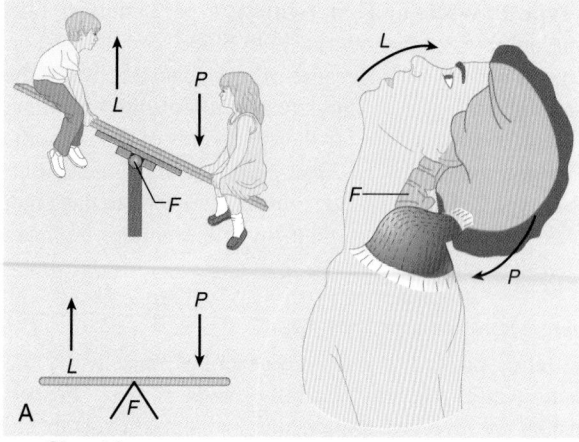

A Class 1 lever

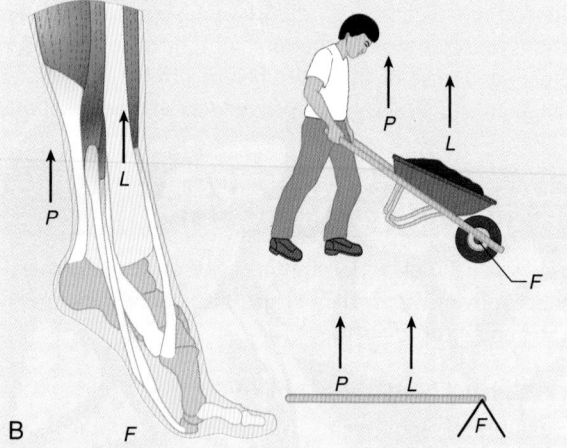

B Class 2 lever

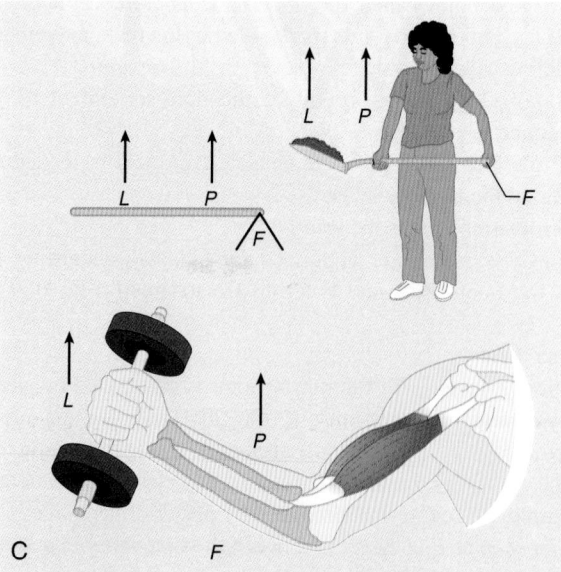

C Class 3 lever

FIG. 20.9 Muscle classification by lever system. Lever systems have three parts: load or L (weight of the body or object to be moved), pull or P (effort or muscle contraction needed to move the bone or lever), and fulcrum or F (the joint). Levers are organized into three classes according to how the L, P, and F are arranged. (A) Class 1 lever. (B) Class 2 lever. (C) Class 3 lever. (From Patton, K., & Thibodeau, G. [2014]. *The human body in health and disease* [6th ed.]. St. Louis, MO: Mosby.)

Class 3 Lever

Class 3 levers have the load at one end, the pull in the middle, and the fulcrum at the other end, or L−P−F. This arrangement, which is the most common in the body, resembles using a shovel. An example of a class 3 lever is bending the elbow during a bicep curl. The *fulcrum* or **F** is the elbow joint, the *pull* or **P** is the bicep muscle, and the *load* or **L** is the weight of the barbell.

Classifying Muscles by Shape

Muscles can be classified by their shape or architecture (Fig. 20.10). Some muscles fall into several categories. For example, pectoralis major in the chest can be classified as convergent or as spiral.

Parallel

Parallel muscles have fibers arranged parallel to one another and pull in one direction. Most skeletal muscles are parallel muscles. These muscles vary in length from the smallest muscle in the body (stapedius in the ear) to the longest muscle in the body (sartorius of the thigh). Parallel muscles can be divided into fusiform and nonfusiform according to their shape. *Fusiform parallel muscles* are more spindle shaped and are tapered at both ends with a larger central region or belly. An example is the biceps brachii in the arm that is responsible for flexing the elbow. *Nonfusiform parallel muscles* are more rectangular with a constant diameter. An example is the rectus abdominis in the abdominal wall that flexes the spine.

Convergent

Convergent muscles have fibers joining at one end and spreading out like a fan at the other end to cover a large area, allowing for more varieties of movement. Convergent muscles often have a triangular shape. An example of a convergent muscle is the pectoralis major in the chest, which causes several movements of the shoulder.

Spiral

Spiral muscles twist between their points of attachment. Examples of spiral muscles are latissimus dorsi in the lower back, and levator scapulae of the lateral neck.

Circular

Circular muscles have a rounded fiber arrangement and cause an opening to become smaller, Examples of circular muscles are the orbicularis oris, which controls the opening of the mouth and orbicularis oculi, which closes the eye. Sphincter muscles are also circular muscles, but some are smooth muscles and involuntary compared with skeletal muscles, which are voluntary.

Pennate

Pennate muscles have muscle fibers emerging diagonally from one or more central tendons, giving them a featherlike appearance. Muscle fibers pull on tendons at an angle, not moving as far as parallel muscles during contraction. However, pennate muscles tend to have more fibers than simi-

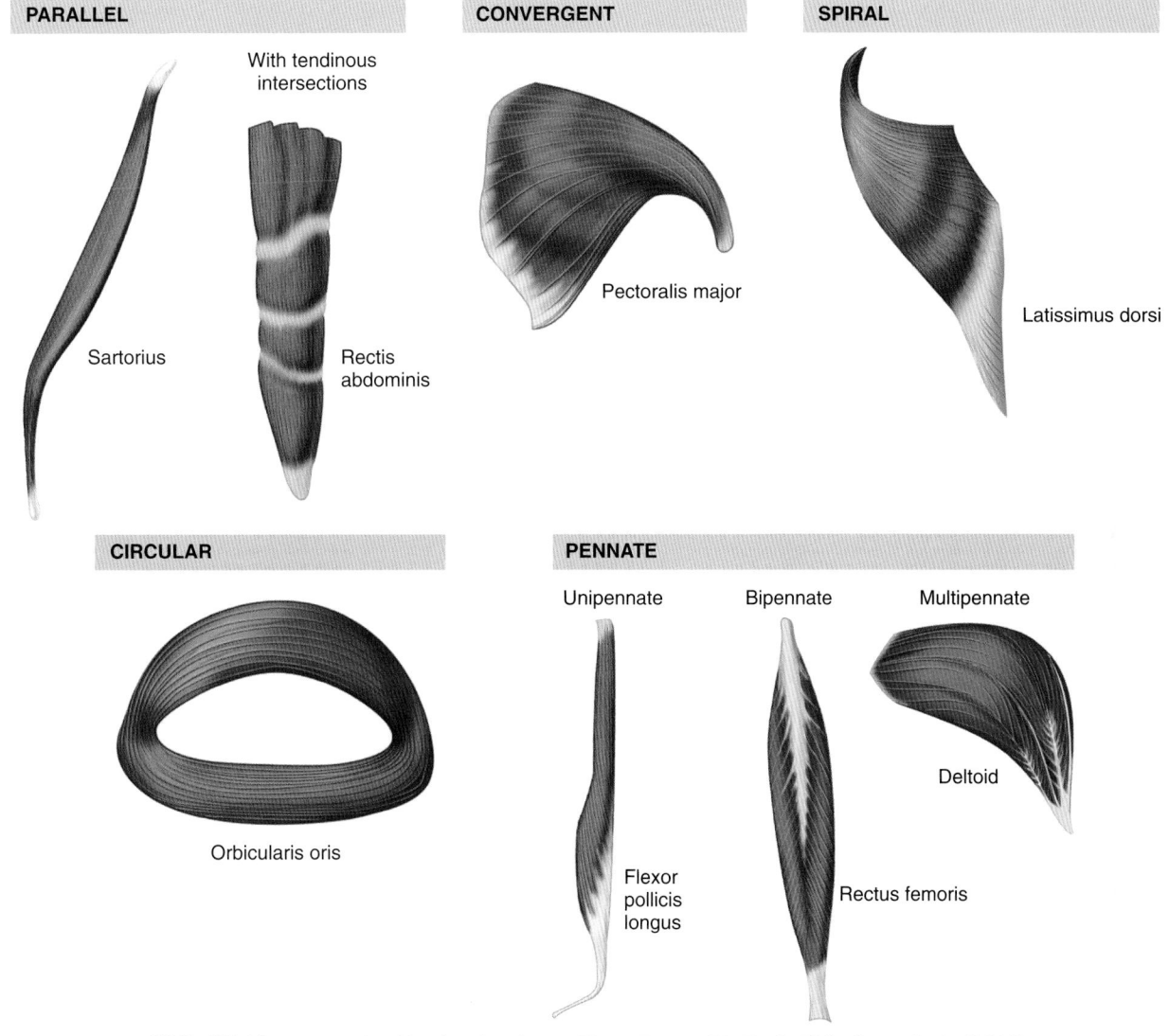

FIG. 20.10 Muscle classification by shape. (From Patton, K. T., & Thibodeau, G. A. [2010]. *Anatomy & physiology* [7th ed.]. St. Louis, MO: Mosby.)

larly sized parallel muscles, so they generate more force. Types of pennate muscles are listed next.

- **Unipennate.** If fibers of a pennate muscle are on the same side of the tendon, the pennate muscle is called unipennate. An example of a unipennate muscle is flexor pollicis longus in the forearm.
- **Bipennate.** These muscles have fibers arranged on both sides of a tendon. An example of a bipennate muscle is the rectus femoris in the thigh.
- **Multipennate.** These muscles have several tendon branches within the muscle with fibers running diagonally between them. Examples of multipennate muscles are the deltoid and subscapularis in the shoulder region.

Classifying Muscles by Action

Most skeletal muscles work in functional groups instead of separately and can assume different roles depending on the required task. When muscles are arranged in opposing pairs, some muscles contract to perform specific actions, while others offer support by either lengthening or stabilizing joints. These same muscles previously shortening can suddenly lengthen while opposing muscles contract and shorten (Fig. 20.11).

Agonists (Prime Movers)

Agonists cause the desired action. For example, a muscle causing the desired action of elbow flexion is brachialis.

Synergists

Synergists assist prime movers by performing the same movement at the same time. For example, pronator teres is a synergist to biceps brachialis because they both cause elbow flexion (see Fig. 20.11B). Synergists tend to be near prime movers and smaller in size.

Fixators (Stabilizers)

Fixators are specialized synergists that stabilize joints or help maintain posture so prime movers can exert their action. An example of a fixator is the deltoid stabilizing

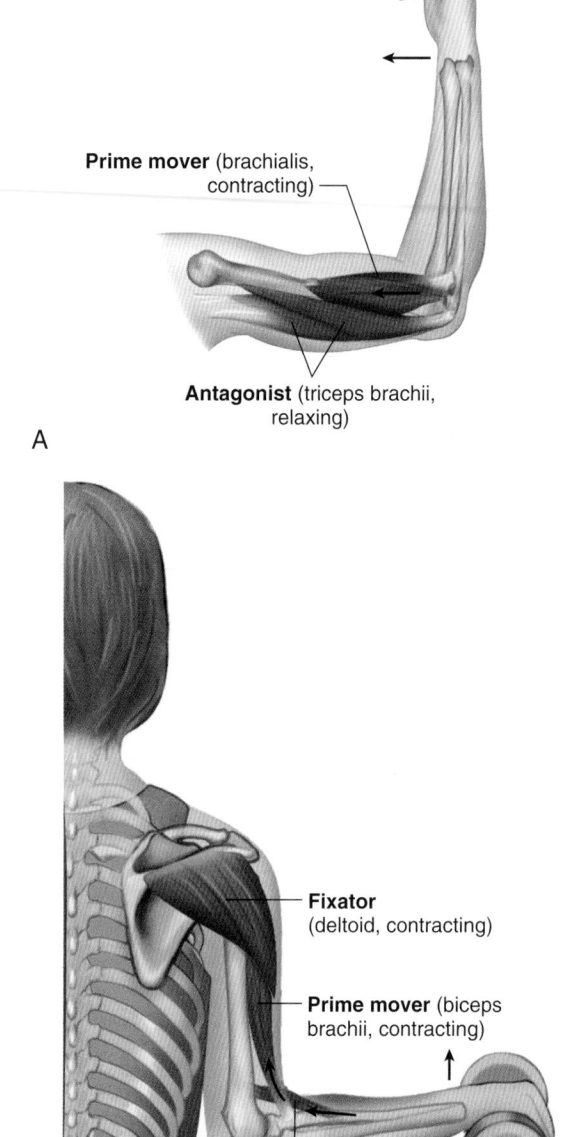

FIG. 20.11 Muscle classification by action. (A) Relationship between prime movers and their antagonists (brachialis [prime mover] shortens to flex the elbow while triceps brachii [antagonist] lengthens). (B) Relationship between prime movers, synergists, and fixators (deltoid [fixator] stabilizes the shoulder while the biceps brachii [prime mover] and pronator teres [synergist] shorten to flex the elbow) (*posterior views*). (From Muscolino, J. E. [2006]. *Kinesiology.* St. Louis, MO: Mosby.)

the shoulder so the biceps brachii can flex the elbow (see Fig. 20.11B). Fixators are also called **stabilizers.**

Antagonists

Antagonists lengthen while prime movers and their synergists contract and shorten to produce movement. Antagonists usually lie on the opposite side of the moving joint and create the opposite action when they reverse roles with prime movers (see Fig. 20.11A). Examples of prime mover-antagonist relationships are the brachialis-triceps brachii and quadriceps-hamstrings (see Chapter 21).

Classifying Muscles by Number of Joints Crossed

Muscles can be classified by the number of joints they cross. When muscles cross a joint, they can act on the joint to create movements.

Uniarticular

Uniarticular muscles cross only one joint. Examples of uniarticular muscles are the deltoid crossing the shoulder joint, brachialis crossing the elbow joint, and soleus crossing the ankle joint.

Biarticular

Biarticular muscles cross two joints. Examples of biarticular muscles are the triceps brachii, which crosses the shoulder and elbow joints, and rectus femoris, which crosses the hip and the knee joints.

Multiarticular

Multiarticular muscles cross three or more joints. Examples of multiarticular muscles are the transversospinalis and the erector spinae groups, which cross multiple vertebral joints.

> *Pain is inevitable. Suffering is optional.*
> ~ **Kathleen Casey Theisen**

MUSCULAR PATHOLOGIES, DISORDERS, AND INJURIES

Featured next are common pathologies, disorders, and injuries of the muscular system listed alphabetically. Each item includes a brief description and their massage-related modifications. Many injuries in this section undergo stages of inflammation; this topic is discussed in Chapter 14. A more extensive list and related research is found in the current edition of *Mosby's Pathology for Massage Professionals* (2022).

Fibromyalgia Syndrome

Fibromyalgia syndrome (FMS) is a chronic condition characterized by widespread pain and joint stiffness, restless sleep, and chronic fatigue. "Widespread" is defined as pain on both sides of the body, and above and below the waist. Individuals with FMS also experience headaches, lack of concentration, bowel dysfunction, temporomandibular disorders, and mood problems ranging from anxiety to depression. Diagnosis is made after a 3-month history of widespread pain and presence of other symptoms with no underlying medical condition that could cause the pain. In the past, the person would be checked for pain elicited by firmly pressing 11 of 18 specific points on the body called tender points. Newer diagnostic guidelines do not require a tender point examination.

In a person with FMS, there are no signs of inflammation or degeneration in the tissues. The affected person experiences periods of exacerbation and remission. People with FMS experience pain at a lower pressure pain threshold. Pressure pain threshold is the minimum applied force that induces pain in a person. This may result from an imbalance in the way the autonomic nervous system responds to physical, chemical, and psychosocial stress. One notable finding in people with FMS is elevated levels of substance P, a neuroreceptor, and neuromodulator associated with pain signal transmission.

Massage and Fibromyalgia Syndrome

Massage should be tailored to how the client is feeling at the time of the treatment because symptoms vary daily. The National Institutes of Health (2016) recommends using light pressure during the initial treatment, with a gradual increase in pressure intensity from session to session, but never to the point of pain. Post-treatment discomfort can be avoided by keeping the discomfort level of applied pressure below 5 on a numeric scale of 0 to 10 (Goodman & Fuller, 2017). Coexisting conditions (temporomandibular disorders, rheumatoid arthritis, lupus) should be factored into the treatment plan.

Headaches (Tension, Migraines, and Cluster)

Headaches are a pain or discomfort in the face, head, or neck. The International Headache Society classifies headaches as primary and secondary. Primary headaches are not caused by an underlying condition, disorder, or pathology. Tension headaches, migraine headaches, and cluster headaches are primary headaches.

- **Tension Headaches.** This is the most common type and usually has a band-like or bilateral pattern with nonthrobbing pain ranging from mild to moderate. Tension headache pain may occur frequently and does not worsen during routine daily activities such as bending over or walking upstairs.
- **Migraine Headaches.** Migraines are the second most common type of primary headaches. Migraine pain is moderate to severe, often described as pounding, pulsing, or throbbing. Migraines are often accompanied by nausea, vomiting, and extreme sensitivity to light, smells, and sounds. Migraine attacks can last from 4 to 72 hours, and the pain can be so severe it interferes with daily activities. Females are affected more than males (4:1). The average age of onset is between 25 and 55 years, but migraines can occur in children. Migraine headaches are also called vascular headaches.
- **Cluster Headaches.** Cluster headaches are rare and occur in cluster periods, which can last from 2 weeks to 3 months. Cluster headache pain starts suddenly and is unilateral (behind the eye or in the eye region). The pain is severe and often described as burning or stabbing; pain

can be throbbing or constant. Cluster headaches occur one to eight times per day during a cluster period, and then go into remission. The remission period may last months or years before recurring.

Secondary headaches are caused by conditions, disorders, or pathologies. Other causes of secondary headaches include sinus infections, allergies, premenstrual syndrome, or increases in altitude. Secondary headaches are also symptoms of serious conditions such as meningitis, intracranial hemorrhage, or tumors.

Massage and Headaches

Screen headache clients for the presence of secondary headache red flags using SNOOP. If a client states the headache is different from a typical headache, including migraines, and has one or more red flags described in the acronym, urge the client to seek medical attention.

- **S: S**ystemic symptoms or disease (fever, weight loss, cancer, human immunodeficiency virus [HIV] infection)
- **N: N**eurologic symptoms (mental confusion, impaired alertness, lack of coordination, visual disturbances)
- **O: O**nset that is sudden or after recent head trauma
- **O: O**lder age of 50+ years
- **P: P**revious headache history (first, worst, change in frequency, or different kind of headache)

For tension headaches, treat soft tissues of the scalp, suboccipitals, posterior neck, and shoulders. Use moderate-to-deep pressure.

For migraine and cluster headaches, massage is postponed until the client's headache has subsided. In addition, a client with a migraine or a cluster headache is not likely to want a massage. Afterward, focus on soft tissues of the scalp, suboccipitals, posterior neck, and shoulders. Use moderate-to-deep pressure.

Myofascial Pain Syndrome

Myofascial pain syndrome (MPS) is a chronic pain disorder characterized by the presence of myofascial trigger points and muscular pain. Trigger points are hyperirritable tender spots in taut palpable bands within skeletal muscle or its associated fascia. When pressed, trigger points cause pain and/or motor dysfunction and autonomic phenomena. Examples of motor dysfunction are muscle stiffness, weakness, or limited movement. Examples of autonomic phenomena are pallor, sweating, and watering eyes. Trigger points are discussed in Chapter 14.

Females and males are equally affected. In addition, MPS is common in people with FMS. This syndrome typically occurs after a muscle has been contracted repetitively. This can be caused by direct trauma or overuse from repetitive motions occurring while doing a job, a sport, or hobby (e.g., playing a musical instrument). Other factors which may contribute to trigger point formation include diseases and disorders such as arthritis and temporomandibular disorders; nutritional deficiencies, including vitamins C, D, and B-complex; iron and magnesium; and miscellaneous factors such as structural asymmetry, insufficient strength, lack of flexibility, loss of electrolytes, or emotional trauma. One theory states people may be more likely to develop MPS who chronically clench their muscles, a form of repeated strain that leaves muscles susceptible to trigger point formation.

Massage and Myofascial Pain Syndrome

Incorporate the application of direct pressure on trigger points to improve treatment outcomes (not in endangerment sites). It is important the client gives feedback on the level of discomfort, any referral patterns, and how the tissue is responding to the applied pressure. Adjust pressure according to the client's preference. Coexisting conditions (arthritis, temporomandibular disorders) should be factored into the treatment plan.

When deciding whether to work on trigger points in the area, consider their purpose and usefulness. If trigger points result from activity such as use of inefficient body mechanics while raking leaves, the client would benefit from trigger point release. However, if trigger points are limiting range of motion (ROM) to protect a hypermobile joint or herniated disc, they might be serving a useful purpose. In this and similar cases, the underlying cause needs to be assessed and corrected before trigger point massage.

Plantar Fasciitis

Plantar fasciitis is chronic inflammation of the plantar fascia, a thick band of tissue on the bottom of the foot, which connects the calcaneus (heel bone) to the toes. The plantar fascia acts like a bowstring to maintain the foot arches and to absorb shock while the body is in motion. If tension and stress on plantar fascia become too great, it can become irritated and inflamed, and even tear. Plantar fasciitis is the most common orthopedic complaint relating to the foot with approximately 2 million people treated for this condition every year. It is a frequent problem for people who participate in sports involving running or jumping. The typical patient with this condition is an active male between the ages of 40 and 70 years. If the affected person changes a gait pattern to compensate for foot pain, plantar fasciitis may lead to knee, hip, or back pain. Plantar fasciitis is also called plantar heel pain. The most common cause of plantar fasciitis is prolonged repetitive motion.

Massage and Plantar Fasciitis

While acute inflammation is present, treat the area as a local contraindication. Elevate the affected area during the massage, which may help reduce swelling. While the client is prone, use a higher-than-normal (8 inches) bolster in front of the ankles to prevent pain from uncomfortable foot/ankle positions.

Once acute inflammation has resolved or entered the subacute phase, local massage can begin. Include techniques of compression, transverse friction, and myofascial techniques applied over the plantar surface of the foot and at the insertion of the plantar fascia near the calcaneus. Consider using gentle passive dorsiflexion to stretch the plantar fascia. Inquire about pressure sensitivity over affected areas and adjust it below the client's pain tolerance. Recommend self-massage and self-stretching to help clients maintain or improve their treatment goals.

Shin Splints (Medial Tibial Stress Syndrome)

Shin splints are pain along the medial tibia or shin bone. This condition is often bilateral and is more common among people who participate in sports and exercises of running and jumping such as runners, dancers, and military recruits. This condition may occur during the first few weeks of a new exercise program or after a sudden increase in the amount of exercise in an ongoing fitness program. The most common cause of shin splints is repetitive use of tibial neighboring muscles and connective tissues (including the tibial periosteum).

Massage and Shin Splints

If acute inflammation is present, treat the affected area as a local contraindication. You can elevate the affected area during the massage, which may help reduce swelling. While the client is prone, use a higher-than-normal (8 inches) bolster in front of the ankles to prevent pain from uncomfortable foot/ankle positions.

Once acute inflammation has resolved or entered the subacute phase, local massage can begin. Include techniques of compression, transverse friction, and sustained myofascial techniques (applied parallel to the tibia) along with gentle passive dorsiflexion and plantarflexion (Fogarty, 2015). Inquire about pressure sensitivity over affected areas and adjust it below the client's pain tolerance. Ice massage can also be used to reduce pain and recovery time.

Strain

A **strain** is an injury caused by an overstretched or torn muscle and/or tendon. The most common locations for strains are the hands, thighs (hamstrings), and lower back. Strains are also called pulled muscles. Strains are caused by trauma from excessive mechanical force (e.g., lifting, vehicular accident) and/or excessive tension by extreme elongation of a given length of tissue (landing from fall while the ankle or knee is rotated in an unnatural or unstable position), or a combination of the two events. Strains can be classified into three grades or degrees of severity: first, second, and third.

- **Grade 1 (1st Degree).** Affected musculotendinous units are overstretched and damaged microscopically but are not torn. The joint is stable, and the person is usually able to move or continue with an activity, but with slight discomfort.
- **Grade 2 (2nd Degree).** Affected musculotendinous units are torn. Swelling is noted, and the surrounding muscles

splint to restrict movement. Joint instability is moderate, and the area is painful without movement.

- **Grade 3 (3rd Degree).** Affected musculotendinous units are completely ruptured and swelling is significant. A snapping sound is often heard at the time of injury and there is a palpable depression in the rupture. Joints are unstable, and a piece of the bone may be torn away (avulsion fracture). Person is unable to move or continue with an activity. Grade 3 strains may require surgical intervention to correct.

Massage and Strains

While acute inflammation is present, treat the area as a local contraindication. If on a limb, elevate the affected area to help reduce swelling during the massage. If the client is wearing a cast or splint, do not apply heat to distal areas to prevent swelling.

Once acute inflammation has resolved or is in the subacute phase, local massage can begin. Massage, especially friction massage, may promote healing of muscles and tendons. Inquire about pressure sensitivity over affected areas and adjust it below the client's pain tolerance. Avoid overstretching the injured area.

Tendinopathies: Tendinitis, Tendinosis, Tenosynovitis (De Quervain Tenosynovitis), and Epicondylitis

Tendinopathy is a term to describe acute or chronic conditions involving tendons, their synovial sheaths, or attachment sites. Tendinopathies include tendinitis, tendinosis, tenosynovitis, and epicondylitis. Tendinopathies can occur in any tendon, but the most common are overuse tendinopathies involving the rotator cuff, medial and lateral humeral epicondyles, patellar tendon, and Achilles tendon.

- **Tendinitis.** Inflammation of a tendon(s). Tendinitis is also called *tendonitis.*
- **Tendinosis.** Degeneration of a tendon(s). Tendinosis is often mislabeled as tendinitis, but inflammation is not present in tendinosis.
- **Tenosynovitis.** Inflammation of the synovial sheath surrounding a tendon.
  - **De Quervain Tenosynovitis.** The most common type and involves inflammation of the synovial sheath on the radial or thumb side of the wrist.
- **Epicondylitis.** Inflammation of a tendon where it attaches to an epicondyle. The most commonly affected epicondylar region is the elbow.
  - **Lateral Epicondylitis** (*tennis elbow*) is inflammation of the common extensor tendons at their origin on the lateral humeral epicondyle.
  - **Medial Epicondylitis** (*golfer's elbow*) is inflammation of the common flexor tendons at the medial humeral epicondyle.

Common causes of *inflammatory tendinopathies* are repetitive motion and or direct trauma related to injury.

Underlying conditions such as RA, gout, psoriatic arthritis, thyroid disorders, or unusual medication reactions can also cause or contribute to the development of tendinopathies. The aging process (changes in collagen cause tendons to lose elasticity) can cause *degenerative tendinopathies.*

Massage and Tendinopathies

While acute inflammation is present, treat the area as a local contraindication. If on a limb, elevate the affected area to help reduce swelling during the massage.

Once acute inflammation has resolved or has entered the subacute phase, local massage can begin. Massage, especially friction massage, may promote tendon healing, reduce pain, and improve function (Chaves et al., 2019; Gehlsen et al., 1999), especially when combined with other methods such as trigger point massage, myofascial techniques, PROM, conventional physical therapy, and home care. Inquire about pressure sensitivity over affected areas and adjust it below the client's pain tolerance. Avoid overstretching the affected area.

Keep in mind the average healing time for tendinitis ranges from a few days up to 6 weeks; average healing time for tendinosis is between 3 and 6 months because degenerated tendons require over 100 days to produce new collagen (Khan et al., 2000). Factor these timelines into your treatment plans.

Rotator Cuff Tears and Impingement Syndrome

Rotator cuff tears occur when one or more rotator cuff muscles is partially or completely torn from its attachment on the humerus. Rotator cuff muscles include the supraspinatus, infraspinatus, subscapularis, and teres minor. The rotator cuff muscle most often torn is supraspinatus. Whereas individuals who perform repetitive shoulder motions are at increased risk for rotator cuff tears, most cases are from normal wear and tear, with people over 40 years at the greatest risk for rotator cuff problems.

Impingement syndrome, or *shoulder impingement syndrome,* occurs when the supraspinatus tendon and the subacromial bursa become compressed between the narrow space beneath the acromion process and the humeral head. This compression leads to pain and dysfunction during shoulder adduction.

Massage and Rotator Cuff Tears/Impingement Syndrome

For trauma-related cases, the affected area is a local contraindication while acute inflammation is present. If the client is wearing a cast or splint, do not apply heat to distal areas to prevent swelling.

When acute inflammation has resolved, is in the subacute phase, or is degenerative, local massage can be applied. Inquire about pressure sensitivity over affected areas and adjust it below the client's pain tolerance. Massage, especially friction massage, over shoulder muscles may reduce pain and improve mobility. These effects may be enhanced with gentle shoulder PROM and traction. Avoid overstretching the affected area.

Torticollis

Torticollis is a group of disorders involving spasms of the sternocleidomastoid muscle. This causes the head to turn and tilt to one side. Other muscles, such as the trapezius, and splenius muscles, also may be involved. Two main categories of torticollis are featured next.

- **Congenital Muscular Torticollis** (CMT): Occurs from birth trauma; this condition is rare.
- **Spasmodic Torticollis** (ST): Occurs after injury or repetitive motion. ST is more common than CMT. ST is also called acquired torticollis.

Massage and Torticollis

If acute inflammation is present, treat the area as a local contraindication.

Once acute inflammation has resolved or entered the subacute phase, massage can begin. Position the client for comfort, which may include avoiding the prone position. Address tension in the posterior neck muscles (e.g., trapezius, splenii, paraspinals, levator scapulae) and attachment sites of sternocleidomastoid (mastoid process and clavicular/sternal attachments). Inquire about pressure sensitivity over affected areas and make adjustments according to the client's preference. Do not use massage techniques over the anterior neck (anterior and posterior triangles) as this area is an endangerment site. Avoid overstretching the injured area. Discussions about neutral sleeping postures may be helpful with some clients.

Whiplash-Associated Disorders

Whiplash-associated disorder (WAD) is a collective term describing neck injuries caused by rapid forceful back-and-forth movements of the cervical spine, similar to cracking a whip. The most injured neck area is the junction between the fourth and fifth cervical vertebrae. Surrounding muscles are stretched beyond their normal range, may incur a strain, and there may be joint trauma, fractures, herniated discs and cervical radiculopathy, and traumatic brain injuries. The head motion may also be side-to-side (lateral) or in any degree of rotation, depending on the direction of impact. The most frequent cause of WAD is traumatic injury from being pushed or struck from behind, such as by a rear-end motor vehicle accident.

Massage and Whiplash-Associated Disorders

If acute inflammation is present, treat the area as a local contraindication.

Once acute inflammation has resolved or entered the subacute phase, massage can begin. Position the client for comfort, which may include avoiding the prone position. Address tension in the posterior neck muscles (e.g., trapezius, splenii, paraspinals, levator scapulae) and attachment sites of sternocleidomastoid (mastoid process and clavicular/sternal attachments). Inquire about pressure sensitivity over affected areas and make adjustments according to the client's preference. Do not use massage techniques over the anterior neck (anterior and posterior triangles) as this area is an endangerment site. Avoid overstretching the injured area. Discussions about neutral sleeping postures may be helpful with some clients.

E-RESOURCES

http://evolve.elsevier.com/Salvo/MassageTherapy

- Chapter challenge
- Flash cards

JUDITH DELANY

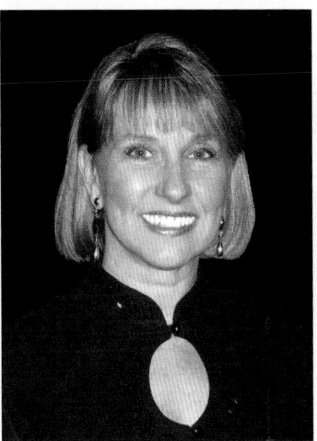

Clinical reasoning, the ability to accurately assess a client's needs, provide treatment, and reflect on the results, is a vital skill for any massage practitioner. These skills can be learned in massage school, of course; they are a central component of any good curriculum. Even so, the attitudes involved in high-quality clinical reasoning are often formed earlier in life. "Observant," "curious," and "precise" are not always the first words a person thinks of with respect to massage practitioners, but these are qualities characterizing some of the greatest massage practitioners of our time.

Judith DeLany was born in 1956 to parents who had little formal education but believed strongly in acquiring and applying knowledge. Her father had never studied beyond fifth grade but could fix anything using the tools at hand. Her mother read the encyclopedia the way other people read novels. She used to ask her children questions like, "Do you know how your finger works?" and then encourage them to find out by looking up the information for themselves. DeLany absorbed this well, and as a result she excelled in school, graduating second in her high school class in 1974.

In 1981, DeLany injured her neck and back falling from a ladder. The pain was not very bad—at first. But over the course of the next year, her symptoms became worse. She could no longer dance or run, a huge blow to the athletic young woman. Even walking became difficult, and she developed a significant limp from the pain, which began radiating into her leg and foot. It was this limp that caught the eye of a massage practitioner, who suggested neuromuscular therapy might help. He was right: DeLany's pain improved so much after a few treatments she could move freely and easily. Not long after, she enrolled in massage school.

At the time, DeLany had no intention of being a full-time massage practitioner. She was happily employed at a real estate company, and she planned to use massage exclusively as a way of helping family and friends. But just as she graduated from massage school in 1982, the company she worked for closed, leaving her out of work. And so DeLany turned to her newfound skills to build herself a new career.

Quite naturally, DeLany focused her work on neuromuscular therapy, the technique that had done so much for her own pain. She was offered a position working in the clinical practice of Paul St. John, a noted neuromuscular practitioner and innovator. This massage practitioner position turned into a teaching position, and soon DeLany became the first person besides St. John to be permitted to teach his methods. In 1990, DeLany began teaching her own style of neuromuscular therapy, separate from St. John.

In 1994, renowned osteopath Leon Chaitow asked DeLany to contribute to a book comparing neuromuscular therapy practiced in the United States with techniques commonly practiced in Europe. The two found the partnership quite fruitful and continued to collaborate, coauthoring *Clinical Application of Neuromuscular Techniques.* DeLany also helped Chaitow develop the *Journal of Bodywork and Movement Therapies,* the first peer-reviewed journal of its kind. She served as an associate editor of the journal for many years and is still a member of its international advisory board.

While DeLany's work today still involves writing and teaching extensively, she's branching out to embrace new technology. She was the lead contributor of the computer study program "3D Anatomy of Massage and Manual Therapies," published in 2012, and has also developed her first webinar series. "The very core of education has changed dramatically over the last 30 years," she notes. But in education, just as in massage, she notes it is important to adapt the method to the need, rather than relying on preconceived notions of what should be effective.

Judith DeLany's career has been so successful because she found ways to harness her inherent strengths: curiosity, determination, and a keen eye. Find your strengths, develop them, and build your work around them. That way, you will create a practice nobody else can, because at its heart is something irreplaceable: you.

REFERENCES

Chaves, P., Simões, D., Paço, M., Silva, S., Pinho, F., Duarte, J. A., & Ribeiro, F. (2019). Deep friction massage in the management of patellar tendinopathy in athletes: Short-term clinical outcomes. *Journal of Sport Rehabilitation, 30,* 1–6.

Fogarty, S. (2015). Massage treatment and medial tibial stress syndrome: a commentary to provoke thought about the way massage therapy is used in the treatment of MTSS. *Journal of Bodywork and Movement Therapies, 19*(3), 447–452.

Gehlsen, G. M., Ganion, L. R., & Helfst, R. (1999). Fibroblast responses to variation in soft tissue mobilization pressure. *Medicine and Science in Sports and Exercise, 31*(4), 531–535.

Goodman, C. C., & Fuller, K. S. (2017). *Pathology for the physical therapist assistant* (2nd ed.). St Louis: Elsevier.

Janda, V. (1983). On the concept of postural muscles and posture in man. *Australian journal of Physiotherapy*Aust J Physiother, 29(3), 83–84.

Khan, K. M., Cook, J. L., Taunton, J. E., & Bonar, F. (2000). Overuse tendinosis, not tendinitis—Part 1: A new paradigm for a difficult clinical problem. *The Physician and Sportsmedicine*, 28(5), 38–48.

National Institutes of Health. (2016). *National center for complementary and integrative health: Fibromyalgia in depth*. Retrieved from https://nccih.nih.gov/health/pain/fibromyalgia.htm#hed3

Salvo, S. G. (2022). *Mosby's pathology for massage professionals* (5th ed.). St Louis: Mosby.

BIBLIOGRAPHY

Abrahams, P. H., Spratt, J. D., Loukas, M., & van Schoor, A. N. (2003). *Abrahams' and McMinn's clinical atlas of human anatomy* (8th ed.). St Louis: Elsevier.

Applegate, E. (2010). *The anatomy and physiology learning system* (4th ed.). Philadelphia: Saunders.

Como, D. (Ed.). (2016). *Mosby's dictionary of medicine, nursing, and health professions* (10th ed.). St Louis: Elsevier.

Frazier, M. S., & Drzymkowski, J. W. (2015). *Essentials of human diseases and conditions* (6th ed.). St Louis: Elsevier.

Hubert, R. J., & VanMeter, K. C. (2018). *Gould's pathophysiology for the health professions* (6th ed.). Philadelphia: Saunders.

Haubrich, W. S. (2003). *Medical meanings: A glossary of word origins* (2nd ed.). New York: American College of Physicians.

Herlihy, B. (2017). *The human body in health and illness* (6th ed.). St Louis: Saunders.

Huether, S. E., McCance, K. L., & Brashers, V. L. (2019). *Understanding pathophysiology* (7th ed.). St Louis: Mosby.

Kalat, J. W. (2013). *Biological psychology* (11th ed.). Belmont, Calif: Cengage Learning.

Kapit, W., & Elson, L. M. (2013). *The anatomy coloring book* (4th ed.). New York: Benjamin Cummings.

Kumar, V., Abbas, A. K., & Aster, J.C. (2015). *Robbins & Cotran pathologic basis of disease* (9th ed.). St Louis: Mosby.

Lauderstein, D. (2012). *The deep massage book: How to combine structure and energy in bodywork*. Taos: Redwing Book Company.

Marieb, E. N., & Keller, S. M. (2018). *Essentials of human anatomy and physiology* (12th ed.). New York: Benjamin Cummings.

McCance, K. L., & Huether, S. E. (2019). *Pathophysiology: The biological basis for disease in adults and children* (8th ed.). St Louis: Mosby.

Myers, T. W. (2014). *Anatomy trains: Myofascial meridians for manual and movement therapists* (3rd ed.). Churchill Livingstone: Elsevier.

Netter, F. H. (2018). *Atlas of human anatomy* (7th ed.). St Louis: Mosby.

Patton, K. T (2019). *Anatomy and physiology* (10th ed.). St Louis: Elsevier.

Patton, K. T., Thibodeau, G. A., & Douglas, M. M. (2012). *Essentials of anatomy and physiology* (4th ed.). New York: Pearson.

Porter, R. S. (2011). *The Merck manual of diagnosis and therapy* (19th ed.). Whitehouse Station, NJ: Merck Sharp and Dohme Corp.

REVIEW AND APPLY YOUR KNOWLEDGE

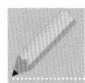 **MATCHING ONE: CONCEPT REVIEW**

Place the letter of the answer next to the number of the term or phrase that best describes it.

A. Acetylcholine
B. Aponeurosis
C. Excitability
D. Posture
E. Motor end plate
F. Muscle fibers
G. Insertion
H. Sarcolemma
I. Sarcomere
J. Myosin
K. Thin filaments
L. Tendons

_____   1. Structures made up of proteins called actin, tropomyosin, and troponin.
_____   2. Thick filaments in the center of the sarcomere.
_____   3. Basic unit of muscle contraction.
_____   4. Muscle fiber property enabling it to respond to a stimulus.
_____   5. Dense cordlike connective tissue that attach muscles to bones.
_____   6. Term synonymous with muscle cells.
_____   7. Broad, flat tendon.
_____   8. Tendinous attachment on the bone that moves during contraction.
_____   9. Folded sections of the sarcolemma within the neuromuscular junction.
_____ 10. Body positions maintained by muscle contraction; examples are standing and sitting.
_____ 11. Cell membrane surrounding muscle fibers.
_____ 12. Principal neurotransmitter involved in muscle contraction.

MATCHING TWO: CONCEPT REVIEW

Place the letter of the answer next to the number of the term or phrase that best describes it.

A. All-or-none law
B. Agonist
C. Antagonist
D. Class 3
E. Isotonic
F. Motor unit
G. Isometric
H. Origin
I. Recruitment
J. Pennate
K. Adenosine triphosphate
L. Type 1

_____   1. Muscle fibers containing large amounts of myoglobin and mitochondria; also called red muscle.
_____   2. A single motor neuron and all muscle fibers it innervates.
_____   3. Main source of energy for muscle contraction.
_____   4. Process of motor unit activation based on need.
_____   5. Term to describe a muscle with fibers emerging diagonally from one or more central tendon.
_____   6. Tendinous attachment on the less moveable bone during muscle contraction.
_____   7. Type of contraction in which muscle length remains the same and movement does not occur.
_____   8. Type of contraction in which muscle length changes.
_____   9. Most common lever arrangement in the body— the load at one end, the pull in the middle, and the fulcrum at the other end.
_____ 10. Term used to describe the muscle that lengthens while prime movers and their synergists contract and shorten to produce the desired action.
_____ 11. Principle stating when a muscle fiber receives a stimulus to contract, it either will contract to its fullest ability or it will not contract at all.
_____ 12. Prime mover or muscle causing the desired action.

MULTIPLE CHOICE: TEST YOUR KNOWLEDGE

Place the letter of the answer next to the number of the term or phrase that best describes it.

_____ 1. The continuous and partial contraction of muscles is called:
A. posture
B. tonus
C. stance
D. position

_____ 2. The ability of muscle fibers to return to precontraction after lengthening or stretching is:
A. excitability
B. contractility
C. extensibility
D. elasticity

_____ 3. Which is the intracellular fluid in a muscle fiber?
A. Sarcolemma
B. Sarcoplasm
C. Sarcomere
D. Sarcoma

_____ 4. Which are the borders of the sarcomeres and where thin filaments attach?
A. I bands
B. H zone
C. Z lines
D. A band

_____ 5. Which is the thick outer layer of connective tissue that surrounds the entire muscle or muscle group?
A. Epimysium
B. Perimysium
C. Endomysium
D. Retinaculum

_____ 6. Which part of the neuromuscular junction contains the receptor sites for acetylcholine?
A. Motor neuron
B. Synaptic gap
C. Motor end plate
D. Transverse tubules

_____ 7. Which is the red respiratory pigment that stores oxygen in muscles?
A. Adenosine triphosphate
B. Acetylcholine
C. Hemoglobin
D. Myoglobin

_____ 8. Which phrase describes the cycle that begins with excitation by a motor neuron that causes the thick filaments to attach to the thin filaments?
A. Cross bridging
B. Power stroke
C. Excitation-contraction coupling
D. All-or-none response

_____ 9. Which is another term for static contractions because it does not involve movement?
A. Concentric contractions
B. Eccentric contractions
C. Isotonic contractions
D. Isometric contractions

_____ 10. Which type of muscles has fibers joining at one end and spreading out like a fan at the other end?
A. Circular
B. Parallel
C. Convergent
D. Pennate

_____ 11. Smaller muscles that are near prime movers and assist them by performing the same movement are:
A. agonists
B. antagonists
C. fixators
D. synergists

_____ 12. Which is a chronic pain disorder characterized by the presence of trigger points and muscular pain?
A. Fibromyalgia syndrome
B. Myofascial pain syndrome
C. Plantar fasciitis
D. Spasmodic torticollis

CRITICAL THINKING

Good Posture

Which type of muscle fibers make up postural muscles? Why do you think so?

Answers can include but are not limited to:

Postural muscles are made up of type 1, slow twitch fibers. Muscle fibers containing large amounts of myoglobin and mitochondria and have copious amounts of blood capillaries are called type 1. Because type 1 contains a larger amount of myoglobin and blood vessels, they take on a deeper red appearance and are called red muscle fibers. Muscles in the back and lower extremities possess more type 1 fibers. Type 2 muscle fibers contain less myoglobin and mitochondria and fewer blood capillaries compared with type 1. Because of these characteristics, type 2 muscle fibers are lighter in color and are called white muscle fibers. Muscles of the upper extremity contain several type 2 muscle fibers.

Slow twitch fibers contract more slowly, for longer periods, and they take longer to fatigue. Type 1 or red fibers are also classified as slow twitch fibers. Marathon runners tend to have more type 1 or slow twitch fibers in their lower extremities than other athletes such as tennis players or sprinters. Fast twitch fibers contract more quickly and for shorter periods. These fibers possess a type of myosin that moves faster, and their systems of T tubules and sarcoplasmic reticulum are more efficient at delivering stored Ca. The price of rapid contraction is a quick depletion of ATP, resulting in fatigue occurring more quickly compared with slow twitch muscle.

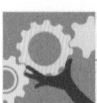

PROFESSIONAL PRACTICE

Evidence-Informed Practice

Christine is a 58-year-old woman diagnosed with fibromyalgia 5 years ago. She takes yoga classes three times a week and pain management medication daily. A few days ago, she decided to stop drinking coffee to reduce caffeine intake and has caffeine withdrawal headaches. Christine has an appointment with you today. She has never had a massage before. During the intake, she states her neighbor receives deep massage and finds it beneficial. She would like a deep massage today. Should Christine receive this type of massage? Why or why not? What techniques are appropriate for her? Cite research studies to support your choice of techniques.

DISCUSSION

Weighing Risks Versus Benefits

Many clients seek out massage to help manage pain. These same clients may also be taking pain-reducing medications. Medication effects, both therapeutic effects and side effects, may alter your treatment plan with a particular client. Pick two commonly used pain relievers and look up their effects. Which effect should you be concerned with and why? How would you modify your massage session for a particular medication effect? Weigh the possible benefits of massage with any potential risks.

CHAPTER 21

Kinesiology

LEARNING OBJECTIVES

After completing this chapter, the student should be able to:

1. Define kinesiology, bony markings, and identify bones and relevant bony markings of the upper extremity.
2. Identify bones and relevant bony markings of the lower extremity.
3. Identify bones and relevant bony markings of the axial skeleton.
4. Identify muscles of scapular movement including their origins, insertions, and actions.
5. Identify muscles of shoulder joint movement including their origins, insertions, and actions.
6. Identify muscles of elbow and radioulnar joint movement including their origins, insertions, and actions.
7. Identify muscles of wrist and hand movement, including their origins, insertions, and actions.
8. Identify muscles of hip and knee movement, including their origins, insertions, and actions.
9. Identify muscles of ankle and foot movement, including their origins, insertions, and actions.
10. Identify muscles of neck and facial movement, including their origins, insertions, and actions.
11. Identify muscles of trunk and vertebral column movement, including their origins, insertions, and actions.
12. Identify muscles of respiration, including their origins, insertions, and any secondary actions.

http://evolve.elsevier.com/Salvo/MassageTherapy

INTRODUCTION

Kinesiology is the study of human motion. Learning kinesiology requires knowledge of bones, skeletal muscles, joints, and their movements. Most bones come together at joints. Muscles cross joints, and they shorten or lengthen to pull on bones, changing their relative positions to create movement. Joints and joint movements are discussed in Chapter 19. Muscles and types of contractions are discussed in Chapter 20.

This chapter begins with bones of the skeletal system and lists bones, associated joints, and bony markings; these are useful when locating muscles on clients. As you are learning kinesiology, it is helpful to make flash cards and write the name of the bone, joint, or muscle on the front of the card and information about the structure on the back. Drawing bones, joints, or muscles on a real body is helpful; recruit a classmate, friend, or family member and use water-soluble markers. Use anatomical terms, such as "scapula" instead of "shoulder blade," or "olecranon process" instead of "tip of the elbow," to reinforce new vocabulary. For example, instead of thinking, "I am massaging the arm," say to yourself silently, or aloud, the specific structures of the arm, such as humerus, triceps brachii, biceps brachii, and brachialis.

This chapter contains 12 lessons: The first three lessons feature bones, bony markings, and their significance, such as joint formation or muscle attachment. Also included in the Notes section of featured bones are their joints and the applicable palpable surface landmarks. The next nine lessons include individual muscles and common muscle groups; their origins, insertions, actions, nerve innervations, and a Notes section. Specific lessons for this chapter are:

1. Lesson One: Bones and Joints of the Upper Extremity
2. Lesson Two: Bones and Joints of the Lower Extremity
3. Lesson Three: Bones and Joints of the Axial Skeleton
4. Lesson Four: Muscles of Scapular Movement
5. Lesson Five: Muscles of Shoulder Joint Movement
6. Lesson Six: Muscles of the Elbow and Radioulnar Joint Movement
7. Lesson Seven: Muscles of Wrist and Hand Movement
8. Lesson Eight: Muscles of Hip and Knee Movement
9. Lesson Nine: Muscles of Ankle and Foot Movement
10. Lesson Ten: Muscles of the Neck and Facial Movement
11. Lesson Eleven: Muscles of Trunk and Vertebral Column Movement
12. Lesson Twelve: Muscles of Respiration

BONES AND BONY MARKINGS

Bones are the hard connective tissues that make up the skeletal system. When two or more bones come together, or *join*, a joint is formed. Most joints allow the body to move in response to muscular forces or external forces. Bones contain **bony markings**, projections and depressions on bones where muscles, tendons, and ligaments attach and where nerves and blood vessels pass (Fig. 21.1). Bony markings are also called *surface markings* or *bony landmarks*. Muscles usually attach to bony markings. Muscle attachments are called origins or insertions. *Origins* are the attachments on the less movable bone. Origins are usually more medial or proximal compared with insertions and are also called proximal attachments. Origins are red when featured on skeletons in classrooms and textbooks. *Insertions* are the attachments on the bone that moves during contraction. Insertions are usually more lateral or distal compared with origins and are also called distal attachments. Insertions are blue when featured on skeletons in classrooms and textbooks. Insertions usually move toward origins. However, the opposite can occur; this is called functional reversibility. Because bones are among the hardest substances in the body, bony markings are usually easy to locate through palpation. Learning bony markings is important for massage practitioners, as they represent ways to locate muscles and other structures. Not all bones, bony markings, joints, or muscles are featured—just those important to a massage practice.

Bony Markings: Projections and Processes

Listed next are bony markings representing projections and processes, along with their descriptions and an example or two.

Angle
An angle is a projecting corner of a bone. Examples: mandibular angle and superior angle of the scapula.

Border
A border is the linear edge of a bone. Examples: lateral border of the scapula and superior border of the rib.

Condyle
A condyle is a large, rounded, knuckle-shaped projection that usually articulates with another bone to form a joint. Examples: occipital condyles and femoral condyles.

Crest
A crest is a linear elevation on a bone. Examples: iliac crest and pubic crest.

Epicondyle
An epicondyle is an enlargement near, or above, a condyle. Examples: epicondyle of the humerus and epicondyle of the femur.

Head
A head is the enlarged and rounded end of a bone. Examples: femoral head and fibular head.

Line
A line is a narrow elevation on a bone and is less prominent than a crest. Examples: nuchal line and gluteal line.

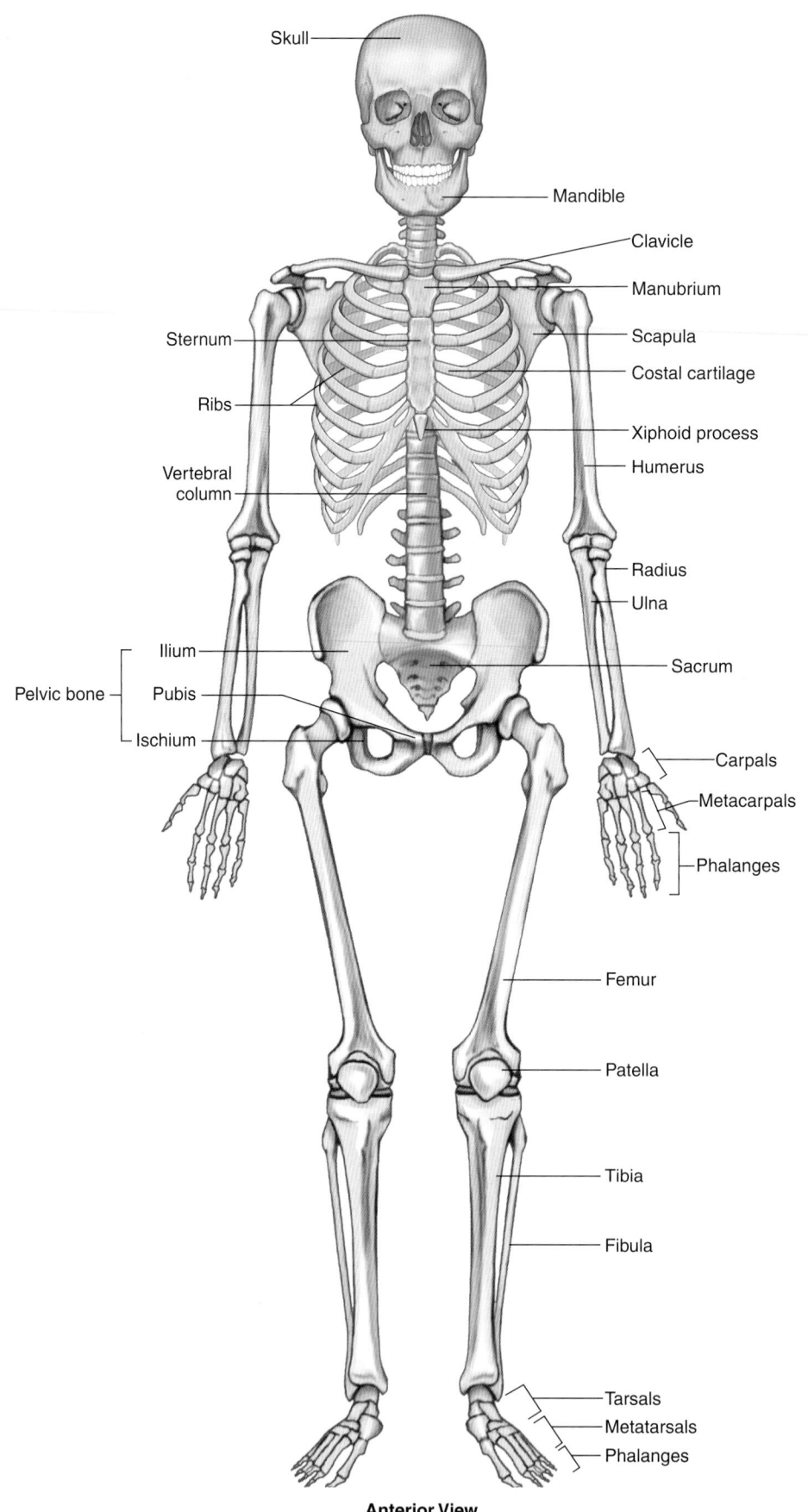

Anterior View

FIG. 21.1 Bones in the human axial skeleton (*blue*) and upper and lower extremities (*brown*). (From Patton, K. T., & Thibodeau, G. A. [2014]. *The human body in health and disease* [6th ed.]. St. Louis, MO: Elsevier.)

Process

A process is a prominent projection, or prolongation, extending from a bone. Examples: styloid process and the olecranon process.

Protuberance

A protuberance is a knob-like protrusion from a bone. Example: external occipital protuberance.

Ramus

A ramus is a long, branch-like prolongation of a bone. Examples: pubic ramus and mandibular ramus.

Ridge

A ridge is an elongated projection of a bone. Example: supracondylar ridge.

Spine

A spine is a sharp, slender projection from a bone. Examples: scapular spine and iliac spine.

Trochanter

A trochanter is a large, rounded projection found only on the femur. Examples: greater trochanter and lesser trochanter.

Tubercle

A tubercle is a rounded projection from a bone, usually blunt and irregular. Examples: pubic tubercle and adductor tubercle.

Tuberosity

A tuberosity is a large and rounded, or roughened, projection on a bone. Examples: deltoid tuberosity and ischial tuberosity.

Bony Markings: Depressions and Openings

Listed next are bony markings representing depressions and openings, along with their descriptions and an example or two.

Foramen

A foramen is an opening through a bone(s) and usually serves as a passage for blood vessels, nerves, or ligaments. Examples: intervertebral foramen and foramen magnum.

Facet

A facet is a small, flattened, shallow depression articulating with another bone. Examples: costal facet and articular facet.

Fossa

A fossa is a shallow depression. Examples: subscapular fossa and iliac fossa.

Groove

A groove is a linear depression accommodating another structure. Examples: intertubercular groove and laminar groove.

Notch

A notch is a deep indentation, or a narrow gap, in the bone. Examples: radial notch and sciatic notch.

Sinus

A sinus is a cavity or hollow space in a bone. Examples: frontal sinus and maxillary sinus.

Lesson One: Bones and Joints of the Upper Extremity

The upper extremity bones include the clavicle, scapula, humerus, ulna, radius, carpals, metacarpals, and phalanges. Associated joints and other structures are listed as bullets in the Notes section (Fig. 21.2).

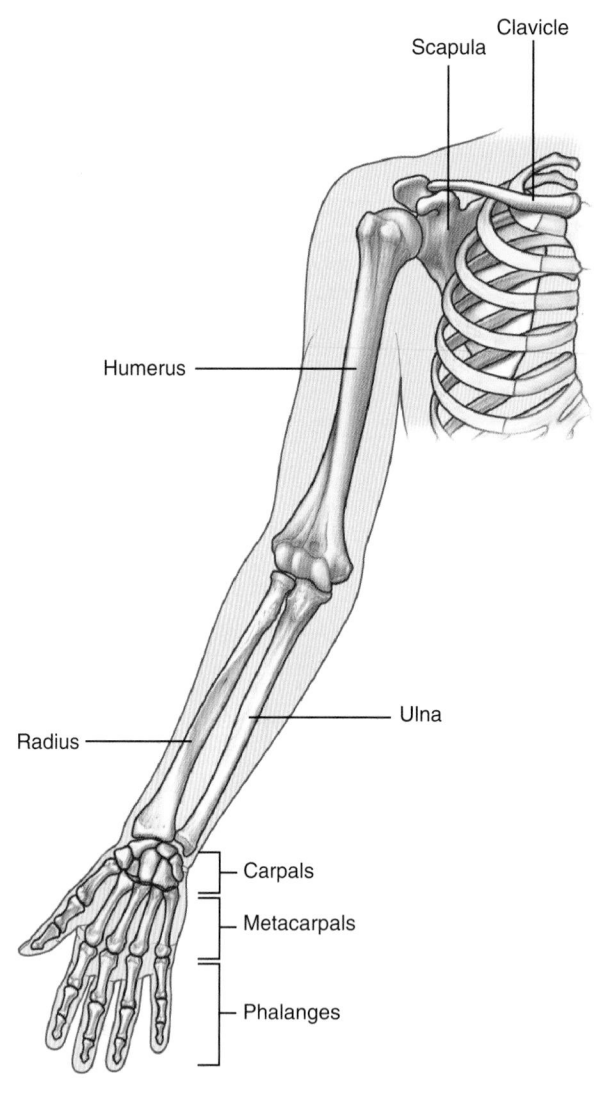

Anterior View

FIG. 21.2 Bones of the right upper extremity. (Modified from Drake, R. L., Vogl, A. W., & Mitchell, A. W. M. [2010]. *Gray's anatomy for students* [2nd ed.]. Philadelphia, PA: Churchill Livingstone.)

CLAVICLE (FIG. 21.3)

Latin: Little key

BONY MARKING	SIGNIFICANCE
Medial (sternal) end	Joint formation
Lateral (acromial) end	Joint formation

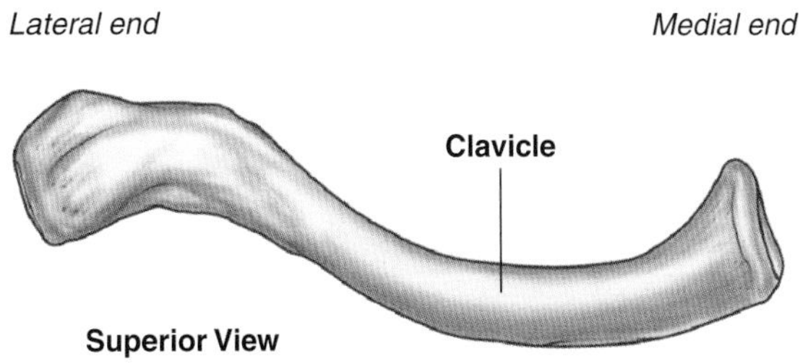

FIG. 21.3 Right clavicle. (Modified from Drake, R. L., Vogl, A. W., & Mitchell, A. W. M. [2010]. *Gray's anatomy for students* [2nd ed.]. Philadelphia, PA: Churchill Livingstone.)

NOTES: The clavicle is the collarbone. It is the most commonly fractured bone in the body. The clavicle and the scapula (featured next) make up the *shoulder girdle,* or the *pectoral girdle.* The clavicle and its medial and lateral ends can easily be palpated. ***LEARNING TIP:*** To help you remember the **C**lavicle is the **C**ollarbone, remember both words begin with the letter **C**.

- **Acromioclavicular (AC) Joints.** The acromion process of the scapula articulates with the lateral end of the clavicle at the AC joint. This gliding joint moves a short distance to mimic the motions of the scapula, similar to the SC joint discussed next. The AC's joint capsule is weak, making it prone to injury by separation and dislocation.
- **Sternoclavicular (SC) Joints.** The medial end of the clavicle articulates with the manubrium of the sternum at the SC joint. This gliding joint moves a short distance to mimic the motions of the scapula, similar to the AC joint mentioned previously. Ligament reinforcements and an articular disc provide strength, often resulting in a clavicular fracture before a SC joint dislocation. The SC joints are the only joints connecting the upper extremities to the axial skeleton.

SCAPULA (FIG. 21.4)

Latin: Shoulder

BONY MARKING	SIGNIFICANCE
Medial (vertebral) border	Muscle attachment
Lateral (axillary) border	Muscle attachment
Superior angle	Muscle attachment
Inferior angle	Muscle attachment
Scapular spine	Muscle attachment
Root of spine	Muscle attachment
Acromion (process)	Muscle attachment and joint formation
Coracoid process	Muscle attachment
Glenoid cavity (fossa)	Joint formation
Supraspinous fossa	Muscle attachment
Infraspinous fossa	Muscle attachment
Subscapular fossa	Muscle attachment
Supraglenoid tubercle	Muscle attachment
Infraglenoid tubercle	Muscle attachment

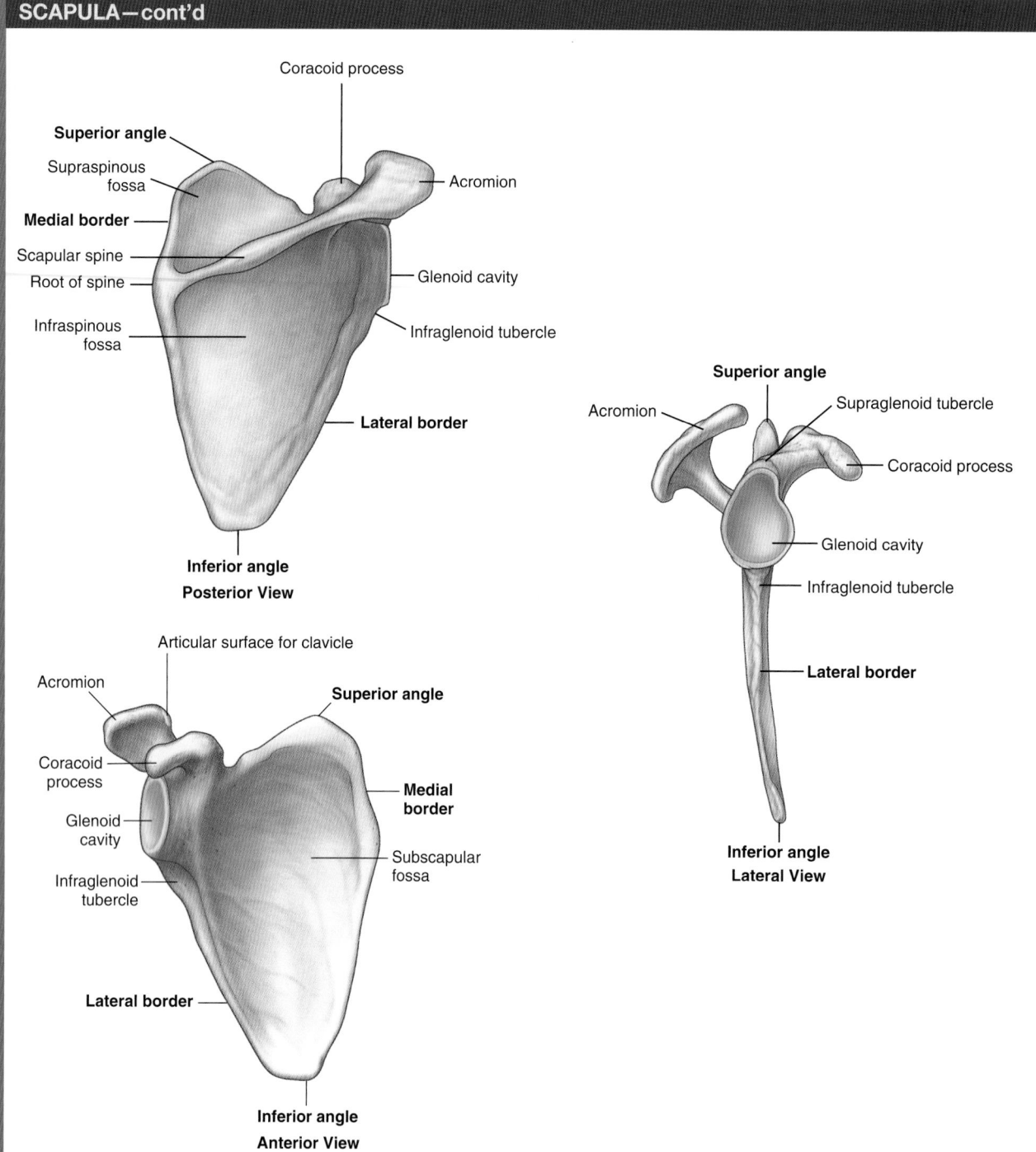

FIG. 21.4 Right scapula. (Modified from Drake, R. L., Vogl, A. W., & Mitchell, A. W. M. [2010]. *Gray's anatomy for students* [2nd ed.]. Philadelphia, PA: Churchill Livingstone.)

NOTES: The scapula is the shoulder blade. This triangular-shaped bone is posterior to ribs 2 through 7, and it slides against the ribcage as it moves. The medial and lateral borders, superior and inferior angles, acromion and coracoid processes, supraspinous and infraspinous fossae, and scapular spine are easily palpated. ***LEARNING TIP:*** To help you remember the **S**capula is the **S**houlder blade, remember both words begin with the letter **S**.

- **Glenohumeral (Shoulder) Joints.** The glenoid cavity of the scapula articulates with the humeral head at the glenohumeral joint. This ball-and-socket joint provides flexion, extension, adduction, abduction, internal (medial) rotation, external (lateral) rotation, and circumduction. The shoulder is one of the most mobile joints in the body, partly because the glenoid cavity is shallow. Although this anatomic feature gives the shoulder mobility, it sacrifices stability, making the shoulder prone to injury by separation and dislocation.

- **Acromioclavicular (AC) Joints.** See Notes section under "Clavicle."

HUMERUS (FIG. 21.5)

Latin: Shoulder

BONY MARKING	SIGNIFICANCE
Humeral head	Joint formation
Anatomic neck	Landmark
Surgical neck	Most fractured area
Greater tubercle	Muscle attachment
Lesser tubercle	Muscle attachment
Intertubercular (bicipital) groove	Muscle attachment (medial and lateral lips)
Deltoid tuberosity	Muscle attachment
Olecranon fossa	Joint formation
Coronoid fossa	Joint formation
Capitulum	Joint formation
Trochlea	Joint formation
Medial epicondyle	Muscle attachment
Lateral epicondyle	Muscle attachment
Supracondylar ridge	Muscle attachment (medial and lateral sections)

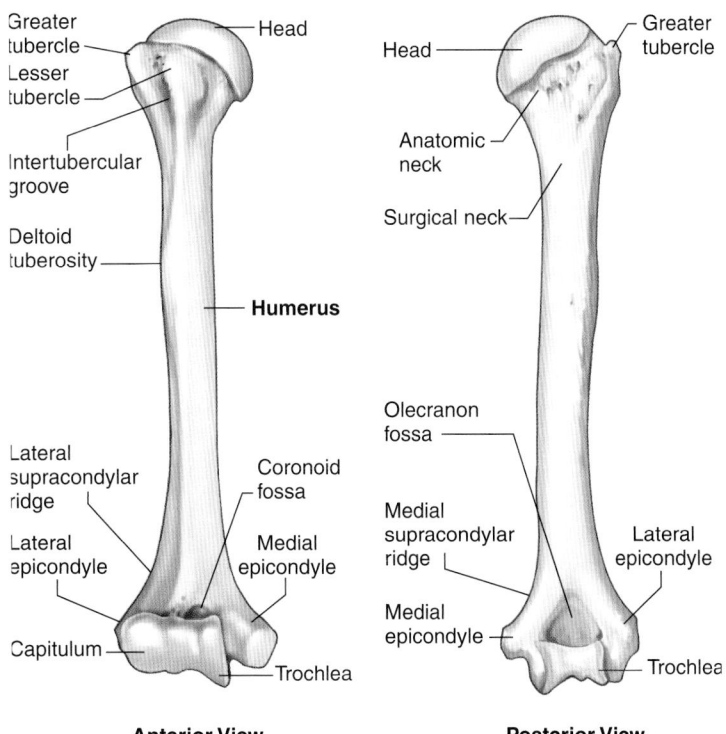

FIG. 21.5 Right humerus. (From Patton, K. T., & Thibodeau, G. A. [2010]. *Anatomy & physiology* [7th ed.]. St. Louis, MO: Mosby.)

NOTES: The humerus is the arm bone. The humerus is named the "funny bone" because hitting a region at its distal end at the elbow makes it feel funny or humorous; these odd sensations originate from pressure on the ulnar nerve, which passes posterior to the medial epicondyle of the humerus. The humeral head and medial/lateral epicondyles are easily palpated.

- **Glenohumeral (Shoulder) Joints.** See Notes section under "Scapula."

- **Elbow Joints.** The elbow joints are a three-bone articulation between the humerus of the arm and the radius and ulna of the forearm. This hinge joint provides flexion and extension. The elbow joint gives rise to two joints.
  - **Humeroulnar Joint.** This is between the distal medial end of the humerus and the proximal end of the ulna.
  - **Humeroradial Joint.** This is between the distal lateral end of the humerus and the proximal end of the radius.

ULNA (FIG. 21.6)

Latin: Elbow

BONY MARKING	SIGNIFICANCE
Olecranon (process)	Muscle attachment
Trochlear (semilunar) notch	Joint formation
Radial notch	Joint formation
Ulnar tuberosity	Muscle attachment
Coronoid process	Muscle attachment
Styloid process	Landmark
Ulnar head	Landmark

NOTES: The ulna is the medial forearm bone on the little finger or pinky side of the forearm. The olecranon (tip of the elbow), ulnar shaft, and ulnar head are easily palpated. **_LEARNING TIP:_** To help you remember which forearm bone is the ulna, the **U**lna has a **U** at its proximal end.

- **Humeroulnar Joints (Part of the Elbow Joints).** See Notes section under "Humerus."
- **Radioulnar (Proximal and Distal) Joints.** The proximal and distal ends of the ulna articulate with the radius at its proximal and distal ends to form the proximal and distal radioulnar joints. The proximal radioulnar joint is distal to the elbow and the distal radioulnar joint is proximal to the wrist. Both radioulnar joints are pivot joints, allowing the forearm to pronate (turn down) and supinate (turn up) (i.e., rotation of the radius over the ulna).

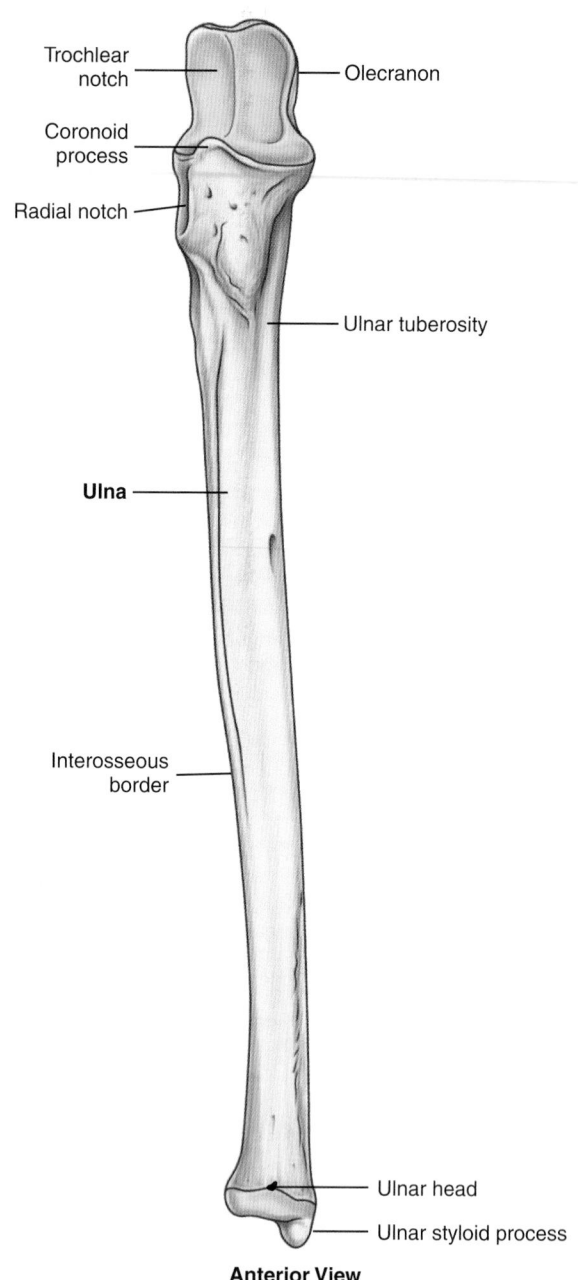

Anterior View

FIG. 21.6 Right ulna. (Modified from Drake, R. L., Vogl, A. W., & Mitchell, A. W. M. [2010]. *Gray's anatomy for students* [2nd ed.]. Philadelphia, PA: Churchill Livingstone.)

RADIUS (FIG. 21.7)

Latin: Staff or spoke of a wheel

BONY MARKING	SIGNIFICANCE
Radial head	Joint formation
Radial neck	Landmark
Radial (bicipital) tuberosity	Muscle attachment
Ulnar notch	Joint formation
Styloid process	Muscle attachment

NOTES: The radius is the lateral forearm bone on the thumb side of the forearm. The radial head and the styloid process can be palpated. ***LEARNING TIP:*** To help you remember which forearm bone moves during pronation and supination, the **R**adius **R**otates over the ulna, and both words begin with the letter **R**.

An *interosseous membrane* connects the radius and the ulna (Fig. 21.8). This anatomic arrangement gives the forearm lightness and mobility, and provides attachment sites for many muscles of the forearm and hand. An interosseous membrane is also between the tibia and fibula (see Lesson Two).

- **Humeroradial Joints (Part of the Elbow Joints).** See Notes section under "Humerus."
- **Radioulnar (Proximal and Distal) Joints.** See the Notes section under "Ulna."
- **Radiocarpal (Wrist) Joints.** The distal ends of the radius in the forearm articulate with the proximal carpal bones in the wrist at the radiocarpal joints. The carpal bones articulating with the radius are the scaphoid, lunate, and triquetral bones. This condyloid (ellipsoidal) joint provides flexion, extension, abduction (radial deviation), and adduction (radial deviation).

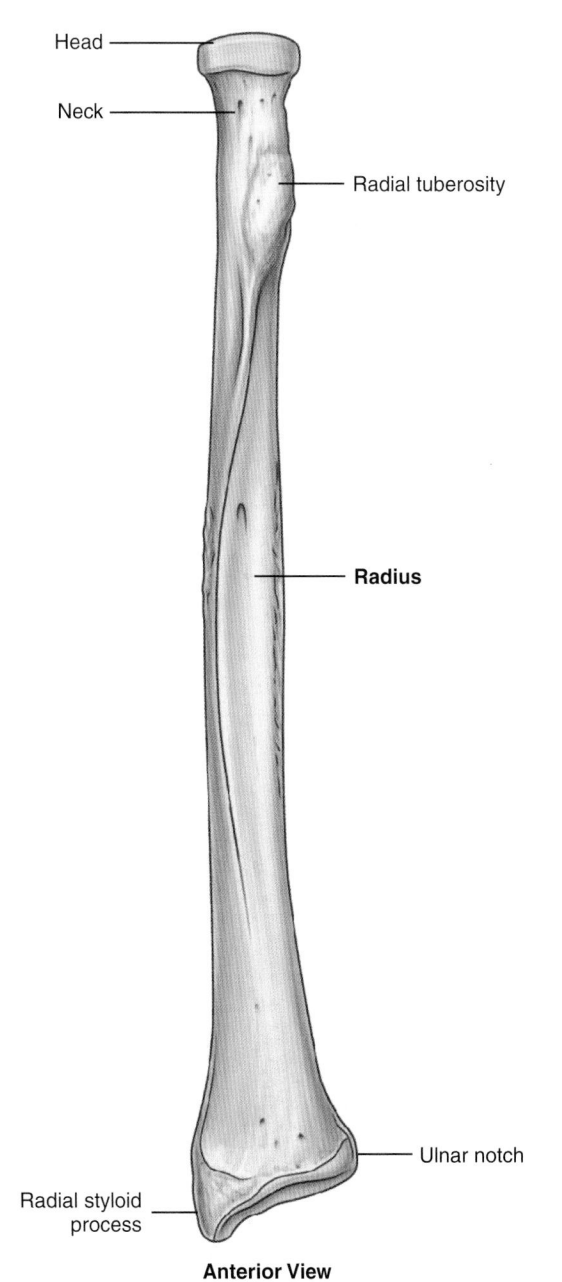

Anterior View

FIG. 21.7 Right radius. (Modified from Drake, R. L., Vogl, A. W., & Mitchell, A. W. M. [2010]. *Gray's anatomy for students* [2nd ed.]. Philadelphia, PA: Churchill Livingstone.)

Anterior View

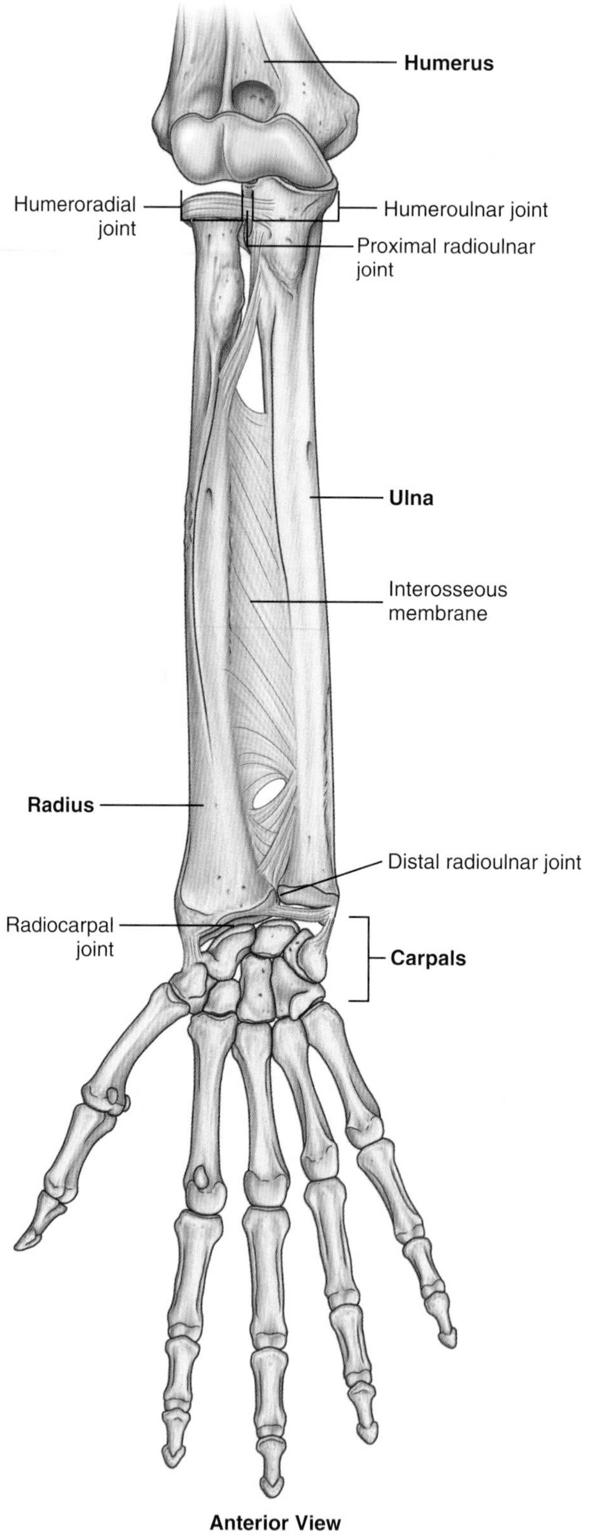

FIG. 21.8 Right forearm, wrist, and hand. Associated forearm bones, interosseous membrane, and joints identified. (Modified from Drake, R. L., Vogl, A. W., & Mitchell, A. W. M. [2010]. *Gray's anatomy for students* [2nd ed.]. Philadelphia, PA: Churchill Livingstone.)

CARPALS (FIG. 21.9)

Greek: Wrist

BONE	SIGNIFICANCE
Scaphoid	Largest carpal bone in some individuals and most fractured carpal bone
Lunate	Crescent-shaped bone; most dislocated carpal bone
Triquetrum	Triangular- or pyramid-shaped bone
Pisiform	Pea-shaped and smallest carpal bone; attaches to the transverse carpal ligament
Trapezium	Triangular-shaped bone; part of the thumb's saddle joint
Trapezoid	Four-sided bone with two parallel sides
Capitate	Largest carpal bone in some individuals and possesses a round head
Hamate	Possesses a hook-like projection called the hook of hamate; attaches to the transverse carpal ligament

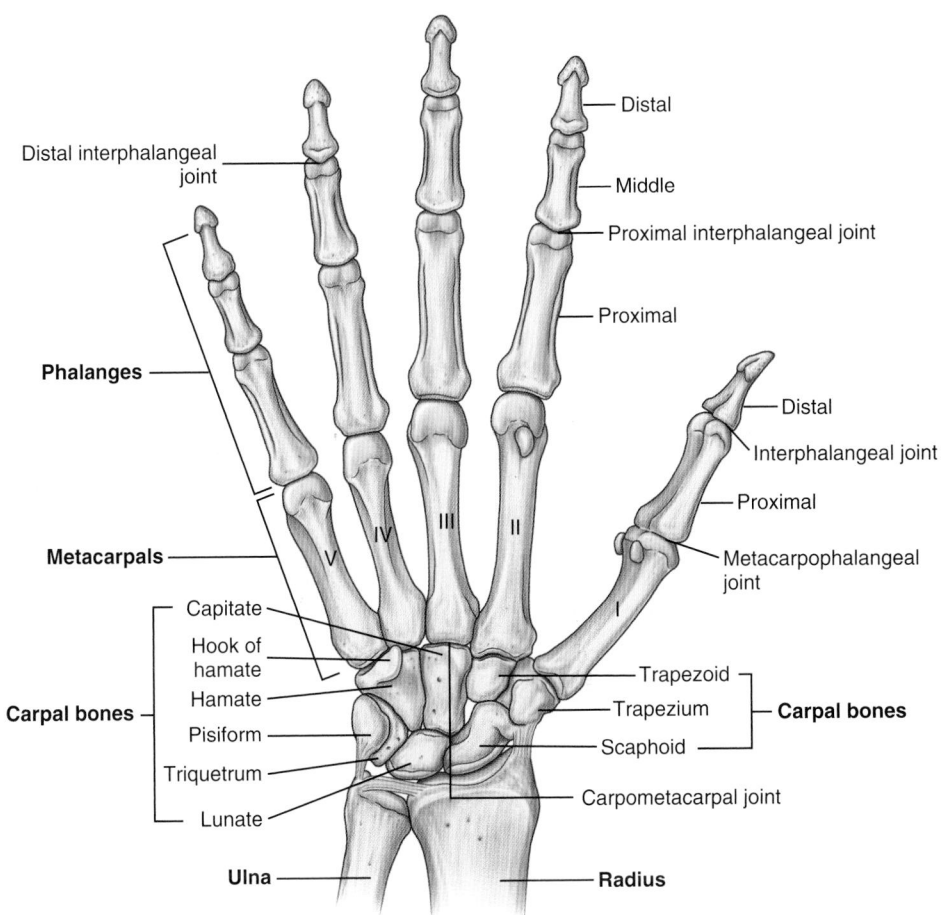

Anterior View

FIG. 21.9 Right hand and wrist with carpals, metacarpals, phalanges, and joints identified. (Modified from Drake, R. L., Vogl, A. W., & Mitchell, A. W. M. [2010]. *Gray's anatomy for students* [2nd ed.]. Philadelphia, PA: Churchill Livingstone.)

NOTES: The carpal bones are the wrist bones. Eight carpal bones in each wrist are bound by ligaments and arranged in two rows, a proximal and a distal row. The bones in the proximal row are the scaphoid, lunate, triquetrum, and pisiform (lateral to medial). The bones in the distal row are the trapezium, trapezoid, capitate, and hamate (lateral to medial). **LEARNING TIP:** To help you remember the names of the carpal bones, use the phrase **S**teve **L**eft **T**he **P**arty **T**o **T**ake **C**athy **H**ome for Scaphoid—Lunate—Triquetrum—Pisiform—Trapezium—Trapezoid—Capitate—Hamate or the phrase **S**o **L**ong **T**o **P**inky, **H**ere **C**omes **T**he **T**humb for Scaphoid—Lunate—Triquetrum—Pisiform—Hamate—Capitate—Trapezoid—Trapezium.

The **carpal tunnel** is a passageway surrounded on three sides by carpal bones and on one side by the transverse carpal ligament

Continued

CARPALS—cont'd

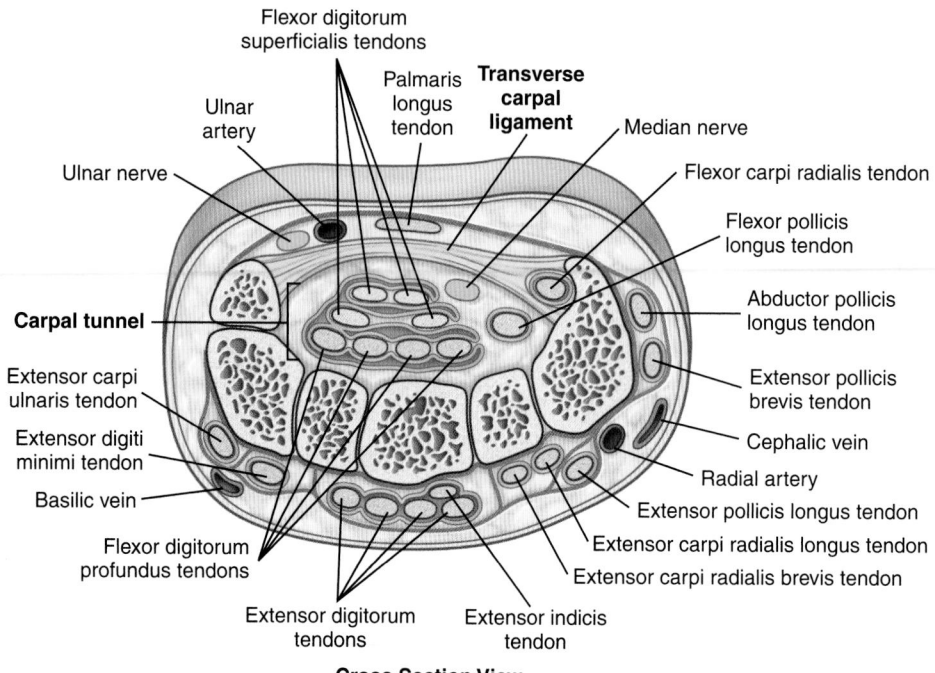

Flexor digitorum
superficialis tendons

Palmaris
longus
tendon

**Transverse
carpal
ligament**

Median nerve

Ulnar
artery

Ulnar nerve

Flexor carpi radialis tendon

Flexor pollicis
longus tendon

Carpal tunnel

Abductor pollicis
longus tendon

Extensor carpi
ulnaris tendon

Extensor pollicis
brevis tendon

Extensor digiti
minimi tendon

Cephalic vein

Basilic vein

Radial artery

Extensor pollicis longus tendon

Flexor digitorum
profundus tendons

Extensor carpi radialis longus tendon

Extensor carpi radialis brevis tendon

Extensor digitorum
tendons

Extensor indicis
tendon

Cross Section View

FIG. 21.10 Right carpal tunnel with associated tendons and median nerve identified. (Modified from Drake, R. L., Vogl, A. W., & Mitchell, A. W. M. [2010]. *Gray's anatomy for students* [2nd ed.]. Philadelphia, PA: Churchill Livingstone.)

(Fig. 21.10). The transverse carpal ligament (TCL) is a fibrous band on the anterior or palmar side of the hand at the wrist. The TCL is attached to the pisiform and hook of the hamate on the ulnar (medial) side and to the scaphoid and trapezium on the radial (lateral) side. The TCL forms the roof of the carpal tunnel. The TCL is also called the *flexor retinaculum* and *anterior annular ligament*. The carpal tunnel contains nine tendons: one for *flexor pollicis longus,* four for *flexor digitorum superficialis*, and four for *flexor digitorum profundus*. The carpal tunnel also contains the median nerve. Because the carpal tunnel is a nonyielding compartment, its contents can become compressed, under certain circumstances, causing carpal tunnel syndrome. See Chapter 23 for more information about carpal tunnel syndrome.
- **Radiocarpal (Wrist) Joints.** See Notes section under "Radius."

- **Carpometacarpal (CMC) Joints.** The distal row of carpals in the wrist articulates with the proximal metacarpals of the hands at the carpometacarpal joints. There are five CMC joints in each hand— the first CMC joint of the thumb is the most specialized. The remaining four CMC joints are condyloid (ellipsoidal) joints that provide flexion, extension, abduction, and adduction. The CMC joint also permits palmar cupping and object grasping.
- **Carpometacarpal of the Thumb (First CMC Joints or Trapeziometacarpal Joints).** The CMC joint of the thumb is between the trapezium carpal bone and the first metacarpal. This saddle joint plays an important role in the normal functioning of the hand. Movements permitted at this joint are flexion, extension, abduction, adduction, circumduction, opposition, and reposition.

METACARPALS (SEE FIG. 21.9)

Greek: After or beyond; wrist

NOTES: The metacarpals are in each hand and are numbered I through V, starting with the thumb (metacarpal I) and ending with the little finger (metacarpal V). The distal ends are the metacarpal heads, or *knuckles*, which can be easily palpated when the hand is clenched in a fist.

- **Carpometacarpal (CMC) Joints.** See Notes section under "Carpals."

- **Metacarpophalangeal (MCP) Joints.** The distal ends of the metacarpals of the hands articulate with the proximal phalanges of the fingers at the metacarpophalangeal joints. These five condyloid (ellipsoidal) joints provide flexion, extension, abduction, adduction, and circumduction.

PHALANGES (SEE FIG. 21.9)

Greek: A line of soldiers

NOTES: Phalanges are in the fingers and thumb. They are also called *digits*. Each hand contains 14 phalanges. Each finger has three phalanges, while the thumb has two. Fingers contain a proximal phalanx, a middle phalanx, and a distal phalanx. The thumb contains only a proximal and a distal phalanx.

- **Metacarpophalangeal (MCP) Joints.** See Notes section under "Metacarpals."

- **Interphalangeal (IP) Joints.** These are between adjacent phalanges in the fingers and the thumb. The thumb has a single IP joint, while the second to fifth fingers have a proximal and a distal interphalangeal joint. These hinge joints provide flexion and extension, along with supporting fine motor movements of the hand.

- **Proximal Interphalangeal (PIP) Joints.** The distal ends of the proximal phalanges articulate with their middle phalanges at the PIP joints.

- **Distal Interphalangeal (DIP) Joints.** The middle phalanges articulate with their distal phalanges at the DIP joints.

Lesson Two: Bones and Joints of the Lower Extremity

Bones of the lower extremity are the pelvic bone, femur, patella, tibia, fibula, tarsals, metatarsals, and phalanges. Associated joints and other structures are listed as bullets the Notes section (Fig. 21.11).

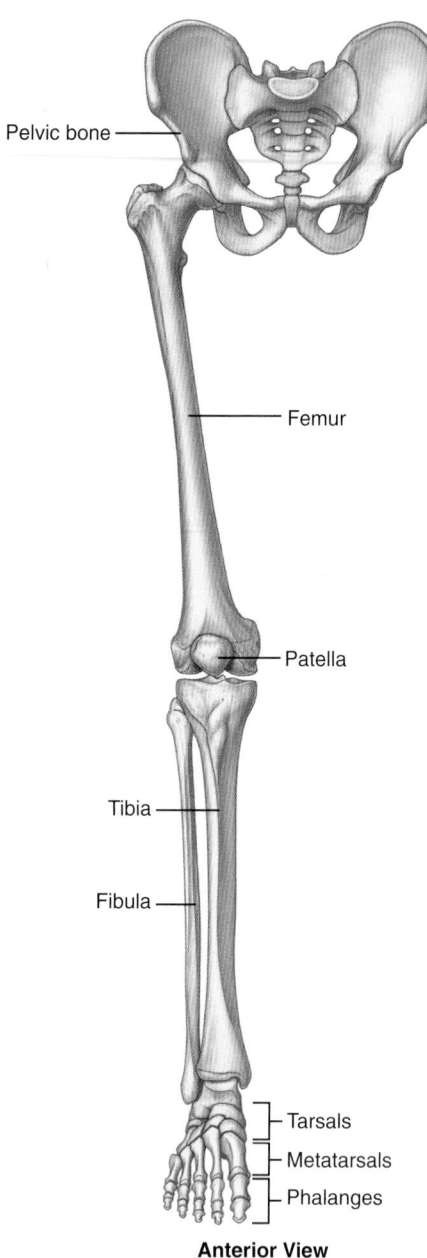

Pelvic bone

Femur

Patella

Tibia

Fibula

Tarsals

Metatarsals

Phalanges

Anterior View

FIG. 21.11 Bones of the right lower extremity. The two pelvic bones and the pelvic spine (sacrum and coccyx) comprise the circle of bones called the *pelvis*. (Modified from Drake, R. L., Vogl, A. W., & Mitchell, A. W. M. [2010]. *Gray's anatomy for students* [2nd ed.]. Philadelphia, PA: Churchill Livingstone.)

PELVIC BONES (FIG. 21.12)

Latin: A basin

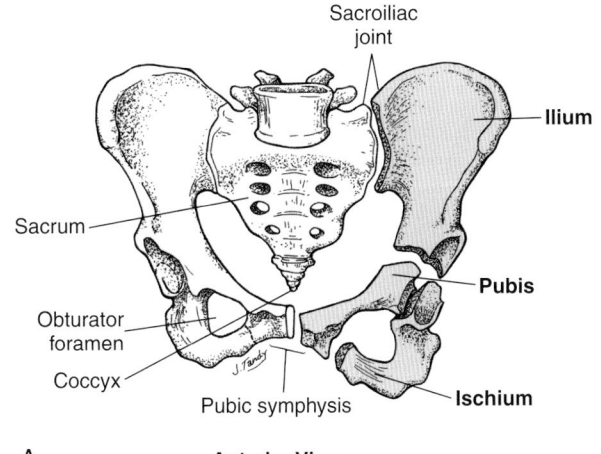

A   **Anterior View**

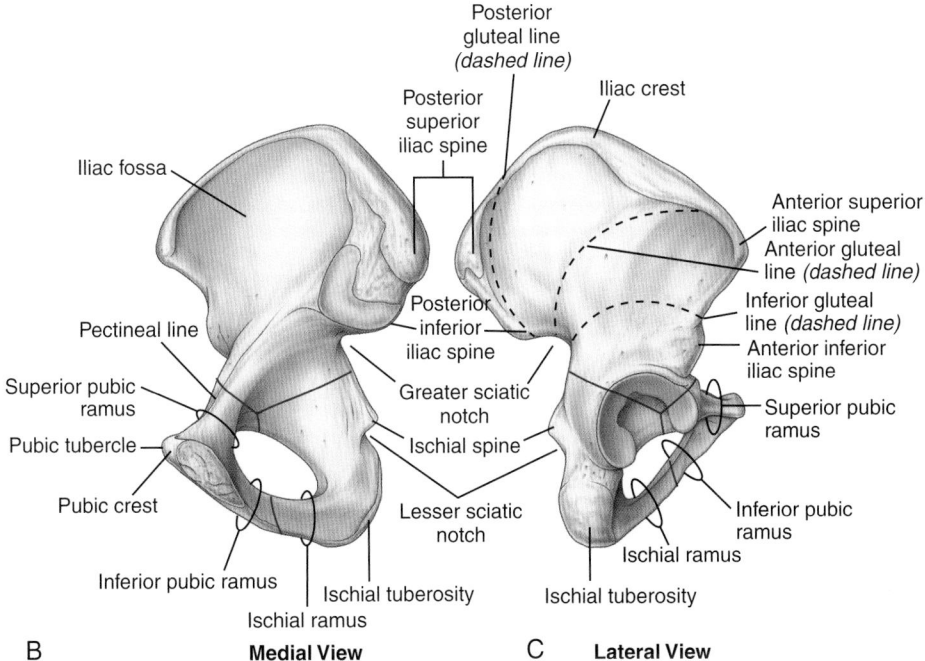

B   **Medial View**   **C**   **Lateral View**

FIG. 21.12 The pelvis with right and left pelvic bones, the sacrum, and the coccyx (*A*) (Modified from Ball, J. [2019]. *Seidel's Guide to Physical Examination* [9th ed.]. St. Louis, MO: Mosby.) The right pelvic bone (*B, medial view; C, lateral view*). (Modified from Drake, R. L., Vogl, A. W., & Mitchell, A. W. M. [2010]. *Gray's anatomy for students* [2nd ed.]. Philadelphia, PA: Churchill Livingstone.)

NOTES: There are two pelvic bones in the abdominopelvic region of the body. Each pelvic bone consists of three paired fused bones: the ilium, ischium, and pubis. The right and left pelvic bones make up the *pelvic girdle*; these structures are also called the *os coxa, coxal bones, appendicular hip bones,* or just *hip bones.*

The pelvic bones and the pelvic spine (sacrum and coccyx) comprise a circle of bones of the *pelvis.* The pelvis can assume several positions as it rests on the femurs. Most positions are described by the direction of their tilt (Fig. 21.13).

- **Anterior Pelvic Tilt.** Pelvis tilts anteriorly or forward. This action increases lumbar lordosis.
- **Posterior Pelvic Tilt.** Pelvis tilts posteriorly or backward. This action decreases lumbar lordosis.
- **Neutral Pelvis (No Tilt).** Anterior superior iliac spines (ASIS) and posterior superior iliac spines (PSIS) are level in the

Continued

PELVIC BONES—cont'd

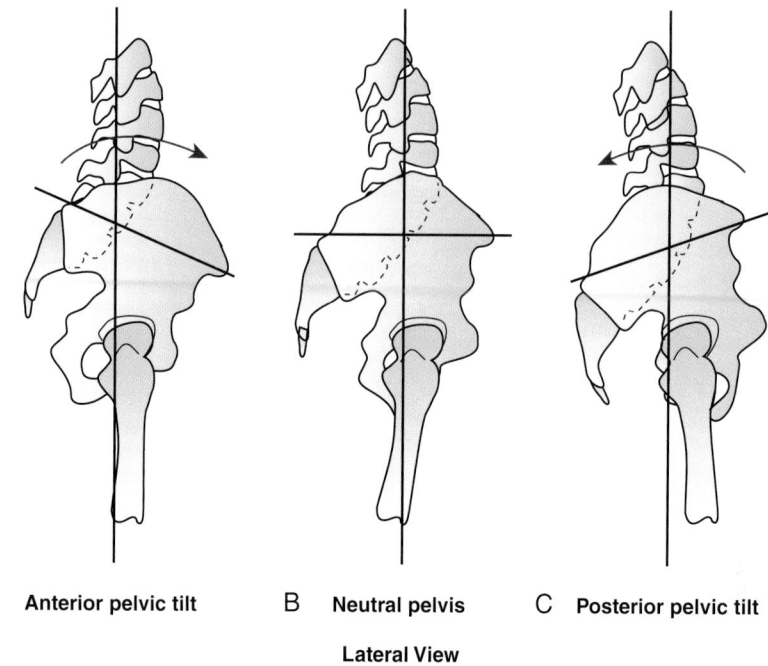

A **Anterior pelvic tilt**   B **Neutral pelvis**   C **Posterior pelvic tilt**

Lateral View

FIG. 21.13 Pelvic tilts. Comparing a neutral pelvis (*B, middle image*), an anterior pelvic tilt (*A, left image*), and a posterior pelvic tilt (*C, right image*). The vertical lines represent the approximate center of gravity. The horizontal lines represent the positions of the anterior and posterior superior iliac spines. The red arrow represents the direction of tilt. (From Fritz, S. [2017]. *Mosby's essential sciences for therapeutic massage* [5th ed.]. St. Louis, MO: Elsevier.)

transverse/horizontal plane. Essentially a balanced position between exaggerated anterior and posterior tilts.
- **Right Pelvic Tilt.** Pelvis tilts toward the right.
- **Left Pelvic Tilt.** Pelvis tilts toward the left.
  The *acetabulum*, or acetabular cavity, is the deep hip socket made from portions of all three pelvic bones (Fig. 21.14).
  The *obturator foramen* is inferior to the acetabulum. It provides attachment sites for several muscles and a passageway for blood vessels and nerves. In a living skeleton, the *obturator membrane* "obstructs" most of the obturator foramen and provides attachment sites for several muscles.
- **Acetabulofemoral (Hip) Joints.** The acetabulum articulates with the femoral head at the acetabulofemoral joint. This ball-socket joint provides flexion, extension, adduction, abduction, internal (medial) rotation, external (lateral) rotation, and circumduction. The hip joint is mobile but not as mobile as the ball-and-socket joint of the shoulder because the acetabulum is deeper compared with the glenoid cavity. This anatomic feature gives the hip joint greater stability but sacrifices some mobility.

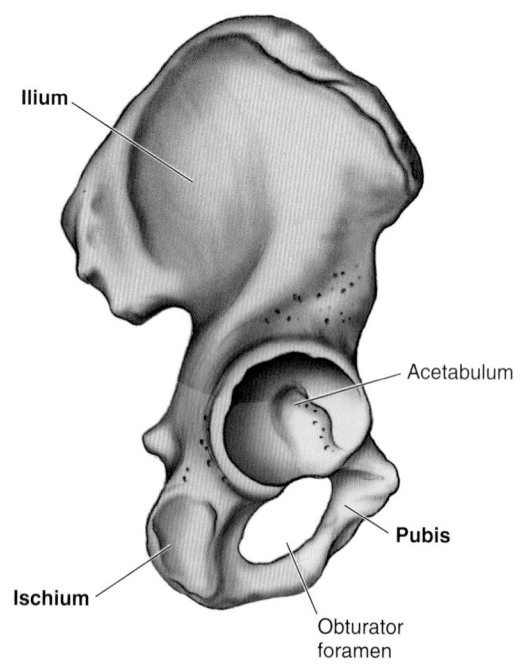

Ilium

Acetabulum

Pubis

Ischium

Obturator foramen

Lateral View

FIG. 21.14 Right pelvic bone. The ilium (*purple*), ischium (*blue*), pubis (*green*), acetabulum, and obturator foramen are identified. (From Hagen-Ansert, S. L. [2018]. *Textbook of diagnostic sonography* [8th ed.]. Philadelphia, PA: Elsevier.)

ILIUM (SEE FIG. 21.12)

Latin: Flank

BONY MARKING	SIGNIFICANCE
Iliac crest	Muscle attachment
Iliac fossa	Muscle attachment
Anterior superior iliac spine (ASIS)	Muscle attachment
Anterior inferior iliac spine (AIIS)	Muscle attachment
Posterior superior iliac spine (PSIS)	Muscle attachment
Posterior inferior iliac spine (PIIS)	Muscle attachment
Posterior gluteal line	Muscle attachment
Anterior gluteal line	Muscle attachment
Inferior gluteal line	Muscle attachment
Greater sciatic notch	Passage of sciatic nerve

NOTES: The ilium bones are the most superior pelvic bones and resemble a broad, expanding blade. The PSIS can be seen between the buttocks and the waist and is nicknamed the "dimples of Venus." The iliac crest and all iliac spines are easily palpated.
- **Sacroiliac (SI) Joints.** The sacrum of the spine articulates with the right and left ilia of the pelvis at the SI joints (see Fig. 21.12A). These gliding joints provide a small degree of sliding and rotational movements. This joint is unique because it contains fibrocartilage as well as hyaline cartilage, the latter is typical of synovial joints. Functions of the SI joint are to provide stability and to transfer weight from the axial skeleton to the lower extremities. The SI joints are the only joints connecting the lower extremities to the axial skeleton.

ISCHIUM (SEE FIG. 21.12)

Latin: Hip

BONY MARKING	SIGNIFICANCE
Ischial spine	Muscle attachment
Ischial tuberosity	Muscle attachment
Ischial ramus	Muscle attachment

NOTES: The ischium bones are the most inferior and posterior pelvic bones. These bones are the *sitz bones* because correct seated posture involves the weight of the upper body resting on these bones (the ischial tuberosities) rather than on the sacrum and coccyx (part of the pelvic spine). The ischial tuberosity is easily palpated.

The *sacrotuberous ligament* is a triangular-shaped ligament extending from the ischial tuberosity to the sacrum and provides pelvic stability (see Fig. 21.67).

PUBIS (SEE FIG. 21.12)

Latin: Grownup

BONY MARKING	SIGNIFICANCE
Superior pubic ramus	Muscle attachment
Inferior pubic ramus	Muscle attachment
Pubic tubercle	Muscle attachment
Pubic crest	Muscle attachment
Pectineal line	Muscle attachment

NOTES: The pubic bones are the most anterior pelvic bones.
- **Pubic Symphysis.** This cartilaginous joint is between the right and left pubic bones and has very little movement (see Fig. 21.12A).

Hormonal changes such as increased levels of relaxin during the last trimester of pregnancy cause the pubic symphysis to widen slightly so the baby can pass through the pelvis during childbirth.

FEMUR (FIG. 21.15)

Latin: Thigh

BONY MARKING	SIGNIFICANCE
Femoral head	Joint formation
Femoral neck	Landmark (where most femoral fractures occur)
Greater trochanter	Muscle attachment
Lesser trochanter	Muscle attachment
Intertrochanteric line	Muscle attachment
Intertrochanteric crest	Muscle attachment
Linea aspera	Muscle attachment (medial and lateral lips)
Gluteal tuberosity	Muscle attachment
Adductor tubercle	Muscle attachment
Medial condyle	Joint formation
Lateral condyle	Joint formation
Intercondylar fossa	Ligament attachment (cruciate ligaments)
Medial epicondyle	Muscle attachment
Lateral epicondyle	Muscle attachment

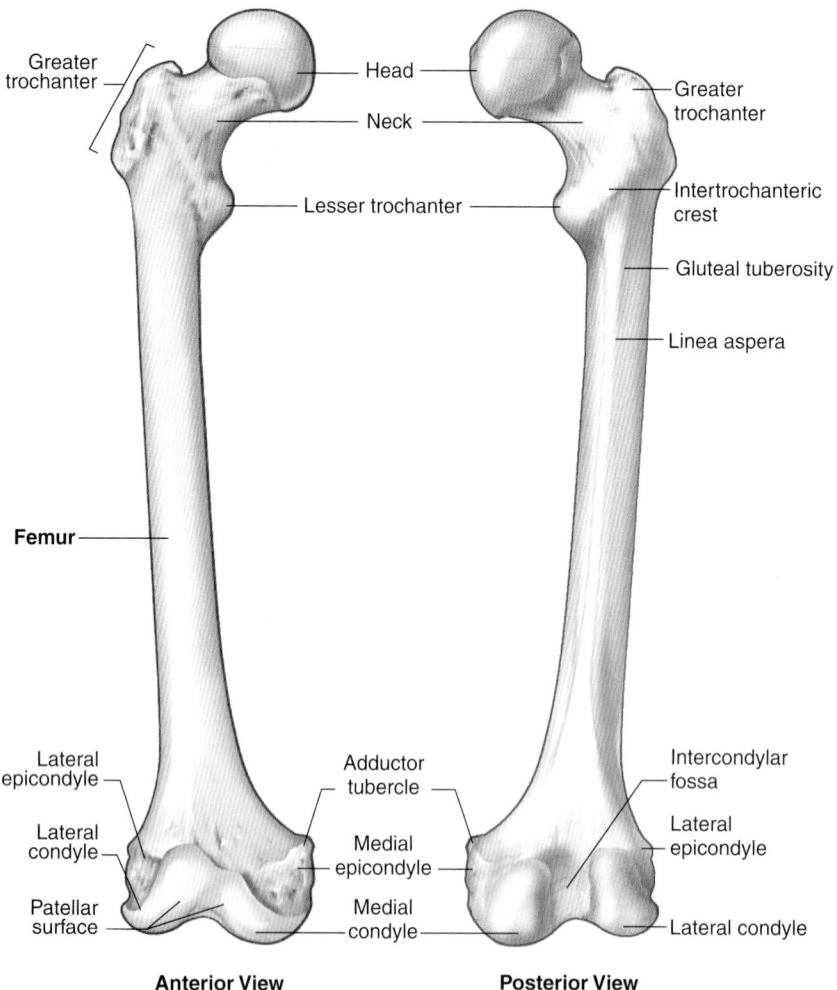

Anterior View **Posterior View**

FIG. 21.15 Right femur. (From Patton, K. T., & Thibodeau, G. A. [2010]. *Anatomy & physiology* [7th ed.]. St. Louis, MO: Mosby.)

FEMUR—cont'd

NOTES: The femur is the thigh bone. It is the longest, heaviest, and strongest bone in the body. The greater trochanter and medial/lateral condyles are easily palpated.

- **Acetabulofemoral (Hip) Joints.** See the Notes section under "Pelvic Bones."
- **Tibiofemoral (Knee) Joints.** The distal end of the femur of the thigh articulates with the tibia of the leg at the tibiofemoral joint. This hinge joint permits flexion and extension of the knee. The knee is the most complex joint in the body and contains several important structures (Fig.21.16). Most knee ligaments keep the tibia from sliding out from under the femur.
  - **Medial and Lateral Meniscus.** These half-ringed fibrocartilage discs are on the proximal ends of the tibia. The femoral condyles slide over the menisci during knee flexion and extension.
  - **Anterior Cruciate Ligament (ACL) and Posterior Cruciate Ligaments (PCL).** These are inside the knee. The ACL is toward the front of the knee and helps prevent anterior or forward motion of the tibia; the ACL is the most commonly injured knee ligament. The PCL is toward the back of the knee and helps prevent posterior or backward motion of the tibia.
  - **Tibial (Medial) Collateral Ligament (TCL) and Fibular (Lateral) Collateral Ligament (LCL).** The TCL is on the medial, or inner, side of the knee. The LCL is on the lateral, or outer, side of the knee. Both ligaments help prevent side-to-side motions of the tibia.
  - **Patellar Ligament.** Connects the patella to the tibial tuberosity.
  - **Infrapatellar Fat Pad.** Beneath the patellar ligament and helps reduce friction between it and the tibia during knee flexion and extension.
- **Patellofemoral Joints.** See Notes section under "Patella."

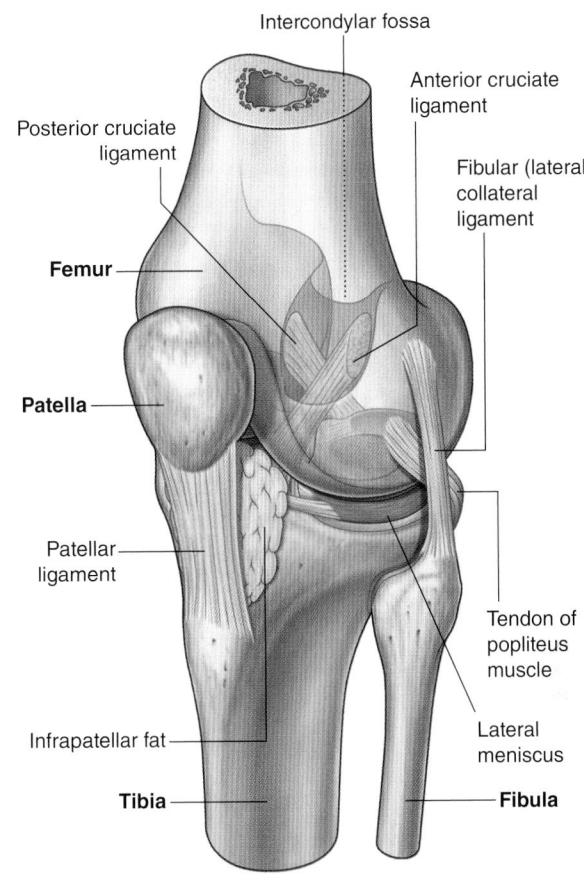

Anterolateral View

FIG. 21.16 Left knee. (Modified from Drake, R. L., Vogl, A. W., & Mitchell, A. W. M. [2010]. *Gray's anatomy for students* [2nd ed.]. Philadelphia, PA: Churchill Livingstone.)

PATELLA (SEE FIG. 21.16)

Latin: A little dish

NOTES: The patella is the kneecap and the largest sesamoid bone in the body. The patella is embedded in the tendon of the quadriceps. The main function of the patella is to assist knee extension by increasing leverage in the quadriceps tendon.

- **Patellofemoral Joints.** The patella of the knee articulates with the distal anterior portion of the femur at the patellofemoral joint. This gliding joint slides inferiorly during knee flexion and superiorly during knee extension.

TIBIA (FIG. 21.17)

Latin: Shinbone

BONY MARKING	SIGNIFICANCE
Medial condyle	Joint formation
Lateral condyle	Joint formation
Tibial tuberosity	Muscle attachment
Gerdy tubercle	Attachment of the iliotibial band
Crest (anterior border)	Landmark
Soleal line	Muscle attachment
Medial malleolus	Landmark

NOTES: The tibia is the medial leg bone and is larger in diameter compared with the fibula. The tibia is also called the *shinbone*. The tibial tuberosity, tibial crest, and medial malleolus are easily palpated. ***LEARNING TIP:*** To help you remember the tibia is the larger or thicker leg bone, remember **T**ibia and **T**hick both begin with the letter **T**.

- **Tibiofemoral (Knee) Joints.** See Notes section under "Femur."
- **Tibiofibular (Proximal and Distal) Joints.** The proximal and distal ends of the tibia articulate with the fibula to form the proximal and distal tibiofibular joints. The proximal tibiofibular joint is distal to the knee and the distal tibiofibular joint is proximal to the ankle. Both tibiofibular joints are gliding joints and permit only a small amount of anterior and posterior movement. This is to accommodate flexion and extension of the knee, as well as the dorsiflexion and plantar flexion of the ankle.
- **Talocrural (Ankle) Joints.** See Notes section under "Tarsals."

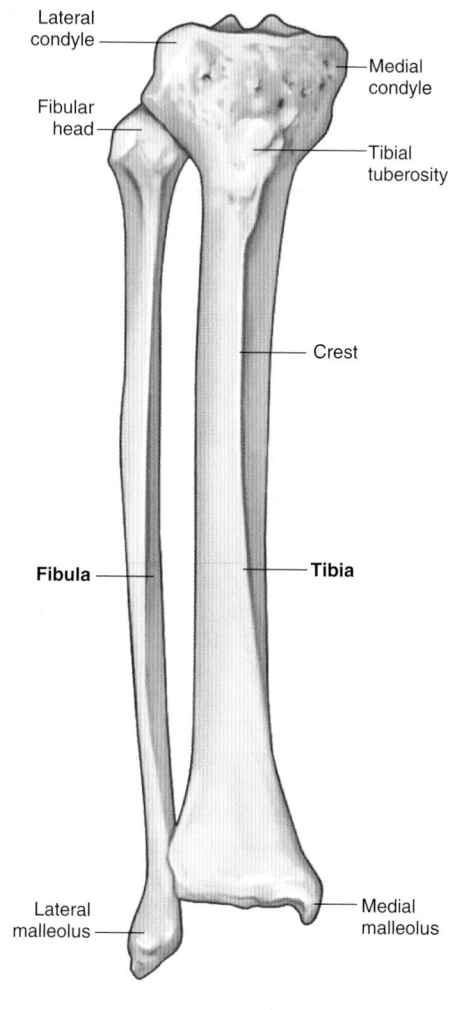

Anterior View

FIG. 21.17 Right tibia and fibula. (From Patton, K. T., & Thibodeau, G. A. [2014]. *The human body in health and disease* [6th ed.]. St. Louis, MO: Elsevier.)

FIBULA (SEE FIG. 21.17)

Latin: Clasp or pin of a brooch

BONY MARKING	SIGNIFICANCE
Fibular head	Muscle attachment
Lateral malleolus	Landmark

NOTES: The fibula is the lateral leg bone. It is smaller in diameter compared with the tibia and the fibula supports only 10% of the body's weight. The fibular head and the lateral malleolus are easily palpated. ***LEARNING TIP:*** To help you remember which leg bone is lateral, fibu**LA** and **LA**teral both have the letters **LA**. To help you remember the fibula is the smaller of the two leg bones, use the phrase "Never tell a little fib."

An *interosseous membrane* connects the tibia and the fibula. This anatomic arrangement helps stabilize the leg bones, separates the leg muscles into compartments, and provides attachment sites for many muscles. An interosseous membrane is also between the ulna and radius (see Lesson One).

- **Tibiofibular (Proximal and Distal) Joints.** See Notes section under "Tibia."
- **Talocrural (Ankle) Joints.** See Notes section under "Tarsals."

TARSALS (FIG. 21.18)

Latin: Broad, flat surface; foot

BONES	SIGNIFICANCE
Talus	Ankle bone, second largest tarsal bone, and transfers the weight of the body from the legs to the foot; no muscle attachments
Calcaneus	Heel bone, largest tarsal bone, transfers the weight of the body to the ground, and contains the calcaneal tuberosity, which is the most posterior and inferior part of the bone
Cuneiforms: medial (I), intermediate (II), lateral (III)	Wedge-shaped bone on the medial side of the foot
Navicular	Boat-shaped bone on the medial side of the foot
Cuboid	Cube-shaped bone on the lateral side of the foot

NOTES: The tarsal bones are in the proximal foot between the leg bones (tibia and fibula) and the metatarsals. The seven tarsal bones are the talus, calcaneus, cuboid, navicular, and the medial, intermediate, and lateral cuneiforms. ***LEARNING TIP:*** To help you remember the names of the tarsal bones, use the phrase **T**he **C**ircus **N**eeds **M**ore **I**nteresting **L**ittle **C**lowns for Talus—Calcaneus—**N**avicular—**M**edial cuneiform—**I**ntermediate cuneiform—**L**ateral cuneiform—**C**uboid. Thinking about a clown's big feet will help you remember this mnemonic phrase for tarsal bones of the foot.

The foot can be divided into three regions; the rearfoot, the midfoot, and the forefoot (Fig. 21.19). The *rearfoot*, or hindfoot, contains the talus and calcaneus; the *midfoot* contains the navicular, cuboid, and cuneiforms. The *forefoot* contains the metatarsal and phalanges that are discussed later.

The foot has three arches: two longitudinal (medial and lateral) arches and one anterior transverse arch. They are formed by the tarsal and metatarsal bones and are supported by ligaments and tendons of the foot. The arches resemble a geodesic dome and help the foot bear weight, absorb shock, and assist in propulsive movements such as walking, running, and jumping. The *medial arch* is the higher of the two longitudinal arches and is found on the inner edge of the foot. The *lateral arch* is the flatter of the two longitudinal arches and is found on the outer edge of the foot. The *transverse (metatarsal) arch* is in the forefoot and runs side-to-side across the bases of the metatarsals (Fig. 21.20).

- **Talocrural (Ankle) Joints.** The talus of the foot articulates with the distal ends of the tibia and the fibula of the leg at the talocrural joint (crural is *Latin* for leg). This hinge joint allows for dorsiflexion and plantar flexion.
- **Talocalcaneal (Subtalar) Joints.** The talus articulates with the calcaneus at the talocalcaneal joint. Commonly referred to as a gliding joint, this joint is saddle-shaped and provides inversion and eversion. Inversion sprains are more common than eversion sprains and the most common ligament injured from an inversion sprain is the *anterior talofibular ligament* (ATFL).
- **Tarsometatarsal (TMT) Joints.** The tarsal bones (cuboid and all cuneiforms) articulate with the proximal ends of the metatarsals at the tarsometatarsal joints. This gliding joint permits a slight sliding of these bones over each other.

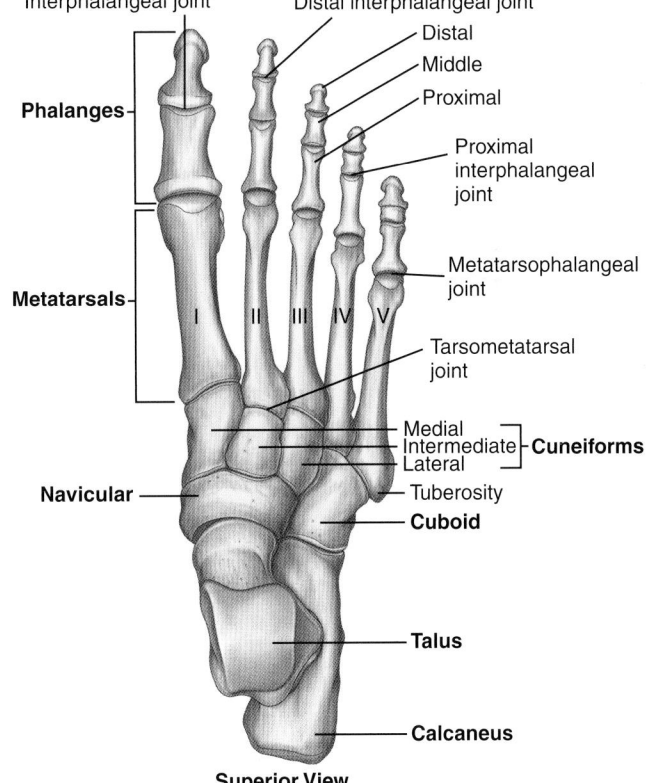

Superior View

FIG. 21.18 Right foot with tarsals, metatarsals, phalanges, and joints identified. (Modified from Drake, R. L., Vogl, A. W., & Mitchell, A. W. M. [2010]. *Gray's anatomy for students* [2nd ed.]. Philadelphia, PA: Churchill Livingstone.)

METATARSALS (SEE FIG. 21.18)

Greek: After or beyond; foot

NOTES: The metatarsals are in the distal foot and numbered I through V, starting with the great toe (metatarsal I) and ending with the little toe (metatarsal V). The distal ends are the metatarsal heads and are easily palpated when the toes are flexed. The fifth metatarsal has a tuberosity on its distal surface, which can be palpated on the lateral border of the foot. The length of the metatarsals determines your shoe size. *Morton foot* (Morton toe) occurs when metatarsal II is longer than metatarsal I.

- **Tarsometatarsal (TMT) Joints.** See the Notes section under "Tarsals."
- **Metatarsophalangeal (MTP) Joints.** The distal ends of the metatarsals of the foot articulate with the corresponding proximal phalanges of the toes at the MTP joints. These condyloid (ellipsoidal) joints permit flexion, extension, abduction, and adduction.

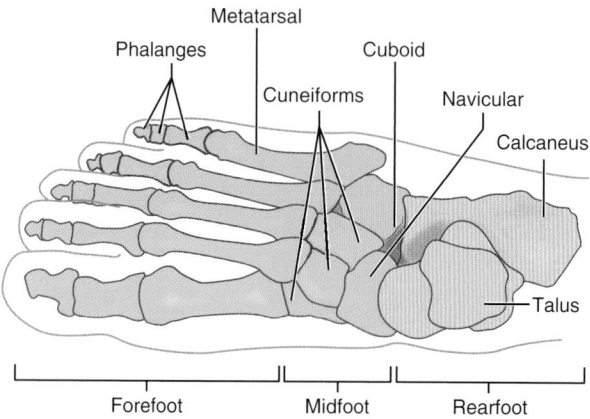

FIG. 21.19 Right foot regions and associated bones. The forefoot, the midfoot, and the rearfoot (*superior view*).

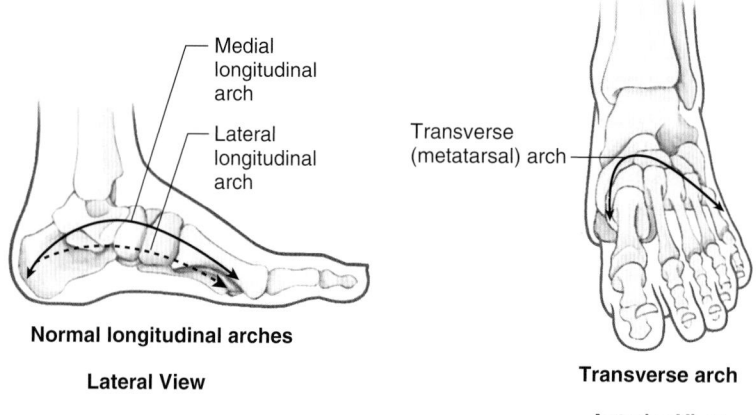

FIG. 21.20 Arches on the left foot. (From Patton, K. T., & Thibodeau, G. A. [2014]. *The human body in health and disease* [5th ed.]. St. Louis, MO: Elsevier.)

PHALANGES (SEE FIG. 21.18)

Greek: A line of soldiers

NOTES: The phalanges are in the toes. They are also called *digits.* Each foot contains 14 phalanges. Each toe has three phalanges except the great toe, which has two. Toes contain a proximal phalanx, a middle phalanx, and a distal phalanx. The great toe has only a proximal and a distal phalanx.

- **Metatarsophalangeal (MTP) Joints.** See Notes section under "Metatarsals."
- **Interphalangeal (IP) Joints.** These are between adjacent phalanges in the toes. The great toe has a single IP joint, and the second

to fifth toes have a proximal and a distal interphalangeal joint. These hinge joints provide flexion and extension.

- **Proximal Interphalangeal (PIP) Joints.** The distal ends of the proximal phalanges articulate with their middle phalanges at the PIP joints.
- **Distal Interphalangeal (DIP) Joints.** The middle phalanges articulate with their distal phalanges at the DIP joints.

LESSON THREE: BONES AND JOINTS OF THE AXIAL SKELETON

The axial skeleton bones are the skull, ribcage, sternum, and vertebral column. Associated joints and other structures are listed as bullets in the Notes section.

SKULL (FIG. 21.21)

Greek: Skull

CRANIAL BONES	BONY MARKING/SIGNIFICANCE
Frontal bone	No significant bony markings
Parietal bones	No significant bony markings
Temporal bones	Styloid process (ligament attachment and muscle attachment)
	Mastoid process (muscle attachment)
	Zygomatic process (muscle attachment)
Ethmoid bone	No significant bony markings
Sphenoid bone	Sella turcica (pituitary location)
	Medial and lateral pterygoid plates (muscle attachment)
	Greater wings (muscle attachment)
Occipital bone	Foramen magnum (passage for spinal cord)
	Superior nuchal line (muscle attachment)
	Inferior nuchal line (muscle attachment)
	External occipital protuberance (landmark and muscle attachment)
	Occipital condyles (joint formation)

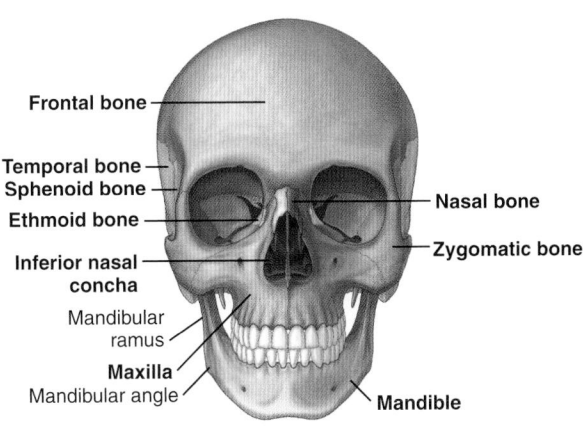

A   **Anterior View**

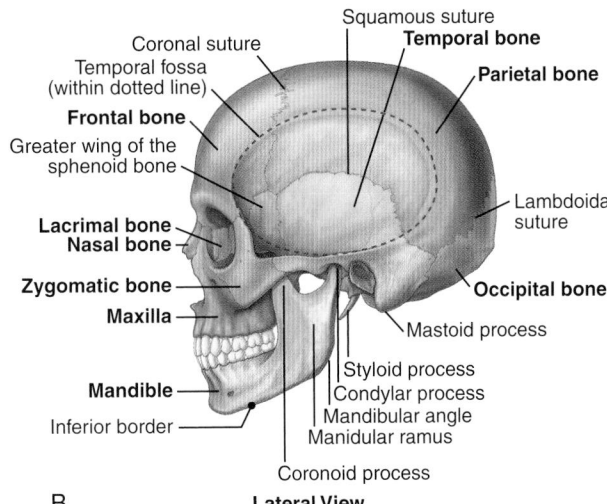

B   **Lateral View**

FIG. 21.21 The skull (*A, anterior view; B, lateral view; C, posterior view; D. inferior view*). The inferior view (*D*) is shown without the mandible. (Modified from Drake, R. L., Vogl, A. W., & Mitchell, A. W. M. [2010]. *Gray's anatomy for students* [2nd ed.]. Philadelphia, PA: Churchill Livingstone.)

Continued

SKULL—cont'd

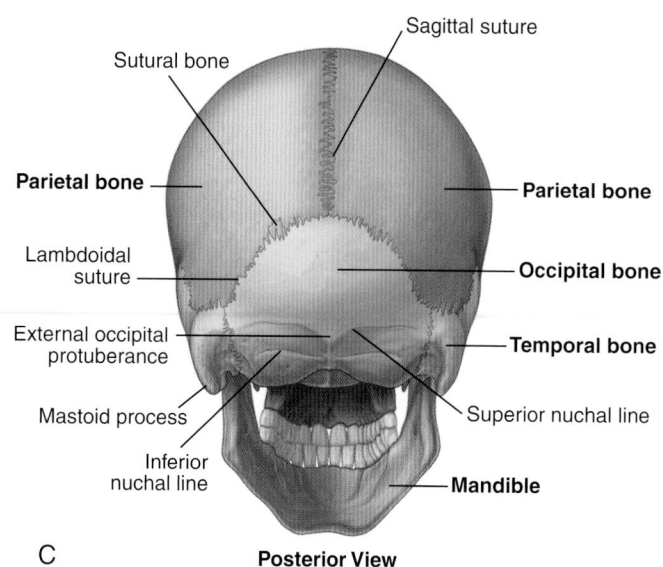

C   **Posterior View**

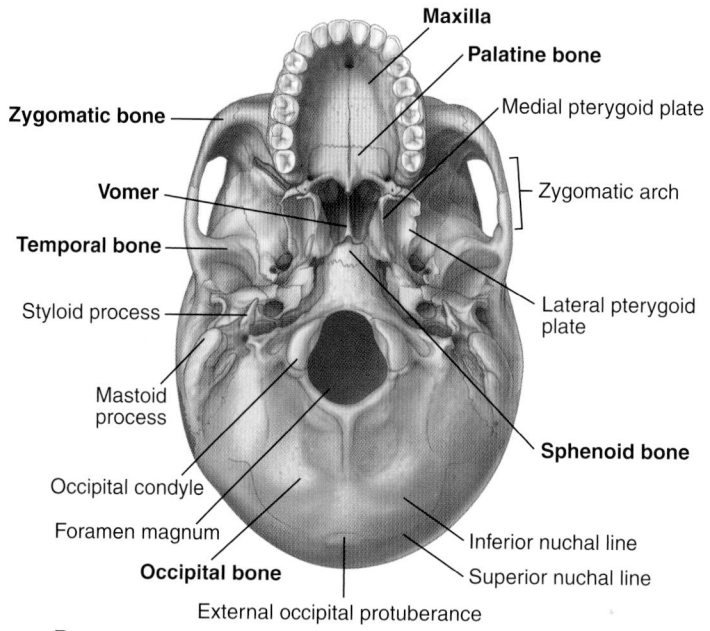

D   **Inferior View**

FIG. 21.21, CONT'D

NOTES: The skull includes the bones of the head. These bones can be divided into *cranial bones* and *facial bones*. The cranial bones are the frontal bone, two parietal bones, two temporal bones, the ethmoid bone, the sphenoid bone, and the occipital bone. The hyoid is often considered a skull bone because its main suspensory ligament joins the temporal bones. The mastoid process, posterior rim of the foramen magnum, and external occipital protuberance can be easily palpated. **LEARNING TIP:** To help you remember the names of the cranial bones, use the phrase **F**luffy **P**uppies **O**n **E**very **T**hird **S**treet for **F**rontal—**P**arietal—**O**ccipital—**E**thmoid—**T**emporal—**S**phenoid.

Paranasal sinuses are in the skull and include the frontal, sphenoidal, ethmoidal, and maxillary sinuses. The sinuses are discussed in Chapter 28.

Sutures are fibrous joints connecting the cranial bones in the skull.
LEARNING TIP: To help you remember the names of the sutures, use the phrase **C**ome **S**ing **L**ove **S**ongs for **C**oronal—**S**agittal—**L**ambdoidal—**S**quamosal.

• **Sagittal Suture.** Between the parietal bones
• **Coronal Suture.** Between the frontal bone and the parietal bones
• **Lambdoidal (Lambdoid) Suture.** Between the parietal bones and the occipital bone
• **Squamosal Suture.** Between the parietal bones and the temporal bones.

Sutural (Wormian) bones are irregular bones found within sutures. The number of sutural bones varies from person to person.

Fontanels, or soft spots, are in the sutural regions of the fetal or infant skull. These membrane-covered spaces allow the skull to

SKULL—cont'd

become compressed slightly during vaginal childbirth and permit subsequent rapid brain growth. Two prevalent fontanels are the anterior and posterior fontanels. The *anterior fontanel* is between the sagittal and coronal sutures. This diamond-shaped landmark is the largest fontanel and ossifies between the ages of 18 and 24 months. The *posterior fontanel* is between the sagittal and lambdoidal sutures. This fontanel ossifies within 3 months of age.

- **Temporomandibular Joint (TMJ).** The temporal bones of the skull articulate with the mandible of the jaw at the temporomandibular joint. This bilateral joint functions as a unit and is both a hinge joint and a gliding joint, permitting depression (mouth opening), elevation (mouth closing), protraction, retraction, and lateral movements called deviation or excursion. As the mouth opens wide, translation occurs, which is an inferior and anterior sliding motion combined with a slight rotational motion. These actions allow eating, drinking, talking, singing, respiratory movements such as breathing and blowing, and nonrespiratory movements such as laughing and yawning. The TMJ is one of the few synovial joints with an articular disc—the other being the knee and SC joints. The resting position of the TMJ is a combination of muscular balance and proprioceptive feedback, with a distance of 2–4 mm between teeth and lips, usually together.

- **Atlantooccipital (Yes-Yes) Joint.** The atlas, or C1, of the spine articulates with the occipital condyles at the base of the skull to form the atlantooccipital joint. This gliding joint permits up-and-down or nodding movements of the head (i.e., agreement gestures).

FACIAL BONES	MARKING/SIGNIFICANCE
Nasal bones	No significant bony markings
Vomer bone	No significant bony markings
Zygomatic bones	Temporal process (muscle attachment)
Lacrimal bones	No significant bony markings
Inferior nasal concha	No significant bony markings
Palatine bones	No significant bony markings
Maxillae	No significant bony markings
Mandible	Mandibular ramus (muscle attachment)
	Mandibular angle (muscle attachment)
	Inferior border (landmark)
	Coronoid process (muscle attachment)
	Condylar process (muscle attachment and joint formation)

NOTES: The facial bones are the vomer bone, two nasal bones, two zygomatic bones, two lacrimal bones, two inferior nasal concha bones, two palatine bones, two fused maxillae, and one mandible (jawbone). The mandibular ramus, mandibular angle, inferior border, and coronoid process can be easily palpated.

The *zygomatic arch* (cheekbone) is the palpable bony arch on the outer border of the eye sockets, formed by the union of two processes: the temporal process of the zygomatic bone and the zygomatic process of the temporal bone.

HYOID (FIG. 21.22)

Greek: U-shaped

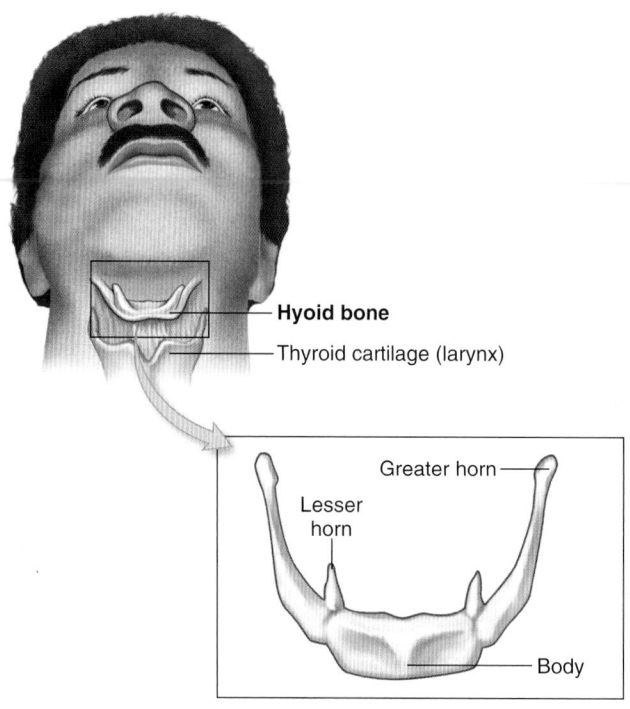

Anterior View

FIG. 21.22 Hyoid bone. The relationship of the hyoid to the thyroid cartilage of the larynx (*upper image*) and a detailed view of the hyoid (*lower image*). (From Patton, K. T., & Thibodeau, G. A. [2010]. *Anatomy & physiology* [7th ed.]. St. Louis, MO: Mosby.)

NOTES: The hyoid is a U-shaped bone between the chin and the thyroid cartilage. The hyoid does not articulate directly with any other bone; it is suspended by ligaments originating from the styloid process of the temporal bone. Some anatomists classify the hyoid as an irregular bone due to its shape, and others as a sesamoid bone, because it is embedded in tendons and ligaments.

At rest, the hyoid lies at the level of the mandible, positioned anterior to the third cervical vertebra, or C3. It is shaped like a miniature mandible with two canine teeth (i.e., *lesser horns*). It serves as an anchoring structure for the tongue above, an attachment site for several small anterior neck muscles.

The lateral portions of the mandible can be palpated by placing your thumb and index finger under the inferior border of the mandible and applying gentle side-to-side pressure. This hyoid almost always breaks during strangulation or when a person is hanged, which is a vital piece of information when performing an autopsy.

RIBCAGE (FIG. 21.23)

Old English: To roof, cover

BONES	SIGNIFICANCE
True ribs (seven pairs)	Connects with the sternum directly
False ribs (five pairs)	Connects with the sternum indirectly or not at all

NOTES: The ribcage is the bony structure in the chest and upper back consisting of bony and cartilaginous tissues. It includes the ribs, sternum, and thoracic vertebrae.

Ribs are long, flat, curved bones. There are 24 individual, or 12 pairs of ribs. The *intercostal space* is the space between two ribs. The *costal border* is formed by the lower costal cartilages of several ribs (ribs 7–10). Ribs can be classified as true ribs or false ribs. *True ribs* (ribs 1–7) connect anteriorly to the sternum. *False ribs* (ribs 8–12) do not connect directly to the sternum. Ribs 8, 9, and 10 are indirectly connected by borrowing the costal cartilages of rib 7. Ribs 11 and 12 are *floating ribs* because they do not connect to the sternum at all. The ribs are easily palpated.

- **Costovertebral Joints**. Ribs articulate posteriorly with the thoracic vertebrae of the spine at the costovertebral joints. The ribs attach to the thoracic vertebrae at two places—the costal facets on the transverse processes and the costal demifacets on the vertebral bodies (see Fig. 21.26). Ribs 2–10 articulate with two vertebrae, and ribs 1, 11, and 12 articulate with one vertebra. These gliding joints provide an up-and-down "pump-handle" or "bucket-handle" action, sliding and rotating slightly to accommodate changes in the size of the thoracic cavity during breathing.
- **Sternocostal Joints**. The sternum articulates with ribs 1–7 (true ribs) anteriorly at the sternocostal joints. The first sterno-costal joint attaches to the manubrium of the sternum and is a cartilaginous joint. The remaining ribs attach to the sternal body, or xiphoid process—these gliding joints facilitate movements that occur during breathing.
- **Costochondral Joints**. The ribs attach to their respective hyaline cartilages at the costochondral joints. There are 10 pairs of costochondral joints between ribs 1 and 10. These cartilaginous joints are relatively immobile, providing only slight movements during breathing.

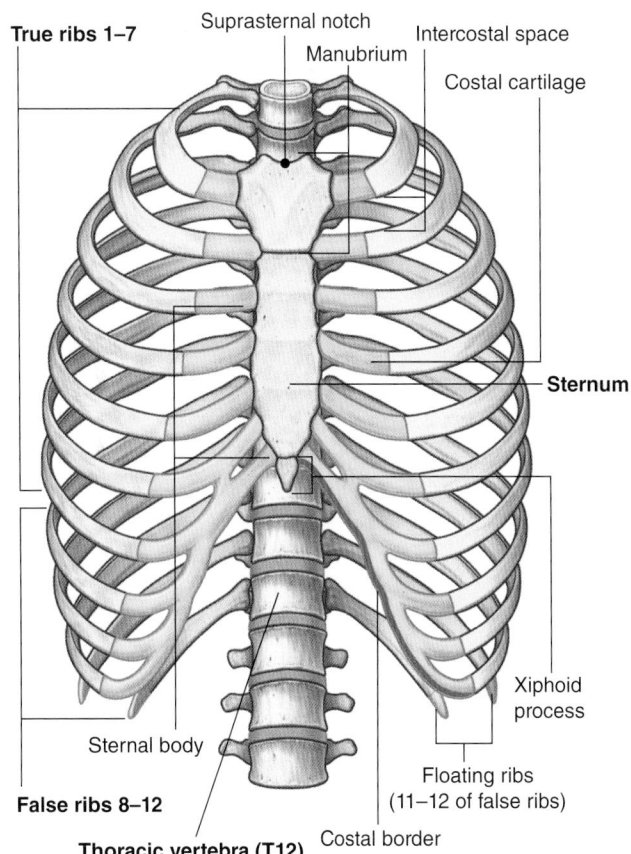

FIG. 21.23 Ribcage. The ribs, sternum, and vertebrae. (Modified from Drake, R. L., Vogl, A. W., & Mitchell, A. W. M. [2010]. *Gray's anatomy for students* [2nd ed.]. Philadelphia, PA: Churchill Livingstone.)

STERNUM (SEE FIG. 21.23)

Greek: Chest, breast, breastbone

BONY MARKING	SIGNIFICANCE
Manubrium	Muscle attachment and joint formation
Suprasternal notch	Landmark
Sternal body	Muscle attachment and joint formation
Xiphoid process	Muscle attachment and joint formation

NOTES: The sternum is the breastbone. This flat bone forms the central portion of the anterior chest wall. The sternum contains three regions: manubrium, sternal body, and xiphoid process. These structures, as well as the suprasternal notch, are easily palpated.

- **Sternoclavicular (SC) Joints**. See Notes section under "Clavicle."
- **Sternocostal Joints**. See Notes section under "Ribcage."

VERTEBRAL COLUMN (FIG. 21.24)

Latin: Turning joint

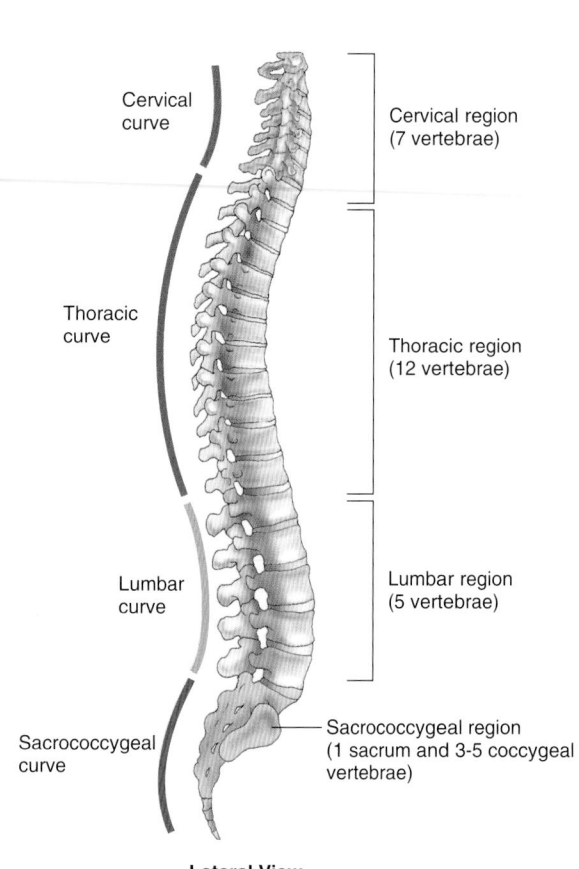

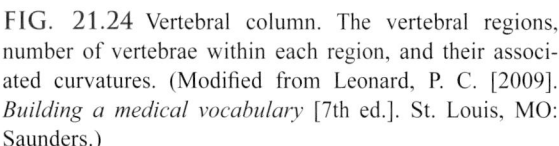

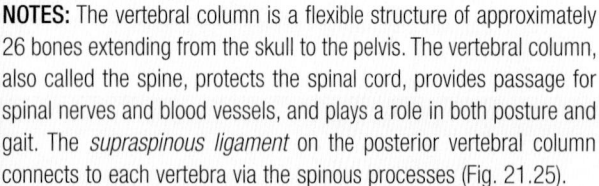

Lateral View

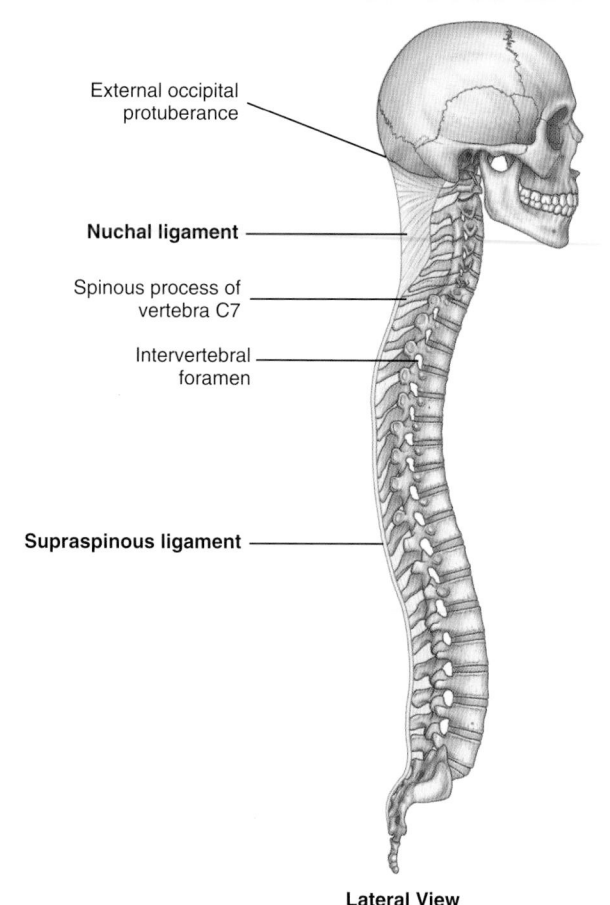

Lateral View

FIG. 21.24 Vertebral column. The vertebral regions, number of vertebrae within each region, and their associated curvatures. (Modified from Leonard, P. C. [2009]. *Building a medical vocabulary* [7th ed.]. St. Louis, MO: Saunders.)

FIG. 21.25 Vertebral ligaments. The intervertebral foramen and attachments of the nuchal ligament are identified. (Modified from Drake, R. L., Vogl, A. W., & Mitchell, A. W. M. [2010]. *Gray's anatomy for students* [2nd ed.]. Philadelphia, PA: Churchill Livingstone.)

NOTES: The vertebral column is a flexible structure of approximately 26 bones extending from the skull to the pelvis. The vertebral column, also called the spine, protects the spinal cord, provides passage for spinal nerves and blood vessels, and plays a role in both posture and gait. The *supraspinous ligament* on the posterior vertebral column connects to each vertebra via the spinous processes (Fig. 21.25).

The vertebral column is divided into several regions: cervical, thoracic, lumbar, and sacrococcygeal. Individual vertebrae are named by their region and placement in the region from top to bottom. For example, the first vertebra in the cervical region is C1. The vertebral column curves forward and backward to help maintain an upright posture (see Fig. 21.24).

- **Cervical Region (C1-C7)**. Contains seven vertebrae and is in the neck area. The *nuchal ligament* extends from the external occipital protuberance to C7 and attaches to all spinous processes of the cervical vertebrae. The nuchal ligament is continuous with the supraspinous ligament mentioned previously and can be palpated when the neck is flexed. The cervical region curves anteriorly.

- **Thoracic Region (T1-T12)**. Contains 12 vertebrae and is part of the ribcage. These structures make the thoracic region more stable than the cervical or lumbar regions. Thoracic vertebrae have costal facets on the transverse process and costal demifacets on the sides of the vertebral bodies for attaching ribs (see Fig. 21.26). The thoracic region curves posteriorly.

- **Lumbar Region (L1-L5)**. Contains five vertebrae and is in the lower back. The lumbar region curves anteriorly.

- **Sacrococcygeal Region**. The sacrococcygeal region contains one sacrum, with five fused vertebrae, and one coccyx, with three to five fused vertebrae. The sacrococcygeal region curves posteriorly.

LEARNING TIP: To help you remember how many vertebrae are in the cervical, thoracic, and lumbar regions, use this phrase; Breakfast **C**ereal at 7 (7 **C**ervical vertebrae)—lunch with **T**ea at 12 (12 **T**horacic vertebrae)—dinner with **L**asagna at 5 (5 **L**umbar vertebrae).

Latin: Turning joint

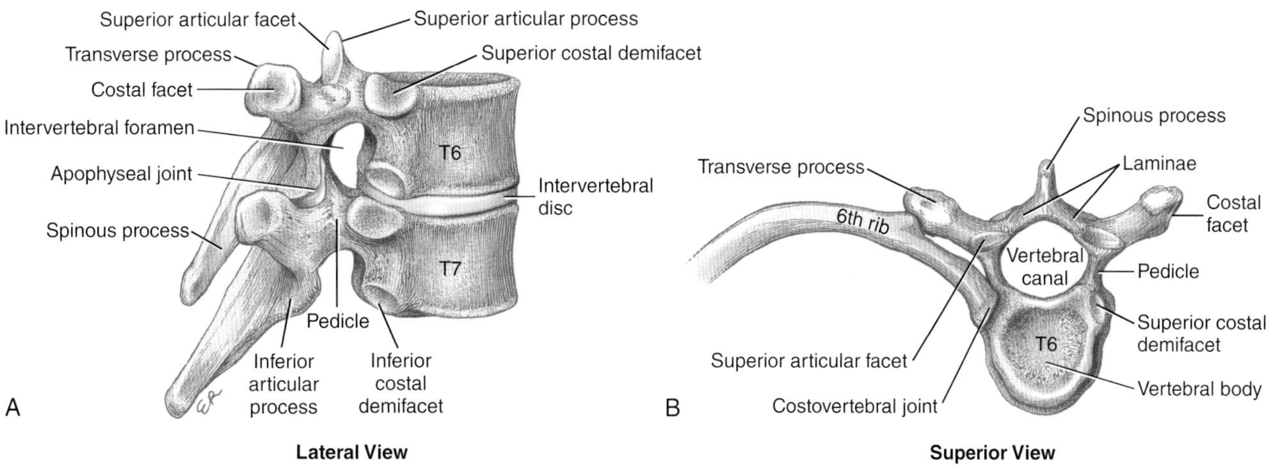

FIG. 21.26 Typical vertebrae. Characteristics of two thoracic vertebrae (*A, lateral view*). A thoracic vertebra and its associated rib (*B, superior view*). (Modified from Neumann, D. A. [2010]. *Kinesiology of the musculoskeletal system: Foundations for physical rehabilitation* [2nd ed.]. St. Louis: Mosby; Figure 9.5).

NOTES: Vertebrae are individual bones of the vertebral column. They provide attachment sites for muscles and ligaments, as well as passageways for nerves and blood vessels. A typical vertebra has two main parts.

- **Vertebral Body**. The anterior weight-bearing region. Vertebral bodies gradually increase in size from the cervical region to the lumbar region. The upper and lower surfaces of the vertebral bodies attach to intervertebral discs.
- **Vertebral Arch**. The posterior portion extends from the vertebral body and forms a semicircle around the spinal cord. The vertebral arch is formed by a pair of pedicles, a pair of laminae, and seven processes: four articular, two transverse, and one spinous process.
  - **Pedicles**. Anchors the vertebral arch to the vertebral body.
    - **Intervertebral Foramen (IVF)**. Openings between the pedicles of neighboring vertebrae and allows passage of spinal nerves.

- **Spinous Process**. Project posteriorly, and sometimes inferiorly. This structure is easily palpated.
- **Transverse Processes**. Project laterally.
- **Laminae**. Short spans of bones that run laterally from the base of the spinous process to the transverse processes.
  - **Laminar Groove**. Depression in the lamina of several stacked vertebrae between the spinous and transverse processes.
- **Superior and Inferior Articular Processes**. Between the pedicles and lamina of the same vertebra. This is where the vertebra articulates with the adjacent vertebrae.

The *vertebral (spinal) canal* is the large central hole formed by the vertebrae and contains the spinal cord.

- **Intervertebral Joints**. Joints between each vertebra. These contain several joints: one intervertebral disc joint, two right apophyseal joints, and two left apophyseal joints. The intervertebral joints connect the vertebrae into a single mobile structure.

Continued

VERTEBRAE—cont'd

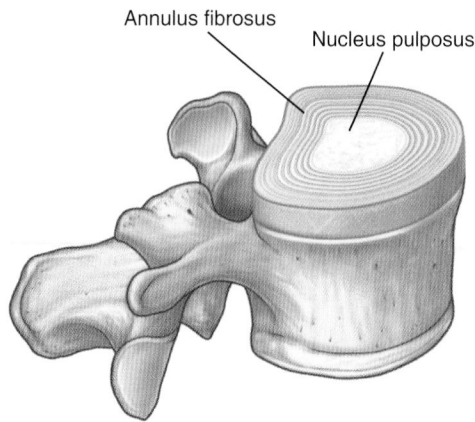

Superolateral View

FIG. 21.27 Intervertebral disc of a lumbar vertebra. (Modified from Drake, R. L., Vogl, A. W., & Mitchell, A. W. M. [2010]. *Gray's anatomy for students* [2nd ed.]. Philadelphia, PA: Churchill Livingstone.)

- **Intervertebral Disc Joints**. These cartilaginous joints are between adjacent vertebral bodies and their intervertebral discs. Each intervertebral disc (IVD) contains two regions: the annulus fibrosus and the nucleus pulposus. *Annulus fibrosus* is the tough outer ring, and *nucleus pulposus* is the gel-like center (Fig. 21.27). IVDs help maintain joint spaces, absorb vertical shock, allow the presence of spinal curvatures, and permit movements of flexion, extension, lateral flexion, and rotation.
- **Apophyseal (Facet, Zygapophyseal [Z]) Joints**. These gliding joints are where one vertebra articulates with another vertebra. Each joint is composed of a superior articular facet and an inferior articular facet. Apophyseal joints are named by their spinal region (i.e., cervical, thoracic, lumbar).

- **Atlantooccipital (Yes-Yes) Joint**. See the Notes section under "Skull."
- **Atlantoaxial (No-No) Joint**. The atlas, or C1, articulates with the dens (odontoid process) of C2 at the atlantoaxial joint, near the top of the spine. This pivot joint permits rotational, side-to-side, or shaking movements of the head (i.e., disagreement gestures).
- **Lumbosacral Joint**. The fifth lumbar vertebra (L5) articulates with the sacrum of the spine at the lumbosacral joint. This joint has the same characteristics as other lumbar intervertebral joints. Movements of the lumbosacral joint are limited to flexion and extension, with a small amount of lateral flexion.
- **Sacroiliac (SI) Joints**. See the Notes section under "Ilium."

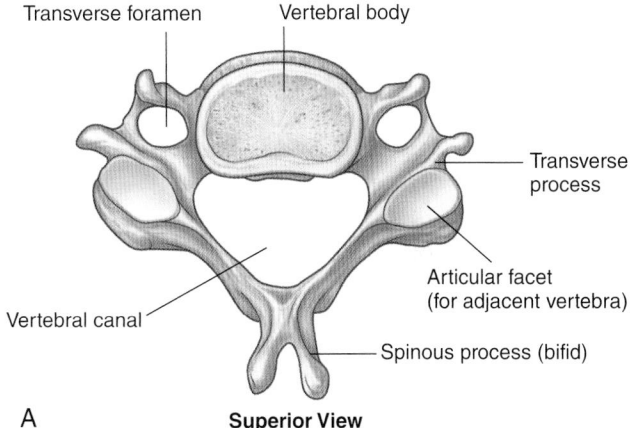

A **Superior View**

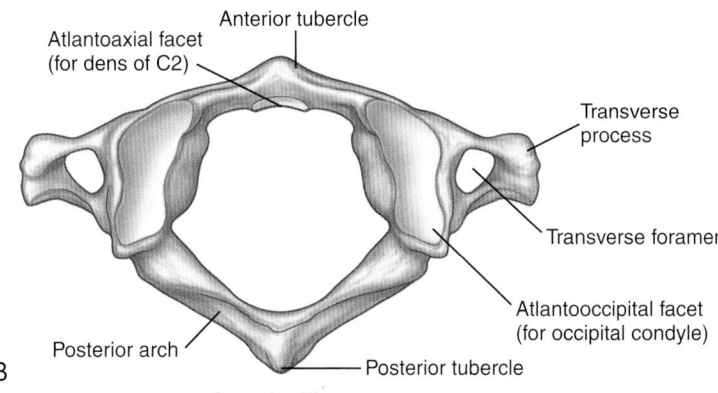

B **Superior View**

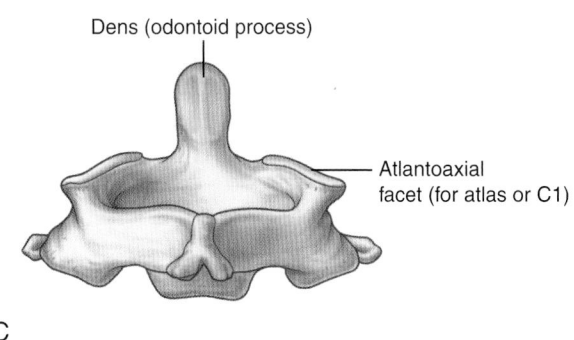

C **Posterior View**

FIG. 21.28 Atypical vertebrae and differences between cervical, sacral, and coccygeal vertebrae. (*A*) Cervical vertebra. (*B*) Atlas or C1. (*C*) Axis or C2. (*D*) Sacrum. (*E*) Coccyx. (Modified from Drake, R. L., Vogl, A. W., & Mitchell, A. W. M. [2010]. *Gray's anatomy for students* [2nd ed.]. Philadelphia, PA: Churchill Livingstone.)

ATYPICAL VERTEBRAE—cont'd

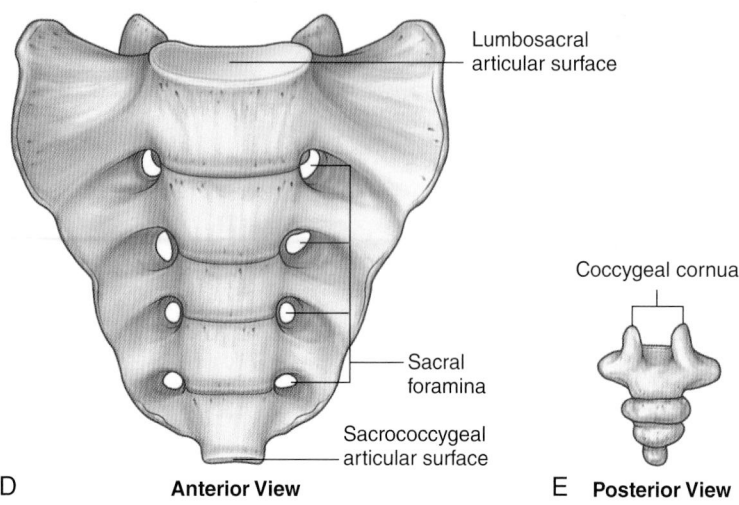

FIG. 21.28, CONT'D

NOTES: Some vertebrae have unique characteristics compared with the typical vertebrae described previously.

Cervical vertebrae are characterized by their small shape. Cervical vertebrae often possess a foramen, or hole, in their transverse processes called the *transverse foramen,* which allows for the passage of blood vessels and nerves. Spinous processes of most cervical vertebrae are bifid or fork-shaped (see Fig. 21.28A). The following are specific atypical vertebrae.

Atlas (C1). This ring-shaped lacks a vertebral body and pedicles. Its spinous process is reduced to a posterior tubercle, and its laminae are reduced to posterior arches (see Fig. 21.28B). The atlas has an anterior tubercle, two facets which articulate with the occipital condyles above, and a facet which articulates with the axis below.

Axis (C2). This bone possesses the *dens (odontoid process),* a bony protrusion projecting superiorly and articulates with the atlas (see Fig. 21.28C).

C7 (Vertebral Prominens). This bone contains a long, prominent spinous process, which is visible and easily palpable at the back of the neck.

Sacrum. This triangular-shaped bone is between the two pelvic bones (see Fig. 21.28D). The sacrum represents five fused vertebrae and contains anterior and posterior *sacral foramina* for the passage of sacral nerves.

Coccyx (Tailbone). This small triangular-shaped bone is at the base of the vertebral column (see Fig. 21.28E). The coccyx represents three to five fused bones and contains the paired coccygeal cornua projecting superiorly where the coccyx articulates with the sacrum.

SKELETAL MUSCLES

Skeletal muscles are groups of contractile tissue surrounded by connective tissue, attached to bones, and can produce movement at joints (Fig. 21.29). Muscles can also attach to ligaments (e.g., nuchal), fascia (e.g., iliotibial band), membranes (e.g., obturator, interosseous), specialized tendinous structures (e.g., galea aponeurotica), and to deep layers of skin and fascia, such as several muscles of facial expression. Prime movers, or agonists, are muscles causing the desired action. Synergists assist prime movers by performing the same movement at the same time. Fixators, or stabilizers, are specialized synergists that stabilize joints or help maintain posture so prime movers can exert their action. Antagonists lengthen while prime movers and their synergists contract and shorten to produce movement.

To understand muscle actions, you need to know where they attach and which joints they cross. The action, or "A," of a muscle occurs when its insertion, or "I," moves toward its origin, or "O." The following information is helpful when learning muscle actions.

- Muscle origins are generally medial, or proximal, to their insertions.
- Muscles on the anterior side of the trunk and the upper extremity generally flex.
- Muscles on the posterior side of the lower extremity generally flex.
- Muscles on the posterior side of the trunk and the upper extremity generally extend.
- Muscles on the anterior side of the lower extremity generally extend.
- Muscles on the medial side of the body generally adduct.
- Muscles on the lateral side of the body generally abduct.
- Muscles with fibers running superior to inferior generally flex or extend.
- Muscles with oblique running fibers generally rotate.
- If a muscle crosses two joints, it acts on both joints.
- Most muscles have at least two actions.
- Prime movers and antagonists are generally opposite each other.

Naming Muscles

The names of skeletal muscles can be difficult to remember. The key to learning this vocabulary is to understand why muscles are named, including their Latin and Greek meanings. The ways muscles are named are listed next.

Origins and Insertions

A muscle's origins and insertions, or attachment sites, can be used to name muscles. For example, the sternocleidomastoid attaches to the sternum, clavicle, and the mastoid process. Typically origins are listed first, then insertions.

Number of Origins

Muscles can be named by the numbers of their origins. The number of muscle origins is usually listed first, followed by the region of the body where they are located. For example, biceps brachii has two origins, and it is in the brachial region. Triceps brachii has three origins and is in the brachial region. Quadriceps femoris has four origins, and it is in the femoral region.

Relative Shape and Size

Muscles can be named for their shape and size. For example, gluteus maximus is a large muscle, and gluteus minimus is a smaller muscle. The adductor longus is a long muscle, and the deltoid is triangular-shaped.

Location and/or Direction of Fibers

Muscles can be named for their location and direction of fibers. For example, temporalis lies in the temporal fossa. Frontalis is over the frontal bone. Rectus femoris has straight muscle fibers and is over the femur. Internal obliques have slanted fibers. Latissimus dorsi is on the dorsum or posterior side of the body. Transverse abdominis has crosswise fibers and is over the abdomen.

Actions or Functions

Muscles can be named by their primary action or function, followed by where the action occurs. For example, flexor pollicis longus flexes the thumb. Levator scapula elevates the scapula.

Combinations

Many muscles are named using a combination of methods. For example, extensor digitorum longus is a long muscle that extends the digits or fingers. Flexor digitorum profundus is a deep muscle that flexes the digits or fingers.

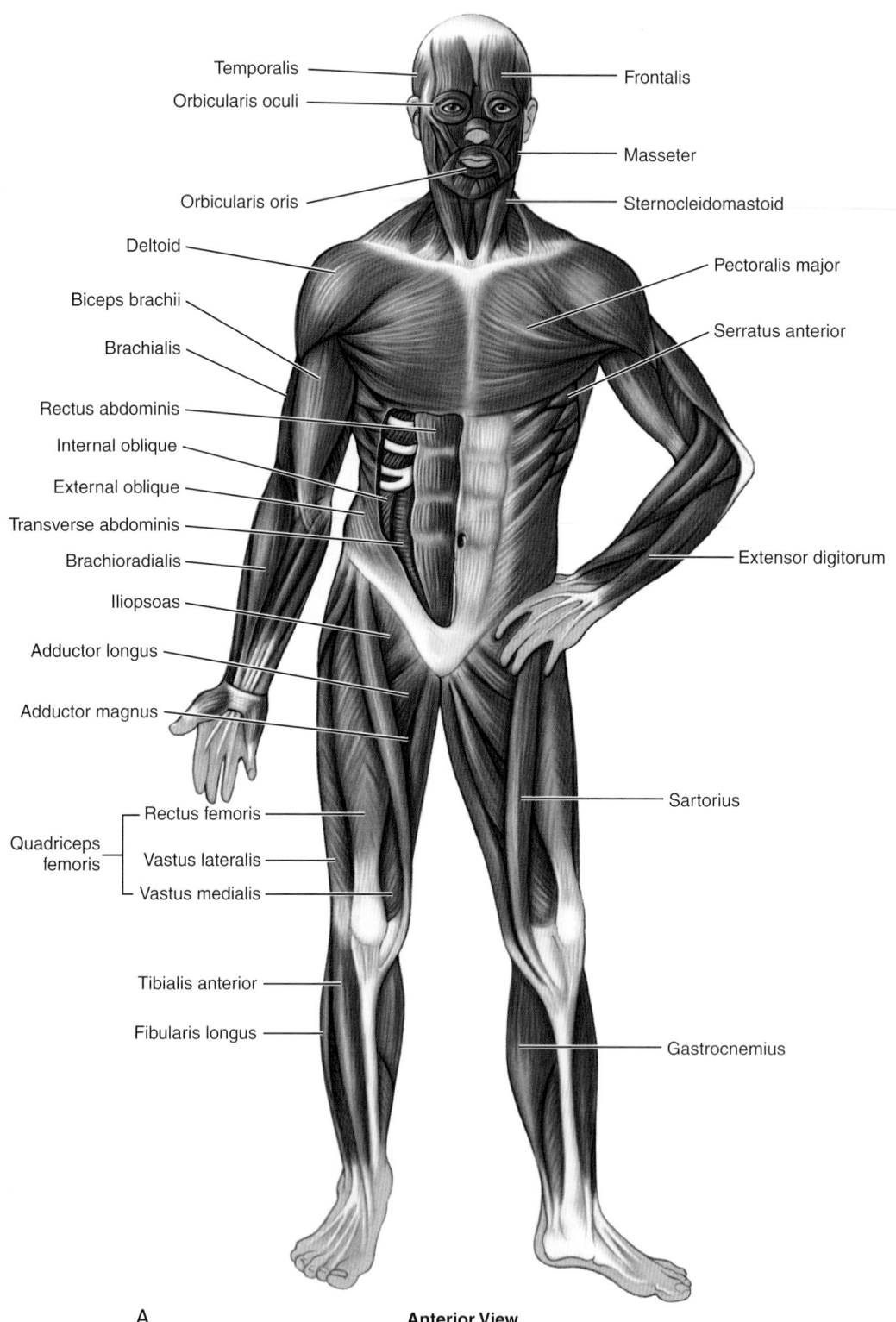

A   **Anterior View**

FIG. 21.29 Skeletal muscles of the body with several muscles labeled (*A, anterior view; B, posterior view*).

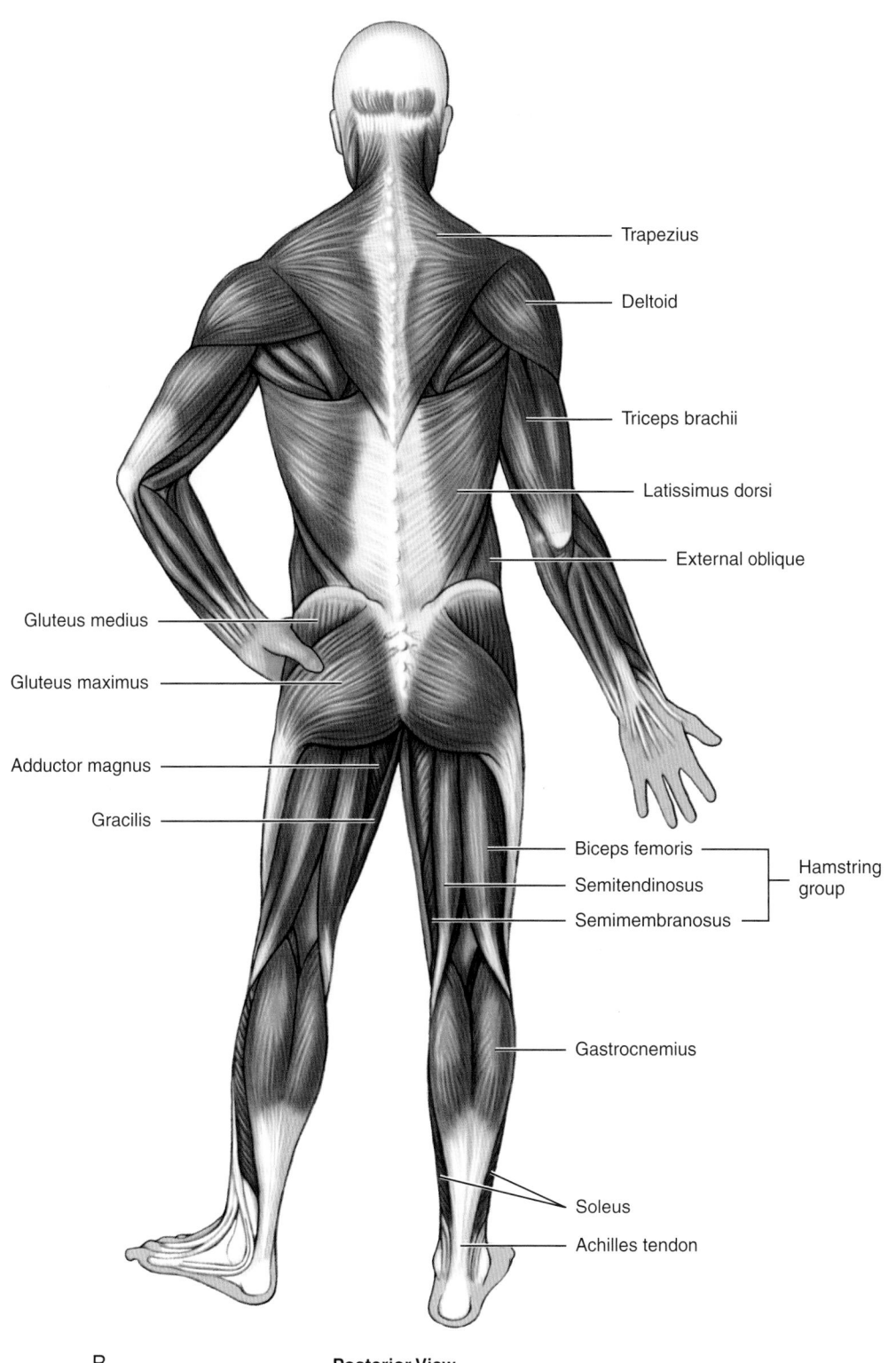

B
Posterior View
FIG. 21.29, CONT'D

Lesson Four: Muscles of Scapular Movement

Movements of the scapula are elevation, depression, upward rotation, downward rotation, protraction (aka abduction), and retraction (aka adduction). Muscles creating scapular movements are trapezius, levator scapulae, rhomboids, serratus anterior, and pectoralis minor (Fig. 21.30).

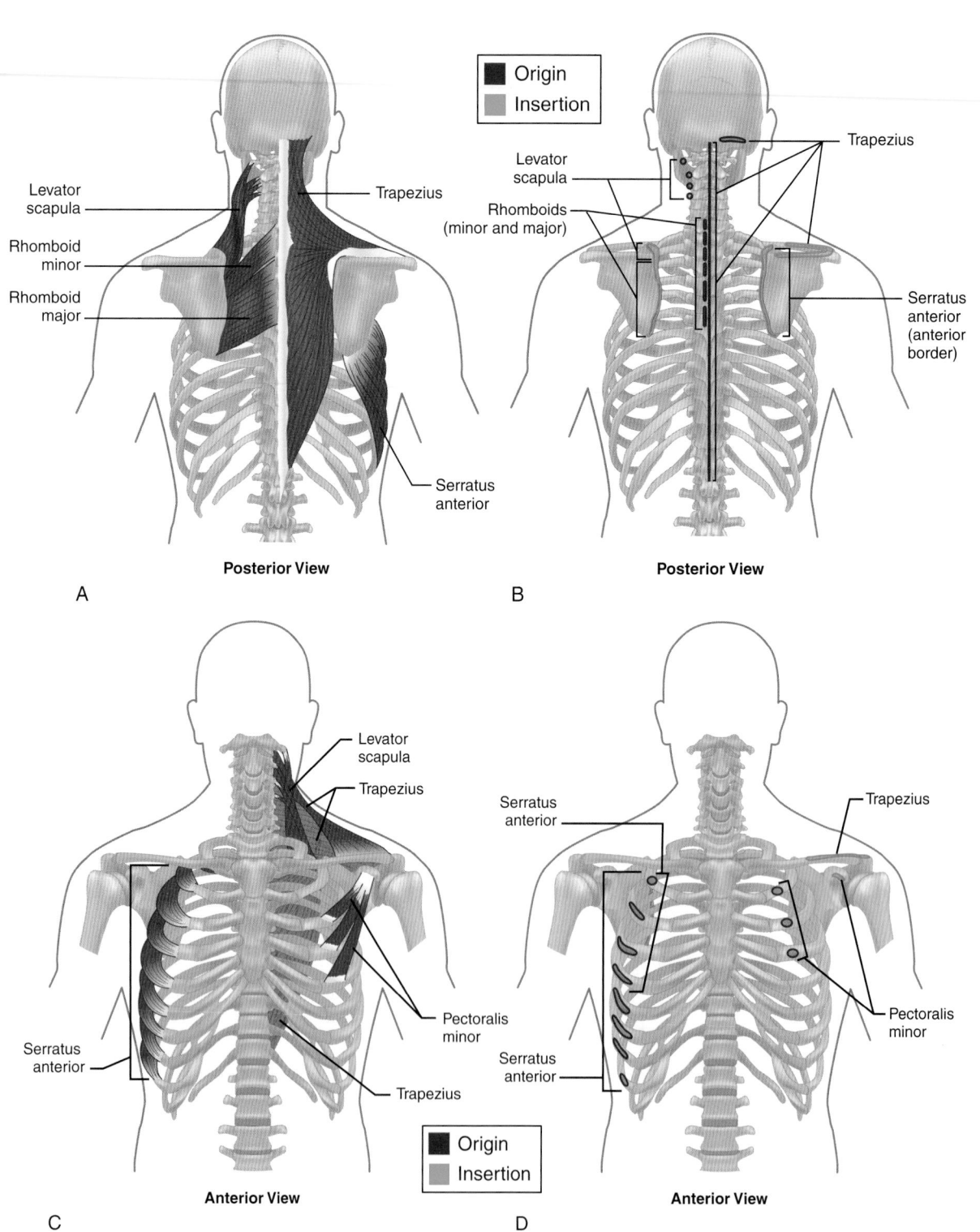

FIG. 21.30 Muscles of scapular movement (*A and C*) their associated origins (*red*) and insertions (*blue; B and D*).

TRAPEZIUS (FIG. 21.31)

Greek: trapezoeidestrapeza—four-legged table

ORIGINS
External occipital protuberance
Superior nuchal line
Nuchal ligament
Spinous processes of C7–T12

INSERTIONS
Lateral third of the clavicle
Acromion process
Scapular spine

ACTIONS
Extends the neck and head (upper fibers)
Elevates the scapula (upper fibers)
Upwardly rotates the scapula (upper fibers)
Retracts the scapula (middle fibers)
Depresses the scapula (lower fibers)
Laterally flexes the neck (unilateral contraction)
Rotates the head (unilateral contraction)

NERVES
Spinal accessory nerve (cranial nerve XI)
Midcervical nerves

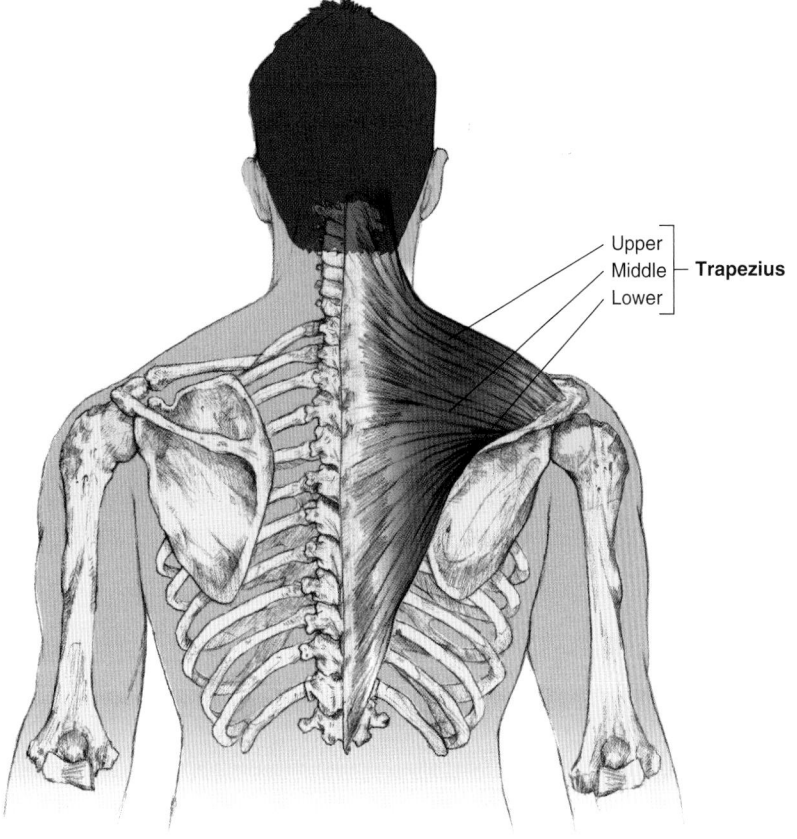

A   **Posterior View**

FIG. 21.31 (A) Right trapezius and its upper, middle, and lower fibers. (Modified from Mansfield, P. [2014]. *Essentials of kinesiology for the physical therapist assistant* [2nd ed.]. St. Louis, MO: Mosby.) (B) Right trapezius and its positional relationship to the right deltoid. (From Drake, R., Vogel, A. W., & Mitchell, A. [2015]. *Gray's anatomy for students* [3rd ed.]. Philadelphia, PA: Elsevier.)

Continued

TRAPEZIUS—cont'd

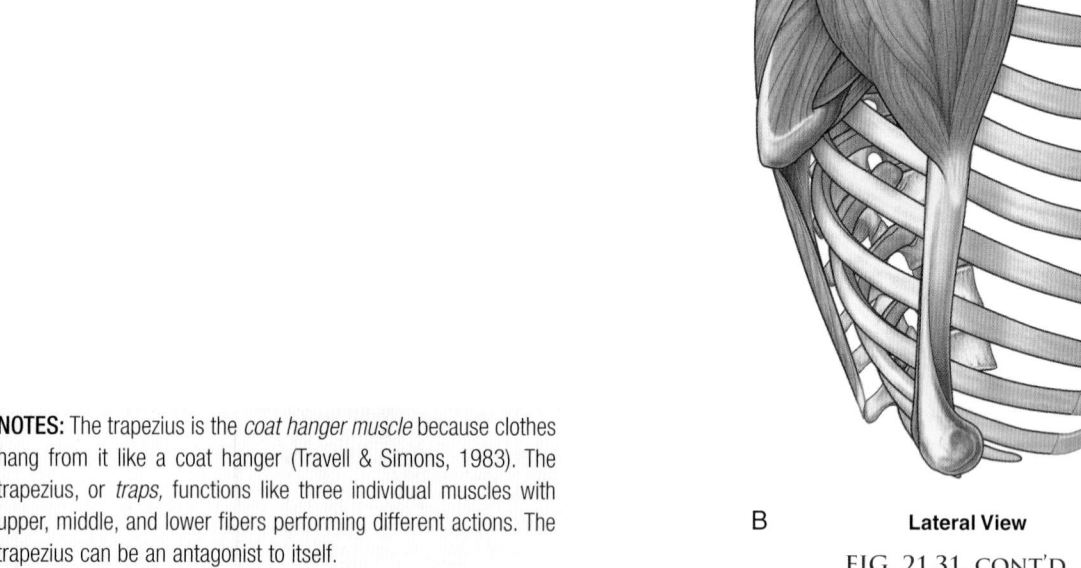

Trapezius

Scapular spine

Acromion process

Clavicle

Deltoid

B   **Lateral View**

FIG. 21.31, CONT'D

NOTES: The trapezius is the *coat hanger muscle* because clothes hang from it like a coat hanger (Travell & Simons, 1983). The trapezius, or *traps,* functions like three individual muscles with upper, middle, and lower fibers performing different actions. The trapezius can be an antagonist to itself.

LEVATOR SCAPULAE (FIG. 21.32)

Latin: levator—a lifter
scapulae—shoulder blade

ORIGINS
Transverse processes of C1–C4

INSERTION
Medial border of the scapula (from superior angle to root of spine)

ACTIONS
Elevates the scapula
Downwardly rotates the scapula
Laterally flexes the neck

NERVES
Dorsal scapular nerve
Midcervical nerves

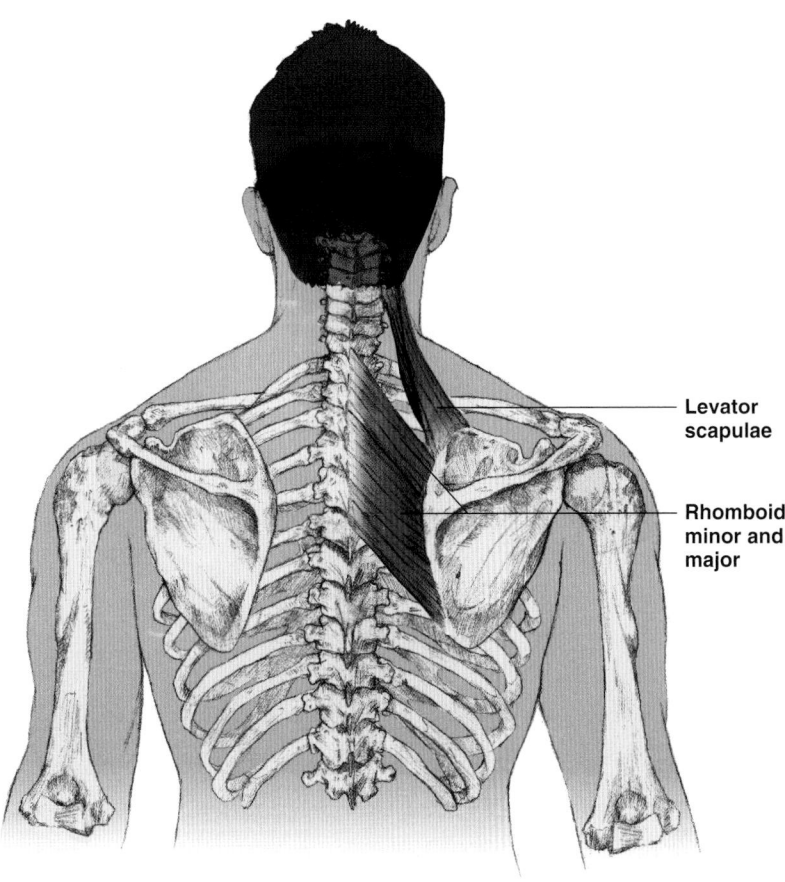

Levator
scapulae

Rhomboid
minor and
major

Posterior View

NOTES: The insertion of the levator scapulae may feel thick and stringy as it is strummed during palpation.

FIG. 21.32 Right levator scapulae with right rhomboid minor (*superior*) and major (*inferior*). (Modified from Mansfield, P. [2014]. *Essentials of kinesiology for the physical therapist assistant* [2nd ed.]. St. Louis, MO: Mosby.)

RHOMBOID MAJOR AND MINOR (SEE FIG. 21.32)

Latin: rhombus—all sides even
major—larger
minor—smaller

ORIGINS
Spinous processes of C7–T1 (minor)
Spinous processes of T2–T5 (major)

INSERTIONS
Medial border of the scapula below the superior angle to the
   root of the scapular spine (minor)
Medial border of the scapula from the root of the scapular
   spine to the inferior angle (major)

ACTIONS
Retracts the scapula
Downwardly rotates the scapula

NERVE
Dorsal scapular nerve

NOTES: Rhomboids are the collective term for rhomboid major and minor. These muscles are rarely referred to by their individual names because they have identical fiber arrangement, therefore having identical lines of pull and identical actions. In fact, the rhomboids occasionally fuse to form a single muscle. Janak (2011) refers to the rhomboids as the *Christmas tree muscle* because of their oblique fiber direction, which resembles Christmas tree branches. The rhomboids lie deep to the trapezius, and rhomboid minor is positioned superior to rhomboid major.

SERRATUS ANTERIOR (FIG. 21.33)

Latin: serratus—notched or jagged, similar to a saw
ante—before

ORIGINS
Ribs 1 through 8 or 9 (lateral to costal cartilage—exterior surface of the ribs)

INSERTION
Medial border of the scapula (anterior aspect)

ACTIONS
Protracts the scapula
Upwardly rotates the scapula
Depresses the scapula

NERVE
Long thoracic nerve

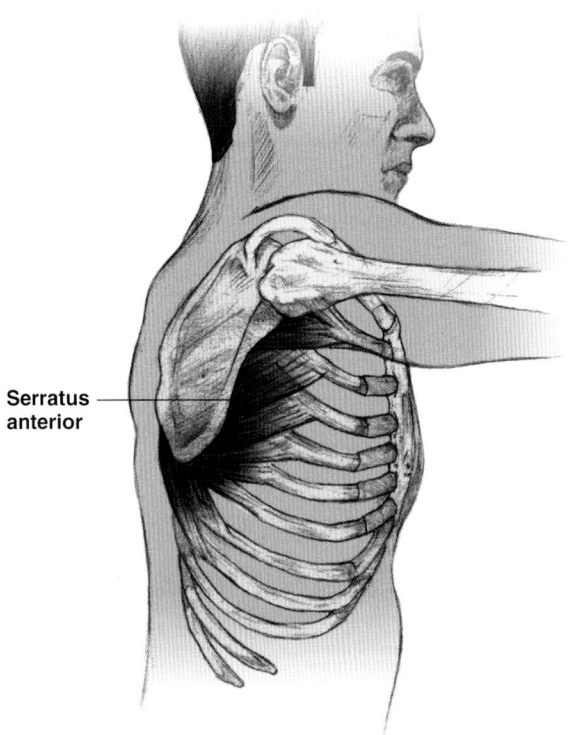

Serratus anterior

Lateral View

FIG. 21.33 Right serratus anterior. (Modified from Mansfield, P. [2014]. *Essentials of kinesiology for the physical therapist assistant* [2nd ed.]. St. Louis, MO: Mosby.)

NOTES: The serratus anterior is a fan-shaped muscle on the lateral ribcage. Most of this muscle lies beneath the scapula. The serratus anterior and triceps brachii (Lesson Six) are the *boxer's muscles* because they protract the scapula and extend the elbow, the movements that occur to throw a boxer's punch (Lung et al., 2020). Serratus anterior and the rhomboids are antagonists to each other. Fibers of serratus anterior and external obliques (Lesson Eleven) may interlace on the lateral trunk. *Winged scapula* occurs from serratus anterior paralysis, which causes the scapula to lift off the ribcage like a wing (Martin & Fish, 2008).

PECTORALIS MINOR (FIG. 21.34)

Latin: pectoralis—pertaining to the chest
minor—smaller

ORIGINS
Ribs 3 through 5 (lateral to costal cartilage)

INSERTION
Coracoid process of the scapula

ACTIONS
Depresses the scapula
Protracts the scapula
Downwardly rotates the scapula
Assists in forced inhalation (elevates ribs)

NERVES
Medial pectoral nerves (C8 and T1)

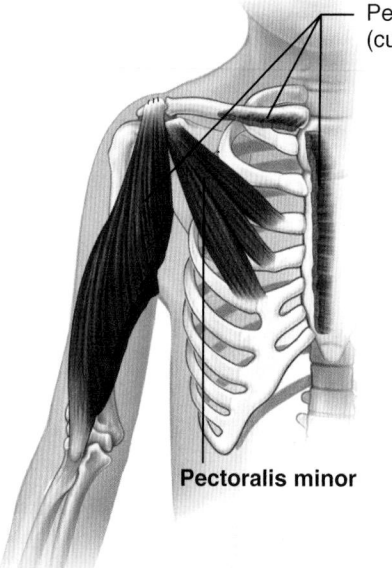

Pectoralis major
(cut and reflected)

Pectoralis minor

Anterior View

FIG. 21.34 Right pectoralis minor with right pectoralis major cut and reflected. (From Herring, J. A. [2014]. *Tachdjian's pediatric orthopaedics: From the Texas Scottish Rite Hospital for Children* [5th ed.]. Philadelphia, PA: Elsevier.)

NOTES: Pectoralis minor lies deep to pectoralis major (Lesson Five). Pectoralis minor is the *neurovascular entrapper* because it can entrap the brachial plexus and axillary artery when it is tense (Travell & Simons, 1983). Entrapment of these structures can cause thoracic outlet syndrome-like symptoms (pain, tingling, and numbness down the arm into the affected hand). See Chapter 23 for more information about thoracic outlet syndrome.

Lesson Four Review: Muscles of Scapular Movement

ELEVATION	DEPRESSION	PROTRACTION	RETRACTION	UPWARD ROTATION	DOWNWARD ROTATION
Trapezius (upper fibers) Levator scapulae	Trapezius (lower fibers) Serratus anterior Pectoralis minor	Serratus anterior Pectoralis minor	Trapezius (middle fibers) Rhomboids	Trapezius (upper fibers) Serratus anterior	Levator scapulae Rhomboids Pectoralis minor

Posterior view   Posterior view   Anterior view   Posterior view   Anterior view   Posterior view   Posterior view   Posterior view   Anterior view

Lesson Five: Muscles of Shoulder Joint Movement

Movements of the humerus at the shoulder joint are flexion, extension, adduction, abduction, internal (medial) rotation, external (lateral) rotation, and circumduction. Muscles that cause these movements are latissimus dorsi, teres major, supraspinatus, infraspinatus, teres minor, subscapularis, deltoid, pectoralis major, coracobrachialis, biceps brachii, and triceps brachii. Biceps and triceps brachii also move the elbow joint; these muscles are featured in Lesson Six (Fig. 21.35).

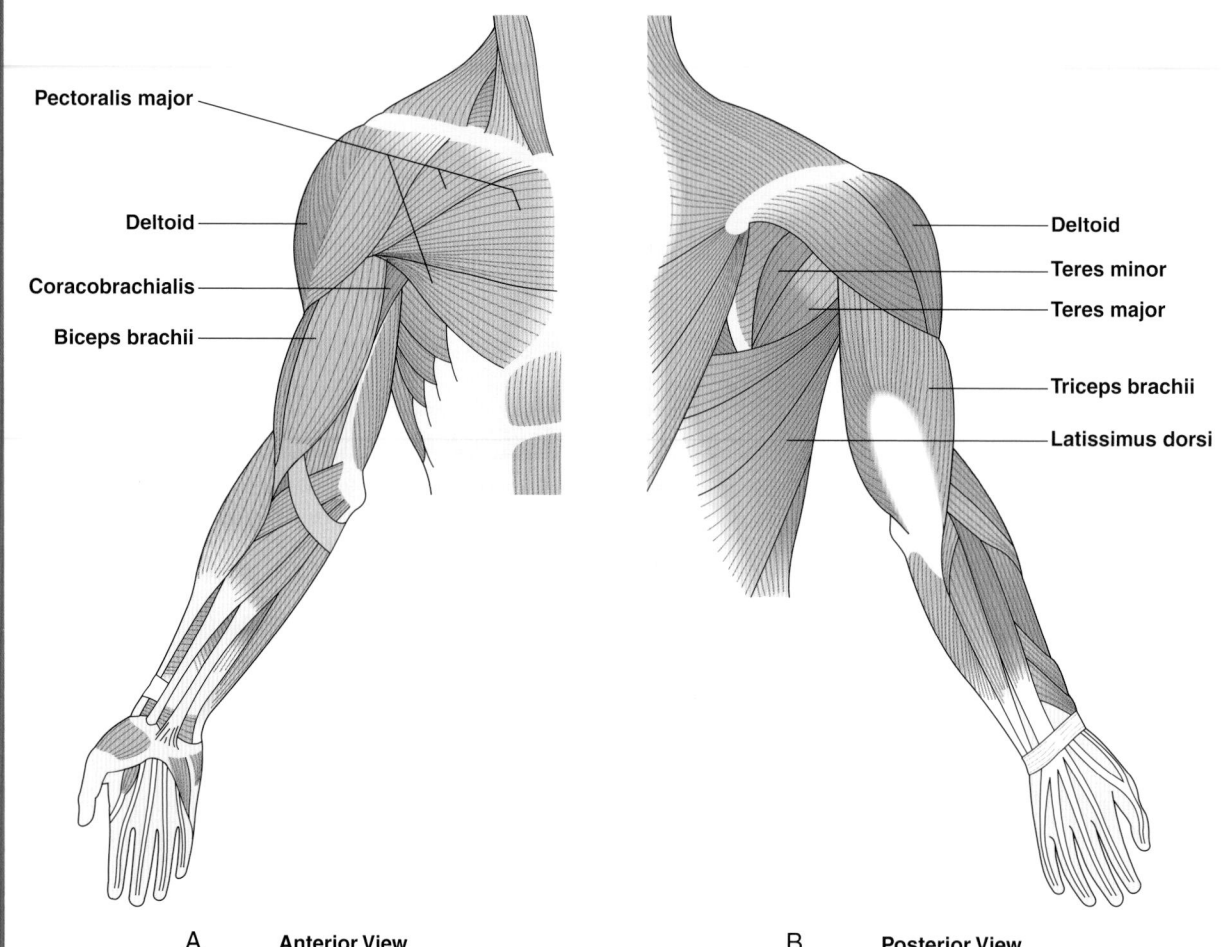

A   **Anterior View**   B   **Posterior View**

FIG. 21.35 Muscles of right shoulder joint movement (*A and B*) with their associated origins (*red*) and insertions (*blue, C-F*). Not all muscles, origins, and insertions in Lesson Five are featured. Biceps and triceps brachii muscles are in Lesson Six because of their primary actions on the elbow. (From Jenkins, D. B. [1991]. *Hollinshead's functional anatomy of the limbs and back* [6th ed.]. Philadelphia, PA: Saunders.)

Lesson Five: Muscles of Shoulder Joint Movement—cont'd

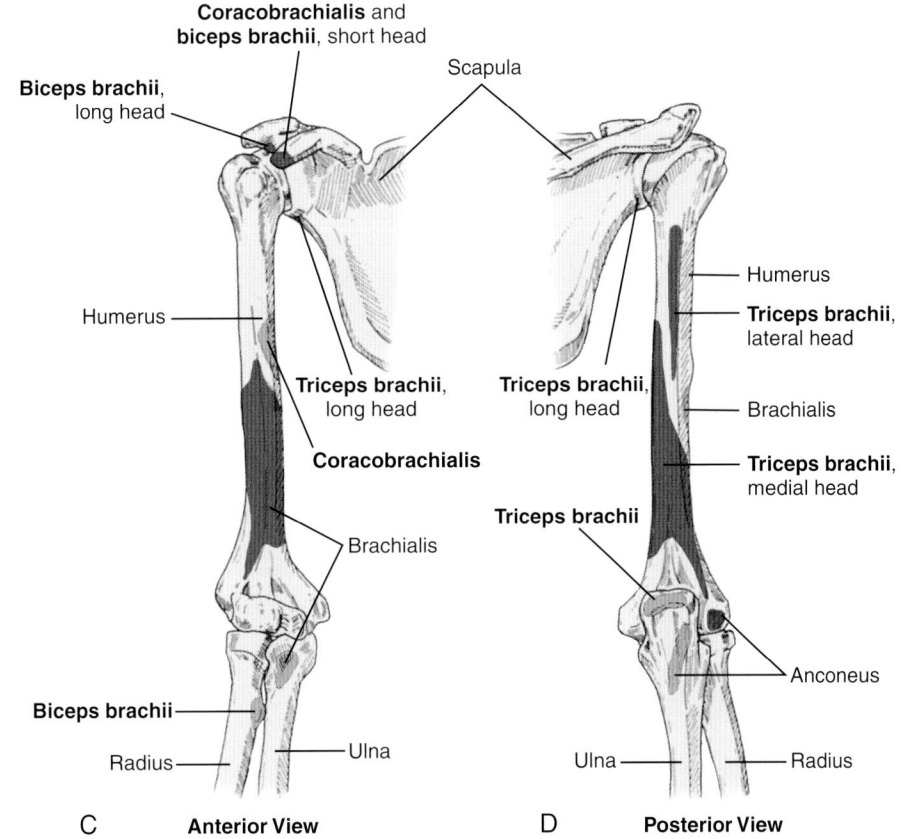

C   **Anterior View**   D   **Posterior View**

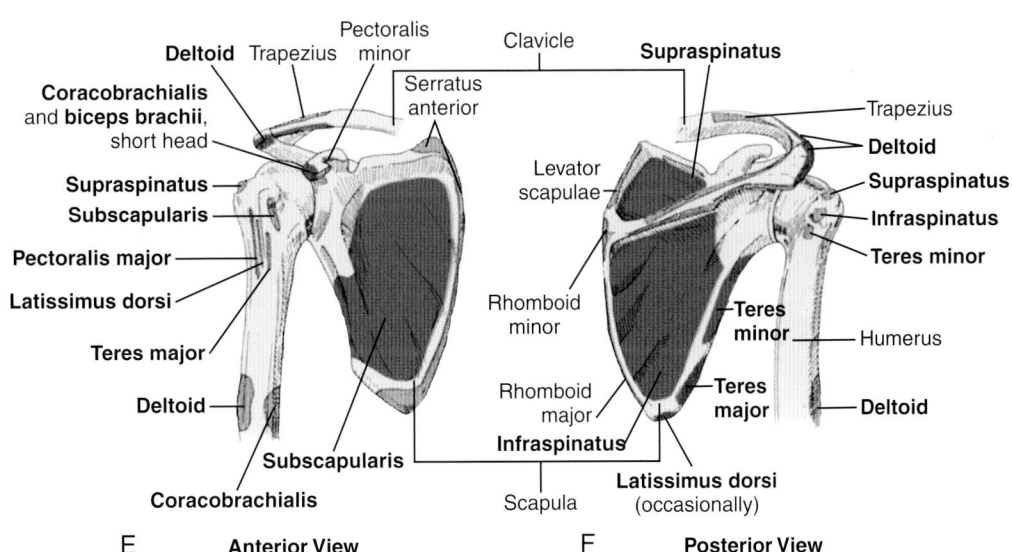

E   **Anterior View**   F   **Posterior View**

FIG. 21.35, CONT'D

LATISSIMUS DORSI (FIG. 21.36)

Latin: latus—broad
dorsum—back

ORIGINS
Spinous processes of T7–L5
Ribs 9 through 12 (posterior surface)
Posterior iliac crest
Posterior sacrum

INSERTION
Intertubercular groove of the humerus (medial lip)

ACTIONS
Extends the humerus
Internally/medially rotates the humerus
Adducts the humerus (posteriorly)

NERVE
Thoracodorsal nerve

NOTES: Latissimus dorsi, or lats, is the *swimmer's muscle* because many of its actions are involved in swimming (Herlihy, 2018). The lats are the widest muscles in the body and form the posterior axillary folds (the pecs form the anterior axillary folds). Fibers of the latissimus dorsi and external obliques (Lesson Eleven) may interlace on the lateral trunk.

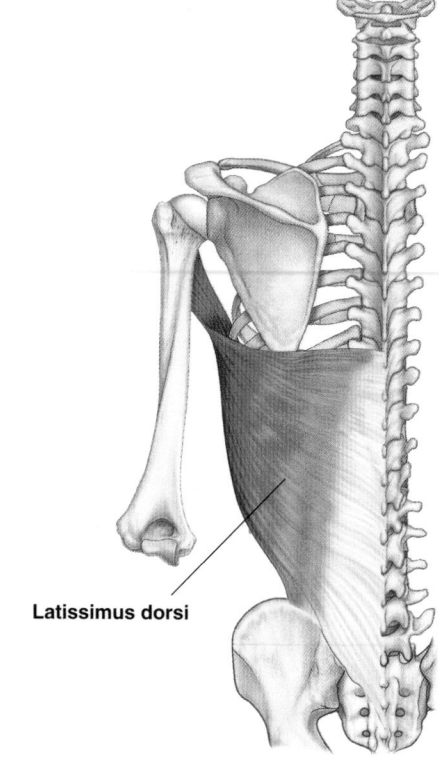

Latissimus dorsi

Posterior View

FIG. 21.36 Left latissimus dorsi. (Modified from Soames, R., & Palastanga, N. [2019]. *Anatomy and human movement: Structure and function* [7th ed.]. Philadelphia, PA: Elsevier.)

TERES MAJOR (FIG. 21.37)

Latin: teres—round
major—larger

ORIGIN
Inferior third of the lateral border of the scapula

INSERTION
Intertubercular groove of the humerus (medial lip)

ACTIONS
Extends the humerus
Internally/medially rotates the humerus
Adducts the humerus

NERVE
Lower subscapular nerve

NOTES: Teres major is lat's little helper or lat's twin because it performs the same action as the lats and is its synergist (Travell & Simons, 1983).

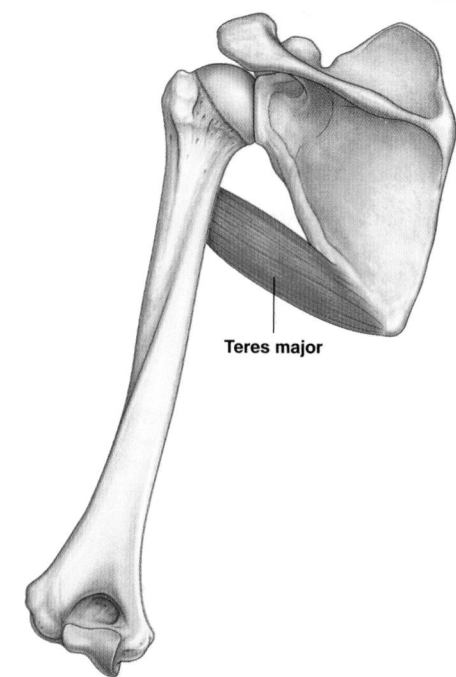

Teres major

Posterior View

FIG. 21.37 Left teres major. (Modified from Soames, R., & Palastanga, N. [2019]. *Anatomy and human movement: Structure and function* [7th ed.]. Philadelphia, PA: Elsevier.)

ROTATOR CUFF (FIG. 21.38)

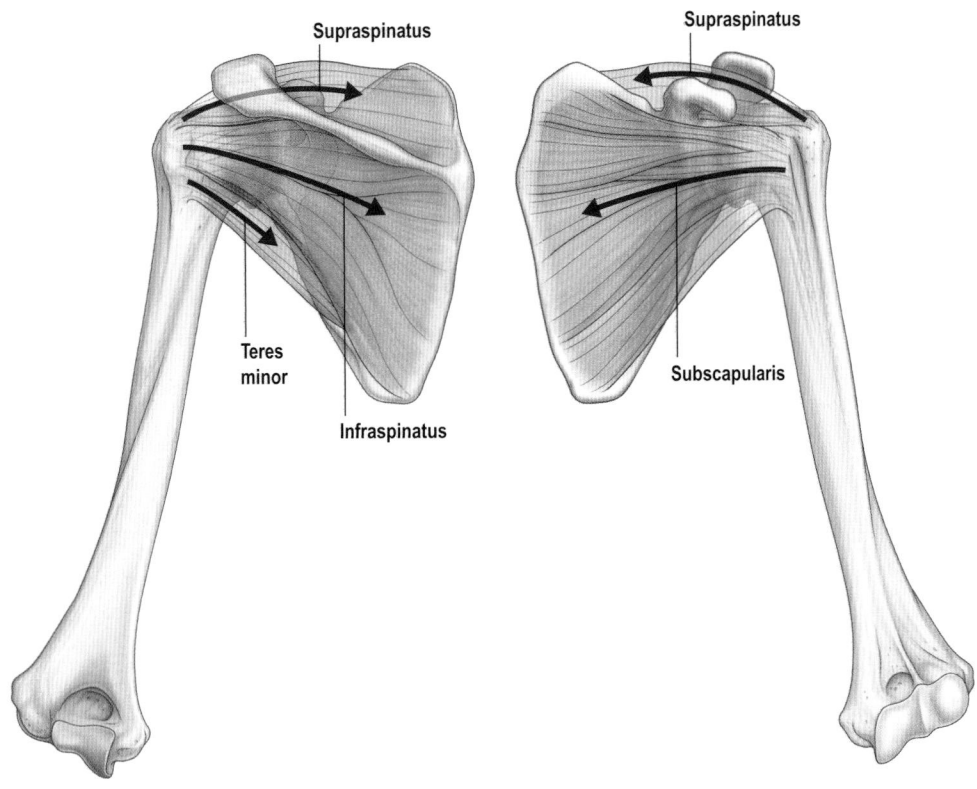

Posterior View

Anterior View

FIG. 21.38 Left muscles of the rotator cuff. The red arrows represent their actions or direction of pull. (Modified from Soames, R., & Palastanga, N. [2019]. *Anatomy and human movement: Structure and function* [7th ed.]. Philadelphia, PA: Elsevier.)

NOTES: The rotator cuff, or musculotendinous cuff, is a group of four muscles, deep to the deltoids. The rotator cuff muscles are supraspinatus, infraspinatus, teres minor, and subscapularis. Most of these muscles provide rotation as their primary action; the supraspinatus does not but instead provides abduction. Origins of three rotator cuff muscles are in fossae of the same name. Supraspinatus originates in the supraspinous fossa; infraspinatus originates in the infraspinatus fossa; and subscapularis originates in the subscapular fossa. Three rotator cuff muscles insert on the greater tubercle: supraspinatus, infraspinatus, and teres minor. Subscapularis inserts on the lesser tubercle. **LEARNING TIP**: To help you remember the names of the rotator cuff muscles, use the word **SItS** for **S**upraspinatus—**I**nfraspinatus—**t**eres minor—**S**ubscapularis. The lowercase "t" helps you remember teres "*minor*" and not teres major.

SUPRASPINATUS (FIG. 21.39)

Latin: supra—above
spinatus—spine

ORIGIN
Supraspinous fossa of the scapula

INSERTION
Greater tubercle of the humerus

ACTION
Abducts the humerus

NERVE
Suprascapular nerve

NOTES: The tendon of the supraspinatus passes beneath the acromion process of the scapula. The supraspinatus is the only rotator cuff muscle that does not rotate the humerus. Instead, it initiates the first 10–15 degrees of abduction; the deltoid then takes over to complete abduction. Supraspinatus also helps prevent downward dislocation of the humerus when lifting and carrying a heavy object, such as a portable massage table. It is also the most commonly injured rotator cuff muscle and is susceptible to shoulder impingement syndrome (Maruvada et al., 2021). See Chapter 20 for more information about shoulder impingement syndrome.

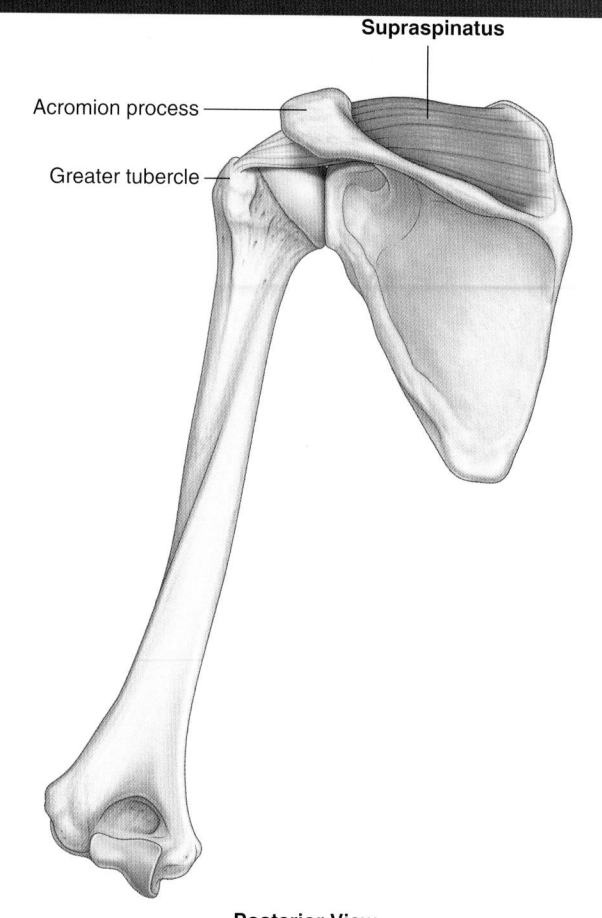

Posterior View

FIG. 21.39 Left supraspinatus. Note how this muscle passes beneath the acromion process before attaching to the greater tubercle. (Modified from Soames, R., & Palastanga, N. [2019]. *Anatomy and human movement: Structure and function* [7th ed.]. Philadelphia, PA: Elsevier.)

INFRASPINATUS (FIG. 21.40)

Latin: infra—beneath
spinatus—spine

ORIGIN
Infraspinous fossa of the scapula

INSERTION
Greater tubercle of the humerus

ACTION
Externally/laterally rotates the humerus

NERVE
Suprascapular nerve

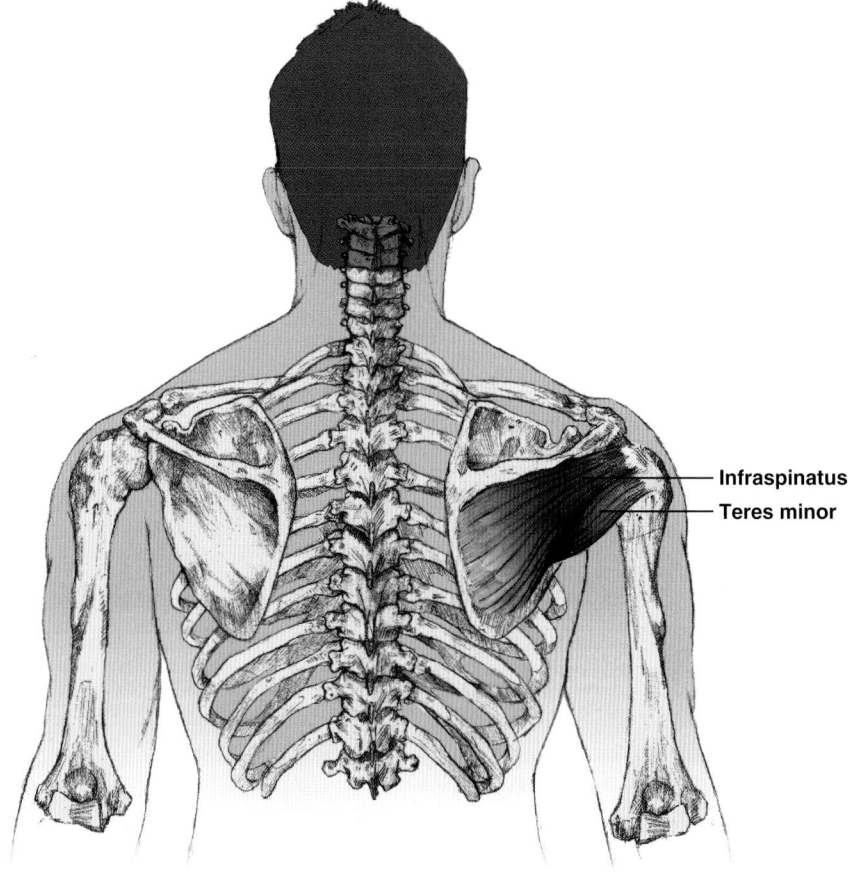

Infraspinatus
Teres minor

Posterior View

FIG. 21.40 Right infraspinatus and right teres minor. (Modified from Mansfield, P. [2014]. *Essentials of kinesiology for the physical therapist assistant* [2nd ed.]. St. Louis, MO: Mosby.)

TERES MINOR (SEE FIG. 21.40)

Latin: teres—round
minor—smaller

ORIGIN
Superior two-thirds of the lateral border of the scapula

INSERTION
Greater tubercle of the humerus

ACTIONS
Externally/laterally rotates the humerus
Adducts the humerus

NERVE
Axillary nerve

NOTES: Teres minor and infraspinatus are synergists, and their fibers may fuse.

SUBSCAPULARIS (FIG. 21.41)

Latin: sub—below
scapulae—shoulder blade

ORIGIN
Subscapular fossa of the scapula

INSERTION
Lesser tubercle of the humerus

ACTION
Internally/medially rotates the humerus

NERVE
Subscapular nerve

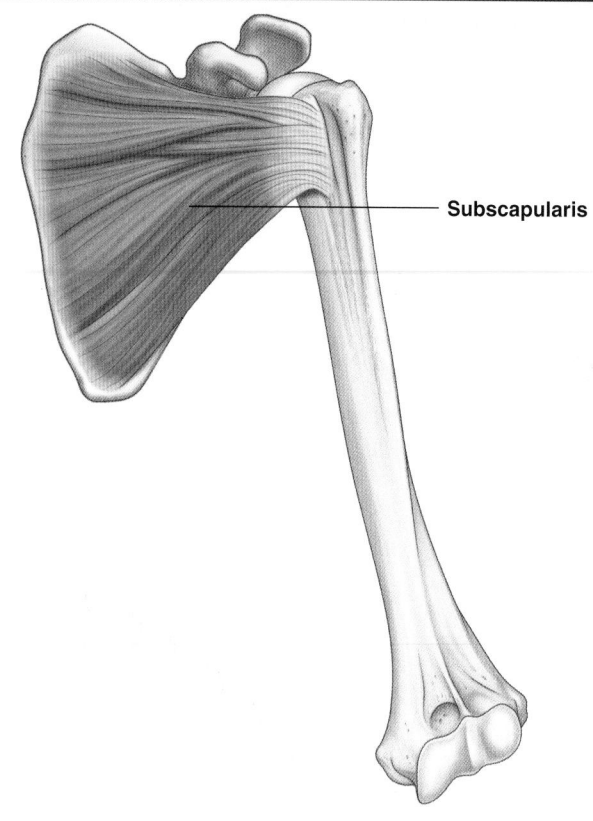

Subscapularis

Anterior View

NOTES: Subscapularis lies on the anterior scapula and is the *frozen shoulder muscle,* as myofascial trigger points may lead to shoulder immobility (Travell & Simons, 1983). Frozen shoulder is also called adhesive capsulitis. See Chapter 19 for more information about frozen shoulder.

FIG. 21.41 Left subscapularis. (From Soames, R. W. [2019]. *Anatomy and human movement* [7th ed.]. Philadelphia, PA: Elsevier.)

DELTOID (FIG. 21.42)

Greek: delta—triangular

ORIGINS
Lateral third of the clavicle
Acromion process
Scapular spine

INSERTION
Deltoid tuberosity

ACTIONS
Flexes the humerus (anterior fibers)
Internally/medially rotates the humerus (anterior fibers)
Abducts the humerus (middle fibers)
Extends the humerus (posterior fibers)
Externally/laterally rotates the humerus (posterior fibers)

NERVE
Axillary nerve

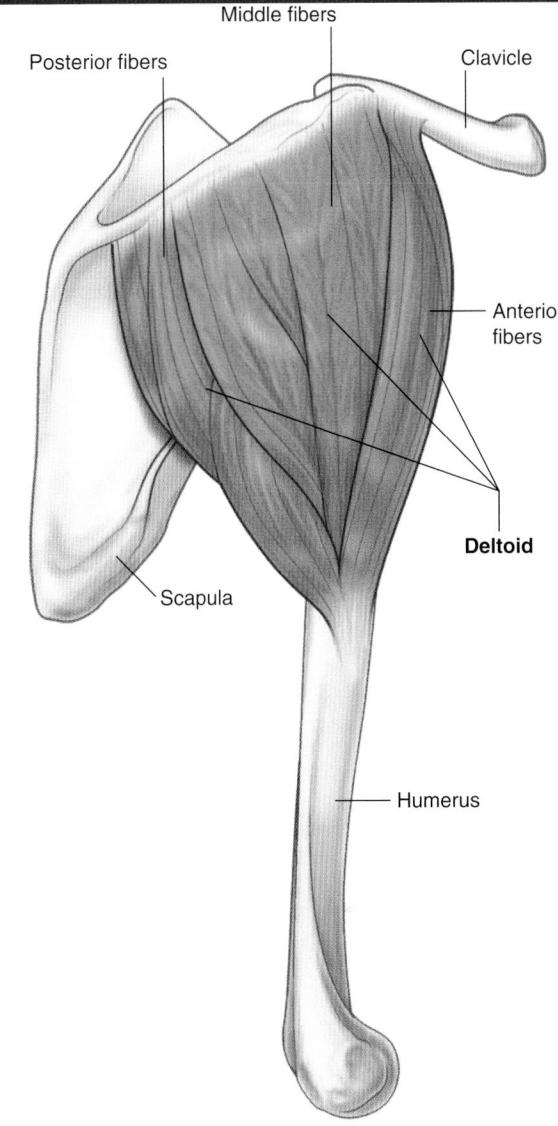

Lateral View

FIG. 21.42 Right deltoid with its anterior, middle, and posterior fibers identified. (Modified from Soames, R., & Palastanga: N. [2019]. *Anatomy and human movement: Structure and function* [7th ed.]. Philadelphia, PA: Elsevier.)

NOTES: The deltoid, or *delts,* can be divided into three regions for performing separate actions. *Anterior deltoid* flexes and internally/medially rotates the humerus. *Middle deltoid* abducts the humerus. *Posterior deltoid* extends and externally/laterally rotates the humerus. The deltoid can be an antagonist to itself.

PECTORALIS MAJOR (FIG. 21.43)

Latin: pectoralis—pertaining to the chest
major—larger

ORIGINS
Medial half of the clavicle
Edge of the sternal body
Ribs 1 through 7 (costal cartilages)

INSERTION
Intertubercular groove of the humerus (lateral lip)

ACTIONS
Adducts the humerus (anteriorly)
Internally/medially rotates the humerus
Flexes the humerus
Extends the humerus

NERVE
Medial and lateral pectoral nerves

NOTES: Pectoralis major, or *pecs,* forms the anterior axillary folds (the lats form the posterior axillary folds). This muscle possesses clavicular, sternal, and costal regions. Excessive muscle tension in the pecs may cause postural distortions, such as rounded shoulders as well as angina-like pain (Simons et al., 1998). See Chapter 26 for more information about angina.

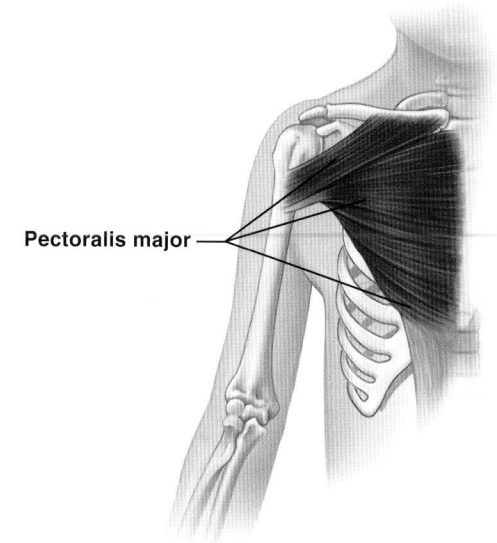

Pectoralis major

Anterior View

FIG. 21.43 Right pectoralis major. (From Herring, J. A. [2014]. *Tachdjian's pediatric orthopaedics: From the Texas Scottish Rite Hospital for Children* [5th ed.]. Philadelphia, PA: Elsevier.)

CORACOBRACHIALIS (FIG. 21.44)

Greek: korax—crow's beak
Latin: bracchium—arm

ORIGIN
Coracoid process of the scapula

INSERTION
Medial humeral shaft (middle region)

ACTIONS
Flexes the humerus
Adducts the humerus

NERVE
Musculocutaneous nerve

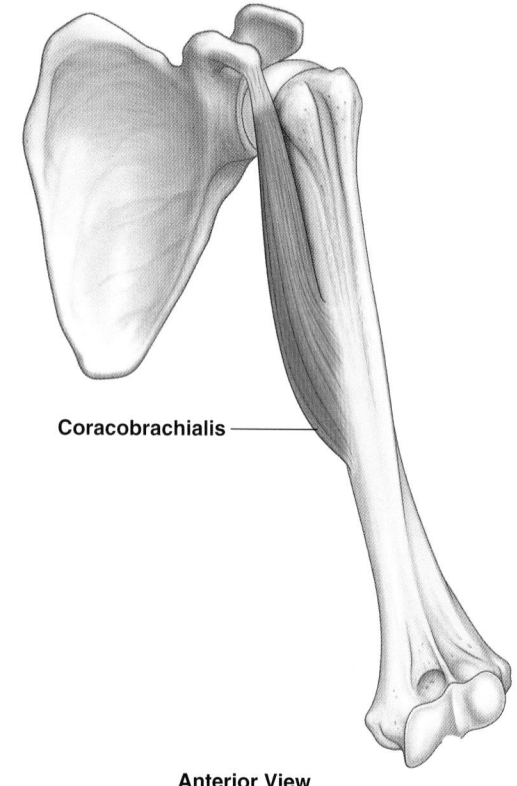

Coracobrachialis

Anterior View

FIG. 21.44 Left coracobrachialis. (Modified from Soames, R., & Palastanga N. [2019]. *Anatomy and human movement: Structure and function* [7th ed]. Philadelphia, PA: Elsevier.)

Lesson Five Review: Muscles of Shoulder Joint Movement

FLEXION	EXTENSION	ABDUCTION	ADDUCTION	INTERNAL (MEDIAL) ROTATION	EXTERNAL (LATERAL) ROTATION
Pectoralis major	Latissimus dorsi	Supraspinatus	Latissimus dorsi	Latissimus dorsi	Infraspinatus
Anterior deltoid	Teres major	Middle deltoid	Teres major	Teres major	Teres minor
Coracobrachialis	Posterior deltoid		Teres minor	Subscapularis	Posterior deltoid
Biceps brachii	Pectoralis major		Pectoralis major	Anterior deltoid	
	Triceps brachii		Coracobrachialis	Pectoralis major	
			Triceps brachii		

| Anterior view | Anterior/Posterior view | Anterior/Posterior view | Anterior/Posterior view | Anterior/Posterior view | Posterior view |

Lesson Six: Muscles of Elbow and Radioulnar Joint Movement

Movements of the elbow are flexion and extension. Movements of the radioulnar joints are supination and pronation. Muscles of elbow and radioulnar joint movements are biceps brachii, brachialis, brachioradialis, triceps brachii, anconeus, pronator teres, pronator quadratus, supinator, and flexor carpi radialis. Flexor carpi radialis also moves the wrist and is featured in Lesson Seven (Fig. 21.45).

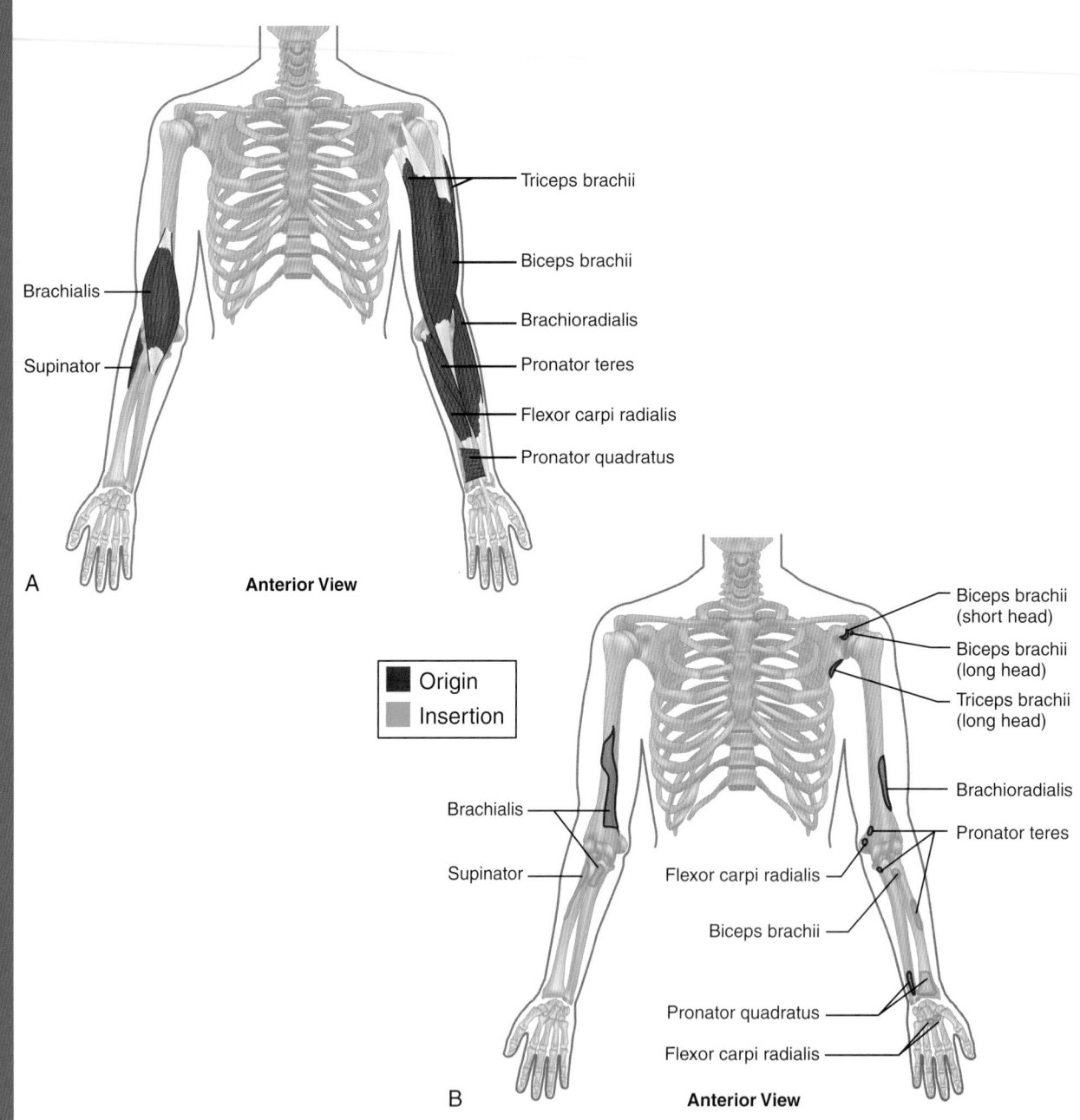

FIG. 21.45 Muscles of elbow and radioulnar joint movement (*A and C*) with their associated origins (*red*) and insertions (*blue, B and D*).

Lesson Six: Muscles of Elbow and Radioulnar Joint Movement—cont'd

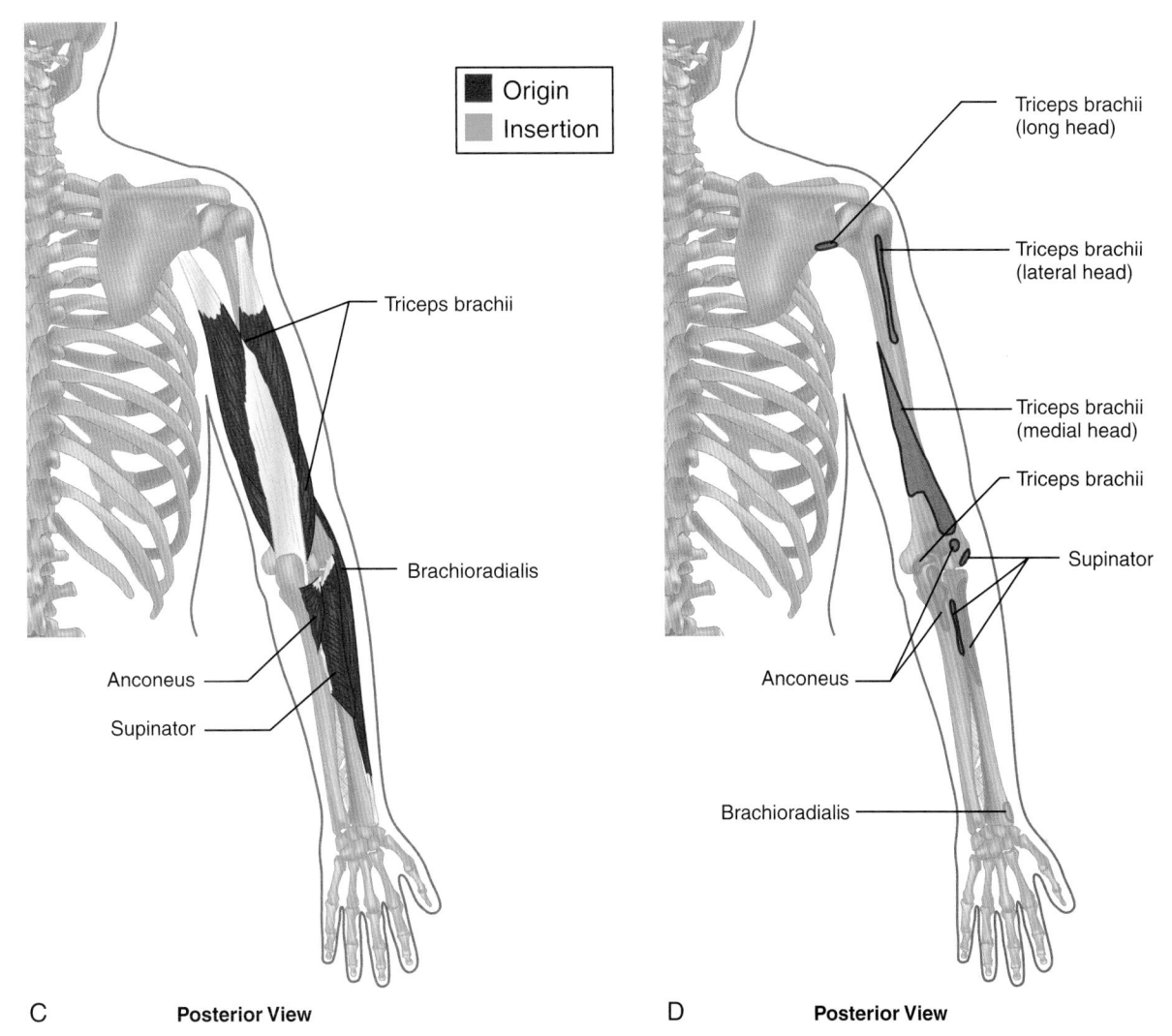

FIG. 21.45, CONT'D

BICEPS BRACHII (FIG. 21.46)

Latin: bis—twice + caput—head
bracchium—arm

ORIGINS
Supraglenoid tubercle of the scapula (long head)
Coracoid process of the scapula (short head)

INSERTIONS
Radial tuberosity
Bicipital aponeurosis

ACTIONS
Flexes the elbow
Supinates the forearm
Flexes the humerus

NERVE
Musculocutaneous nerve

NOTES: Biceps brachii is the *corkscrew muscle,* because two of its actions are used when opening a bottle with a corkscrew. First, forearm supination unscrews the cork, then elbow flexion pulls the cork out of the bottle (Lippert, 2006). The long head tendon is within the intertubercular groove of the humerus and extends through the joint capsule of the shoulder. The biceps brachii has actions at three joints (shoulder, elbow, and radioulnar joints). Biceps brachii may have an additional origin on the midshaft of the humerus (approximately 10% of cadavers).

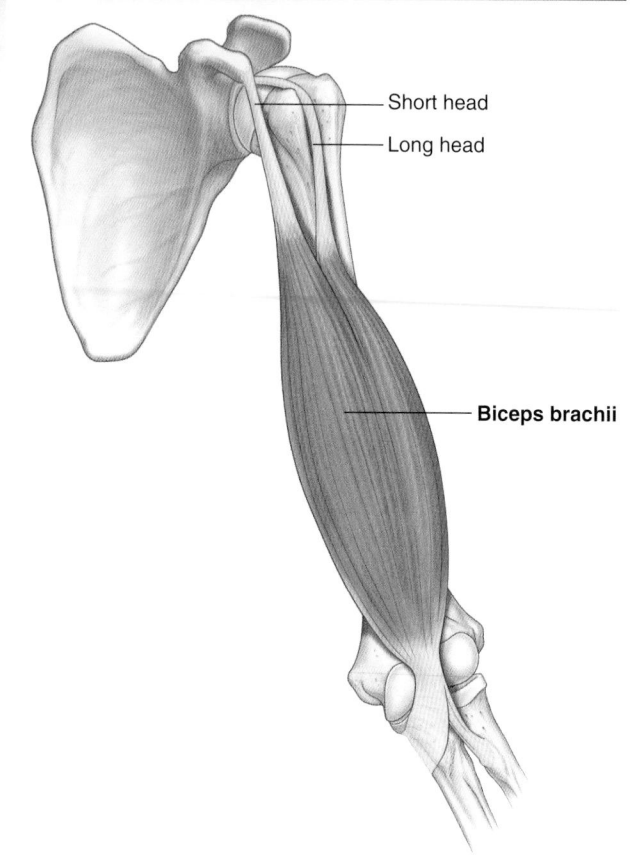

Short head
Long head

Biceps brachii

Anterior View

FIG. 21.46 Left biceps brachii with the long and short heads identified. (From Soames, R. W. [2019]. *Anatomy and human movement* [7th ed.]. Philadelphia, PA: Elsevier.)

BRACHIALIS (FIG. 21.47)

Latin: bracchium—arm

ORIGIN
Distal half of anterior humeral shaft

INSERTIONS
Ulnar tuberosity
Coronoid process of the ulna

ACTION
Flexes the elbow

NERVE
Musculocutaneous nerve

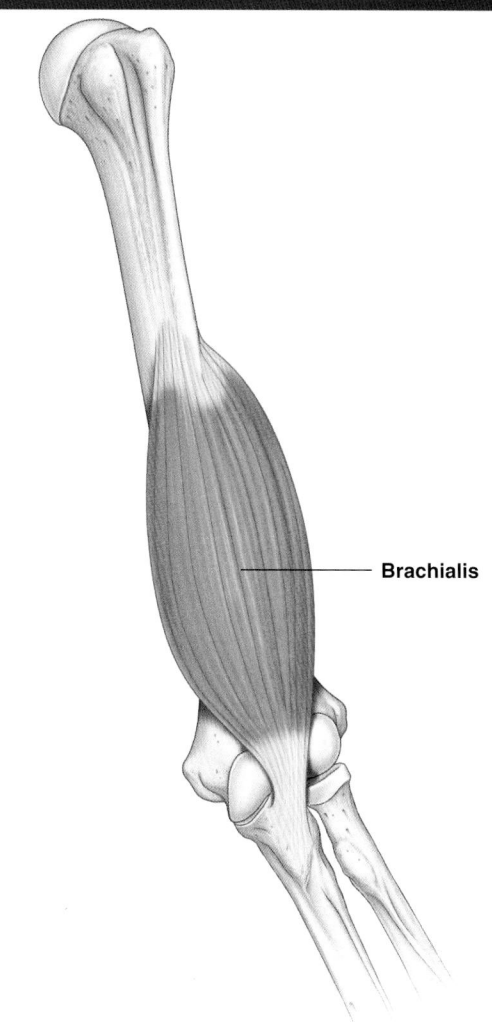

Brachialis

Anterior View

FIG. 21.47 Left brachialis. (From Soames, R. W. [2019]. *Anatomy and human movement* [7th ed.]. Philadelphia, PA: Elsevier.)

NOTES: Brachialis is beneath biceps brachii and is the *workhorse elbow flexor* because it is the most effective elbow flexor due to its mechanical advantage (Travell & Simons, 1983). When you flex your elbow to show off your biceps brachii, brachialis is pushing the biceps up, making it appear larger than it really is.

BRACHIORADIALIS (FIG. 21.48)

Latin: bracchium—arm
radialis—spoke of a wheel

ORIGIN
Lateral supracondylar ridge of the humerus

INSERTION
Styloid process of the radius

ACTION
Flexes the elbow

NERVE
Radial nerve

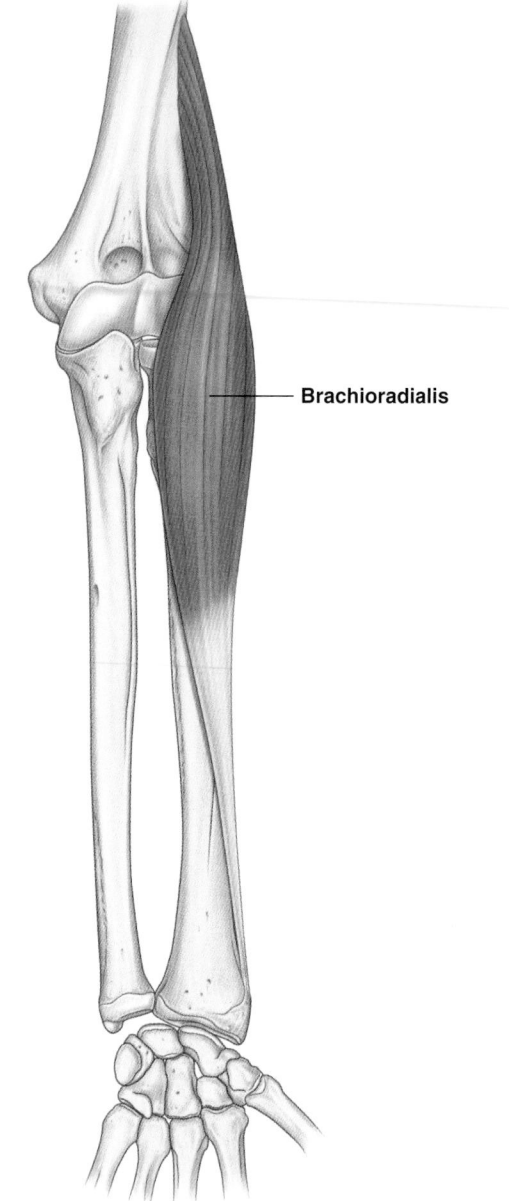

Brachioradialis

Anterior View

NOTES: Brachioradialis can be palpated as the fleshy prominence in the upper region of the lateral forearm. The radial pulse is between the tendons of the brachioradialis and flexor carpi radialis (Lesson Seven).

FIG. 21.48 Left brachioradialis. (From Soames, R. W. [2019]. *Anatomy and human movement* [7th ed.]. Philadelphia, PA: Elsevier.)

TRICEPS BRACHII (FIG. 21.49)

Greek: treis—three
Latin: bracchium—arm

ORIGINS
Infraglenoid tubercle of the scapula (long head)
Posterior proximal humeral shaft (lateral head)
Posterior distal humeral shaft (medial head)

INSERTION
Olecranon process

ACTIONS
Extends the elbow
Extends the humerus
Adducts the humerus

NERVE
Radial nerve

NOTES: Triceps brachii and serratus anterior (Lesson Four) are the *boxer's muscles* because they work simultaneously to extend the elbow to throw a boxer's punch (Herlihy, 2018).

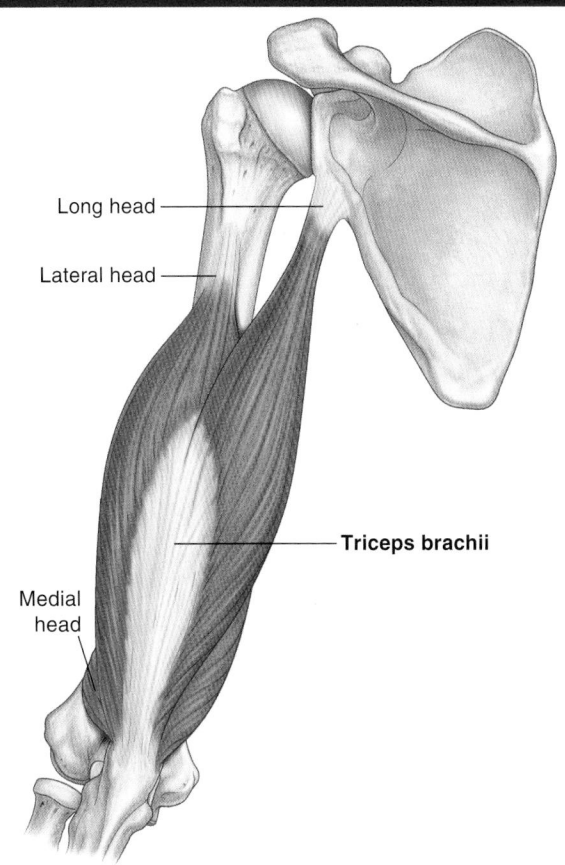

Posterior View

FIG. 21.49 Left triceps brachii with the long, lateral, and medial heads identified. (From Soames, R. W. [2019]. *Anatomy and human movement* [7th ed.]. Philadelphia, PA: Elsevier.)

ANCONEUS (FIG. 21.50)

Greek: angkon—elbow

ORIGIN
Lateral epicondyle of the humerus

INSERTIONS
Olecranon process
Superior eighth of the posterior ulnar shaft

ACTION
Extends the elbow

NERVE
Radial nerve

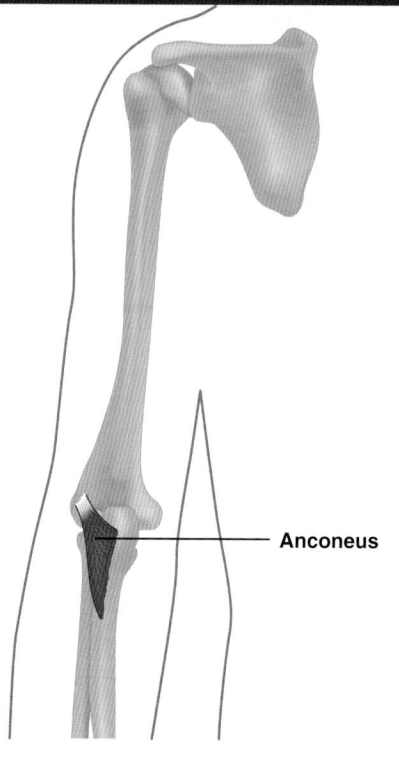

Anconeus

Posterior View

FIG. 21.50 Left anconeus.

PRONATOR TERES (FIG. 21.51)

Latin: pronus—downward
teres—round

ORIGINS
Medial epicondyle of the humerus via the common flexor tendon
Coronoid process of the ulna

INSERTION
Midlateral radial shaft

ACTIONS
Pronates the forearm
Flexes the elbow

NERVE
Median nerve

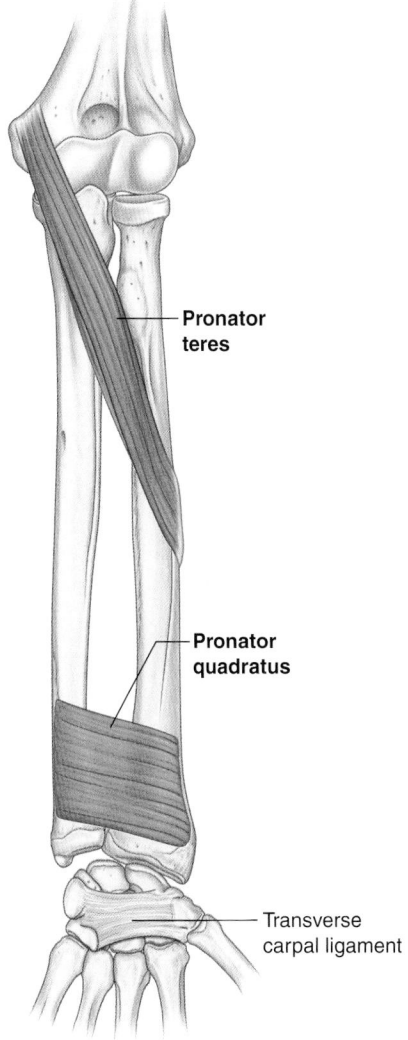

Anterior View

FIG. 21.51 Left pronator teres and pronator quadratus. (From Soames, R. W. [2019]. *Anatomy and human movement* [7th ed.]. Philadelphia, PA: Elsevier.)

NOTES: The *common flexor tendon* listed in the origins section is the proximal attachment for five muscles—pronator teres, flexor carpi radialis, palmaris longus, flexor carpi ulnaris, and flexor digitorum superficialis (Lesson Seven).

PRONATOR QUADRATUS (SEE FIG. 21.51)

Latin: pronus—downward
quadratus—four-sided

ORIGIN
Anterior distal quarter of the ulnar shaft

INSERTION
Anterior distal quarter of the radial shaft

ACTION
Pronates the forearm

NERVE
Median nerve

SUPINATOR (FIG. 21.52)

Latin: supinatus—bent backward

ORIGINS
Lateral epicondyle of the humerus
Proximal eighth of the ulnar shaft
Radial collateral ligament
Annular ligament

INSERTION
Proximal lateral radial shaft

ACTION
Supinates the forearm

NERVE
Radial nerve

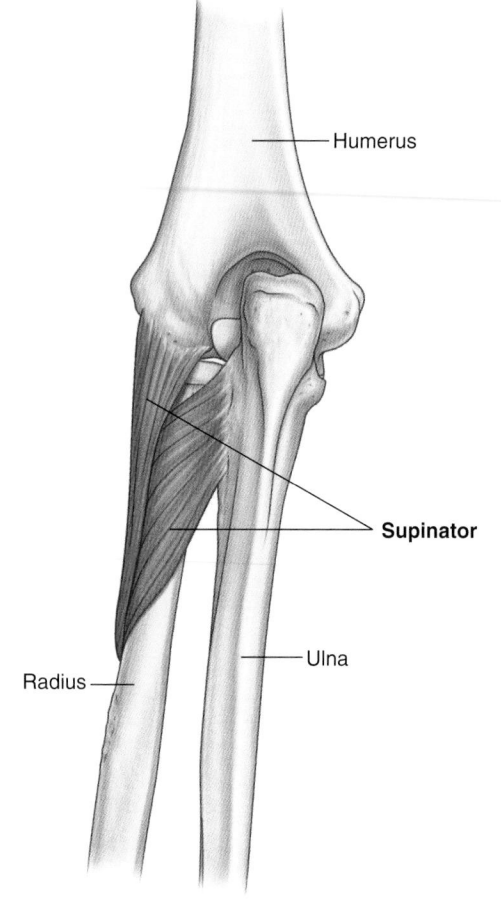

Posterior View

FIG. 21.52 Left supinator with arm and forearm bones identified. (From Soames, R. W. [2019]. *Anatomy and human movement* [7th ed.]. Philadelphia, PA: Elsevier.)

Lesson Six Review: Muscles of Elbow and Radioulnar Joint Movement

FLEXION	EXTENSION	PRONATION	SUPINATION
Biceps brachii	Triceps brachii	Pronator teres	Biceps brachii
Brachialis	Anconeus	Pronator quadratus	Supinator
Brachioradialis			
Pronator teres			
Flexor carpi radialis			

Anterior
view

Anterior
view

Anterior
view

Anterior
view

Lesson Seven: Muscles of Wrist and Hand Movement

Movements of the wrist and fingers are flexion, extension, adduction, and abduction. The thumb and little finger can be moved into opposition. Muscles that control the wrist and hand movements are the flexor carpi radialis, flexor carpi ulnaris, palmaris longus, flexor digitorum superficialis, flexor digitorum profundus, extensor carpi radialis longus and brevis, extensor carpi ulnaris, extensor digitorum, extensor digiti minimi, extensor indicis, extensor pollicis longus and brevis, flexor pollicis longus and brevis, opponens pollicis, abductor pollicis longus and brevis, flexor digiti minimi, abductor digiti minimi, and opponens digiti minimi (Fig. 21.53).

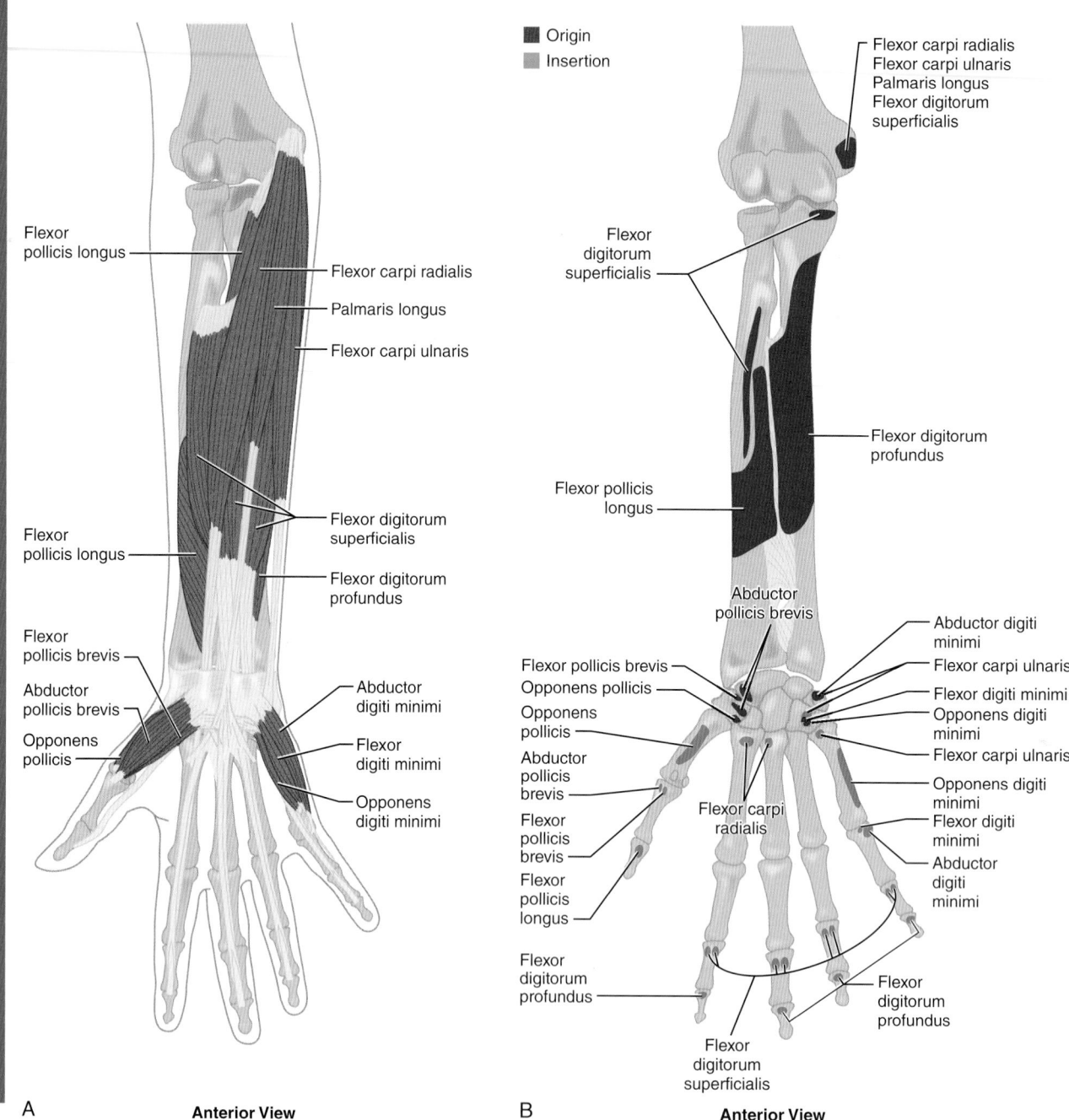

FIG. 21.53 Muscles of wrist and hand movement (*A and C*) and their associated origins (*red*) and insertions (*blue, B and D*).

Lesson Seven: Muscles of Wrist and Hand Movement—cont'd

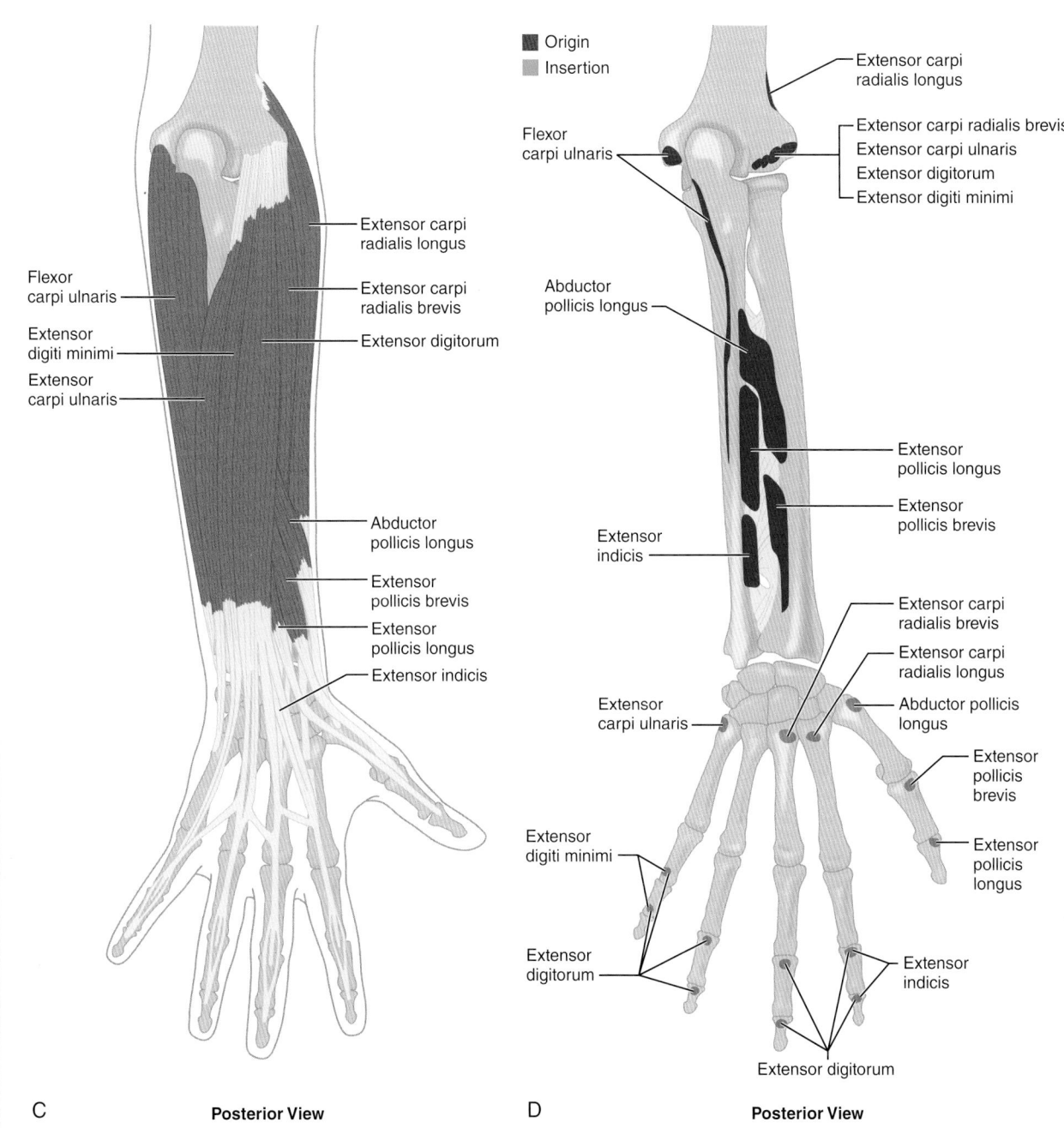

■ Origin
■ Insertion

Panel C labels:
Flexor carpi ulnaris
Extensor digiti minimi
Extensor carpi ulnaris
Extensor carpi radialis longus
Extensor carpi radialis brevis
Extensor digitorum
Abductor pollicis longus
Extensor pollicis brevis
Extensor pollicis longus
Extensor indicis

C **Posterior View**

Panel D labels:
Flexor carpi ulnaris
Extensor carpi radialis longus
Extensor carpi radialis brevis
Extensor carpi ulnaris
Extensor digitorum
Extensor digiti minimi
Abductor pollicis longus
Extensor pollicis longus
Extensor pollicis brevis
Extensor indicis
Extensor carpi radialis brevis
Extensor carpi radialis longus
Abductor pollicis longus
Extensor pollicis brevis
Extensor pollicis longus
Extensor carpi ulnaris
Extensor digiti minimi
Extensor digitorum
Extensor indicis
Extensor digitorum

D **Posterior View**

FIG. 21.53, CONT'D

NOTES: The hands possess four small worm-like muscles called *lumbricals* (see Fig, 21.55). These deep muscles assist with gripping movements. The feet also contain these muscles and have similar actions on the toes.

FLEXOR CARPI RADIALIS (FIG. 21.54)

Latin: flexus—bent
karpos—wrist
radialis—spoke of a wheel

ORIGIN
Medial epicondyle of the humerus via the common flexor tendon

INSERTIONS
Bases of metacarpals II and III

ACTIONS
Flexes the wrist
Abducts the wrist
Flexes the elbow

NERVE
Median nerve

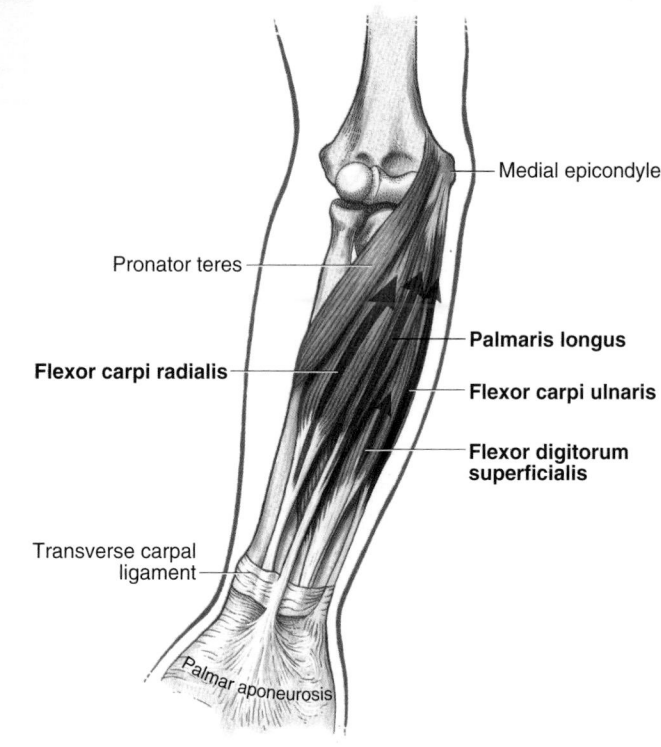

Anterior View

FIG. 21.54 Right flexor carpi radialis, flexor carpi ulnaris, palmaris longus, and flexor digitorum superficialis. The arrows represent their common action of wrist flexion. (Modified from Mansfield, P. [2014]. *Essentials of kinesiology for the physical therapist assistant* [2nd ed.]. St. Louis, MO: Mosby.)

NOTES: Flexor carpi radialis and the following three muscles (flexor carpi ulnaris, palmaris longus, and flexor digitorum superficialis) originate on the medial epicondyle of the humerus. *Medial epicondylitis (golfer's elbow)* can occur with forceful repetitive wrist flexion. The radial pulse is between the tendons of flexor carpi radialis and brachioradialis (Lesson Six).

FLEXOR CARPI ULNARIS (SEE FIG. 21.54)

Latin: flexus—bent
karpos—wrist
ulna—elbow

ORIGINS
Medial epicondyle of the humerus via the common flexor tendon
Medial olecranon
Posterior proximal two thirds of the ulna

INSERTIONS
Base of metacarpal V
Pisiform
Hook of hamate

ACTIONS
Flexes the wrist
Adducts the wrist

NERVE
Ulnar nerve

PALMARIS LONGUS (SEE FIG. 21.54)

Latin: palma—hand
longus—long

ORIGIN
Medial epicondyle of the humerus via the common flexor tendon

INSERTION
Palmar aponeurosis

ACTIONS
Flexes the wrist
Cups (tenses) the palm

NERVE
Median nerve

NOTES: Palmaris longus is present in approximately 75% of the population. Its long tendon can be used to repair injuries of the hand and wrist; removal or absence of this tendon does not decrease hand function, including grip strength. Tendon of palmaris longus can be seen by touching the pads of the fourth finger and thumb, and flexing the wrist. If present, the tendon will be visible in the middle of the anterior wrist.

Palmar aponeurosis (palmar fascia) is a triangular-shaped structure occupying the central portion of the palm. Its proximal region joins the lower border of the transverse carpal ligament and receives the expanded tendon of palmaris longus. The distal region of palmar aponeurosis has four small openings to allow passage of the flexor tendons.

FLEXOR DIGITORUM SUPERFICIALIS (SEE FIG. 21.54)

Latin: flexus—bent
digitus—finger
superficialis—toward the surface

ORIGINS
Medial epicondyle of the humerus via the common flexor tendon
Anterior proximal radial shaft
Coronoid process of the ulna

INSERTIONS
Middle phalanges of digits II through V

ACTIONS
Flexes the wrist
Flexes the fingers at the proximal interphalangeal (PIP) and metacarpophalangeal (MCP) joints

NERVE
Median nerve

FLEXOR DIGITORUM PROFUNDUS (FIG. 21.55)

Latin: flexus—bent
digitus—finger
profundus—deep

ORIGINS
Proximal three-fourths of the anterior ulnar shaft
Interosseous membrane

INSERTIONS
Distal phalanges of digits II through V

ACTIONS
Flexes the wrist
Flexes the fingers at the distal interphalangeal (DIP),
    PIP, and MCP joints

NERVES
Ulnar nerve
Median nerve

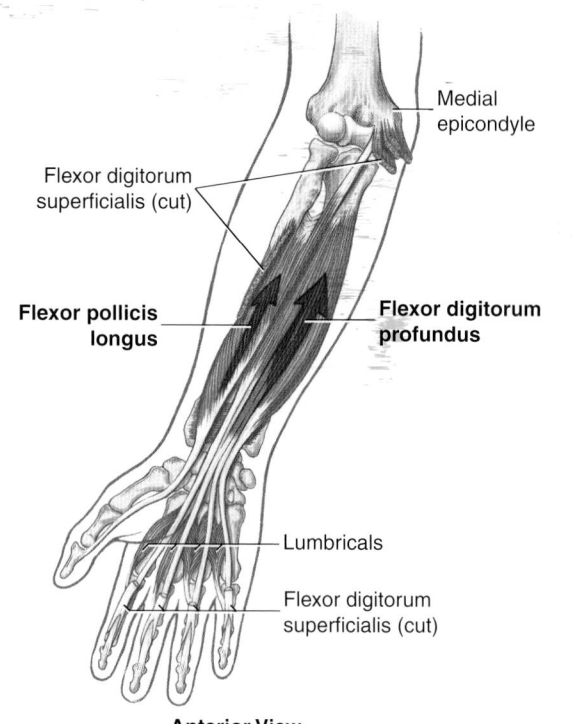

Anterior View

FIG. 21.55 Right flexor digitorum profundus and flexor pollicis longus. The arrows represent their common action of flexion. (Modified from Mansfield, P. [2014]. *Essentials of kinesiology for the physical therapist assistant* [2nd ed.]. St. Louis, MO: Mosby.)

EXTENSOR CARPI RADIALIS LONGUS (FIG. 21.56)

Latin: extensio—to extend
karpos—wrist
radialis—spoke of a wheel
longus—long

ORIGIN
Lateral supracondylar ridge of the humerus

INSERTION
Posterior base of metacarpal II

ACTIONS
Extends the wrist
Abducts the wrist

NERVE
Radial nerve

Posterior View

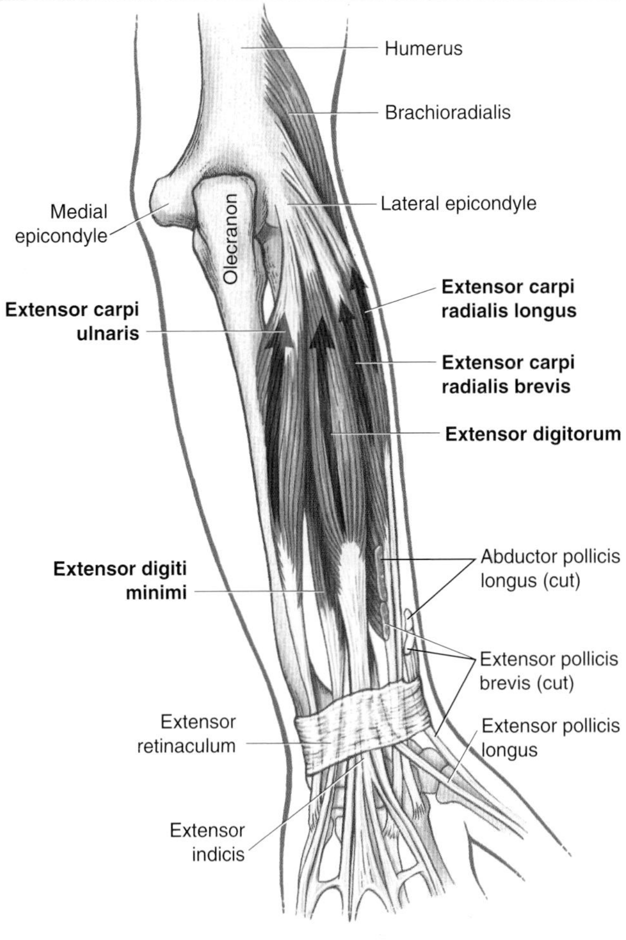

FIG. 21.56 Right extensor carpi radialis longus, extensor carpi radialis brevis, extensor carpi ulnaris, extensor digitorum, and extensor digiti minimi. The arrows represent their common action of extension. (Modified from Mansfield, P. [2014]. *Essentials of kinesiology for the physical therapist assistant* [2nd ed.]. St. Louis, MO: Mosby.)

NOTES: *Extensor retinaculum (dorsal carpal ligament)* is a fibrous band on the posterior side of the hand near the wrist that holds the extensor tendons in place.

EXTENSOR CARPI RADIALIS BREVIS (SEE FIG. 21.56)

Latin: extensio—to extend
karpos—wrist
radialis—spoke of a wheel
brevis—brief

ORIGIN
Lateral epicondyle of the humerus via the common extensor tendon

INSERTION
Posterior base of metacarpal III

ACTIONS
Extends the wrist
Abducts the wrist

NERVE
Radial nerve

NOTES: Extensor carpi radialis brevis and the following muscles (extensor carpi ulnaris, extensor digitorum, and extensor digiti minimi) originate on the lateral epicondyle of the humerus. *Lateral epicondylitis (tennis elbow)* can occur with forceful repetitive extension of the wrist.

EXTENSOR CARPI ULNARIS (SEE FIG. 21.56)

Latin: extensio—to extend
karpos—wrist
ulna—elbow

ORIGIN
Lateral epicondyle of the humerus via the common extensor tendon

INSERTION
Metacarpal V

ACTIONS
Extends the wrist
Adducts the wrist

NERVE
Radial nerve

EXTENSOR DIGITORUM (SEE FIG. 21.56)

Latin: extensio—to extend
digitus—finger

ORIGIN
Lateral epicondyle of the humerus via the common extensor tendon

INSERTIONS
Middle and distal phalanges of digits II through V

ACTIONS
Extends the wrist
Extends the fingers at the DIP, PIP, and MCP joints

NERVE
Radial nerve

EXTENSOR DIGITI MINIMI (SEE FIG. 21.56)

Latin: extensio—to extend
digitus—finger
minimum—least

ORIGIN
Lateral epicondyle of the humerus via the common extensor tendon

INSERTIONS
Posterior middle and distal phalanges of digit V via the tendon of the extensor digitorum

ACTION
Extends the little finger (digit V)

NERVE
Radial nerve

EXTENSOR INDICIS (FIG. 21.57)

Latin: extensio—to extend
indicis—forefinger

ORIGINS
Posterior distal ulnar shaft
Interosseous membrane

INSERTIONS
Middle and distal phalanges of the index finger (digit II)

ACTION
Extends the index finger (digit II)

NERVE
Radial nerve

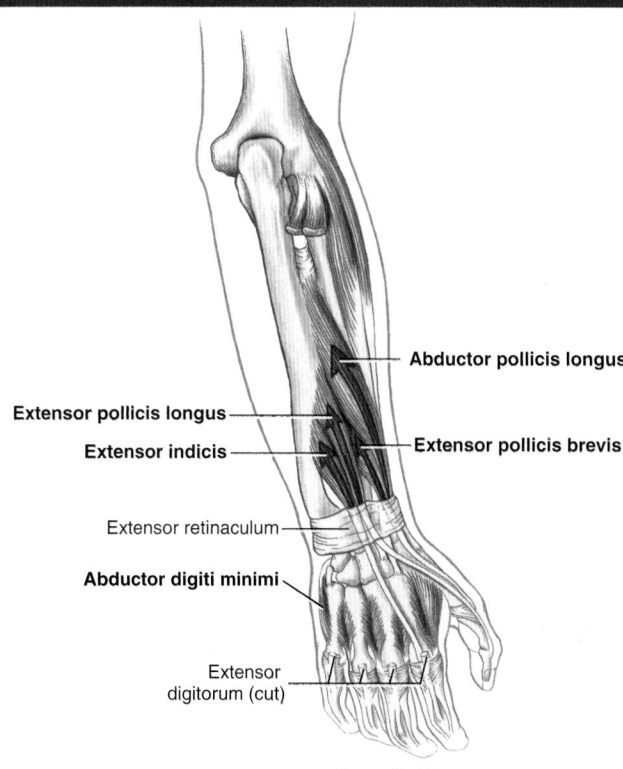

FIG. 21.57 Right extensor indicis, extensor pollicis longus, extensor pollicis brevis, abductor pollicis longus, and abductor digiti minimi. The arrows represent their action of extension or abduction. (Modified from Mansfield, P. [2014]. *Essentials of kinesiology for the physical therapist assistant* [2nd ed.]. St. Louis, MO: Mosby.)

EXTENSOR POLLICIS LONGUS AND BREVIS (SEE FIG. 21.57)

Latin: extensio—to extend
pollex—thumb
longus—long
brevis—brief

ORIGINS
Posterior ulnar shaft—middle region (longus)
Posterior radial shaft—distal region (brevis)
Interosseous membrane (brevis and longus)

INSERTIONS
Posterior distal phalanx of the thumb (longus)
Posterolateral proximal phalanx of the thumb (brevis)

ACTION
Extends the thumb (digit I)

NERVE
Radial nerve

NOTES: The *anatomic snuffbox* is a triangular depression on the back of the hand at the base of the thumb (Hallett & Ashurst, 2021). It is formed medially by tendons of extensor pollicis longus, and laterally by tendons of extensor pollicis brevis and abductor pollicis longus. The floor of the anatomical snuffbox is formed by the scaphoid and trapezium bones. This depression is visible when the wrist is adducted and the thumb is extended and abducted. The name "anatomic snuffbox" was derived by using it as a placement for snuff (powdered tobacco) before it was inhaled through the nose. Extensor pollicis longus may assist in wrist extension. Extensor pollicis brevis may assist in wrist abduction.

FLEXOR POLLICIS LONGUS (SEE FIG. 21.57) AND BREVIS (FIG. 21.58)

Latin: flexus—bent
pollex—thumb
longus—long
brevis—brief

ORIGINS

Anterior radial shaft—middle region (longus)
Interosseous membrane (longus)
Trapezium (brevis)
Transverse carpal ligament (brevis)

INSERTIONS

Anterior distal phalanx of the thumb (longus)
Proximal phalanx of the thumb (brevis)

ACTION

Flexes the thumb

NERVES

Median nerve (longus)
Median and ulnar nerves (brevis)

NOTES: The *thenar eminence* (thumb pad) is the fleshy bulge at the base of the thumb formed by flexor pollicis brevis, opponens pollicis, and abductor pollicis brevis.

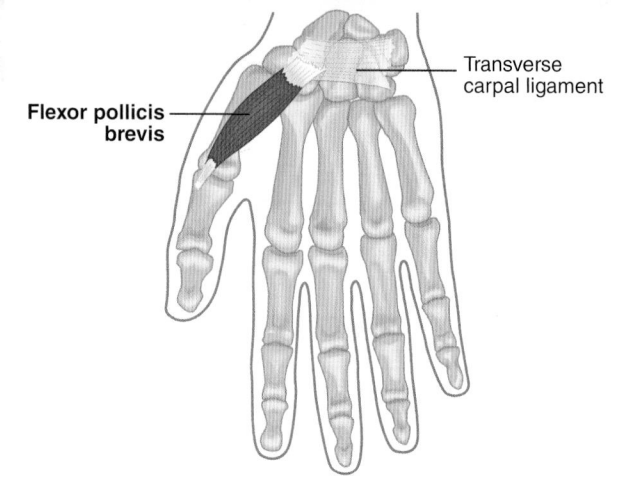

Anterior Views

FIG. 21.58 Right flexor pollicis brevis (see Fig. 21.55). Flexor pollicis longus is featured in Fig. 21.57.

OPPONENS POLLICIS (FIG. 21.59)

Latin: opponens—opposing
pollex—thumb

ORIGINS

Trapezium
Transverse carpal ligament

INSERTION

Anterior metacarpal I

ACTIONS

Opposes the thumb (adduction)
Flexes the thumb

NERVE

Median nerve

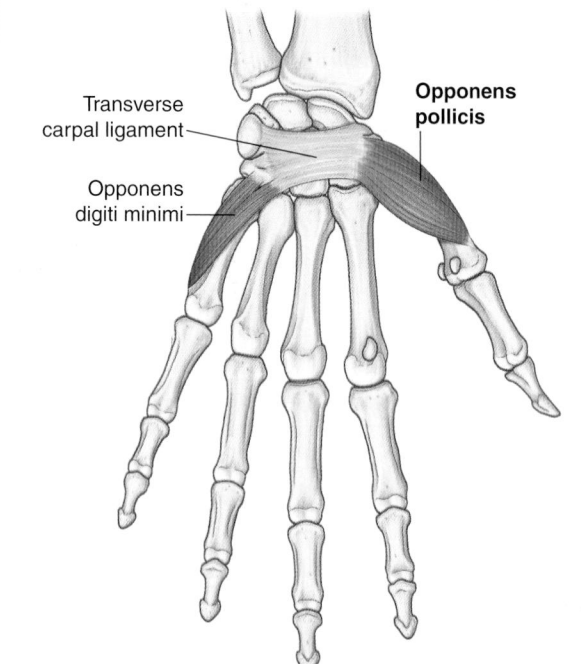

Anterior View

FIG. 21.59 Left opponens pollicis. Opponens digiti minimi is also featured in Fig. 21.62.

ABDUCTOR POLLICIS LONGUS (SEE FIG. 21.57) AND BREVIS (FIG. 21.60)

Latin: abductus—led away
pollex—thumb
longus—long
brevis—brief

ORIGINS
Posterior ulnar and radial shaft—middle region (longus)
Interosseous membrane (longus)
Trapezium (brevis)
Scaphoid (brevis)
Transverse carpal ligament (brevis)

INSERTIONS
Lateral metacarpal I (longus)
Lateral proximal phalanx of the thumb (brevis)

ACTION
Abducts the thumb (longus and brevis)

NERVES
Radial nerve (longus)
Median nerve (brevis)

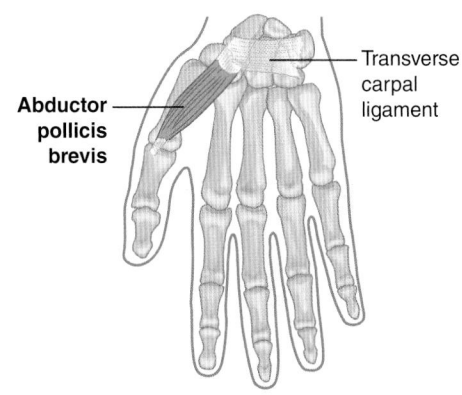

Abductor pollicis brevis

Transverse carpal ligament

Anterior View

FIG. 21.60 Right abductor pollicis brevis. Abductor pollicis longus is featured in Fig. 21.57.

FLEXOR DIGITI MINIMI (FIG. 21.61)

Latin: flexus—bent
digitus—finger
minimum—least

ORIGINS
Hook of hamate
Transverse carpal ligament

INSERTION
Proximal phalanx of digit V

ACTION
Flexes digit V (little finger)

NERVE
Ulnar nerve

NOTES: The *hypothenar eminence* is the fleshy bulge at the base of the fifth digit (little finger) formed by flexor digiti minimi, abductor digiti minimi, and opponens digiti minimi.

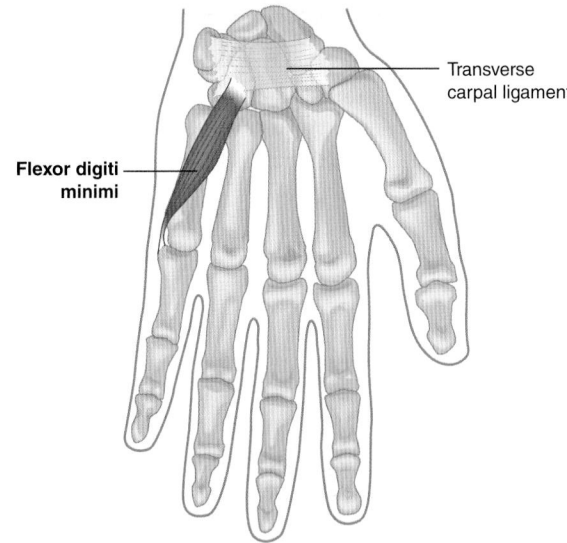

Flexor digiti minimi

Transverse carpal ligament

Anterior View

FIG. 21.61 Left flexor digiti minimi.

ABDUCTOR DIGITI MINIMI (SEE FIG. 21.57)

Latin: abductus—led away
digitus—finger
minimum—least

ORIGINS
Pisiform
Tendon of flexor carpi ulnaris

INSERTION
Proximal phalanx of digit V (little finger)

ACTION
Abducts digit V (little finger)

NERVE
Ulnar nerve

OPPONENS DIGITI MINIMI (FIG. 21.62)

Latin: opponens—opposing
digitus—finger
minimum—least

ORIGINS
Hamate
Transverse carpal ligament

INSERTION
Metacarpal V

ACTION
Adducts digit V (moves little finger into opposition)

NERVE
Ulnar nerve

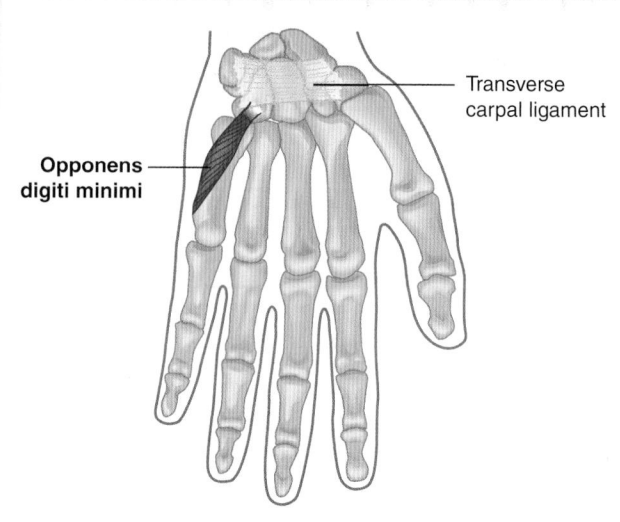

Anterior View

FIG. 21.62 Left opponens digiti minimi. This muscle is also featured in Fig. 21.59.

Lesson Seven Review: Muscles of Wrist and Hand Movement

FLEXION	EXTENSION	ABDUCTION	ADDUCTION
Flexor carpi radialis	Extensor carpi radialis longus	Flexor carpi radialis	Flexor carpi ulnaris
Flexor carpi ulnaris	Extensor carpi radialis brevis	Extensor carpi radialis longus	Extensor carpi ulnaris
Palmaris longus	Extensor carpi ulnaris	Extensor carpi radialis brevis	
Flexor digitorum superficialis	Extensor digitorum		
Flexor digitorum profundus			

Anterior view   Posterior view   Anterior view   Anterior view

Lesson Eight: Muscles of Hip and Knee Movement

Movements of the hip are flexion, extension, abduction, adduction, internal (medial) rotation, external (lateral) rotation, and circumduction. Movements of the knee are flexion and extension. Muscles of hip and knee movements are psoas major, iliacus, piriformis, gemellus superior, gemellus inferior, obturator internus, obturator externus, quadratus femoris, gluteus maximus, gluteus medius, gluteus minimus, tensor fasciae latae, gracilis, adductor magnus, adductor longus, adductor brevis, pectineus, rectus femoris, vastus intermedius, vastus medialis, vastus lateralis, sartorius, semimembranosus, semitendinosus, biceps femoris, gastrocnemius, plantaris, and popliteus. Gastrocnemius and plantaris also move the ankle; these muscles are featured in Lesson Nine (Fig. 21.63).

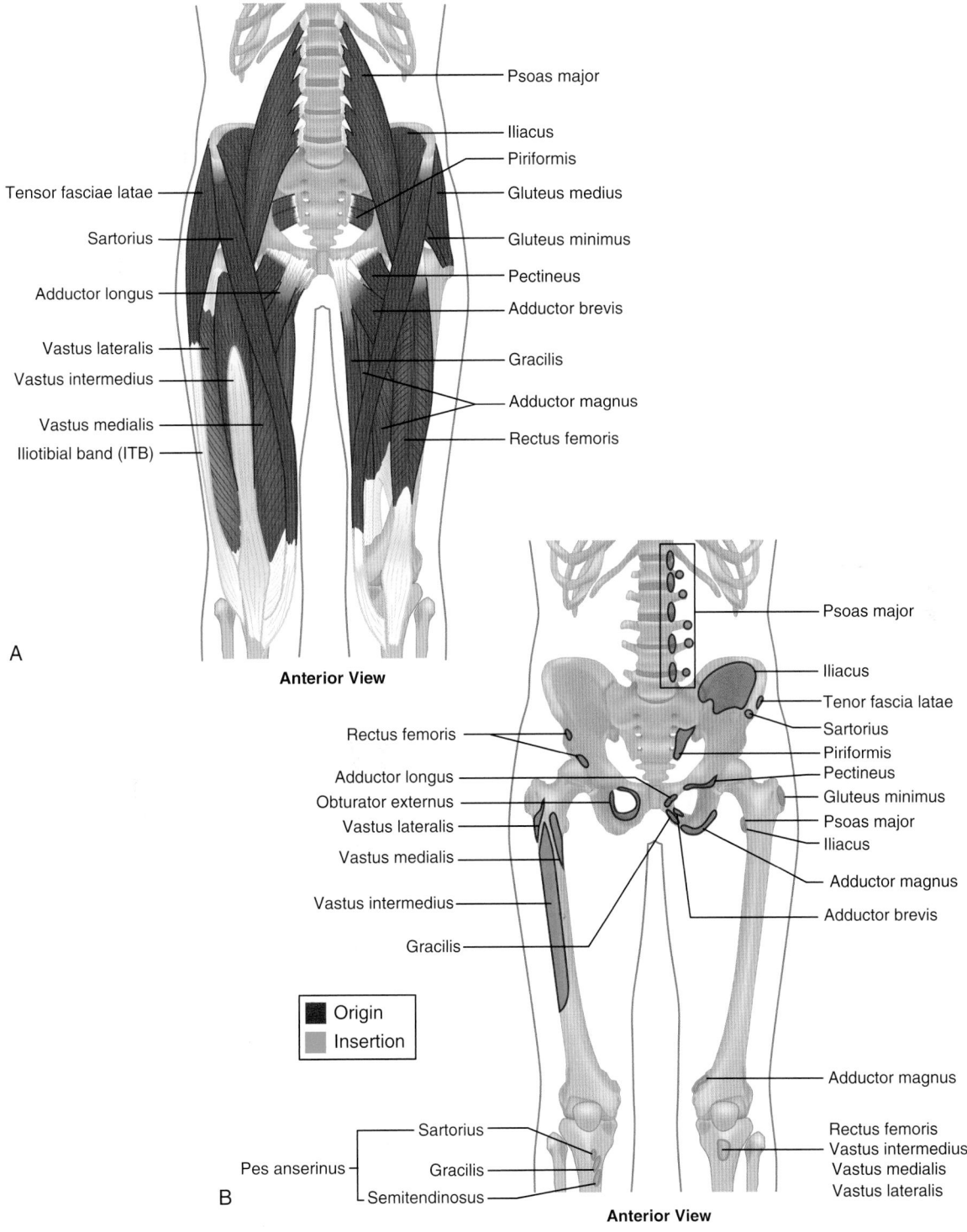

FIG. 21.63 Muscles of hip and knee movement (*A and C*) with their associated origins (*red*) and insertions (*blue, B and D*).

Continued

Lesson Eight: Muscles of Hip and Knee Movement—cont'd

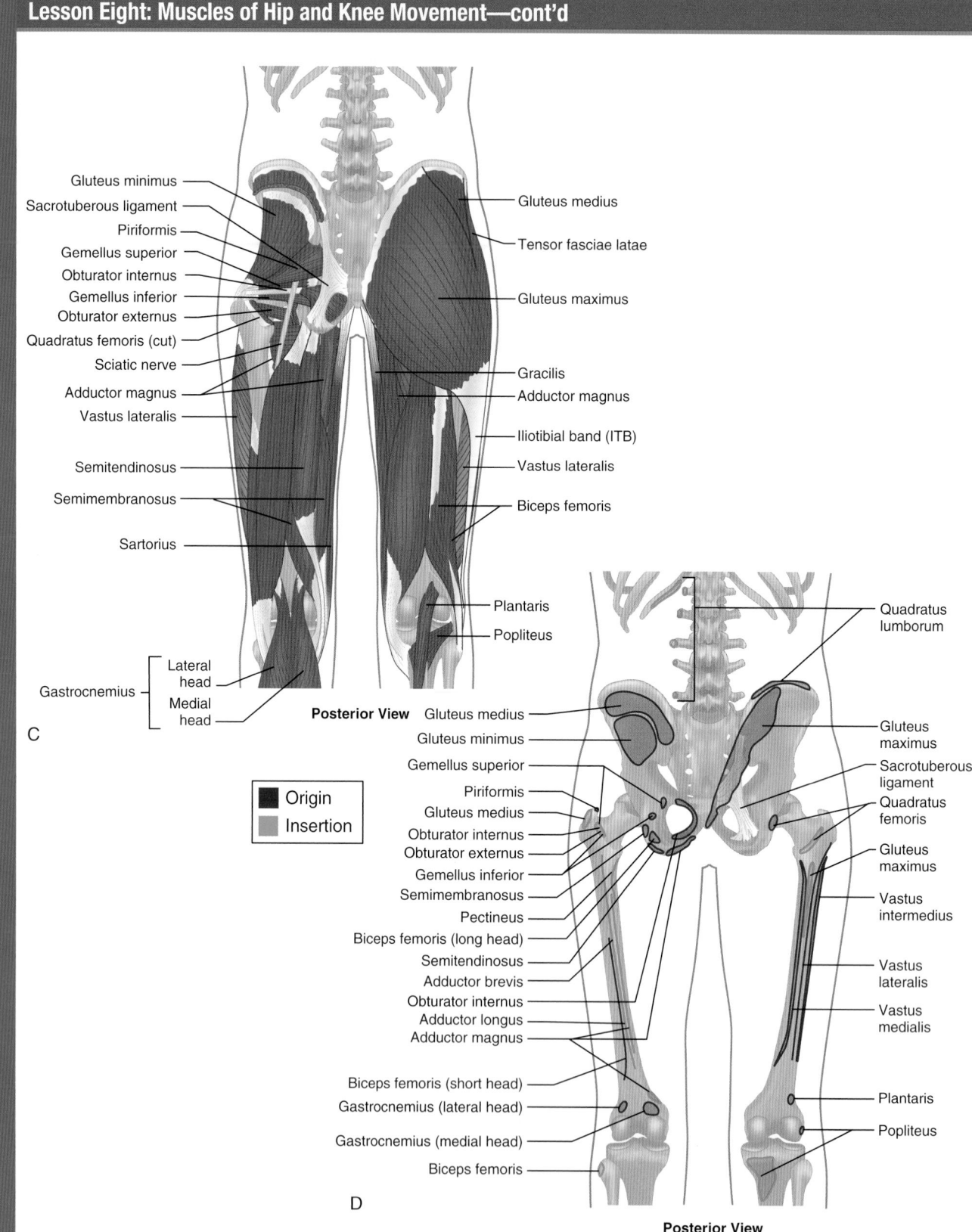

C

Posterior View

Origin
Insertion

D

Posterior View

FIG. 21.63, CONT'D

ILIOPSOAS (FIG. 21.64)

Latin: ilium—flank
Greek: psoa—muscle of the loin

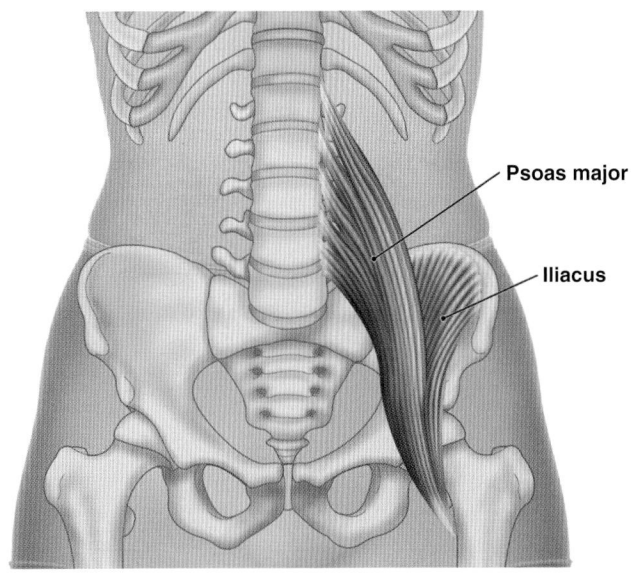

Anterior View

FIG. 21.64 Left iliopsoas. (Modified from Muscolino, J. [2010]. *Muscular system manual: The skeletal muscles of the human body* [3rd ed.]. St. Louis, MO: Mosby.)

NOTES: Iliopsoas consists of psoas major and iliacus. These muscles attach to the lesser trochanter. Psoas minor is present in approximately 50% of cadavers and is not included in this discussion.

PSOAS MAJOR (FIG. 21.65)

Greek: psoa—muscle of the loin
major—larger

ORIGINS
Transverse processes of T12–L5 (anterior surface)
Vertebral bodies of T12–L5
Intervertebral discs of lumbar vertebrae

INSERTION
Lesser trochanter

ACTIONS
Flexes the hip
Externally/laterally rotates the hip
Flexes the vertebral column (bilateral contraction)
Anteriorly tilts the pelvis (bilateral contraction)

NERVES
Lumbar plexus

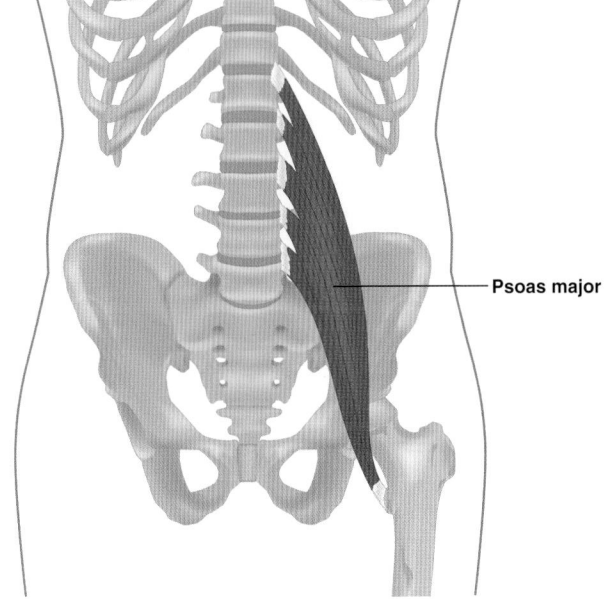

Anterior View

FIG. 21.65 Left psoas major.

NOTES: Psoas major is the strongest hip flexor. Beef tenderloin steak is the psoas major muscle of a cow. *Filet mignon* is a cut of steak from the smaller end of psoas major.

ILIACUS (FIG. 21.66)

Latin: iliacus—ilium

ORIGINS
Iliac fossa

INSERTION
Lesser trochanter

ACTIONS
Flexes the hip
Externally/laterally rotates the hip
Anteriorly tilts the pelvis (bilateral contraction)

NERVE
Femoral nerve

NOTES: The *inguinal ligament* extends from the anterior superior iliac spine to the pubic tubercle. The inferolateral portions of the internal obliques and the transverse abdominis (discussed later) attach to the inguinal ligament. Iliacus, psoas major, pectineus (discussed later), and structures such as nerves, blood vessels, and lymphatics pass beneath the inguinal ligament.

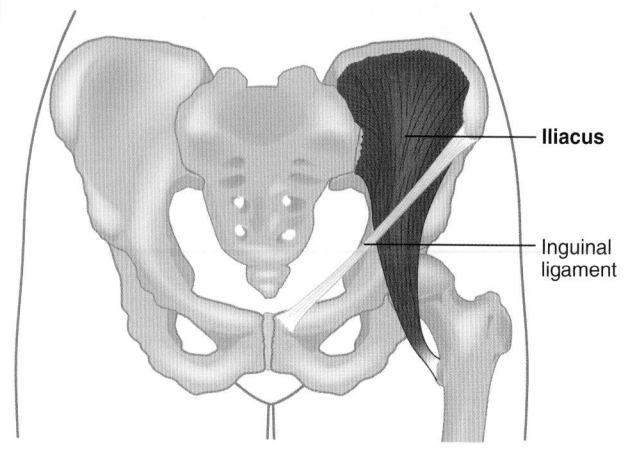

Anterior View

FIG. 21.66 Left iliacus.

LATERAL ROTATORS OF THE HIP (FIG. 21.67)

NOTES: The lateral (external) hip rotators are a group of six individual muscles that include piriformis, gemellus superior and inferior, obturator internus and externus, and quadratus femoris. These muscles are deep to the gluteus maximus. Most of the lateral rotators attach on the greater trochanter. These muscles are not the only ones involved with hip external (lateral) rotation, but it is their primary action.
LEARNING TIP: To help you remember the names of the lateral hip rotators, use the phrase **P**atched **G**oods **O**ften **G**o **O**n **Q**uilts for **P**iriformis—**G**emellus superior—**O**bturator internus—**G**emellus inferior—**O**bturator externus—**Q**uadratus femoris. The sciatic nerve generally exits the pelvis inferior to the piriformis muscle; however, other exit routes do exist and are discussed under the next entry, titled "Piriformis."

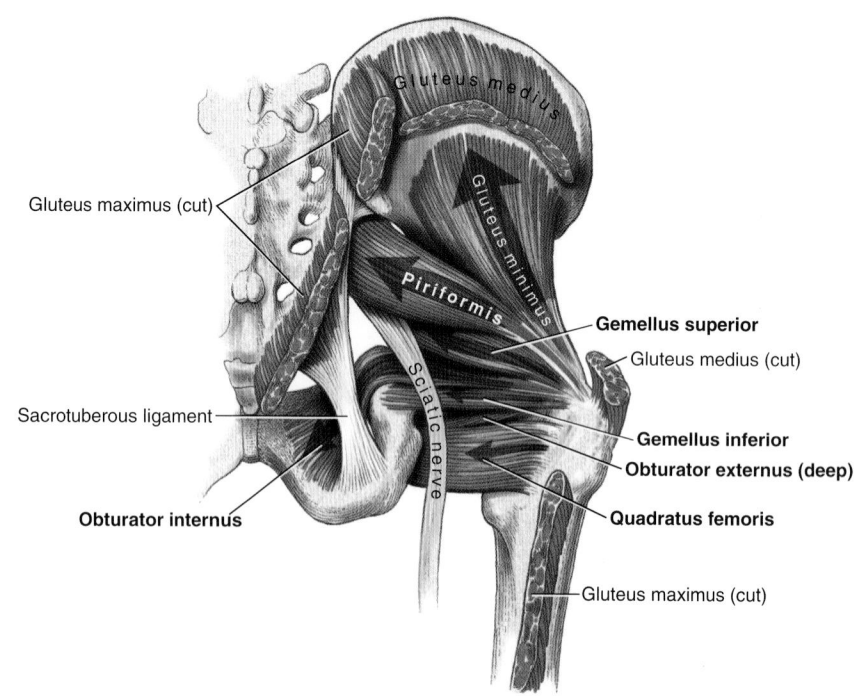

Posterior View

FIG. 21.67 Lateral rotators of the hip; right side. Also featured is the right gluteus minimus, the right sacrotuberous ligament, and the right sciatic nerve. The arrows represent their common action of hip lateral rotation. (From Neumann, D. A. [2010]. *Kinesiology of the musculoskeletal system: Foundations for physical rehabilitation* [2nd ed.]. St. Louis: Mosby.)

PIRIFORMIS (SEE FIG. 21.67)

Latin: pirum—pear
forma—shape

ORIGIN
Anterior sacrum

INSERTION
Greater trochanter

ACTIONS
Externally/laterally rotates the hip
Abducts the hip

NERVE
Sciatic nerve

NOTES: Piriformis is the largest lateral rotator of the hip. As stated previously, the sciatic nerve often exits the pelvis inferior to this muscle, but it can also pass superiorly. In approximately 15% of the population, all or part of the sciatic nerve passes through the muscle (Travell & Simons, 1993). These occurrences may lead to piriformis syndrome and sciatica, with accompanying pain and paresthesia, along the sciatic nerve. However, most cases of sciatica are not from piriformis syndrome but are symptoms of another condition, such as herniated disc.

GEMELLUS SUPERIOR (SEE FIG. 21.67)

Latin: gemellus—twin
superus—upper

ORIGIN
Ischial spine

INSERTION
Greater trochanter

ACTION
Externally/laterally rotates the hip

NERVE
Sciatic nerve

GEMELLUS INFERIOR (SEE FIG. 21.67)

Latin: gemellus—twin
inferus—beneath

ORIGIN
Superior ischial tuberosity

INSERTION
Greater trochanter

ACTION
Externally/laterally rotates the hip

NERVE
Sciatic nerve

OBTURATOR INTERNUS (SEE FIG. 21.67)

Latin: obturare—obstruct
internus—within

ORIGINS
Obturator membrane
Obturator foramen (interior border)

INSERTION
Greater trochanter

ACTION
Externally/laterally rotates the hip

NERVE
Sciatic nerve

OBTURATOR EXTERNUS (SEE FIG. 21.67)

Latin: obturare—obstruct
externus—outside

ORIGINS
Obturator membrane
Superior pubic ramus
Inferior pubic ramus
Ischial ramus

INSERTION
Greater trochanter

ACTION
Externally/laterally rotates the hip

NERVE
Obturator nerve

QUADRATUS FEMORIS (SEE FIG. 21.67)

Latin: quadratus—four-sided
femoralis—pertaining to the femur

ORIGIN
Lateral ischial tuberosity

INSERTION
Intertrochanteric crest

ACTIONS
Externally/laterally rotates the hip
Adducts the hip

NERVE
Sciatic nerve

GLUTEALS (FIG. 21.68)

Greek: gloutous—buttock

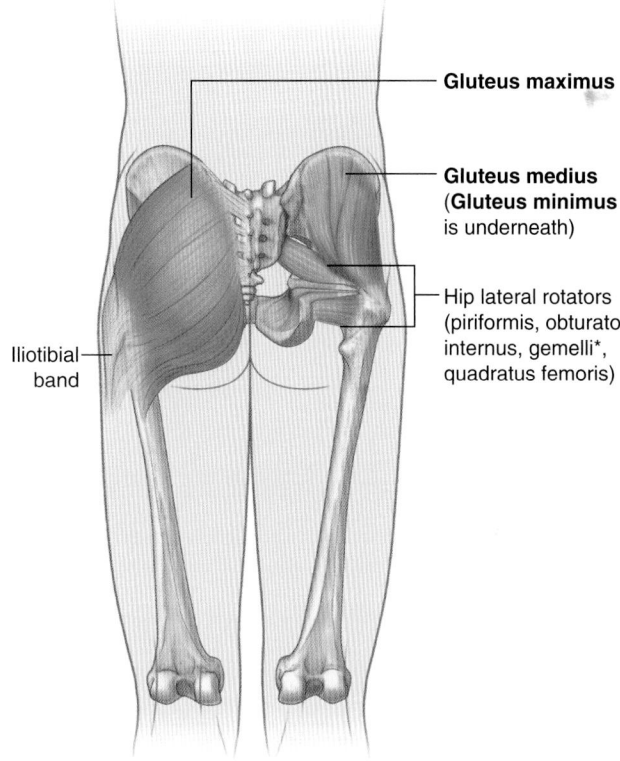

Posterior View

FIG. 21.68 Left gluteus maximus, right gluteus medius, and right gluteus minimus with nearby muscles. *Gemelli is used to describe gemellus superior and inferior. (From Drake, R., Vogel, A. W., & Mitchell, A. [2015]. *Gray's anatomy for students* [3rd ed.]. Philadelphia, PA: Elsevier.)

NOTES: Gluteal muscles (glutes) are a group of buttock muscles consisting of gluteus maximus, gluteus medius, and gluteus minimus. These muscles can be antagonists to each other.

GLUTEUS MAXIMUS (FIG. 21.69)

Greek: gloutos—buttock
Latin: maximus—greatest

ORIGINS
Posterior sacrum
Posterior coccyx
Posterior iliac crest
External ilium to the posterior gluteal line

INSERTIONS
Gluteal tuberosity (25% of fibers)
Iliotibial band (75% of fibers)

ACTIONS
Extends the hip
Externally/laterally rotates the hip
Abducts the hip
Posteriorly tilts the pelvis

NERVE
Inferior gluteal nerve

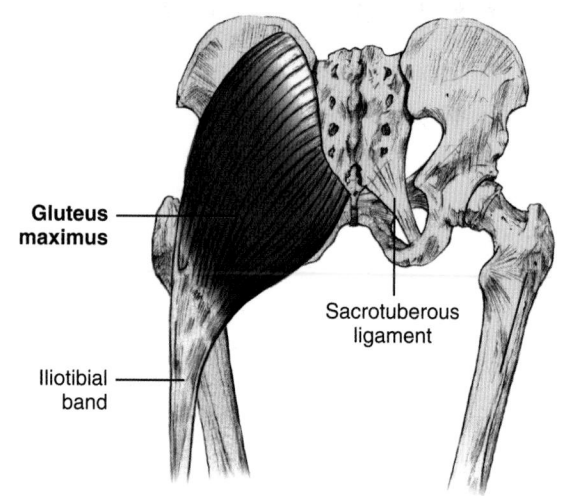

Posterior View

FIG. 21.69 Left gluteus maximus. (Modified from Mansfield, P. [2019]. *Essentials of kinesiology for the physical therapist assistant* [3rd ed.]. St. Louis, MO: Mosby.)

NOTES: Gluteus maximus is the strongest hip extender and one of the strongest muscles in the body. This muscle is active during climbing stairs, rising from a seated position, or running instead of walking. Most of gluteus maximus inserts on the iliotibial band (ITB).

The *ITB (iliotibial tract)* is a thickened band of the fascia lata on the lateral thigh. The *fascia lata* is a deep fascial structure surrounding the thigh, like a tight stocking, and forms the outer regions of several fascial compartments. The anterior compartment contains extensors of the knee, or quadriceps; the medial compartment contains adductors of the hip, and the posterior compartment contains flexors of the knee or hamstrings. ITB extends from the iliac crest to the Gerdy tubercle on the lateral proximal tibia and helps stabilize the hip and knee.

GLUTEUS MEDIUS (FIG. 21.70)

Greek: gloutos—buttock
Latin: medius—middle

ORIGIN
External ilium between the anterior and posterior gluteal lines

INSERTION
Greater trochanter

ACTIONS
Abducts the hip
Internally/medially rotates the hip (anterior fibers)
Externally/laterally rotates the hip (posterior fibers)
Anteriorly and posteriorly tilts the pelvis

NERVE
Superior gluteal nerve

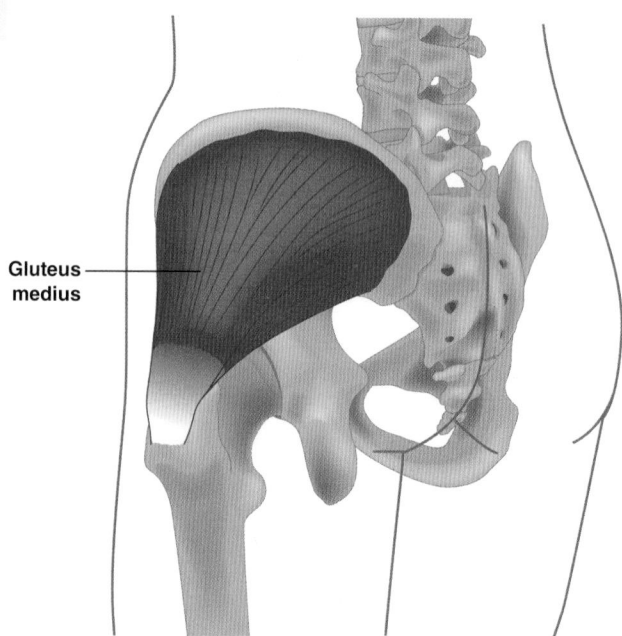

Posterolateral View

FIG. 21.70 Left gluteus medius.

GLUTEUS MINIMUS (FIG. 21.71)

Greek: gloutos—buttock
Latin: minimum—least

ORIGIN
External ilium between the anterior and inferior gluteal lines

INSERTION
Greater trochanter

ACTIONS
Abducts the hip
Internally/medially rotates the hip (anterior fibers)
Externally/laterally rotates the hip (posterior fibers)
Anteriorly and posteriorly tilts the pelvis

NERVE
Superior gluteal nerve

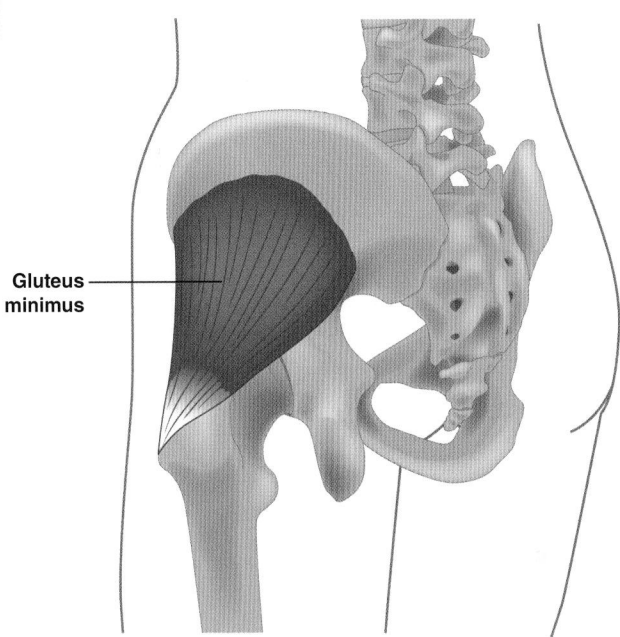

Gluteus minimus

Posterolateral View

FIG. 21.71 Left gluteus minimus.

TENSOR FASCIAE LATAE (FIG. 21.72)

Latin: tensor—stretching
fascia—band
lata—broad

ORIGINS
Anterior iliac crest
Anterior superior iliac spine (ASIS)

INSERTION
Iliotibial band (ITB)

ACTIONS
Abducts the hip
Flexes the hip
Internally/medially rotates the hip

NERVE
Superior gluteal nerve

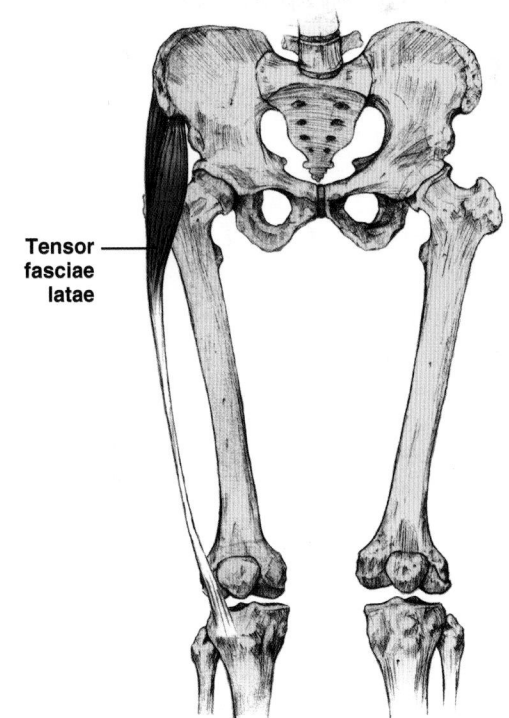

Tensor fasciae latae

Anterior View

FIG. 21.72 Right tensor fasciae latae. (Modified from Mansfield, P. [2019]. *Essentials of kinesiology for the physical therapist assistant* [3rd ed.]. St. Louis, MO: Mosby.)

NOTES: Tensor fasciae latae inserts into the ITB and tenses the fascia lata.

ADDUCTORS (FIG. 21.73)

Latin: adductus—brought forward

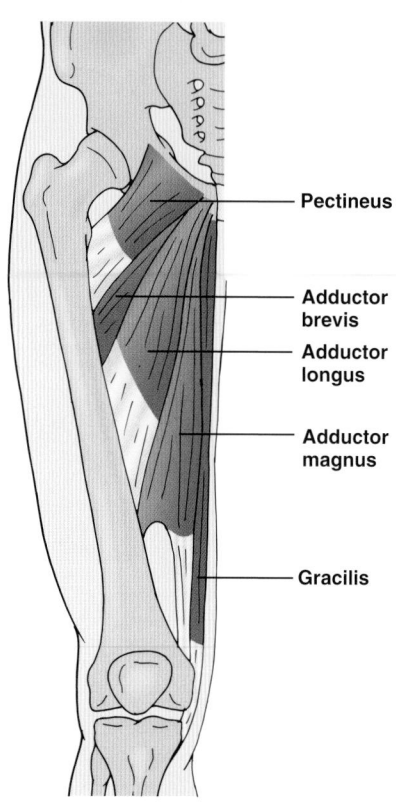

Anterior View

FIG. 21.73 Adductors of the hip; right side. (From Frontera, W. R., Silver, J. K., & Rizzo Jr., T. D. [2019]. *Essentials of physical medicine and rehabilitation*. Philadelphia, PA: Elsevier.)

NOTES: Adductors are a group of muscles in the medial thigh and includes gracilis, adductor magnus, longus, and brevis, and pectineus. These muscles originate on the pubis and ischium bones and insert mainly on the linea aspera, on the posterior femur. ***LEARNING TIP***: To help you remember the names of the adductors from medial to lateral, use the phrase **G**irls **M**ostly **L**ike **B**ig **P**ecs for **G**racilis—adductor **M**agnus—adductor **L**ongus—adductor **B**revis—**P**ectineus.

GRACILIS (FIG. 21.74)

Latin: gracilis—slender

ORIGIN
Inferior pubic ramus

INSERTION
Medial proximal tibial shaft (at pes anserinus)

ACTIONS
Adducts the hip
Flexes the hip
Flexes the knee
Internally/medially rotates the knee (when the knee is flexed)

NERVE
Obturator nerve

NOTES: Gracilis is the most medial adductor, the only adductor crossing the hip and knee, and is part of the *pes anserinus*. The pes anserinus is the conjoined tendons of three muscles attaching to the medial proximal tibial shaft—gracilis, semitendinosus, and sartorius.

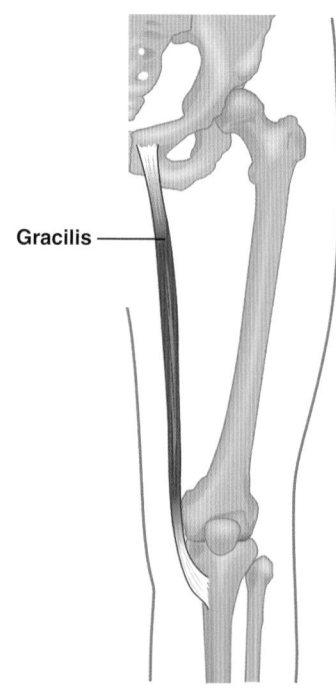

Anterior View

FIG. 21.74 Left gracilis.

ADDUCTOR MAGNUS (FIG. 21.75)

Latin: adductus—brought toward
magnum—large

ORIGINS
Ischial tuberosity
Inferior pubic ramus
Ischial ramus

INSERTIONS
Linea aspera (medial lip)
Adductor tubercle of the femur

ACTIONS
Adducts the hip
Flexes the hip
Extends the hip

NERVES
Sciatic and obturator nerves

NOTES: Adductor magnus is a large triangular muscle deep to the hamstrings. It consists of two sections with a gap between them—one section attaches on the linea aspera and the other on the adductor tubercle. The gap, or *adductor hiatus,* allows passage of blood vessels from the anterior thigh to the posterior thigh and toward the popliteal fossa (a shallow depression behind the knee). Adductor magnus is sometimes considered part of the hamstrings because of its common origin in the ischial tuberosity and its common action of hip extension.

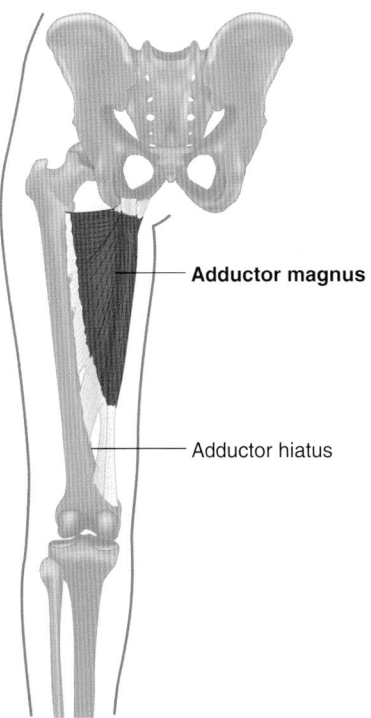

Adductor magnus

Adductor hiatus

Posterior View

FIG. 21.75 Left adductor magnus.

ADDUCTOR LONGUS (FIG. 21.76)

Latin: adductus—brought toward
longus—long

ORIGIN
Anterior pubic body

INSERTION
Middle third of the linea aspera (medial lip)

ACTION
Adducts the hip

NERVE
Obturator nerve

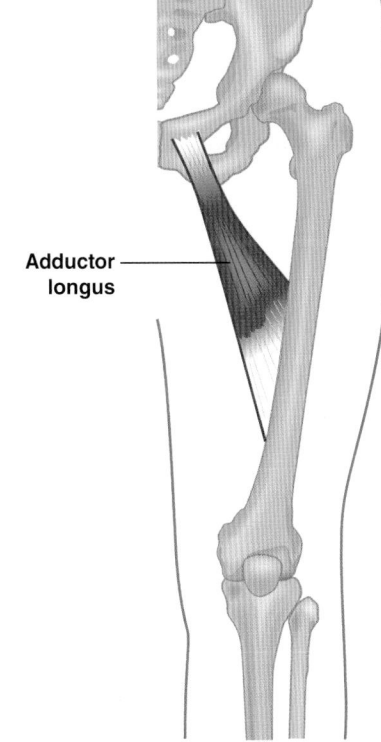

Adductor longus

Anterior View

FIG. 21.76 Left adductor longus.

ADDUCTOR BREVIS (FIG. 21.77)

*Latin: adductus—brought toward
brevis—brief*

ORIGIN
Inferior pubic ramus

INSERTION
Proximal third of the linea aspera (medial lip)

ACTION
Adducts the hip

NERVE
Obturator nerve

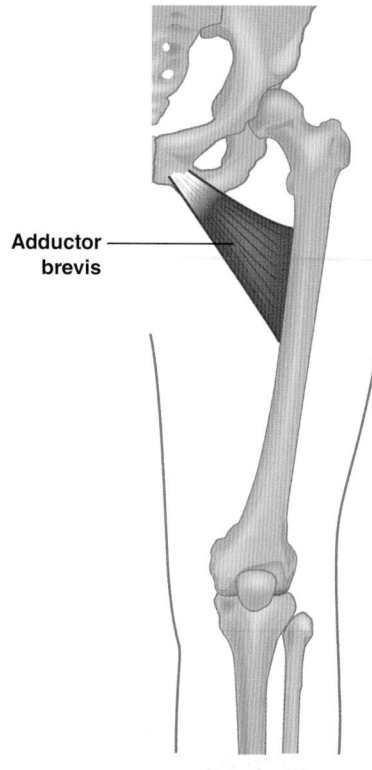

Adductor brevis

Anterior View

FIG. 21.77 Left adductor brevis.

PECTINEUS (FIG. 21.78)

Latin: pecten—comb

ORIGINS
Superior pubic ramus
Pectineal line on pubis

INSERTION
Posterior proximal femoral shaft (inferior to lesser trochanter)

ACTIONS
Flexes the hip
Adducts the hip

NERVE
Femoral nerve

NOTES: Pectineus can be regarded as an extension of the iliopsoas because its common insertion near the lesser trochanter and its common action of hip flexion.

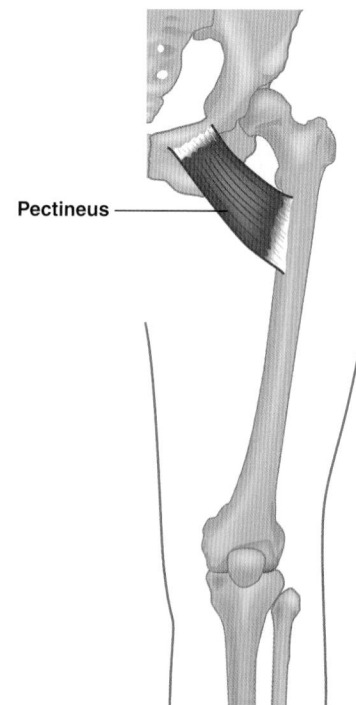

Pectineus

Anterior View

FIG. 21.78 Left pectineus.

QUADRICEPS FEMORIS (FIG. 21.79)

Latin: quattuor—four
caput—head
femoralis—pertaining to the femur

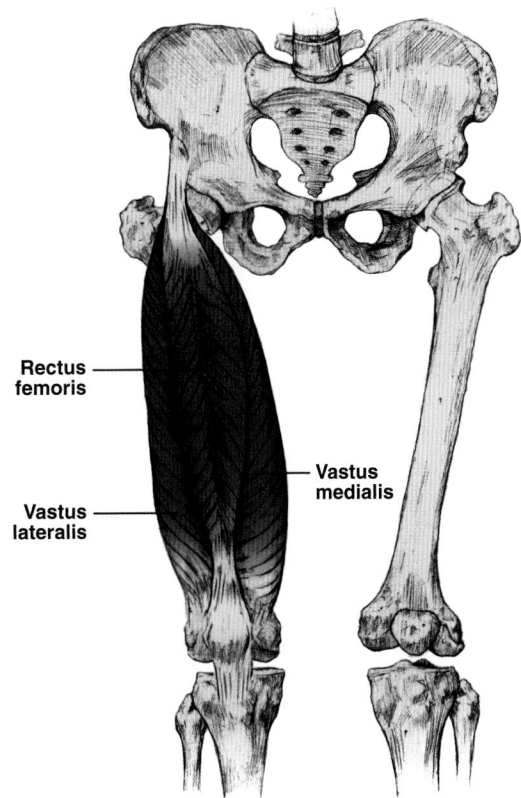

FIG. 21.79 Quadriceps femoris; right side. Vastus intermedius is beneath the rectus femoris. (Modified from Mansfield, P. [2019]. *Essentials of kinesiology for the physical therapist assistant* [3rd ed.]. St. Louis, MO: Mosby.)

Anterior View

Rectus femoris
Vastus medialis
Vastus lateralis

NOTES: Quadriceps femoris (quads) is a group of four muscles, which include rectus femoris, vastus lateralis, intermedius, and medialis. These muscles are on the anterolateral thigh and largely extend the knee. The quads insert on the tibial tuberosity via the patella, where the quadriceps tendon becomes part of the patellar ligament. ***LEARNING TIP***: To help you remember the names of the quads, use the phrase **RV3** for **R**ectus femoris and three vasti muscles of **V**astus lateralis—**V**astus intermedius—**V**astus medialis.

RECTUS FEMORIS (FIG. 21.80)

Latin: rectus—straight
femoralis—pertaining to the femur

ORIGINS
Anterior inferior iliac spine (AIIS)
External ilium just superior to the acetabulum

INSERTION
Tibial tuberosity

ACTIONS
Flexes the hip
Extends the knee
Anteriorly tilts the pelvis

NERVE
Femoral nerve

NOTES: Rectus femoris is a channel formed by the three vastus muscles and is the only quad muscle crossing two joints—the hip and knee.

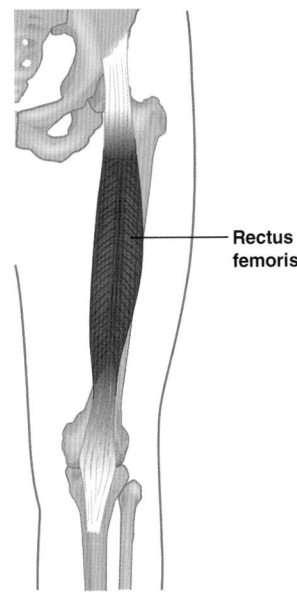

Rectus femoris

Anterior View

FIG. 21.80 Left rectus femoris.

VASTUS INTERMEDIUS (FIG. 21.81)

Latin: vastus—immense
inter—internal
medius—middle

ORIGIN
Anterior lateral femoral shaft

INSERTION
Tibial tuberosity

ACTION
Extends the knee

NERVE
Femoral nerve

NOTES: Vastus intermedius is beneath rectus femoris.

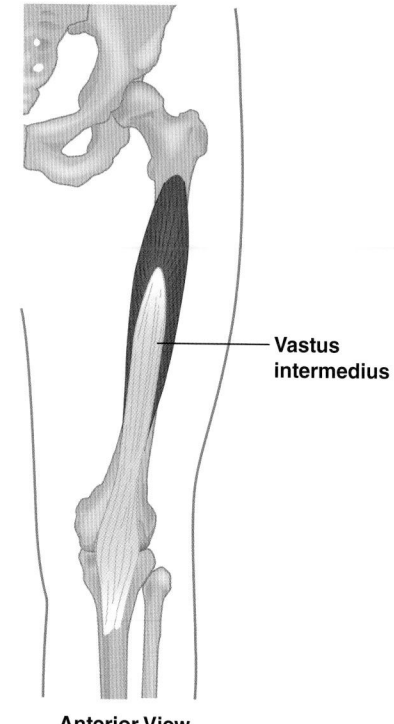

Anterior View

FIG. 21.81 Left vastus intermedius.

VASTUS MEDIALIS (FIG. 21.82)

Latin: vastus—immense
medius—middle

ORIGINS
Linea aspera (medial lip)
Intertrochanteric line

INSERTION
Tibial tuberosity

ACTION
Extends the knee

NERVE
Femoral nerve

NOTES: Vastus medialis is the *teardrop muscle* because of its teardrop shape on the medial anterior thigh. Vastus medialis is also called *vastus internus*. The vastus medialis has two distinct sections with different fiber orientations: *vastus medialis longus (VML)* and *vastus medialis oblique (VMO)* (Smith et al., 2009).

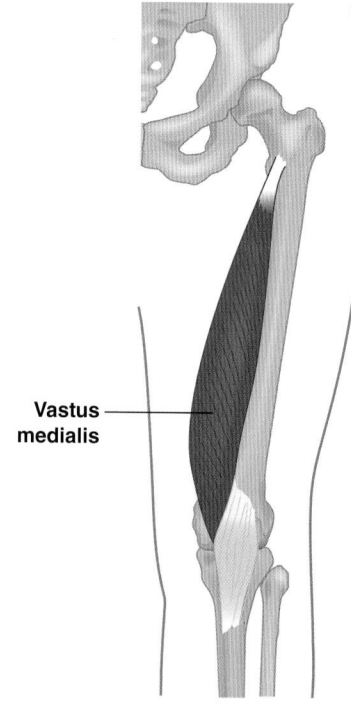

Anterior View

FIG. 21.82 Left vastus medialis.

VASTUS LATERALIS (FIG. 21.83)

Latin: vastus—immense
lateralis—toward the side

ORIGINS
Linea aspera (lateral lip)
Gluteal tuberosity

INSERTION
Tibial tuberosity

ACTION
Extends the knee

NERVE
Femoral nerve

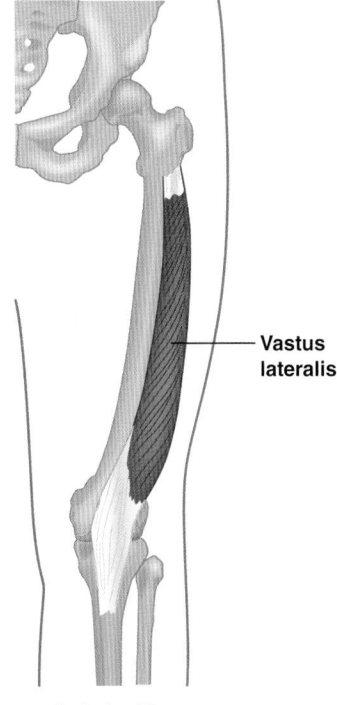

Vastus
lateralis

Anterior View

NOTES: Vastus lateralis is also called *vastus externus.*

FIG. 21.83 Left vastus lateralis.

SARTORIUS (FIG. 21.84)

Latin: sartor—tailor

ORIGIN
Anterior superior iliac spine (ASIS)

INSERTION
Medial proximal tibial shaft (at pes anserinus)

ACTIONS
Flexes the hip
Externally/laterally rotates the hip
Abducts the hip
Flexes the knee

NERVE
Femoral nerve

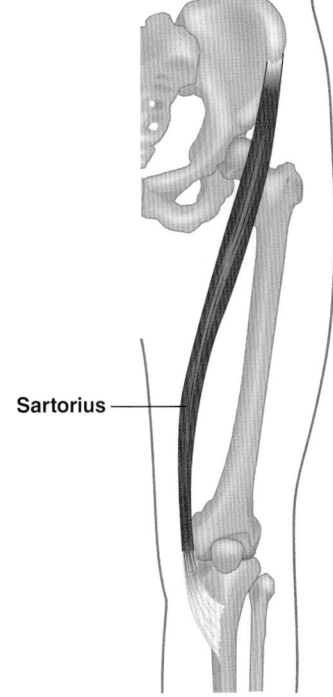

Sartorius

Anterior View

NOTES: Actions of sartorius—hip flexion, abduction, external rotation, and knee flexion—allow us to sit cross-legged. Sartorius is the *tailor's muscle* because tailors sat in a cross-legged position as they sewed (Herlihy, 2018). Sartorius is the longest muscle in the body and lies obliquely over the thigh, crossing both the hip and the knee. Sartorius is part of the *pes anserinus*, conjoined tendons of three muscles attaching to the medial proximal tibial shaft—sartorius, semitendinosus, and gracilis.

FIG. 21.84 Left sartorius.

POPLITEUS (FIG. 21.85)

Latin: poples—hollow behind the knee

ORIGIN
Lateral condyle of femur

INSERTION
Posterior proximal tibial shaft

ACTIONS
Flexes the knee
Internally/medially rotates the knee (when the knee is flexed)

NERVE
Tibial nerve

NOTES: Popliteus is the *key that unlocks the knee* because it unlocks an extended knee and begins the first few degrees of flexion (Centeno, 2015).

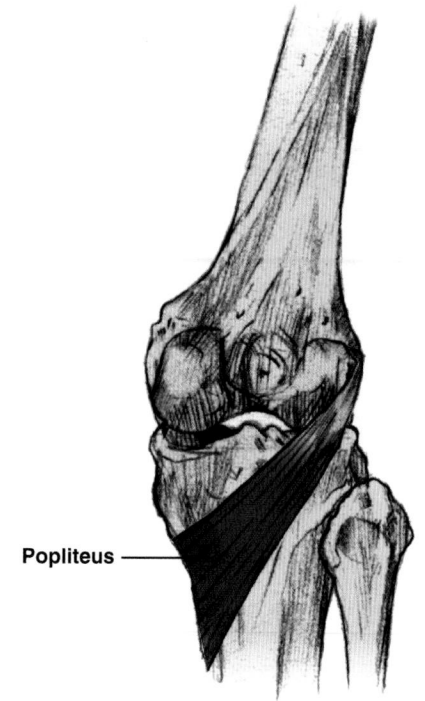

Posterior View

FIG. 21.85 Right popliteus. (Modified from Mansfield, P. [2019]. *Essentials of kinesiology for the physical therapist assistant* [3rd ed.]. St. Louis, MO: Mosby.)

HAMSTRINGS (FIG. 21.86)

Anglo-Saxon: haun—haunch

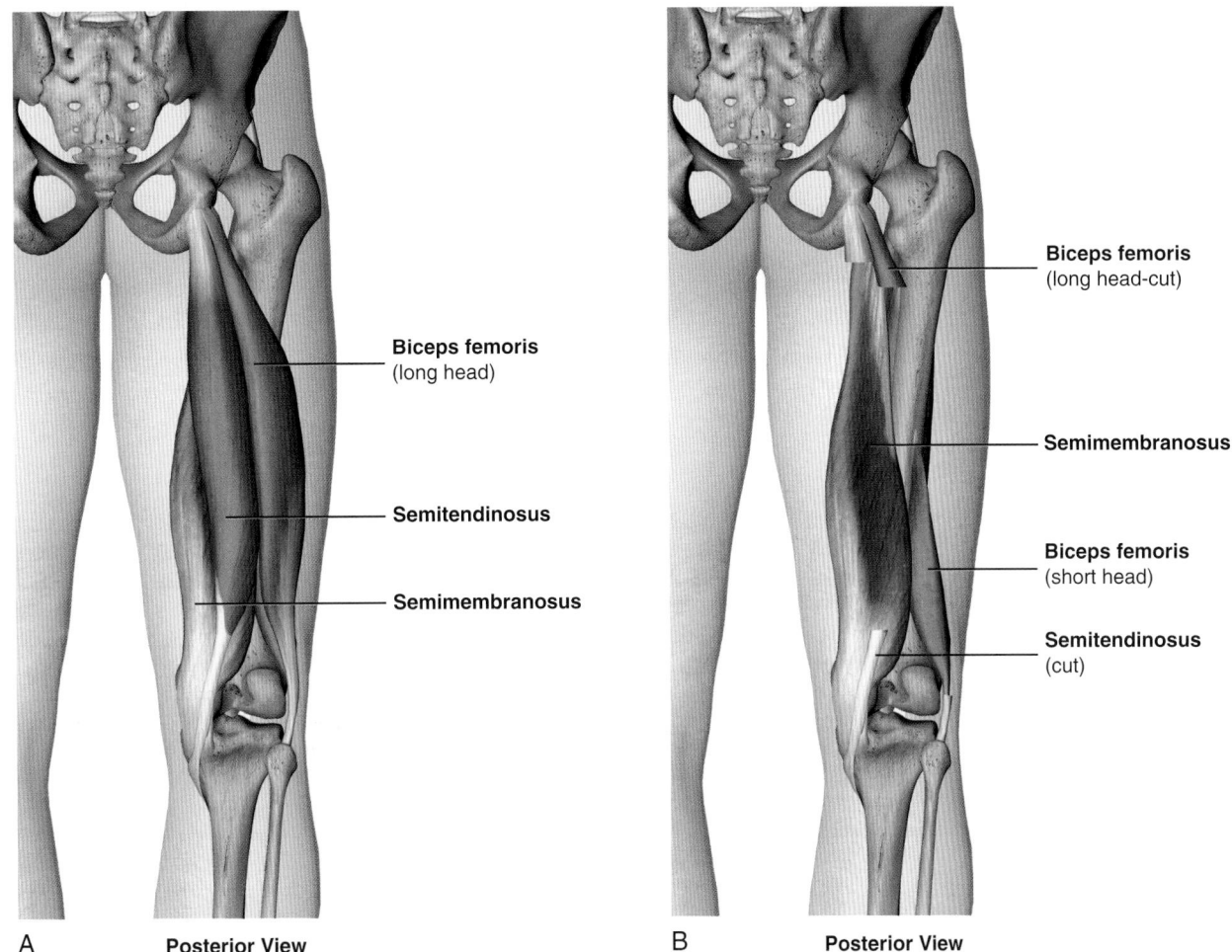

A   **Posterior View**

B   **Posterior View**

Biceps femoris
(long head)

Semitendinosus

Semimembranosus

Biceps femoris
(long head-cut)

Semimembranosus

Biceps femoris
(short head)

Semitendinosus
(cut)

FIG. 21.86 Right hamstrings featuring its superficial (*A*) and deep (*B*) muscle layers. (From Liebgott, B. [2018]. *The anatomical basis of dentistry* [4th ed.]. St. Louis, MO: Elsevier.)

NOTES: Hamstrings are three posterior thigh muscles—biceps femoris, semimembranosus, and semitendinosus. Hamstrings get their name because butchers hang ham by their tendons, which look like strings (Herlihy, 2018). All hamstring muscles attach to the ischial tuberosity and largely flex the knee and extend the hip.

The hamstrings have four heads, which lie either on the medial or lateral side of the thigh and are either deep or superficial. Semitendinosus and semimembranosus lie on the medial side, with semimembranosus positioned most medially. The two heads of biceps femoris are on the lateral side. Semimembranosus and the short head of biceps femoris are the deepest hamstrings, and semitendinosus and the long head of biceps femoris are the superficial hamstrings. ***LEARNING TIP***: To help you remember the names of the hamstrings, use the letters **B-M-T** for **B**iceps femoris, semi**M**embranosus, and semi**T**endinosus.

SEMIMEMBRANOSUS (FIG. 21.87)

Latin: semis—half
membrana—membrane

ORIGIN
Ischial tuberosity

INSERTION
Medial condyle of the tibia

ACTIONS
Flexes the knee
Internally/medially rotates the knee (when the knee is flexed)
Extends the hip
Posteriorly tilts the pelvis

NERVE
Tibial nerve

NOTES: Semimembranosus attaches to the medial condyle of the tibia by a flat membranous tendon. ***LEARNING TIP****:* To help you remember the medial location of semimembranosus on the posterior thigh, remember **M**edial starts with the letter **M** and **M** is in the word semi**M**embranosus.

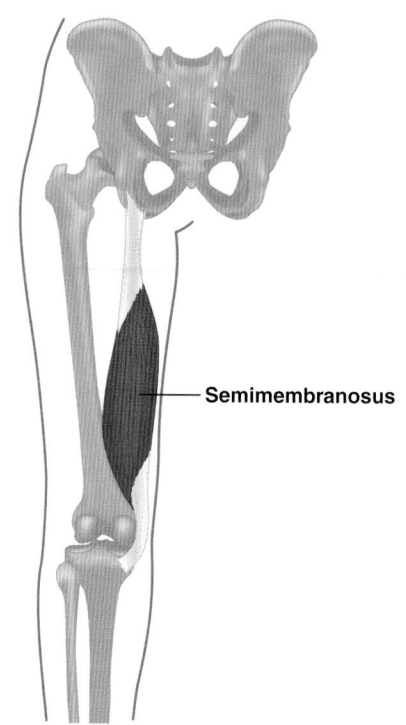

Posterior View

FIG. 21.87 Left semimembranosus.

SEMITENDINOSUS (FIG. 21.88)

Latin: semis—half
tendinosus—tendinous

ORIGIN
Ischial tuberosity

INSERTION
Medial proximal tibial shaft (at pes anserinus)

ACTIONS
Flexes the knee
Internally/medially rotates the knee (when the knee is flexed)
Extends the hip
Posteriorly tilts the pelvis

NERVE
Tibial nerve

NOTES: Semitendinosus has a long, slender, and round tendon. It attaches to the medial proximal tibial shaft at the *pes anserinus* or *pes*. The pes is the conjoined tendons of three muscles attaching to the medial proximal tibial shaft—semitendinosus, gracilis, and sartorius. ***LEARNING TIP****:* To help you remember the superficial (top) location of the semitendinosus on the medial aspect of the posterior thigh, remember **T**op starts with the letter **T** and **T** is in the word semi**T**endinosus.

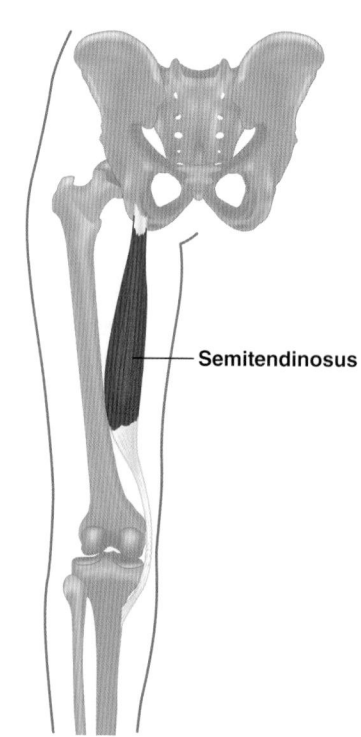

Posterior View

FIG. 21.88 Left semitendinosus.

BICEPS FEMORIS (FIG. 21.89)

Latin: bi—twice
caput—head
femoralis—pertaining to the femur

ORIGINS
Ischial tuberosity (long head)
Sacrotuberous ligament (long head)
Linea aspera; lower lateral lip (short head)

INSERTION
Fibular head

ACTIONS
Flexes the knee
Externally/laterally rotates the knee (when the knee is flexed)
Extends the hip
Posteriorly tilts the pelvis

NERVES
Tibial nerve (long head)
Common fibular/peroneal nerve (short head)

NOTES: Biceps femoris is on the lateral posterior thigh and consists of two heads. The long head crosses the hip and knee, while the short head crosses only the knee.

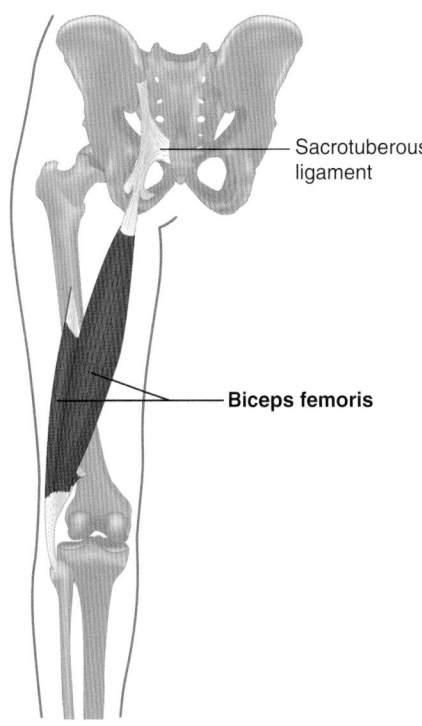

Posterior View

FIG. 21.89 Left biceps femoris with the nearby sacrotuberous ligament.

PES ANSERINUS (FIG. 21.90)

Latin: pes—foot
French: anser—a goose

NOTES: The *pes anserinus (pes)* is on the medial proximal tibial shaft and is the conjoined tendinous attachment of three muscles—sartorius, gracilis, and semitendinosus. ***LEARNING TIP***: To help you remember the names of the pes, use the phrase **S**ay **G**race before **T**ea or **S**hiny **G**reen **T**omatoes for **S**artorius, **G**racilis, and semi**T**endinosus.

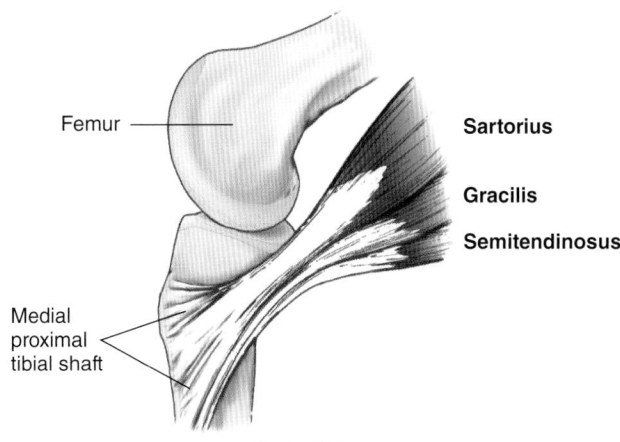

Medial View

FIG. 21.90 Right pes anserinus and its insertion on the medial proximal tibia. (From Donatelli, R. A. [2010]. *Orthopedic physical therapy* [4th ed.]. St. Louis, MO: Churchill Livingstone.)

Lesson Eight Review: Muscles of Hip Movement

FLEXION	EXTENSION	ABDUCTION	ADDUCTION	INTERNAL (MEDIAL) ROTATION	EXTERNAL (LATERAL) ROTATION
Psoas major	Gluteus maximus	Piriformis	Adductor magnus	Gluteus medius	Psoas major
Iliacus	Semimembranosus	Gluteus medius	Gracilis	Gluteus minimus	Iliacus
Tensor fasciae latae	Semitendinosus	Gluteus minimus	Adductor longus	Tensor fasciae latae	Gluteus medius
Rectus femoris	Biceps femoris	Tensor fasciae latae	Adductor brevis		Gluteus minimus
Sartorius	Adductor magnus	Sartorius	Pectineus		Piriformis
Gracilis		Gluteus maximus	Quadratus femoris		Gemellus superior
Adductor magnus					Gemellus inferior
Pectineus					Obturator internus
					Obturator externus
					Quadratus femoris
					Gluteus maximus
					Sartorius

Lateral views   Posterior view   Anterior view   Anterior view   Anterior view   Posterior view   Anterior view   Posterior view

Lesson Eight Review: Muscles of Knee Movement

FLEXION	EXTENSION
Semimembranosus	Rectus femoris
Semitendinosus	Vastus medialis
Biceps femoris	Vastus lateralis
Sartorius	Vastus intermedius
Gracilis	
Gastrocnemius	
Plantaris	
Popliteus	

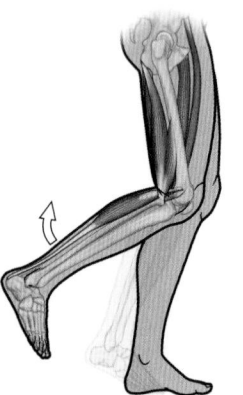
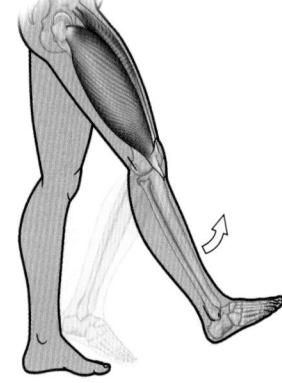

Lateral views

Lesson Nine: Muscles of Ankle and Foot Movement

Movements of the ankle are plantar flexion and dorsiflexion. Movements of the foot are inversion and eversion. Muscles of ankle and foot movements are tibialis anterior, extensor digitorum longus and brevis, extensor hallucis longus, fibularis longus, fibularis brevis, fibularis tertius, gastrocnemius, plantaris, soleus, tibialis posterior, flexor digitorum longus, and flexor hallucis longus (Fig. 21.91). Retinacula surround the ankle; tendons of several muscles pass beneath these structures.

NOTES: The plantar aspect of the foot contains four muscle layers. The *first layer,* or most superficial layer, contains the abductor hallucis, flexor digitorum brevis, and abductor digiti minimi. The *second layer* contains the quadratus plantae, lumbricals, and the tendons of the flexor hallucis longus and flexor digitorum longus. The *third layer* contains the flexor hallucis brevis, adductor hallucis, and flexor digiti minimi brevis. The *fourth layer,* or deepest layer, contains the dorsal interossei, plantar interossei, and tendons of the fibularis longus and tibialis posterior.

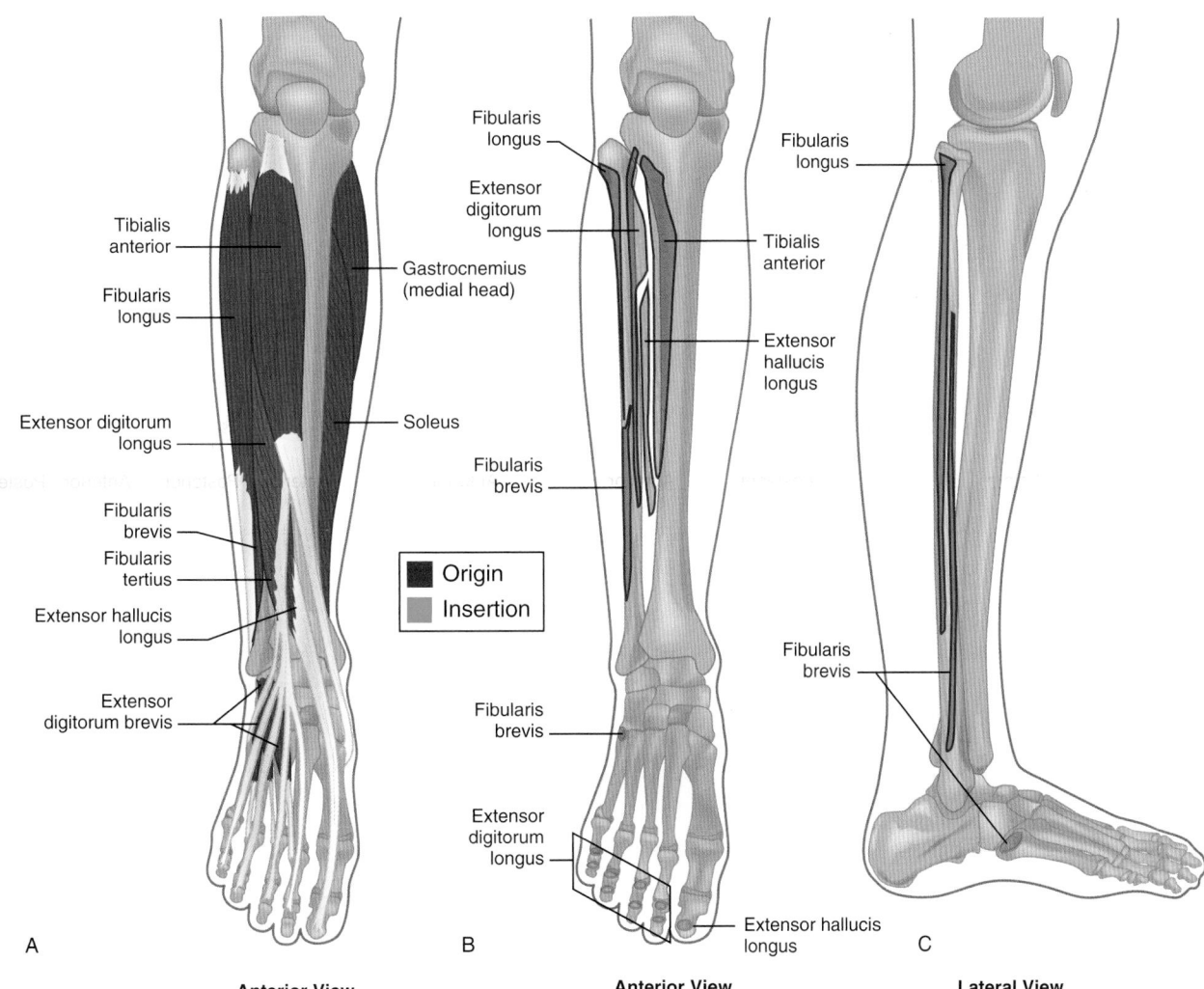

FIG. 21.91 Muscles of ankle and foot movement (*A and D*) with their associated origins (*red*) and insertions (*blue, B, C. and E*).

Continued

Lesson Nine: Muscles of Ankle and Foot Movement—cont'd

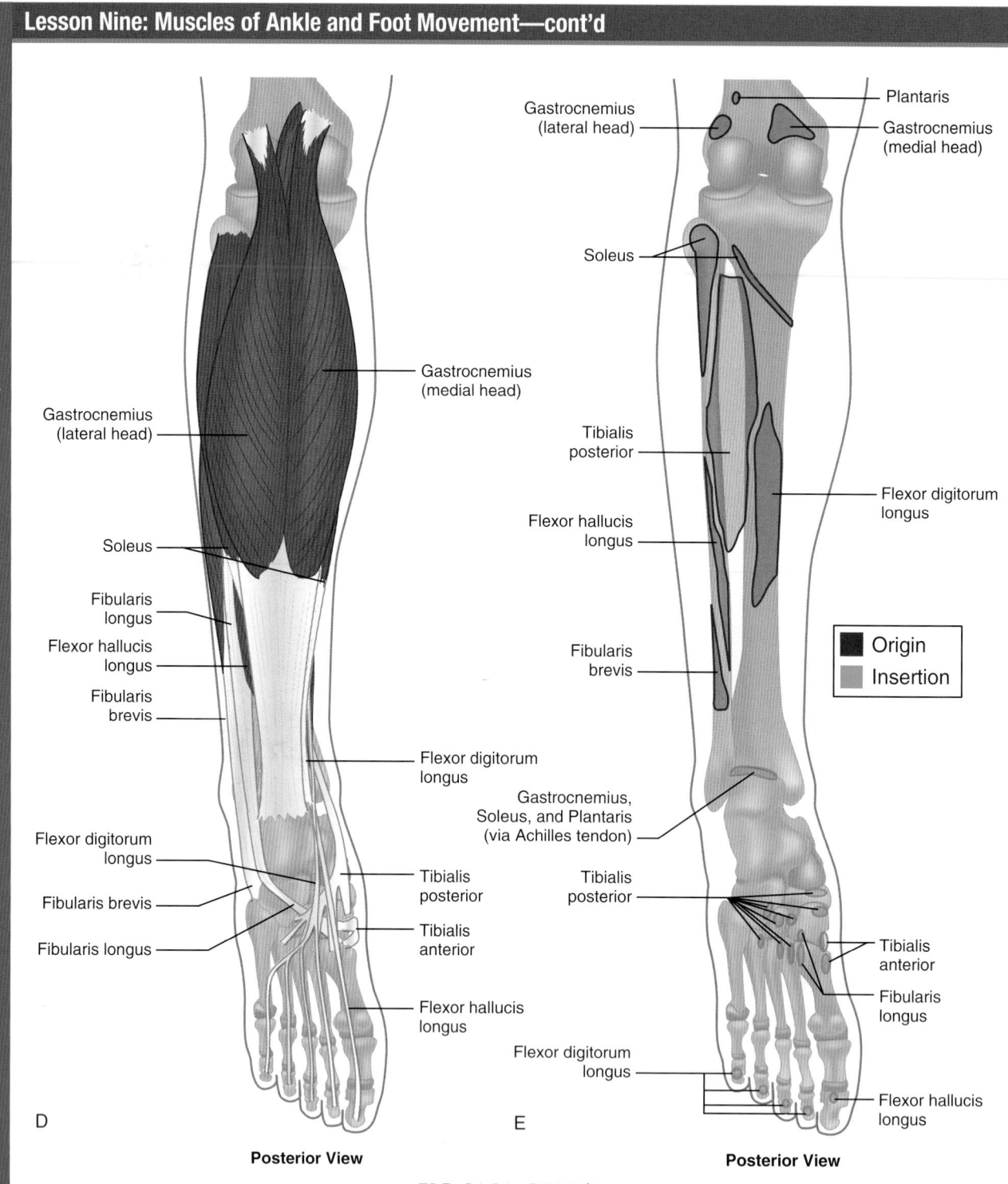

Gastrocnemius (lateral head)

Plantaris

Gastrocnemius (medial head)

Soleus

Gastrocnemius (medial head)

Gastrocnemius (lateral head)

Soleus

Tibialis posterior

Flexor hallucis longus

Fibularis brevis

Fibularis longus

Flexor hallucis longus

Fibularis brevis

Flexor digitorum longus

Flexor digitorum longus

Origin

Insertion

Flexor digitorum longus

Fibularis brevis

Fibularis longus

Tibialis posterior

Tibialis anterior

Flexor hallucis longus

Gastrocnemius, Soleus, and Plantaris (via Achilles tendon)

Tibialis posterior

Tibialis anterior

Fibularis longus

Flexor digitorum longus

Flexor hallucis longus

D

Posterior View

E

Posterior View

FIG. 21.91, CONT'D

TIBIALIS ANTERIOR (FIG. 21.92)

Latin: tibialis—shinbone
ante—before

ORIGINS
Proximal half of the lateral tibial shaft
Interosseous membrane

INSERTIONS
Metatarsal I
Medial cuneiform

ACTIONS
Dorsiflexes the ankle
Inverts the foot

NERVE
Deep fibular nerve

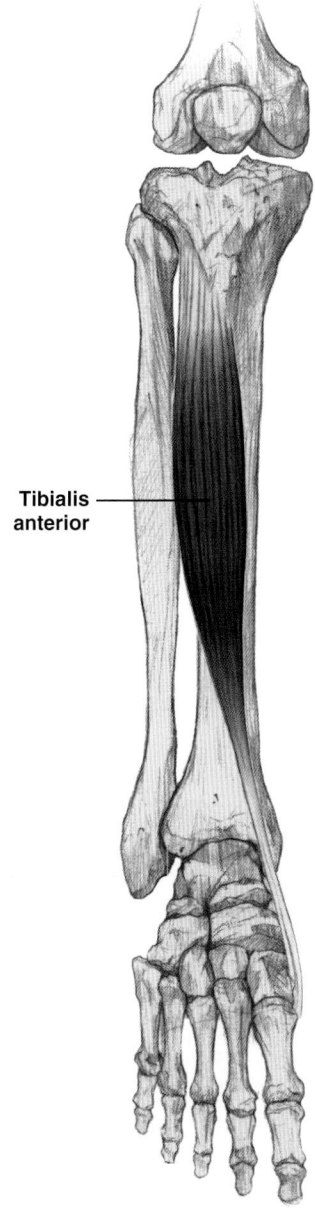

Tibialis anterior

Anterior View

FIG. 21.92 Right tibialis anterior. (Modified from Mansfield, P. [2014]. *Essentials of kinesiology for the physical therapist assistant* [2nd ed.]. St. Louis, MO: Mosby.)

NOTES: Tibialis anterior is also called *anterior tibialis*. Tibialis anterior and fibularis longus are the *stirrup muscles* because their tendons attach to the medial cuneiform and the first metatarsal, forming a stirrup, or sling, under the foot (O'Rahilly et al., 2008).
LEARNING TIP: To help you remember the names of the stirrup muscles, use the word **FLAT** for **F**ibularis **L**ongus—**A**nterior **T**ibialis.

EXTENSOR DIGITORUM LONGUS AND BREVIS (FIG. 21.93)

Latin: extensio—to extend
digitus—finger or toe
longus—long
brevis—brief

ORIGINS
Fibular head (longus)
Proximal two-thirds of the anterior fibular shaft (longus)
Lateral condyle of the tibia (longus)
Anterior surface of the interosseous membrane (longus)
Calcaneus (brevis)

INSERTIONS
Middle phalanges of digits II through V (longus)
Distal phalanges of digits II through V (longus)
Tendons of extensor digitorum longus to digits II through IV (brevis)

ACTIONS
Extends digits II through V (longus)
Dorsiflexes the ankle (longus)
Everts the foot (longus)
Extends digits II through IV (brevis)

NERVE
Deep fibular nerve (longus and brevis)

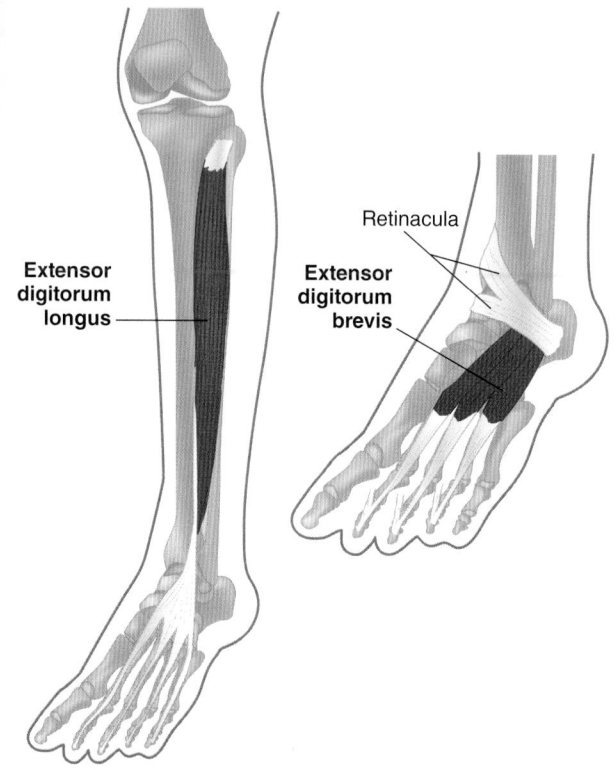

Anterolateral Views

FIG. 21.93 Left extensor digitorum longus and brevis.

EXTENSOR HALLUCIS LONGUS (FIG. 21.94)

Latin: extensio—to extend
hallux—large toe
longus—long

ORIGINS
Anterior fibular shaft (middle region)
Interosseous membrane

INSERTION
Distal phalanx of the great toe

ACTIONS
Extends the great toe
Dorsiflexes the ankle

NERVE
Deep fibular nerve

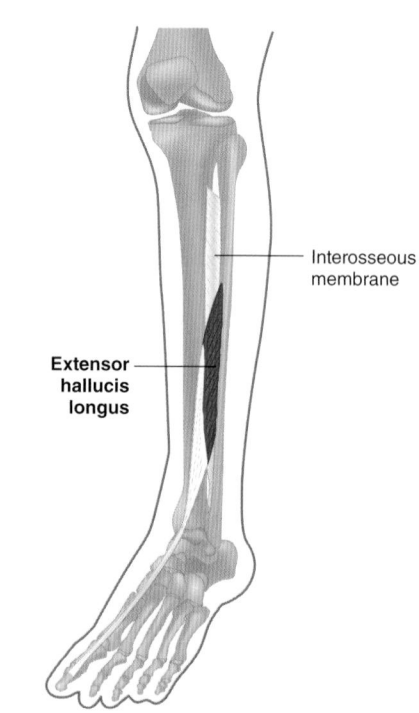

Anterolateral View

FIG. 21.94 Left extensor hallucis longus.

FIBULARIS LONGUS (FIG. 21.95)

Greek: fibula—pin
Latin: longus—long

ORIGINS
Fibular head
Lateral proximal half of the fibular shaft

INSERTIONS
Metatarsal I
Medial cuneiform

ACTIONS
Everts the foot
Plantarflexes the ankle

NERVE
Superficial fibular nerve

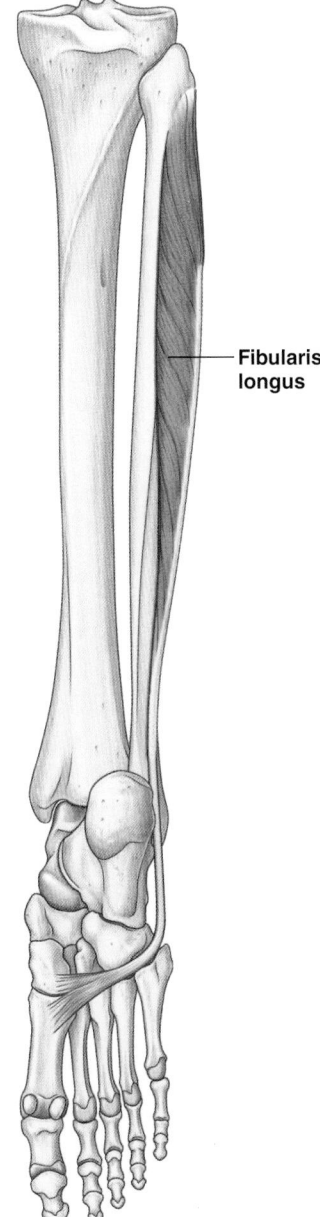

Fibularis longus

Posterior View

NOTES: Fibularis longus is also called *peroneus longus*. Fibularis longus and tibialis anterior are *stirrup muscles,* as both their tendons attach to the medial cuneiform and the first metatarsal, forming a stirrup, or sling, under the foot (O'Rahilly et al., 2008).
***LEARNING TIP*:** To help you remember the names of the stirrup muscles, use the word **FLAT** for **F**ibularis **L**ongus—**A**nterior **T**ibialis.

FIG. 21.95 Right fibularis longus. (From Soames, R., & Palastanga, N. [2019]. *Anatomy and human movement: Structure and function* [7th ed.]. Philadelphia, PA: Elsevier.)

FIBULARIS BREVIS (FIG. 21.96)

Greek: fibula—pin
Latin: brevis—brief

ORIGIN
Lateral distal half of the fibular shaft

INSERTION
Metatarsal V

ACTIONS
Everts the foot
Plantarflexes the ankle

NERVE
Superficial fibular nerve

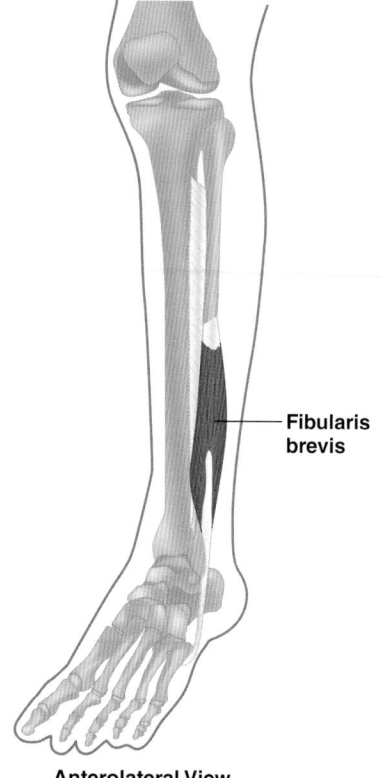

Anterolateral View

NOTES: Fibularis brevis is also called *peroneus brevis.*

FIG. 21.96 Left fibularis brevis.

FIBULARIS TERTIUS (FIG. 21.97)

Greek: fibula—pin
Latin: tertiarius—third

ORIGINS
Lateral distal third of the fibular shaft
Interosseous membrane

INSERTION
Metatarsal V

ACTIONS
Everts the foot
Dorsiflexes the ankle

NERVE
Deep fibular nerve

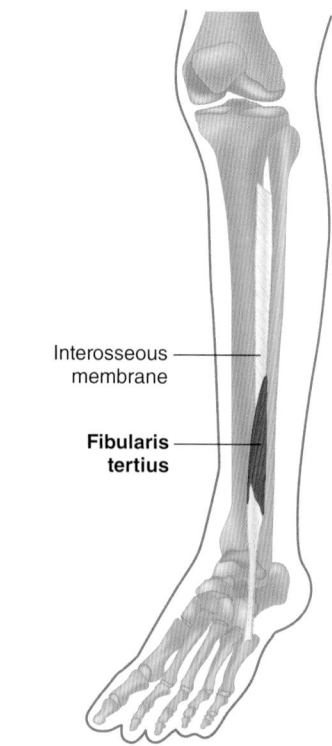

Anterolateral View

NOTES: Fibularis tertius is also called *peroneus tertius.*

FIG. 21.97 Left fibularis tertius.

GASTROCNEMIUS (FIG. 21.98)

Greek: gaster—belly
kneme—leg

ORIGINS
Medial epicondyle of the femur (medial head)
Lateral epicondyle of the femur (lateral head)

INSERTION
Calcaneus via the Achilles tendon

ACTIONS
Plantarflexes the ankle
Flexes the knee

NERVE
Tibial nerve

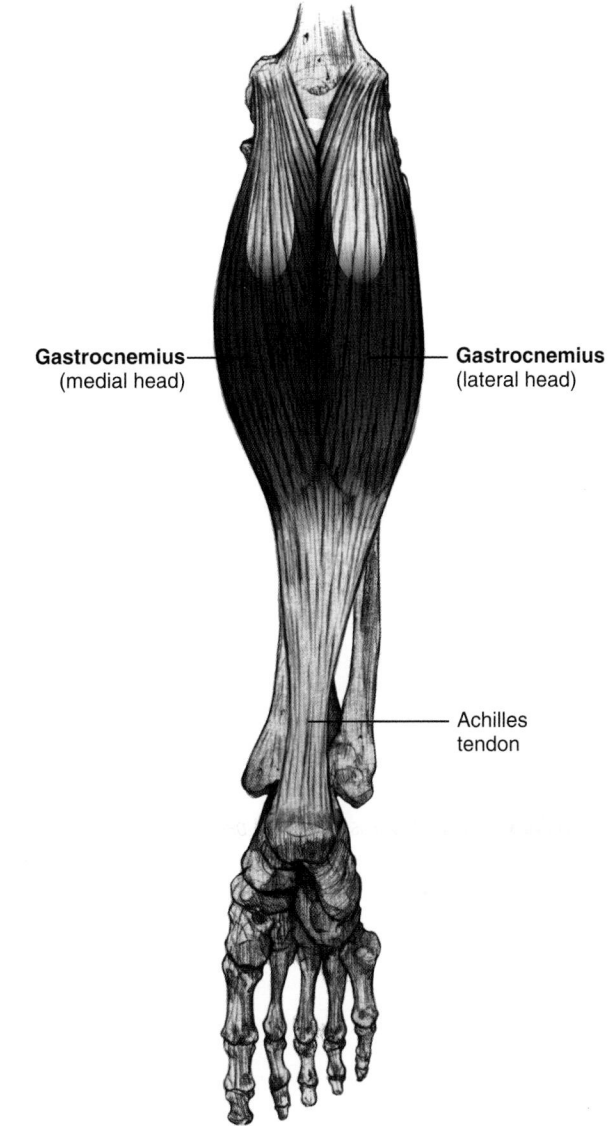

Gastrocnemius (medial head)

Gastrocnemius (lateral head)

Achilles tendon

Posterior View

FIG. 21.98 Right gastrocnemius. (Modified from Mansfield, P. [2019]. *Essentials of kinesiology for the thysical therapist assistant* [3rd ed.]. St. Louis, MO: Mosby.)

NOTES: The gastrocnemius is the most superficial muscle of the calf that forms the bulk of the calf. This muscle has two heads—a medial head and a lateral head. The gastrocnemius and other calf muscles insert on the *Achilles (calcaneal) tendon*, a tough band of fibrous tissue, attaching to the calcaneus, or heel bone. The Achilles tendon is the largest and strongest tendon in the body. Actions of gastrocnemius are an either/or situation—it can provide plantar flexion or knee flexion, but not at the same time. Gastrocnemius is the *toe dancer's muscle* because it helps ballet dancers stand on pointe (Herlihy, 2018).

PLANTARIS (FIG. 21.99)

Latin: planta—sole

ORIGIN
Lateral epicondyle of the femur

INSERTION
Calcaneus via the Achilles tendon (distal portion)

ACTIONS
Plantarflexes the ankle
Flexes the knee

NERVE
Tibial nerve

NOTES: The plantaris has the longest tendon in the body (between 30–45 cm [12–18"] in length) and is sometimes used for reconstructive surgeries.

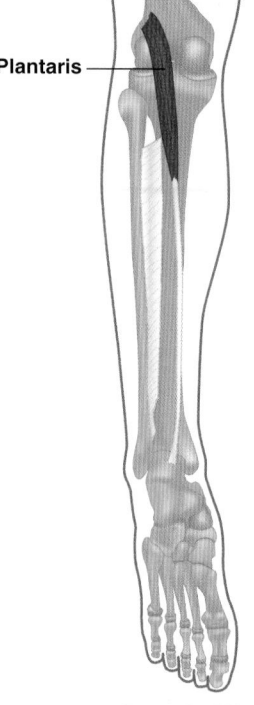

Plantaris

Posterior View

FIG. 21.99 Left plantaris.

SOLEUS (FIG. 21.100)

Latin: solea—sole of the foot or sandal

ORIGINS
Superior posterior third of the fibular shaft
Soleal line of the tibia

INSERTION
Calcaneus via the Achilles tendon

ACTION
Plantarflexes the ankle

NERVE
Tibial nerve

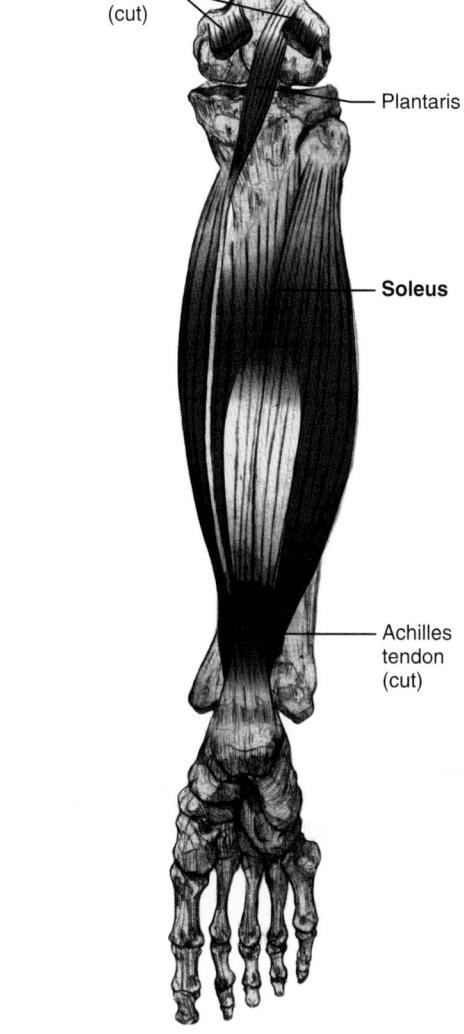

Posterior View

FIG. 21.100 Right soleus. (Modified from Mansfield, P. [2019]. *Essentials of kinesiology for the physical therapist assistant* [3rd ed.]. St. Louis, MO: Mosby.)

NOTES: The soleus is palpable on the sides of the Achilles tendon.

TIBIALIS POSTERIOR (FIG. 21.101)

Latin: tibialis—shinbone
posterus—behind

ORIGINS
Posterior tibial shaft
Posterior fibular shaft
Interosseous membrane

INSERTIONS
Plantar surfaces of most tarsals (navicular, cuneiforms, cuboid, and calcaneus)
Bases of metatarsals II, III, and IV

ACTIONS
Inverts the foot
Plantarflexes the ankle

NERVE
Tibial nerve

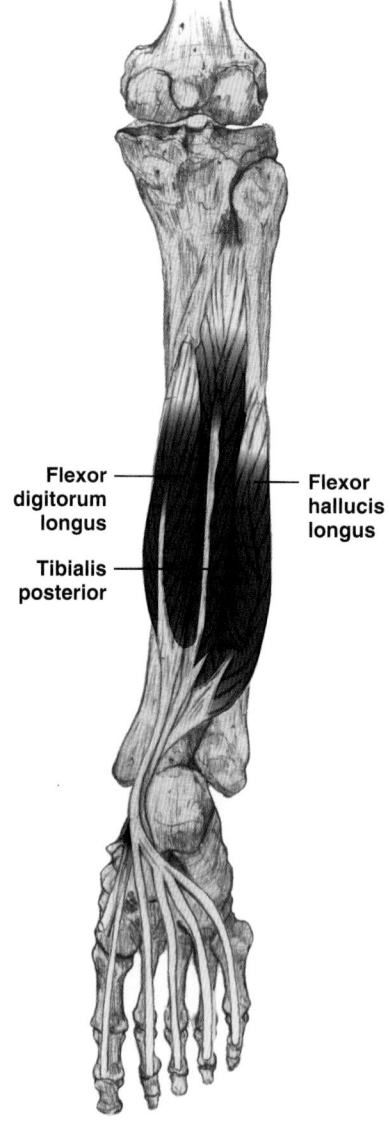

Flexor
digitorum
longus

Flexor
hallucis
longus

Tibialis
posterior

Posterior View

FIG. 21.101 Right tibialis posterior, flexor digitorum longus, and flexor hallucis longus. (Modified from Mansfield, P. [2019]. *Essentials of kinesiology for the physical therapist assistant* [3rd ed.]. St. Louis, MO: Mosby.)

FLEXOR DIGITORUM LONGUS (SEE FIG. 21.101)

Latin: flexus—bent
digitus—finger or toe
longus—long

ORIGIN
Posterior tibial shaft—middle region

INSERTIONS
Distal phalanges of digits II through V (plantar surface)

ACTIONS
Flexes digits II through V at the DIP, PIP, and MTP joints
Plantarflexes the ankle
Inverts the foot

NERVE
Tibial nerve

FLEXOR HALLUCIS LONGUS (SEE FIG. 21.101)

Latin: flexus—bent
hallux—large toe
longus—long

ORIGINS
Posterior fibular shaft—middle region
Interosseous membrane

INSERTION
Distal phalanx of the great toe (plantar surface)

ACTIONS
Flexes the great toe
Plantarflexes the ankle
Inverts the foot
Supports the longitudinal arch

NERVE
Tibial nerve

Lesson Nine Review: Muscles of Ankle and Foot Movement

PLANTAR FLEXION	DORSIFLEXION	INVERSION	EVERSION
Gastrocnemius	Tibialis anterior	Tibialis anterior	Fibularis longus
Soleus	Extensor hallucis longus	Tibialis posterior	Fibularis brevis
Plantaris	Fibularis tertius	Flexor digitorum longus	Fibularis tertius
Fibularis longus	Extensor digitorum longus	Flexor hallucis longus	Extensor digitorum longus
Fibularis brevis			
Tibialis posterior			
Flexor digitorum longus			
Flexor hallucis longus			

Lateral view

Lateral view

Anterior view

Anterior view

Lesson Ten: Muscles of Neck and Facial Movement

Movements of the neck are flexion, extension, rotation, and lateral flexion. Mandibular movements are depression, elevation, protraction, retraction, and excursion or lateral deviation. Muscles of the neck and facial movements are occipitofrontalis, orbicularis oculi, orbicularis oris, platysma, temporalis, masseter, lateral pterygoid, medial pterygoid, sternocleidomastoid, scalenus anterior, scalenus medius, scalenus posterior, splenius capitis, splenius cervicis, rectus capitis posterior major, rectus capitis posterior minor, oblique capitis superior, oblique capitis inferior, levator scapulae, trapezius, spinalis, and longissimus. Levator scapulae and trapezius also move the shoulder; these muscles are featured in Lesson Five. Spinalis and longissimus also move the vertebral column; these muscles are featured in Lesson Eleven (Fig. 21.102).

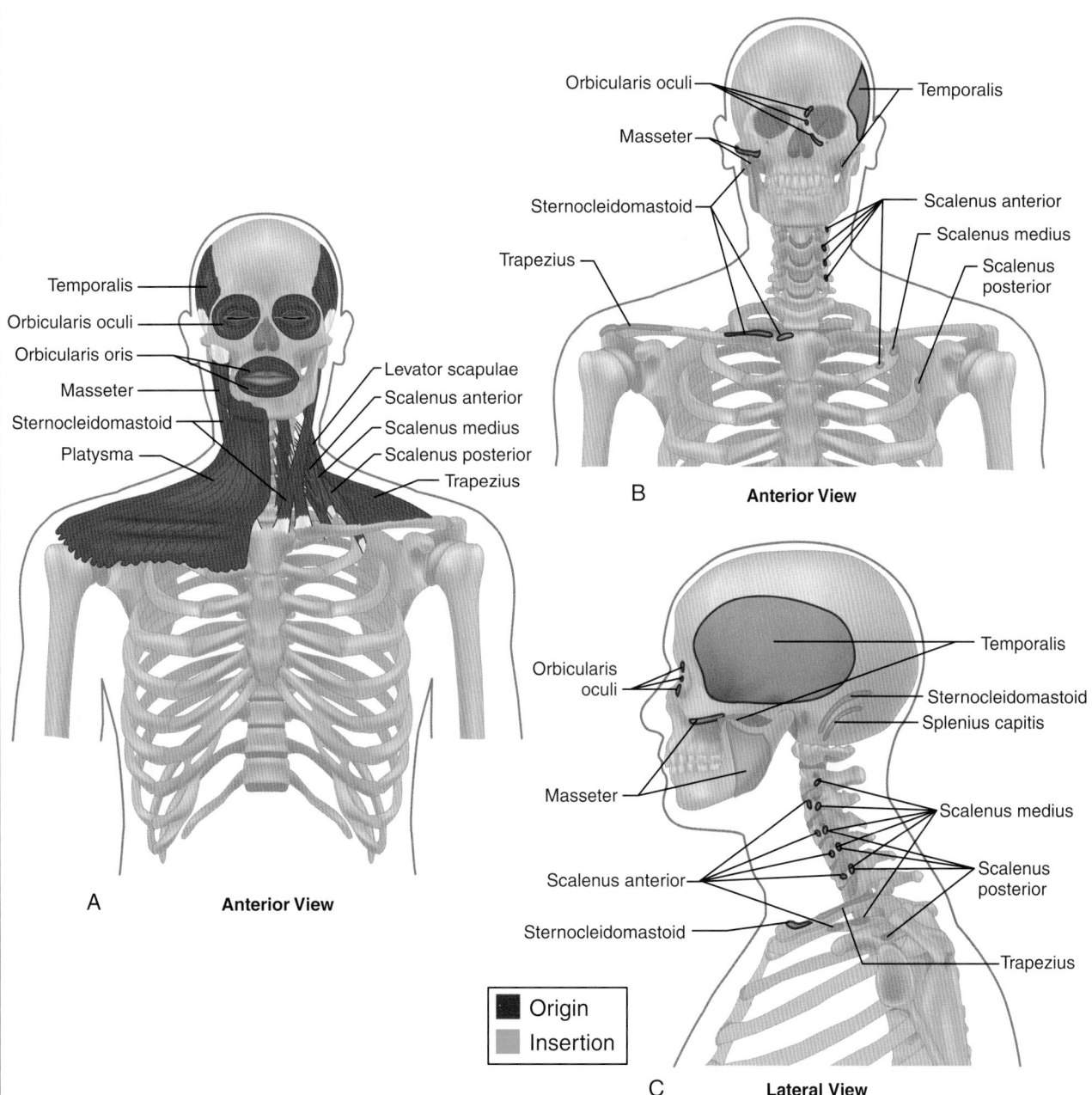

FIG. 21.102 Muscles of neck and facial movement (*A and D*) with their associated origins (*red*) and insertions (*blue, B, C, and E*).

Continued

Lesson Ten: Muscles of Neck and Facial Movement—cont'd

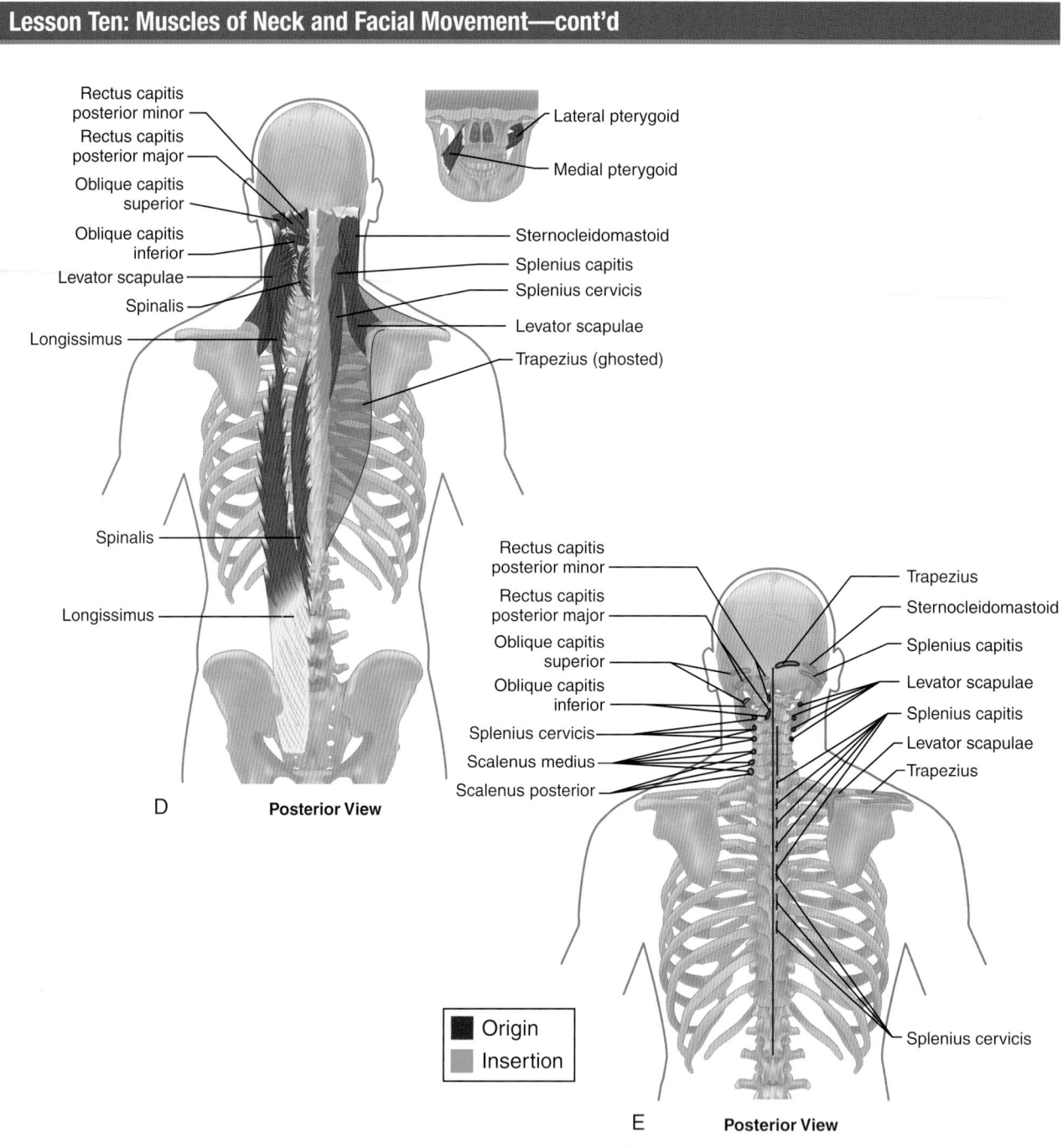

Rectus capitis posterior minor
Rectus capitis posterior major
Oblique capitis superior
Oblique capitis inferior
Levator scapulae
Spinalis
Longissimus

Lateral pterygoid
Medial pterygoid

Sternocleidomastoid
Splenius capitis
Splenius cervicis
Levator scapulae
Trapezius (ghosted)

Spinalis
Longissimus

D **Posterior View**

Rectus capitis posterior minor
Rectus capitis posterior major
Oblique capitis superior
Oblique capitis inferior
Splenius cervicis
Scalenus medius
Scalenus posterior

Trapezius
Sternocleidomastoid
Splenius capitis
Levator scapulae
Splenius capitis
Levator scapulae
Trapezius

Splenius cervicis

■ Origin
■ Insertion

E **Posterior View**

FIG. 21.102, CONT'D

OCCIPITOFRONTALIS (FIG. 21.103)

*Latin: occipitalis—pertaining to the back of the head
frons—brow or referring to the frontal bone*

ORIGINS
Lateral two-thirds of the superior nuchal line (occipitalis)
Galea aponeurotica (frontalis)

INSERTIONS
Galea aponeurotica (occipitalis)
Superficial fascia beneath the eyebrows (frontalis)

ACTIONS
Moves the scalp over the cranium (occipitalis)
Elevates the eyebrows (frontalis)
Horizontally wrinkles the skin over the forehead (frontalis)

NERVE
Facial nerve (cranial nerve VII)

NOTES: Occipitofrontalis (*epicranius*) covers the top of the skull and consists of two muscles—occipitalis, which lies over the occipital bone; and frontalis, which lies over the frontal bone. These muscles are connected by a tough fibrous sheet of connective tissue on top of the cranium called *galea aponeurotica (epicranial aponeurosis).*

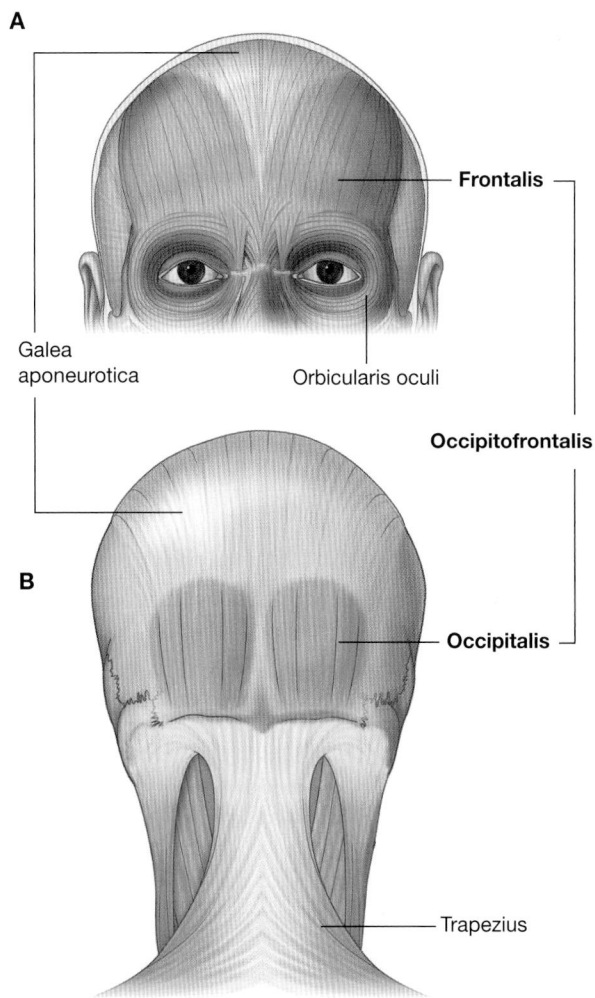

FIG. 21.103 Occipitofrontalis and connecting aponeurosis showing frontalis (*A, anterior view*) and occipitalis (*B, posterior view*). (Modified from Drake, R. L., Vogl, W., Mitchell, A. W. M. [2010]. *Gray's anatomy for students* [2nd ed.]. St Louis: Churchill Livingstone.)

ORBICULARIS OCULI (FIG. 21.104)

Latin: orbiculus—little circle
oculus—eye

ORIGIN
Orbital margin

INSERTION
Superficial fascia beneath the upper eyelids

ACTIONS
Closes the eyelids
Folds the skin around the orbit (to protect eyeball)
Squints the eyelids

NERVE
Facial nerve (cranial nerve VII)

NOTES: Orbicularis oculi is a sphincter-type muscle encircling the eye. It is the *winking muscle,* or *blinking muscle,* because it closes one or both eyelids (Herihy, 2018).

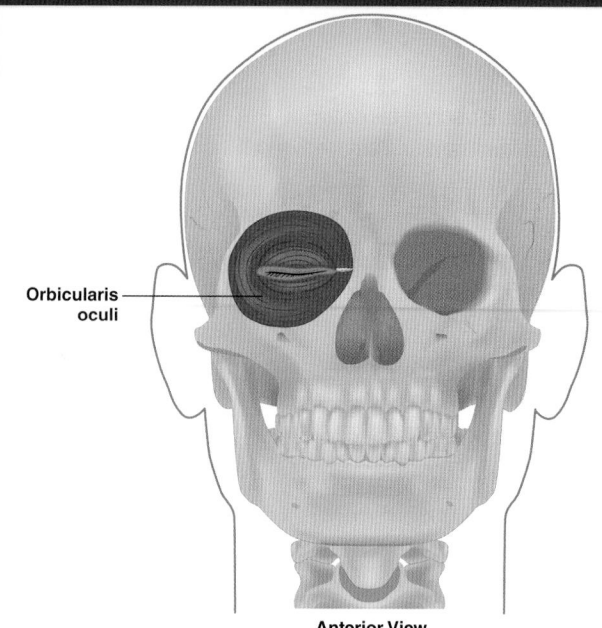

Anterior View

FIG. 21.104 Right orbicularis oculi.

ORBICULARIS ORIS (FIG. 21.105)

Latin: orbiculus—little circle
oris—mouth

ORIGINS
Maxillae
Mandible

INSERTIONS
Mucous membranes of the lips
Muscles inserting into the lips

ACTIONS
Closes the lips
Protrudes and protracts the lips
Assists in dozens of activities such as eating, drinking, and speaking

NERVE
Facial nerve (cranial nerve VII)

NOTES: Orbicularis oris is a sphincter-type muscle encircling the mouth. It is the *kissing muscle* because it protrudes the lips for a kiss (Herlihy, 2018).

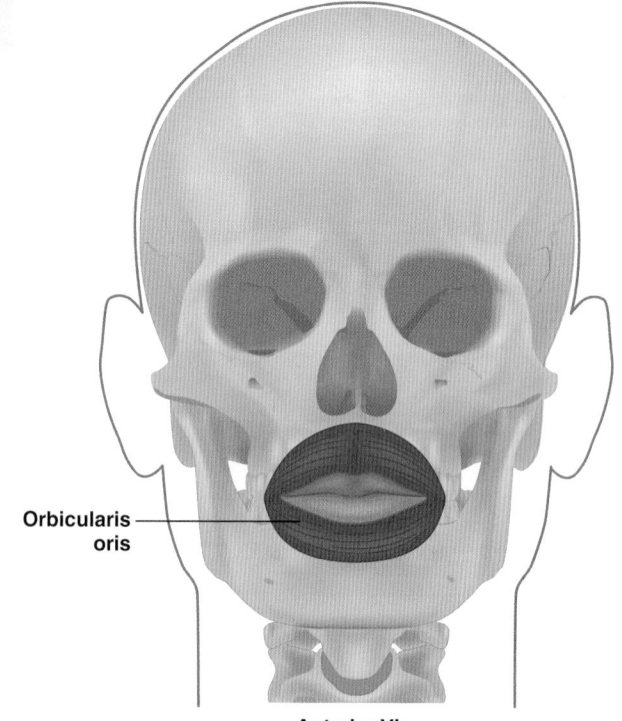

Anterior View

FIG. 21.105 Orbicularis oris.

PLATYSMA (FIG. 21.106)

Greek: platysma—plate

ORIGINS
Superficial fascia of the deltoid
Superficial fascia of pectoralis major

INSERTIONS
Mandible
Muscles around the angle of the mouth
Superficial fascia of the lower face

ACTIONS
Tenses the skin of the anterior neck (creating ridges)
Pulls the corner of the mouth downward and backward
Depresses the mandible

NERVE
Facial nerve (cranial nerve VII)

NOTES: Platysma is the *pouting muscle* because it pulls the corners of the mouth downward and backward as in pouting (Herlihy, 2018). It is the most superficial muscle of the anterior neck.

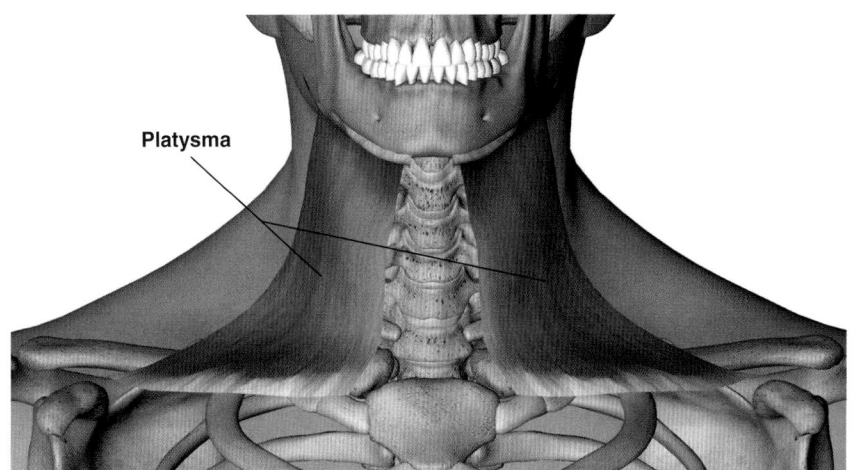

Anterior View

FIG. 21.106 Platysma. (From Liebgott, B. [2018]. *The anatomical basis of dentistry* [4th ed.]. St. Louis, MO: Elsevier.)

MUSCLES OF MASTICATION (FIG. 21.107)

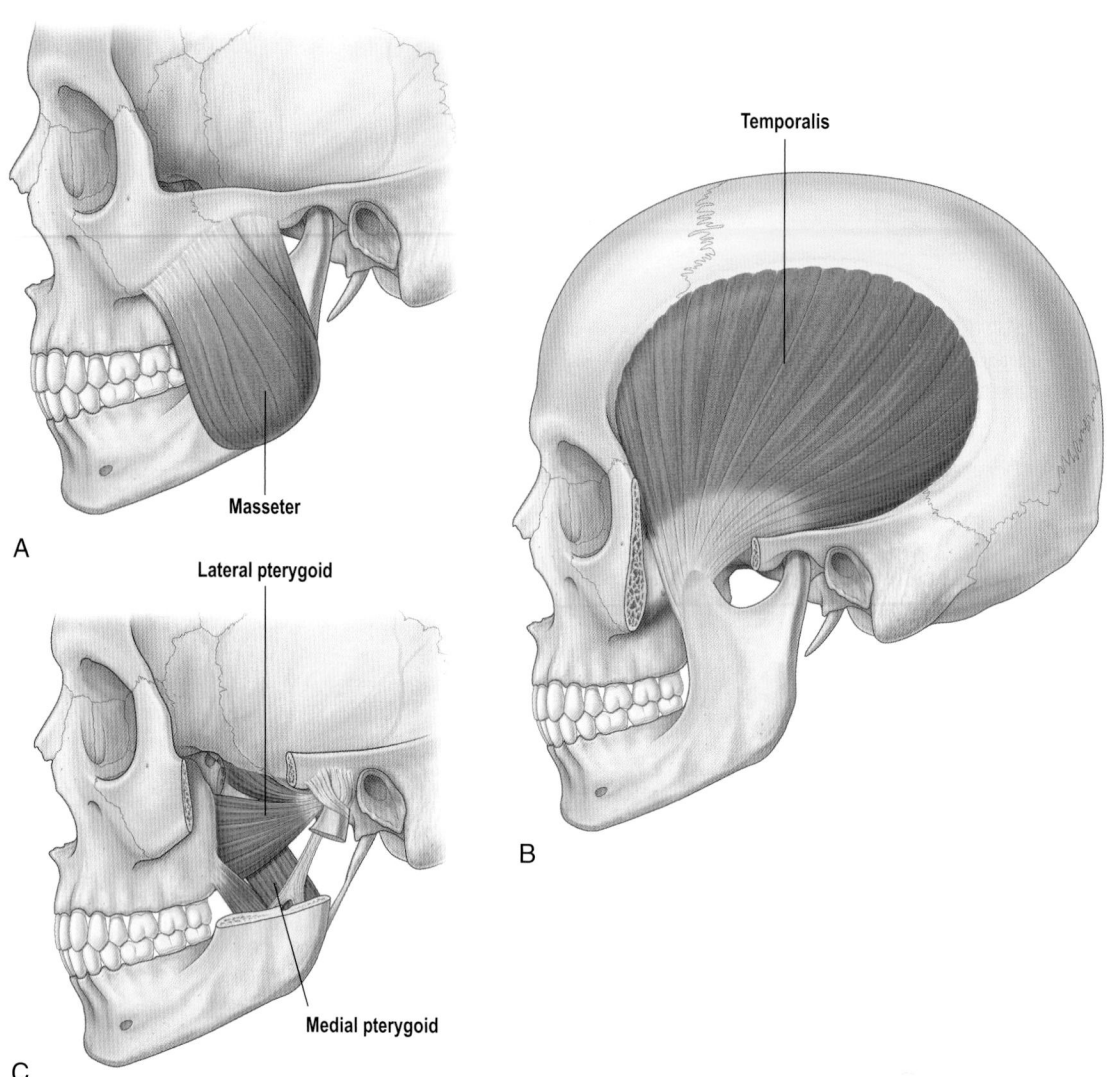

Lateral Views

FIG. 21.107 Muscles of mastication; left side. (*A*) Masseter. (*B*) Temporalis. (*C*) Medial and lateral pytergoids (*parts of the mandible, maxilla, and zygomatic bones are removed to show these muscles*). (Modified from Soames, R., & Palastanga, N. [2019]. *Anatomy and human movement: Structure and function* [7th ed.]. Philadelphia, PA: Elsevier.)

NOTES: These muscles attach to the mandible, or jaw, and produce movements involved in mastication, or chewing. The muscles of mastication are temporalis, masseter, medial, and lateral pterygoids.

TEMPORALIS (FIG. 21.108)

Latin: temporalis—pertaining to the temporal bone

ORIGIN
Temporal fossa

INSERTION
Coronoid process

ACTIONS
Elevates the mandible
Retracts the mandible

NERVE
Trigeminal nerve (cranial nerve V)

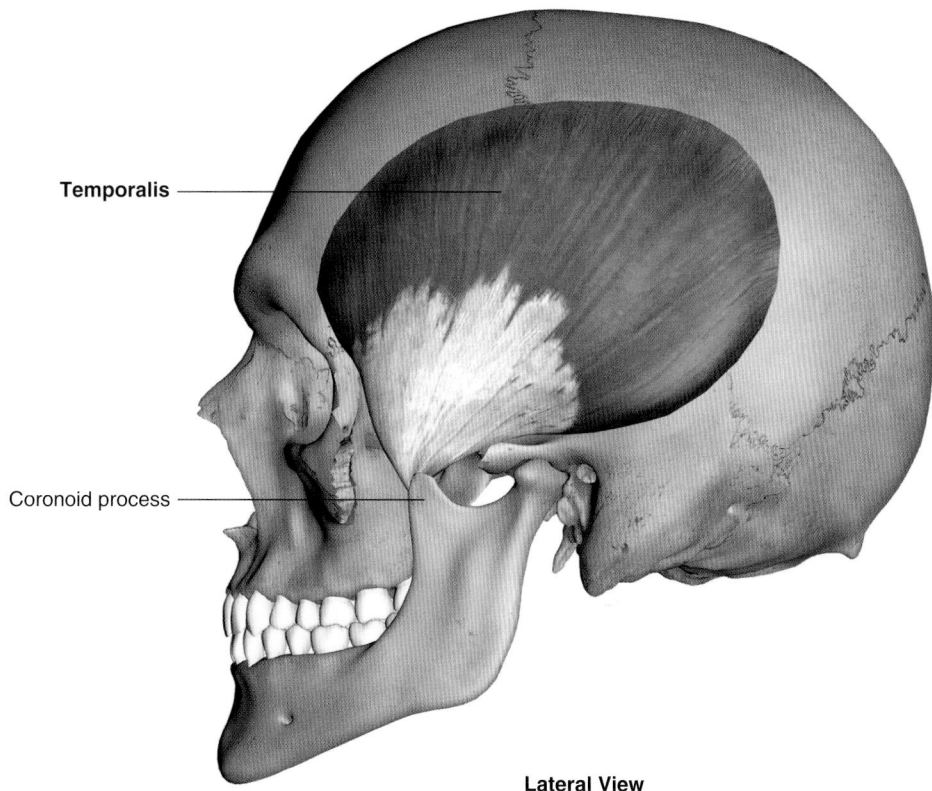

Lateral View

FIG. 21.108 Left temporalis (*the zygomatic arch is removed to show the entire muscle*). (From Liebgott, B. [2018]. *The anatomical basis of dentistry* [4th ed.]. St. Louis, MO: Elsevier.)

NOTES: Temporalis arises from the *temporal fossa*, a shallow depression on the sides of the skull in the temporal region. The temporal fossa is formed by the temporal lines and terminates below the level of the zygomatic arch. Temporalis passes beneath the zygomatic arch before it attaches to the mandible at the coronoid process.

MASSETER (FIG. 21.109)

Greek: masseter—chewer

ORIGIN
Zygomatic arch

INSERTIONS
Mandibular angle (superficial head)
Mandibular ramus (deep head)

ACTIONS
Elevates the mandible
Protracts the mandible

NERVE
Trigeminal nerve (cranial nerve V)

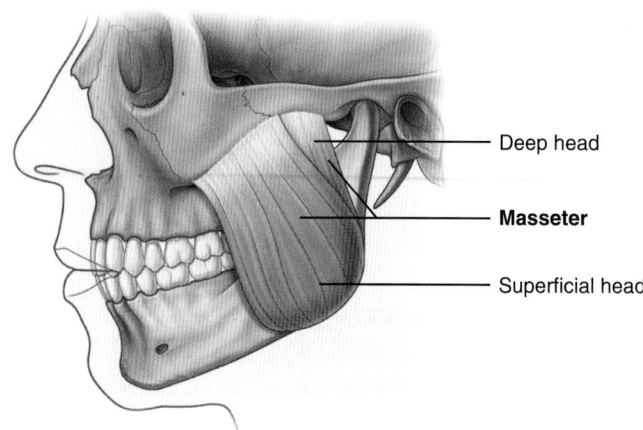

Deep head

Masseter

Superficial head

Lateral View

NOTES: Masseter contains two heads—a superficial head and a deep head. Masseter is a mirror image of the medial pterygoid.

FIG. 21.109 Left masseter. (From Drake, R. L., Vogl, W., & Mitchell, A. W. M.[2010]. *Gray's anatomy for students* [2nd ed.]. St Louis: Churchill Livingstone.)

LATERAL PTERYGOID (FIG. 21.110)

Latin: lateralis—toward the side
Greek: pterygodes—shaped like a wing

ORIGINS
Lateral pterygoid plate of the sphenoid bone
Greater wing of the sphenoid bone (lateral portion)

INSERTIONS
Condylar process of the mandible
Temporomandibular joint capsule

ACTIONS
Excursion or laterally deviates the mandible (unilateral contraction)
Depresses the mandible (bilateral contraction)
Protracts the mandible (bilateral contraction)

NERVE
Trigeminal nerve (cranial nerve V)

NOTES: Lateral pterygoid is also called *external pterygoid.*

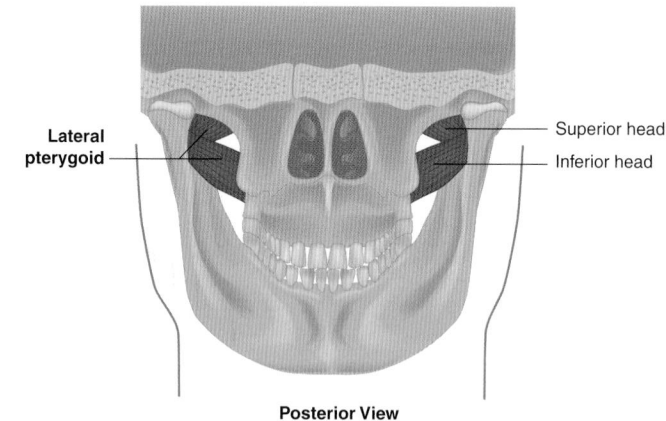

Lateral pterygoid

Superior head
Inferior head

Posterior View
FIG. 21.110 Lateral pterygoid.

MEDIAL PTERYGOID (FIG. 21.111)

Latin: medialis—toward the midline
Greek: pterygodes—shaped like a wing

ORIGIN
Medial pterygoid plate of the sphenoid bone

INSERTIONS
Mandibular angle (interior surface)
Mandibular ramus (interior surface)

ACTIONS
Excursion or laterally deviates the mandible (unilateral contraction)
Elevates the mandible (bilateral contraction)
Protracts the mandible (bilateral contraction)

NERVE
Trigeminal nerve (cranial nerve V)

NOTES: Medial pterygoid is also called *internal pterygoid*. It is the mirror image of the masseter.

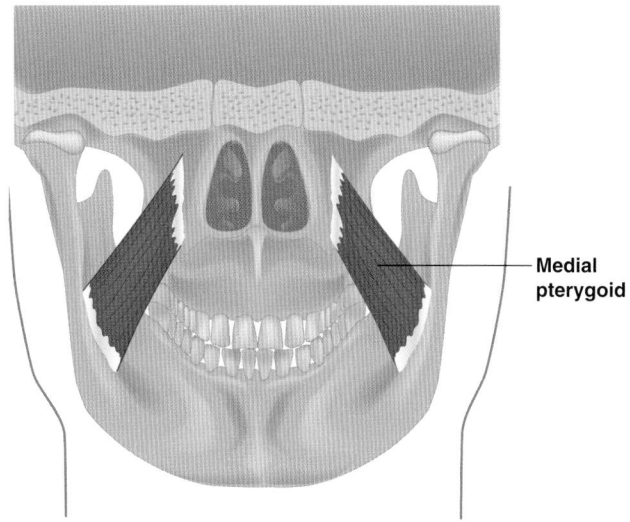

Posterior View

FIG. 21.111 Medial pterygoid.

STERNOCLEIDOMASTOID (FIG. 21.112)

Greek: sternon—sternum
cleido—clavicle
mastos—breast-like

ORIGINS
Manubrium of the sternum (sternal head)
Medial third of the clavicle (clavicular head)

INSERTIONS
Mastoid process
Superior nuchal line

ACTIONS
Laterally flexes the neck (unilateral contraction)
Rotates the head to the opposite side (unilateral contraction)
Flexes the neck (bilateral contraction)
Elevates the sternum during forced inhalation (bilateral contraction)

NERVE
Spinal accessory nerve (cranial nerve XI)

NOTES: Sternocleidomastoid (SCM) serves as a neck landmark, by dividing it into anterior and posterior cervical triangles (see Fig. 8.1). SCM is the *praying muscle* because bilateral contraction flexes the neck to lower, or bow, the head to demonstrate respect or reverence while praying (Herlihy, 2018). The SCM is the mirror image of splenius capitis. *Torticollis (wryneck or cervical/spasmodic dystonia)* occurs when SCM is in a spasm.

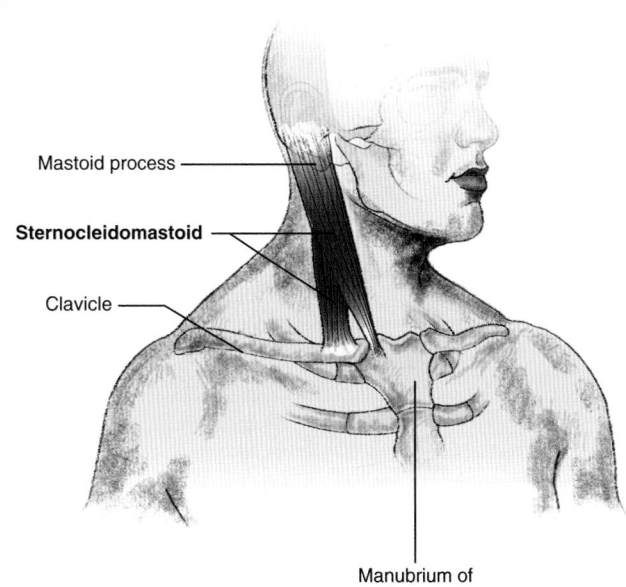

Anterior View

FIG. 21.112 Right sternocleidomastoid with attachment sites. (Modified from Mansfield, P. [2019]. *Essentials of kinesiology for the physical therapist assistant* [3rd ed.]. St. Louis, MO: Mosby.)

SCALENES (FIG. 21.113)

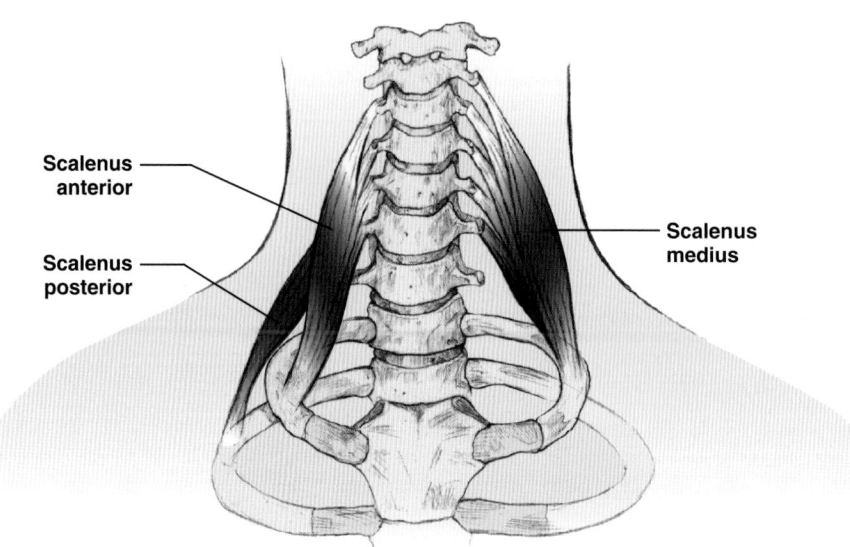

Anterior View

FIG. 21.113 Scalenes with right scalenus anterior, left scalenus medius, and right scalenus posterior identified. (Modified from Mansfield, P. [2019]. *Essentials of kinesiology for the physical therapist assistant* [3rd ed.]. St. Louis, MO: Mosby.)

NOTES: Scalenes are a group of muscles consisting of scalenus anterior, scalenus medius, and scalenus posterior. Scalenes are the *entrappers* because tense scalenus anterior and medius can entrap the brachial plexus, causing thoracic outlet syndrome-like symptoms (pain, tingling, and numbness down the arm into the affected hand) (Travell & Simons, 1983). See Chapter 23 for more information about thoracic outlet syndrome.

SCALENUS ANTERIOR (SEE FIG. 21.113)

Greek: skalenos—uneven
Latin: ante—before

ORIGINS
Transverse processes of C3–C6 (anterior surface)

INSERTION
Rib 1 (superior surface)

ACTIONS
Flexes the neck (bilateral contraction)
Laterally flexes the neck (unilateral contraction)
Rotates the head (unilateral contraction)
Elevates the first rib during forced inhalation (bilateral contraction)

NERVES
Anterior rami of the cervical nerves

NOTES: Scalenus anterior is also called *anterior scalene.*

SCALENUS MEDIUS (SEE FIG. 21.113)

Greek: skalenos—uneven
Latin: medialis—toward the midline

ORIGINS
Transverse processes of C2–C7 (posterior surface)

INSERTION
Rib 1 (superior surface)

ACTIONS
Flexes the neck (bilateral contraction)
Laterally flexes the neck (unilateral contraction)
Rotates the head (unilateral contraction)
Elevates the first rib during forced inhalation (bilateral contraction)

NERVES
Anterior rami of the cervical nerves

NOTES: Scalenus medius is also called *middle scalene.*

SCALENUS POSTERIOR (SEE FIG. 21.113)

Greek: skalenos—uneven
Latin: posterus—behind

ORIGINS
Transverse processes of C5–C7 (posterior surface)

INSERTION
Rib 2 (superior lateral surface)

ACTIONS
Laterally flexes the neck (unilateral contraction)
Elevates the second rib during forced inhalation (bilateral contraction)

NERVES
Anterior rami of cervical nerves

NOTES: Scalenus posterior is also called *posterior scalene.*

SPLENIUS CAPITIS (FIG. 21.114)

Greek: splenion—splint or bandage
caput—head

ORIGINS
Nuchal ligament (level of C3)
Spinous processes of C7–T4

INSERTIONS
Mastoid process
Superior nuchal line—lateral region

ACTIONS
Rotates the head (unilateral contraction)
Laterally flexes the neck (unilateral contraction)
Extends the head (bilateral contraction)

NERVES
Posterior rami of the middle cervical nerves

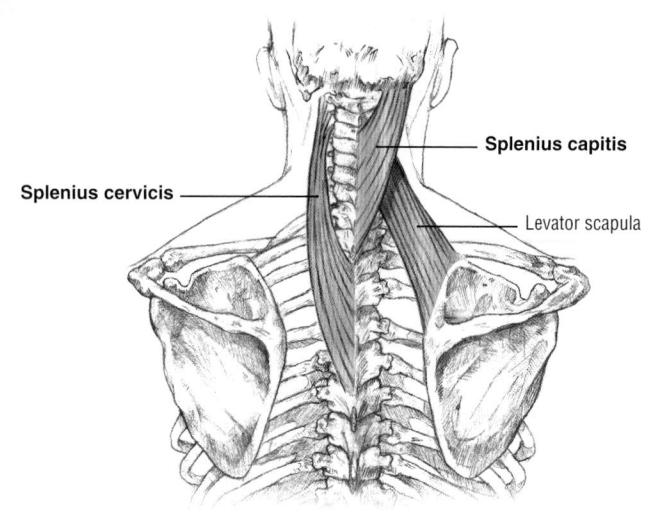

Splenius capitis
Splenius cervicis
Levator scapula

Posterior View

FIG. 21.114 Right splenius capitis and left splenius cervicis with neighboring right levator scapula. (From Mansfield, P., Neumann, D. [2008]. *Essentials of Kinesiology for the Physical Therapist Assistant*. Elsevier Health Sciences (US): Elsevier, p 211.)

NOTES: Splenius capitis is a mirror image of SCM.

SPLENIUS CERVICIS (SEE FIG. 21.114)

Greek: splenion—splint or bandage
cervicalis—neck

ORIGINS
Spinous processes of T3–T6

INSERTIONS
Transverse processes of C1–C3

ACTIONS
Rotates the head (unilateral contraction)
Laterally flexes the neck (unilateral contraction)
Extends the head (bilateral contraction)

NERVES
Posterior rami of the lower cervical nerves

SUBOCCIPITALS (FIG. 21.115)

Latin: sub—below
occipitalis—pertaining to the back of the head

NOTES: The suboccipital muscles are beneath the occipital bone. They include the rectus capitis posterior major, rectus capitis posterior minor, oblique capitis inferior, and oblique capitis superior. Suboccipitals are the *headache ghosts* because their referred pain patterns are "ghostly" and may radiate from the base of the skull through the head to the back of the eyes (Travell & Simons, 1983).

The suboccipitals are part of the *prevertebral muscles*. Other prevertebral muscles are *longus capitis* and *longus colli*, which act to flex and laterally flex the neck, provide some rotation, and help stabilize the neck during swallowing. Longus capitis and longus colli are not massaged as they are deep within the anterior neck, which is an endangerment site. Anterior neck massage has been reported to cause injury (see Chapter 8 for a list of case reports and systematic reviews).

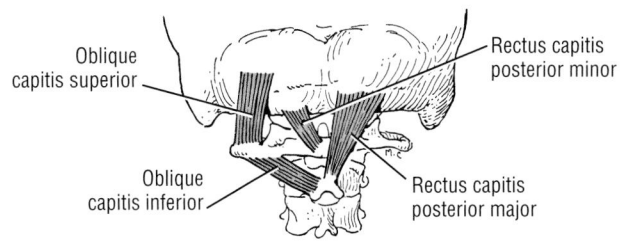

Posterior View

FIG. 21.115 Suboccipitals with right rectus capitis posterior major, left rectus capitis posterior minor, left oblique capitis inferior, and left oblique capitis superior identified. (From Porterfield, J. A., DeRosa, C. [1995]. *Mechanical Neck Pain: Perspectives in Functional Anatomy.* Philadelphia: Saunders.)

RECTUS CAPITIS POSTERIOR MAJOR (SEE FIG. 21.115)

Latin: rectus—straight
caput—head
posterus—behind
major—larger

ORIGIN
Spinous process of C2

INSERTION
Lateral inferior nuchal line

ACTIONS
Extends the head
Rotates the head

NERVE
Suboccipital nerve

RECTUS CAPITIS POSTERIOR MINOR (SEE FIG. 21.115)

Latin: rectus—straight
caput—head
posterus—behind
minor—smaller

ORIGIN
Posterior tubercle of C1

INSERTION
Medial inferior nuchal line

ACTION
Extends the head

NERVE
Suboccipital nerve

OBLIQUE CAPITIS SUPERIOR (SEE FIG. 21.115)

Latin: obliquus—slant
caput—head
superus—upper

ORIGIN
Transverse process of C1

INSERTION
Inferior nuchal line

ACTIONS
Extends the head
Laterally flexes the head

NERVE
Suboccipital nerve

OBLIQUE CAPITIS INFERIOR (SEE FIG. 21.115)

Latin: obliquus—slant
caput—head
infra—beneath

ORIGIN
Spinous process of C2

INSERTION
Transverse process of C1

ACTION
Rotates the head

NERVE
Suboccipital nerve

NOTES: Oblique capitis inferior is the only "capitis" muscle that does not attach to the skull.

Lesson Ten Review: Muscles of Mandibular Movement

ELEVATION	DEPRESSION	PROTRACTION	RETRACTION	EXCURSION
Temporalis	Lateral pterygoid	Masseter	Temporalis	Lateral pterygoid
Masseter	Platysma	Lateral pterygoid		Medial pterygoid
Medial pterygoid		Medial pterygoid		

Lateral views

Anterior view

Lesson Ten Review: Muscles of Head and Neck Movement

FLEXION	EXTENSION	LATERAL FLEXION	ROTATION
Sternocleidomastoid	Trapezius	Trapezius	Trapezius
Scalenus anterior	Splenius capitis	Levator scapulae	Sternocleidomastoid
Scalenus medius	Splenius cervicis	Sternocleidomastoid	Scalenus anterior
	Rectus capitis posterior major	Scalenes	Scalenus medius
	Rectus capitis posterior minor	Splenius capitis	Splenius capitis
	Oblique capitis superior	Splenius cervicis	Splenius cervicis
	Longissimus	Oblique capitis superior	Rectus capitis posterior major
			Oblique capitis inferior

Lateral views

Anterior views

Lesson Eleven: Muscles of Trunk and Vertebral Column Movement

Movements of the trunk and vertebral column are flexion, extension, lateral flexion, and rotation. Muscles of the trunk and vertebral column are rectus abdominis, external obliques, internal obliques, transverse abdominis, quadratus lumborum, semispinalis, rotatores, multifidus, spinalis, longissimus, and iliocostalis (Fig. 21.116).

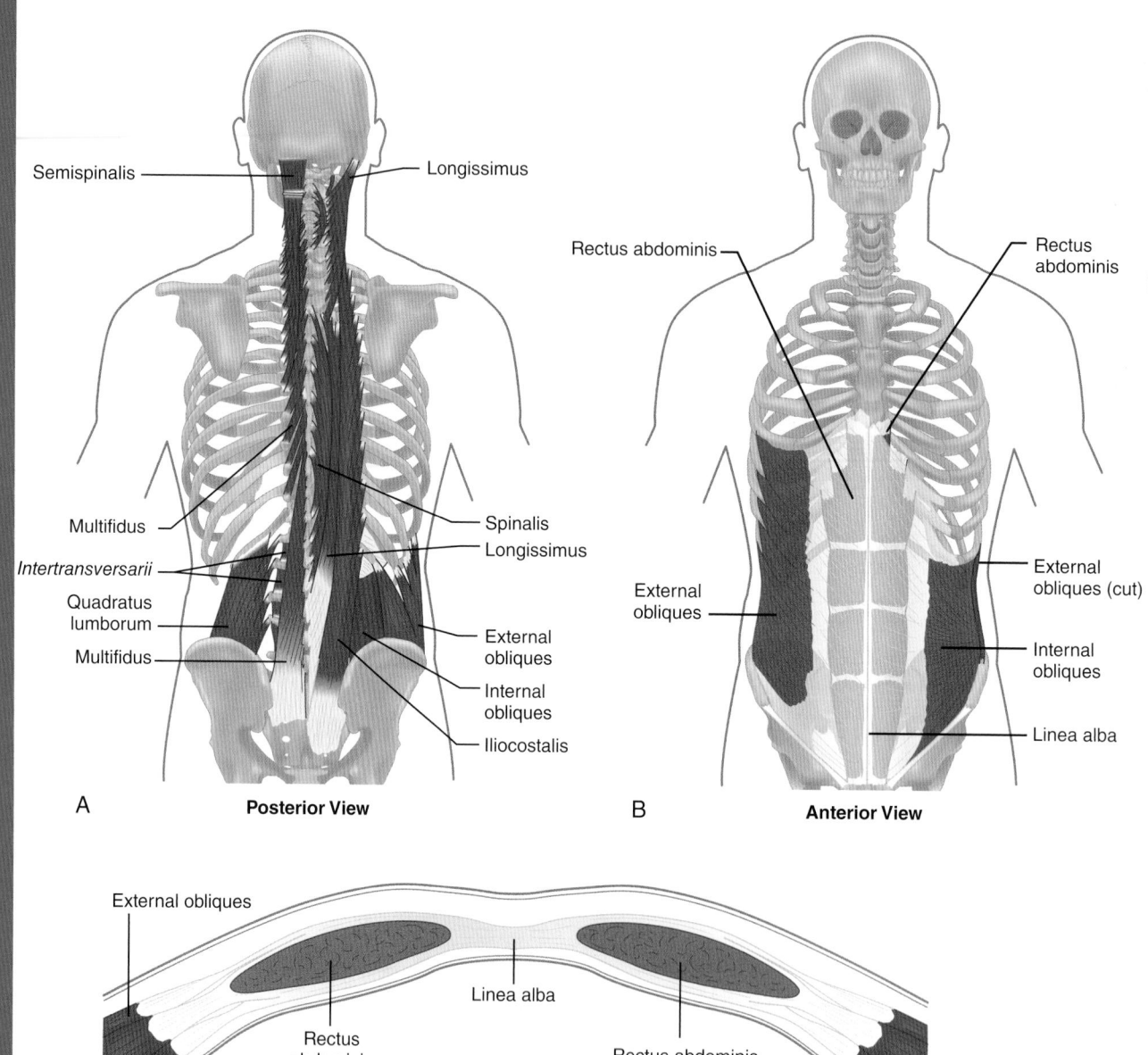

FIG. 21.116 Muscles of trunk and vertebral column movement (*A and B, upper images*) and the rectus sheath (*C, lower image*).

ABDOMINALS

NOTES: The abdominal muscles are a group of four individual muscles—rectus abdominis, transverse abdominis, external obliques, and internal obliques. Contraction of the abdominal muscles facilitates forceful exhalation by forcing abdominal organs upward against the diaphragm. This action pushes the diaphragm further into the thoracic cavity, forcing more air out of the lungs. **LEARNING TIP:** To help you remember the names of the abdominal muscles, use the phrase **TIRE** (as in "I have a spare *tire* around my abdomen") for **T**ransverse abdominis, **I**nternal obliques, **R**ectus abdominis, and **E**xternal obliques.

The *rectus sheath* is formed by the aponeuroses of the lateral abdominal muscles and encloses the rectus abdominis. The *linea alba* is a fibrous structure in the central abdomen extending from the xiphoid process to the pubic symphysis between the left and right rectus abdominis muscles (see Fig. 21.144; *superior view*).

RECTUS ABDOMINIS (FIG. 21.117)

Latin: rectus—straight
abdomen—belly

ORIGINS
Pubic symphysis
Pubic tubercle

INSERTIONS
Ribs 5–7 (costal cartilage—anterior surface)
Xiphoid process

ACTIONS
Flexes the vertebral column
Laterally flexes the vertebral column
Compresses abdominal contents
Posteriorly tilts the pelvis

NERVES
Anterior rami of intercostal nerves (T7–T12)

NOTES: Rectus abdominis is enclosed in the rectus sheath (mentioned previously). Rectus abdominis contains *tendinous intersections*, fibrous horizontal bands of connective tissue to help keep its length relatively constant because the distance between skeletal attachment sites is wide (e.g., ribcage to pelvic bone). Rectus abdominis is the *six-pack muscle* because it looks like someone has a six-pack in their abs when left and right sections are tone. However, rectus abdominis actually contains eight to ten sections, but usually only six sections can be seen.

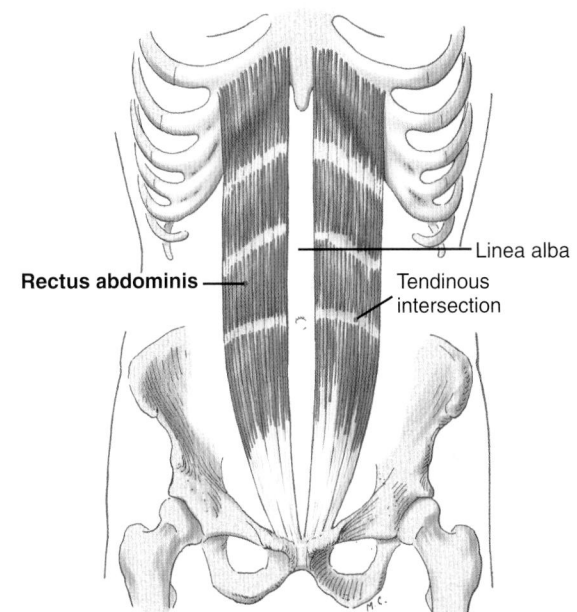

Anterior View

FIG. 21.117 Rectus abdominis with its linea alba and left tendinous intersections identified. (Modified from Mansfield, P. [2014]. *Essentials of kinesiology for the physical therapist assistant* [2nd ed.]. St. Louis, MO: Mosby.)

EXTERNAL OBLIQUES (FIG. 21.118)

Latin: externus—outside
obliquus—slant

ORIGINS
Ribs 5–12 (anterior lateral surface)

INSERTIONS
Anterior iliac crest
Aponeurosis of rectus sheath
Pubic crest

ACTIONS
Laterally flexes the vertebral column
Rotates the vertebral column
Flexes the vertebral column
Compresses abdominal contents
Posteriorly tilts the pelvis

NERVES
Anterior rami of intercostal nerves (T7–T12)

NOTES: External obliques are also called *external abdominal obliques*. External obliques have a fiber arrangement similar to the direction of your fingers when your hands are in the pockets of a jacket. The pockets of most jackets do not reach the midline. Similarly, the external obliques do not reach the midline but join the rectus sheath instead.

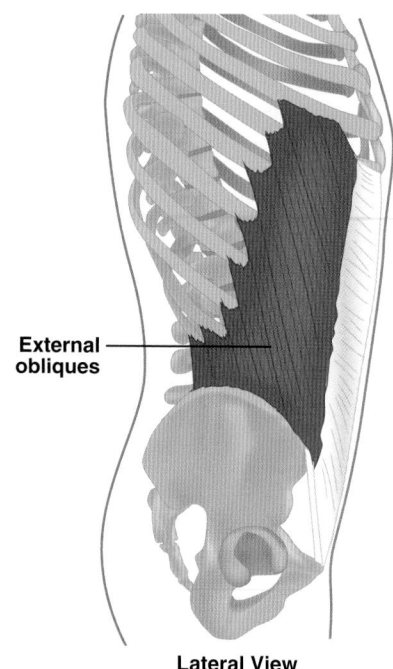

External obliques

Lateral View

FIG. 21.118 Right external obliques.

INTERNAL OBLIQUES (FIG. 21.119)

Latin: internus—within
obliquus—slant

ORIGINS
Iliac crest (anterior portion)
Thoracolumbar fascia
Aponeurosis of rectus sheath
Inguinal ligament (lateral half)

INSERTIONS
Ribs 9–12 (anterior lateral surface)

ACTIONS
Laterally flexes the vertebral column
Rotates the vertebral column
Flexes the vertebral column
Compresses abdominal contents
Posteriorly tilts the pelvis

NERVES
Anterior rami of the intercostal nerves

NOTES: Internal obliques are also called *internal abdominal obliques.*

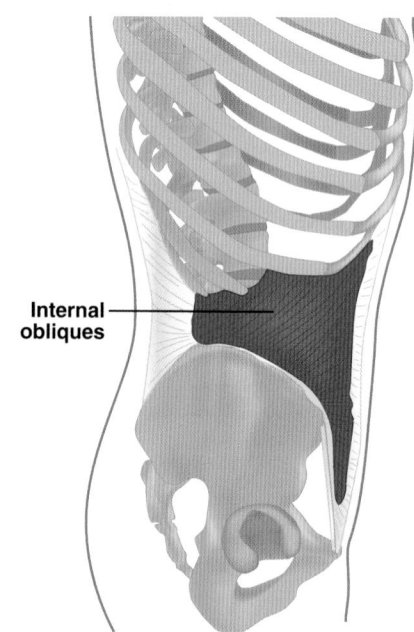

Internal obliques

Lateral View

FIG. 21.119 Right internal obliques.

TRANSVERSE ABDOMINIS (FIG. 21.120)

Latin: transversus—lying across
abdomen—belly

ORIGINS
Ribs 7–12 (costal cartilage—inner surface)
Iliac crest
Aponeurosis of rectus sheath
Thoracolumbar aponeurosis
Inguinal ligament

INSERTIONS
Abdominal aponeurosis

ACTION
Compresses abdominal contents

NERVES
Anterior rami of intercostal nerves

NOTES: Transverse abdominis is the deepest abdominal muscle and wraps around the internal organs like a cummerbund. The lower fibers of rectus abdominis are tucked beneath transverse abdominis, presumably for added strength.

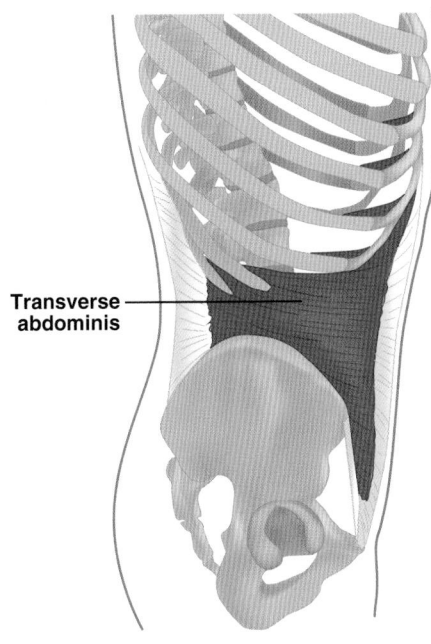

Lateral View

FIG. 21.120 Right transverse abdominis.

QUADRATUS LUMBORUM (FIG. 21.121)

Latin: quadratus—four-sided
lumbus—loins

ORIGIN
Posterior iliac crest

INSERTIONS
Rib 12 (inferior surface)
Transverse processes of L1–L4

ACTIONS
Laterally flexes the vertebral column (unilateral contraction)
Elevates the hip (unilateral contraction)
Extends the lumbar spine (bilateral contraction)
Anteriorly tilts the pelvis (bilateral contraction)

NERVES
Lumbar plexus

NOTES: Quadratus lumborum (QL) is the *hip hiker muscle* because unilateral contraction elevates, or "hikes," the hip. Travell and Simons (1993) called QL the *joker of lower back pain,* as chronic contraction of this muscle may lead to a diagnosis of spinal nerve root compression, but the cause may be QL.

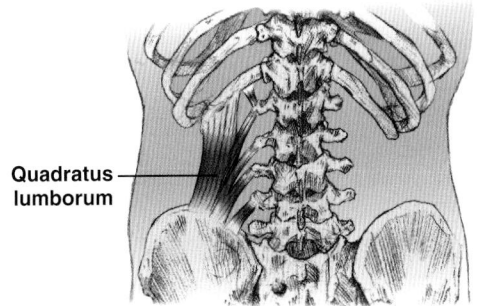

Posterior View

FIG. 21.121 Left quadratus lumborum. (Modified from Mansfield, P. [2014]. *Essentials of kinesiology for the physical therapist assistant* [2nd ed.]. St. Louis, MO: Mosby.)

PARASPINALS (FIG. 21.122)

Greek: para—beside
Latin: spinatus—spine

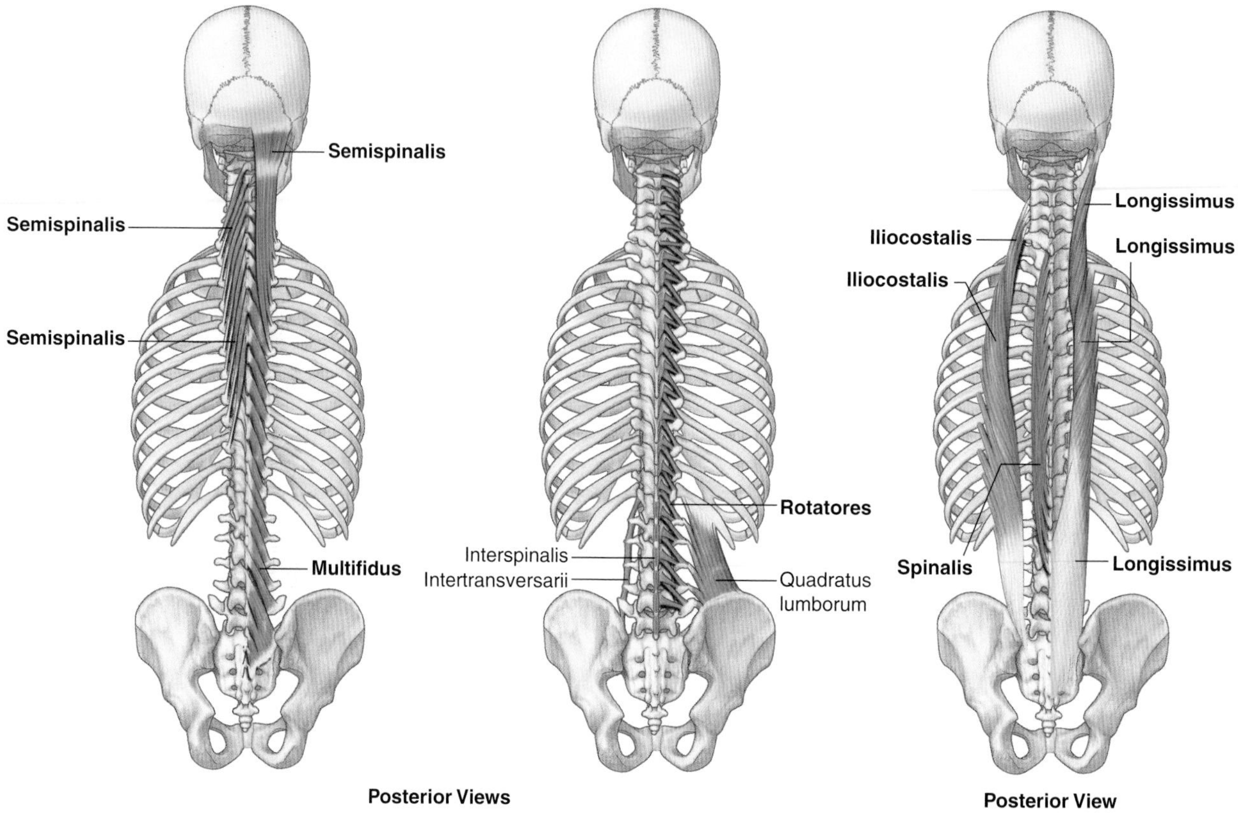

Semispinalis

Semispinalis

Semispinalis

Multifidus

Rotatores

Interspinalis
Intertransversarii

Quadratus lumborum

Iliocostalis
Iliocostalis

Longissimus
Longissimus

Spinalis

Longissimus

Posterior Views

Posterior View

A   B   C

FIG. 21.122 Paraspinals. Transversospinalis group with neighboring segmental muscles (interspinales, intertransversarii) and quadratus lumborum (*A and B, left and middle images*) and erector spinae group (*C, right image*). (Modified from Soames, R., & Palastanga, N. [2019]. *Anatomy and human movement: Structure and function* [7th ed.]. Philadelphia, PA: Elsevier.)

NOTES: *Paraspinals* is the term for a group of back muscles that consists of deep and superficial sections (Fig. 21.123)

- Transversospinalis (Deep Paraspinals)
  - Semispinalis
  - Rotatores
  - Multifidus
- Erector Spinae (Superficial Paraspinals)
  - Spinalis
  - Longissimus
  - Iliocostalis

Segmental muscles include interspinales and intertransversarii. These lie deep to transversospinalis and span a single vertebral segment. *Interspinales* attach to the spinous processes. *Intertransversarii* attach to the transverse processes.

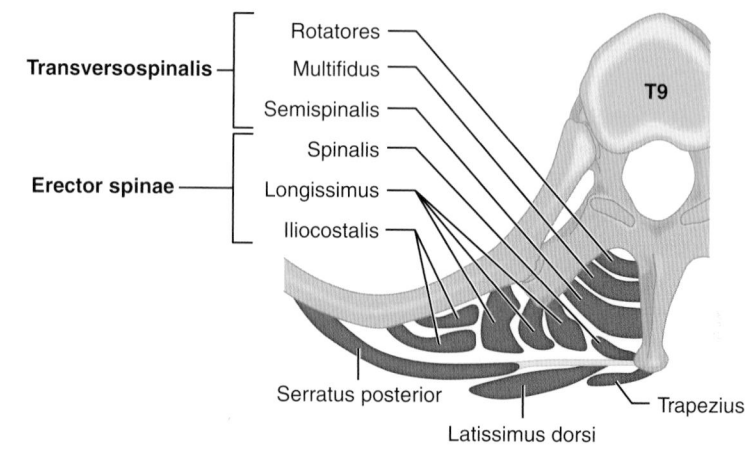

Rotatores
Multifidus
Semispinalis

Transversospinalis

Spinalis
Longissimus
Iliocostalis

Erector spinae

T9

Serratus posterior

Latissimus dorsi

Trapezius

Cross-section, Superior View

FIG. 21.123 Paraspinals, left side.

TRANSVERSOSPINALIS

Latin: transversus—lying across
spinatus—spine

NOTES: Transversospinalis consists of semispinalis, multifidus, and rotatores. This muscle group lies in the laminar groove between the transverse and spinous processes of each vertebrae. These muscles are arranged anterior to posterior, unlike those in the erector spinae muscle group, which are arranged medial to lateral. ***LEARNING TIP***: To help you remember the muscles of the transversospinalis from anterior to posterior, use the phrase **R**ed **M**eat **S**auce for **R**otatores, **M**ultifidus, and **S**emispinalis.

SEMISPINALIS (FIG. 21.124)

Latin: semis—half
spinatus—spine

ORIGINS
Transverse process of one vertebral segment (cervical and thoracic regions)

INSERTIONS
Between superior and inferior nuchal lines
Spinous processes of the fifth, sixth, and seventh vertebral segments above (cervical and thoracic regions except C1)

ACTIONS
Laterally flexes the vertebral column (unilateral contraction)
Rotates the vertebral column (unilateral contraction)
Extends the vertebral column (bilateral contraction)

NERVES
Posterior rami of the cervical and thoracic spinal nerves

NOTES: Semispinalis is the most superficial muscle in the transversospinalis group. Semispinalis extends partway over the spine and contains several subgroupings: *semispinalis capitis, semispinalis cervicis,* and *semispinalis thoracis.* ***LEARNING TIP***: To help you remember the superficial placement of semispinalis in relation to other transversospinalis muscles, both **S**emispinalis and **S**uperficial begin with the letter **S**.

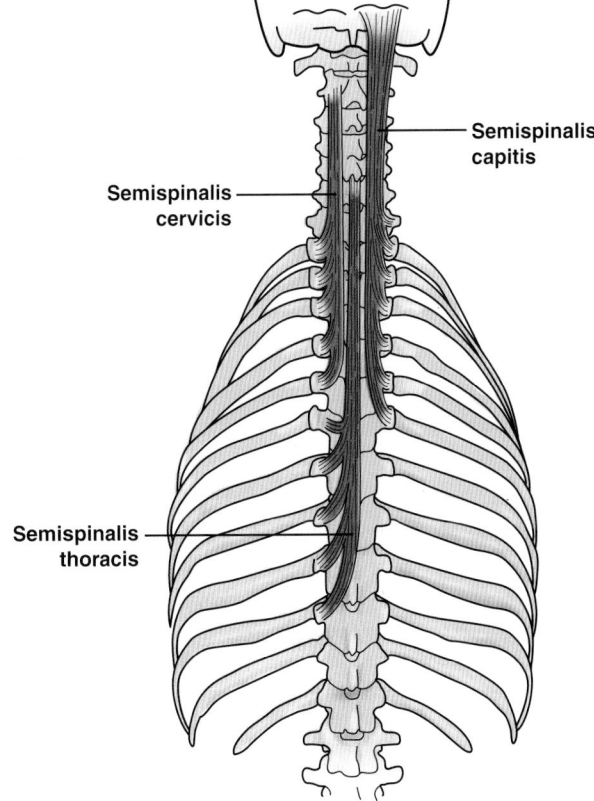

Posterior View

FIG. 21.124 Semispinalis; semispinalis capitis is on the right and semispinalis cervicis/thoracis is on the left. (From Fritz, S., Fritz, L. [2021]. *Mosby's Essential Sciences for Therapeutic Massage.* (6th ed., p 359]. Elsevier Health Sciences (US): Elsevier.)

MULTIFIDUS (FIG. 21.125)

Latin: multus—many
fidus—to split

ORIGINS
Transverse process of one vertebral segment

INSERTIONS
Spinous processes of the second, third, and fourth
   vertebral segments above

ACTIONS
Rotates the vertebral column (unilateral contraction)
Laterally flexes the vertebral column (unilateral contraction)
Extends the vertebral column (bilateral contraction)

NERVES
Posterior rami of spinal nerves

NOTES: Multifidus lies between semispinalis and rotators. It does
not have subgroups. ***LEARNING TIP***: To help you remember the
middle placement of multifidus in relation to other transversospinalis muscles, both **M**ultifidus and **M**iddle begin with the letter **M**.

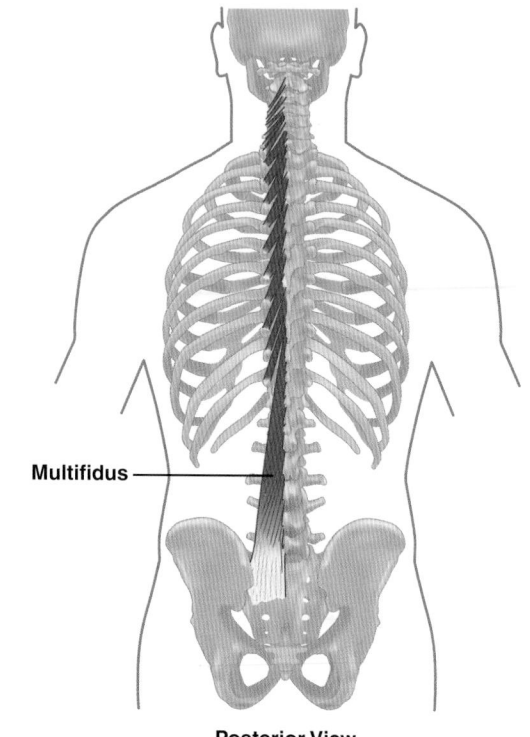

Posterior View

FIG. 21.125 Left multifidus.

ROTATORES (FIG. 21.126)

Latin: rotare—to turn

ORIGINS
Transverse process of one vertebral segment

INSERTIONS
Spinous process of the first or second vertebral segment above

ACTIONS
Rotates the vertebral column

NERVES
Posterior rami of spinal nerves

NOTES: Rotatores are the deepest muscles in the transversospinalis group. They contain two subgroupings: *rotatores longus*
and *rotatores brevis.*

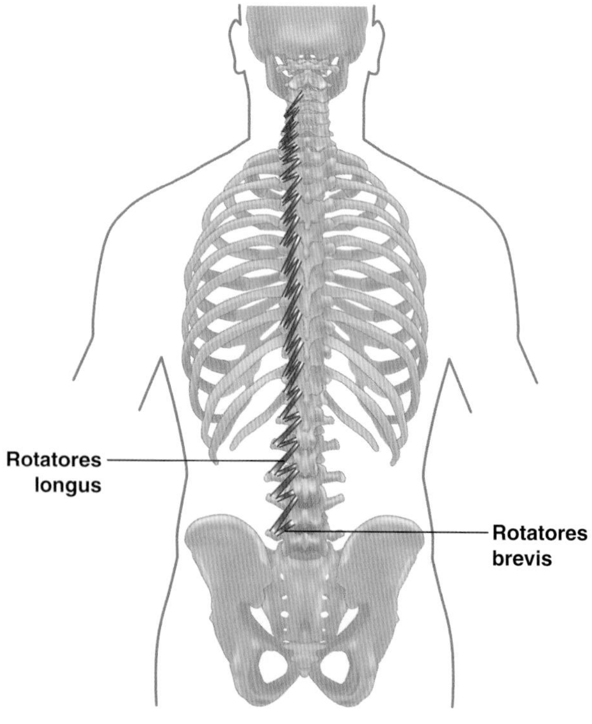

Posterior View

FIG. 21.126 Left rotatores.

ERECTOR SPINAE

Latin: erigere—to erect
spinatus—spine

NOTES: Erector spinae consist of spinalis, longissimus, and iliocostalis. Erector spinae extend vertically up the length of the back, parallel to the spine. ***LEARNING TIP:*** To help you remember the muscles of erector spinae from lateral to medial, use the phrase **I** Love **S**paghetti for **I**liocostalis, **L**ongissimus, and **S**pinalis.

SPINALIS (FIG. 21.127)

Latin: spinatus—spine

ORIGINS
Spinous process of C7 and nuchal ligament
Spinous process of upper lumbar and lower thoracic vertebrae

INSERTIONS
Spinous process of C2–C7
Spinous process of mid-thoracic and lumbar vertebrae

ACTIONS
Laterally flexes the vertebral column (unilateral contraction)
Extends the vertebral column (bilateral contraction)

NERVES
Posterior rami of thoracic and lower cervical spinal nerves

NOTES: Spinalis is the smallest and the most medial muscle of the erector spinae group and lies in the laminar groove. It contains three subgroupings: *spinalis capitis, spinalis cervicis,* and *spinalis thoracis.*

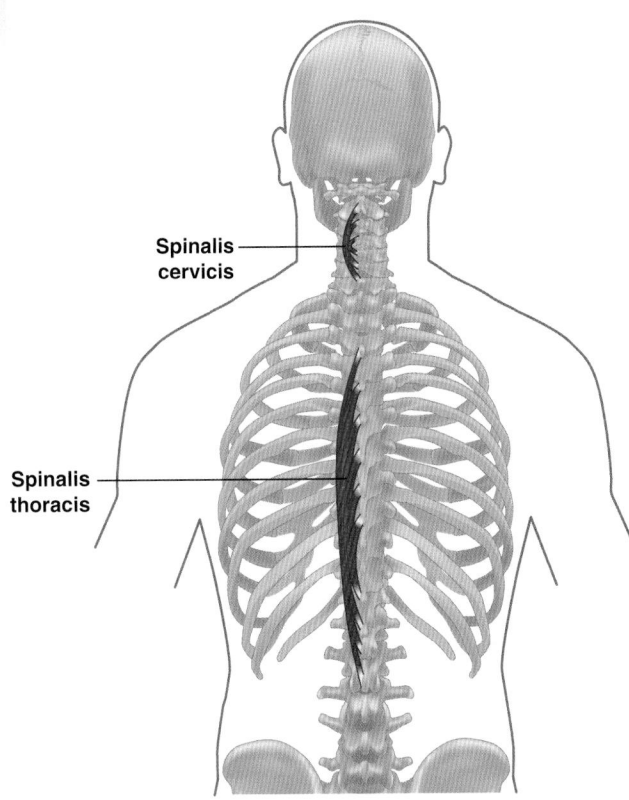

Posterior View

FIG. 21.127 Left spinalis. Spinalis capitis is not shown.

LONGISSIMUS (FIG. 21.128)

Latin: longus—long

ORIGINS
Posterior sacrum
Transverse processes of T1–T5 and L1–L5
Transverse processes of C5–C7

INSERTIONS
Mastoid process
Transverse processes of C2–T12
Ribs 4–12 (posterior surface)

ACTIONS
Laterally flexes the vertebral column (unilateral contraction)
Extends the vertebral column (bilateral contraction)
Extends the head (bilateral contraction)

NERVE
Posterior rami of lumbar, thoracic, and lower cervical spinal nerves

NOTES: Longissimus lies between spinalis and iliocostalis. Longissimus covers a "long" territory, extending from the sacrum to the skull, and contains three subgroupings: *longissimus capitis, longissimus cervicis,* and *longissimus thoracis.*

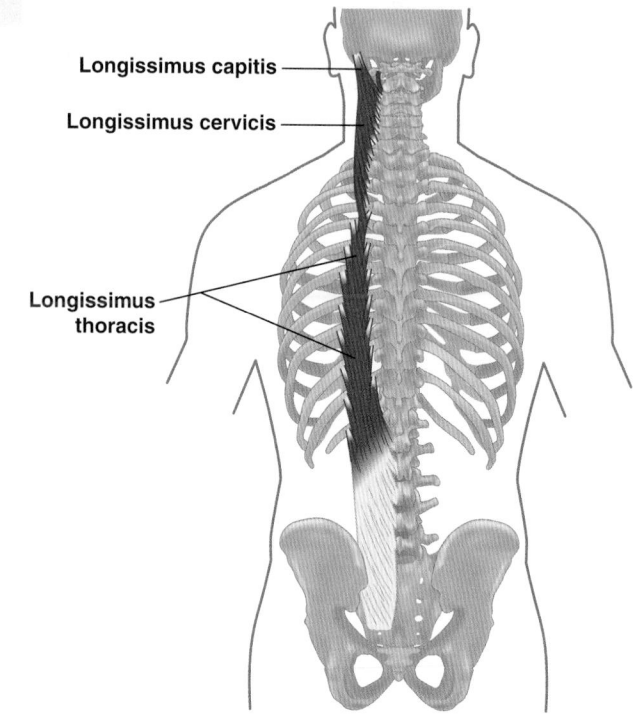

Posterior View

FIG. 21.128 Left longissimus.

ILIOCOSTALIS (FIG. 21.129)

Latin: ilium—flank
costae—rib

ORIGINS
Posterior iliac crest
Posterior sacrum
Ribs 3–12 (posterior surface)

INSERTIONS
Ribs 1–12 (posterior surface)
Transverse processes of C4–C7

ACTIONS
Laterally flexes the vertebral column (unilateral contraction)
Extends the vertebral column (bilateral contraction)

NERVES
Posterior rami of upper lumbar, thoracic, and lower cervical
    spinal nerves

NOTES: Iliocostalis is the lateral muscle of the erector spinae group. Iliocostalis lies over the costals, or ribs, and contains three subgroups: *iliocostalis cervicis, iliocostalis thoracis,* and *iliocostalis lumborum.*

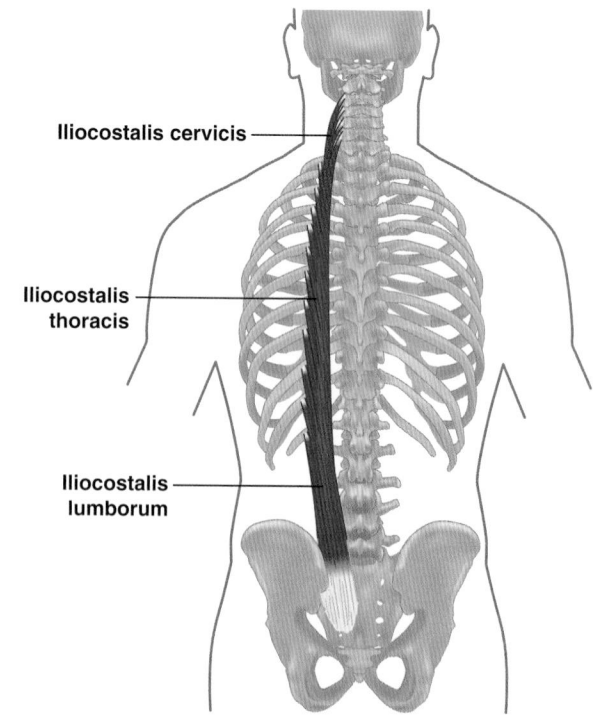

Posterior View

FIG. 21.129 Left iliocostalis.

Lesson Eleven Review: Muscles of Trunk and Vertebral Movement

FLEXION	EXTENSION	LATERAL FLEXION	ROTATION
Psoas major	Quadratus lumborum	Rectus abdominis	External obliques
Rectus abdominis	Semispinalis	External obliques	Internal obliques
External obliques	Multifidus	Internal obliques	Transversospinalis
Internal obliques	Erector spinae	Quadratus lumborum	
		Semispinalis	
		Multifidus	
		Erector spinae	

Lateral views   Anterior view   Posterior view   Anterior view   Posterior view

Lesson Twelve: Muscles of Respiration

Muscles of respiration include the diaphragm, external intercostals, internal intercostals, serratus posterior superior, serratus posterior inferior, pectoralis minor, scalenes, sternocleidomastoid, and the abdominals. Pectoralis minor also moves the scapula; this muscle is featured in Lesson Four. Scalenes and SCM also move the neck; these muscles are featured in Lesson Ten. The abdominals also move the trunk; these muscles are featured in Lesson Eleven (Fig. 21.130).

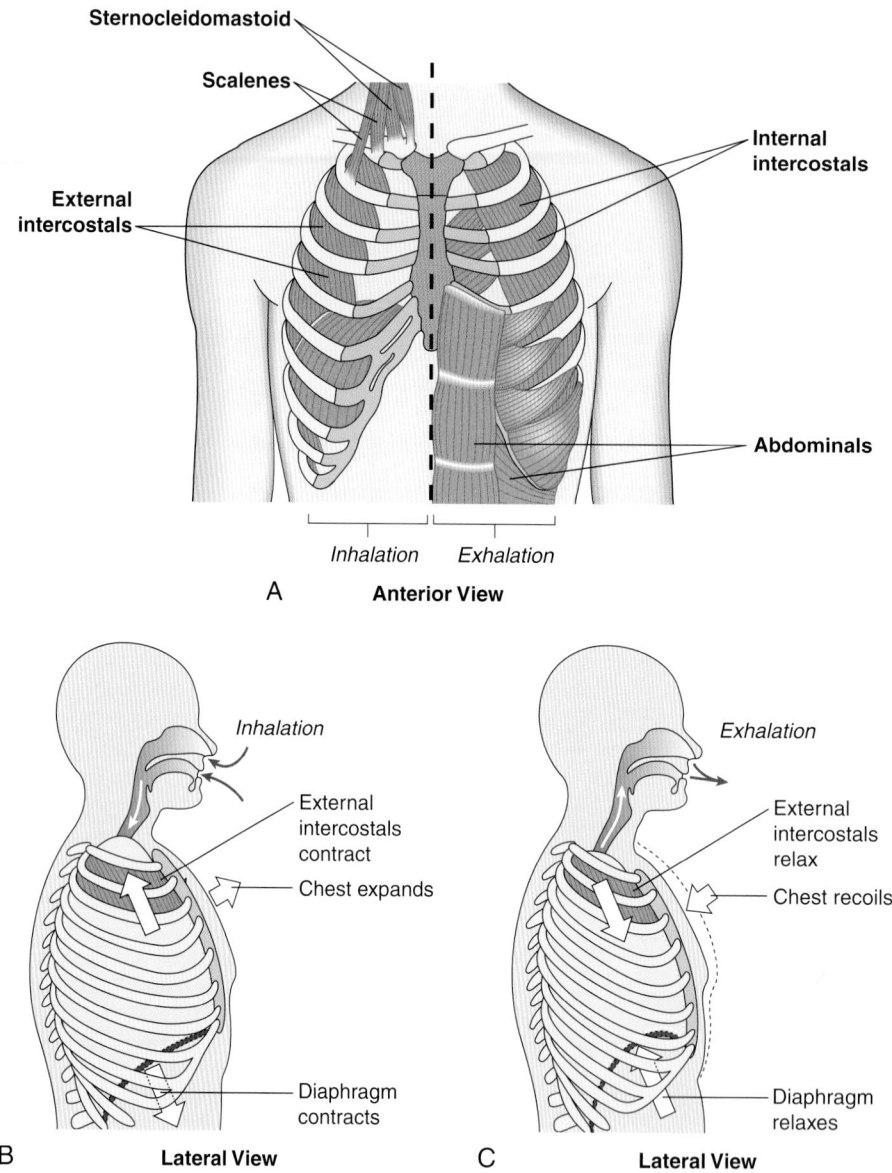

FIG. 21.130 Muscles of respiration with muscles of inhalation (*A, top image; left half*), exhalation (*A, top image; right half*), and thoracic changes featured (*B and C, bottom images*). (From Waugh, A., & Grant, A. [2014]. *Ross and Wilson anatomy and physiology in health and illness* [12th ed.]. Edinburgh, Scotland: Churchill Livingstone.)

DIAPHRAGM (FIG. 21.131)

Greek: diaphragma—a partition

ORIGINS
L1–L3
Ribs 6–12
Xiphoid process of the sternum

INSERTION
Central tendon (cloverleaf-shaped aponeurosis)

ACTION
Descends or moves inferiorly during inhalation, which helps move air into the lungs
Increases intraabdominal pressure

NERVE
Phrenic nerve

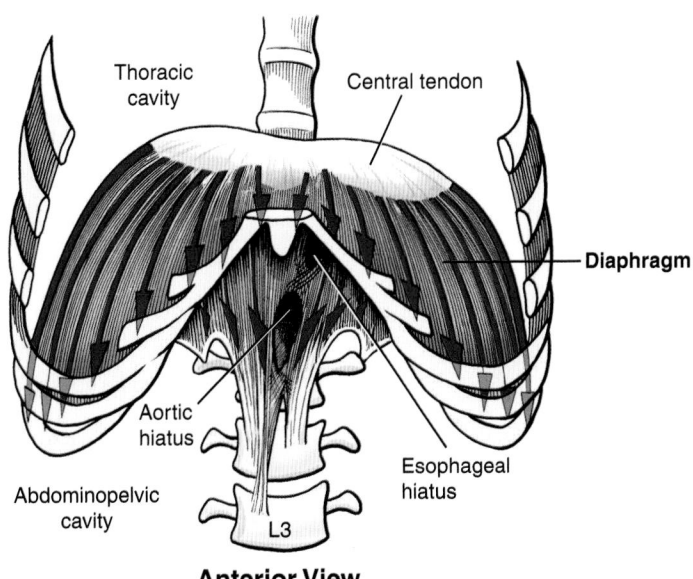

Anterior View

FIG. 21.131 Diaphragm with the esophageal hiatus and the aortic hiatus identified. The caval opening is not shown. The arrows represent the descending or inferior movement of this muscle during inhalation. (From Neumann, D. A. [2017]. *Kinesiology of the musculoskeletal system: Foundations for physical rehabilitation* [3rd ed.]. St Louis: Mosby).

NOTES: The diaphragm is a broad muscle extending across the inferior ribcage that separates the thoracic cavity from the abdominopelvic cavity. The diaphragm contains three openings. The *caval opening* passes through the central tendon and contains the inferior vena cava and the phrenic nerve. The *esophageal hiatus* contains the esophagus. The *aortic hiatus* contains the aorta and the thoracic duct. The diaphragm is also called the *respiratory* or *thoracic diaphragm*.

The diaphragm is the main muscle of respiration. When it contracts and moves in an inferior direction, it increases the volume of the thoracic cavity and helps move air into the lungs to fill the void. The diaphragm is also involved in nonrespiratory movements such as helping to vomit, urinate, defecate, and even push a fetus from the body by increasing intraabdominal pressure.

EXTERNAL INTERCOSTALS (FIG. 21.132)

Latin: externus—outside
internus—within
costae—rib

ORIGINS
Inferior border of rib (above)

INSERTIONS
Superior border of rib (below)

ACTIONS
Elevates the ribcage during inhalation
Maintains the intercostal spaces

NERVES
Intercostal nerves

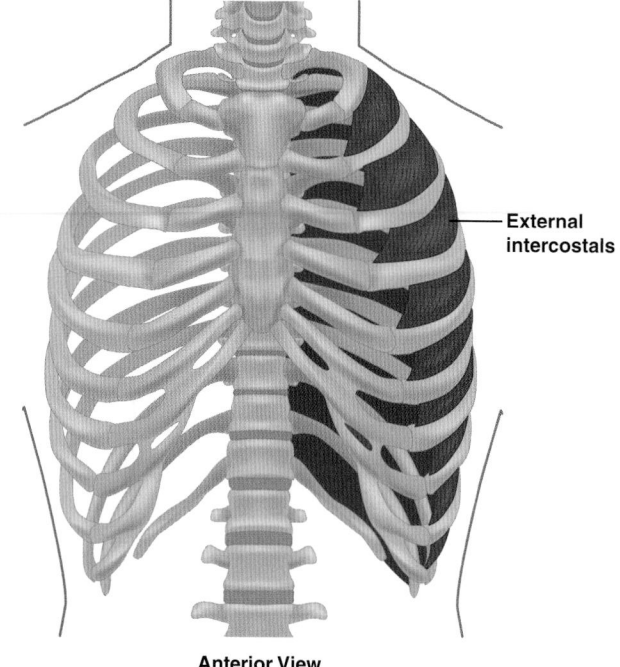

Anterior View

FIG. 21.132 Left external intercostals.

INTERNAL INTERCOSTALS (FIG. 21.133)

Latin: internus—within
costae—rib

ORIGINS
Superior border of rib (below)

INSERTIONS
Inferior border of rib (above)

ACTIONS
Depresses the ribcage during exhalation (forced)
Maintains the intercostal spaces

NERVES
Intercostal nerves

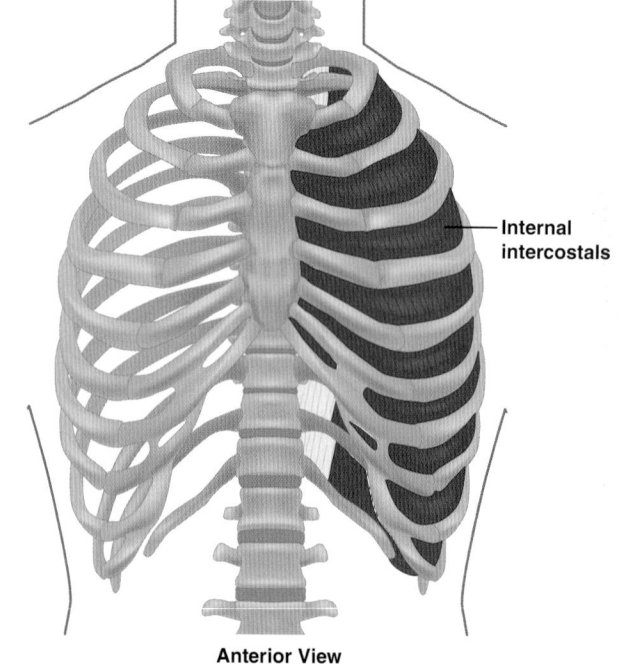

Anterior View

FIG. 21.133 Left internal intercostals.

SERRATUS POSTERIOR SUPERIOR (FIG. 21.134)

Latin: serratus—notched or jagged, as a saw
posterus—behind
superus—upper

ORIGINS
Spinous processes of C7–T3

INSERTIONS
Ribs 2–5 (posterior surface)

ACTION
Elevates the ribs during inhalation

NERVES
Intercostal nerves

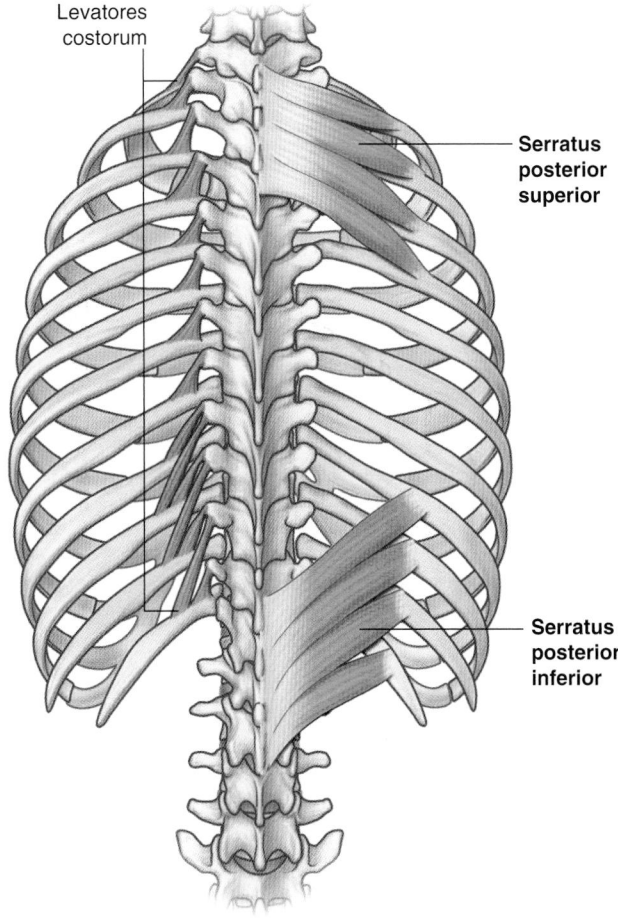

Levatores costorum

Serratus posterior superior

Serratus posterior inferior

Posterior View

NOTES: Serratus posterior superior is deep to the rhomboids.

FIG. 21.134 Right serratus posterior superior, right serratus posterior inferior, and nearby muscles on the left called levatores costorum. These small muscles arise from the transverse processes of C7–T11, insert onto the posterior surfaces of the rib below, and can assist in forceful inhalation. (From Soames, R. W. [2019]. *Anatomy and human movement* [7th ed.]. Philadelphia, PA: Elsevier.)

SERRATUS POSTERIOR INFERIOR (SEE FIG. 21.134)

Latin: serratus—notched or jagged, as a saw
posterus—behind
infra—beneath

ORIGINS
Spinous processes of T11–L2

INSERTIONS
Ribs 9–12 (posterior surface)

ACTION
Depresses the ribs during exhalation

NERVES
Intercostal nerves (T9–T12)

E-RESOURCES

http://evolve.elsevier.com/Salvo/MassageTherapy
- Chapter challenge
- Flash cards

REFERENCES

Centeno, C. (2015). *Knee locking up? Get to know the popliteus muscle*. Retrieved from https://www.regenexx.com/knee-locking-up/.

Hallett, S., & Ashurst, J. V. (2021). *Anatomy, shoulder, and upper limb, hand anatomical snuff box*. Retrieved from https://www.ncbi.nlm.nih.gov/books/NBK482228/.

Herlihy, B. (2018). *The human body in health and illness* (6th ed.). St Louis, MO: Saunders.

Janak, T. (2011). *The Christmas tree muscle: Rhomboids*. Retrieved from http://theweekly-muscle.blogspot.com/2011/12/christmas-tree-muscle-rhomboids.html.

Lippert, L. S. (2006). *Clinical kinesiology and anatomy* (4th ed.). Philadelphia, PA: F. A. Davis Company.

Lung, K., St Lucia, K., & Lui, F. (2020). *Anatomy, thorax, and serratus anterior muscles*.

Retrieved from https://www.ncbi.nlm.nih.gov/books/NBK531457/.

Martin, R. M., & Fish, D. E. (2008). Scapular winging: Anatomical review, diagnosis, and treatments. *Current Reviews in Musculoskeletal Medicine*, *1*(1), 1–11.

Maruvada, S., Madrazo-Ibarra, A., & Varacallo, M. (2021). *Anatomy: Rotator cuff*. Retrieved from https://www.ncbi.nlm.nih.gov/books/NBK441844/

O'Rahilly, R., Müller, F., Carpenter, S., & Swenson, R. (2008). *Basic human anatomy: A regional study of human structure*. Philadelphia, PA: W. B. Saunders Co.

Simons, D. G., Travell, J. G., & Simons, L. S. (1998). *Myofascial pain and dysfunction, the trigger point manual* (2nd ed., Vol. 1.). Baltimore, MD: Lippincott Williams & Wilkins.

Smith, T. O., Nichols, R., Harle, D., & Donell, S. T. (2009). Do the vastus medialis obliquus and vastus medialis longus really exist? A systematic review. *Clinical Anatomy*, *22*(2), 183–99.

Travell, J. G., & Simons, D. G. (1983). *Myofascial pain and dysfunction, the trigger point manual, the upper extremities*. Baltimore, MD: Williams & Wilkins.

Travell, J. G., & Simons, D. G. (1993). *Myofascial pain and dysfunction, the trigger point manual, the lower extremities*. Baltimore, MD: Lippincott Williams & Wilkins.

REVIEW AND APPLY YOUR KNOWLEDGE

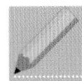

MATCHING ONE: BONES AND JOINTS OF THE UPPER EXTREMITY: CONCEPT

REVIEW *Place the letter of the answer next to the term or phrase that best describes it.*

A. Acromioclavicular joint
B. Clavicle
C. Glenohumeral joint
D. Humerus
E. Phalanges
F. Radiocarpal joint
G. Radius
H. Scaphoid
 I. Scapula
J. Shoulder girdle
K. Sternoclavicular joint
L. Ulna

_____   1. Composed of the clavicle and scapula.
_____   2. Medial forearm bone.
_____   3. Bone containing the supraglenoid and infraglenoid tubercles.
_____   4. Bone containing the deltoid tuberosity.
_____   5. Joint connecting the upper extremity with the axial skeleton.
_____   6. Lateral forearm bone.
_____   7. Shoulder joint.
_____   8. Carpal bone.
_____   9. Joint between the clavicle and the scapula.
_____ 10. Wrist joint.
_____ 11. Most commonly fractured bone.
_____ 12. Bones in the fingers and thumb.

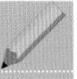

MATCHING TWO: BONES AND JOINTS OF THE LOWER EXTREMITY: CONCEPT

REVIEW *Place the letter of the answer next to the term or phrase that best describes it.*

A. Acetabulofemoral joint
B. Acetabulum
C. Calcaneus
D. Femur
E. Fibula
F. Obturator foramen
G. Patella
H. Sacroiliac joint
 I. Ischium
J. Talocrural joint
K. Tibia
L. Tibiofemoral joint

_____   1. Most inferior and posterior pelvic bone.
_____   2. Ankle joint.
_____   3. Largest sesamoid bone.
_____   4. Lateral leg bone.
_____   5. Bone containing the linea aspera.
_____   6. Deep hip socket made from portions of all three pelvic bones.
_____   7. Joint connecting the lower extremity with the axial skeleton.
_____   8. Tarsal bone.
_____   9. Hip joint.
_____ 10. Medial leg bone.
_____ 11. Knee joint.
_____ 12. Pelvic structure inferior to the acetabulum.

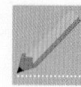

MATCHING THREE: BONES AND JOINTS OF THE AXIAL SKELETON: CONCEPT REVIEW *Place the letter of the answer next to the term or phrase that best describes it.*

A. Atlantooccipital joint
B. Axis
C. Hyoid
D. Intercostal
E. Laminae
F. Intervertebral foramen
G. Sagittal
H. Sternum
I. Sutures
J. Temporomandibular joints
K. Apophyseal joint
L. Zygomatic arch

_____ 1. Suture between the parietal bones.
_____ 2. Space between the ribs.
_____ 3. Bilateral joints of the skull and functions as hinge and gliding joints.
_____ 4. Joint between the skull and the first cervical vertebra.
_____ 5. Section of the vertebral arch at the base of the spinous process to the transverse processes.
_____ 6. Fibrous joints between the cranial bones.
_____ 7. Openings between the pedicles of neighboring vertebrae and allows passage of spinal nerves.
_____ 8. Bone containing the dens.
_____ 9. U-shaped bone between the chin and the thyroid cartilage.
_____ 10. Bone containing the manubrium and the xiphoid process.
_____ 11. Term synonymous with cheek bone.
_____ 12. Joint where one vertebra articulates with another vertebra.

MATCHING FOUR: MUSCLES OF SCAPULAR AND SHOULDER MOVEMENTS: CONCEPT REVIEW *Place the letter of the answer next to the term or phrase that best describes it.*

A. Deltoid
B. Infraspinatus
C. Latissimus dorsi
D. Levator scapulae
E. Pectoralis major
F. Pectoralis minor
G. Rhomboids
H. Rotator cuff
I. Serratus anterior
J. Subscapularis
K. Supraspinatus
L. Trapezius

_____ 1. Forms the posterior axillary folds.
_____ 2. Attaches to the transverse processes of C1–C4.
_____ 3. Forms the anterior axillary folds.
_____ 4. Attaches to the lesser tubercle of the humerus; rotator cuff muscle.
_____ 5. Muscle involved with "winged scapula."
_____ 6. Attaches to the external occipital protuberance, superior nuchal line, nuchal ligament, and spinous processes of C7–T12.
_____ 7. Externally rotates the humerus; rotator cuff muscle.
_____ 8. Attaches to the coracoid process.
_____ 9. Only rotator cuff muscle that does not rotate the humerus.
_____ 10. Attaches to the deltoid tuberosity.
_____ 11. Collective term for supraspinatus, infraspinatus, teres minor, and subscapularis.
_____ 12. Attaches to the medial border of the scapula; retracts the scapula.

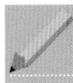 **MATCHING FIVE: MUSCLES OF ELBOW, RADIOULNAR JOINT, WRIST, AND HAND MOVEMENTS: CONCEPT REVIEW** *Place the letter of the answer next to the term or phrase that best describes it.*

A. Coracoid process of the scapula
B. Anatomic snuffbox
C. Biceps brachii
D. Brachialis
E. Infraglenoid tubercle of the scapula
F. Anconeus
G. Extensor indicis
H. Hypothenar eminence
I. Medial epicondyle of the humerus
J. Pronator teres and pronator quadratus
K. Thenar eminence
L. Triceps brachii

_____ 1. Corkscrew muscle.
_____ 2. Muscles that pronate the forearm.
_____ 3. Attaches to the olecranon process and the lateral epicondyle of the humerus.
_____ 4. Boxer's muscle.
_____ 5. Fleshy bulge at the base of the fifth digit formed by flexor digiti minimi, abductor digiti minimi, and opponens digiti minimi.
_____ 6. Attachment for most wrist flexors.
_____ 7. Attachment for the long head of triceps brachii.
_____ 8. Workhorse elbow flexor.
_____ 9. Attachment for the short head of biceps brachii.
_____ 10. Muscle extending the second finger.
_____ 11. Fleshy bulge at the base of the thumb formed by flexor pollicis brevis, opponens pollicis, and abductor pollicis brevis.
_____ 12. Triangular depression on the back of the hand at the base of the thumb.

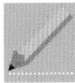 **MATCHING SIX: MUSCLES OF HIP, KNEE, ANKLE, AND FOOT MOVEMENTS: CONCEPT REVIEW** *Place the letter of the answer next to the term or phrase that best describes it.*

A. Calcaneus via the Achilles tendon
B. Biceps femoris
C. Fibularis longus and tibialis anterior
D. Gastrocnemius
E. Hamstrings
F. Iliotibial band
G. Pes anserinus
H. Piriformis
I. Popliteus
J. Iliopsoas
K. Quadriceps femoris
L. Sartorius

_____ 1. Tailor's muscle.
_____ 2. Attaches to the lesser trochanter.
_____ 3. Attaches to the medial and lateral epicondyles of the femur.
_____ 4. Thickened fascial band on the lateral thigh.
_____ 5. Key that unlocks the knee.
_____ 6. Muscles that attach to the medial cuneiform and the first metatarsal.
_____ 7. Muscle group attaching to the ischial tuberosity.
_____ 8. Lateral hip rotator attaching to the anterior sacrum.
_____ 9. Common attachment of gastrocnemius, plantaris, and soleus.
_____ 10. Hamstring muscle attaching to the fibula.
_____ 11. Muscle group attaching to the tibial tuberosity.
_____ 12. Three conjoined tendons attaching to the medial proximal tibial shaft.

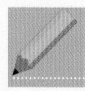

MATCHING SEVEN: MUSCLES OF NECK, FACIAL, TRUNK, AND VERTEBRAL COLUMN MOVEMENTS: CONCEPT REVIEW *Place the letter of the answer next to the term or phrase that best describes it.*

A. Galea aponeurotica
B. Orbicularis oculi
C. Platysma
D. Quadratus lumborum
E. Rectus abdominis
F. Scalenes
G. Semispinalis, rotatores, and multifidus
H. Spinalis, longissimus, and iliocostalis
I. Sternocleidomastoid
J. Suboccipitals
K. Temporalis
L. Temporalis, masseter, medial, and lateral pterygoids

_____ 1. Attaches to rib 12 and the posterior iliac crest.
_____ 2. Sphincter-type muscle encircling the eye.
_____ 3. Pouting muscle.
_____ 4. Headache ghosts.
_____ 5. Can entrap the brachial plexus.
_____ 6. Passes beneath the zygomatic arch before attaching to the coronoid process.
_____ 7. Attachment for occipitofrontalis.
_____ 8. Erector spinae muscles.
_____ 9. Muscles of mastication.
_____ 10. Transversospinalis muscles.
_____ 11. Muscle containing tendinous intersections.
_____ 12. Primary landmark of the neck, dividing it into anterior and posterior cervical triangles.

MATCHING EIGHT: MUSCLES OF RESPIRATION: CONCEPT REVIEW *Place the letter of the answer next to the term or phrase that best describes it.*

A. Aortic hiatus
B. Phrenic nerve
C. Lower six ribs, L1–L3, and the xiphoid process
D. External intercostals
E. Inferior border of rib
F. Central tendon
G. Internal intercostals
H. Serratus posterior superior
I. Caval opening
J. Serratus posterior inferior
K. Diaphragm
L. Esophageal hiatus

_____ 1. Main muscle of respiration.
_____ 2. Elevates the ribcage during inhalation and maintains intercostal spaces.
_____ 3. Diaphragmatic passageway for the inferior vena cava and the phrenic nerve.
_____ 4. Muscle originating on the spinous processes of C7-T3 and is deep to the rhomboids.
_____ 5. Origin of external intercostals.
_____ 6. Origins of the diaphragm.
_____ 7. Diaphragmatic passageway that does not contain blood vessels.
_____ 8. Innervates the diaphragm.
_____ 9. Depresses the ribcage during forced exhalation and maintains intercostal spaces.
_____ 10. Attaches to T11–L2 and ribs 9–12.
_____ 11. Insertion for the diaphragm.
_____ 12. Diaphragmatic passageway for the aorta and the thoracic duct.

MULTIPLE CHOICE ONE: TEST YOUR KNOWLEDGE: BONES AND JOINTS

Place the letter of the answer next to the term or phrase that best describes it.

_____ 1. On which bone would you find an acromial end?
   A. Scapula
   B. Clavicle
   C. Humerus
   D. Sternum

_____ 2. Which bone rotates during pronation?
   A. Humerus
   B. Hamate
   C. Radius
   D. Ulna

_____ 3. What is the anatomical term for the tip of the elbow?
   A. Capitulum
   B. Olecranon
   C. Capitate
   D. Trapezium

_____ 4. Which joint is classified as ball-and-socket?
   A. Acromioclavicular
   B. Radioulnar
   C. Carpometacarpal
   D. Glenohumeral

_____ 5. On which bone would you find the greater trochanter?
   A. Humerus
   B. Femur
   C. Radius
   D. Tibia

_____ 6. Which of these are known as the "sitz bones?"
   A. Ilium
   B. Ischium
   C. Pubis
   D. Sacrum

_____ 7. What is the most commonly injured knee ligament?
   A. Anterior cruciate ligament
   B. Posterior cruciate ligament
   C. Medial collateral ligament
   D. Lateral collateral ligament

_____ 8. On which bone would you find the soleal line?
   A. Femur
   B. Tibia
   C. Fibula
   D. Patella

_____ 9. Which is the suture that is between the frontal bone and the parietal bones?
   A. Sagittal
   B. Coronal
   C. Lambdoidal
   D. Squamosal

_____ 10. On which bone would you find the sella turcica?
   A. Temporal
   B. Ethmoid
   C. Occipital
   D. Sphenoid

_____ 11. True ribs contain how many pairs?
   A. 5
   B. 6
   C. 7
   D. 12

_____ 12. The thoracic region contains _____ vertebrae.
   A. 3
   B. 5
   C. 7
   D. 12

MULTIPLE CHOICE TWO: TEST YOUR KNOWLEDGE: MUSCLES OF THE UPPER EXTREMITIES

Place the letter of the answer next to the term or phrase that best describes it.

_____ 1. Which muscle can be an antagonist to itself?
   A. Trapezius
   B. Rhomboids
   C. Levator scapulae
   D. Serratus anterior

_____ 2. Which muscle retracts the scapula?
   A. Levator scapulae
   B. Rhomboids
   C. Serratus anterior
   D. Pectoralis minor

_____ 3. Which is a "boxer's muscle?"
   A. Levator scapulae
   B. Rhomboid major
   C. Serratus anterior
   D. Pectoralis minor

_____ 4. Which muscle attaches to the sacrum and the humerus?
   A. Supraspinatus
   B. Infraspinatus
   C. Teres major
   D. Latissimus dorsi

_____ 5. Which rotator cuff muscle may be involved with "frozen shoulder"?
   A. Supraspinatus
   B. Infraspinatus
   C. Teres minor
   D. Subscapularis

_____ 6. Angina-like pain can be attributed to excessive tension in the:
   A. Pectoralis major
   B. Pectoralis minor
   C. Levator scapulae
   D. Latissimus dorsi

_____ 7. The radial pulse can be found between the tendons of the flexor carpi radialis and the:
   A. Brachialis
   B. Brachioradialis
   C. Anconeus
   D. Supinator

_____ 8. Which muscle flexes both the shoulder and the elbow?
   A. Biceps brachii
   B. Triceps brachii
   C. Brachialis
   D. Brachioradialis

_____ 9. Which muscle is a synergist to the pronator quadratus?
   A. Anconeus
   B. Pronator teres
   C. Supinator
   D. Teres minor

_____ 10. Golfer's elbow is another term for:
A. Medial epicondylitis
B. Lateral epicondylitis
C. Carpal tunnel syndrome
D. Thoracic outlet syndrome

_____ 11. "Pollicis" means:
A. Forearm
B. Wrist
C. Pinky toe
D. Thumb

_____ 12. Which attaches to the hook of hamate?
A. Transverse carpal ligament
B. Sacrotuberous ligament
C. Deltoid ligament
D. Anterior cruciate ligament

MULTIPLE CHOICE THREE: TEST YOUR KNOWLEDGE: MUSCLES OF THE LOWER EXTREMITIES _Place the letter of the answer next to the term or phrase that best describes it._

_____ 1. Which muscle attaches to the lumbar vertebrae and the lesser trochanter?
A. Psoas major
B. Iliacus
C. Piriformis
D. Pectineus

_____ 2. What is the strongest hip extender?
A. Piriformis
B. Gluteus maximus
C. Quadratus femoris
D. Iliacus

_____ 3. Which is NOT a lateral hip rotator?
A. Quadratus lumborum
B. Quadratus femoris
C. Obturator internus
D. Obturator externus

_____ 4. Which attaches to the iliotibial band?
A. Gluteus medius
B. Gluteus minimus
C. Quadratus femoris
D. Tensor fasciae latae

_____ 5. Which adductor muscle attaches to the ischial tuberosity?
A. Gracilis
B. Pectineus
C. Adductor magnus
D. Adductor longus

_____ 6. What adductor muscle is part of the pes anserinus?
A. Adductor magnus
B. Adductor longus
C. Gracilis
D. Pectineus

_____ 7. Which quadricep muscle flexes the hip?
A. Rectus femoris
B. Vastus intermedius
C. Vastus medialis
D. Vastus lateralis

_____ 8. Which is a hamstring muscle?
A. Biceps brachii
B. Biceps femoris
C. Quadratus femoris
D. Quadratus lumborum

_____ 9. Which muscles attach to an interosseous membrane?
A. Fibularis longus
B. Fibularis brevis
C. Gastrocnemius
D. Tibialis posterior

_____ 10. Which is a "stirrup muscle?"
A. Tibialis anterior
B. Tibialis posterior
C. Fibularis brevis
D. Fibularis tertius

_____ 11. Which is the "toe dancer's muscle?"
A. Gastrocnemius
B. Soleus
C. Plantaris
D. Sartorius

_____ 12. Which muscle extends the big toe?
A. Plantaris
B. Soleus
C. Flexor hallucis longus
D. Extensor hallucis longus

MULTIPLE CHOICE FOUR: TEST YOUR KNOWLEDGE: MUSCLES OF THE HEAD AND TRUNK _Place the letter of the answer next to the term or phrase that best describes it._

_____ 1. Which muscle protrudes the lips?
A. Occipitofrontalis
B. Orbicularis oculi
C. Orbicularis oris
D. Platysma

_____ 2. What muscle attaches to the sphenoid bone?
A. Medial pterygoid
B. Levator scapulae
C. Temporalis
D. Masseter

_____ 3. The sternocleidomastoid is the mirror image of:
A. Rectus capitis posterior major
B. Rectus capitis posterior minor
C. Splenius cervicis
D. Splenius capitis

_____ 4. Torticollis is a condition that occurs with _____ spasms.
A. Suboccipital
B. Temporalis
C. Sternocleidomastoid
D. Masseter

_____ 5. Which is a masticatory muscle?
A. Suboccipitals
B. Temporalis
C. Platysma
D. Frontalis

_____ 6. Which can cause thoracic outlet syndrome-like symptoms when they are tense?
A. Suboccipitals
B. Scalenes
C. Hamstrings
D. Adductors

_____ 7. On which muscle would you find the linea alba?
A. Rectus abdominis
B. Transverse abdominis
C. External obliques
D. Internal obliques

_____ 8. What is the "hip hiker muscle?"
   A. Quadratus femoris
   B. Quadratus lumborum
   C. Rectus femoris
   D. Rectus abdominis

_____ 9. Which is the most superficial transversospinalis muscle?
   A. Piriformis
   B. Semispinalis
   C. Rotatores
   D. Multifidus

_____ 10. Which muscle extends from the sacrum to the skull?
   A. Spinalis
   B. Iliocostalis
   C. Latissimus dorsi
   D. Longissimus

_____ 11. Which muscle attaches to the spinous processes of T11-L2 and ribs 9-12?
   A. External intercostals
   B. Iliocostalis
   C. Serratus posterior inferior
   D. Serratus anterior

_____ 12. Which direction does the diaphragm move in when it contracts?
   A. Inferior
   B. Superior
   C. Medial
   D. Lateral

CRITICAL THINKING

So Many Muscles!

Monique and Sam have been attending massage school for a while and are now studying kinesiology. Monique is very flustered. She had no idea there were so many muscles in the body and there would be a dizzying amount of information for each one—not to mention the agonist and antagonist pairs. Sam, however, doesn't seem to be too upset about learning the muscles. Monique is dumbfounded about this and asks Sam what his secret is to learning muscles without going crazy. What steps is Sam most likely using to learn muscles?

Answers can include but are not limited to:

To understand muscle actions, you need to know where they attach and which joints they cross. The action of a muscle occurs when its insertion, or "I," moves toward its origin, or "O." The following information is helpful when learning muscle actions:

- Origins are generally medial or proximal to their insertions.
- Muscles on the anterior side of the trunk and the upper extremity generally create flexion.
- Muscles on the posterior side of the lower extremity generally create flexion.
- Muscles on the posterior side of the trunk and the upper extremity generally create extension.
- Muscles on the anterior side of the lower extremity generally create extension.
- Muscles on the medial side of the body generally create adduction.

- Muscles on the lateral side of the body generally create abduction.
- Muscles with fibers running superior to inferior generally create flexion or extension.
- Muscles with oblique running fibers generally create rotation.
- If a muscle crosses two joints, it acts on both joints.
- Most muscles have at least two actions (primary action and secondary action).
- Prime movers and antagonists are generally opposite each other.

Muscle names are usually derived from Latin or Greek words. A muscle's attachment sites can be used to name muscles. A muscle can be named by the number of origins or heads. The number is usually listed first, followed by the region of the body where these muscles are located. Muscles are named for their shape and size, or for their actions or functions. A muscle's primary action is usually listed first, followed by where the action takes place. Finally, muscles are named using a combination of these methods. Organizing movements of major muscles into a table format is helpful for some students.

Movements	Agonists/Prime Movers	Antagonists
Neck Flexion	Sternocleidomastoid	Trapezius
Trunk Extension	Erector Spinae	Rectus Abdominis
Scapula Retraction	Rhomboids	Serratus Anterior
Shoulder Flexion	Pectoralis Major	Latissimus Dorsi
Shoulder External/ Lateral Rotation	Infraspinatus/Teres Minor	Subscapularis
Shoulder Abduction	Supraspinatus/ Middle Deltoid	Latissimus Doris
Elbow Extension	Triceps Brachii/ Anconeus	Biceps Brachii/ Brachialis
Forearm Supination	Supinator/Biceps Brachii	Pronator Teres/ Pronator Quadratus
Hip Extension	Gluteus Maximus	Iliopsoas
Hip Adduction	Adductor Magnus	Gluteus Medius/ Gluteus Minimus
Knee Flexion	Hamstrings	Quadriceps
Plantar Flexion	Gastrocnemius/ Soleus	Tibialis Anterior
Inversion	Tibialis Anterior	Fibularis Longus/ Fibularis Brevis

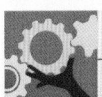

PROFESSIONAL PRACTICE

Heal the Pain

Erik completed a continuing education course in clinical massage a month ago. Jackie, one of Erik's regular clients, is scheduled for a 90-minute massage today. When Jackie arrives, she appears agitated and is rubbing a sore neck. Erik notices postural imbalances in her lower extremity. Jackie explains it has been a difficult week and all she wants is to slip away while Erik provides a relaxation massage. Erik begins to explain what he has learned, and he thinks massage targeting her neck pain is more beneficial.

How should Erik proceed? What consequences may result if Erik assesses her posture and does a clinical massage even though Jackie does not seem overly interested? If Erik decides to do clinical massage, could it also address the goals of relaxation? If Erik does a relaxation massage, which massage techniques should he use and which should he avoid?

DISCUSSION

Myofascial Release Techniques

How effective are myofascial release techniques compared with other massage techniques? Conduct a brief research on myofascial release to locate a definition, history, basic techniques, case reports, or studies. Pay special attention to randomized control trials and systematic reviews. If available, post your reflections on an internet-based discussion board monitored by your instructor.

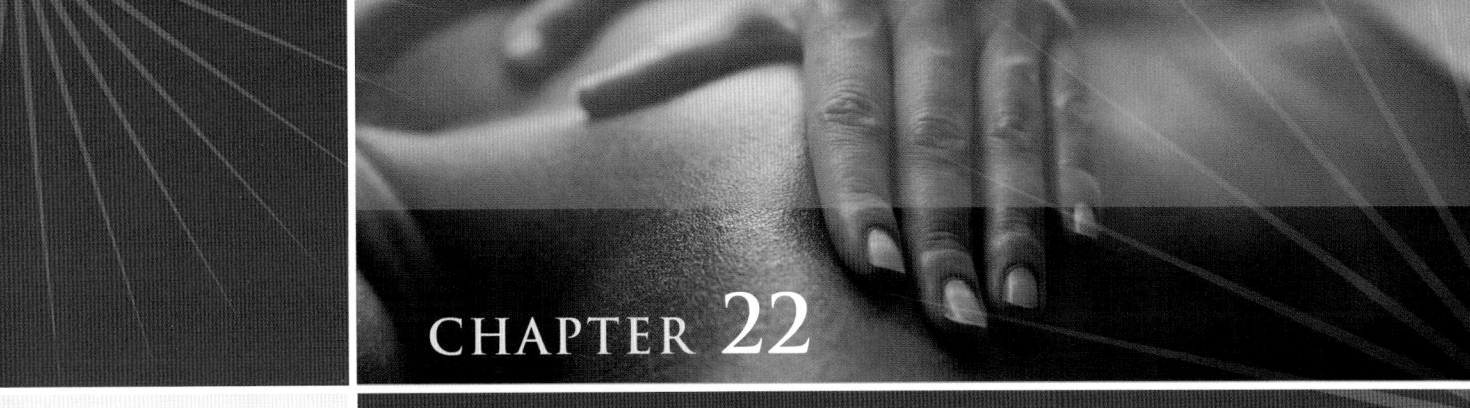

CHAPTER 22

Integumentary System, Pathologies, Conditions, and Injuries

The skin is no more separate from the brain than the surface of a lake is separate from its depths. They are two different locations in a continuous medium. To touch the surface is to stir the depths.

—Deane Juhan

LEARNING OBJECTIVES

After completing this chapter, the student should be able to:

1. List anatomic structures and physiologic processes related to the integumentary system, and describe the epidermis, dermis, and subcutaneous layer.
2. Discuss skin color, hair, nails, skin glands, thermoregulation, and skin receptors.
3. Describe dermatologic pathologies, conditions, and injuries and state their massage modifications.

INTRODUCTION

The integumentary system includes the skin and its appendages such as hair, nails, and glands. The integumentary system is the largest and heaviest organ system, making up 7% of the body's weight. The skin is our contact with the external environment and receives much personal attention. No other organ system is scrubbed, polished, or covered with products such as lotions, cremes, and gels compared with skin. Hair is cut, colored, and styled; nails are trimmed and painted.

Skin is a self-repairing and protective barrier between the internal and external environments. Natural openings, such as the mouth, nose, urethra, vagina, and anus, create passageways to the digestive, respiratory, urinary, and reproductive systems. Although the integumentary system is more easily exposed to infections, disease, pollution, or injury than any other system, it also is one of the body's defenses against these affronts. Skin is strong and flexible and permits a wide variety of changes as we move.

The appearance of the skin reflects the inner workings of our organs and cellular processes. Information about nutrition, hygiene habits, circulation, age, immunity, genetics, and environmental factors can be noted from the skin. Not only does skin reveal possible pathology (e.g., fever), but it also mirrors our thoughts and emotions through nerve impulses and muscle contractions. What we think and how we feel are often reflected on the surface of the skin. The skin is assessed by massage practitioners, noting areas flushed, warm, swollen, cyanotic, pale, or containing lesions, which may denote contraindications.

Skin is classified as a cutaneous membrane. *Dermatology* is the study of the integumentary system. See Table 22.1 to help you understand the terms associated with the integumentary system.

Skin is composed of two regions: the epidermis and dermis. An epidermal-dermal junction joins these two regions together. The subcutaneous tissue layer is beneath the skin and attaches the skin to underlying muscles and bones.

ANATOMY

The basic anatomy of the integumentary system is:
- Skin
- Hair
- Nails
- Glands

PHYSIOLOGY

Important functions of the integumentary system are:
- Protection—Skin acts as a physical barrier and protects underlying tissues. Skin also provides limited protection from ultraviolet (UV) radiation such as found in sunlight through the darkening effects of melanin produced by *melanocytes*.

TABLE 22.1 Word Meanings

WORD	MEANING
Acne vulgaris	*Gr.* point; common or ordinary common acne
Boil	*AS.* sore
Bruise	*O. Fr.* to break
Corium	*L.* leather, skin
Cutaneous	*L.* skin
Cuticle	*L.* little skin
Decubitus	*L.* lying down
Dermis	*Gr.* skin
Eczema	*L.* to boil out
Epidermis	*Gr.* upon or over skin
Follicle	*L.* sac, small
Granulosum	*L.* grain, small
Integument	*L.* a covering
Krause	German anatomist (1833–1910)
Lacrimal	*L.* tear
Lucidum	*L.* clear
Meissner	German histologist (1829–1905)
Melano	*Gr.* black
Pacini	Italian anatomist (1812–1883)
Palpate	*L.* stroke or touch
Psoriasis	*Gr.* itching
Ruffini	Italian anatomist (1864–1929)
Scleroderma	*Gr.* hard, skin
Seborrhea	*L.* tallow, to flow
Sebum	*L.* grease, tallow
Stratum	*L.* a layer, cover, or spread
Sudoriferous	*L.* sweat, to carry or bear
Verruca	*L.* wart

AS., Anglo Saxon; *Fr.,* French; *Gr.,* Greek; *L.,* Latin; *O.Fr.,* Old French.

- Immunity—Skin acts as a biologic and chemical barrier through immunologic responses. As a biologic barrier, intact skin resists pathogenic invasion. Skin secretions (oil and sweat) combine to form an *acid mantle,* a slightly acidic film that acts as a chemical barrier to bacteria, viruses, and other potentially harmful agents that might penetrate the skin. Epidermal cells stimulate immunologic responses when skin is damaged.
- Absorption—Skin has limited properties of absorption. Substances absorbed by skin are fat-soluble molecules (e.g., oxygen, carbon dioxide), fat-soluble vitamins (e.g., A, D, E, K), steroids, resins of certain plants (e.g., poison ivy, poison oak), and salts of heavy metals (e.g., lead, mercury, nickel). The use of medicated patches is based on the absorptive properties of skin.
- Sensation—Skin is a sophisticated sensory organ and houses receptors for touch, pressure, and temperature.
- Temperature regulation—Skin plays a role in temperature regulation through changes in blood flow and activity of sweat glands.
- Excretion—Skin plays a minor role in excretion through the elimination of water, salt, and wastes such as urea through sweating.
- Vitamin D synthesis—Skin helps synthesize vitamin D, a nutrient necessary for the absorption of calcium by the gastrointestinal tract.

EPIDERMIS

The **epidermis** is the thin outer region of skin and is composed of epithelial tissue. The epidermis itself is relatively avascular; therefore nutrients are provided by tissue fluids from the underlying dermis. The epidermis contains small openings, which allow the passage of hair and products from skin glands to the surface of the skin. The epidermis is derived from *ectoderm,* the same embryonic cell layer that becomes the brain, spinal cord, and special senses.

Epidermal Layers

The epidermis contains several layers. These are featured next from the deepest to the most superficial layer (Fig. 22.1).

- **Stratum Basale.** This is the deepest layer and where cells develop, grow, and divide. The stratum basale is so named because it adheres to the basement membrane, a membrane that connects the epidermis to the dermis below. The stratum basale is also called the *stratum germinativum* or "growth layer."
- **Stratum Spinosum.** The next layer is the stratum spinosum and nicknamed the "spiny layer" because it contains slender or spiny projections. These projections connect this layer to the stratum granulosum, which is the layer above.
- **Stratum Granulosum.** This layer is where keratinization occurs, giving it a granular appearance. More about keratinization in the next section.

- **Stratum Lucidum.** This layer is translucent and only present in the thick skin of the palms and soles.
- **Stratum Corneum.** This is the most superficial epidermal layer and is nicknamed the "horny layer" because its cells are toughened like an animal's horn.

When epidermal cells reach the surface of the stratum corneum, they are completely keratinized, dead, and begin to slough off, or *desquamate.* Cells in the stratum basale are forming at approximately the same rate as cells in the stratum corneum are sloughing off, which allows the skin to maintain a constant thickness. This entire process occurs approximately every 21 to 27 days over the person's lifetime. ***LEARNING TIP:*** To help remember the names of the epidermal layers, use the phrase Babies Smell Good Like Cookies for Stratum Basale—Spinosum—Granulosum—Lucidum—Corneum.

Epidermal Cells

The epidermis contains several cells including keratinocytes, melanocytes, and dendritic or Langerhans cells.

- **Keratinocytes.** Keratinocytes constitute 90% of all cells in the epidermis. As new keratinocytes are produced in the stratum basale, they push older keratinocytes toward the skin's surface. Older keratinocytes receive fewer nutrients, stop dividing, and begin to die. During this process, they secrete **keratin,** which mixes with skin oils and forms an *epidermal water barrier,* essentially waterproofing and preventing dehydration from the loss of body water.

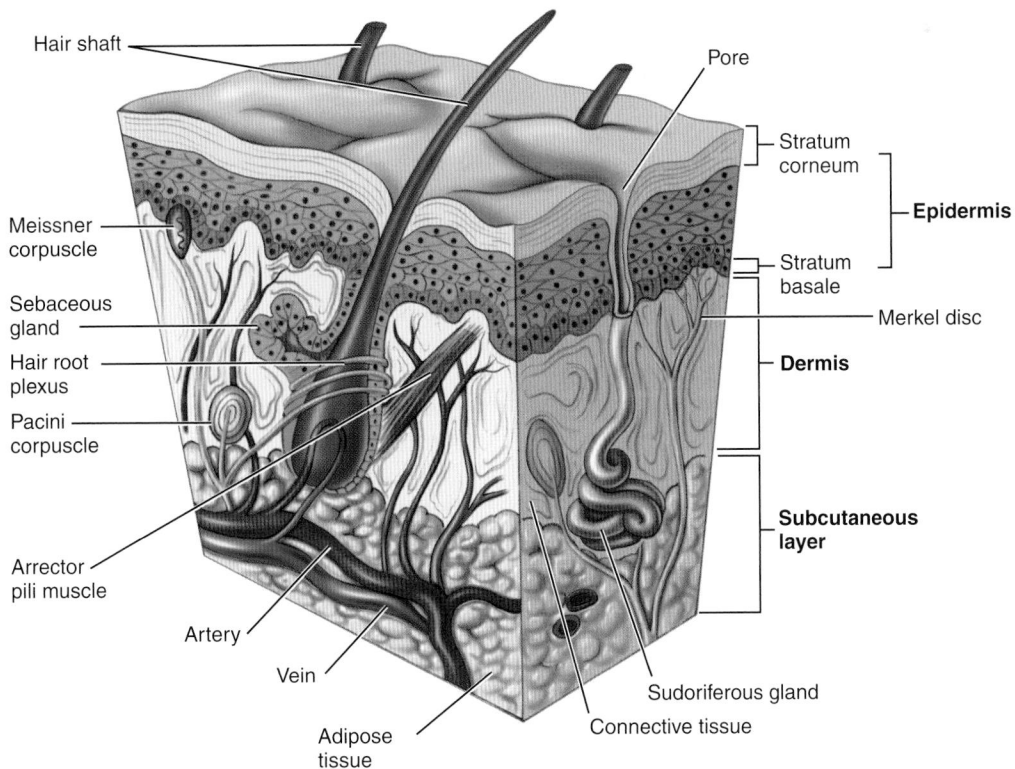

FIG. 22.1 Microscopic cross-section view of the skin with its regions and structures. (Modified from Herlihy, H. [2011]. *The human body in health and disease* [4th ed.]. St. Louis: Mosby; Elsevier..)

- **Melanocytes.** Approximately one-fourth of cells in the stratum basale are melanocytes, which produce a brown or black pigment called **melanin**. All individuals have the same distribution of melanocytes, but the amount of melanin produced differs according to genetics, ethnicity, hormones, and environmental factors, including exposure to sunlight. Melanin production stimulated by sunlight darkens the skin, creating a semiprotective shield against UV radiation in sunlight. Melanocytes are also found in hair and the iris and retina of the eyes.
- **Dendritic (Langerhans) Cells.** Dendritic cells stimulate immunologic responses when skin is injured or invaded by pathogens.

Epidermal-Dermal Junction

Between the epidermis and the dermis is the epidermal-dermal junction. These two regions are separated by a basement membrane. The epidermal-dermal junction also provides support for the epidermis and nutrient exchange between the two regions.

DERMIS

The **dermis** is the thick, deeper region, or "true skin." The dermis is derived from *mesoderm,* the same embryonic cell layer that gives rise to muscles and connective tissue. Connective tissue within the dermis is mainly collagen and elastin. Collagen constitutes approximately 70% to 90% of the dermis and offers structural support to nerves, blood vessels, hair follicles, muscles, and glands. Elastin constitutes approximately 10% of the dermis and gives skin its pliability and resiliency. These two proteins work together to give skin its shape and firmness—collagen provides rigidity and elastin allows stretch.

Dermal Growth and Repair

Cells within the dermis do not continually grow and shed as cells do in the epidermis. However, when the dermis is injured, fibroblasts quickly form a dense collection of new connective tissue called a *scar.* If elastic fibers in the dermis are overstretched, such as skin over the abdomen during advanced pregnancy, these fibers may weaken and tear, resulting in a *stretch mark.* See the "Dermatologic Pathologies, Conditions, and Injuries" section for more information.

SUBCUTANEOUS LAYER

The subcutaneous layer is deeper into the dermis and is not a true layer of skin, but anchors skin to the underlying structures. It is also called the *hypodermis* or *superficial fascia.* When this layer extends inward and surrounds deeper structures, it is called *deep fascia.* The subcutaneous layer consists of loose connective tissue, including adipose tissue as well as nerves and blood vessels. Several areas of the body do not contain subcutaneous tissue, and skin attaches directly to the bone (e.g., knuckles and anterior tibia [medial leg bone]).

Adipose tissue or fat in the subcutaneous layer is also called the *panniculus adiposus.* The thickness of panniculus adiposus varies with age, gender, and health. Infants and children have a uniform layer under the skin. Females have extra fat over the breasts, hips, and inner thighs. Males have extra fat on the nape of the neck, deltoid and triceps muscles, and abdomen.

SKIN COLOR

Skin color ranges from almost black to nearly colorless and is determined by several factors, including diet, emotions, physiology, and disease processes. Skin color is influenced by a number of pigments including brown/black (melanin), yellow (carotene), and red (hemoglobin).

The brown or black pigment of the skin is melanin. As mentioned previously, the amount of melanin produced is influenced by exposure to sunlight, genetics, ethnicity, and hormones. Skin pigmentation affects the color of skin and areas affected by pigmentations may be small or cover the entire skin surface of the body. Several types of pigmentation are featured next.

- **Freckles.** These are small tan-to-brown spots on sunlight-exposed skin, especially in children. Freckles tend to fade in adult life. The propensity to develop freckles is inherited and is seen most frequently in fair-skinned individuals.
- **Birthmarks and Moles.** These are a dense collection of melanocytes appearing as small oval or round brown or black spots. Birthmarks are also called nevi. Moles are the most common type of birthmark; some moles may become cancerous. Other types of birthmarks include blue spots, café-au-lait spots, and hemangiomas.
  - **Hemangiomas.** These are vascular birthmarks present at birth (30% of cases) or appear within a few years after birth. Most hemangiomas are shades of red or purple and may be slightly raised with a rough surface. Types of hemangiomas are cherry hemangiomas, strawberry hemangiomas, port-wine stains, stork bites, and angel kisses.
- **Melasma.** These are tan-to-brown spots, particularly on the nose, cheeks, chin, and forehead of females caused by hormonal fluctuations. This condition is most common in pregnant clients or clients taking female oral contraceptives and disappears after childbirth or when oral contraceptive use is discontinued. This can produce a linea nigra, or pregnancy line, between the navel and pubic area or the mask of pregnancy, a darkening of the skin on the face and neck.
- **Age Spots.** These are flat brown-to-black patches on the skin of older individuals and are usually on sunlight-exposed areas such as the face, hands, arms, back, and feet. Age spots are also called solar lentigo, senile lentigo, or liver spots.
- **Vitiligo.** This is the partial or total loss of pigmentation occurring in patches; irregular patches of depigmented skin that appear milky white. These patches tend to grow

larger and spread over time. Common areas of involvement are the face, lips, hands, arms, and legs. Vitiligo is also called leukoderma. Although the exact cause of vitiligo is unknown, there is strong evidence to suggest it is genetic in origin.

- **Albinism.** This is a rare genetic condition in which individuals produce little or no melanin. Individuals with albinism have pale skin, white hair, and typically pale blue or pink eyes from visible blood vessels.
- **Tattoos.** These are usually elective and involve indelible ink injected into the dermis of the skin by needles to create an image, a design, or a word(s).

The yellow pigment of the skin is from carotene, and gives the skin a golden color. In most individuals, the skin color of carotene is dominated by the skin color of melanin. However, individuals of Asian descent produce less melanin, giving their skin a yellow hue. The skin may appear yellow because of disease processes. For example, individuals with liver diseases are unable to excrete a pigment called *bilirubin.* This substance becomes deposited in the skin and mucous membranes, causing *jaundice.* Skin color may change in response to diet. For example, individuals who consume large amounts of carotene-rich vegetables, such as carrots, may experience yellowing skin.

The red pigment of the skin is from hemoglobin in the blood, and gives skin a rosy color, usually in fair-skinned people. These individuals produce small amounts of melanin, so the blood in the dermis is more visible. Skin reddening from vasodilation and increased blood flow is called **hyperemia** and can be seen in cases of fever, inflammation, increased physical activity, or hot flashes common during menopause. During hyperemia, the skin may redden and feel warm. Blue or purple-tinted skin is called **cyanosis,** and pale or ashen skin is called **pallor.** Both cyanosis and pallor may occur from low oxygen levels in the blood or decreased blood flow, from emotional reactions such as embarrassment or fright, from diseases such as anemia or Raynaud disease, or from ischemia. **Ischemia** is decreased blood flow from vasoconstriction or other causes. During ischemia, the skin may feel cool.

HAIR

Hair is composed of keratinized filaments arising from pouchlike hair follicles in the dermis. The hair shaft protrudes through a pore in the epidermis. The main function of hair is to protect skin and body orifices. Hair shields the scalp from injury and UV radiation. Eyebrows and eyelashes guard the eyes against foreign particles; hair in the nostrils and external ear canals protect the nose and ears, respectively. Hairs also function in our sense of touch: A receptor is stimulated when hair is moved (see the section titled "Skin Receptors" for more information).

Hair covers most of the body. Only a few areas of skin are hairless (i.e., palms, soles, lips, nipples, and some genital areas). *Terminal hair,* or mature hair, is found on the scalp,

the axillae, and the external genitalia develops in males and females. Males generally will develop terminal hair in additional areas such as the face, chest, abdomen, and feet. Hair characteristics, including natural color and texture, are genetically determined.

Hair color originates from one or a combination of several color pigments: brown/black, yellow, and black. Red hair is a combination of brown/black and yellow pigment. White or gray hair lacks pigment and occurs with advancing age. Psychosocial stress, medical treatments such as chemotherapy and radiation therapy, excessive vitamin A, and certain fungal diseases can cause changes in hair color, hair growth, and hair loss.

Arrector Pili

Arrector pili are muscles attached to hair follicles. These muscles contract to pull the hair shaft upright. This action may occur when cold or during emotions such as fright or anxiety. During muscular contraction, skin may dimple, causing the appearance of *goosebumps* or *gooseflesh.* If an animal is cold or frightened, upright hair shafts create an insulating layer of air in the animal's fur. This increased fur volume makes the animal appear larger, which may deter an unpleasant encounter with an opponent. Humans do not have fur, so this effect is relatively useless except to recognize the feeling of having hair rise on the back of one's neck which may be a warning sign of danger or a strong emotional response to an event.

NAILS

Nails are compact keratinized cells forming the thin hard plates on distal surfaces of fingers and toes. The main functions of nails are protecting the ends of fingers and toes, and a tool for tasks such as digging, scratching, and manipulating objects.

The *nail body* is the largest and most visible part of the nail. Nail production takes place in the *nail root.* The *nailbed* is the skin beneath the nail; it can be seen through the clear nail. The *lateral nail folds* are the side edges of the nail where they meet the skin; this area is where most hangnails occur. The *cuticle* is the tough ridge of skin growing over the nail from its base. Also located here is the *lunula,* which is the crescent-shaped white area at the base of the nail. The most distal portion of the nail is the *free edge,* which is trimmed as a result of nail growth (Fig. 22.2).

Nails are typically transparent but appear pinkish because of blood vessels present in the dermis below. Nail changes, such as ridges, white spots, or clubbing, may occur as a result of poor nutrition, advancing age, or disease processes.

SKIN GLANDS

Skin glands secrete substances onto the surface of the skin by way of ducts. There are three major skin glands: sebaceous, sudoriferous, and ceruminous.

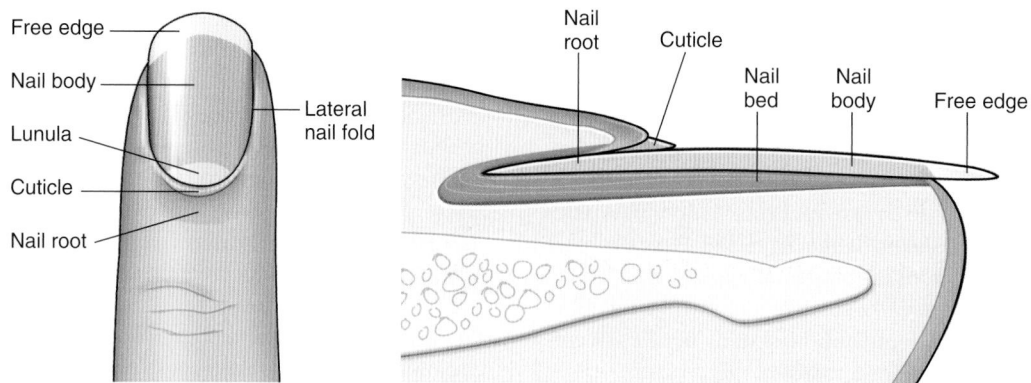

FIG. 22.2 Nail and its structures viewed dorsally (*left image*) and in a lateral cross-section (*right image*).

Sebaceous (Oil) Glands

Sebaceous glands secrete sebum into a duct connected to a hair follicle (see Fig. 22.1). Sebum is an oily, waxy substance that lubricates the hair and the epidermis, and helps protect the skin as it has antibacterial and antifungal properties. Overproduction of sebum can make skin appear oily; this can be caused by hormones (e.g., androgens) or disease (e.g., seborrheic dermatitis). Underproduction of sebum can make skin dry; this can be caused by nutritional factors (e.g., deficiencies of vitamins A, D, E) and UV radiation in sunlight.

Sudoriferous (Sweat) Glands

Sudoriferous glands secrete a watery fluid called sweat or perspiration. Their functions are regulation of body temperature through evaporation and the elimination of wastes. The skin possesses approximately 2 million sweat glands (see Fig. 22.1). Nearly 1 pint of fluids and impurities are lost in each 8-hour period when a person is visibly sweating. When sweat production is high, the replacement of lost minerals is essential. When sweat production is low, most sodium chloride present in perspiration is reabsorbed and mineral depletion is negligible. Sweat is a liquid made from 99% water and 1% salt and fat.

Female breasts, or *mammary glands,* are modified sweat glands. These glands are part of the reproductive system because of their function of feeding the newborn.

Sudoriferous glands can be classified into groups depending on the type of secretion, their location, and their association with the nervous system. These are eccrine glands and apocrine glands (Fig. 22.3).

- **Eccrine Glands.** These are the most numerous and are all over the skin except the lips, ear canal, penis, and nailbeds. Eccrine glands secrete watery perspiration directly on the skin's surface and help regulate body temperature through evaporative cooling.
- **Apocrine Glands.** These are larger than eccrine glands and open into hair follicles in the axilla, anogenital region, and areola of the breast. Apocrine glands begin to function during puberty and secrete a strong-smelling perspiration; this odor is largely caused by the breakdown of skin bacteria. Apocrine secretions may contain

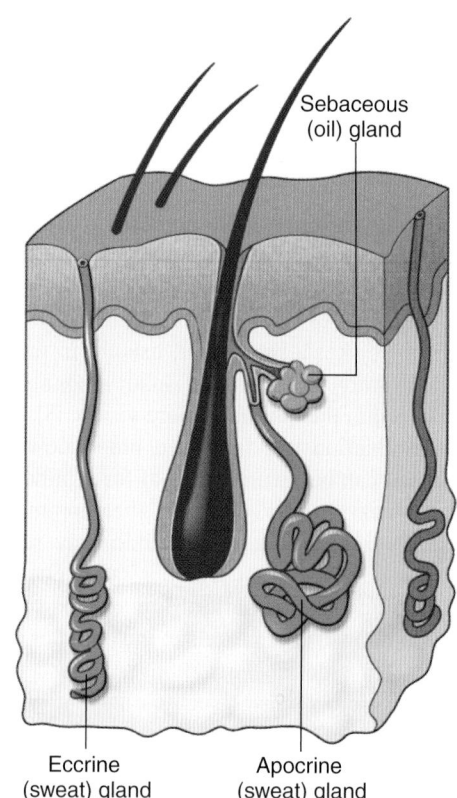

FIG. 22.3 Skin glands. Sebaceous (oil) glands and sudoriferous (sweat) glands. Sebaceous gland and apocrine gland secretions are released into hair follicles. Eccrine gland secretions are released directly on the skin's surface.

pheromones, chemical substances used in communication between organisms of the same species. Pheromones in the areola of female breasts may stimulate the sucking reflexes in infants.

Ceruminous Glands

Ceruminous glands are specialized sudoriferous glands and secrete cerumen, or earwax. These glands are found in the external auditory or ear canal. Wax is sticky and traps particles and pathogens as they enter the ear.

It's not the age; it's the mileage.
~ **Harrison Ford as Indiana Jones in *Raiders of the Lost Ark***

THERMOREGULATION

Thermoregulation is the constant maintenance of internal body temperature independent of the external environmental temperature. Normal body temperature of 37°C (98.6°F) is sustained by balancing heat production with heat loss. The body's thermostat is in the hypothalamus of the brain. If the hypothalamus senses an increase or decrease in body temperature, it responds by sending signals to the nervous system to move it back to homeostasis. The skin plays a vital role in thermoregulation by (1) activity or inactivity of sweat glands, and by (2) dilation or constriction of blood vessels (Fig. 22.4).

When body temperature rises above normal, blood vessels in the dermis begin to dilate. This action increases blood flow to the skin, moves body heat to the surface, and releases it into the surrounding air. The dermis can contain as much as 5% of total blood volume. In addition, sudoriferous glands become active and release sweat, which evaporates to help reduce body temperature.

When body temperature falls below normal, blood vessels in the dermis begin to constrict. This action decreases blood flow to skin and reduces the amount of body heat moving to the surface. However, if a region of skin becomes too cold (below 15°C [59°F]), local blood vessels dilate to move blood and heat to the area. In addition, sweat glands become inactive. Adipose tissue in the subcutaneous layer can also act as an insulator.

Failure of the body to thermoregulate may cause *hypothermia,* excessive decreases in body temperature, or *hyperthermia,* excessive increases in body temperature. Extremes in body temperature are often fatal.

SKIN RECEPTORS

Touch is the ability to perceive objects or forces through physical contact. Touch is mediated by receptors on or near the surface of the body. Touch receptors are generally classified as *exteroceptors* because they receive stimuli from the external environment. Information gathered by these receptors travels to the somatosensory cortex, which is the primary sensory area in the brain's parietal lobe (see Chapter 23). This area determines the type of sensation felt (i.e., pressure, temperature, pain), and where the sensation is located. Certain areas of the body are more richly innervated, and therefore has more sensory activity, compared with other areas of the body. In fact, 80% of the real estate in the somatosensory cortex is dedicated to the hands and fingers, face, lips, and tongue, which is represented by a homunculus or "little man." (Fig. 22.5). Receptors in the skin and mucosae can be structurally classified as free nerve endings or encapsulated nerve endings (Fig. 22.6).

Free Nerve Endings: Merkel Discs, Nociceptors, and Hair Root Plexuses

These receptors have no covering and are the simplest, most common, and most widely distributed receptors.

- **Merkel (Tactile) Discs.** These detect light pressure as well as subtle changes in surface topography such as depressions and elevations or contours. Merkel discs are

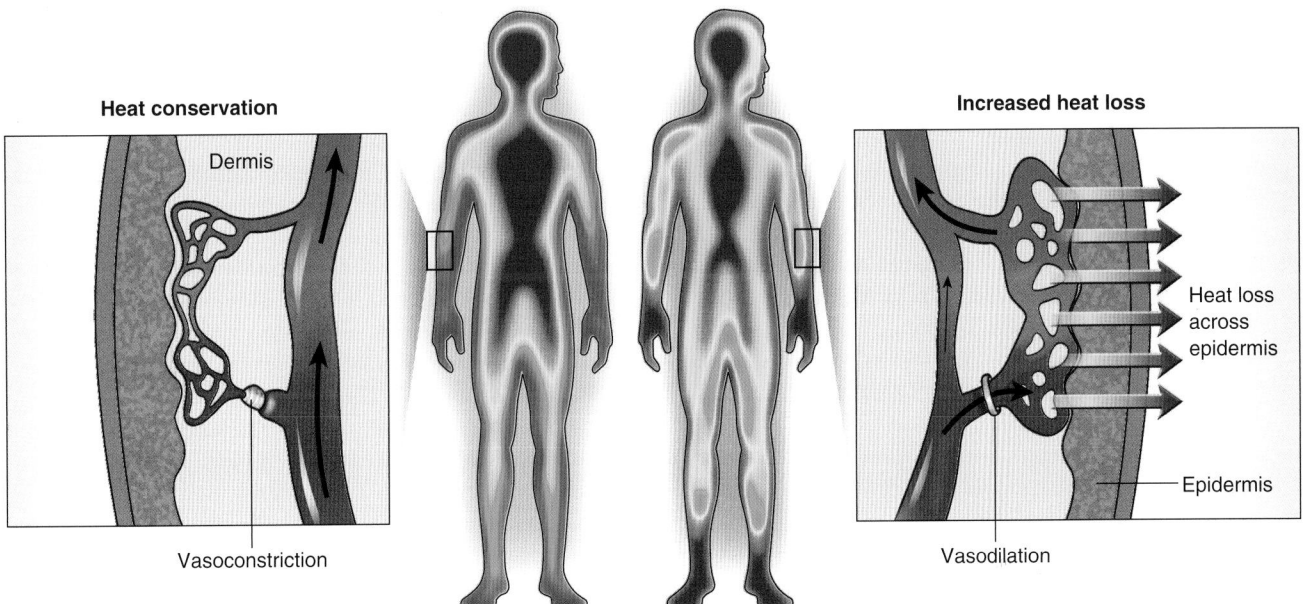

FIG. 22.4 Thermoregulation by blood vessels. Vasoconstriction in the skin conserves body heat (*left image*) and vasodilation increases heat loss by moving blood and heat to the skin's surface, so heat can radiate into the surrounding air (*right image*).

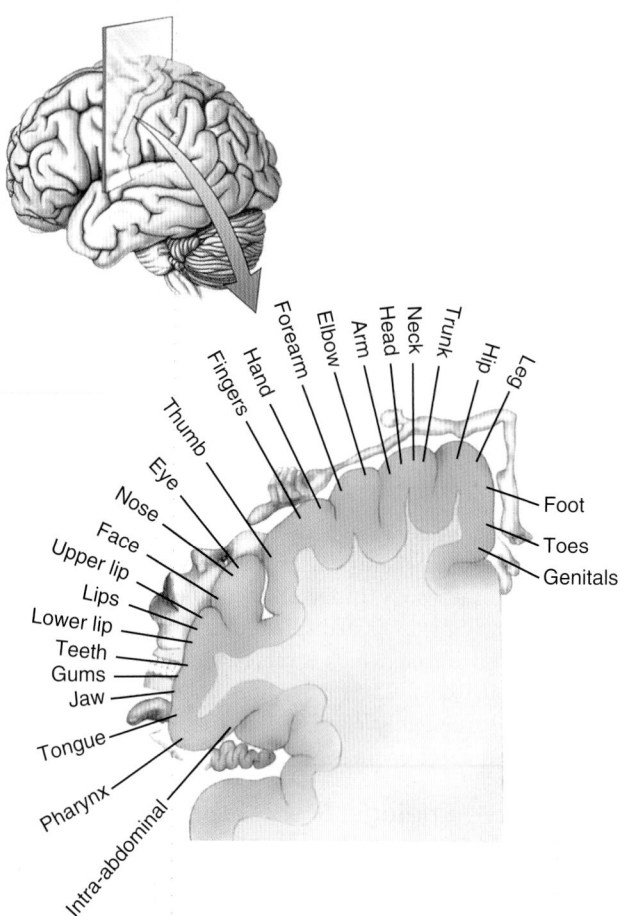

FIG. 22.5 The somatosensory cortex or primary sensory area in the brain's parietal lobe. Eighty percent of this area is used to detect sensations in the hands and fingers, face, lips, and tongue, which is represented by a homunculus or "little man." (From Cramer, G. D., & Darby, S. A. [2014]. *Clinical anatomy of the spine, spinal cord, and ANS* [3rd ed.]. St. Louis, MO: Mosby.)

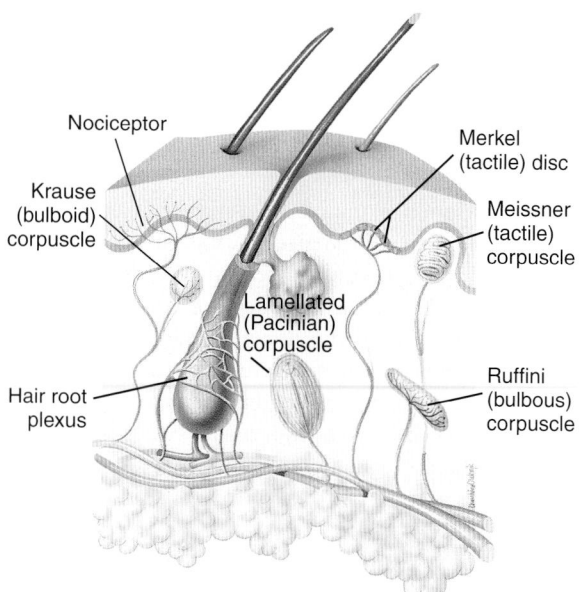

FIG. 22.6 Skin receptors receive stimuli from the external environment. (Modified from Thibodeau, G. A., & Patton, K. T. [2007]. *Anatomy and physiology* [6th ed.]. St Louis: Mosby.)

specialized for *discriminative touch,* or touch that is easy to locate on the skin. They are in the epidermis, have small receptive fields, and adapt slowly so they continually send information to the central nervous system for relatively long periods of time. *Receptive fields* are areas of the body where a sensory nerve can detect sensations.

- **Nociceptors.** These detect actual or potential tissue damage, are sensitive to pain, and serve a protective function by sending signals of a possible threat. The largest concentrations are found in the skin, but they are in almost every tissue of the body.
- **Hair Root Plexus (Hair Follicle Receptor).** These respond to hair movement and resemble netting wrapped around the hair follicle.

Encapsulated Nerve Endings: Meissner, Krause, Ruffini, and Pacini Corpuscles

These receptors have capsules at their terminal end. Most are mechanoreceptors, specialized nerve endings detecting mechanical sensation. Pressure must mechanically change their shape before they are activated. Encapsulated receptors vary in size and in body distribution.

- **Meissner (Tactile) Corpuscles.** These detect light pressure, textural sensations, and low-frequency vibrations. Although their encapsulated surfaces require slightly more deforming pressure compared with Merkel discs (free nerve endings). Meissner corpuscles adapt quickly and have small receptive fields. An example of the function of Meissner corpuscles is their use in reading Braille. These are in the dermis beneath the epidermal-dermal junction and are abundant in hairless skin such as the fingertips, lips, eyelids, nipples, and genitals.
- **Krause (Bulboid) Corpuscles**. These detect deep pressure, cold or reduced temperatures, low-frequency vibrations, and textural sensations. Krause corpuscles are found in skin and mucous membranes.
- **Ruffini (Bulbous) Corpuscles**. These detect deep pressure, continuous or persistent pressure, skin stretching, and warmth. Ruffini corpuscles have wide receptive fields, adapt slowly, and provide valuable feedback for gripping objects, controlling finger position, and movement. Ruffini corpuscles are thought to inhibit sympathetic activity. Ruffini corpuscles are found in the dermis.
- **Pacini (Lamellar) Corpuscles**. Also called *Pacinian corpuscles,* these detect deep pressure, vibrations, and stretch, usually detecting only sudden disturbances. Pacini corpuscles adapt quickly to stimuli; for this reason, they respond only when the stimulus is first applied. Pacini corpuscles have wide receptive fields. Like Ruffini, Pacini corpuscles respond to pressure changes, such as when grasping or releasing an object. Pacini corpuscles are found in the dermis, especially in the hands and feet, as well joint capsules, viscera, and the periosteum of bone.

Everybody is a genius. But if you judge a fish by its ability to climb a tree, it will live its whole life believing that it is stupid.

~ **Albert Einstein**

DERMATOLOGIC PATHOLOGIES, CONDITIONS, AND INJURIES

Featured next are common pathologies, conditions, and injuries of the integumentary system listed alphabetically. Each item includes a brief description and its massage-related modifications. A more extensive list and related research can be found in the current edition of *Mosby's Pathology for Massage Professionals* (2022).

Acne

Acne is a bacterial infection in which skin containing hair follicles and sebaceous glands become clogged producing lesions called *comedones* (e.g., whiteheads and blackheads or pimples). Acne is most commonly found on the face, but it also can appear on the V of the chest and upper back, neck, and shoulders. Although not life-threatening, acne can be distressing and disfiguring.

Acne is most common among adolescents, affecting 85% of the population between 12 and 20 years of age. However, people in their 30s and 40s also may have acne. Males and females are affected, but males tend to have more severe acne. Factors contributing to acne development are bacteria and hormones, mainly androgens.

Massage and Acne

Avoid affected areas because the pressure and friction from massage and massage lubricants may cause acne to worsen (American Academy of Dermatology [AAD], 2018; Sutaria & Schlessinger, 2018). Avoid the use of table warmers or hot packs over affected areas (AAD, 2018).

Athlete's Foot

Athlete's foot is a fungal infection of the foot or feet, most often the soles and between the toes. It is most prevalent among teenagers and adult males, as well as people with weakened or impaired immune responses, such as individuals with diabetes. Athlete's foot can be transmitted by contact with infected skin or contaminated objects such as flooring, towels, and shoes or socks. This condition is more common in warm and humid climates. A fungal toenail infection often coexists. The infection can spread to the hands, especially if the person scratches the infected area. Athlete's foot is also called *tinea pedis*. Athlete's foot is caused by several species of fungi called *dermatophytes*.

Massage and Athlete's Foot

Athlete's foot is a local contraindication or contact precaution. **Contact precautions** are methods to reduce or prevent disease transmission that is spread by direct or indirect contact. Contact precautions require the use of barriers and disinfecting of contaminated surfaces. The feet can be massaged if the practitioner wears gloves or massaged through a barrier if the feet do not contain broken skin. Massage linens are treated as contaminated. See Chapter 9 for recommended protocols.

Boils and Methicillin-Resistant *Staphylococcus aureus*

Boils are infected hair follicles that manifest as a painful pus-filled mass or abscess. Boils are also called furuncles. Boils can occur anywhere on the body, but they are most common on the face, neck, axillae, back, buttocks, and thighs. A collection or cluster of boils that coalesce to form a larger mass is called a *carbuncle*. Although anyone can develop boils and carbuncles, people who have diabetes or suppressed immunity are at increased risk. Some boils and carbuncles are MRSA infections, which are more difficult to treat.

Methicillin-resistant *Staphylococcus aureus* (MRSA) infections are caused by staph bacteria resistant to antibiotics commonly used to treat ordinary staph infections. Most MRSA infections occur in the healthcare settings and are called healthcare-associated MRSA (HA-MRSA). Another type of MRSA infection can occur among healthy individuals and is called community-associated MRSA (CA-MRSA). The five Cs of spreading MRSA are:

1. **C**rowding
2. **C**ontact
3. **C**ompromised skin
4. **C**ontaminated items
5. **C**leanliness, lack of

MRSA infections can spread and sometimes become life-threatening. The most common cause of boils and carbuncles is staphylococcal bacteria, but they may be caused by bacteria such as MRSA.

Massage and Boils/Methicillin-Resistant *Staphylococcus aureus*

Boils, carbuncles, and MRSA infections are local contraindications. Skin lesions must be covered during the massage. Use gloves or other barriers such as the sheet for massaging the hands as they may become contaminated by clients touching their own lesions (Centers for Disease Control and Prevention [CDC], 2019). Massage linens are treated as contaminated. See Chapter 9 for recommended protocols. If working in healthcare settings, follow the institution's policies for MRSA.

Bruises

Bruises, or contusions, are injuries from broken capillaries; leaked blood collecting in interstitial spaces often creates skin discoloration. There are several types of bruises: those beneath the skin's surface are called *subcutaneous bruises*, those within a muscle belly are called *intramuscular bruises*, and those on bone are called *periosteal* or *bone bruises*. Most subcutaneous bruises are caused by trauma such as a slip or fall, impact with a person or an object, injury such as from a motor vehicle accident, or a physical attack. Bruises usually appear within 24 hours of the causative event. Other types of bruising are caused by blood disorders, medications such as platelet inhibitors, cancer treatments including chemotherapy and radiation therapy, skin and blood vessels fragility common in older adults (called *senile purpura*), and diseases such as leukemia, hepatitis, and scurvy.

Massage and Bruises

Subcutaneous bruises are local contraindications until they begin to turn greenish-yellow (this color change is difficult to determine on darker skin). This time frame can range from 4 to 7 days after the first appearance of the bruise. Light pressure massage can be applied over bruises caused by aging and blood disorders. An example of light pressure is 3 on a 10-point pressure scale. Discontinue massage over any bruise (including well-healed subcutaneous bruises) if the pressure causes pain. Senile purpura is common in older adults. These may be perceived by the client as unattractive, and may be a source of embarrassment, anxiety, and psychosocial distress. When working with these clients, display loving kindness, acceptance, empathy, and nonjudgment. Underlying conditions and diseases causing nontraumatic bruises, such as blood disorders, medication use (i.e., aspirin, ibuprofen), leukemia, cancer treatments, hepatitis, and advancing age should be factored into the treatment plan.

Burns

Burns are tissue damage from heat (including fire, hot liquid, steam, and hot objects including metal or glass), extreme cold, radiation (including sunlight exposure, tanning beds, and radiation therapy), chemicals (strong acids, drain openers, toilet bowl cleaners, and paint thinner), electricity, or friction. Tissue damage depth ranges from superficial to deep, which is used as a criterion for burn classification.

- **First-Degree Burn.** Also called a superficial thickness burn, a first-degree burn damages only the epidermis. An example of a first-degree burn is mild sunburn.
- **Second-Degree Burn.** Also called a partial-thickness burn, a second-degree burn is deeper and more severe than first-degree burns and involves both the epidermis and upper layers of the dermis. Hair follicles and sweat glands are spared and remain functional. After the burn heals, a scar may remain.
- **Third-Degree Burn.** Also called a full-thickness burn, a third-degree burn destroys the epidermis, dermis, hair follicles, and associated glands and possibly extends into the subcutaneous tissue and underlying soft tissue.
- **Fourth-Degree Burn.** A fourth-degree burn is a full-thickness burn that extends to the muscle or bone.

Massage and Burns

Burned areas are a local contraindication until the area has completely healed. Healing time depends on many factors, such as degree of severity, and ranges from several weeks to several months. Massage over unburned areas is permitted while affected areas are healing. Once healed, massage and scar mobilization are permissible. Use moderate pressure and include friction and skin rolling petrissage over the affected area applied in all directions. Consider using cocoa butter or a cocoa butter blend as a massage lubricant.

Before massaging the affected area, obtain verbal consent. Some clients with disfiguring burns or scarring may feel self-conscious. If consent is granted, ask the client how sensitive the affected area is and adjust the pressure accordingly. Large burns can be devastating to the client. Provide positive reinforcement, being aware each client will progress through different stages of grief during the recovery processes. Massage may help reduce anxiety and depression in this population.

Teach clients how to massage their own scars if in easily accessible areas. Or teach a caregiver a few massage techniques to be used on the person with burn scars. Ask them to follow the same precautions licensed practitioners follow.

Cold Sores

Cold sores are recurrent viral infections affecting the skin and mucous membranes. The lesions can appear anywhere on the body, but most are found around the mouth. Cold sores can also occur around the nose, over the chin, or on the fingers (called herpetic whitlow). Cold sores may be found inside the mouth and are often confused with canker sores. However, canker sores are not caused by viruses and are not contagious. Cold sores are also called *fever blisters* and *oral herpes simplex*. Cold sores are a common disease; most people in the United States are infected by age 20. Cold sores are spread by contact with infected skin and indirectly by contact with contaminated items such as razors, towels, and eating utensils. Lesions tend to recur because the virus lies dormant in sensory nerve cells corresponding to the site of infection. Reactivation of the virus can be triggered by exposure to sunlight, wind, or the presence of another infection such as the common cold (hence the name "cold" sores). Fever ("fever" blisters), hormonal changes occurring during menstruation or pregnancy, stress, anxiety; and chapped lips can also trigger reactivation of the virus.

Massage and Cold Sores

Cold sores are local contraindications. Use gloves or other barriers such as the sheet when massaging the hands as they may become contaminated by clients touching their own lesions (CDC, 2019). Massage linens are treated as contaminated. See Chapter 9 for recommended protocols. Bear in mind that healthcare-associated transmission of cold sores is rare (Goodman & Fuller, 2014). If the massage practitioner has a cold sore on the fingers (herpetic whitlow), gloves are worn during the massage.

Contact Dermatitis

Contact dermatitis is inflammation of the skin that develops at the site of contact with the causative agent. The characteristic rash develops within minutes to hours of contact exposure and can last 2 to 4 weeks. Contact dermatitis is caused by contact with either an irritant (causing irritant dermatitis) or an allergen (causing allergic dermatitis). Irritant dermatitis accounts for 80% of cases, and allergic dermatitis accounts for 20% of cases.

Massage and Contact Dermatitis

The affected area is a local contraindication because it is often hypersensitive; contact dermatitis cannot be transmitted by contact.

The practitioner should always consider the client's skin reaction to the products used. Inquire about past skin reactions from chemicals in laundry detergents and eliminate contact with linens washed in the detergent identified, if applicable. Also, inquire about allergies to latex and wool. If the client is allergic to these, they may have allergic reactions to shea butter or lanolin, respectively. In these cases, avoid products containing these ingredients or use a hypoallergenic product. Avoid latex gloves on clients who have latex allergies.

Latex allergies have been linked to shea butter hypersensitivity because of cross-reactivity (Grier, 2012). Also, essential oils used in massage products have been linked to contact dermatitis (Lakshmi, 2014) including laurel (Adişen & Onder, 2007) and turmeric (Lopez-Villafuerte & Clores, 2016), as well as ayurvedic oils, particularly Dhanwantharam thailam and Eladi thailam (Eladi coconut oil); so caution is warranted.

Practitioners who use essential oils in their practice are at increased risk for occupational contact dermatitis (Crawford et al., 2004; Trattner et al., 2008). Crawford et al. (2004) found that 15% to 23% of massage practitioners had contact dermatitis on their hands and risks were greater among practitioners with a history of eczema or atopic dermatitis.

Decubitus Ulcers

Decubitus ulcers, or decubiti, are injuries to the skin and underlying tissues from prolonged pressure and are usually found over bony prominences. Areas of involvement can extend to underlying bones and joints. At-risk individuals have a medical condition that impairs mobility, sensation, or blood flow or who spend most of their time in a bed or chair. Tissue death can occur in as little as 12 hours. Decubiti are major threats to a person's health. Decubitus ulcers are also called *bedsores*, *pressure sores*, and *pressure ulcers*.

Massage and Decubitus Ulcers

Areas containing ulcers or areas at risk for ulcer formation are local contraindications. Massage does not prevent decubiti and massage may contribute to tissue damage by promoting inflammatory reactions, especially in frail older adults (Buss et al., 1997: National Institute for Health and Care Excellence, 2014; National Pressure Ulcer Advisory Panel, 2014; Shahin et al., 2009). The practitioner cannot rely on assessment to determine the presence of developing decubiti because the client may have inflammation manifesting as nonblanching skin which is difficult to observe, particularly in clients with darker skin. At-risk areas are featured next.

- **Bedridden Clients: At-Risk Areas.** Back of the head, over the scapulae, the elbows, the sacrum, and over the heels.
- **Chair-Bound Clients: At-Risk Areas.** Over the scapulae, the sacrum, the ischial tuberosities, the popliteal areas, and the plantar surfaces of the feet.

Massage is postponed if the ulcer is emitting a discharge or has a foul odor because these are hallmarks of infection, which could be life-threatening. Refer clients to their healthcare provider immediately for evaluation and treatment.

Eczema (Atopic Dermatitis)

Eczema is an inflammatory skin condition. It is not contagious. Eczema is more common in children and most often found on the hands, wrists, scalp, face, nape of the neck, upper chest, creases of the elbows and knees, ankles, feet, and in infants, the face and scalp. Between 25% and 30% of children have at least one episode of eczema by age 5. Adult cases tend to be more chronic with periods of exacerbation. Exacerbation frequency is related to stress, anxiety, and sudden or extreme changes in temperature and high humidity. Eczema is also called *eczematous dermatitis*. Eczema has no known cause, but it may be related to allergies and can be hereditary. Between 75% and 80% of affected individuals have a personal or family history of asthma or hay fever (allergic rhinitis). In children, food allergies may play a role in causing eczema.

Massage and Eczema

Eczema is a local contraindication if it contains broken skin. Before massaging affected areas that do not contain broken skin, obtain verbal consent. Some clients with disfiguring eczema may feel self-conscious. If consent is granted, ask the client how sensitive the affected area is and adjust the pressure accordingly. Affected skin should never be rubbed vigorously. Use emollient lubricants to combat dry skin and avoid products containing alcohol or essential oils as the latter was found to worsen eczema, especially with repeated use (Anderson et al., 2000). Some clients do best with a hypoallergenic product. The National Eczema Association (2015) recommends that parents of children with eczema massage moisturizers into their skin, rather than simply applying moisturizers.

Impetigo

Impetigo is a common bacterial infection seen primarily in children. Lesions occur mainly around the mouth, nose, and skin folds such as the axillae. This skin condition is highly contagious and can spread by contact with an infected person or by handling contaminated objects such as eating utensils, toothbrushes, towels, and bed linens. The most common causes of impetigo are staphylococci or streptococci bacteria.

Massage and Impetigo

Impetigo is a local contraindication. Skin lesions must be covered during the massage. Use gloves or other barriers such as the sheet for massaging the hands as they may become contaminated by clients touching their own lesions (CDC, 2019). Massage linens are treated as contaminated (see Chapter 9 for recommended protocols).

Lice Infestation

Lice infestation is the presence of lice on the body or in fabrics. Lice (*louse is singular*) are wingless parasites that live their entire life cycle on a single human host and depend on its blood for survival. Three forms of human lice are head lice, body lice, and pubic lice, or crabs. The female louse reproduces approximately every 2 weeks. She prefers to lay eggs on hair shafts, cementing her egg sacs close to the skin, but she will also lay eggs in folds of clothing. Eggs hatch in about 1 week. Lice can spread by direct or indirect contact with either lice or their eggs. Close contact with infected individuals or with infected items, such as pillows, blankets, combs, clothing, hats, or contaminated furniture can increase the risk of cross-infestation. Lice can live for 1 to 2 days off the body. Pubic lice usually spread through sexual contact.

Massage and Lice Infestation

Massage is postponed until the lice infestation is eradicated because lice are highly contagious.

Psoriasis

Psoriasis is a chronic inflammatory skin condition in which the proliferation rate of skin cells accelerates, causing them to build up in thick patches. Instead of skin renewing approximately every 28 days, it occurs every few days. Psoriasis typically affects the scalp and skin over the elbows, knees, back, chest, and buttocks. Psoriasis may spread to nails, causing pitting, discoloration, and nail separation. Psoriasis affects between 1% and 3% of the U.S. population. It can occur at any age but is more common between the ages of 10 and 30 years and again between the ages of 57 and 60 years. *Psoriatic arthritis* is a form of arthritis that develops in approximately 30% of people with moderate to severe psoriasis. Both psoriasis and psoriatic arthritis are marked by periods of exacerbation alternating with periods of remission; exacerbations are related to trauma and psychosocial stress. The tendency to acquire psoriasis seems to be related to a weakened or impaired immune response. Risk factors include genetics, the environment, and systemic inflammation.

Massage and Psoriasis

Psoriasis is a local contraindication if it contains broken skin. Before massaging affected areas that do not contain broken skin, obtain verbal consent. Some clients with disfiguring psoriasis may feel self-conscious. If consent is granted, ask the client how sensitive the affected area is and adjust the pressure accordingly. Use emollient lubricants to combat dry skin; some clients do best with a hypoallergenic product. Affected skin should never be rubbed vigorously. Because emotional stress was found to play a role in the onset and exacerbation of psoriasis (Devrimci-Ozguven et al., 2000), massage using techniques that promote relaxation are indicated.

For clients with psoriatic arthritis, avoid swollen or tender areas (i.e., fingers and toes), or use only light pressure. An example of light pressure is 3 on a 10-point pressure scale. Avoid forceful passive range of motion on affected joints.

Ringworm

Ringworm is a fungal infection of the skin. Ringworm can be transmitted by direct skin-to-skin contact with an infected person or contact with domestic animals or with objects. Ringworm usually affects nonhairy areas of the face, trunk, and limbs. This condition occurs more frequently in warm and humid climates. Ringworm gets its name from its ringlike appearance; a worm is not involved. Ringworm is also called *tinea corporis*.

Massage and Ringworm

Ringworm is a local contraindication or contact precaution. Use gloves or other barriers such as the sheet when massaging the hands as they may become contaminated by clients touching their own lesions (CDC, 2019). Massage linens are treated as contaminated. See Chapter 9 for recommended protocols.

Rosacea

Rosacea is a progressive, inflammatory skin condition causing facial redness. Typically, only the middle third of the face is involved (e.g., nose, cheeks, chin); however, it can also affect the forehead and around the eyes. Rosacea is seen more frequently in fair-skinned middle-aged females. Approximately 14 million people in the United States have rosacea. Rosacea is also called acne rosacea and adult-onset acne. The cause of rosacea is unknown. Hereditary and environmental factors, such as overexposure to sunlight, may play a role in its development.

Massage and Rosacea

Inquire about sensitivity over affected areas and adjust pressure accordingly. Avoid techniques that generate heat, such as friction. Also, avoid areas containing pustules.

Scabies Infestation

Scabies infestation is the presence of human itch mites or scabies on the body or in fabrics. Scabies are microscopic parasitic mites that burrow under the skin. Areas most affected by scabies are the webbing between the fingers, creases of the wrists, elbows, and knees, waistline, axillae, under the breasts, lower buttocks, groin, and feet. Scabies infestations are highly contagious. Secondary bacterial skin infections are common.

Massage and Scabies Infestation

Massage is postponed until the scabies infestation is eradicated because scabies are highly contagious.

Scars

A **scar** is a mark left on the skin after the body repairs wounds caused by surgery, injuries, or diseases such as shingles. Scars are the result of collagen production which occurs during the healing process. Location of the scar, skin type, and age affect scar formation. Older skin tends to leave less visible scars whereas younger skin tends to over-heal, resulting in larger and thicker scars. Scars can extend into deeper layers causing adhesions. **Adhesions** are bands of scar tissue that bind together two or more previously separated structures. Abnormal scars are elevated and do not flatten like normal scars. Hypertrophic, keloid, and contracture scars are examples of abnormal scars.

- **Hypertrophic Scars.** These scars are elevated but do not spread beyond the boundaries of the original wound. Hypertrophic scars are more common than keloid or contracture scars.
- **Keloid Scars.** Keloids are elevated scars and spread beyond the boundaries of the original wound. Keloids are more common in darker skin types.
- **Contracture Scars.** These scars are caused by skin tightening or contracting, and are more common in burn scars, especially second- or third-degree burns.

Massage and Scars

The scar over the wound or incision is a local contraindication until the area is dry and in the remodeling (maturation) phase. This time frame is 8 weeks or longer. Use deep friction and skin-rolling techniques near and directly over the scar with or without lubricant. Massage tissues in several directions (superior, inferior, medial, lateral, clockwise, anticlockwise) because scar tissue is arranged haphazardly. Begin with light pressure and progress to deeper pressure. Inquire about pressure sensitivity and make adjustments according to the client's preference. Discontinue scar tissue massage and refer clients to their healthcare provider if the scar is redder, warmer, or more painful upon subsequent sessions (Moffitt Cancer Center [MCC], 2008). Teach clients how to massage their own scars if they are in accessible areas, and to follow the same precautions licensed practitioners follow.

Scleroderma

Scleroderma is a chronic disease characterized by hardening and tightening of the skin and connective tissues. Scleroderma is caused by overproduction and accumulation of collagen, a protein found in connective tissues, which leads to fibrosis accompanied by inflammation. Fibrosis may remain localized and just affect the skin and superficial fascia, or it may extend to the deep fascia, become systemic, and affect internal organs.

When the latter occurs, the individual may experience cardiac arrhythmias, respiratory failure, kidney failure, or esophageal or intestinal obstruction. If damage occurs to blood vessel walls, Raynaud disease may develop; this is often the first indicator of scleroderma. Scleroderma is most common in middle-aged females. The cause of scleroderma is unknown, but it is likely related to autoimmune, genetics, and/or environmental factors.

Massage and Scleroderma

Keep the client warm because they may be prone to cold intolerance. This modification may include the use of a blanket, an electric table warmer, raising the room temperature, asking the client to wear socks during the massage, or a combination of these. Before massaging the affected area, obtain verbal consent. Some clients with disfiguring scleroderma may feel self-conscious while they are on the massage table. If consent is granted, ask the client how sensitive the skin is and adjust pressure accordingly. Clients with highly sclerosed skin may be extremely sensitive to pressure. Use emollient lubricants to combat dry skin; some clients do best with a hypoallergenic product.

If the client is frail, use slowly applied light pressure. An example of light pressure is 3 on a 10-point pressure scale. Coexisting medical conditions (Raynaud disease, carpal tunnel syndrome, respiratory disease) should be factored into the treatment plan.

Seborrheic Dermatitis

Seborrheic dermatitis is a chronic inflammatory condition affecting skin that contains numerous sebaceous glands such as the scalp, face (i.e., eyebrows, eyelids, sides of the nose, behind the ears), axillae, chest, and groin. Seborrheic dermatitis on the scalp is called *dandruff*. In infants, it is called *cradle cap*. Between 10% and 20% of the population is affected by this condition in their lifetime, with people experiencing periods of exacerbation and remission. Seborrhea has no known cause, but it is associated with a yeast (fungus) called malassezia sometimes found in sebum, weakened immune responses, and the skin's reaction to stress or medications. Heredity may play a role in its development.

Massage and Seborrheic Dermatitis

Inquire about past skin reactions from chemicals in laundry detergents and eliminate contact with linens washed in the detergent identified, if applicable. Also, inquire about sensitivity over affected areas and adjust pressure accordingly. Use thin, water-based lubricants rather than oil-based lubricants over affected areas or perform techniques that do not require lubricant.

Shingles

Shingles is an acute, localized viral infection of the skin, caused by the varicella-zoster virus (VZV). It is essentially a reactivation of the chickenpox virus. After chickenpox resolves, the virus travels down a dermatome (areas of skin supplied by a single sensory spinal nerve) and is kept inactive by healthy immune responses. However, if immune responses become weakened, the virus can be reactivated and cause the lesions of shingles. The dermatome the virus previously retreated determines the area where skin lesions appear. The lesions are usually unilateral and typically affect only a small area of the body, usually the torso. However, the rash can appear on the face, and both sides of the body may be involved. Shingles is also called herpes zoster.

Shingles are fairly common, with about one million shingles cases occurring in the U.S. every year; almost one in three U.S. adults will get shingles in their lifetime. People most likely to acquire shingles are adults older than 50 years of age and people who are immunosuppressed, such as those who are positive for HIV, have diabetes, are taking immunosuppressant medications, or are under extreme psychosocial stress.

Massage and Shingles

For most practitioners, shingles is a local contraindication because lesions are painful. Use gloves or other barriers such as the sheet when massaging the hands as they may become contaminated by clients touching their own lesions (CDC, 2019). Massage linens are treated as contaminated to protect at-risk individuals. See Chapter 9 for recommended protocols. Table warmers and thermotherapy such as hot packs should not be used on affected areas.

Practitioners who have not had chickenpox, who have not received the chickenpox vaccine, or who are pregnant should not massage a client who has shingles. Even with prior immunity, VZV can be activated in the unborn, possibly causing shingles in the first few years of life (Royal College of Obstetricians and Gynaecologists [RCOG], 2015); this risk to the unborn increases after 28 weeks gestation. These precautions remain in effect until the shingles blisters scab over.

Stretch Marks

Stretch marks are indented lines or bands from overstretched skin. Common areas of the body affected are the breasts, hips, thighs, buttocks, and abdomen. Some marks cover large areas of the body. Stretch marks are also called *striae*. Stretch marks are caused by the rapid expansion of connective tissue leading to skin thinning and atrophy. This can occur from advanced pregnancy, breast enlargement surgery, or sudden weight gain. Their severity may be affected by genetic factors.

Massage and Stretch Marks

Use light pressure over stretch marks as they are weaknesses in the skin. An example of light pressure is 3 on a 10-point pressure scale. Massage will not reduce or minimize stretch marks because they are not caused by a build-up of collagen as occurs in scar tissue.

Warts

Warts are small, rough, raised, viral-induced skin growths. They may occur anywhere on the body, but most warts are on the hands, feet (called plantar warts), face and legs (called flat warts), and genitals (called genital warts). Warts may appear singularly or as multiple growths. Warts are contagious and are mainly spread by direct skin contact, but they may also be spread by touching objects like towels or razors. People who have warts in one location of the body can also spread the infection to other body parts. Warts are also called *verrucas*. Warts are caused by the human papillomavirus virus (HPV). Certain strains of HPV are responsible for cervical cancer.

Massage and Warts

Warts are local contraindications or contact precautions because they can be transmitted by contact. Use gloves or other barriers such as the sheet when massaging the hands as they may become contaminated by clients touching their own lesions (CDC, 2019). Massage linens are treated as contaminated. See Chapter 9 for recommended protocols.

E-RESOURCES

http://evolve.elsevier.com/Salvo/MassageTherapy

- Chapter challenge
- Flash cards

ASHLEY MONTAGU

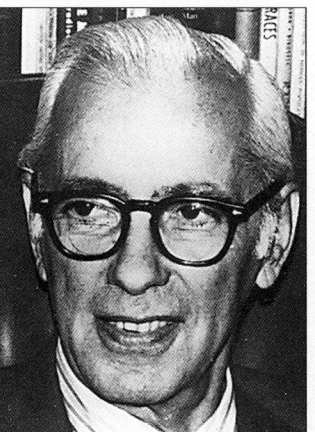

All massage practitioners bring their skills and talents from their lives before massage school to the table. Former accountants may keep well-organized records. Former teachers may find it easy to explain scientific research to clients in a way that is clear and easy to understand. Even those who choose massage as a first career bring their own unique skills to massage. Whether your passion in school was for chemistry or choir, you can use those strengths for the benefit of your clients and your practice.

In many cases, a person who has had a major impact on the massage field was not even a massage practitioner at all. This was the case with Ashley Montagu, an anthropologist who changed the way the medical profession thought about touch.

Montagu was born in London and moved to the United States to earn his doctorate in anthropology at Columbia University. He did extensive research and published widely, writing more than 60 books over the course of his lifetime. He is best known outside of the manual therapies for his work debunking the idea of distinct races among the human species. He helped write the United Nations Educational, Scientific and Cultural Organization (UNESCO) Statement on Race, as well as the book, *Man's Most Dangerous Myth: The Fallacy of Race.*

Less known to the wider world, however, is another aspect of the human experience Montagu researched: the role of touch. A professor of anatomy and anthropology, he read an article on the effects of thyroid surgery on two groups of rodents. Seventy-five percent of the first group survived, whereas none of the second group did. As an aside, it was mentioned the first group had been cuddled and stroked at feeding time by their caretaker, whereas the caretaker of the second group simply threw food into the cage. The authors of the study did not find this significant. Montagu did. When Montagu shared the study with a class he was teaching, one student said everyone from his farming hometown knew newborn animals must be licked by their mothers or else die. This propelled Montagu's research into physical nurturing.

Montagu's studies show mental health, as well as physical health, require effective nurturing and touch. The only thing about his research he found terribly surprising "was doctors had rarely understood this." He wrote a book on the subject called *Touching: The Human Significance of the Skin,* which is a must-read for massage practitioners who want to understand the deeper importance of what they do.

Montagu was not universally loved. He received abuse at the hands of anti-Semites in his younger years and anti-Communists later in his career. (His work with the United Nations was not without controversy, and he was dismissed from his teaching position at Rutgers University over it.) Still, his research into various aspects of the human condition has been validated time and again by further studies. He's received more than a dozen major awards and two honorary doctoral degrees.

When thinking about how you can contribute to the advancement of the massage community, do not limit yourself to the work of your hands. Researchers, writers, artists, engineers, teachers, and all kinds of people have done much to improve the experience, spread awareness, build community, and grow knowledge. Ashley Montagu was an anthropologist who never thought about what a boon his work would be to the massage community, and yet it was. What will you do?

REFERENCES

Adişen, E., & Onder, M. (2007). Allergic contact dermatitis from *Laurus nobilis* oil induced by massage. *Contact Dermatitis, 56*(6), 360–361.

American Academy of Dermatology. (2018). *Help stop pimples*. Retrieved from https://www.aad.org/public/kids/skin/acne-pimples-zits/helping-stop-pimples

Anderson, C., Lis-Balchin, M., & Kirk-Smith, M. (2000). Evaluation of massage with essential oils on childhood atopic eczema. *Phytotherapy Research, 14*(6), 452–456.

Buss, I. C., Halfens, R. J., Abu-Saad, H. H. (1997). The effectiveness of massage in preventing pressure sores: A literature review. *Rehabilitation Nursing, 22*(5), 229–234,

Centers for Disease Control and Prevention. (2019). *Type and duration of precautions recommended for selected infections and conditions: Appendix A updates*. Retrieved from https://www.cdc.gov/infectioncontrol/guidelines/isolation/appendix/type-duration-precautions.html?fbclid=IwAR0wKVWUgn6H5Gf34X2wCMI38mknFejJzjCPXicGZaKLlwrk8w6hHvfdaHI#I

Crawford, G. H., Katz, K. A., Ellis, E., & James, W. D. (2004). Use of aromatherapy products and increased risk of hand dermatitis in massage therapists. *Archives of Dermatology, 140*(8), 991–996.

Devrimci-Ozguven, H., Kundakci, T. N., Kumbasar, H., & Boyvat, A. (2000). The depression, anxiety, life satisfaction and affective expression levels in psoriasis patients. *Journal of the European Academy of Dermatology and Venereology, 14*(4), 267–271.

Goodman, C. C., & Fuller, K. S. (2014). *Pathology: Implications for the physical therapist* (4th ed.). St Louis: Elsevier.

Grier, T. (2012). *Is there cross-reactivity between shea butter and natural rubber latex?* http://www.latexallergyresources.org/sites/default/files/newsletter-attachments/The%20ALERT%20Dec%202012.pdf.

Lakshmi, C. (2014). Allergic contact dermatitis (type IV hypersensitivity) and type I hypersensitivity following aromatherapy with ayurvedic oils (Dhanwantharam thailum, Eladi coconut oil) presenting as generalized erythema and pruritus with flexural eczema. *Indian Journal of Dermatology, 59*(3), 283–286.

Lopez-Villafuerte, L., & Clores, K. H. (2016). Contact dermatitis caused by turmeric in a massage oil. *Contact Dermatitis, 75*(1), 52–53.

Moffitt Cancer Center. (2008). *Managing your scar*. Retrieved from https://moffitt.org/media/1086/managing_your_scar.pdf

National Eczema Association. (2015). *Natural and alternative treatments for eczema, what works, what doesn't*. Retrieved from https://nationaleczema.org/alternative-treatments/

National Institute for Health and Care Excellence (2014). *The prevention and management of pressure ulcers in primary and secondary care*. Retrieved from https://www.ncbi.nlm.nih.gov/books/NBK333138/

National Pressure Ulcer Advisory Panel, European Pressure Ulcer Advisory Panel, and Pan Pacific Pressure Injury Alliance. (2014). *Prevention and treatment of pressure ulcers: Quick reference guide*. Retrieved from http://www.npuap.org/wp-content/uploads/2014/08/Updated-10-16-14-Quick-Reference-Guide-DIGITAL-NPUAP-EPUAP-PPPIA-16Oct2014.pdf.

Royal College of Obstetricians and Gynaecologists. (2015). *Chickenpox and pregnancy*. Retrieved from https://www.rcog.org.uk/globalassets/documents/patients/patient-information-leaflets/pregnancy/pi-chickenpox-and-pregnancy.pdf

Salvo, S. G. (2022). *Mosby's pathology for massage professionals* (5th ed.). St Louis: Mosby.

Shahin, E. S., Dassen, T., & Halfens, R. J. (2009). Pressure ulcer prevention in intensive care patients: guidelines and practice. *Journal of Evaluation in Clinical Practice, 15*(2), 370–374.

Sutaria, A. H., & Schlessinger, J. (2018). *Acne vulgaris*. Retrieved from https://www.ncbi.nlm.nih.gov/books/NBK459173/.

Trattner, A., David, M., & Lazarov, A. (2008). Occupational contact dermatitis due to essential oils. *Contact Dermatitis, 58*(5), 282–284.

BIBLIOGRAPHY

Abrahams, P. H., Spratt, J. D., Loukas, M., & van Schoor, A. N. (2003). *Abrahams' and McMinn's clinical atlas of human anatomy* (8th ed.). St Louis: Elsevier.

Applegate, E. (2010). *The anatomy and physiology learning system* (4th ed.). Philadelphia: Saunders.

Como, D. (Ed.). (2016). *Mosby's dictionary of medicine, nursing, and health professions* (10th ed.). St Louis: Elsevier.

Frazier, M. S., & Drzymkowski, J. W. (2015). *Essentials of human diseases and conditions* (6th ed.). St Louis: Elsevier.

Hubert, R. J., & VanMeter, K. C. (2018). *Gould's pathophysiology for the health professions* (6th ed.). Philadelphia: Saunders.

Haubrich, W. S. (2003). *Medical meanings: A glossary of word origins* (2nd ed.). New York: American College of Physicians.

Herlihy, B. (2017). *The human body in health and illness* (6th ed.). St Louis: Saunders.

Huether, S. E., McCance, K. L., & Brashers, V. L. (2019). *Understanding pathophysiology* (7th ed.). St Louis: Mosby.

Kalat, J. W. (2013). *Biological psychology* (11th ed.). Belmont, Calif: Cengage Learning.

Kapit, W., & Elson, L. M. (2013). *The anatomy coloring book* (4th ed.). New York: Benjamin Cummings.

Kumar, V., Abbas, A. K., & Aster, J. C. (2015). *Robbins & Cotran pathologic basis of disease* (9th ed.). St Louis: Mosby.

Lauderstein, D. (2012). *The deep massage book: How to combine structure and energy in bodywork*. Taos: Redwing Book Company.

Marieb, E. N., & Keller, S. M. (2018). *Essentials of human anatomy and physiology* (12th ed.). New York: Benjamin Cummings.

McCance, K. L., & Huether, S. E. (2019). *Pathophysiology: The biological basis for disease in adults and children* (8th ed.). St Louis: Mosby.

Montagu, A. (1986). *Touching: The human significance of the skin* (3rd ed.). New York: HarperCollins.

Myers, T. W. (2014). *Anatomy trains: myofascial meridians for manual and movement therapists* (3rd ed.). Churchill Livingstone: Elsevier.

Netter, F. H. (2018). *Atlas of human anatomy* (7th ed.). St Louis: Mosby.

Patton, K. T (2019). *Anatomy and physiology* (10th ed.). St Louis: Elsevier.

Patton, K. T., Thibodeau, G. A., & Douglas, M.M. (2012). *Essentials of anatomy and physiology* (4th ed.). New York: Pearson.

Porter, R. S., (2011). *The Merck manual of diagnosis and therapy* (19th ed.) Whitehouse Station, NJ: Merck Sharp and Dohme Corp.

Taber, C. W. (2021). *Taber's cyclopedic medical dictionary* (24nd ed.). Philadelphia: FA Davis.

REVIEW AND APPLY YOUR KNOWLEDGE

 **MATCHING ONE: CONCEPT REVIEW**

Place the letter of the answer next to the number of the term or phrase that best describes it.

A. Arrector pili
B. Dermis
C. Epidermis
D. Hair root plexus
E. Subcutaneous layer
F. Integumentary
G. Keratinocyte
H. Meissner corpuscle
I. Melanocyte
J. Pacini corpuscle
K. Sebaceous
L. Sudoriferous

_____   1. Receptor detecting light pressure, low-frequency vibrations, and textural sensations.
_____   2. Epidermal cell secreting a substance that waterproofs skin.
_____   3. Body system that includes skin, hair, nails, and glands.
_____   4. Sweat-producing glands that help regulate body temperature and eliminate wastes.
_____   5. Epidermal cell that produces dark pigment.
_____   6. Muscle attached to hair follicles and contracts to pull the hair shaft upright.
_____   7. Thick, deeper region of the skin.
_____   8. Layer beneath the dermis containing loose connective tissue, adipose tissue, nerves, and blood vessels.
_____   9. Receptor detecting deep pressure, high-frequency vibrations, and stretch.
_____ 10. Oil-producing glands connected to hair follicles.
_____ 11. Thin, outer region of the skin.
_____ 12. Receptor detecting hair movement.

MATCHING TWO: CONCEPT REVIEW

Place the letter of the answer next to the number of the term or phrase that best describes it.

A. Apocrine
B. Carotene
C. Ceruminous
D. Cyanosis
E. Ischemia
F. Hair
G. Hyperemia
H. Melanin
I. Pallor
J. Somatosensory cortex
K. Ruffini corpuscle
L. Eccrine

_____   1. Skin reddening from vasodilation and increased blood flow.
_____   2. Type of sudoriferous gland that secretes watery perspiration which can help regulate body temperature.
_____   3. Decreased blood flow from vasoconstriction or other causes.
_____   4. Area of brain receiving stimuli from the external environment and determines the type of sensation felt (i.e., pressure, temperature, pain), and where the sensation is located
_____   5. Pale or ashen skin.
_____   6. Yellow pigment giving skin a golden color.
_____   7. Keratinized filaments arising from pouchlike follicles in the dermis.
_____   8. Pigment that darkens to create a semiprotective shield against UV radiation in sunlight.
_____   9. Receptor that detects deep pressure, continuous pressure, and warmth.
_____ 10. Skin gland producing earwax.
_____ 11. Blue or purple-tinted skin.
_____ 12. Type of sudoriferous gland that begins to function during puberty and secretes a strong-smelling perspiration.

MULTIPLE CHOICE: TEST YOUR KNOWLEDGE

Place the letter of the answer next to the number of the term or phrase that best describes it.

_____ 1. The use of medicated patches is based on which function of the integumentary system?
A. Protection
B. Immunity
C. Absorption
D. Sensation

_____ 2. The deepest epidermal layer where cells develop, grow, and divide is the:
A. stratum basale.
B. stratum lucidum.
C. stratum corneum.
D. stratum spinosum.

_____ 3. The translucent epidermal layer and is only present in the thick skin of the palms and soles is the:
A. stratum basale.
B. stratum lucidum.
C. stratum corneum.
D. stratum spinosum.

_____ 4. Another term for the subcutaneous layer is the:
A. dermis.
B. epidermis.
C. ectodermis.
D. hypodermis.

_____ 5. The panniculus adiposus is another term for:
A. the epidermal-dermal junction.
B. epidermis.
C. dermis.
D. the subcutaneous layer.

_____ 6. A port-wine stain is which type of skin pigmentation?
A. Freckle
B. Hemangioma
C. Melasma
D. Mole

_____ 7. The area where most hangnails occur is the:
A. nail root.
B. lateral nail folds.
C. cuticle.
D. free edge.

_____ 8. Mammary glands are a modified type of which gland?
A. Sebaceous
B. Ceruminous
C. Sudoriferous
D. Hypothalamus

_____ 9. Receptors that detect actual or potential tissue damage and are sensitive to pain are called:
A. nociceptors.
B. mechanoreceptors.
C. Merkel discs.
D. Krause corpuscles.

_____ 10. Burn classification that is also called a full-thickness burn and extends to the muscle or bone.
A. First-degree
B. Second-degree
C. Third-degree
D. Fourth-degree

_____ 11. Which is contagious and requires postponement of massage until the condition has resolved?
A. Impetigo
B. Ringworm
C. Warts
D. Scabies

_____ 12. Which type of scar is elevated and spreads beyond the boundaries of the original wound?
A. Adhesion
B. Hypertrophic
C. Keloid
D. Contracture

CRITICAL THINKING

Can Massage Trigger a Shingles Outbreak?

Do you think it is possible to activate the herpes zoster virus through the application of deep pressure, causing the client to have a shingles outbreak?

Answers to this question can include but are not limited to:

Although it is theoretically possible to activate the herpes zoster virus through the application of deep pressure, it is highly unlikely. In people who have had chickenpox, the immune system keeps the herpes zoster virus in check unless the immune system is depleted in some way. Deep pressure applied during a massage treatment does not deplete the immune system. If a client does develop shingles after receiving a massage, it is most likely because they are older than 50 years of age; is immunosuppressed, such as being positive for HIV or having diabetes; is taking immunosuppressant medications; or is under extreme psychosocial stress.

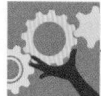

PROFESSIONAL PRACTICE

If It Itches, Scratch It

Contessa had been working at a very chic salon for approximately 4 years. One of her regulars was Julia, wife of a prominent local attorney and stay-at-home mom. Julia, who also receives other salon services, came in faithfully every week for a 90-minute massage.

Contessa usually spent the first hour massaging Julia's back while Julia was prone and then turned her supine for the last 30 minutes. Julia usually napped when she was face down, but she liked to spend the last 30 minutes chatting. As they were talking about parenting, Julia exclaimed, "Oh! I almost forgot, please save the last 5 minutes or so for a scalp massage. My daughter, Jill, came home with head lice, and ever since then, I can't stop thinking about it, and the very thought makes my head itch."

As Contessa began to comply with Julia's request for a scalp massage, she realized nits were attached to some of Julia's own hair shafts. Contessa finished the massage without saying anything. She knew she should tell Julia, but she was afraid of ruining the relaxation effect of the massage, afraid of Julia's reaction, and afraid of losing her as a client.

If you were Contessa, how might you have approached Julia with the news?

Should Contessa share the information with the other employees at the salon, especially Julia's hairdresser?

What steps does Contessa need to take as far as sanitizing her table, linens, and face rest?

If you were Julia, how might you have received the news you were infested with head lice?

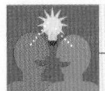 **DISCUSSION**

Got the Herp?

Cold sores are contagious viral infections and can be spread by direct contact. Some practitioners believe they should not work if they have one, whereas others think it is okay. What do you think? What would you do if/when you looked in the mirror and saw a cold sore on your lower lip? If available, post your reflections on an Internet-based discussion board monitored by your instructor.

CHAPTER 23

Nervous System, Pathologies, Disorders, and Injuries

LEARNING OBJECTIVES

After completing this chapter, the student should be able to:

1. List anatomic structures and physiologic processes related to the nervous system and discuss its basic organization.
2. Outline types of cells, neural structures, and their function, including neuroglia, neurons, reflexes, reflex arcs, nerves and nerve impulses, synapses, and synaptic transmission.
3. List structures, functions, and characteristics of the central and peripheral nervous systems, including the brain, spinal cord, cranial and spinal nerves, and the autonomic nervous system and its divisions.
4. Identify the senses and their receptors.
5. Describe neurologic pathologies and disorders and state their massage modifications.

INTRODUCTION

Every thought, action, and sensation, including pain and pleasure, is a reflection of nervous system activity. We are what our brains experience. The nervous system is the body's primary communication and regulation system; the nervous system detects stimuli inside and outside the body, interprets them, determines a response, and then executes the response, usually by muscle contraction or glandular secretion. To accomplish this, the body must be able to interact and communicate with both the internal and external environments. As stated in Chapter 18, *homeostasis* is the constant and stable internal environment within a narrow range despite changes that occur in the external environment. *Allostasis* is the process of achieving homeostasis and is regulated primarily by the nervous and endocrine systems. The endocrine system, discussed in the next chapter, responds more slowly and uses hormones as chemical messengers. The nervous system responds more rapidly and uses neurotransmitters as chemical messengers as well as electrical signals called impulses to transmit information along nerve cells. The nervous and endocrine systems are interrelated and, in some instances, even regulate each other. For example, nerve impulses can cause hormonal secretions, and hormones can stimulate parts of the brain. The nervous and endocrine systems can be referred to as the *neuroendocrine system* because of their shared regulatory functions.

This chapter examines the structures and functions of the nervous system. It begins with a brief look at how this system is organized, neurons and nerves, progresses to nerve impulses and synaptic transmissions, and then examines specialized divisions of the nervous system. Finally, the chapter reviews the senses and their receptors and conditions of the nervous system, some of which may affect the application of massage. Use Table 23.1 to help you understand terms of the nervous system. *Neurology,* or *neuroscience,* is the study of the nervous system.

ANATOMY

Basic structures and components of the nervous system are:
- Brain
- Spinal cord
- Cranial and spinal nerves
- Sense organs
- Neurotransmitters

PHYSIOLOGY

Important functions of the nervous system are:
- Sensory input—Nerve cells detect internal or external stimuli and transmit this information to the brain and spinal cord.
- Interpretive functions—The brain and spinal cord interpret the information, store some of it, and may issue a response such as motor output.

TABLE 23.1 Word Meanings

WORD	MEANING
arachnoid	*Gr.* spider; shaped
autonomic	*Gr.* self; law
axon	*Gr.* axis
baroreceptor	*Gr.* weight; *L.* to receive
Broca area	Broca, French surgeon (1824–1880)
cauda equina	*L.* tail-like; horse
cerebellum	*L.* little brain
cerebrum	*L.* brain
chemoreceptor	*Gr.* chemical; *L.* to receive
cochlea	*L.* snail shell
conduction	*L.* to lead together
corpus callosum	*L.* body; hard or callused
cortex	*L.* bark or rind
cyton	*Gr.* cell
dendrites	*Gr.* treelike
diencephalon	*Gr.* two or second; brain
dura mater	*L.* hard or tough; mother
encephalic	*Gr.* brain
filum terminale	*L.* threadlike; at the end
ganglion	*Gr.* knot
gyri	*Gr.* circle
incus	*L.* anvil
intrafusal	*L.* within; spindle
macula	*L.* spot
mechanoreceptor	*Gr.* machine; *L.* to receive
medulla oblongata	*L.* marrow or middle; long
meninges	*Gr.* membrane
myelin	*Gr.* marrow
neurilemma	*Gr.* sinew; husk
neuro	*Gr.* sinew
neuroglia	*Gr.* sinew; glue
neurotransmitter	*Gr.* sinew; *L.* a sending across
nociceptor	*L.* hurt; to receive
node of Ranvier	Ranvier, French pathologist (1835–1922)
oligodendrocyte	*Gr.* little; tree; cell
parasympathetic	*Gr.* by the side of, sympathetic
photoreceptor	*Gr.* light; *L.* to receive
pia mater	*L.* tender, soft; mother
plexus	*L.* braid
proprioceptor	*L.* one's own; a receiver
pons	*L.* bridge
reciprocal inhibition	*L.* to move backward; to restrain
reflex	*L.* bent back
retina	*L.* a net
saltatory	*L.* to dance or leap
Schwann cell	Schwann, German anatomist (1810–1882)
soma	*Gr.* body
stapes	*L.* stirrup
stimuli	*L.* to incite
sulci	*L.* groove or furrow
summation	*L.* total
sympathetic	*Gr.* to feel with
synapse	*Gr.* to join
thalamus	*Gr.* chamber
thermoreceptor	*Gr.* heat; *L.* to receive
tympanic	*Gr.* drum
vagus	*L.* wandering
Wernicke area	Wernicke, German neurologist (1848–1905)

Gr., Greek; *L.,* Latin.

- Motor output—Nerve cells send impulses to muscles and glands. Motor output includes muscle contractions and reflexes, glandular secretions, which can lead to changes in hormone levels or activation of immune reactions such as inflammation.
- Higher mental functioning and emotional responsiveness—The nervous system is responsible for mental processes including **cognition** or thinking, memory, and learning, as well as emotional responses such as joy, fear, sadness, and anger.

ORGANIZATION OF THE NERVOUS SYSTEM

The nervous system is divided into systems, subsystems, and divisions.

Central and Peripheral Nervous Systems

The **central nervous system** (CNS) occupies a central or medial position in the body and includes the brain, spinal cord, meninges, and cerebrospinal fluid (CSF). These structures are surrounded by bones of the skull and spinal column. The CNS interprets sensory information and issues instructions in the form of motor output (Fig. 23.1).

The **peripheral nervous system** (PNS) extends beyond the skull and vertebral column and includes the cranial and spinal nerves. Cranial nerves exit the brain and spinal nerves exit the spinal cord. The PNS carries sensory information to the CNS, which issues instructions to muscles and glands, and regulates autonomic functions such as blood pressure or sweating.

Somatic and Autonomic Nervous Systems

The PNS is subdivided into the somatic and autonomic nervous systems. The **somatic nervous system** (SNS) transmits sensory input (vision, hearing, taste, smell, and touch) and controls the voluntary function of skeletal muscles. The exceptions are cranial and spinal reflexes, which are involuntary.

The **autonomic nervous system** (ANS) regulates the involuntary activities of organs, glands, and smooth muscle. The exception is breathing, which is both voluntary and involuntary.

Sympathetic and Parasympathetic Divisions

The ANS contains sympathetic and parasympathetic subdivisions. The **sympathetic division** controls energy expenditure, and the **parasympathetic division** controls energy conservation. These two divisions are discussed later in this chapter.

NEURONS, NEUROTRANSMITTERS, REFLEXES, REFLEX ARCS, AND NEUROGLIA

The nervous system contains cells called *neurons* and *neuroglia.* Neurons transmit nerve impulses. Neuroglia do not generate nerve impulses but instead supports neurons.

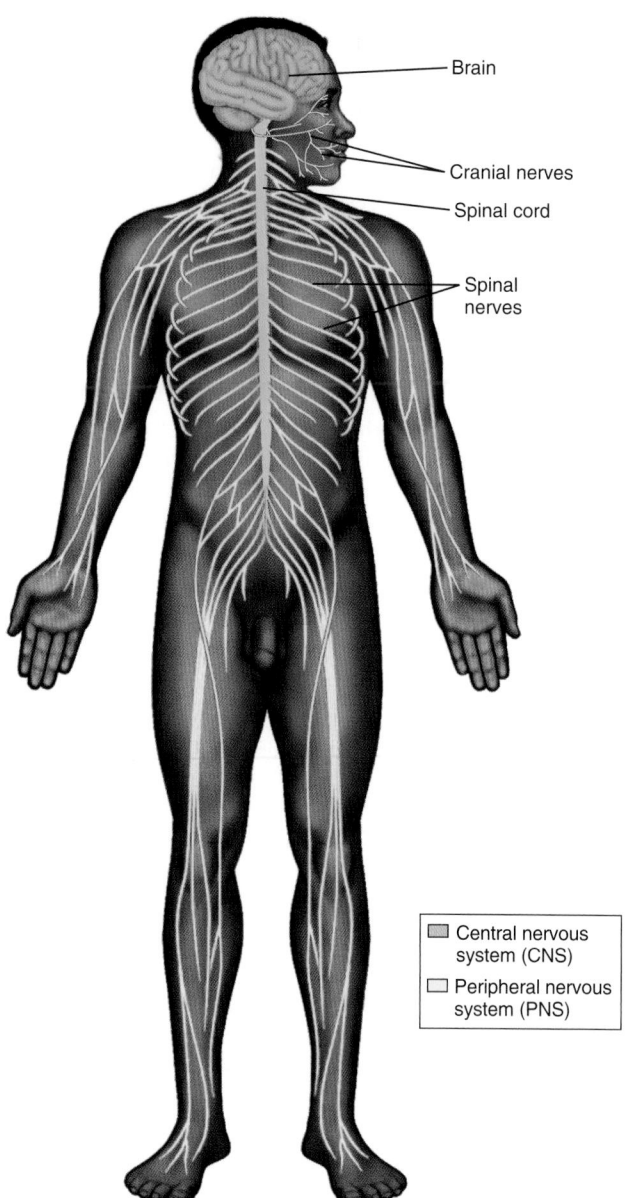

FIG. 23.1 Central and peripheral nervous systems, anterior view. The central nervous system occupies a central position in the body and includes the brain and spinal cord *(green).* The peripheral nervous system includes cranial and spinal nerves *(yellow).* (From Patton, K., & Thibodeau, G. [2014]. *The human body in health and disease* [6th ed.]. St. Louis, MO: Mosby.)

Neurons

Neurons are impulse-conducting cells and are the simplest structural units of the nervous system. Neurons also produce and secrete neurotransmitters that assist in the transmission of nerve impulses. To accomplish this task, neurons possess properties of excitability or irritability, conductivity, and secretion.

- **Excitability/Irritability.** Ability to respond to a stimulus and produce an impulse, which is a tiny electrical current. Neurons can respond to electrical, chemical, thermal, visual, or mechanical stimuli.

- **Conductivity.** Ability to transmit an impulse along the length of their axons and then on to other neurons, muscles, or glands.
- **Secretion.** Ability to release a chemical called a neurotransmitter.

Neurons vary in shape and size. However, they all have three basic parts: cell body, dendrite, and axon (Fig. 23.2). Dendrites and axons are collectively referred to as *nerve fibers*.

- **Cell Body.** Contains the nucleus and other organelles. The cell body is also known as the *soma*.
  - **Nuclei.** Cell bodies in the CNS.
  - **Ganglia.** Cell bodies in the PNS.
- **Dendrites.** Projections that receive and transmit the impulse toward the cell body. Dendrites are usually short and narrow.
- **Axon.** Projection that transmits the impulse away from the cell body. Axons usually extend from the hillock, which is the narrow region of the cell body. The ends of the axon are called *telodendria,* or *axon terminals*, which contain *synaptic bulbs*. Each bulb possesses multiple synaptic vesicles, which contain neurotransmitters and are discussed next (see Fig. 23.2). Some axons contain collateral branches, which allow individual neurons to make synaptic connections with other neurons, muscles, or glands. **LEARNING TIP**: To help you remember <u>a</u>xons transmit nerve impulses <u>a</u>way from the cell body, both <u>A</u>xon and <u>A</u>way begin with the letter "A."

Neurotransmitters

Neurotransmitters are chemical messengers that are released by synaptic vesicles upon arrival of a nerve impulse, travel across a synapse, and can transfer the impulse to another neuron, muscle, or gland. Neurotransmitters are excitatory or inhibitory. Excitatory neurotransmitters allow the impulse to be transferred, and inhibitory neurotransmitters prevent impulse transmission.

The most common neurotransmitter is acetylcholine, and is needed for muscle contraction. Other neurotransmitters include serotonin, dopamine, and gamma-aminobutyric acid (GABA). Some neurotransmitters are also hormones, such as epinephrine, norepinephrine, and endorphins. In addition, many cells have receptors for both neurotransmitters and hormones and therefore can be regulated by both.

See Table 23.2 for a list of common neurotransmitters.

Classifying Neurons by Impulse Direction

Neurons can be classified structurally by the number of poles or processes that extend from the cell body (e.g., unipolar [not found in humans], bipolar, pseudounipolar, and multipolar). Neurons can be classified functionally by the direction the nerve impulse is traveling.

- **Afferent (Sensory) Neuron.** Transmit impulses toward the CNS and are found in the skin, joints, and muscles; these neurons are also called *receptors*.
- **Efferent (Motor) Neuron.** Transmit impulses away from the CNS toward muscles or glands; these neurons are also called *effectors*.
- **Interneuron.** Transmit impulse between the sensory and motor segments of the nervous system. Interneurons have integrative functions and are the "decision-making" neurons. These are found in the brain and spinal cord and are also called *association neurons*.

LEARNING TIP: Use the word <u>**SAME**</u> to help you remember <u>S</u>ensory neurons are <u>A</u>fferent neurons and <u>M</u>otor neurons are <u>E</u>fferent neurons.

More About Receptors – Receptors generally respond to specific stimuli (e.g., light, sound, pressure). Some receptors adapt to stimuli rapidly. **Sensory adaptation** is the gradual decrease in receptor responsiveness to a constant or

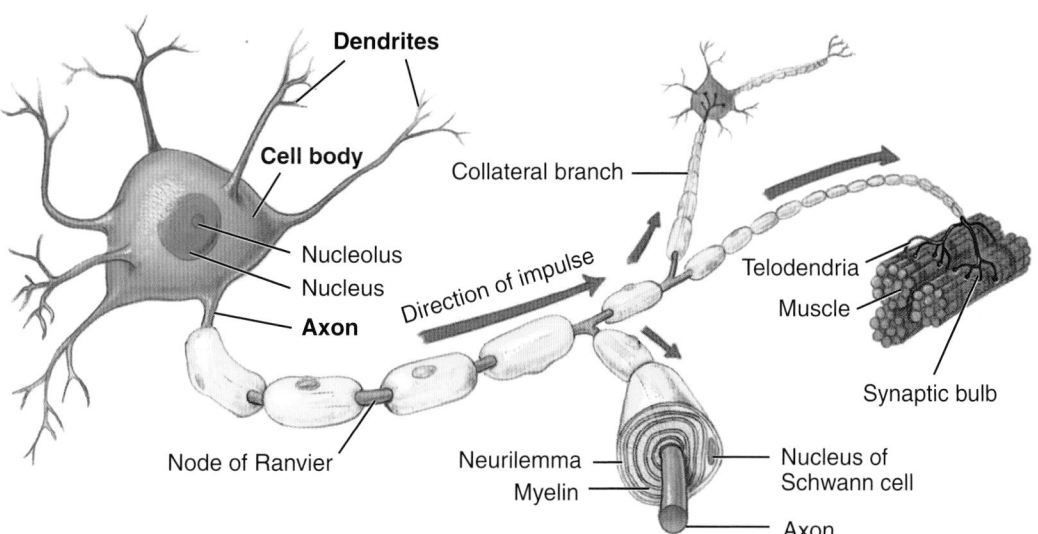

FIG. 23.2 A neuron, the impulse-conducting cell of the nervous system. An axon may contain collateral branches. (From Applegate, E. [2011]. *The anatomy and physiology learning system* [4th ed.]. St. Louis, MO: Saunders.)

TABLE 23.2 Neurotransmitters

NEUROTRANSMITTER	LOCATION	FUNCTION
Acetylcholine	Found in the CNS and PNS and neuromuscular junctions	Can be excitatory or inhibitory; vital for stimulating muscle contraction and the parasympathetic division of the autonomic nervous system; also involved with memory and motivation
Epinephrine	Found in several areas of the CNS and the sympathetic division of the ANS	Can be excitatory or inhibitory; hormone-like action when secreted by the adrenal medulla; stimulates the sympathetic division of the autonomic nervous system, or "fight-or-flight" response; involved in long-term memory, especially of stressful events
Norepinephrine	Found in several areas of the CNS and the sympathetic division of the ANS	Similar to epinephrine, can be excitatory or inhibitory; also a hormone secreted by the adrenal medulla; mediates several physiologic and metabolic responses of the autonomic nervous system or "fight-or-flight" response; also increases arousal and alertness, promotes vigilance, enhances formation and retrieval of memory, and focuses attention
Dopamine	Found in the brain and ANS	Can be excitatory or inhibitory; involved in motor control regulation and reward-motivated behaviors, especially those involving pleasure. Nicknamed "the pleasure hormone."
Serotonin	Found in several regions of the CNS and other tissues such as the digestive tract, bones, and blood vessels	Mostly inhibitory and important for sensory perception, mood regulation (contributes to feelings of well-being and happiness), and sleep. Nicknamed "the happy hormone."
Histamine	Found in the brain and other tissues such as the digestive tract, blood vessels, and skin	Mostly excitatory; involved in sleep–wake regulation, body temperature regulation, pain perception, endocrine regulation, and appetite regulation; histamine stimulates inflammatory responses when not acting as a neurotransmitter
Enkephalins	Found in the CNS and adrenal glands	Mostly inhibitory; action is similar to opiates, a pain-reducing agent
Endorphins	Found in the CNS and pituitary gland	Mostly inhibitory; action is similar to opiates; a pain-reducing agent
Gamma-aminobutyric acid (GABA)	Found in the brain	Mostly inhibitory; reduces neuronal excitability, and regulates muscle tone
Substance P	Found in the CNS and other tissues such as blood vessels and skin	Mostly excitatory; transmits pain information and associated with regulation of mood disorders, anxiety, and stress; associated with inflammatory processes

ANS, autonomic nervous system; CNS, central nervous system; PNS, peripheral nervous system.

prolonged stimulus. For example, the feeling of clothing against the skin diminishes over time. Receptors that detect movement and position adapt slowly. Receptors that detect pain rarely adapt.

Some receptors are distributed over small areas of the body (e.g., tongue, nose, eyes, and ears) and others are distributed over larger areas (e.g., skin, mucosa, muscles, and joints). Furthermore, the area of receptor distribution varies. For example, there are more receptors in the skin of the face and fingertips compared with the skin covering the back and the hips. Some receptors have wide **receptive fields,** which are areas of the body where a single sensory nerve can detect stimuli.

Classifying Receptors by Location

Receptors can be classified by where they are located and include exteroceptors, interceptors, and proprioceptors.

- **Exteroceptors.** Receive stimuli from the external environment, are distributed in the skin and mucosa, and are largely associated with the five senses (sight, smell, hearing, taste, and skin). Exteroceptors also include pain receptors located in the skin and mucosa. Chapter 22 contains a list of skin receptors.

- **Interoceptors (Visceroceptors).** Receive stimuli from the internal environment, and they are distributed throughout various organs. Interoceptors are involved with self-awareness and the detection of internal sensations such as heartbeat, breathing, hunger, satiety, thirst, and the urge to defecate or urinate. There is a growing body of research that suggests interoception is critical for homeostasis and is central to cognition, memory, decision-making, emotional processing, body ownership, and a general sense of self. Interoception is mediated by the glossopharyngeal and vagus nerves (cranial nerves 9 and 10).

- **Proprioceptors.** A type of interoceptor in muscles, tendons, and joints. These detect body movement and body position. Proprioceptors are discussed in the section titled "Spinal Nerves."

Classifying Receptors by Stimulus

Receptors can be classified by the stimuli they detect and include chemoreceptors, photoreceptors, thermoreceptors, nociceptors, mechanoreceptors, and osmoreceptors.

- **Chemoreceptors.** Detect chemical stimuli and include receptors on the tongue for taste, receptors in the nose for smell, and receptors in arterial walls for levels of oxygen, carbon dioxide, and pH.

- **Photoreceptors.** Detect light stimuli and include rods and cones in the retina of the eye.
- **Thermoreceptors.** Detect changes in environmental temperature and are found in the skin and mucosae.
- **Nociceptors.** Detect actual or potential tissue damage and are sensitive to pain; these serve a protective function by sending signals of a possible threat. The largest concentration of nociceptors is found in the skin, but they are in almost every tissue of the body.
- **Mechanoreceptors.** Detect mechanical stimuli such as pressure and soundwaves. The stimuli must change or deform their shape before they are activated. Mechanoreceptors are found in the skin, blood vessels, ears, muscles, and joints. Mechanoreceptors associated with reflexes (e.g., muscle spindles, Golgi tendon organs) are discussed in the section titled "Reflexes."
- **Osmoreceptors.** Detect changes in electrolyte concentrations in blood plasma. They are found in high concentration in the hypothalamus. They can stimulate the secretion of antidiuretic hormone by the pituitary and contribute to thirst.

Nerve Tracts, Nerves, and Connective Tissue Layers

Both nerves and nerve tracts are bundles of nerve fibers, but in different locations. **Nerve tracts** are bundles of nerve fibers in the CNS. Tracts are discussed in the spinal cord section of this chapter. **Nerves** are bundles of nerve fibers in the PNS. These structures are surrounded by connective tissue layers (Fig. 23.3).

- **Endoneurium.** The innermost connective tissue layer and surrounds the neuron.
- **Perineurium.** The middle connective tissue layer and surrounds bundles of neurons called fascicles. The perineurium provides vascularization. Fat fills the spaces between blood vessels and neighboring fasciculi.
- **Epineurium.** The outermost connective tissue layer surrounds groups of fascicles within the nerve.

Neuroglia

Neuroglia, or *glial cells,* are connective tissues that support, nourish, protect, and insulate neurons. Neuroglia do not transmit impulses, but they play an active role in many neurologic processes including memory, cognition, emotions, and pain regulation. Neuroglia are smaller and more

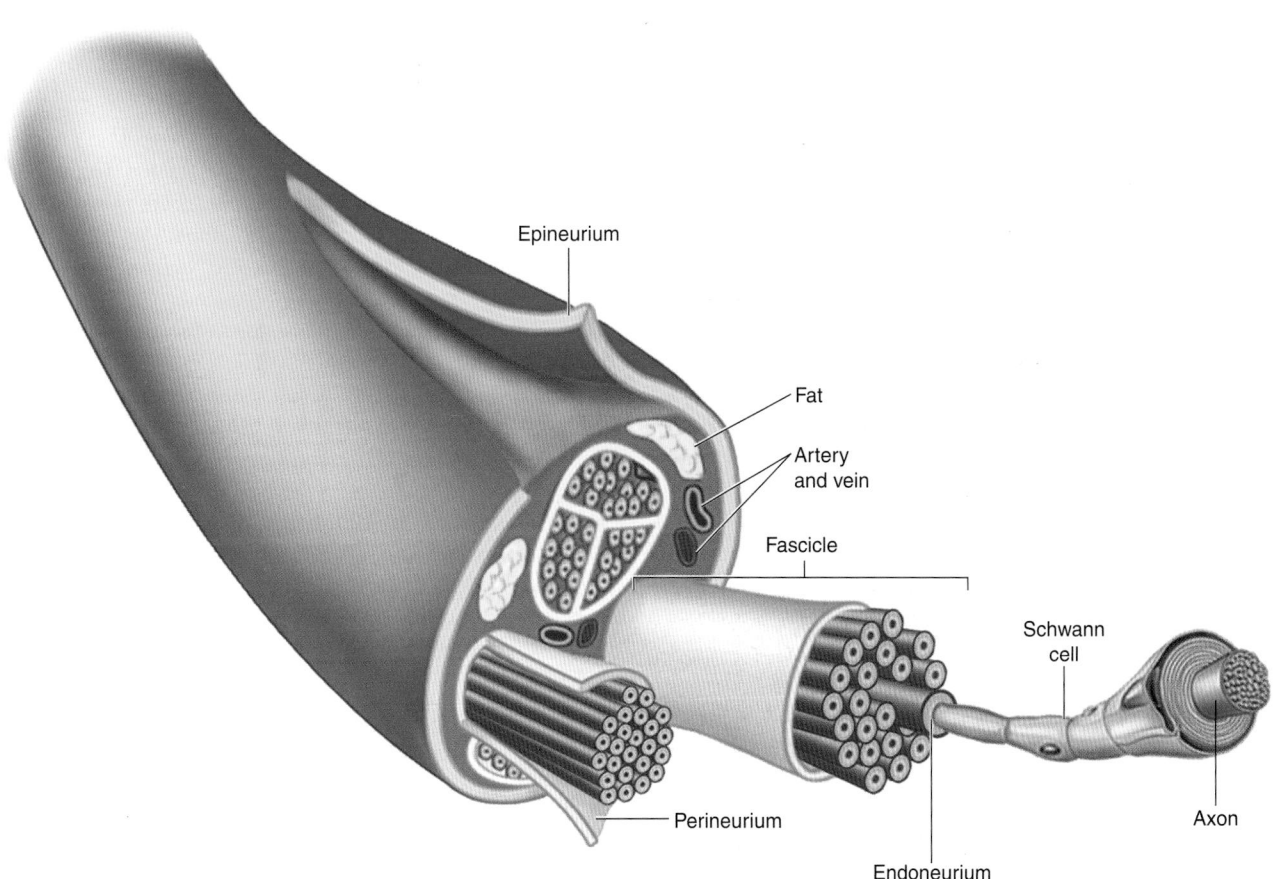

FIG. 23.3 A nerve with connective tissue layers identified, including the epineurium surrounding the nerve, the perineurium surrounding the fascicle, and the endoneurium surrounding the neuron *(cross-section view).* (From Patton, K., & Thibodeau, G. [2016]. *Structure and function of the body* [15th ed.]. St. Louis: Mosby.)

numerous compared with neurons. In fact, more than 50% of the CNS is composed of neuroglia. Neuroglia in the CNS includes astrocytes, ependymocytes, microglia, and oligodendrocytes.

- **Astrocytes.** Anchors neurons to capillaries, plays an important role in the exchange of nutrients, in stimulation of immune responses, and helps form the blood–brain barrier. Astrocytes are the largest and most numerous glial cells.
- **Ependymocytes (Ependymal Cells).** Lines ventricles in the CNS that helps circulate CSF.
- **Microglia.** Monitors the health of the neuron and can destroy and remove cellular debris and harmful microorganisms. These cells become hyperactive during disease-related processes, including Alzheimer disease.
- **Oligodendrocytes.** Produce the insulating myelin sheath around axons within the CNS.

Neuroglia in the PNS or those located outside the central nervous system include Schwann cells and satellite cells.

- **Schwann Cells.** Produce the fatty myelin sheath around axons in the PNS and are similar to oligodendrocytes of the CNS. The outer layer of myelin sheaths is called the **neurilemma**. In fact, Schwann cells are also called *neurolemmocytes.*
- **Satellite Cells.** Surrounds some neurons and plays an important role in the inflammation process and in repairing damage to the PNS following injury.

Myelin, myelin sheaths, and spaces between myelin sheaths called nodes of Ranvier are discussed in the section titled "Types of Nerve Impulse Conduction."

NERVE IMPULSES, SYNAPSES, AND SYNAPTIC TRANSMISSION

This section discusses nerve impulses, synapses, types of synapses, and synaptic transmission.

Nerve Impulses

A **nerve impulse** is a response to a stimulus that causes a neuron to depolarize, so it can transmit nerve impulses to other neurons, muscles, or glands. Some stimuli originate from external sources (e.g., pressure, light, smell). Other stimuli originate from neurotransmitters released by nearby neurons. Nerve impulses occur because the cell membrane of a neuron can conduct an electrical charge and polarize, depolarize, and repolarize.

Polarization

A polarized membrane has a positive electrical charge on one side and a negative charge on another side, which produces the resting state—not conducting an impulse. The cell membrane maintains this polarization through a mechanism called the **sodium–potassium pump,** which actively transports sodium out of the cell and potassium into the cell at unequal rates (for every three sodium ions [Na+] that move out of the cell, two potassium ions [K+] move into the cell [3:2]). The higher concentration of Na+ outside the cell creates a positive (+) charge, and the lower concentration of K+ inside the cell membrane creates a negative (−) charge.

Depolarization

When a neuron receives a stimulus, gates on the cell membrane open. Because Na+ outside the cell is electrically attracted to the negative charge inside the cell, Na+ rushes inside the cell. This action reverses the polarity—outside the cell becomes negative and inside the cell becomes positive. This reversal of cell membrane polarity is called depolarization, causing the generated nerve impulse to travel down the axon in segments, much like a line of dominoes. This action will continue until it reaches the end of the neuron. The impulse always moves in one direction and does not re-stimulate the segment from which it came (Fig. 23.4). Once the nerve impulse begins, it will be conducted at maximum capacity and is referred to as the **all-or-none response**.

Repolarization

After the cell membrane depolarizes, it quickly reverses back to its resting (polarized) state in a process called *repolarization.* During repolarization, K+ gates open and allow potassium to flow out. Next, the sodium–potassium pump (mentioned previously) pumps Na+ out of the cell and K+ into the cell. Neurons must be repolarized before they can conduct another nerve impulse. Within the brief span of time in which the membrane is repolarizing, it cannot respond to another stimulus. This time frame is referred to as the **refractory period**.

Synapse and Synaptic Transmission

The space between two neurons, or between a neuron and a muscle, or a gland where nerve impulses are transmitted, is called a **synapse**. A synapse has three main parts.

- **Synaptic Bulbs of the Presynaptic Neuron.** Tiny budlike structures are on the axon terminal ends of the presynaptic neuron. Each bulb contains numerous synaptic vesicles filled with neurotransmitters.
- **Synaptic Gap (Cleft).** Small space between the synaptic bulb on the presynaptic neuron and the cell membrane on the postsynaptic cell membrane of a neuron, muscle, or gland.
- **Postsynaptic Cell Membrane**. Contains binding sites on the cell membrane of a neuron, muscle, or gland.

Synaptic transmission is the process of transferring nerve impulses from one neuron across a synapse to another neuron, a muscle, or a gland. The process occurs in three steps.

1. A nerve impulse travels down the axon of a presynaptic neuron. When the impulse reaches the synaptic bulbs, neurotransmitters are released into the synapse.
2. Neurotransmitters travel across the synaptic gap from a presynaptic neuron to a postsynaptic cell membrane. The actions of neurotransmitters do not persist because they are continuously removed from the synapse by enzymes or **reuptake**, which is the reabsorption of neurotransmitters by the presynaptic neuron. Some drugs used to treat mood

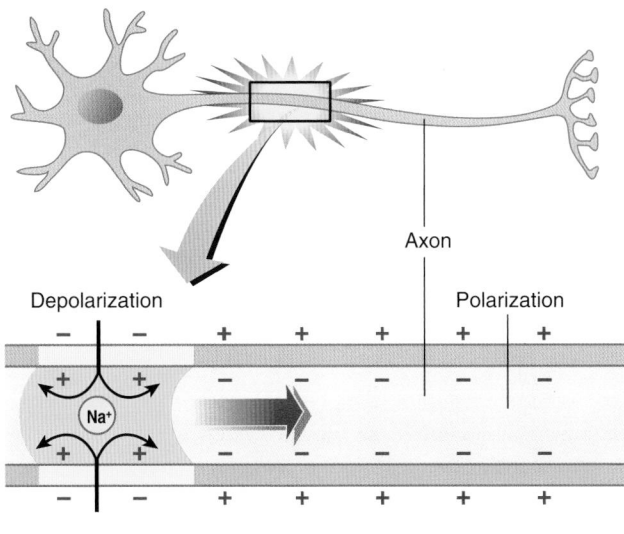

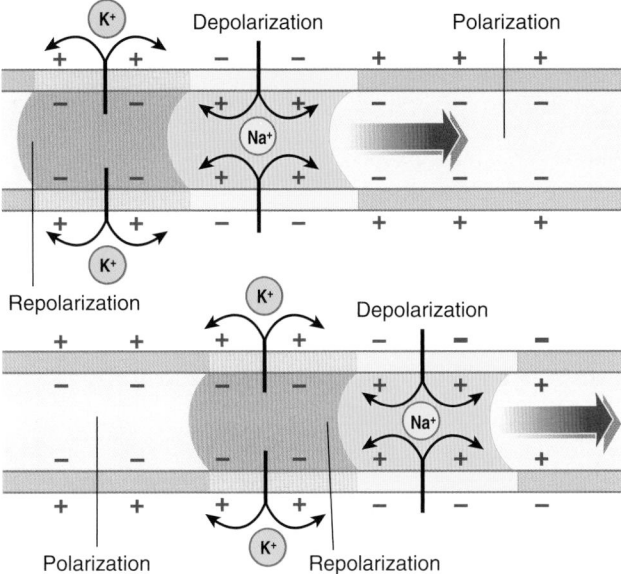

FIG. 23.4 Nerve impulse. Polarization or the neuron's resting state *(blue)*. Depolarization occurs when the neuron receives a stimulus and transmits a nerve impulse down the axon *(yellow)*. Sodium (Na+) moves inside the cell. Repolarization occurs as the neuron resumes its resting state *(purple)*. Potassium (K+) moves outside the cell.

disorders block or inhibit reabsorption of certain neurotransmitters to increase their concentration or prolong their action (e.g., selective serotonin reuptake inhibitors [SSRIs]; serotonin-norepinephrine reuptake inhibitors [SNRIs]).

3. Neurotransmitters attach to binding sites on the postsynaptic cell membrane (Fig. 23.5).

Types of Nerve Impulse Conduction: Saltatory and Continuous

Nerve impulse transmission can be classified by the speed of the impulse and whether or not the axon contains myelin.

- **Saltatory Conduction.** Nerve impulse conduction along myelinated axons. **Myelin** is a white fatty material that insulates axons and prevents impulse "leakage" to adjacent neurons. Unmyelinated spaces between myelinated sheaths are called **nodes of Ranvier**, which increase the speed of the nerve impulse because they literally jump from one unmyelinated space to the next (or node-to-node). The term *saltatory* comes from the Latin word *saltare,* meaning "to leap."

- **Continuous Conduction.** Nerve impulse conduction along unmyelinated axons. Nerve impulses are moved down the entire length of the axon, and more time is needed for this to occur.

More on Myelinated and Unmyelinated Axons: White and Gray Matter

As mentioned previously, myelin is white in color, which distinguishes myelinated axons from unmyelinated axons. Bundles of myelinated axons are called *white matter*. Bundles of unmyelinated axons and their associated cell bodies and dendrites are called *gray matter*.

CENTRAL NERVOUS SYSTEM

The CNS consists of the brain and spinal cord. These two structures are among the most important organs in the body, and they have several structures that protect them from damage. The most obvious is the bony protection of the skull and vertebral column. Other protective structures are the meninges, CSF, and the blood–brain barrier.

Meninges, Cerebrospinal Fluid, and the Blood–Brain Barrier

Meninges are connective tissue membranes that line the internal surfaces of the skull and vertebral column and surround the brain and spinal cord. The meninges help protect the CNS from physical injury. It does this by anchoring and cushioning the CNS, which helps reduce the impact during traumatic events. There are several meningeal layers (Fig. 23.6).

- **Pia Mater.** Innermost layer and attaches to the surface of the brain and spinal cord. This layer is thin and delicate and contains a rich supply of blood vessels. This layer also produces and helps circulate CSF. CSF is discussed in the next section.
    - **Subarachnoid Space.** Between the pia mater and the arachnoid mater and filled with CSF.
- **Arachnoid Mater.** Middle layer and composed of loosely arranged collagen fibers, which give it a weblike appearance.
    - **Subdural Space.** This is a potential space between the arachnoid mater and the dura mater. This space does not exist under normal circumstances, but it can be opened because of trauma or disease as it fills fluid (e.g., subdural hematoma).
- **Dura Mater.** Outermost layer and lies against the skull and vertebral column. The dura is thick and dense and creates partitions within the brain. The *falx cerebri* is between the right and left cerebral hemispheres. The

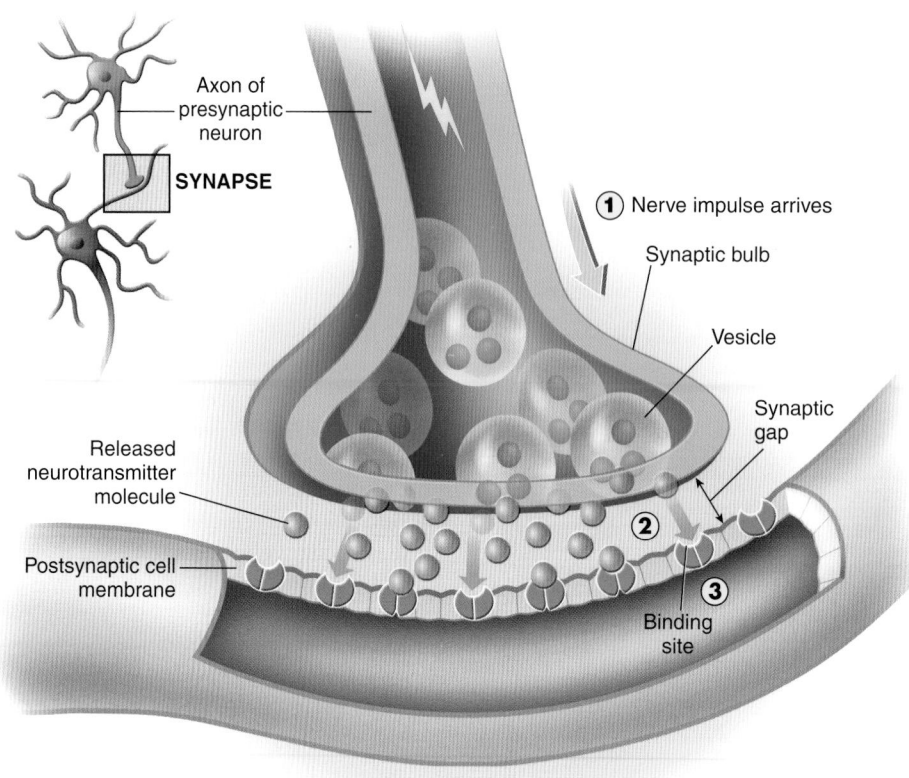

FIG. 23.5 Synaptic transmission. (1) A nerve impulse travels down an axon of the presynaptic neuron and reaches the synaptic bulb. Neurotransmitters are released from synaptic vesicles. (2) Neurotransmitters travel across the synaptic gap. (3) Neurotransmitters attach to binding sites on the postsynaptic cell membrane.

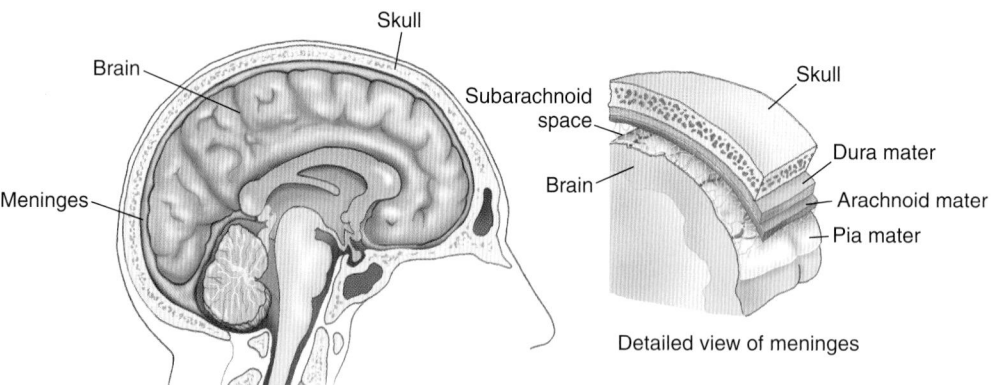

FIG. 23.6 Meninges. Locations of the meninges in relationship to the skull and the brain (*left image, lateral view*). Meningeal layers (*right image, detailed view*). (From Leonard, P. [2009]. *Building a medical vocabulary* [7th ed.]. St. Louis, MO: Saunders.)

tentorium cerebelli is between the cerebrum and cerebellum. The *falx cerebelli* is between the cerebellar hemispheres.

- **Epidural Space.** Between the dura and the vertebral canal. This space contains fat and blood vessels; this is where epidural injections are administered (i.e., anesthesia and nerve blockers, steroids).

LEARNING TIP: To help you remember the position of the meninges from the innermost to the outermost layer, use the word **PAD** for **P**ia mater, **A**rachnoid mater, and **D**ura mater.

Cerebrospinal fluid is the clear, colorless fluid surrounding the brain and spinal cord or CNS. It is found in the subarachnoid space. CSF is produced by the *choroid plexus*, a network of capillaries and ependymal (neuroglia) cells within the pia mater that line the cerebral ventricles. The CSF cushions the CNS and serves as a shock absorber, supplies the CNS with oxygen and nutrients, and helps remove metabolic wastes (i.e., amyloid-beta) during sleep. After CSF circulates through the CNS, it is reabsorbed into the bloodstream. CSF is sensitive to glucose and electrolyte balance and to changes in carbon dioxide levels.

The **blood–brain barrier** (BBB) refers to a tightly packed group of cells in the lining of blood vessels that supply the CNS. This allow the passage of certain molecules (e.g., oxygen, glucose) but prevents the passage of some harmful molecules (e.g., viruses, drugs, and even blood itself, as blood contains chemicals harmful to neurons). Cells of the BBB include astrocytes (glial cells), endothelial cells of blood capillaries, and a basement membrane. Just beyond the BBB are clusters of microglial cells. Although they are not part of the BBB, they also serve a protective function by looking for and destroying pathogens they encounter.

Brain

The **brain** is located in the skull, and consists of the cerebrum, the diencephalon, the cerebellum, and the brainstem (Fig. 23.7). It is one of the largest organs in the body, containing an estimated 86 billion neurons and storing trillions of bytes of information. The brain depends on glucose as its main source of energy. Glucose cannot be stored as glycogen, unlike glucose stored in the liver or in muscle cells, and needs a consistent supply. Glucose breaks down only by

aerobic respiration; thus the brain also needs a continuous supply of oxygen. Indeed, the brain uses approximately 20% of the body's oxygen intake.

Cerebrum

The **cerebrum** is the largest and most superior portion of the brain. The cerebrum controls somatosensory information (e.g., pressure, warmth, pain), motor responses, cognition, memory, language, intelligence, emotions, vision, smell, taste, and hearing. The surface of the brain is highly convoluted and consists of sulci (depressions or fissures) and gyri (elevations or ridges). The thin outermost layer of the cerebrum is the *cerebral cortex*. This layer is often referred to as gray matter. White matter, which comprises most of the cerebrum, lies beneath the cerebral cortex. The first two cranial nerves discussed later in the chapter emerge from the cerebrum.

The cerebrum is divided into the left and right hemispheres by the longitudinal fissure. The *left hemisphere* specializes in processing language (both receptive and expressive), analytic skills, and abstract thinking. The *right hemisphere* specializes in visual and spatial relationships, musical abilities, and emotional expression. The two hemispheres remain in contact and in communication with each other through a bundle of transverse fibers called the *corpus callosum*. Each hemisphere is further subdivided into regions called *lobes*. They are named for their overlying bone (Fig. 23.8).

- **Frontal Lobe.** Regulates executive functions such as judgment, problem-solving, planning, concentration,

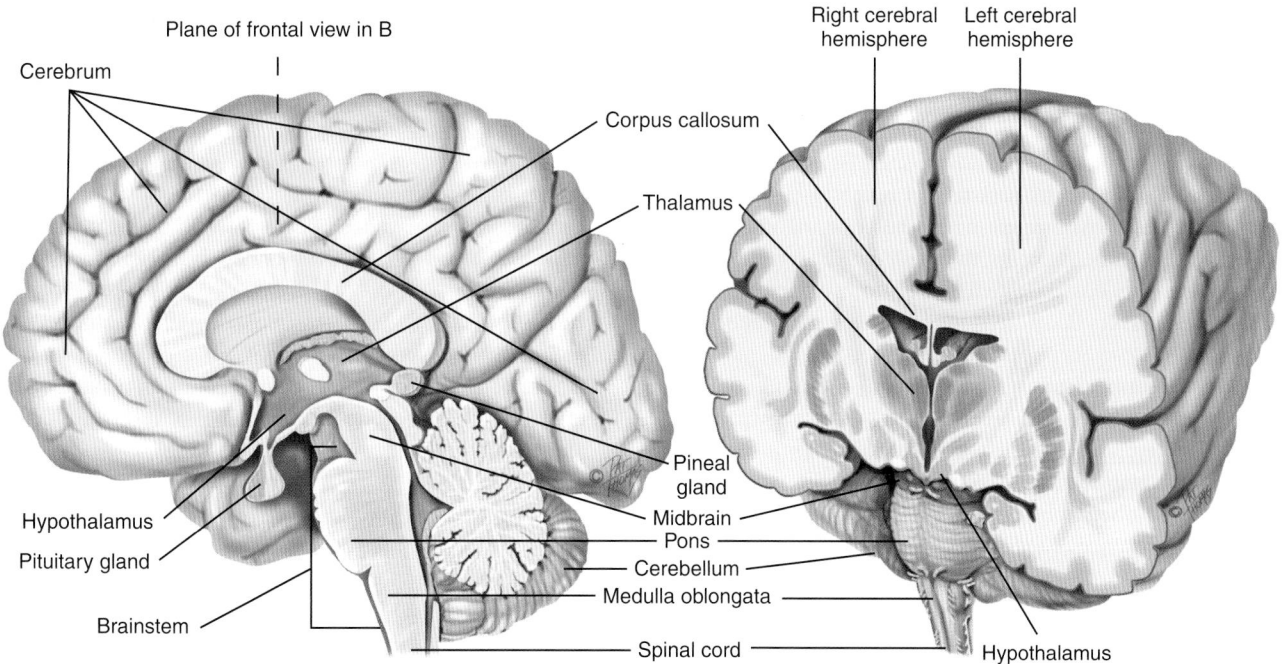

A. Cross section view of right hemisphere.

B. Frontal view

FIG. 23.7 Main regions of the brain (*lateral view [A] and frontal view [B]*). (Modified from Forbes, H. [2021]. *Jarvis's physical examination and health assessment* [3rd ed.]. Sydney: Elsevier.)

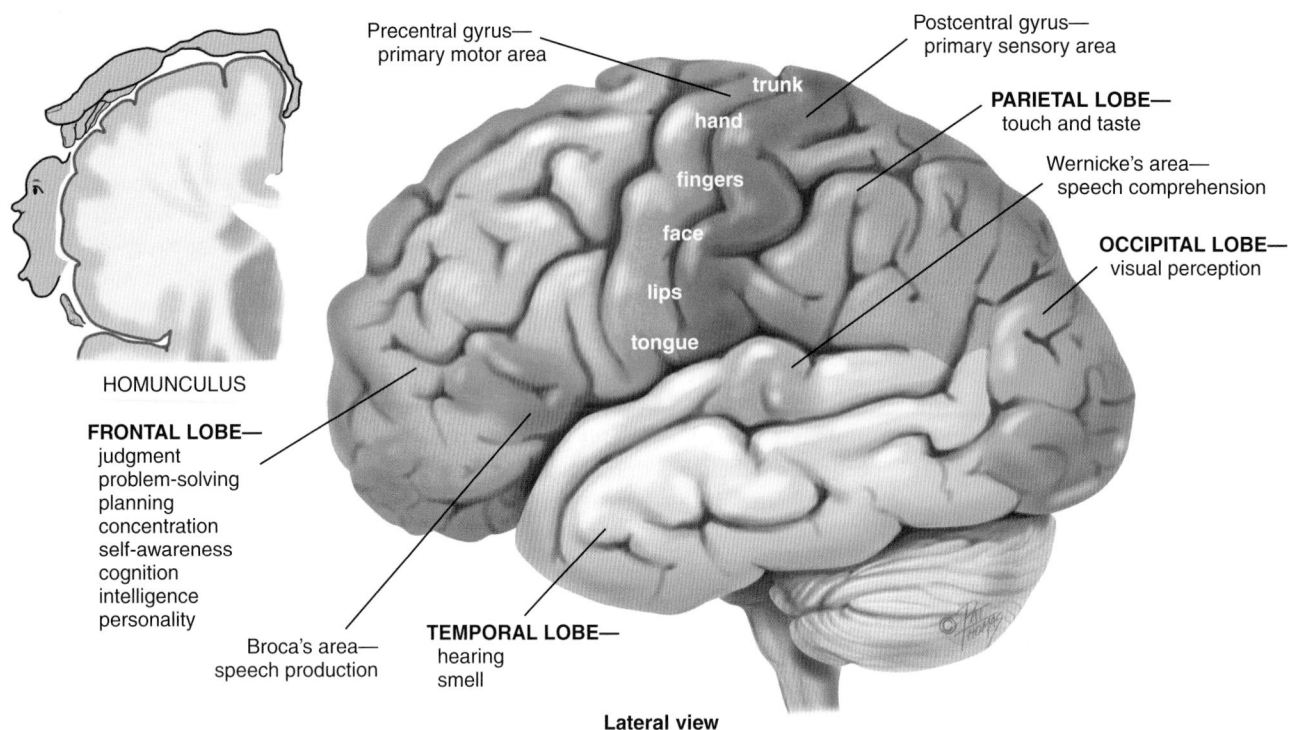

Precentral gyrus— primary motor area

Postcentral gyrus— primary sensory area

trunk

hand

fingers

face

lips

tongue

PARIETAL LOBE— touch and taste

Wernicke's area— speech comprehension

OCCIPITAL LOBE— visual perception

HOMUNCULUS

FRONTAL LOBE— judgment problem-solving planning concentration self-awareness cognition intelligence personality

Broca's area— speech production

TEMPORAL LOBE— hearing smell

Lateral view

FIG. 23.8 Cerebral lobes (*lateral view*). Locations of the frontal, parietal, temporal, and occipital lobes and their functions. (From Forbes, H. [2021]. *Jarvis's physical examination and health assessment* [3rd ed.]. Sydney: Elsevier).

self-awareness, cognition, intelligence, as well as personality. The frontal lobe also contains the Broca area, which is critical for speech production. The primary motor area in the *precentral gyrus* controls movements in the contralateral body. Certain parts of the body are more richly innervated compared with others. In fact, about 80% of the primary motor area is used to control muscles of the hands and fingers, face, lips, and tongue, which is represented by a homunculus, or "little man."

- **Parietal Lobe.** Controls taste and touch (i.e., pressure, temperature, pain) originating in the contralateral body. The parietal lobe contains the *postcentral gyrus* or the somatosensory cortex, which is the primary sensory area. This area mirrors body areas innervated by the precentral gyrus.
- **Temporal Lobe.** Controls hearing and smell. It contains the Wernicke area, which is critical to speech comprehension. The temporal lobe also helps to form memories and integrates them with taste, sound, sight, and touch.
- **Occipital Lobe.** Contains centers for visual perception including distance, depth, color, form, motion, and facial recognition.

A fifth lobe called the *insula* is hidden by parts of the frontal, parietal, and temporal lobes. This area is believed to be involved in consciousness, self-awareness, and interpersonal experience. The insula also plays a role in maintaining homeostasis by regulating the sympathetic and parasympathetic divisions of the ANS systems and may play a role in immune reactions.

Brainwaves

Brainwaves are rhythmic patterns of cerebral electrical activity displayed by an electroencephalogram (EEG). Brainwaves correlate with specific states of consciousness. Brainwaves are measured in cycles per second or hertz (Hz), and the lower the Hz value, the slower the brainwave activity. Names of EEG patterns are identified by Greek letters (Fig. 23.9).

- **Delta ($\leq$4 Hz).** The slowest and associated with sleep.
- **Theta (4 to 7 Hz).** Associated with deep relaxation, daydreaming, and is sometimes called the "twilight zone" because it is experienced between waking and sleeping.
- **Alpha (8 to 13 Hz).** Associated with calmness and relaxation.
- **Beta (14 to 38 Hz).** Associated with alertness and outwardly-focused concentration.
- **Gamma ($\geq$39 Hz).** The fastest and associated with inwardly-focused concentration, high-level information processing, problem-solving, and learning.

Diencephalon

The **diencephalon**, in the center of the brain and contains the thalamus, the hypothalamus, the pituitary gland, and the pineal gland (see Fig. 23.7). This region encloses a cavity called the *third ventricle*. The diencephalon governs many important bodily functions.

The **thalamus** is the largest region of the diencephalon and relays sensory information (except olfaction, the sense of smell) to appropriate areas of the cerebrum. The thalamus also regulates consciousness, sleep, and alertness. The

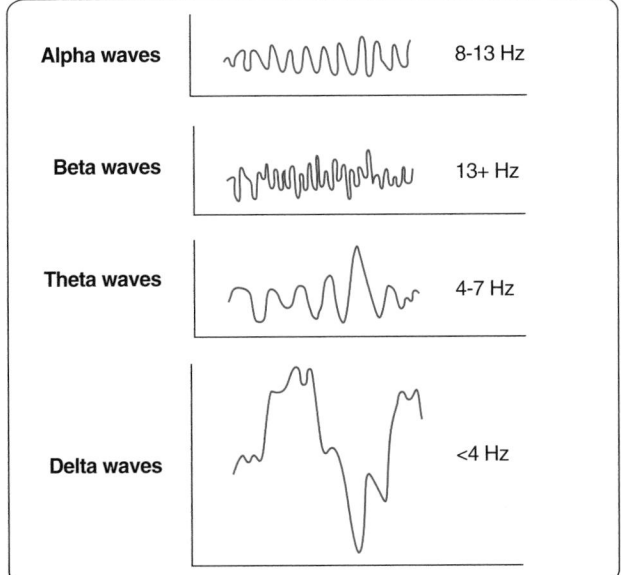

Alpha waves		8-13 Hz
Beta waves		13+ Hz
Theta waves		4-7 Hz
Delta waves		<4 Hz

FIG. 23.9 Brainwaves and their associated states of consciousness depicted by an electroencephalogram. Alpha waves are associated with calmness and relaxation; beta waves are associated with alertness and mental activity; theta waves are related to deep relaxation and sometimes called the "twilight state" because they are experienced while falling sleep or upon waking; and delta waves occur during sleep. Gamma waves are not shown. (From Patton, K. T., & Thibodeau, G. A. [2010]. *Anatomy & physiology* [7th ed.]. St. Louis, MO: Mosby.)

hypothalamus regulates the ANS and controls hunger, thirst, anger, hormones, sexual behavior, body temperature, and sleep patterns. The hypothalamus is part of the hypothalamic–pituitary–adrenal (HPA) axis, which plays a role in the stress response. The **pituitary gland** is connected to the hypothalamus by a slender stalk (infundibulum) and sits in the sella turcica of the sphenoid bone. This gland helps regulate energy, mood, reproduction, growth, and metabolism. The **pineal gland** is below the corpus callosum and, with the help of other hormones, maintains the body's circadian rhythm (sleep-wake cycle). The pituitary gland and the pineal gland are discussed in Chapter 24.

Cerebellum

The **cerebellum** is a cauliflower-shaped structure between the cerebrum and the brainstem. The cerebellum is the second largest region of the brain and is responsible for balance, posture, coordination, equilibrium, and muscle tone (see Fig. 23.7).

Brainstem

The **brainstem** is the inferior stalk-like region of the brain. It connects the cerebrum to the spinal cord. The brainstem contains the midbrain, the pons, and the medulla oblongata (see Fig. 23.7). This region helps regulate functions essential to life, such as breathing, heart rate, and blood pressure. Ten of the 12 cranial nerves discussed later in the chapter emerge from the brainstem (nerves 2 to 12).

The **midbrain** is the superior portion of the brainstem and conducts impulses from the cerebrum to the pons and from the spinal cord to the thalamus. The midbrain helps control movements of the eyes, head, and neck in response to visual and auditory stimuli and assists in the regulation of circadian rhythms and temperature regulation.

The **pons** is located between the midbrain and the medulla oblongata and functions like a highway, transporting signals between the cerebellum and the cerebrum.

The **medulla oblongata** is the inferior portion of the brainstem and transmits sensory and motor impulses between parts of the brain and the spinal cord. The medulla oblongata, often considered the most vital part of the brain, contains the respiratory, cardiovascular, and vasomotor centers. The medulla regulates autonomic functions such as blood pressure, gastric secretions, sweating, sneezing, swallowing, and vomiting. The medulla, along the uppermost region of the spinal cord, contains the crossing-over of fibers, or *decussation*, causing the left cerebral hemisphere's association with the right side of the body and vice versa. Decussation is the reason why brain injuries and strokes on one side of the brain typically cause paralysis on the other side of the body.

Limbic system – The **limbic system** regulates behavioral and emotional responses, especially those needed for survival. Structures of the limbic system include the hypothalamus, thalamus, amygdala, hippocampus, and olfactory bulbs. The limbic system was originally called the rhinencephalon (meaning "smell brain") because it was thought to be primarily involved with olfaction. It is now known that the limbic system is involved in the processing and regulating of emotions, learning and the formation and storage of memories, reproduction, and caring for young. The limbic system is important in the body's response to stress, being highly connected to the endocrine and ANS. Its activation causes chemicals such as dopamine, serotonin, oxytocin, endorphins, adrenaline, and adrenocorticotrophic hormone to increase or decrease, which influences bodily functions.

Spinal Cord

The **spinal cord** is a cylindrical bundle of nerve fibers that extends from the brainstem, through the foramen magnum of the skull, down the vertebral column, and ends in the lower back (approximately L2). The ends of the spinal cord fan out like a horse's tail, forming the *cauda equina*. Beneath the cauda equina is the *filum terminale*, which stabilizes the spinal cord by anchoring it to the coccyx. The spinal cord serves as an information highway and an integrating center, transporting impulses from the brain to the body and vice versa. Two notable enlargements in the spinal cord are in the cervical and lumbar regions (Fig. 23.10).

A cross-section of the spinal cord reveals white matter on the periphery, gray matter inside shaped like the letter "H" or "butterfly," and a tiny *central canal* filled with CSF. The sides of the H are called *horns*, and are divided into the anterior, lateral, and posterior horns. The white matter is

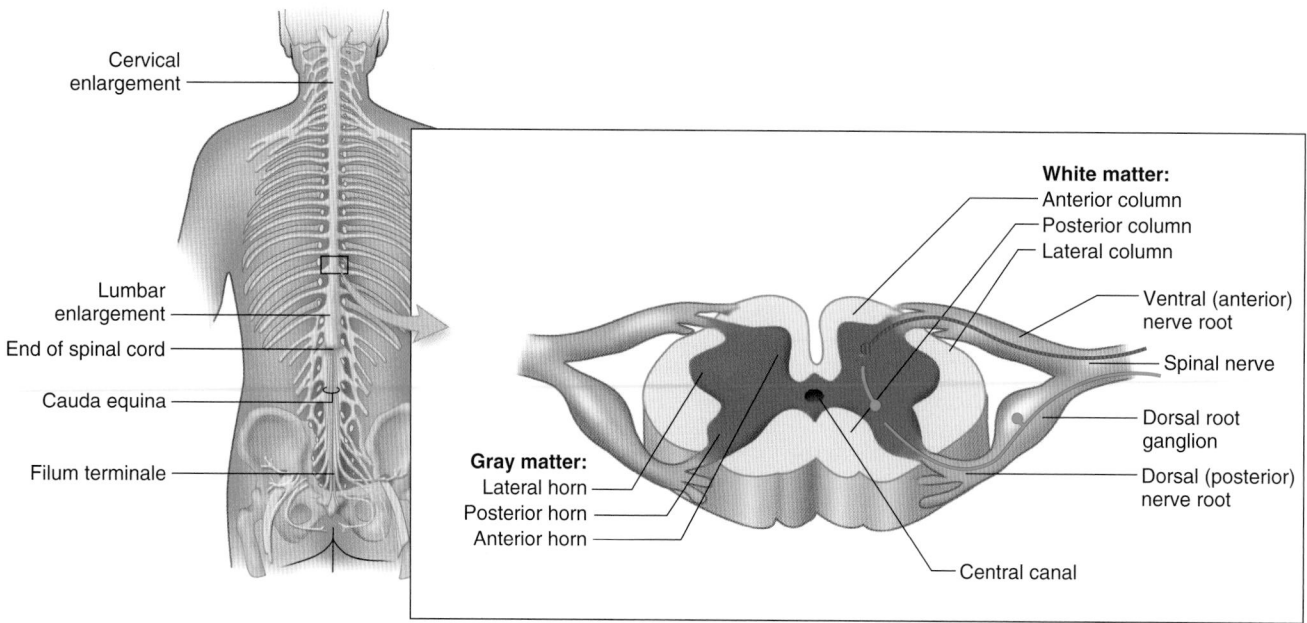

FIG. 23.10 Spinal cord. Enlargements and inferior segments of the cord *(left image, posterior view)*. Columns, horns, and spinal nerves emerging from the sides of the cord *(right image, cross-section view)*. (From Patton, K. T., & Thibodeau, G. A. [2010]. *Anatomy & physiology* [7th ed.]. St. Louis, MO: Mosby.)

organized into regions called *columns*, and is divided into the anterior, lateral, and posterior columns. Within the spinal cord are collections of nerves running up and down in columns called *tracts*. They are divided into the ascending and descending tracts. Afferent impulses travel on ascending tracts, and efferent impulses travel on descending tracts.

> *I happen to feel that the degree of a person's intelligence is directly reflected by the number of conflicting attitudes she can bring to bear on the same topic.*
> ~ **Lisa Alter**

PERIPHERAL NERVOUS SYSTEM

The PNS is composed of cranial and spinal nerves. Nerves from the brain are called *cranial nerves* and nerves from the spinal cord are called *spinal nerves*. Primary functions of the PNS include carrying sensory impulses to the CNS (except vision), carrying motor impulses to skeletal muscles and glands, and regulating autonomic functions such as heart rate and blood pressure by using sympathetic and parasympathetic responses within the ANS.

Cranial Nerves

The **cranial nerves** (CN) emerge from the brain and control much of the sensory and motor functions of the head and neck. There are 12 pairs of cranial nerves, and they are named after Roman numerals, for areas they supply or for their function (Fig. 23.11). As stated previously, the first 2 cranial nerves emerge from the cerebrum and the last 10 emerge from the brainstem. The numbering of the cranial nerves is based on the order in which they emerge from the brain, from superior to inferior.

- **CN I (Olfactory).** Detects smell and is sensory.
- **CN II (Optic).** Detects visual information and is sensory.
- **CN III (Oculomotor).** Moves the eyeballs, constricts the pupils, maintains an open eyelid, and is motor.
- **CN IV (Trochlear).** Moves the eyeballs and is motor.
- **CN V (Trigeminal).** Contains three branches and is both sensory and motor.
  - **Ophthalmic Branch.** Innervates areas around the nose, eyes, and forehead.
  - **Maxillary Branch.** Innervates areas of the upper lip and cheeks.
  - **Mandibular Branch.** Innervates sides of the tongue, lower lip, areas near the cheek and the ear, and the jaw.
- **CN VI (Abducens).** Moves the eyeballs and is motor.
- **CN VII (Facial).** Controls muscles of facial expression, detects taste, produces saliva and tears, and is both sensory and motor.
- **CN VIII (Vestibulocochlear).** Detects hearing and balance/equilibrium from the inner ear and is sensory.
- **CN IX (Glossopharyngeal).** Detects taste, produces saliva, controls swallowing, and is both sensory and motor.
- **CN X (Vagus).** The longest cranial nerve, part of the ANS. It is one of the most important nerves in the body. The vagus nerve establishes one of the connections between the brain and the gastrointestinal tract (sometimes called the gut-brain axis) and regulates heart rate, respiration rate, blood pressure, sweating, and helps keep the larynx open for breathing. The vagus nerve is both sensory and motor.

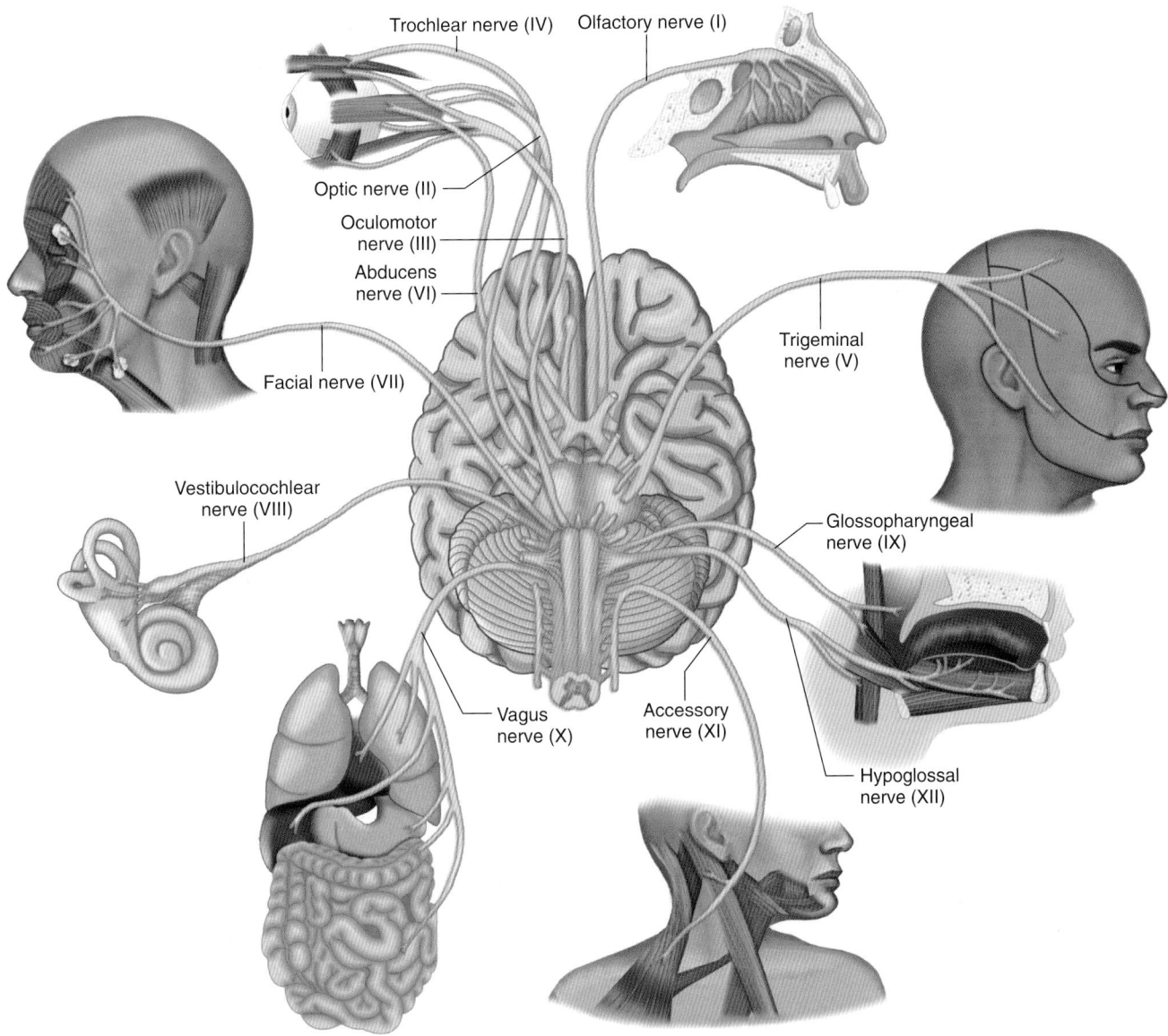

FIG. 23.11 Cranial nerves and areas that they supply *(inferior view)*. (From Patton, K., & Thibodeau, G. [2014]. *The human body in health and disease* [6th ed.]. St. Louis, MO: Mosby.)

- **CN XI (Accessory or Spinal Accessory).** Innervates muscles of the neck and shoulder, such as the trapezius and sternocleidomastoid, and is motor.
- **CN XII (Hypoglossal).** Moves the tongue for speech, chewing, and swallowing, and is motor.

LEARNING TIP: To help you remember the names of the cranial nerves, use the phrase "**O**n **O**ld **O**lympus' **T**owering **T**op, **A** **F**inn **A**nd **G**erman **V**iewed **S**ome **H**ops" or "**O**h, **O**h, **O**h! **T**o **T**ouch **A**nd **F**eel **V**ery **G**reen **V**egetables, **AH**!" for **O**lfactory, **O**ptic, **O**culomotor, **T**rochlear, **T**rigeminal, **A**bducens, **F**acial, **V**estibulocochlear, **G**lossopharyngeal, **V**agus, **A**ccessory, and **H**ypoglossal.

Spinal Nerves

The **spinal nerves** emerge from the right and left sides of the spinal cord, pass through the intervertebral foramen

(except the first pair), and regulate sensory input and motor output (Fig. 23.12). The 31 pairs of spinal nerves are numbered by their location along the spine (Fig. 23.13).

- **Cervical Nerves (C1–C8).** Emerge from the cervical region. The first pair exits between the occipital bone and the first cervical vertebra.
- **Thoracic Nerves (T1–T12).** Emerge from the thoracic vertebrae.
- **Lumbar Nerves (L1–L5).** Emerge from the lumbar vertebrae.
- **Sacral Nerves (S1–S5).** Emerge from the sacrum.
- **Coccygeal Nerve (Co1).** Emerge from the coccyx.

Spinal Nerve Roots, Rami, and Nerve Plexus

Each spinal nerve is formed by two spinal nerve roots that emerge from the same segment of the cord—one dorsal root

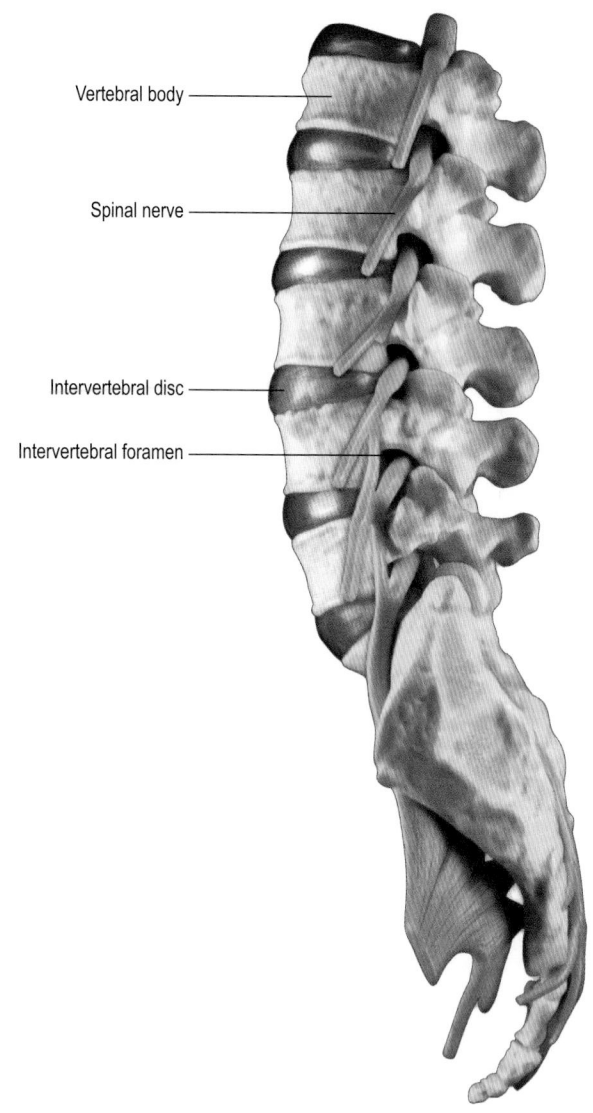

Vertebral body

Spinal nerve

Intervertebral disc

Intervertebral foramen

FIG. 23.12 The lumbar spine with emerging spinal nerves through the intervertebral foramen (*lateral view*). (From Crossman, A. & Neary, D. [2016]. *Neuroanatomy: An illustrated color text* [6th ed.]. Oxford: Elsevier.)

and one ventral root. The **dorsal (posterior) root** comes from the back of the cord and carries sensory information. The dorsal root is easily recognized because it contains a bulge called the *dorsal root ganglion*, a cluster of nerve cell bodies responsible for the transmission of sensory information (see Fig. 23.10). The **ventral (anterior) root** comes from the front of the cord and carries motor impulses to muscles and glands.

After the dorsal and ventral roots join to form a spinal nerve, the nerve divides into branches called **rami.** The *dorsal rami* supplies the skin and muscles on the back of the body. The larger *ventral rami* supplies the skin and muscles on the front and sides of the trunk, as well as the upper and lower extremities. Some ventral rami join to form a network of nerves called a **nerve plexus.** Plexuses are named by where they originate or where the nerves are leading to (see Fig. 23.13).

- **Cervical Plexus (C1–C5).** Passes from the neck and supplies the head, neck, and shoulders.
- **Brachial Plexus (C5–T1).** Passes from the neck to the axilla and supplies the chest, shoulders, and upper extremities.
- **Lumbosacral Plexus (T12–S4).** Passes from the lower back and supplies the abdomen, back, groin, and lower extremities.

In addition to the aforementioned plexuses, there are several that serve an autonomic function. One of these is the **celiac (solar) plexus,** which is between the diaphragm and the stomach (celiac is Latin for abdomen). The celiac plexus regulates many vital functions such as digestion and the release of adrenal secretions.

Dermatomes and Myotomes

A **dermatome** is an area of skin supplied by a single sensory spinal nerve. Dermatomes overlap, which is a form of biologic insurance. That is to say, if one nerve is severed, most sensations can be transmitted by the spinal nerve above and the spinal nerve below. The body can be divided into regions supplied by spinal nerves called a *dermatome map*. For example, C6 dermatome is innervated by spinal nerve C6 (Fig. 23.14).

A **myotome** is a group of skeletal muscles supplied by a single motor spinal nerve. A myotome is the motor equivalent of a dermatome, and therefore the body can be similarly divided into regions supplied by a single motor nerve called a *myotome map* (Fig. 23.15). Like dermatomes, some overlap exists among myotomes.

Reflexes

A **reflex** is a rapid, often protective, involuntary response to a stimulus. A **reflex arc** is the pathway a reflex uses, which is toward and away from the CNS. Reflex arcs are the simplest functional units of the nervous system and consist of at least two neurons—an afferent neuron and an efferent neuron. Some reflex arcs use three neurons—an afferent neuron, an interneuron, and an efferent neuron.

There are two broad categories of reflexes in the PNS—cranial reflexes and spinal reflexes. **Cranial reflexes** are mediated by cranial nerves and include blinking, changes in pupil diameter, salivation, gagging, and sneezing. **Spinal reflexes** are mediated by spinal nerves and include stretch reflexes, autogenic inhibition reflexes, withdrawal reflexes, and crossed extensor reflexes. Although these reflexes occur in the spinal cord, they can be influenced or modified by the brain to either exaggerate or suppress the reflex.

Stretch reflexes and autogenic inhibition reflexes use specialized afferent neurons called **proprioceptors,** which detect body movements and body position. **Proprioception** is the self-awareness of body movements and body positions. These reflexes, especially autogenic inhibition, can play a role in flexibility because inhibiting muscle contraction can allow the stretched muscle to elongate further and easier. These application methods (e.g., muscle energy techniques, proprioceptive neuromuscular facilitation) are found in Chapter 14.

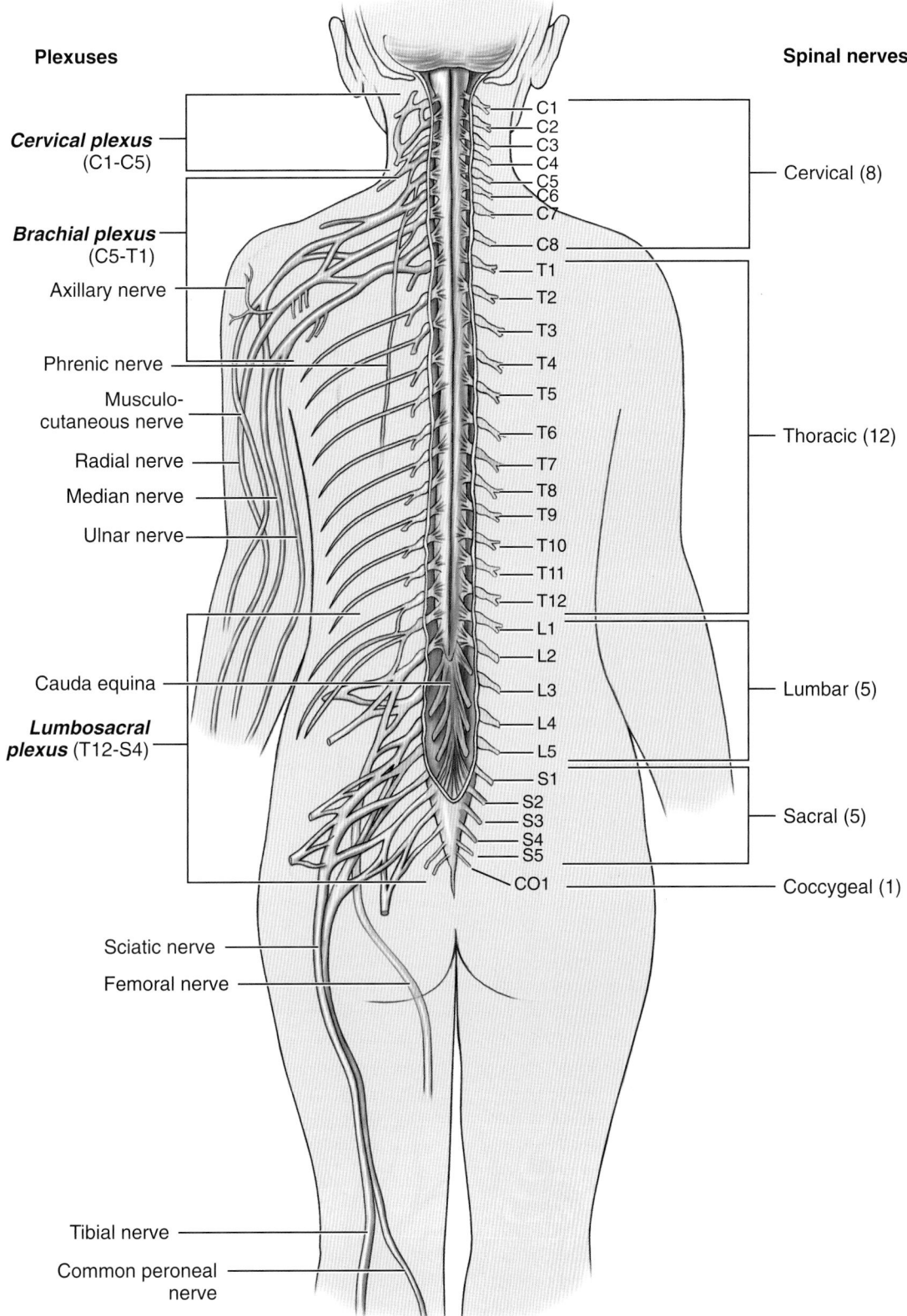

FIG. 23.13 Spinal nerves and their corresponding spinal nerve segments (*right column, posterior view*). Names and locations of plexuses and specific spinal nerves (*left column, posterior view*). (From Herlihy, B. [2011]. *The human body in health and illness* [4th ed.]. St. Louis, MO: Saunders.)

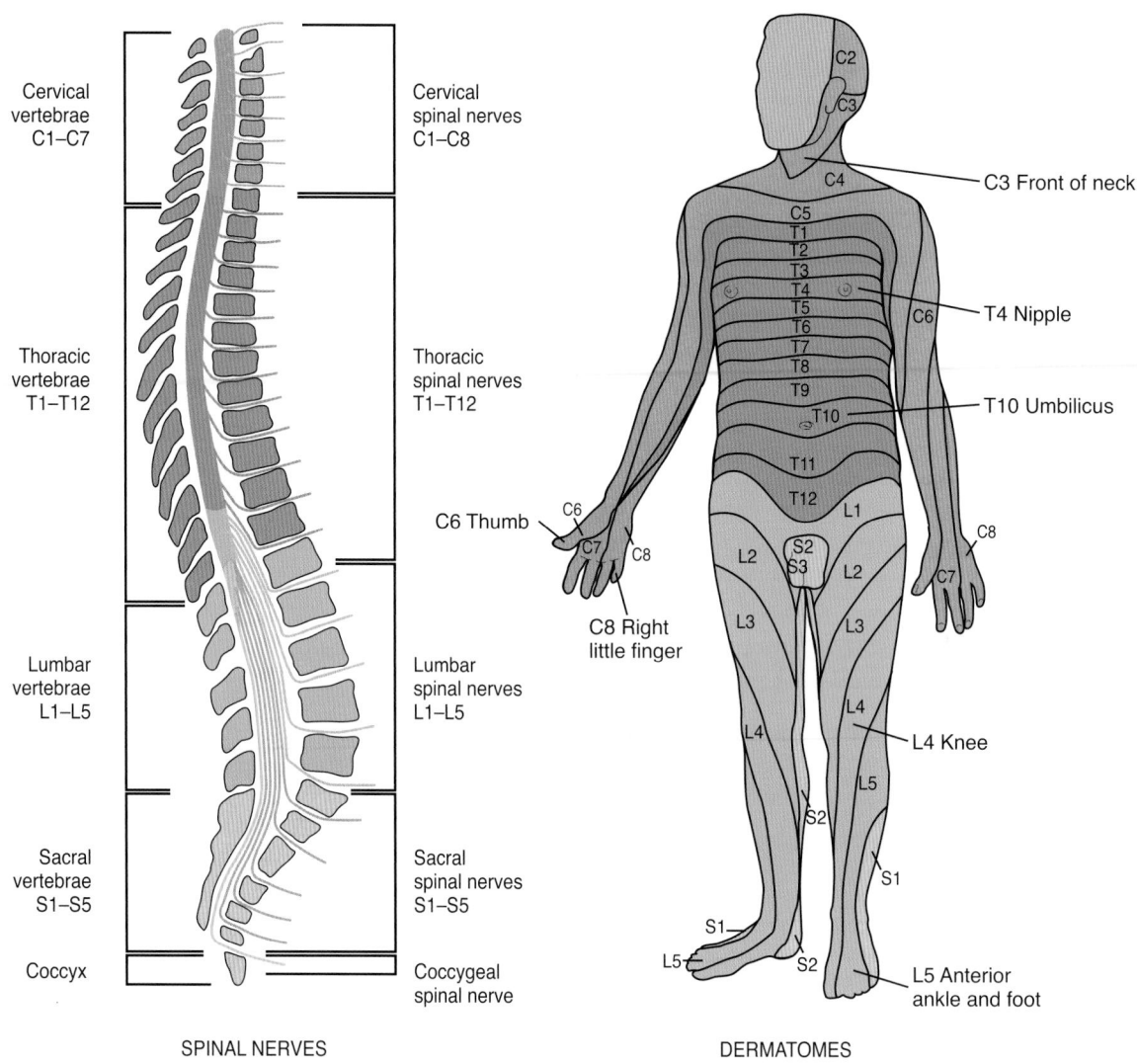

FIG. 23.14 Spinal nerves and dermatomes. A dermatome is an area of skin supplied by a single sensory spinal nerve. Spinal nerves (*image on left-lateral view*) and their associated dermatomes (*image on right-anterior view*). (From Forbes, H. [2021]. *Jarvis's physical examination and health assessment* [3rd ed.]. Sydney: Elsevier).

Stretch (Myotatic) Reflex

A **stretch reflex** is involuntary muscle contraction caused caused by a sudden passive stretch. This action helps protect the muscle from being torn. The receptor that monitors how far and how fast the muscle is being stretched is called a **muscle spindle**. Muscle spindles are wrapped around intrafusal muscle fibers, which are fibers that have lots of sensory and motor innervation. Intrafusal fibers run parallel to extrafusal fibers, which are the muscle's contractile fibers, making up most of the muscle bulk. Even at rest, muscle spindles constantly send motor impulses to help maintain a low level of partial muscle contraction called **muscle tone**. Muscle tone is needed to maintain posture.

Stretch reflexes are usually named for the muscle contracting, with some exceptions such as the patellar/knee-jerk reflex and the Achilles/ankle-jerk reflex. In the case of the patellar/knee-jerk reflex, tapping the patellar tendon with a rubber mallet causes a sudden stretch of the quadriceps. This information travels on an afferent (sensory) neuron to the spinal cord. It activates an efferent (motor) neuron to contract the quadriceps to extend the knee (Fig. 23.16). Another example of the stretch reflex is the sudden contraction of the upper trapezius to pull the head upright after it drops forward after someone begins to fall asleep.

While the muscle spindle is reflexively contracting the stretched muscle, motor activity is inhibited in its antagonist, or opposing muscle, so contraction can occur. This contract/relax neurologic principle is called **reciprocal inhibition** (Box 23.1).

Autogenic Inhibition (Tendon/Inverse Stretch) Reflex

The **autogenic inhibition reflex** is an involuntary reduction of motor activity caused by high levels of tension from either prolonged stretching or excessive contraction. This

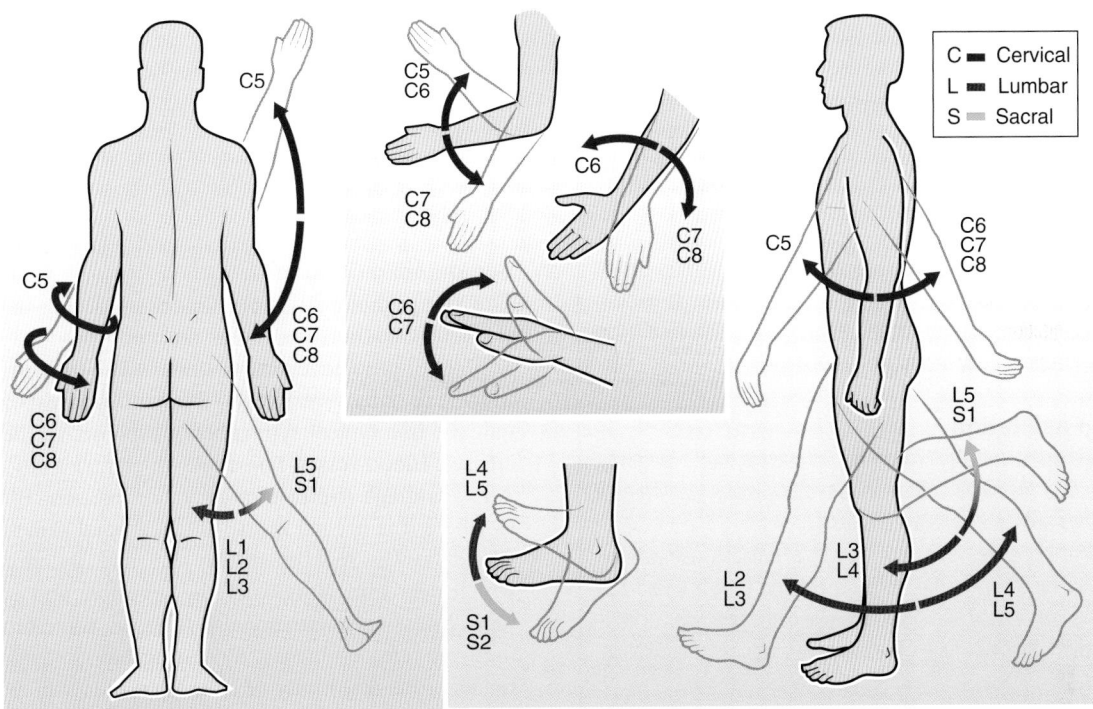

FIG. 23.15 Myotome map. A myotome is a group of skeletal muscles supplied by single motor spinal nerve. Posterior view (*left image*). Lateral view (*right image*). Upper and lower extremities (*middle image*).

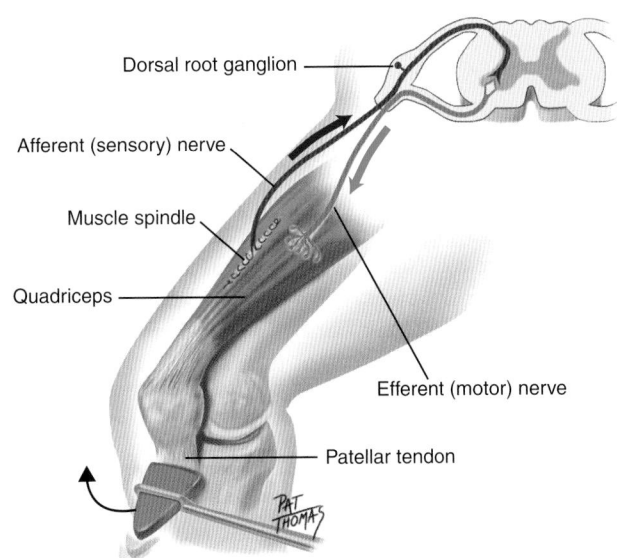

FIG. 23.16 Patellar (knee-jerk) reflex. Tapping the patellar tendon stretches the quadriceps and stimulates muscle spindles. This input travels up an afferent (sensory) neuron to the spinal cord and activates an efferent (motor) neuron to contract the quadriceps and extend the knee. (From Forbes, H. [2021]. *Jarvis's physical examination and health assessment* [3rd ed.]. Sydney: Elsevier.)

decreased motor activity inhibits contraction, which prolongs muscle lengthening and helps protect the muscle from being torn. This reflex is also called the *inverse stretch reflex* because its action is the inverse, or opposite, of the stretch reflex. The receptors responsible for the autogenic inhibition reflex are **Golgi tendon organs** (GTOs), which are at musculotendinous junctions (Fig. 23.17). When GTOs are activated, afferent (sensory) neurons synapse with inhibitory interneurons, which inhibit contraction. This protective action is similar to an electrical circuit breaker. If there is a spike in power coming into your home that could damage electrical devices, the circuit breaker is tripped, and temporarily shuts off electricity.

Whereas muscle spindles respond to stretch, GTOs respond to tension. One might think that stretch and tension are the same thing, but they are not. Have you ever tried to tie shoes really tight and, as you are pulling the laces, one of them snaps from excessive tension? Indeed, muscles are capable of generating enough power to damage tendons or even fracture bones (called an avulsion fracture).

Withdrawal (Flexor) Reflex

The **withdrawal reflex** is the sudden withdrawal of an extremity from a painful stimulus. The receptor stimulated is a nociceptor, which is sensitive to pain. During the withdrawal reflex, a painful signal enters the spinal cord (e.g., standing on a tack) and causes contraction of the hamstring and hip flexors to remove or withdraw from the source of pain (Fig. 23.18).

Neurologic Laws[a]

Sherrington Law of Reciprocal Innervation
Sir Charles Scott Sherrington, English Physician, 1857–1952
When a muscle receives a nerve impulse to contract, impulses are stopped to its antagonist so that it can relax.

Reciprocal innervation states the contraction of a muscle/agonist is accompanied by the simultaneous motor inhibition of the antagonist. This law is the underlying mechanism used to explain reciprocal inhibition, a proprioceptive neuromuscular facilitation (PNF) and muscle energy technique (see Chapter 14).

Law of Facilitation
When an impulse travels through a particular synaptic pathway, it tends to take the same course on future occasions; each time it traverses this path, the resistance is less.

This principle states that activity over a synaptic pathway increases with repetition of the stimulus. Starling (1934) called this principle the *law of habit* and stated it is one of the principles of education. Memory, Starling argued, is essentially a process of facilitation.

Hilton Law
John Hilton, English Surgeon, 1804–1878
The trunk of a nerve not only sends branches to a particular muscle, but also sends branches to the joint moved by that muscle and to the skin overlying the muscle.

Hilton law suggests massage to an area of skin or mobilization of a joint will affect all branches that innervate the areas treated (Thomas, 2013). Hébert-Blouin and colleagues (2014) found Hilton's law to be reliable and applicable to all cranial and peripheral nerves, even 150 years later.

[a]Arndt-Schulz law and Pflüger laws are no longer cited in modern textbooks as they lack evidentiary or scientific support.

Crossed Extensor Reflex
The **crossed extensor reflex** is the reflexive activation of muscles in the contralateral limb to compensate for loss of support when the opposite limb withdraws from a painful stimulus during the withdrawal reflex. For example, after stepping on a tack with one foot, the crossed extensor reflex helps transfer the body's weight to the opposite side, so the foot that stepped on the nail can be withdrawn from the source of pain (see Fig. 23.18).

Autonomic Nervous System

The ANS regulates the involuntary activity of organs, glands, and smooth muscles of the heart and blood vessels, lungs, and intestines. The exception is breathing, which is both voluntary and involuntary. The hypothalamus regulates the ANS by processing sensory and motor impulses, such as heart rate, peristalsis, and contraction of the bladder.

The ANS is part of the PNS. The two divisions of the ANS are sympathetic and parasympathetic. Most organs, glands, and smooth muscles of the body are *dually innervated,* which means they contain nerves from both divisions. The sympathetic and parasympathetic divisions perform complementary functions. For example, if sympathetic nerves increase heart rate, parasympathetic nerves decrease heartbeat and return the heart to its resting rhythm. Some structures, such as the adrenals, have only sympathetic innervation.

Sympathetic Division
The **sympathetic division** dominates during dangerous or stressful situations and helps the body produce the energy needed for physical exertion—this is also called the "fight or flight" or stress response. Sympathetic responses occur quickly. In a typical sympathetic response, the heart rate increases. Blood vessels constrict, which raises blood pressure. Airways dilate and respiration rate increases. Blood travels to where it is needed most—the heart and skeletal muscles. Blood flow is reduced to the skin and abdominal organs, which decreases activity of the digestive and urinary systems. Stress hormones are also released, some of which help the liver release glucose, increasing blood sugar levels and reducing the sensitivity of cells to insulin, which keeps glucose in the bloodstream. In extreme situations, the ANS may illicit the opposite response, such as emptying of the bladder during stressful events. Other sympathetic responses are listed in Fig. 23.19. Sympathetic nerves emerge from thoracic and lumbar segments of the spinal cord (see Fig. 23.19). For this reason, the sympathetic division is also called the *thoracolumbar division.*

Parasympathetic Division
The **parasympathetic division** dominates during restful and calm situations to help the body conserve and restore energy and is referred to as the "housekeeping" division—this is also called the "rest-and-digest" or relaxation response. Typical parasympathetic responses include salivation, digestion, defecation, and urination, as well as reduced heart and respiration rates. Other parasympathetic responses are listed in Fig. 23.19. Parasympathetic nerves emerge from the brain and the sacrum (see Fig. 23.19). For this reason, the parasympathetic division is also called the *craniosacral division.*

SENSES AND THEIR RECEPTORS

The **senses** are organ systems used to gather **sensation**, which is a physical or perceptual experience of the internal or external world. The five basic senses are touch, taste, smell, vision, and hearing. The Greek philosopher Aristotle was the first to discuss the five senses. Receptors in their respective sense organs arise from ectoderm, the embryologic tissue layer that become the brain and spinal cord (see Chapter 18). Four of the five senses reside in the head and are called *special senses.* Touch can be felt throughout the body and is called a *general sense.*

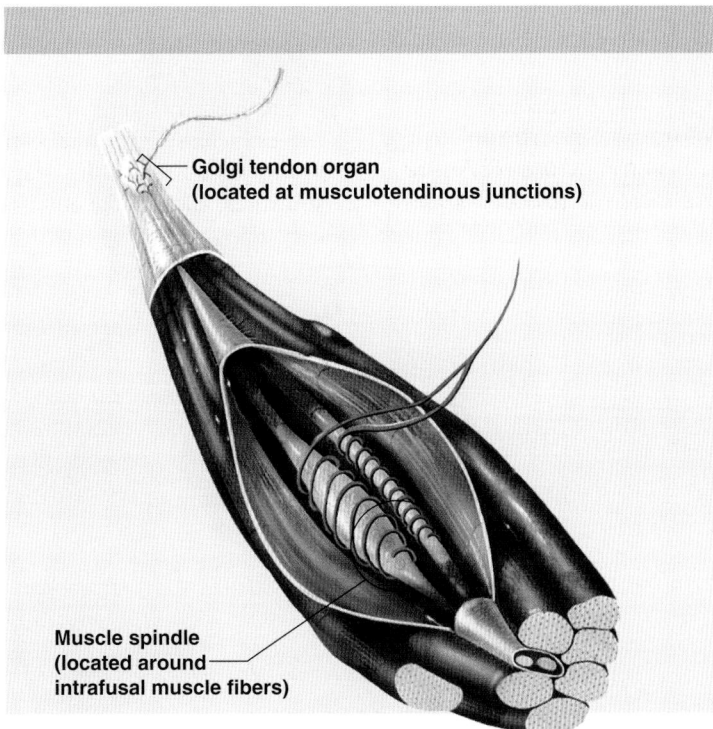

FIG. 23.17 Stretch receptors located at musculotendinous junctions (*Golgi tendon organs*) and around intrafusal muscle fibers (*muscle spindles*). (From Patton, K., & Thibodeau, G. [2014]. *The human body in health and disease* [6th ed.]. St. Louis, MO: Mosby.)

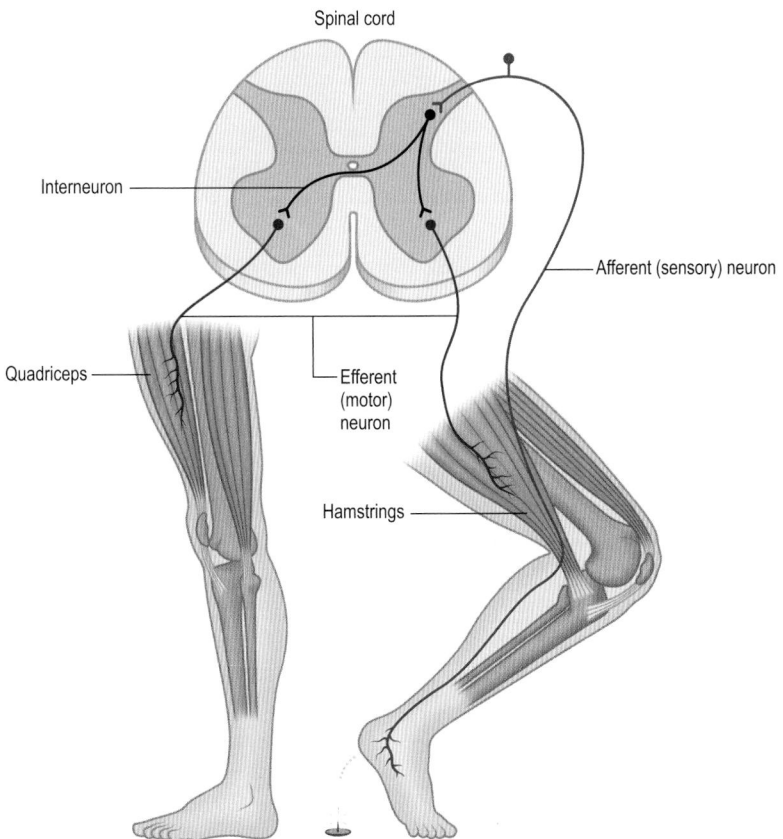

FIG. 23.18 Withdrawal reflex and the crossed extensor reflex. Activation of the flexor reflex by stepping on a tack (*image on the right*) and activation of the crossed extensor reflex causing the contralateral limb to bear the weight of the body. This may involve contraction of the quadriceps and other stabilizing muscles (*image on the left*). (Modified from Crossman, A. & Neary, D. [2016]. *Neuroanatomy: An illustrated color text* [6th ed.]. Oxford: Elsevier.)

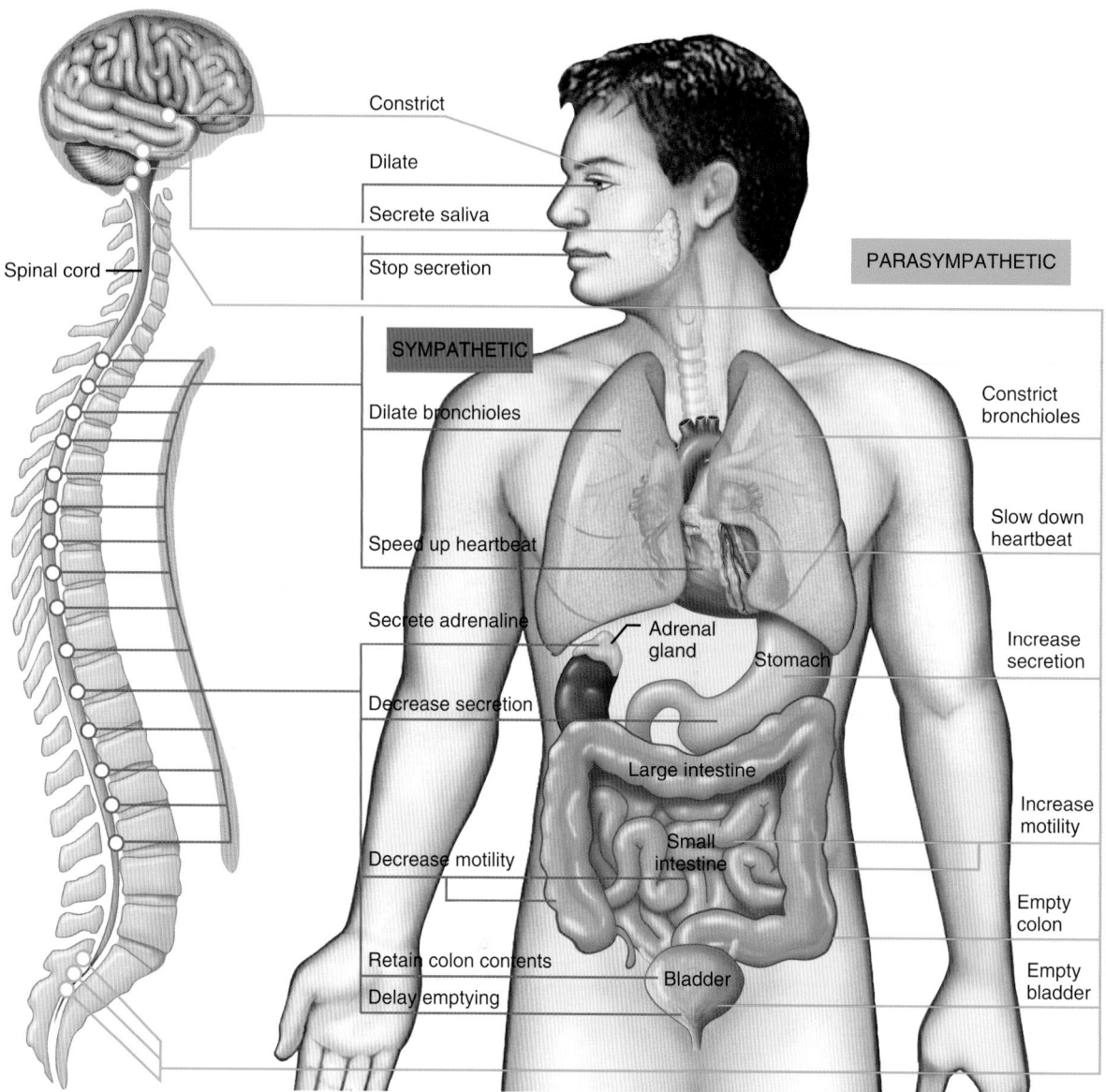

FIG. 23.19 Autonomic nervous system and their complementary functions. Sympathetic *(orange)* and parasympathetic *(green)* divisions. (From Patton, K. & Thibodeau, G. [2014]. *The human body in health and disease* [6th ed.]. St. Louis, MO: Mosby.)

Touch

Touch is the ability to perceive objects or forces through physical contact. Touch is mediated by receptors on or near the surface of the body. Touch is the most primitive of all senses and the first sense to become functional in the human embryo. When an embryo is less than 6 weeks of age and is measuring less than an inch from crown to rump, light stimulation of the upper lip or wings of the nose causes bending of the neck and trunk away from the source of stimulation. At this stage of gestation, neither the eyes nor ears have developed.

Touch receptors are generally classified as *exteroceptors*. Information gathered by these receptors travels to the somatosensory cortex in the parietal lobe. As stated previously, certain areas of the body are more richly innervated, and the hands, fingers, face, lips, and tongue constitute approximately

80% of somatosensory cortex (see Fig. 22.5). Specific touch receptors are discussed in Chapter 22.

Taste

Taste is the ability to detect the chemical composition or the flavors of substances such as salty, sweet, bitter, sour, and/or savory (umami). Receptors responsible for detecting taste are chemoreceptors (gustatory organs) found in papillae (taste buds). Within each papilla are taste hairs extending from a taste pore (Fig. 23.20). Taste receptors are found in highest concentrations on the tongue, but they are also found throughout the oral cavity, in the pharynx, and upper esophagus. These receptors are activated when a molecule of a particular size and shape fits into a specific receptor site, similar to a lock-and-key mechanism. This sensory information travels on the glossopharyngeal nerve (CN 9) to the parietal lobe.

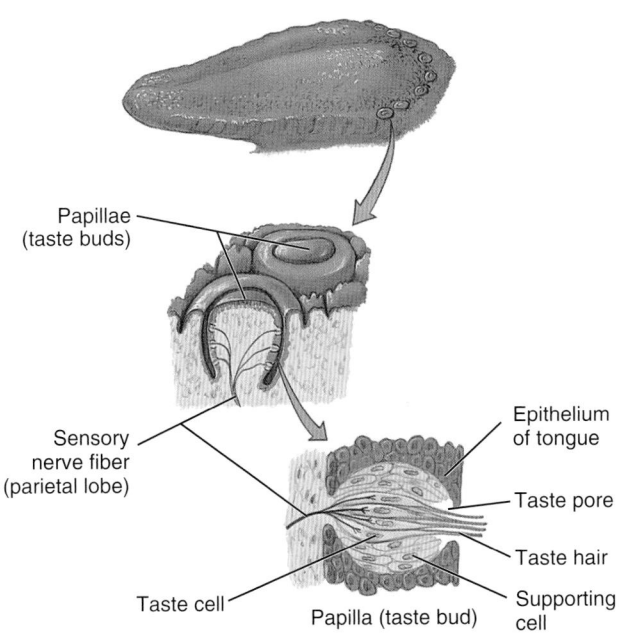

FIG. 23.20 Taste. Papillae or taste buds on the tongue *(cross-section view)*. (From Applegate, E. [2011]. *The anatomy and physiology learning system* [4th ed.]. St. Louis, MO: Saunders.)

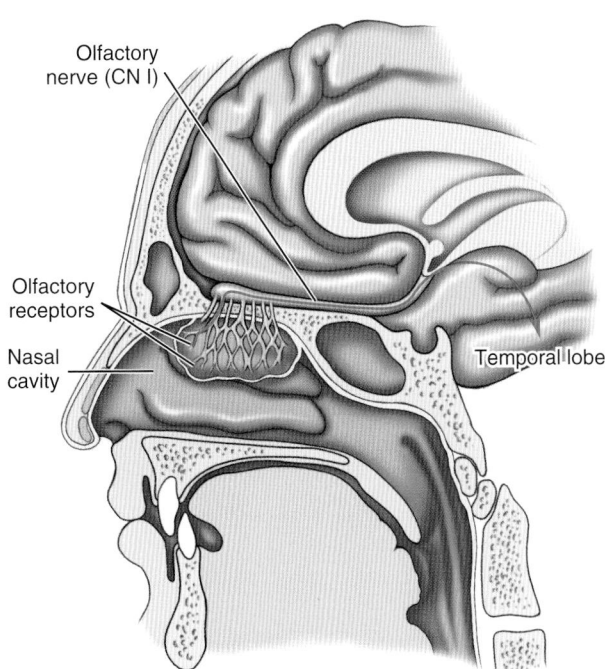

FIG. 23.21 Smell. Olfactory receptors in the nasal cavity *(cross-section view)*. (From Herlihy, B. [2011]. *The human body in health and illness* [4th ed.]. St. Louis, MO: Saunders.)

Taste is largely associated with its smell and its temperature. Hot food is often perceived as tastier compared with cold food because heat disperses scent molecules into the air that we smell as we eat. Conversely, when the sense of smell is impaired, such as during a head cold, even familiar foods can taste differently, or have no taste at all.

Smell

Smell is the ability to detect odors or scents. **Olfaction** is the sense of smell. The receptor responsible for olfaction is the chemoreceptor, the same type of receptor that mediates taste. As we inhale, scent molecules enter the nasal cavity and bind with a chemoreceptor embedded in the nasal mucosa (a mechanism similar to taste). This information travels on the olfactory nerve (CN I) to the temporal lobe (Fig. 23.21).

Research suggests that the human nose can distinguish more than 1000 different pleasant and unpleasant odors. The sense of smell has many functions, including detecting hazards. It is strongly linked to emotions and memories, and plays a role in taste as well as sexual behavior. Loss of the sense of smell is linked to respiratory infections and neurodegenerative diseases such as Alzheimer disease.

Vision (Eyesight)

Vision is the ability to detect the qualities of an object (i.e., shape, size, color) that create its appearance. Vision involves the passage of visible light rays through the pupils, the activation of photoreceptors (i.e., rods and cones) in the retina, and the transmission of visual information on the optic nerve (CN 2) to the occipital lobe (Fig. 23.22). Rods are more active in low-light, are responsible for night vision,

and detect shades of black, gray, and white. Cones require adequate light before becoming active, and they detect color, especially shades of green, red, and blue. A blind spot exists where the optic nerves exit the retina, but this does not affect our ability to see because we have two eyes, and the blind spots do not coincide with each other.

Hearing

Hearing is the ability to detect sounds. It uses mechanoreceptors found in the ear to transmit sound waves or vibrations on the vestibulocochlear nerve (CN 8) to the temporal lobe (Fig. 23.23). Characteristics of sound are pitch and volume. Pitch is the quality of a sound, which depends on vibrational speed; slow vibrations produce deep sounds, while fast vibrations produce high sounds. Volume is the loudness of sound and can change without altering pitch.

When sound waves enter the ear, they travel down the external acoustic meatus within the temporal bone to the tympanic membrane, or the eardrum. This membrane separates the external ear from the middle ear. The vibrations then travel through three small bones (auditory ossicles) in the middle ear: (1) malleus (hammer), (2) incus (anvil), and (3) stapes (stirrup). Ossicles within the ear are the smallest bones in the body. Vibration of the ossicles moves the oval window in the inner ear and then travels to a coiled, fluid-filled cavity called the cochlea, to the vestibulocochlear nerve.

Other structures in the ear are the Eustachian tubes and the semicircular canals. The *Eustachian tubes* are air-containing canals that connect the middle ear to the

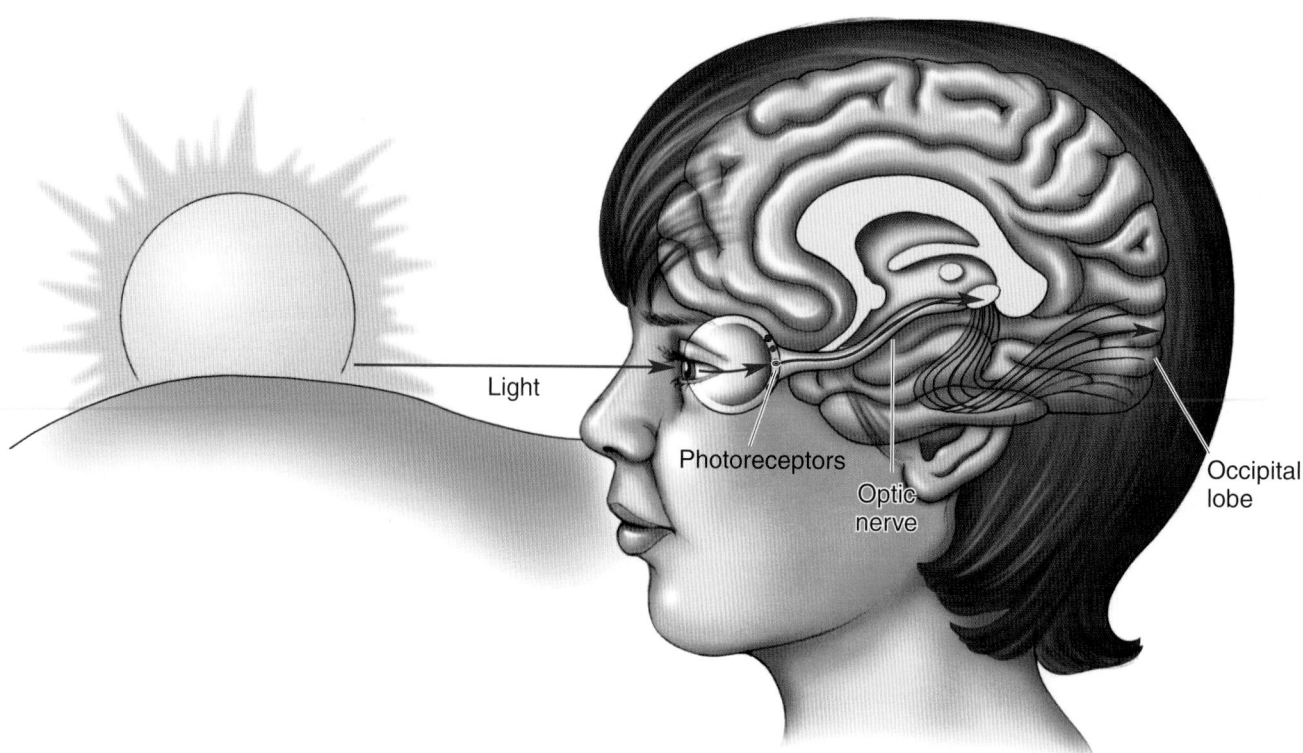

FIG. 23.22 Vision. Visible light rays enter the eye, are detected by photoreceptors, then travel along the optic nerve to the occipital lobe. (Modified from Herlihy, B. [2011]. *The human body in health and illness* [4th ed.]. St. Louis, MO: Saunders.)

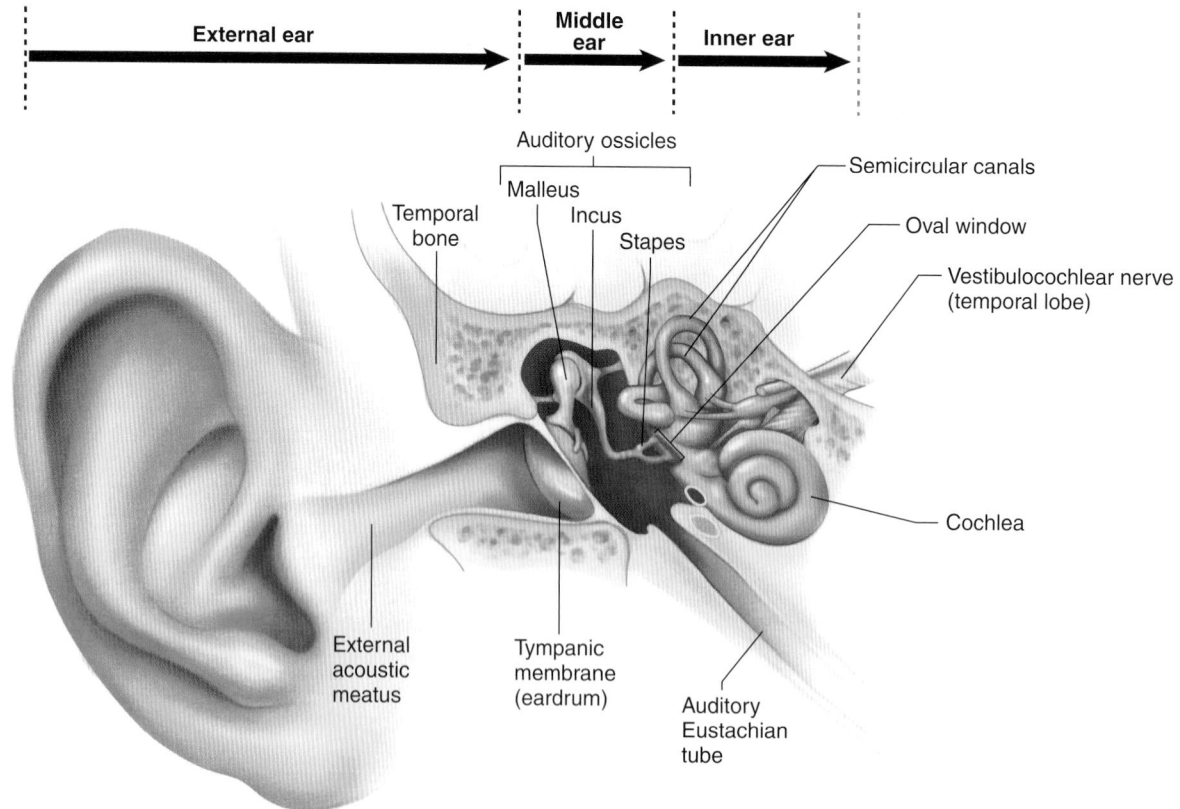

FIG. 23.23 Hearing. Auditory receptors in the inner ear (cross-section view). (Modified from Patton, K., & Thibodeau, G. [2014]. *The human body in health and disease* [6th ed.]. St. Louis, MO: Mosby.

nasopharynx. These tubes help equalize air pressure on both sides of the tympanic membrane. The tube is closed most of the time but opens during swallowing, which permits pressure equalization without conscious effort. However, the tube may remain closed during rapid changes in air pressure (i.e., while ascending or descending in an aircraft). Pressure can be equalized by consciously swallowing, holding the nose and blowing, or by making side-to-side movements of the mandible.

The *semicircular canals* in the inner ear are three fluid-filled tubes lined with cilia. The canals are situated at right angles to each other and provide information about the head position, which helps with spatial orientation and balance.

NEUROLOGIC PATHOLOGIES AND DISORDERS

Featured next are common pathologies, disorders, and injuries of the nervous system, listed alphabetically. Each item includes a brief description and its massage-related modifications. A more extensive list and related research is found in the current edition of *Mosby's Pathology for Massage Professionals* (2022). Migraine headaches are in Chapter 20 under the heading title "Headaches."

Alzheimer Disease

Alzheimer disease (AD) is a disease that slowly destroys memory, thinking, and communicating skills. This decline typically interferes with work, social activities, and the ability to perform activities of daily living. Eventually the person becomes bedridden and dependent on skilled nursing care.

A form of dementia, AD usually begins in late middle life with slight defects in memory and behavior that worsen over time. AD can be classified as mild, moderate, or severe. AD is a common disorder, with 5.8 million people diagnosed in the United States. This number is expected to rise to nearly 14 million by the year 2050. AD is more common in older adults, and studies suggest 50% to 60% of people over the age of 85 have dementia, with most cases being AD. Females are affected more than males, because they generally live longer than males. AD is also called *Alzheimer dementia.*

Massage and Alzheimer Disease

Tailor the massage to the stage of disease, from a few adjustments needed in earlier stages to pressure and positional modifications in later stages. Early-stage adjustments may include massage using slowly applied light pressure. An example of light pressure is 3 on a 10-point pressure scale. Patience and acceptance of behavior are needed, given these individuals experience personality changes. Consider asking a friend or family member of the client for ways to calm the client in case they become argumentative. Many people with AD become agitated when confronted about their confabulations, especially if they are constantly redirected or reoriented. Again, family members or friends of the client are good resources to find ways to handle these situations. Later stage adjustments may include few, if any, changes to the client's position. For example, if you arrive at the client's residence and they are sitting in a recliner, massage the client while in the recliner. Modify your massage technique for application through clothing. These adjustments are even more appropriate when the client's physical condition and ability to communicate deteriorate.

Attention Deficit/Hyperactivity Disorder

Attention deficit/hyperactivity disorder (ADHD) is a disorder in which the affected person displays behaviors associated with inattentiveness, hyperactivity, impulsivity, or a combination of all of these. ADHD is divided into three subtypes, each with different symptoms. They are predominantly inattentive; predominantly hyperactive-impulsive; and a combination of the two. The latter is the most common subtype in the United States. Approximately 9.4% of children 2 to 17 years of age (6.1 million) have been diagnosed with ADHD. Children diagnosed with ADHD usually retain symptoms of the disorder throughout life. Conversely, adults diagnosed with ADHD usually have had traits of the disorder since childhood. Activities that were challenging for a child with ADHD become even more difficult in adulthood as life becomes more demanding and complicated. ADHD is more commonly diagnosed in males than females, but research suggests an almost equal balance during adulthood. ADD, or *attention deficit disorder*, is a term once used for ADHD.

Massage and Attention Deficit/Hyperactivity Disorder

Adapt the length of the session to the client. Shorter sessions, such as 20-minutes in duration, might be more appropriate because individuals with ADHD may have trouble lying still for long periods of time (Allen, 2016). Practitioners will most likely face challenging situations when working with adult clients who have ADHD. These situations range from excessive fidgeting and talking during the massage to missed appointments and forgotten wallets. Consider teaching parents or caregivers how to massage the affected child, making massage more accessible to the child and giving parents/caregivers another way to care for and nurture the child. Limit techniques taught to gliding and kneading and convey the same precautions licensed practitioners follow, such as avoiding skin lesions. Some children and adolescents with ADHD are hypersensitive and may not like to be touched, so be patient and accepting.

Autism Spectrum Disorder

Autism spectrum disorder (ASD) is characterized by difficulty communicating and forming relationships. Although ASD can be diagnosed at any age, autistic-type behaviors usually manifest in the first 3 years of life. ASD can be classified as mild, moderate, or severe, based on presenting signs and symptoms. The diagnosis of ASD is on the rise, which has been attributed to changes in its definition and expansion of the diagnostic criteria. This condition is more common in boys than in girls (4:1). All previous subtypes of ASD, autism, Asperger syndrome, pervasive developmental disorder–not otherwise specified, childhood disintegrative disorder, and Rett syndrome are now diagnosed as ASD.

Massage and Autism Spectrum Disorder

If this is the client's first massage, ask about intolerances to touch and hypersensitivities to sounds, smells, and textures, making modifications to treatment when needed. Shorter sessions ($\geq$20 minutes) may be more appropriate during the first few sessions to learn how the client with ASD tolerates massage. In addition, ask about which position the client uses to calm down or fall asleep and use this as the primary position during the massage (e.g., side lying). It is also helpful to tell the client everything you are doing and why you are doing it throughout the treatment to reduce stress and unpredictability related to social touch (Kuehn, 2016).

If this is not the client's first massage, ask about previous massage experience (as you would with any client), duplicating elements the client enjoyed and avoiding problematic ones. Because of the preference for routine and sameness, whatever routine is established, use the same routine during subsequent sessions. The preference for sameness extends to placement of furniture and fixtures in the massage office.

Individuals diagnosed with ASD may have a preference for deep/strong pressure, which may reduce touch aversion, nervousness, and anxiety (Grandin, 1992). An example of deep/strong pressure is 6 to 7 on a 10-point pressure scale. Furthermore, children diagnosed with ASD favored weighted blankets over non-weighted blankets (Gringras et al., 2014). This suggests that the use of weighted or heavy blankets may be appropriate for these clients. If the client displays any signs of distress while using a heavy or weighted blanket, remove it immediately. In addition, if the client displays any signs of distress during the massage for any reason, discontinue the massage or technique. Consider teaching parents or caregivers how to massage the affected child, making massage more accessible to the child and giving parents/caregivers another way to care for and nurture the child. Limit techniques taught to gliding and kneading and convey the same precautions licensed practitioners follow, such as avoiding skin lesions.

Bell Palsy

Bell palsy is a sudden unilateral facial paralysis in areas supplied by cranial nerve 7, or the facial nerve. The symptoms may be transient, lasting only a few months, or permanent. Bell palsy can recur. Bell palsy is often first noticed in the morning after having developed overnight; symptoms reach their peak within 72 hours. This condition is seen equally in males and females, usually between the ages of 20 and 60. Bell palsy affects about 40,000 U.S. adults and children each year. Unilateral facial paralysis is also a hallmark sign of a stroke. However, a stroke affects more than just facial muscles, so check for other stroke markers such as unilateral arm weakness while making this determination. What causes damage to the facial nerve is often unknown, but viral infections are often implicated (usually herpes simplex). Bell palsy has been associated with pregnancy, with the majority of cases occurring in the second or third trimester and during the early postpartum period.

Massage and Bell Palsy

Massage techniques such as quickly applied effleurage directed upward may improve facial symmetry (Garanhani et al., 2007). These massage techniques may be included in a general massage session for a client with Bell palsy or in a session to specifically address the condition. Obtain permission before applying facial massage, as the client may feel self-conscious and not want the face to be touched. Instruct the client to massage their own face 2 to 3 times a day.

Carpal Tunnel Syndrome

Carpal tunnel syndrome (CTS) is compression of the median nerve within the carpal tunnel, causing numbness, tingling, and other symptoms in the affected hand. The carpal tunnel is formed by the flexor retinaculum (transverse carpal ligament) as it connects to bones on the anterior wrist. The tendons of some wrist flexors and the median nerve pass through the tunnel into the hand. The median nerve serves the palm (anterior) side of the thumb and the index, middle, and lateral half of the ring fingers; it also controls small muscles at the base of the thumb. Because the tunnel is inflexible, it cannot accommodate swelling, which causes compression of its contents. The lifetime risk of CTS is approximately 10% of the adult population. Females are 3 times more likely to develop CTS, compared with males, perhaps because the tunnel itself may be smaller. The dominant hand is usually affected and produces the most severe pain in cases of bilateral CTS.

Double crush syndrome (DCS) is compression of a single peripheral nerve at multiple sites. For example, a person may have both CTS and osteoarthritis of the cervical spine with accompanying radiculopathy.

Massage and Carpal Tunnel Syndrome

Massage the forearm muscles and muscles in the palm of the hand. It should be done below the client's pain tolerance. PROM of the anterior and posterior forearm muscles also may be helpful. Recommend self-massage and self-stretching to help clients maintain or improve their treatment goals. Do not use massage techniques over the anterior neck (anterior and posterior triangles) as this area is an endangerment site.

Intervertebral Disc Disorders

Degenerative disc disease (DDD) is the degeneration and deterioration of the intervertebral discs. Spinal structures including discs change over time, these changes may be of sufficient magnitude to cause symptoms such as pain and dysfunction and conditions such as herniated discs and sciatica (discussed later). Other conditions frequently accompanying DDD are osteoporosis and spinal stenosis, an abnormal narrowing of a passage such as in the central canal or intervertebral foramen. DDD is common and one-third of people aged 40 to 59 years have it, although many are asymptomatic.

A *herniated disc* is a protrusion of the center of a disc (nucleus pulposus) through tears in its outer ring (annulus fibrosus). A herniated disc is also called a ruptured disc. Spinal ligaments will likely be sprained.

A *bulging disc* is similar to a herniated disc but is less severe because the nucleus pulposus remains within the annular wall. Spinal ligaments will likely not be sprained. Compression of neighboring spinal nerves is possible. A bulging disc is also called a slipped disc. Most herniated and bulging discs occur in the lumbar region, but they also occur in the cervical region. A herniation in the thoracic region is rare. Herniated and bulging discs affect males more than females, and incidence rates are highest between the ages of 35 and 60 years.

Massage and Intervertebral Disc Disorders

Pay close attention to the client's level of discomfort. If the client is in severe pain while performing massage-related tasks (e.g., removing a jacket, sitting in a chair, climbing on a massage table), they may not be a good candidate for massage. In this case, it is best to postpone the massage for a day when the client is experiencing less pain. Otherwise, position the client for comfort. If the client is uncomfortable lying prone, opt for a side-lying or seated position to address the back. Muscle spasms along the spine may be serving a protective purpose and may remain or return shortly after the session. If relief from muscle spasms is one of the client's treatment goals, be sure this information is conveyed to the client and reflected in the treatment plan. Avoid forceful PROM to the area of disc herniation.

Multiple Sclerosis

Multiple sclerosis (MS) is a progressive degeneration and demyelination of neurons of the brain, spinal cord, and cranial nerves, especially the optic nerve. Loss of myelin ultimately leads to scarring, or sclerosis, and plaque formation, which interferes with nerve transmission (similar to an electrical wire stripped of its insulation). This process causes sensory and motor abnormalities. Cognitive dysfunction is very common in MS and may appear early in the disease course to include a decrease in information processing speed, word finding, concentration, and attention. MS worsens over time, with periods of remission and exacerbation (called relapses or flare-ups). With each exacerbation, additional areas of the CNS are affected. The interim between exacerbations becomes shorter as the disease advances, often signifying the relapsing pattern has changed to a more progressive course. Many people with MS become incapacitated over a period of 20 to 30 years. MS is the leading neurologic disease in young adults, affecting approximately 1 million people in the United States. Females are more affected than males (3:1), and it is more prevalent in White people than in other ethnic groups. Onset is usually between the ages of 20 and 40 years.

Massage and Multiple Sclerosis

Assess the client thoroughly at every visit because symptoms may change from day to day. During periods of

exacerbation, massage applied slowly using light pressure can be performed. An example of light pressure is 3 on a 10-point pressure scale. Adapt the massage to the client if mobility devices such as wheelchairs are used. Read the massage recommendations in Chapter 11 under the section titled "Clients with Mobility Impairments."

Parkinson Disease

Parkinson disease (PD) is a neurodegenerative disease that causes abnormal movements such as tremors, rigidity, slowness of movements, and postural instability. Neurons deteriorate in a section of the brain that produces dopamine, a neurotransmitter that regulates voluntary movements. Dopamine is also involved in emotions, mood, and motivation. In fact, 50% of people with PD have depression; 20% of people develop dementia (see prior entry). PD is one of the most common neurologic disorders of older adults. Approximately 50,000 people in the United States are diagnosed each year, and about half a million people have the disease. PD can develop in younger people, but this occurrence is rare.

Massage and Parkinson Disease

Allow more time for pre- and post-massage activities such as clothing changes, and getting on/off the massage table. In some situations, massage applied through clothing are best. Consider massaging the client in only one position (prone, supine, seated, or side lying), as rolling over from one position to another can be difficult. Because of possible muscle weakness and increased risk of falls and other injuries, be diligent about safety and provide a barrier-free space in both the office and massage room. This includes setting electric lift tables so clients can place both feet flat on the floor and sit on the tabletop while transferring. This also includes not having supportive cushions such as bolsters on the massage table while the client is transferring on and off the table. Take other safety precautions, including removing throw rugs and securing carpet edges, avoiding waxy floors, removing low furniture and objects on the floor, removing cords and wires on the floor, installing a raised toilet seat if the seat is too low, and checking light sources for adequate illumination.

Sciatica (Piriformis Syndrome)

Sciatica refers to pain radiating down the path of the sciatic nerve. Some cases of sciatica are from **piriformis syndrome,** which is the compression of the sciatic nerve caused by tight or hypertonic piriformis muscle. Part or all of the sciatic nerve runs through the piriformis in approximately 15% of the population (Travell & Simons, 1993). However, piriformis syndrome is rare, and most cases of sciatica are related to other conditions such as herniated disc or stenosis from bone spur. In some cases, the cause of sciatica is unidentified.

Massage and Sciatica/Piriformis Syndrome

Pay close attention to the client's level of pain or discomfort. If the client is in severe pain while performing massage-related tasks (e.g., removing a jacket, sitting in a chair, climbing on a massage table), they may not be a good candidate for massage that day. In this case, it is best to postpone the massage until a day when the client is experiencing less pain.

Otherwise, position the client for comfort. If the client is uncomfortable lying prone, opt for a side-lying or seated position to address the back. Gentle decompression or traction techniques may be used to relieve symptoms. Muscle spasms along the spine may be serving a protective purpose and may remain or return shortly after the session. If relief from muscle spasms is one of the client's treatment goals, be sure this information is conveyed to the client and reflected in the treatment plan. Avoid forceful PROM to the spine or hip. Clients with sciatica are prone to additional nerve injury at pressure points (e.g., behind the knee, the front of the ankle). For this reason, use a soft rather than a stiff bolster in these areas.

For piriformis syndrome, massage may help reduce tension in the piriformis, reducing subsequent sciatic nerve compression. Use deep/strong effleurage and friction over the femoral attachment and along the length of the piriformis. An example of deep/strong pressure is 7 on a 10-point pressure scale. This includes the lateral sacral border and just medial to the greater trochanter. Laterally rotate the hip and flex the knee and massage the muscle in a shortened position. Some practitioners use sustained pressure over the piriformis while moving passively, adducting and abducting the hip by moving the leg in an arc. Recommend self-stretching of the piriformis to help clients maintain or improve their treatment goals.

Seizure Disorders

Seizure disorders are characterized by the presence of *seizures*, which are episodes of uncontrolled and excessive electrical activity in the brain, resulting in a sudden change of behavior and level of consciousness. The event is described as a "lightning storm in the brain." A seizure may be subtle, or it may produce involuntary repetitive movements and loss of consciousness. Epilepsy is a term used to describe recurrent seizures. The two main types of seizures are focal or partial and generalized. *Focal (partial) seizures* are limited to a single area of the brain. *Generalized seizures* involve more areas of the brain. Types of generalized seizures are absence and tonic–clonic.

Massage and Seizure Disorders

If a client has a history of seizures, ask about any known triggers and avoid them during the session. Clients with seizure disorders are more likely to have a seizure if they stop taking their prescribed anti-seizure medications. Ask who to contact first if a seizure occurs. Some clients prefer that you contact a loved one before calling 911. Also ask how long the seizures typically last, as this will inform you how long to wait before making any needed calls. Chapter 9 contains first aid measures for clients experiencing a seizure (more specifically, a tonic–clonic seizure).

Contrasting light/dark patterns and flashing or patterned lights may trigger a seizure in clients who are photosensitive.

Ceiling fans may need to be switched off. Certain odors can trigger a seizure; therefore, aromatherapy may be contraindicated. The Epilepsy Society (2019) recommends avoiding the following essential oils when working with people who have seizure disorders: rosemary, fennel, sage, eucalyptus, hyssop, camphor, and spike lavender. The Epilepsy Society (2019) recommends massage alongside any antiepileptic drugs as a way to reduce stress-induced seizures, decrease tension and pain in muscles, help with poor sleep patterns, improve relaxation, and promote wellness.

Spinal Cord Injuries

Spinal cord injuries (SCIs) occur from direct injury to the spinal cord or indirectly from damage to surrounding bones, tissues, or blood vessels. These events cause paralysis or a complete or total loss of the ability to move or feel sensations in part of the body. In SCIs, paralysis occurs distal to the area of spinal damage in the most mobile regions of the spinal column and manifests as paraplegia or quadriplegia. Paralysis may be temporary, but it usually leads to some degree of permanent disability.

- **Paraplegia.** Paralysis of the lower trunk and legs because of injury to the lumbar region of the spinal cord, usually between T12 and L2.
- **Quadriplegia (Tetraplegia).** Paralysis of the trunk and all four extremities because of injury of the cervical region of the spinal cord, usually between C1 and C7.

Fifty percent of SCIs result in paraplegia and 50% result in quadriplegia. As many as 450,000 people in the United States are living with a spinal cord injury. Every year, an estimated 17,000 new SCIs occur in the United States. Just over half of all SCIs occur in persons aged 16 to 30 years, most of whom are male (80%).

Massage and Spinal Cord Injuries

Massage can be performed during rehabilitation. Use supine, side-lying, or seated positions with the aid of supportive cushions to ensure client comfort (Goldberg et al., 1994). Because most clients with SCIs will be wheelchairbound, adapt the massage to the client. Read the massage recommendations in Chapter 11 under the section titled "Clients with Mobility Impairments." Generally speaking, the longer a client has been inactive, the greater the risk of reduced bone density and blood clots in the legs. Avoid deep pressure over bones and forceful PROM because of the possibility of fracture, which has been reported (Abilash et al., 2017). Also, avoid vigorous massage techniques on the legs because of possible blood clots. Coexisting medical conditions (contractures, decubitus ulcers) should be factored into the treatment plan.

Stroke

A **stroke** is a sudden disruption in cerebral blood flow from an occluded or ruptured blood vessel, leading to irreversible brain damage or, in some cases, death (20% of stroke victims die within the first few days after the attack). Two main types of strokes are ischemic and hemorrhagic. *Ischemic* *strokes* represent 87% of cases and are a result of arterial occlusion from a thrombus or embolus.

Complications of strokes are common and range from mild (these go almost unnoticed) to severe with resultant *hemiplegia* or paralysis of one side of the body. Left-sided brain damage results in right-sided paralysis, and vice versa. Some stroke victims can develop new neural pathways or relearn previous tasks because of neuroplasticity. This development is enhanced by therapy. Strokes are also called cerebrovascular accidents, cerebral infarctions, and brain attacks.

Every year, approximately 795,000 people in the United States have a stroke; about 140,000 of these are fatal. The incidence of stroke increases with age (occurring most often in people aged ≥65 years).

Massage and Strokes

Massage can be performed during rehabilitation. Inquire about positions most comfortable for the client, which may include use of cushions to ensure client comfort or use of alternate positions, such as seated or side-lying. Massage applied slowly using light pressure can be performed. An example of light pressure is 3 on a 10-point pressure scale. Avoid forceful PROM if the client has been inactive for prolonged periods because of possible reduced bone density. Adapt the massage to the client if mobility devices such as a wheelchair are used. Read the massage recommendations in Chapter 11 under the section titled "Clients with Mobility Impairments." If the client has difficulty speaking clearly, ask family members or caregivers for the best communication method. Possible methods include raising a finger or blinking the eyes once to indicate yes, raising two fingers or closing eyes to indicate no, or use of an alphabet board. First aid measures for strokes are in Chapter 9.

Thoracic Outlet Syndrome

Thoracic outlet syndrome (TOS) is a group of disorders caused by compression of nerves or blood vessels (collectively called the neurovascular bundle) in the space between the clavicle and first rib. This space is also called the thoracic outlet. There are several types of TOS, including neurogenic and vascular.
- **Neurogenic (Brachial Plexus Injury).** This involves compression of the brachial plexus and is the most common type (85% to 95% of cases).
- **Vascular.** This involves compression of one or more arteries or veins; this is the least common but most serious type of TOS.

TOS can result from anatomic defects such as a cervical rib (an extra rib above the first rib) or an unusually tight band of fibrous tissues connecting the spine to the first rib. Poor posture or carrying heavy items can compress the area between the clavicle and the first rib. Hypertonicity of the scalenes or pectoralis minor may either pull the first rib upward (reducing the area between the first rib and the clavicle) or compress the neurovascular bundle into the rib cage. Trauma and repetitive motion can cause or contribute to TOS.

Massage and Thoracic Outlet Syndrome

Massage is appropriate for neurogenic cases of TOS, especially using deep/strong pressure. An example of deep/strong pressure is 7 on a 10-point pressure scale. Do not use massage techniques over the anterior neck (anterior and posterior triangles) as this area is an endangerment site. For vascular cases of TOS, the affected area is a local contraindication.

Traumatic Brain Injuries (Concussions, Contusions, Coup-Contrecoup)

Traumatic brain injury (TBI) is an injury from sudden trauma by contact with an object that may or may not penetrate the skull and damage the brain. TBIs range from mild, moderate, to severe. TBIs can be broadly classified as closed (do not break the skull) and open or penetrating (break the skull and enter the brain).

Children and older adults are at the highest risk for TBIs. Approximately 1.7 million cases of TBIs occur in the United States every year, and approximately 5.3 million people live with a disability caused by TBIs.

Massage and Traumatic Brain Injuries

Massage can be performed during rehabilitation. If the client has difficulty communicating, establish the best communication method. Possible methods include raising a finger or blinking the eyes once to indicate yes, raising two fingers or closing the eyes to indicate no, or using an alphabet board.

Adjust the face rest to ensure comfort and obtain verbal consent before touching the client's face and head. If the client is experiencing dizziness, limit positional changes and avoid techniques that cause the client to rock or shake. Coexisting medical conditions should be factored into the treatment plan. For example, if the TBI also caused other injuries such as temporomandibular dysfunction or whiplash-associated disorder, the massage must be modified for those conditions.

Trigeminal Neuralgia

Trigeminal neuralgia (TN) is characterized by excruciating periodic pain in areas supplied by the trigeminal nerve or cranial nerve 5. Any one or all three branches of the trigeminal nerve may be affected. The ophthalmic branch connects to areas near the nose and eyes and over the forehead; the maxillary branch includes areas of the upper lip and cheek; and the mandibular branch involves the side of the tongue, lower lip, area of the cheek closest to the ear, and jaw. TN is also called *tic douloureux*.

Attacks may be spontaneous or triggered by mechanical stimulation such as touching the face while shaving, chewing, drinking, speaking, and brushing teeth. TN tends to be progressive, causing longer and more frequent bouts of intense pain. This pain is so severe that some people with TN are "begging to be killed" to put them out of their misery (Burchiel, 2006). Suicides are not uncommon. TN affects approximately one in 15,000 people, although this number may be higher as a result of frequent misdiagnosis. This condition is more common in females than in males and occurs more frequently in those older than 50 years of age.

Massage and Trigeminal Neuralgia

During severe attacks, it is best to postpone the massage. Otherwise, treat the face and scalp as a local contraindication because mechanical pressure can trigger an attack in susceptible people. In addition, avoid pressure on these areas from the massage table or accessories, which may include using a modified side-lying (do not lay client on their affected side), using a seated position to address the back, or avoiding the prone position.

E-RESOURCES

http://evolve.elsevier.com/Salvo/MassageTherapy

- Chapter challenge
- Flash cards

MOSHE FELDENKRAIS

Given a 50% chance that surgery would help your injury, what would you choose? Some would take the chance and see what happens. Some would decide to tough it out and live with the injury if it were not too debilitating. But Moshe Feldenkrais chose a third possibility, using his experience as an engineer and a martial arts expert to explore how he could heal the injury himself. It was this initial experience that led to Feldenkrais's development of his method of massage.

Feldenkrais was born in what is now Ukraine in 1904. At the age of 14, he moved to what was then Palestine, working as a laborer and finishing high

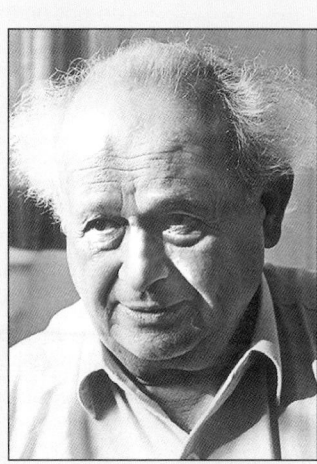

©International Feldenkrais Federation Archive

school. As a teenager, he participated in a self-defense group where he learned basic jiu jitsu. An observant individual, Feldenkrais realized movements taught in jiu jitsu did not take into account those first, instinctive movements people make when first attacked. He wrote an instructional book on the topic, developing a system in which this first spontaneous movement is the initial foundation of the deliberate actions that follow.

This novel idea by a relatively untrained individual attracted the attention of Jigoro Kano, the Japanese minister of education and the creator of judo. Kano asked Feldenkrais to introduce the practice of judo to Europe, but Feldenkrais, who was an engineering student in France by this time, was concerned his studies would suffer if he devoted too much time to martial arts and declined. Eventually, a compromise was reached, and a judo expert traveled to France to work with Feldenkrais in his spare time. Feldenkrais became one of the first Europeans to earn a black belt in judo.

Feldenkrais escaped to the UK during the German invasion of France and experienced a flare-up of an old soccer injury. He was given 50/50 odds that the surgery would successfully repair the injury. However, he decided to use the understanding of efficient movement and reflex developed through judo and the understanding of structures and movement he had developed as an engineer and attempted to rehabilitate himself instead. It worked.

Feldenkrais came to believe habitual patterns of movement become imprinted on the nervous system, for good or ill. In order to break those patterns and establish more effective movement, unusual movements for which there is no established pattern can be used. The Feldenkrais method teaches these movements through the hands-on guidance of a practitioner (called *functional integration*), as well as verbally guided sessions that can be taught in a group setting (called *awareness through movement*). As such, the Feldenkrais method is not a manual technique but rather a method of teaching effective movement. Practitioners receive around 800 hours of training over the course of 4 years, with a focus on body self-awareness.

Feldenkrais moved to the newly created country of Israel in the 1950s, where he remained a resident for the rest of his life, also traveling extensively to teach throughout North America and Europe. He died in 1984, but his methods for empowering people to understand their own bodies and create new, efficient patterns of movement continue to be taught around the globe. In a world intent on selling miracle cures, the teachings of Moshe Feldenkrais put the power solidly in the hands of the people who wish to change an important lesson for anyone who hopes to assist clients in their journeys toward wellness.

REFERENCES

Abilash, K., Mohd, Q., Ahmad, Z., & Towil, B. (2017). Fracture-dislocation at C6–C7 level with quadriplegia after traditional massage in a patient with ankylosing spondylitis: A case report. *Malaysian Orthopaedic Journal, 11*(2), 75–77.

Allen, T. (2016). *ADHD and massage for children.* Retrieved from http://www.liddlekidz.com/adhd-massage-therapy-faqs.html.

Burchiel, K., (2006). *Oregon Health and Science University brings relief to 'suicide disease' sufferers.* Retrieved from https://news.ohsu.edu/2006/04/06/ohsu-brings-relief-to-suicide-disease-sufferers.

Epilepsy Society. (2019). *Complementary therapies.* Retrieved from https://www.epilepsysociety.org.uk/complementary-therapies.

Garanhani, M. R., Rosa Cardoso, J., Capelli Ade, M., & Ribeiro, M. C. (2007). Physical therapy in peripheral facial paralysis: Retrospective study. *Brazilian Journal of Otorhinolaryngology, 73*(1), 106–109.

Goldberg, J., Seaborne, D. E., Sullivan, S. J., & Leduc, B. E. (1994). The effect of therapeutic massage on H-reflex amplitude in persons with a spinal cord injury. *Physical Therapy, 74*(8), 728–737.

Grandin, T. (1992). Calming effects of deep touch pressure in patients with autistic disorder, college students, and animals. *Journal of Child and Adolescent Psychopharmacology, 2*(1), 63–72.

Gringras, P., Green, D., Wright, B., Rush, C., Sparrowhawk, M., Pratt, K., et al. (2014). Weighted blankets and sleep in autistic children—a randomized controlled trial. *Pediatrics, 134*(2), 298–306.

Hébert-Blouin, M. N., Tubbs, R. S., Carmichael, S. W., & Spinner, R. J. (2014). Hilton's law revisited. *Clinical Anatomy, 27*(4), 548–555.

Kuehn, E. (2016). *Research into our sense of touch leads to new treatments for autism.* Retrieved from http://sitn.hms.harvard.edu/flash/2016/research-into-our-sense-of-touch-leads-to-new-treatments-for-autism/.

Salvo, S. G. (2022). *Mosby's Pathology for Massage Professionals* (5th ed.). St Louis: Mosby.

Starling, E. H. (1934). *Principles of human physiology.* Philadelphia: Lea & Lebiger.

Thomas, C. L. (2013). *Taber's Cyclopedic Medical Dictionary* (22th ed.). Philadelphia: FA Davis.

Travell, J. G., & Simons, D. G. (1993). *Myofascial pain and dysfunction: The trigger point manual, the lower extremities.* Baltimore, MD: Lippincott Williams & Wilkins.

BIBLIOGRAPHY

Abrahams, P. H., Spratt, J. D., Loukas, M., & van Schoor, A. N. (2003). *Abrahams' and McMinn's clinical atlas of human anatomy* (8th ed.). St Louis: Elsevier.

Applegate, E. (2010). *The anatomy and physiology learning system* (4th ed.). Philadelphia: Saunders.

Como, D. (Ed.). (2016). *Mosby's dictionary of medicine, nursing, and health professions* (10th ed.). St Louis: Elsevier.

Frazier, M. S., & Drzymkowski, J. W. (2015). *Essentials of human diseases and conditions* (6th ed.). St Louis: Elsevier.

Hubert, R. J., & VanMeter, K. C. (2018). *Gould's pathophysiology for the health professions* (6th ed.). Philadelphia: Saunders.

Haubrich, W. S. (2003). *Medical meanings: A glossary of word origins* (2nd ed.). New York: American College of Physicians.

Herlihy, B. (2017). *The human body in health and illness* (6th ed.). St Louis: Saunders.

Huether, S. E., McCance, K. L., & Brashers, V. L. (2019). *Understanding pathophysiology* (7th ed.). St Louis: Mosby.

Kalat, J. W. (2013). *Biological psychology* (11th ed.). Belmont, CA: Cengage Learning.

Kapit, W., & Elson, L. M. (2013). *The anatomy coloring book* (4th ed.). New York: Benjamin Cummings.

Kumar, V., Abbas, A. K., & Aster, J. C. (2015). *Robbins & Cotran pathologic basis of disease* (9th ed.). St Louis: Mosby.

Marieb, E. N., & Keller, S. M. (2018). *Essentials of human anatomy and physiology* (12th ed.). New York: Benjamin Cummings.

McCance, K. L., & Huether, S. E. (2019). *Pathophysiology: The biological basis for disease in adults and children* (8th ed.). St Louis: Mosby.

Myers, T. W. (2014). *Anatomy trains: Myofascial meridians for manual and movement therapists* (3rd ed.). Churchill Livingstone: Elsevier.

Netter, F. H. (2018). *Atlas of human anatomy* (7th ed.). St Louis: Mosby.

Patton, K. T (2019). *Anatomy and physiology* (10th ed.). St Louis: Elsevier.

Patton, K. T., Thibodeau, G. A., & Douglas, M. M. (2012). *Essentials of anatomy and physiology* (4th ed.). New York: Pearson.

Porter, R. S., (2011). *The Merck manual of diagnosis and therapy* (19th ed). Whitehouse Station, NJ: Merck Sharp and Dohme Corp.

Taber, C. W. (2021). *Taber's cyclopedic medical dictionary* (24nd ed.). Philadelphia: FA Davis.

REVIEW AND APPLY YOUR KNOWLEDGE

MATCHING ONE: CONCEPT REVIEW

Place the letter of the answer next to the number of the term or phrase that best describes it.

A. Autonomic nervous system
B. Axon
C. Central nervous system
D. Dendrites
E. Myelin
F. Nerve
G. Neurons
H. Parasympathetic division
I. Peripheral nervous system
J. Somatic nervous system
K. Sympathetic division
L. Synapse

_____ 1. Bundles of nerve fibers surrounded by several layers of connective tissue.

_____ 2. Subdivision of the ANS that dominates during dangerous or stressful situations and helps the body produce the energy needed for physical exertion.

_____ 3. Impulse-conducting cells of the nervous system and possess properties of excitability or irritability, conductivity, and secretion.

_____ 4. Subdivision of the PNS that transmits sensory input and controls the voluntary function of skeletal muscles.

_____ 5. Projection of the nerve that transmits the impulse away from the cell body.

_____ 6. Nervous system division that includes the brain, spinal cord, meninges, and cerebrospinal fluid and is surrounded by bones of the skull and spinal column.

_____ 7. Subdivision of the PNS that regulates the involuntary activities of organs, glands, and smooth muscle.

_____ 8. Space between two neurons or between a neuron and a muscle or gland where nerve impulses are transmitted.

_____ 9. Projections of the nerve that receives and transmits the impulse toward the cell body.

_____ 10. Subdivision of the ANS that dominates during restful and calm situations and helps the body conserve and restore energy.

_____ 11. White fatty material that insulates axons and prevents impulse "leakage" to adjacent neurons.

_____ 12. Nervous system division that extends beyond the skull and vertebral column and includes the cranial and spinal nerves.

MATCHING TWO: CONCEPT REVIEW

Place the letter of the answer next to the number of the term or phrase that best describes it.

A. Alpha
B. Cerebellum
C. Cerebrum
D. Frontal
E. Hypothalamus
F. Medulla oblongata
G. Meninges
H. Nerve impulse
I. Neurotransmitters
J. Reflex arc
K. Spinal cord
L. Thalamus

_____ 1. Response to a stimulus that causes a neuron to depolarize, so it can transmit impulses to other neurons, muscles, or glands.

_____ 2. Connective tissue membranes that line the internal surfaces of the skull and vertebral column, surround the brain and spinal cord, and help protect the CNS from physical injury.

_____ 3. Area of the brain that regulates the ANS and controls hunger, thirst, anger, hormones, sexual behavior, body temperature, and sleep patterns.

_____ 4. Pathway a reflex uses and is the simplest functional unit of the nervous system.

_____ 5. Largest region of the diencephalon and relays sensory information (except olfaction) to appropriate areas of the cerebrum.

_____ 6. Chemical messengers that are released by synaptic vesicles upon the arrival of a nerve impulse, travel across a synapse, and can transfer the impulse to another neuron, muscle, or gland.

_____ 7. Brain wave pattern associated with calmness and relaxation.

_____ 8. Inferior portion of the brainstem and considered the most vital part of the brain because it contains the respiratory, cardiovascular, and vasomotor centers.

_____ 9. Largest and most superior portion of the brain and is divided into left and right hemispheres.

_____ 10. Cylindrical bundle of nerve fibers that extends from the brainstem, through the foramen magnum of the skull, down the vertebral column, and ends in the lower back.

_____ 11. Cerebral lobe that regulates executive functions such as judgment, problem-solving, planning, concentration, self-awareness, cognition, intelligence, personality, motor output, and speech production.

_____ 12. Part of the brain between the cerebrum and the brainstem and is responsible for balance, posture, coordination, equilibrium, and muscle tone.

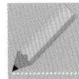

MATCHING THREE: CONCEPT REVIEW

Place the letter of the answer next to the number of the term or phrase that best describes it.

A. Sensory adaptation
B. Schwann cells
C. Dermatome
D. Interoceptors
E. Golgi tendon organs
F. Muscle spindles
G. Cerebrospinal fluid
H. Nociceptors
I. Blood-brain barrier
J. Proprioceptors
K. Nodes of Ranvier
L. Limbic system

_____   1.   Areas of the brain that regulate behavioral and emotional responses, especially those needed for survival.

_____   2.   Clear, colorless fluid surrounding the CNS that serves as a shock absorber, supplies the CNS with oxygen and nutrients, and helps remove metabolic wastes during sleep.

_____   3.   Produces the fatty myelin sheath around axons in the PNS.

_____   4.   Area of skin supplied by a single sensory spinal nerve.

_____   5.   Gradual decrease in receptor responsiveness to a constant or prolonged stimulus.

_____   6.   Tightly packed group of cells in the lining of blood vessels that supply the CNS that allow the passage of some molecules such as oxygen and glucose but prevent the passage of some harmful molecules.

_____   7.   Receptors involved in self-awareness and the detection of sensations such as heartbeat, breathing, hunger, satiety, thirst, and the urge to defecate or urinate.

_____   8.   Unmyelinated spaces between myelinated sheaths that increase the speed of the nerve impulse because it jumps from one unmyelinated space to the next.

_____   9.   Stretch receptors that monitors how far and how fast the muscle is being stretched and can cause involuntary muscle contraction to help protect the muscle from being torn.

_____   10.   Type of interoceptor that detects body movement and body position.

_____   11.   Stretch receptors at musculotendinous junctions that can inhibit muscle contraction to prolong muscle lengthening and help protect the muscle from being torn.

_____   12.   Receptors sensitive to pain and can activate the withdrawal reflex.

MULTIPLE CHOICE: TEST YOUR KNOWLEDGE

Place the letter of the answer next to the number of the term or phrase that best describes it.

_____   1.   Which property describes the ability of a neuron to release neurotransmitters?
A. Excitability
B. Irritability
C. Secretion
D. Conductivity

_____   2.   What is the correct meningeal order from deep to superficial?
A. Arachnoid, pia mater, dura mater
B. Pia mater, arachnoid, dura mater
C. Dura mater, pia mater, arachnoid
D. Dura mater, arachnoid, pia mater

_____   3.   What is a bundle of transverse fibers connecting the right and left cerebral hemispheres called?
A. Gyri
B. Sulci
C. Nerve plexus
D. Corpus callosum

_____   4.   Which is the proper classification for a sensory neuron?
A. Afferent
B. Efferent
C. Motor
D. Association

_____   5.   Receptors in muscles, tendons, and joints are:
A. Exteroreceptors
B. Nociceptors
C. Chemoreceptors
D. Proprioceptors

_____   6.   The reabsorption of neurotransmitters by the presynaptic neuron is called:
A. Homeostasis
B. Allostasis
C. Reuptake
D. Repolarization

_____   7.   Which is nerve impulse conduction along myelinated axons?
A. Transient conduction
B. Saltatory conduction
C. State-dependent conduction
D. Continuous conduction

_____   8.   Which lobe contains the somatosensory cortex, which is the primary sensory area in the brain?
A. Frontal
B. Temporal
C. Parietal
D. Occipital

_____   9.   Which brainwave is associated with day-dreaming?
A. Alpha
B. Beta
C. Theta
D. Delta

_____ 10. Several brain structures involved in processing and regulating of emotions, learning and the formation and storage of memories, reproduction, and caring for young is collectively called the:
   A. Limbic system
   B. Spinal cord
   C. Cauda equine
   D. Medulla oblongata

_____ 11. Which cranial nerve regulates heart rate, respiration rate, and blood pressure.
   A. Facial
   B. Abducens
   C. Assessory
   D. Vagus

_____ 12. The receptor that constantly sends out motor impulses (even at rest) to help maintain muscle tone is called:
   A. Muscle spindle
   B. Golgi tendon organ
   C. Nociceptor
   D. Osmoreceptor

CRITICAL THINKING

Weighty Matters

You greet your next client and notice she is wearing a large purse slung over one shoulder. It appears heavy, and the client even seems to be tilted a bit to one side. Reading over the health history form she has filled out, you discover the client has been having numbness, tingling, and weakness in the arm on the same side she carries her purse. Additionally, during the pretreatment interview, the client says she has a 2-year-old son who she is always running after, which makes her tired. When you ask her which side of her body she holds him on, she indicates the same side she carries her purse.

Which condition is the client most likely experiencing? What is the cause? What would be the most effective massage approach? What recommendations can you give the client?

Answers can include but are not limited to:

It is most likely the client has thoracic outlet syndrome (TOS). TOS is a disorder caused by compression of nerves in the brachial plexus alone or with the subclavian artery and vein (between the base of the neck and axilla). These structures are also called the neurovascular bundle. The term _thoracic outlet_ refers to the area between the first rib and the clavicle where the brachial plexus and the subclavian artery and vein traverse. TOS can be classified according to the structures being compressed. TOS is also called brachial plexus injury. Some causes are from anatomic defects such as a cervical rib (an extra rib above the first rib) or an unusually tight band of fibrous tissue connecting the spine to the first rib. Poor posture or carrying heavy items can compress the area between the clavicle and the first rib. Hypertonus of the scalenes or pectoralis minor may either pull the first rib upward (reducing the area between the first rib and the clavicle) or compress the neurovascular bundle

into the ribcage. Trauma or cumulative stress, such as repetitive activities, can cause or contribute to TOS.

It is most likely the client's TOS is caused by carrying a heavy purse on the same side of her body all the time and carrying her son on the same side of her body all the time.

Massage is helpful for this condition, especially when used in combination with other techniques. For example, massage combined with myofascial release techniques, trigger point massage, cross-fiber friction, muscle stripping, and gentle passive stretching increased shoulder ROM and decreased pain, weakness, and paresthesia. Massage alone or combined with other techniques was seen to relieve numbness. Consider addressing muscles such as the pectoralis minor, the scalenes (only approach laterally), and the muscles of the shoulder girdle and the arm. If the area is swollen, place the affected limb on bolsters or pillows to raise it above the level of the heart. Elevation may help promote dependent drainage (lymph drainage assisted by gravity). Superficial effleurage using light pressure applied centripetally is most beneficial. Massage proximal to the affected area first; for example, massage the arm before the forearm. This approach will help clear the path for lymph from distal areas. Massage practitioners trained in advanced techniques of manual lymphatic drainage may follow appropriate protocols.

Recommendations for the client can include carrying a lighter purse, alternating which shoulder she carries her purse on, alternating the sides of her body she carries her son on, stretching the area on a regular basis, and receiving massage in the area to loosen the affected muscles.

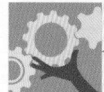

PROFESSIONAL PRACTICE

Roll Up Your Sleeves

Ronald is a regular client who enjoys his weekly massage. A few months ago, he was diagnosed with carpal tunnel syndrome of his right wrist.

When he came for his appointment this week, you noticed he used his left hand rather than his right to open the office door. During the assessment, he states the area is painful and tender to the touch. You ask him to remove his jacket and pull up his right sleeve. You notice the area is slightly swollen. When you palpate the area, it feels overly warm.

How should you proceed? Include your rationale.

DISCUSSION

Dermoneuromodulation

Using a search engine or other resource, locate a description of dermoneuromodulation, or DNM. Does DNM have any relevance to massage? Explain. If available, post your reflections on an internet-based discussion board monitored by your instructor. Include any relevant links to support your ideas.

CHAPTER 24

Endocrine System and Pathologies

LEARNING OBJECTIVES

After completing this chapter, the student should be able to:

1. List anatomic structures and physiologic processes related to the endocrine system and describe its hormones and hormonal regulation systems.
2. Identify specific endocrine glands, their hormonal secretions, and the effects of these hormones.
3. Name types of pathologic conditions of the endocrine system, giving massage modifications for each.

INTRODUCTION

The endocrine system and the nervous system coordinate many body functions. The nervous system uses nerve impulses and chemical messengers called *neurotransmitters,* whereas the endocrine system uses several regulatory mechanisms and chemical messengers called *hormones.* Neurotransmitters are produced by neurons, travel across a space called a synapse, and transmit a nerve impulse to another neuron, muscle, or gland. Most neurologic responses are fast, and neurotransmitter actions are short-lived. Hormones are made by endocrine glands, travel through the bloodstream, and activate target cells (more about target cells later). *Glands* are organs that secrete substances. Hormonal responses are slow and more widespread compared with neurotransmitter responses (Fig. 24.1). However, many cells have receptors for both neurotransmitters and hormones and therefore can be regulated by both. In fact, the nervous and endocrine systems may be referred to as the *neuroendocrine system* because of their shared regulatory functions.

Two types of glands in the body are *endocrine* and *exocrine.* **Endocrine glands** secrete hormones directly into the bloodstream. Endocrine glands do not possess ducts or tubes and are called *ductless glands.* Hormones travel through the bloodstream and affect cells in other parts of the body. Some hormones do not enter the bloodstream and affect neighboring cells only. *Endocrinology* is the study of the endocrine system. In contrast, **exocrine glands** secrete their products into ducts that open to body cavities, the center of a hollow organ, or onto the surface of the body. Examples of exocrine glands are sudoriferous glands that secrete perspiration, sebaceous glands that secrete sebum or oil, and salivary glands that secrete saliva.

Compared with other body systems, which are made up of large and heavy structures, endocrine glands are small, with the total weight of all glands less than 0.5 lb. However, functions of the endocrine glands are vital to the body, which becomes apparent when hormone levels are too low or too high, which cause drastic changes in growth and metabolism (Fig. 24.2). Use Table 24.1 to help you understand the terms of the endocrine system. In this chapter, we will cover only major endocrine glands.

ANATOMY

Basic structures and components of the endocrine system are the:
- Hypothalamus
- Pituitary
- Pineal
- Thyroid
- Parathyroids
- Adrenals
- Pancreas
- Ovaries
- Testes
- Hormones

Several organs, glands, and associated structures possess hormone-secreting cells and include the kidneys, the thymus, the prostate, the heart, the gastrointestinal mucosa, and the placenta. Adipocytes or fat cells also secrete hormones.

PHYSIOLOGY

Important functions of the endocrine system are:
- Hormone production and secretion.
- Regulation of metabolism—Some hormones regulate growth, development, nutrient absorption, and energy metabolism. Some hormones regulate the metabolic activity of other glands and organs.
- Stress adaptation—Some hormones help the body respond or adapt to stress during periods of infection, trauma, dehydration, and anxiety.
- Chemical composition and fluid volume regulation—Some hormones regulate body fluid volume and electrolyte balance.

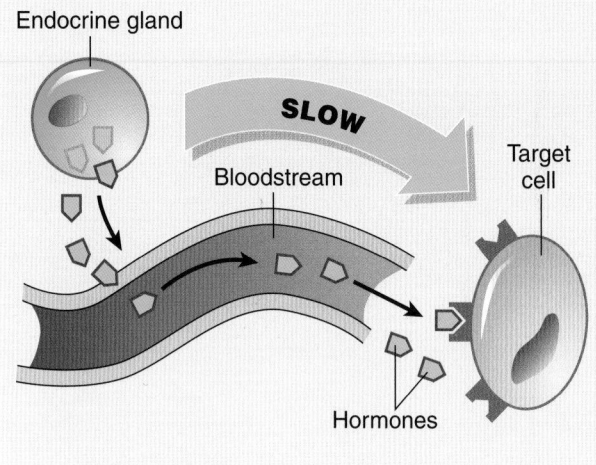

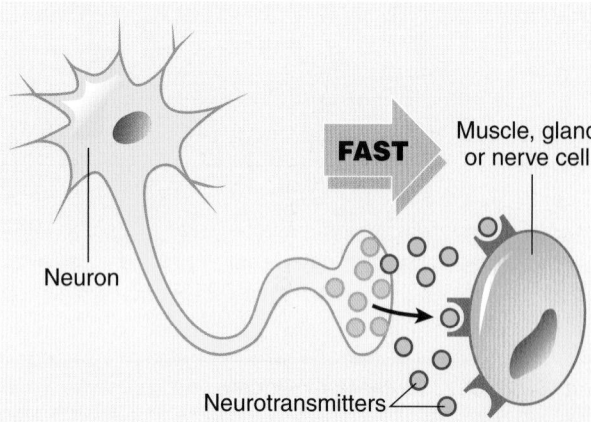

FIG. 24.1 Comparing endocrine system (*top image*) and nervous system (*bottom image*) functions. The endocrine system uses hormones transported through the bloodstream; responses are slow compared with the nervous system. The nervous system uses neurotransmitters and responses are fast compared with the endocrine system.

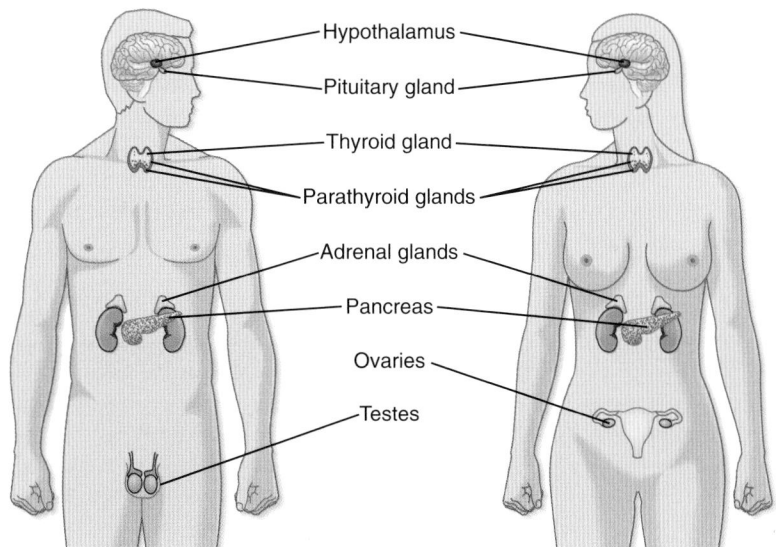

FIG. 24.2 Location of major endocrine glands in males (*left image, anterior view*) and females (*right image, anterior view*). The pineal gland is posterior to the pituitary gland. The parathyroids are on the posterolateral surfaces of the thyroid. (From Koeppen, B. M. [2010]. *Berne & Levy physiology, updated edition* [6th ed.]. St. Louis, MO: Mosby.)

TABLE 24.1 Word Meanings

WORD	MEANING
Adenohypophysis	*Gr.* gland; below; to grow
Adrenal	*L.* kidney
Antidiuretic	*Gr.* against; urine; production
Endocrine	*Gr.* within; to separate
Exocrine	*Gr.* away from; to separate
Hormone	*Gr.* to excite, arouse, urge on
Oxytocin	*Gr.* swift; childbirth
Pancreas	*Gr.* all flesh
Pineal	*L.* pine cone
Suprarenal	*L.* above; kidney
Thyroid	*Gr.* shield; shaped

Gr., Greek; *L.,* Latin.

- Reproductive process regulation—Some hormones regulate the reproductive process, including gamete or sex cell production, fertilization, pregnancy, childbirth, and lactation.

HORMONES AND HORMONAL REGULATION

Hormones are chemical messengers regulating the physiologic activity of other cells. Hormones influence growth, metabolism, digestion, reproduction, and mood. Because most hormones travel through the bloodstream, hormones come into contact with many cells. However, hormones do not affect every cell they encounter. Each hormone is programmed to seek out a **target cell** which contains receptors for the corresponding hormone (see Fig. 24.1). When hormones come into contact with receptors on their target

cells, they fit like puzzle pieces. This action produces an effect, which may be to increase or decrease the target cell's primary function (Table 24.2).

Prostaglandins, *or local hormones*, are secreted by many cells and they generally act only on nearby cells. Prostaglandins regulate smooth muscle contractions and inflammatory responses. Prostaglandins may also increase the sensitivity of nociceptors, which may increase pain. Medications such as aspirin and ibuprofen manage pain partly because they block prostaglandins.

The release of hormones from endocrine glands is regulated by several different mechanisms, including negative feedback regulation, hormonal regulation, and neural regulation.

Negative Feedback Regulation

Negative feedback regulation is the response of an endocrine gland to a stimulus that moves hormone levels in the opposite, or a "negative," direction. This movement brings hormone levels toward homeostasis. For example, the parathyroids regulate calcium levels. When calcium levels are low, the parathyroids secrete a parathyroid hormone (PTH), which releases stored calcium from bones, and increases blood calcium levels. The release of PTH ceases when calcium levels are in normal range. Negative feedback is also called *balancing feedback*. Most hormonal regulation in the body is negative feedback regulation.

Positive feedback systems also regulate hormonal secretion, but these mechanisms are rare compared with other regulatory systems.

Hormonal Regulation

Hormonal regulation involves the release of hormones from one gland regulating the release of hormones from

TABLE 24.2 Major Hormones

HORMONE	GLAND	PRIMARY FUNCTIONS
Adrenocorticotropic hormone (ACTH)	Anterior pituitary	Secreted in response to stress. Stimulates the adrenal cortex to secrete its hormones, namely cortisol
Aldosterone	Adrenal cortex	Maintains sodium levels by causing the kidneys to reabsorb sodium and excrete potassium. The "salt-retaining hormone."
Antidiuretic hormone (ADH)	Posterior pituitary	Decreases urine production and raises blood pressure
Calcitonin (CT)	Thyroid	Decreases blood calcium levels
Cortisol (hydrocortisone)	Adrenal cortex	Helps ensure glucose, lipids, and amino acids are available for energy during times of stress
Endorphins	Anterior pituitary	Inhibits pain during stressful events and promotes the release of the dopamine, which is associated with pleasure
Epinephrine	Adrenal medulla	Enhances and prolongs the fight/flight response (sympathetic arousal)
Estrogens	Ovaries	Development of female secondary sex characteristics; assists in the development and release of the ovum at ovulation; and stimulates proliferation and thickening of the uterine lining in anticipation of implantation of a fertilized ovum
Follicle-stimulating hormone (FSH)	Anterior pituitary	Females: stimulates the ovaries to secrete estrogen to develop an egg in the ovarian follicle
		Males: stimulates the testes to secrete testosterone and to produce sperm
Glucagon	Pancreas (alpha cells)	Increases blood glucose levels
Growth hormone (GH)	Anterior pituitary	Stimulates protein synthesis for muscle and bone growth, maintenance, and repair; plays a role in metabolism
Insulin	Pancreas (beta cells)	Decreases blood glucose levels
Luteinizing hormone (LH)	Anterior pituitary	Females: stimulates the release of estrogens and progesterone, ovulation, and development of the corpus luteum
		Males: stimulates testosterone production
Melanocyte-stimulating hormone (MSH)	Anterior pituitary	Increases skin pigmentation
Melatonin	Pineal	Maintains circadian rhythms, or the body's 24 h cycle
Norepinephrine	Adrenal medulla	Enhances and prolongs the fight/flight response (sympathetic arousal)
Oxytocin (OT)	Posterior pituitary	Stimulates uterine contractions and milk expression from mammary glands
Parathyroid hormone (PTH)	Parathyroids	Increases blood calcium levels
Progesterone	Ovaries; placenta	Maintains the uterine lining for implantation and pregnancy
Prolactin (PRL)	Anterior pituitary	Stimulates milk production from mammary glands
T3 (triiodothyronine)	Thyroid	Regulates metabolism
T4 (tetraiodothyronine or thyroxine)	Thyroid	Regulates metabolism
Testosterone	Testes	Promotes male secondary sex characteristics, libido, and sperm production
Thymopoietin	Thymus	Stimulates T-cell maturation
Thymosin	Thymus	Stimulates T-cell maturation
Thyroid-stimulating hormone (TSH)	Anterior pituitary	Stimulates the thyroid to synthesize and secrete its hormones

another gland. For example, thyroid-stimulating hormone (TSH), secreted by the anterior pituitary stimulates the thyroid gland to secrete its hormones. Hormones that stimulate the release of hormones from other glands are called *tropic hormones*. Most anterior pituitary hormones are tropic hormones.

Neural Regulation

Neural regulation is the release of hormones by nerve impulses. For example, nerve impulses of the sympathetic division of the autonomic nervous system stimulate the adrenal medulla to secrete stress hormones epinephrine and norepinephrine (see Chapter 23). Another example is hypothalamic nerves stimulating the posterior pituitary to secrete its hormones. Neural control systems have a faster response time compared with other hormonal regulatory systems.

HYPOTHALAMUS

The **hypothalamus** is in the diencephalon of the brain and secretes hormones that stimulate or inhibit the release of pituitary hormones. The hypothalamus also regulates the autonomic nervous system, providing a link between the endocrine and nervous systems.

Hypothalamic Hormones

The hypothalamus produces oxytocin and antidiuretic hormone (ADH), which are stored and released by the posterior pituitary. The hypothalamus also produces hormones that stimulate or inhibit the release of anterior pituitary hormones. For example, prolactin-releasing hormone stimulates the release of prolactin. Prolactin-inhibiting hormone inhibits the release of prolactin. Furthermore, hypothalamic hormones travel to the anterior pituitary through a network of capillaries (tiny blood vessels) called the *hypophyseal portal system*. Thus, hormones secreted by the hypothalamus flow through the portal capillaries to the anterior pituitary.

- **Stimulatory Hormones**. These include thyrotropin-releasing hormone, gonadotropin-releasing hormone, growth hormone (GH)–releasing hormone, prolactin-releasing hormone, and corticotropin-releasing hormone.
- **Inhibitory Hormones**. These include GH–inhibiting hormone and prolactin-inhibiting hormone.

I am not afraid of storms for I am learning to sail my ship.

~ **Louisa May Alcott**

PITUITARY GLAND

The **pituitary** is in the diencephalon of the brain and lies in the sella turcica of the sphenoid bone. The pituitary extends from the hypothalamus by a stalk-like structure called the *infundibulum*. The pituitary is about the size of a pea and contains two main regions, called the *anterior lobe* and the *posterior lobe* (Fig. 24.3). These lobes function as separate glands.

- **Anterior Lobe**. This constitutes approximately 75% of the total weight of the pituitary. As stated previously, the secretion of anterior pituitary hormones is regulated by the hypothalamus. The hypophyseal portal system allows hypothalamic hormones to travel to the anterior pituitary without going through the entire cardiovascular system. The anterior lobe is also called the *adenohypophysis*.
- **Posterior Lobe**. This constitutes approximately 25% ° of the total weight of the pituitary. As stated previously, secretion of the posterior pituitary is regulated by the hypothalamus. The posterior pituitary does not manufacture hormones. Instead, it stores and releases hormones produced by the hypothalamus. The posterior pituitary is composed of nervous tissue and is also called the *neurohypophysis*. Nerve impulses originating

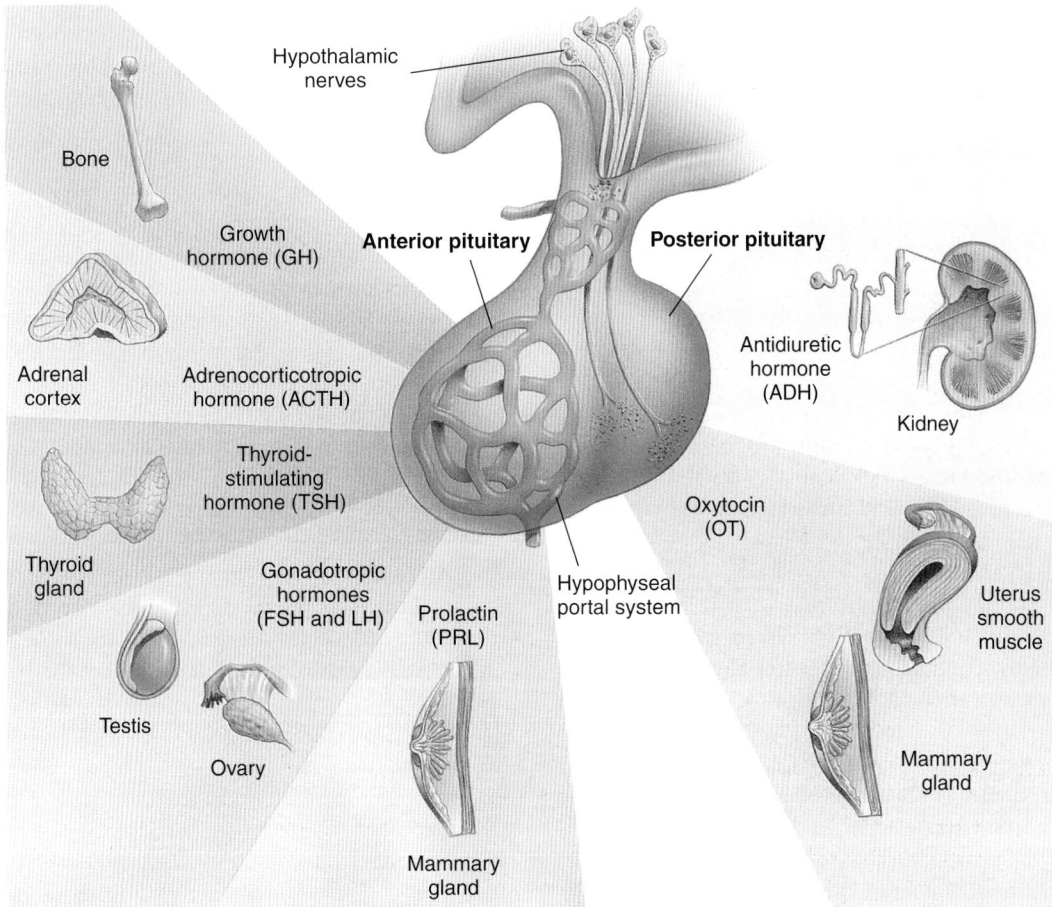

FIG. 24.3 Pituitary hormones and their target organs. Melanocyte-stimulating hormone *(MSH)* is secreted by the anterior pituitary and increases melanin production and hyperpigmentation in skin (not shown). Follicle-stimulating hormone *(FSH)* and luteinizing hormone *(LH)* are collectively called gonadotropins. Hypothalamic hormones travel to the anterior pituitary through the hypophyseal portal system. The hypothalamus stimulates the release of hormones stored in the posterior pituitary through nerve impulses. (From Thibodeau, G. A., & Patton, K. T. [2007]. *Anatomy & physiology* [6th ed.]. St. Louis, MO: Mosby.)

from the hypothalamus release hormones stored in the posterior lobe.

Anterior Pituitary Hormones

Adrenocorticotropic Hormone

The adrenocorticotropic hormone (ACTH) is secreted in response to stress, and stimulates the adrenal cortex to secrete its hormones, namely cortisol. This hormone is part of the hypothalamic-pituitary-adrenal (HPA) axis (see Chapter 23).

Growth Hormone

GH stimulates protein synthesis for muscle and bone growth, maintenance, and repair, and plays a role in metabolism. GH is also called *somatotropin* or STH.

Thyroid-Stimulating Hormone

TSH stimulates the thyroid to secrete its hormones, especially thyroxine.

Follicle-Stimulating Hormone

In females, follicle-stimulating hormone (FSH) stimulates the ovaries to secrete estrogen to develop an egg in the ovarian follicle. In males, FSH stimulates the testes to secrete testosterone and to produce sperm. FSH and luteinizing hormone (LH) are collectively called *gonadotropins*.

Luteinizing Hormone

In females, LH stimulates the release of estrogens and progesterone, ovulation, and development of the corpus luteum in the ovaries. In males, LH stimulates testosterone production in the testes. As stated previously, LH and FSH are collectively called *gonadotropins*.

Prolactin

Prolactin promotes lactation or milk production in mammary glands in the breasts. Prolactin is secreted in larger amounts during pregnancy and breastfeeding the young or lactation.

Melanocyte-Stimulating Hormone

Melanocyte-stimulating hormone (MSH) increases melanin production and hyperpigmentation. Differing levels of MSH do not cause racial variations in skin color.

Endorphins

Endorphins are a group of hormones that inhibit pain and are released during stressful events. Endorphins also promote the release of the neurotransmitter dopamine, which is associated with pleasure. Opioid medications function partly by mimicking endorphins, competing for their receptors. In fact, the word "endorphins" is Greek for "endogenous morphine."

Posterior Pituitary Hormones

Antidiuretic Hormone

ADH regulates fluid balance and helps maintain blood pressure by causing the kidneys to absorb more water, which decreases urine production. ADH also increases blood pressure by stimulating blood vessels to constrict and narrow. Alcohol consumption inhibits the release of ADH, which increases urine production. ADH is also called *vasopressin*.

Oxytocin

Oxytocin stimulates uterine contractions during pregnancy, labor, and childbirth, and stimulates milk expression from mammary glands during lactation. A synthetic version of oxytocin, called Pitocin, is used intravenously to stimulate labor and childbirth in pregnant females.

More recently, oxytocin has been implicated in behaviors, including recognition, trust, feelings of love and attachment, altruism, sexual arousal, and mother-infant bonding. From this research, oxytocin is called the "love hormone" or the "cuddle hormone." Oxytocin may also play a role in mental health and disease, including depression, anxiety, post-traumatic stress disorders, substance use disorders, and eating disorders.

PINEAL GLAND

The **pineal gland** is a small pine-nut shaped structure behind the pituitary in the diencephalon of the brain (see Fig. 24.2). This gland secretes several hormones, but its chief hormone is melatonin.

Pineal Hormone

Melatonin

Melatonin helps to regulate other hormones and to maintain the body's circadian rhythm, which is the body's internal 24-hour sleep-wake cycle. Melatonin plays a critical role in when we fall asleep and when we awaken—melatonin increases production in darkness and decreases production in bright light. Melatonin also regulates the release of female reproductive hormones and appears to regulate immune responses.

THYROID GLAND

The **thyroid** is inferior to the larynx and anterolateral to the trachea. This gland is butterfly-shaped and consists of two lobes connected in the center by the *isthmus* (Fig. 24.4). Occasionally, a third lobe will arise from the isthmus.

Thyroid Hormones

T3 and T4

T3, or *triiodothyronine*, and T4, or *thyroxine*, regulate nearly every process in the body, including metabolism, growth, and development. T3 and T4 are collectively called *thyroid hormones* (TH). These hormones consist of an amino acid bound to iodine; therefore they cannot be made without iodine. Good dietary sources of iodine are seafood and iodized salt. With the exception of seaweed, plant sources are often low in iodine.

Calcitonin

Calcitonin (CT) decreases blood calcium levels (called hypocalcemia) by stimulating osteoblastic activity, which

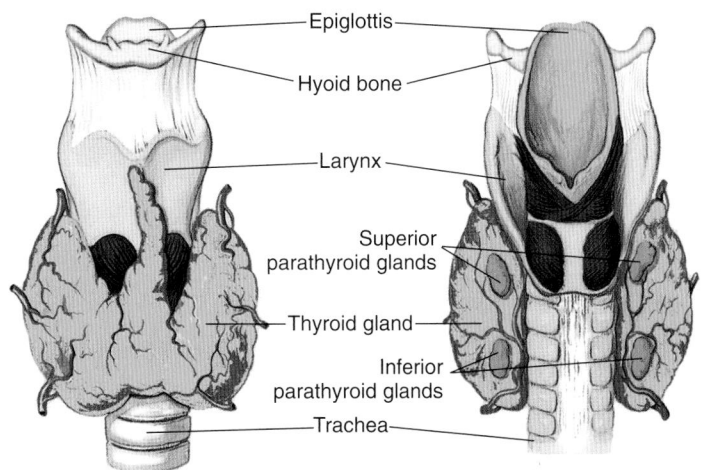

FIG. 24.4 Thyroid gland (*left image, anterior view*) and parathyroid glands (*right image, posterior view*) and their relationship to the larynx and trachea. (From Christensen, B. L. [2010]. *Adult health nursing* [6th ed.]. St. Louis, MO: Mosby.)

increases calcium storage in bones. CT production decreases with advancing age, which may contribute to loss of bone density during advancing age.

PARATHYROID GLANDS

The **parathyroids** are on the posterolateral surfaces of the thyroid and are usually 4 to 5 in number (see Fig. 24.4).

Parathyroid Hormone

Parathyroid Hormone
PTH increases blood calcium levels (called *hypercalcemia*) by stimulating osteoclastic activity, which decreases

calcium storage in bone. PTH also stimulates calcium reabsorption in the kidneys.

ADRENAL GLANDS

The **adrenals** are superior to each kidney and are divided into two regions, called the cortex and medulla (Fig. 24.5). The adrenals are also called the *suprarenals*.
- **Adrenal Cortex**. The gland's outer region.
- **Adrenal Medulla**. The gland's inner region.

Cortical Hormones

Cortical hormones are a group of steroidal hormones collectively called *corticosteroids*. The adrenal cortex contains

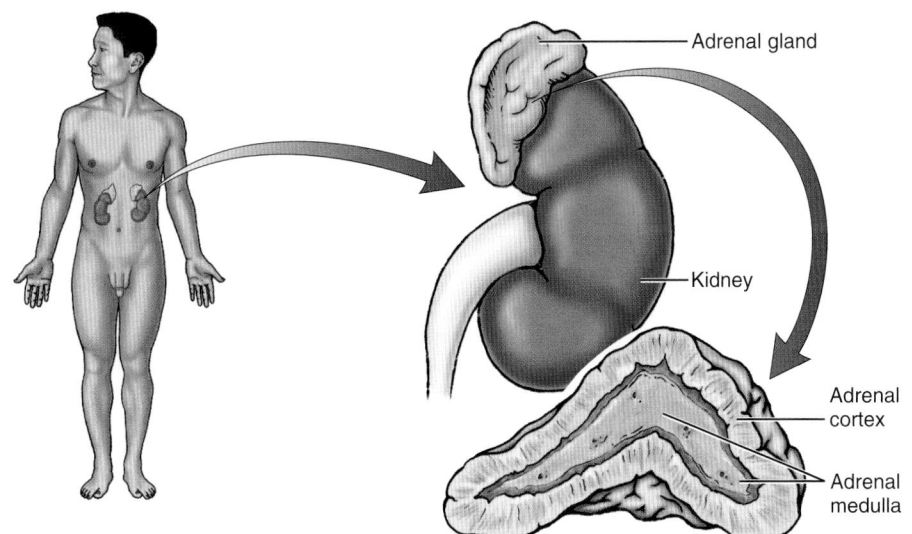

FIG. 24.5 Adrenal glands and their locations in the body (*left image, anterior view*), their locations in relationship to the kidneys (*right image, anterior view*), and a cross-sectional view of the adrenal gland noting the cortex and the medulla. (From Patton, K., & Thibodeau, G. [2014]. *The human body in health and disease* [6th ed.]. St. Louis, MO: Mosby.)

three layers or zones—an outer layer, a middle layer, and an inner layer, each of which secretes different hormones.

- **Mineralocorticoids (Outer Layer)**. Maintain electrolyte and fluid balance in the body by causing the kidneys to reabsorb sodium (salt) and excrete potassium. The principal mineralocorticoid is aldosterone.
- **Glucocorticoids (Middle Layer)**. Promote carbohydrate (sugar) metabolism, and has antistress, antiinflammatory, and immunosuppressive effects. Glucocorticoids also promote the metabolism of proteins and fats. The principal glucocorticoid is cortisol.
- **Gonadocorticoids (Inner Layer)**. Secrete minimal amounts of sex hormones in both males and females (i.e., adrenal estrogens and adrenal androgens). Their effect is usually dominated by hormone production in the testes and ovaries. However, the masculinization effects of adrenal androgens may become evident after menopause, when estrogen levels from the ovaries decline.

LEARNING TIP: To help remember the three hormones of the adrenal cortex, use the 3 S's—**S**alt (mineralocorticoids), **S**ugar (glucocorticoids), and **S**ex (gonadocorticoids).

Aldosterone

Aldosterone increases blood pressure by promoting sodium reabsorption by the kidneys and excreting potassium. These effects increase water retention and blood volume, which causes blood pressure to rise. Aldosterone is called the "salt-retaining hormone."

Cortisol

Cortisol increases blood sugar to fuel antistress, antiinflammatory, and immunosuppressive pathways. This action ensures the body has sufficient energy during demanding situations. Cortisol is widely used in medicine to manage autoimmune conditions such as rheumatoid arthritis.

Medullary Hormones

Medullary hormones are epinephrine and norepinephrine. These two hormones are called *neurohormones* because they act on the sympathetic division of the nervous system. Epinephrine accounts for about 80% of medullary secretions, and norepinephrine accounts for the other 20%. *LEARNING TIP*: To help remember the medullary hormones, think **A-M-E-N**—**A**drenal **M**edulla secretes **E**pinephrine and **N**orepinephrine.

Epinephrine and Norepinephrine

Epinephrine (adrenaline) and norepinephrine (noradrenaline) enhance and prolong the fight or flight response (sympathetic arousal), and provide the energy needed for stressful situations.

PANCREAS

The **pancreas** is inferior to the stomach and possesses both endocrine and exocrine functions. Endocrine functions are provided by specialized cells called **pancreatic islets** or *islets of Langerhans*, which secrete hormones that regulate glucose metabolism. The pancreas contains between 1 and 2 million islets, constituting approximately 2% to 3% of its total mass. Pancreatic islets have several types of cells, including alpha, beta, and delta cells (Fig. 24.6). This section discusses only alpha and beta cells. Exocrine functions of the pancreas and delta cells are discussed in Chapter 29.

- **Alpha Cells**. These cells secrete glucagon.
- **Beta Cells**. These cells secrete insulin.

Pancreatic Hormones

Glucagon

Glucagon increases in blood glucose (hyperglycemia) by stimulating the liver to release stored glucose (called *glycogen*).

Insulin

Insulin decreases in blood glucose (hypoglycemia) by stimulating the liver, skeletal muscle, and fat cells to take in glucose from the blood. Insulin replacement therapy must be administered by injection rather than administered orally, because digestive enzymes deactivate insulin.

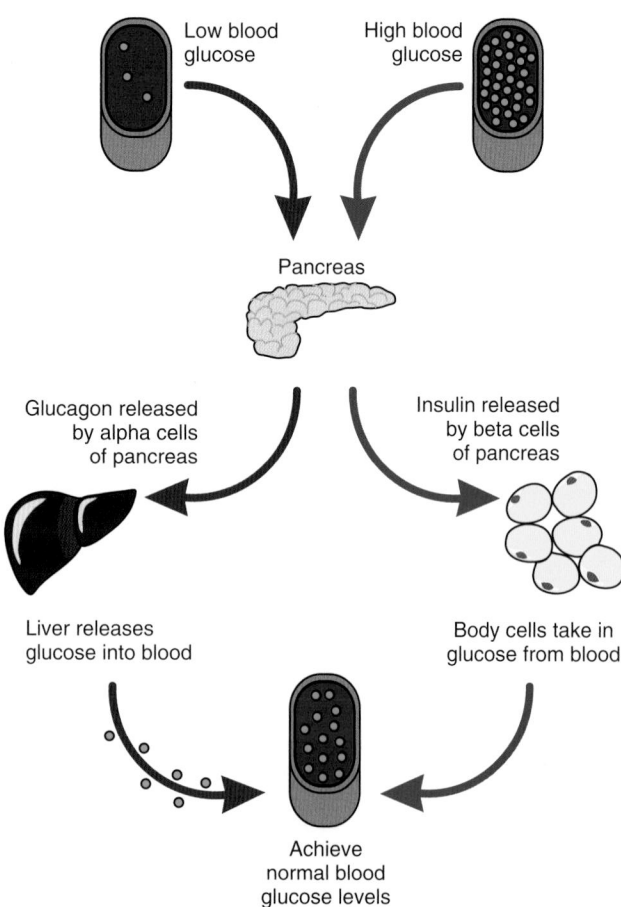

FIG. 24.6 Regulation of blood glucose levels by the pancreatic hormones glucagon (*left image, purple arrows*) and by insulin (*right image, blue arrows*). (From Goodman, C. C. [2011]. *Pathology for the physical therapy assistant*. St. Louis, MO: Saunders.)

OVARIES

Ovaries are paired almond-shaped glands in the abdomino-pelvic cavity of the female body (see Fig. 24.2). The ovaries secrete the hormones *progesterone* and *estrogen*, which are responsible for regulating the menstrual cycle and for female secondary sex characteristics that occur during puberty. Other ovarian hormones are relaxin and inhibin. *Relaxin* facilitates sexual reproduction and childbirth. *Inhibin* suppresses the release of FSH by the anterior pituitary after ovulation.

Ovarian Hormones

Estrogens

Estrogens are responsible for development of female secondary sex characteristics. These characteristics include distribution of adipose or fat tissue in breasts, hips, and abdomen; a wide pelvis; and pubic and axillary hair. During the menstrual cycle, estrogens stimulate proliferation of the uterine endometrium, which is important for implantation of a fertilized ovum and early embryonic life. Estrogens also increase skin blood flow and improve the quality of collagen, which promote skin thickness. Estrogens are linked to improved mental health; reduced estrogen levels are associated with depression.

Progesterone

Progesterone is the "pregnancy-promoting hormone", as it maintains the endometrium and inhibits uterine contractions. Progesterone also increases body temperature slightly, creating an incubating effect during the early weeks of pregnancy. These actions promote embryonic implantation and reduce the risk of miscarriage. Once a fertilized egg successfully implants, the placenta will secrete progesterone for the remainder of the pregnancy. If the ovum is not fertilized, progesterone levels drop, causing the endometrium to detach and slough off during menstruation.

Relaxin

Relaxin is a hormone altering the properties of connective tissues by activating collagenase, an enzyme that breaks down collagen and reduces its strength. In females, relaxin is secreted by the ovaries (corpus luteum) and the placenta during pregnancy; relaxin is also secreted by the prostate in males. In pregnant females, relaxin relaxes the uterine wall to reduce the risk of miscarriage or premature birth. Toward the end of pregnancy, relaxin helps the cervix relax and dilate, and relaxes pelvic ligaments to assist in childbirth.

TESTES

Testes are paired oval glands in the male scrotum (see Fig. 24.2). Scattered between testicular (seminiferous) tubules are the **interstitial cells of Leydig**. These cells secrete androgens, a group of hormones responsible for male secondary sex characteristics that occur during puberty and

play a role in reproduction. The principal androgen is *testosterone*.

Testicular Hormone

Testosterone

Testosterone stimulates sperm production and is responsible for the development of male secondary sex characteristics. These sex characteristics include widening of the shoulders and narrowing of the hips; appearance of facial, axillary, pubic, and chest hair; and the enlargement of the larynx, which contributes to deepening of the male voice. Testosterone also stimulates blood cell production, bone and muscle growth during and after puberty, and enhances libido both in males and females.

> *Every artist was an amateur.*
> ~ **Ralph Waldo Emerson**

ORGANS POSSESSING ENDOCRINE CELLS

Numerous hormone-secreting cells are scattered in organs throughout the body and can be found in the kidneys, the thymus, the prostate, the placenta, the gastrointestinal tract, the heart, and adipocytes.

Kidneys

The kidneys are two reddish-brown organs located bilaterally at or about the spinal level of T11 to L3. Kidneys secrete erythropoietin and renin.

- **Erythropoietin (EPO)**. Stimulates the production of red blood cells in bone marrow. The cells that secrete EPO are sensitive to low levels of oxygen in the blood. When they detect a decline, they release EPO to increase red blood cell count, which increases oxygen levels in the blood.
- **Renin**. Increases blood pressure, leading to restoration of the pressure needed to filter blood. Renin secretion by the juxtaglomerular cells is triggered when blood pressure in the kidneys drops. The release of renin stimulates the renin–angiotensin–aldosterone system, which increases blood pressure.

Thymus

The thymus is posterior to the sternum. Although it is a lymphatic organ (see Chapter 27), the thymus secretes the hormones thymosin and thymopoietin.

- **Thymosin**. Stimulates the development of T lymphocytes.
- **Thymopoietin**. Stimulates the production of B and T lymphocytes and their differentiation.

Prostate

The prostate is a donut-shaped gland inferior to the male urinary bladder and surrounds the urethra. The prostate secretes relaxin. Relaxin is also present in semen but is not found in the bloodstream.

- **Relaxin**. Enhances sperm motility and may enhance fertilization.

Placenta

The placenta is a flattened organ in the pregnant uterus (see Fig. 25.8). The placenta secretes estrogens and progesterone (discussed previously), and it also secretes human chorionic gonadotropin (HCG), placental lactogens, and relaxin.

- **Human Chorionic Gonadotropin.** Called the pregnancy hormone because its presence in blood and urine indicates pregnancy. HCG may also decrease lymphocyte activity, thus protecting the embryo from rejection by the mother's body.
- **Placental Lactogens.** Promote growth of the mammary glands in breasts in preparation for lactation, stimulates maternal and fetal metabolism, and works with GH to promote fetal growth and development.
- **Relaxin.** Works synergistically with progesterone to maintain pregnancy by relaxing the uterus to reduce the risk of miscarriage or premature birth. Toward the end of pregnancy, relaxin helps the cervix relax and dilate, and relaxes the pelvic ligaments to assist in childbirth.

Gastrointestinal Mucosae

The gastric and intestinal mucosae secrete gastrin, cholecystokinin, secretin, ghrelin, and gastric inhibitory polypeptide.

- **Gastrin.** Initiates the secretion of gastric juices in the stomach.
- **Cholecystokinin.** Stimulates bile and pancreatic enzyme emissions into the small intestines.
- **Secretin.** Stimulates the pancreas to secrete an alkaline liquid that neutralizes acidic chyme, thereby facilitating the action of intestinal enzymes. Secretin has a limited effect on bile production.
- **Ghrelin.** Stimulates appetite and is referred to as the "hunger hormone," as high levels of this hormone are found in individuals who are fasting. Ghrelin also stimulates the release of GH from the anterior pituitary gland.
- **Gastric Inhibitory Polypeptide.** Inhibits gastric secretion and potentiates the release of insulin from pancreatic beta cells in response to elevated blood glucose levels.

Adipocytes

Adipocytes, or fat cells, secrete leptin and resistin.

- **Leptin.** Regulates energy by inhibiting hunger and is sometimes called the "fat controller." Leptin is opposed by the action of ghrelin or the "hunger hormone" discussed in the previous section. Body cells become resistant to leptin in cases of obesity (similar to insulin resistance in type 2 diabetes), resulting in a reduced ability to detect satiety or fullness.
- **Resistin.** Increases blood sugar levels by causing body cells, especially liver cells, to be less sensitive to insulin. There is a possible link between obesity and type 2 diabetes mellitus (DM). Resistin has been shown to cause high levels of cholesterol (low-density lipoprotein or LDL), which increases the risk of heart disease.

Heart

The heart secretes atrial natriuretic hormone.

- **Atrial Natriuretic Hormone** (ANH). Increases urine production, which decreases blood pressure. ANH is secreted when pressure-sensitive receptors in the atrium become overstretched. ANH is also called *atrial natriuretic factor*.

ENDOCRINE PATHOLOGIES

Featured next are common pathologies of the endocrine system listed alphabetically. Each item includes a brief description and its massage-related modifications. A more extensive list and related research is found in the current edition of *Mosby's Pathology for Massage Professionals* (2022).

Diabetes Mellitus

Diabetes mellitus (DM) is a group of metabolic diseases characterized by abnormally elevated blood glucose levels called *hyperglycemi*a. There are two main types of DM: type 1 diabetes mellitus (T1DM) and type 2 diabetes mellitus (T2DM). T1DM is caused by insulin deficiency. T2DM is caused by insulin resistance. Gestational diabetes, which occurs during pregnancy, is discussed in Chapter 11.

Insulin is a hormone secreted by pancreatic beta cells. Insulin helps transport glucose into cells. Cells either use glucose for energy immediately or store glucose as glycogen for later use.

To help out, the liver releases glucose into the bloodstream to maintain homeostasis, and this just increases the already elevated blood glucose levels in a person with DM. The kidneys then attempt to restore normal glucose levels by excreting excess glucose in urine. Glucose excreted in the urine causes excretion of increased amounts of water, which causes the person to become extremely thirsty. The lack of glucose can trigger food cravings, which is why these individuals are also often hungry.

People with DM use several methods to monitor and adjust their blood glucose levels. Some individuals monitor their blood glucose levels regularly with a *blood glucose meter* that provides an immediate reading. Some individuals use a test called *glycohemoglobin A1C*, which is administered every 3 to 4 months, to estimate average blood glucose levels. This test measures what percentage of hemoglobin is coated with sugar (glycated). Hemoglobin is a protein in red blood cells that carries oxygen.

It is important to note that the lines between T1DM and T2DM have begun to blur. Hybrid types of DM are starting to emerge; therefore, characteristics of T1DM and T2DM are not mutually exclusive. Indeed, DM may be soon regarded as a spectrum disorder.

Double diabetes is the development of insulin resistance in someone with T1DM. Insulin resistance is a key feature of T2DM. The most common reason for developing insulin resistance in T1DM is obesity.

Type 1 Diabetes Mellitus

Type 1 diabetes mellitus (T1DM) is autoimmune destruction of pancreatic beta cells, resulting in insulin deficiency. Without insulin, glucose cannot leave the bloodstream and enter body cells, which create the condition of hyperglycemia. Individuals with T1DM develop a dependence on insulin. T1DM is also known as *insulin-dependent diabetes mellitus* (IDDM), because individuals with this type of diabetes are dependent on insulin injections. T1DM accounts for approximately 10% of all DM cases and affects approximately 1.25 million Americans. People with T1DM are also prone to other autoimmune diseases, such as Graves disease, Hashimoto disease, and Addison disease.

Hypoglycemia is characterized by abnormally low blood glucose levels, usually below 70 mg/dL. Hypoglycemia is a complication of DM, especially type 1. It occurs most frequently with insulin therapy, and it is associated with injecting too much prescribed insulin, late or skipped meals, or overexertion in physical activity. Although it can occur in people with T2DM, hypoglycemia is usually mild and infrequent side effect of treatment among this population. Signs and symptoms of hypoglycemia include confusion, disorientation, irritability, lack of muscle coordination, slurred speech (resembling drunkenness), visual disturbances, tremors, cold clammy skin, and inability to respond to verbal commands.

Massage and Type 1 Diabetes Mellitus

Query the client about diabetic complications and modify the massage accordingly. Ask if the client carries a blood glucose meter and, if so, where it is in case it is needed during a possible hypoglycemic episode. If the client is wearing a continuous glucose meter (usually on the arm or abdomen), the area around the device is a local contraindication. Clients with T1DM are insulin-dependent. Avoid vigorous massage over sites of recent injection for 24 hours or one-day, as this may increase absorption rates (Berger et al., 1982; Linde, 1986) and thereby decrease blood glucose levels and possibly cause hypoglycemia. In addition, Tosun et al. (2019) found injection site complications were significantly more common in those who massaged the area after injection. Consider teaching parents or caregivers how to massage the child with T1DM, making massage more accessible to the child, and giving parents/caregivers another way to care for and nurture the child. Limit techniques taught to gliding and kneading and convey the same precautions licensed practitioners follow, such as avoiding skin lesions and sites of recent insulin injection.

The practitioner must always be alert for signs of hypoglycemia. When symptoms are present, the practitioner is advised to follow the *15-15 rule.* Give the client glucose/sugar equal to 15 g of carbohydrates (carbs). Ask the client to rest for 15 minutes. If symptoms have not abated, the client should consume 15 more grams of carbs. Examples of foods equal to 15 g of carbs are 4 ounces of fruit juice; 5 to 6 ounces (about 1/2 can) of regular soda (not diet soda); 7 to 8 gummy or regular Life Savers; and 1 tablespoon of honey, sugar, or jelly. To prevent aspiration, fluids should not be forced. Once symptoms abate, ask the client to consume a meal or snack (such as crackers with cheese or peanut butter) to prevent recurrence of hypoglycemia. Use a blood glucose meter to check levels, if possible. This procedure does not harm the hyperglycemic person but could potentially save the life of a hypoglycemic person. The unconscious/unresponsive person needs immediate medical attention. Call 911 (American Diabetes Association [ADA], 2019; Joslin Diabetes Center [JDC], 2019).

Type 2 Diabetes Mellitus

Type 2 diabetes mellitus (T2DM) occurs when cells are resistant to insulin (most common) or from insufficient levels of insulin production by pancreatic beta cells (least common). T2DM is the most common form and accounts for more than 90% of DM cases. T2DM is usually controlled by diet, exercise, and oral hypoglycemics. In some cases, people with T2DM require insulin replacement therapy; this condition is called *insulin-requiring DM* [IRDM].

More than 100 million people in the United States have DM or pre-diabetes (Centers for Disease Control and Prevention [CDC], 2017). This number represents approximately 9.4% of the population. T2DM is often preventable, but the condition is on the rise, fueled largely by the current obesity epidemic. Young people are more likely now than ever to be diagnosed with T2DM, and it is the most common chronic disease in children and adolescents.

Diabetic foot ulcers are wounds that extend through the dermis and are below the ankle on weight-bearing or on exposed surface of the skin. Diabetic foot ulcers are one of the most common complications associated with DM with a lifetime incidence of 19 to 34%. More than 50% of diabetic ulcers become infected, and 20% of these will be severe enough to result in amputation, the surgical removal of a limb such as a foot, leg, or other body area. Eighty-five percent of DM-related amputations are preceded by a foot ulcer. After two decades of declining numbers of lower extremity amputations, there is now an increase of amputations in the United States, particularly among young and middle-aged adults.

Massage and Type 2 Diabetes Mellitus

As with T1DM, query the client about diabetic complications and modify the massage accordingly. Ask if the client carries a blood glucose meter and, if so, where it is in case it is needed during a possible hypoglycemic episode. If the client is wearing a continuous glucose meter (usually on the arm or abdomen), the area around the device is a local contraindication. Some clients with T2DM require insulin via injection.

Avoid vigorous massage over sites of recent injection for 24 hours as this may increase absorption rates and thereby decrease blood glucose levels, and possibly cause hypoglycemia.

Inspect the client's feet during each visit, looking for sores, broken skin, and objects embedded in the skin. Diabetic foot ulcers can occur anywhere pressure or shearing forces are applied to the foot (top, sides, bottom). These may go unnoticed by the client because of loss of sensation, vision, or both. If noted, these areas should be avoided during the massage with a referral made to the client's healthcare provider for a medical evaluation. The practitioner is advised to reinforce client daily self-evaluation at every session.

Safety is an important consideration for people with peripheral neuropathy, which can cause weakness or numbness because of damage to the peripheral nerves. Lack of muscle control and reduced sensation increases the risk of falls and other injuries. Practice safety measures, which include removal of throw rugs, securing of carpet edges, removal of low furniture and objects on the floor, removal of cords and wires on the floor, adequate lighting, and non-waxy flooring. Massage can be performed over areas of neuropathy using light to moderate pressure. Some clients with peripheral neuropathy of the lower extremities are prone to additional nerve injury from pressure; use a soft rather than stiff bolster behind the knees while the client is supine, and in front of the ankles when the client is prone. In addition, avoid the use of hot packs and hot stones over areas affected by peripheral neuropathy, as this may lead to contact burns (Mun et al., 2012).

Although hypoglycemia can occur in T2DM, it is often a mild and infrequent side effect of treatment among this population. Nonetheless, be aware of the symptoms of hypoglycemia listed in T1DM and administer first aid measures when needed.

Graves Disease and Goiters

Graves disease is an overproduction of TH, called hyperthyroidism, causing a generalized increase in the body's metabolism. The affected individual's metabolic rate increases by 60% to 100%. Graves disease affects about one in 200 people in the United States. The disease occurs more often in females than in males (4:1), which may be related to hormonal factors. Graves disease is an autoimmune disorder, and there is a familial predisposition. Disease manifestations include anxiety, hand tremors, weight loss despite increased appetite and food intake, diarrhea, fatigue, insomnia, tachycardia, flushed and warm skin with profuse sweating, heat intolerance (extreme sensitivity to warm temperatures), brittle hair, hair loss, and a goiter. A **goiter** is an enlarged thyroid gland. The most common

cause of goiters worldwide is a lack of dietary iodine. In the United States, where the usage of iodized salt is common, a goiter is usually caused by thyroid diseases. Goiters are usually painless. Large goiters can cause difficulty swallowing or breathing. Other characteristics of Graves disease are bulging eyeballs called *Graves ophthalmopathy* and thick reddened skin usually on the shins and tops of the feet called *Graves dermopathy*.

Massage and Graves Disease/Goiters

Customize the massage according to the client's presenting symptoms. Avoid the use of hot packs, hot immersion baths, and table warmers, because of the likelihood of heat intolerance. Use lightweight draping materials and perhaps uncover the arms and legs during the session. A cool washcloth may be placed over the client's forehead or across the base of the neck if needed. If the client has Graves' dermopathy, use an emollient lubricant to help combat skin dryness; avoid areas of broken skin.

Hashimoto Disease

Hashimoto disease is the underproduction of THs called *hypothyroidism*, causing a generalized decrease in the body's metabolism. Hashimoto disease develops slowly over time and primarily affects middle-aged females, but it can affect adults of any age. It affects 1% to 2% of people in the United States. Hashimoto disease is also called Hashimoto thyroiditis or chronic thyroiditis. Hashimoto disease is an autoimmune disorder, and there is a familial predisposition.

Massage and Hashimoto Disease

Customize the massage according to the client's presenting symptoms. Clients with Hashimoto disease will likely have muscular aches, pains, and stiffness related to hypothyroidism. In fact, some clients are particularly weather conscious and experience increased muscular pain with the onset of cold, rainy weather (Smeltzer & Bare, 2000). Massage may reduce these symptoms, but they will likely return unless the client is also taking thyroid replacement medications. Use an emollient lubricant to help combat skin dryness.

E-RESOURCES

https://evolve.elsevier.com/Salvo/MassageTherapy
- Chapter challenge
- Flash cards

JANET TRAVELL

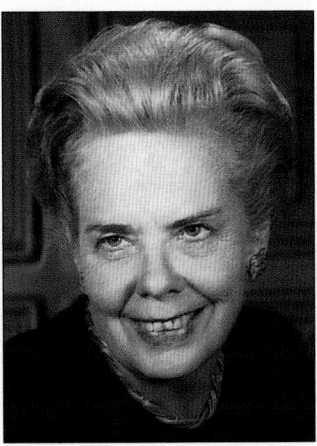

Trigger point therapy is a part of most people's massage education. It is called many names, but all of it comes down to the same idea: there are areas of chronic tension in our muscle tissue creating distinctive patterns of pain, which can be treated manually. It takes many hours of study and practice to learn these pain patterns and how to treat them effectively. Still, it does not compare with the tireless hard work of the woman who first researched them, Janet Travell.

Travell fell in love with science at a very early age. Her father was a physician, and she was determined to follow in his footsteps. He taught her the importance of concentration and efficiency, teaching her to work quickly and with focus, as well as how to think critically. In medical school, this speed and focus were both a blessing and a disadvantage. Her professor constantly accused her of working too quickly during her dissections, assuming she must be missing something in her rush. Finally, Travell started doing all her dissections with her left hand to slow herself to the pace of the other students. This solution kept her occupied and appeased the professor as well.

When she began her medical practice, Travell continued to work hard, long hours. She eventually cut her practice down to part-time, but this did not mean she eased up on herself. Rather, she used her newfound time to research the nature of muscular pain, a topic inspired both by her father's physical medicine experience and a shoulder injury Travell had experienced.

Travell had seen many heart and lung patients during her time working in a cardiac clinic, and many of them had complained of persistent shoulder pain. It took much hard work to find sufficient studies, but she was finally able to begin her research into this muscle pain that would not seem to go away.

Travell tackled the problem from a variety of perspectives. She looked at muscle tissue under a microscope. She poked, sprayed, and injected painful muscles. She talked to her patients and learned how they stood, turned, and moved. She tried therapies in opposition to the norms of the time, including the use of cold. As a result of many devoted hours of research, she discovered that muscles can stay contracted for long periods after trauma or repetitive use. She found evidence that trigger point therapy worked to alleviate myofascial pain from old injuries, developed a method for painless needle injections, and advocated simple lifestyle changes including the use of rocking chairs for people in pain. Through the use of all these techniques, she had excellent success in treating pain other physicians could not. Her reputation spread.

One of the people who heard of her success was the young Senator John F. Kennedy, who credited Travell with reducing his debilitating back pain to the degree he was able to campaign for the presidency. Upon being instated as president, JFK appointed Travell as White House physician, a role she continued to fulfill under Lyndon Johnson, at his request.

Travell left the White House in 1965 but kept up her hard work. Her autobiography, *Office Hours: Day and Night,* was published in 1968. In 1992 she and David G. Simons published *The Trigger Point Manuals,* which are still used by massage practitioners and students of massage today.

Her work ethic remained strong until the end of her life. She didn't stop studying or answering the many questions people posed to her in the mail until a few weeks before she died in 1997, at the age 95. Her passion for bringing relief to those in pain was complemented by a lifetime of constant effort. The remarkable example of Janet Travell shows that an individual who is willing to work with all their might can change the world.

REFERENCES

American Diabetes Association. (2019). *Standards of medical care in diabetes—2019 abridged for primary care providers.* Retrieved from https://clinical.diabetesjournals.org/content/37/1/11

Berger, M., Cüppers, H. J., Hegner, H., Jörgens, V., & Berchtold, P. (1982). Absorption kinetics and biologic effects of subcutaneously injected insulin preparation. *Diabetes Care, 5*(2), 77–91.

Centers for Disease Control and Prevention. (2017). *New CDC report: More than 100 million Americans have diabetes or prediabetes.* Retrieved from https://www.cdc.gov/media/releases/2017/p0718-diabetes-report.html

Joslin Diabetes Center. (2019). *How to treat a low blood glucose.* Retrieved from https://www.joslin.org/info/how_to_treat_a_low_blood_glucose.html

Linde, B. (1986). Dissociation of insulin absorption and blood flow during massage of a subcutaneous injection site. *Diabetes Care, 9*(6), 570–574.

Mun, J. H., Jeon, J. H., Jung, Y. J., Jang, K. U., Yang, H. T., & Lim, H. J., et al. (2012). The factors associated with contact burns from therapeutic modalities. *Annals of Rehabilitation Medicine, 36*(5), 688–695.

Salvo, S. G. (2022). *Mosby's pathology for massage professionals* (5th ed.). St. Louis: Mosby.

Smeltzer, S., & Bare, B. (2000). *Brunner and Suddarth's textbook of medical-surgical nursing.* (9th ed.). Philadelphia, PA: Lippincott.

Tosun, B., Cinar, F. I., Topcu, Z., Masatoglu, B., Ozen, N., & Bağçivan, G., et al. (2019). Do patients with diabetes use the insulin pen properly? *African Health Science, 19*(1), 1628–1637.

BIBLIOGRAPHY

Abrahams, P. H., Spratt, J. D., Loukas, M., & van Schoor, A. N. (2003). *Abrahams' and McMinn's clinical atlas of human anatomy* (8th ed.). St. Louis: Elsevier.

Applegate, E. (2010). *The anatomy and physiology learning system* (4th ed.). Philadelphia, PA: Saunders.

Como, D. (Ed.). (2016). *Mosby's dictionary of medicine, nursing, and health professions* (10th ed.). St. Louis: Elsevier.

Frazier, M. S., & Drzymkowski, J. W. (2015). *Essentials of human diseases and conditions* (6th ed.). St. Louis: Elsevier.

Hubert, R. J., & VanMeter, K. C. (2018). *Gould's pathophysiology for the health professions* (6th ed.). Philadelphia, PA: Saunders.

Haubrich, W. S. (2003). *Medical meanings: A glossary of word origins* (2nd ed.). New York, NY: American College of Physicians.

Herlihy, B. (2017). *The human body in health and illness* (6th ed.). St. Louis: Saunders.

Huether, S. E., McCance, K. L., & Brashers, V. L. (2019). *Understanding pathophysiology* (7th ed.). St. Louis: Mosby.

Juhan, D. (2003). *Job's body: A handbook for bodyworkers* (3rd ed.). Barrington, NY: Station Hill Press.

Kalat, J. W. (2013). *Biological psychology* (11th ed.). Belmont, CA: Cengage Learning.

Kapit, W., & Elson, L. M. (2013). *The anatomy coloring book* (4th ed.). New York, NY: Benjamin Cummings.

Kumar, V., Abbas, A. K., & Aster, J. C. (2015). *Robbins & Cotran pathologic basis of disease* (9th ed.). St. Louis: Mosby.

Marieb, E. N., & Keller, S. M. (2018). *Essentials of human anatomy and physiology* (12th ed.). New York, NY: Benjamin Cummings.

McCance, K. L., & Huether, S. E. (2019). *Pathophysiology: The biological basis for disease in adults and children* (8th ed.). St. Louis: Mosby.

Myers, T. W. (2014). Anatomy trains: Myofascial meridians for manual and movement therapists (3rd ed.). London: Churchill Livingstone; Elsevier.

Netter, F. H. (2018). *Atlas of human anatomy* (7th ed.). St. Louis: Mosby.

Patton, K. T. (2019). *Anatomy and physiology* (10th ed.). St. Louis: Elsevier.

Patton, K. T., Thibodeau, G. A., & Douglas, M. M. (2012). *Essentials of anatomy and physiology* (4th ed.). New York, NY: Pearson.

Porter, R. S. (2011). *The Merck manual of diagnosis and therapy* (19th ed.). Whitehouse Station, NJ: Merck Sharp and Dohme Corp.

Taber, C. W. (2021). *Taber's cyclopedic medical dictionary* (24th ed.). Philadelphia, PA: FA Davis.

REVIEW AND APPLY YOUR KNOWLEDGE

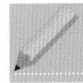 **MATCHING ONE: CONCEPT REVIEW**
Place the letter of the answer next to the number of the term or phrase that best describes it.

A. Adrenal cortex
B. Adrenal medulla
C. Anterior pituitary
D. Adipocytes
E. Hormones
F. Hypothalamus
G. Ovaries
H. Pancreatic alpha cells
 I. Pancreatic beta cells
J. Pituitary
K. Posterior pituitary
L. Thyroid

_____ 1. Cells that secrete insulin.
_____ 2. Chemical messengers that regulate the physiologic activity of other cells.
_____ 3. Gland that extends from the hypothalamus by the infundibulum.
_____ 4. Gland that regulates the autonomic nervous system.
_____ 5. Glandular region that secretes cortisol and aldosterone.
_____ 6. Glandular region that releases antidiuretic hormone and oxytocin.
_____ 7. Cells that secrete glucagon.
_____ 8. Gland that secretes thyroxine and calcitonin.
_____ 9. Cells that secrete leptin and resistin.
_____ 10. Glandular region that secretes adrenocorticotropic hormone and follicle-stimulating hormone.
_____ 11. Glandular region that secretes epinephrine and norepinephrine.
_____ 12. Gland that secretes estrogens and progesterone.

MATCHING TWO: CONCEPT REVIEW
Place the letter of the answer next to the number of the term or phrase that best describes it.

A. Adrenocorticotropic hormone
B. Antidiuretic hormone
C. Calcitonin
D. Cortisol
E. Epinephrine and norepinephrine
F. Estrogens
G. Insulin
H. Glucagon
 I. Melatonin
J. Oxytocin
K. Parathyroid hormone
L. Testosterone

_____ 1. Hormone that increases blood calcium levels.
_____ 2. Hormone responsible for the development of male secondary sex characteristics.
_____ 3. Hormone that activates antistress and antiinflammatory pathways.
_____ 4. Hormone that stimulates uterine contractions in pregnancy and milk expression from the breasts during lactation.
_____ 5. Hormones that enhance and prolong the physiologic effects of stress.
_____ 6. Hormone that decreases urine production.
_____ 7. Hormones responsible for the development of female secondary sex characteristics.
_____ 8. Hormone that maintains the body's circadian rhythm.
_____ 9. Hormone that decreases blood glucose levels.
_____ 10. Hormone that stimulates the adrenal cortex to secrete its hormones.
_____ 11. Hormone that decreases blood calcium levels.
_____ 12. Hormone that increases blood glucose levels.

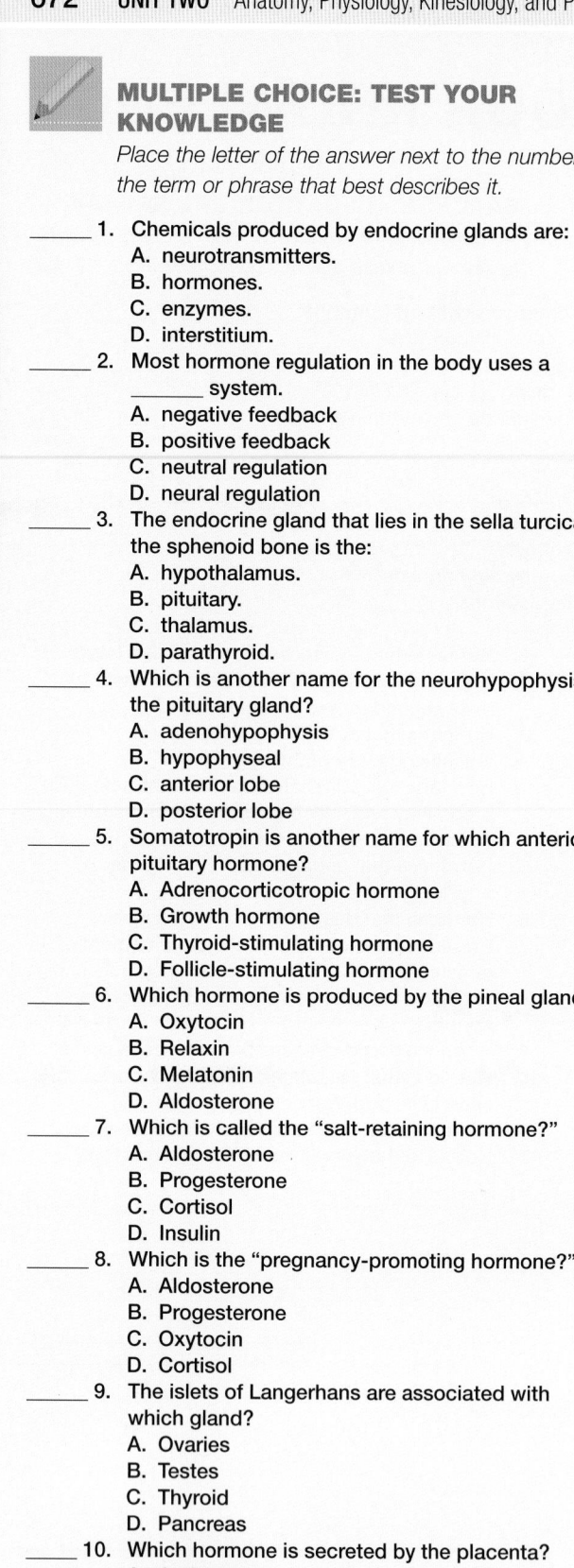

MULTIPLE CHOICE: TEST YOUR KNOWLEDGE

Place the letter of the answer next to the number of the term or phrase that best describes it.

_____ 1. Chemicals produced by endocrine glands are:
A. neurotransmitters.
B. hormones.
C. enzymes.
D. interstitium.

_____ 2. Most hormone regulation in the body uses a _____ system.
A. negative feedback
B. positive feedback
C. neutral regulation
D. neural regulation

_____ 3. The endocrine gland that lies in the sella turcica of the sphenoid bone is the:
A. hypothalamus.
B. pituitary.
C. thalamus.
D. parathyroid.

_____ 4. Which is another name for the neurohypophysis of the pituitary gland?
A. adenohypophysis
B. hypophyseal
C. anterior lobe
D. posterior lobe

_____ 5. Somatotropin is another name for which anterior pituitary hormone?
A. Adrenocorticotropic hormone
B. Growth hormone
C. Thyroid-stimulating hormone
D. Follicle-stimulating hormone

_____ 6. Which hormone is produced by the pineal gland?
A. Oxytocin
B. Relaxin
C. Melatonin
D. Aldosterone

_____ 7. Which is called the "salt-retaining hormone?"
A. Aldosterone
B. Progesterone
C. Cortisol
D. Insulin

_____ 8. Which is the "pregnancy-promoting hormone?"
A. Aldosterone
B. Progesterone
C. Oxytocin
D. Cortisol

_____ 9. The islets of Langerhans are associated with which gland?
A. Ovaries
B. Testes
C. Thyroid
D. Pancreas

_____ 10. Which hormone is secreted by the placenta?
A. Androgen
B. Testosterone
C. Glucagon
D. Human chorionic gonadotropin

_____ 11. Which is the "hunger hormone?"
A. Glucagon
B. Ghrelin
C. Secretin
D. Insulin

_____ 12. Offering a client half a can of regular soda may help with which condition?
A. Graves disease
B. Hashimoto disease
C. Hyperglycemia
D. Hypoglycemia

CRITICAL THINKING

Stressed Out Much?

Massage has been shown to decrease the effects of stress on the body. However, do you think massage can help clients decrease the actual stress in their lives? Why do you answer the way you do?

Answers can include but are not limited to:

By decreasing the effects of stress on the body, clients feel better rested and more clear-minded. This may help them make decisions about how to manage the factors in their lives causing stress. They may be able to see what they need to keep in their lives, what they need to eliminate, and the best way to handle situations they are experiencing. On the other hand, massage is just one aspect of a client's life. It may or may not have enough of an impact for the client to make other life changes. It is hard to know exactly what a client is experiencing, what choices the client is willing or not willing to make, and what choices the client can or cannot make.

PROFESSIONAL PRACTICE

Blood Sugar See-Saw

Steve is a 48-year-old man who works as a business executive for a financial institution. About 4 years ago, he was diagnosed with diabetes. He takes several medications to control his blood sugar, cholesterol levels, and hypertension. Because of some worries he has had on his mind lately, he has been negligent about exercise and eats fast food for most meals.

Steve arrives at 4PM for his weekly appointment. During his intake, he mentions an area on his right foot that is painful. He also mentions that he was extremely busy and he missed lunch, as well as his medication this morning. He is looking forward to his massage today. He stands up and walks toward the massage room, pulling off his necktie as he goes, and says he can't wait for the massage to start. How do you proceed?

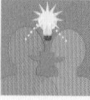

DISCUSSION

Snack Attack

One of your clients is a type 1 diabetic who has recently been placed on an insulin pump. During her massage, she interrupts you and says she needs to take a break to eat something. After having a chance to eat the snack she has brought along and resting for a while, she apologizes for the interruption and says she is feeling much better. What probably happened here? If available, post your reflections on an Internet-based discussion board monitored by your instructor. Include any relevant Internet links to support your ideas.

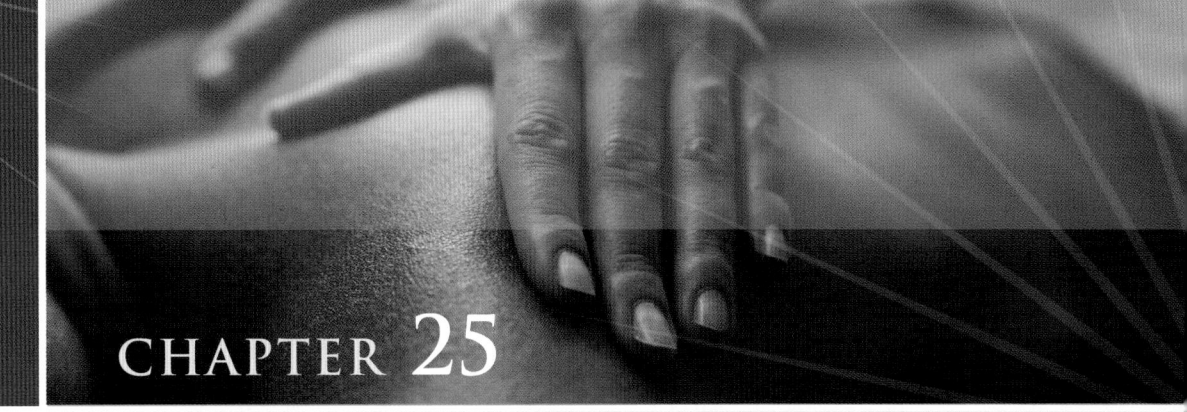

CHAPTER 25

Reproductive System, Pathologies, Conditions, and Disorders

LEARNING OBJECTIVES

After completing this chapter, the student should be able to:

1. List basic anatomic structures and describe physiologic processes of the male and female reproductive systems.
2. Discuss sexual intercourse, fertilization, pregnancy, childbirth, and lactation.
3. Describe reproductive pathologies, conditions, and disorders and state their massage modifications.

http://evolve.elsevier.com/Salvo/MassageTherapy

INTRODUCTION

The reproductive system contains the male and female reproductive organs and glands, sex cells, and fluids needed for sexual reproduction. **Sexual reproduction** is the process by which male sex cells and female sex cells unite. The union of these cells may produce offspring, which passes on hereditary traits from one generation to the next to continue the species. Primary organs called *gonads* produce both male or female sex cells, called *gametes,* and the hormones that assist sexual reproduction. Use Table 25.1 to help you understand terms of the reproductive system.

Although both male and female reproductive systems contribute to these events, the female body is responsible for developing the young, giving birth, and providing nourishment through lactation and breastfeeding. *Gynecology* is the study of the female reproductive system. *Andrology* is the study of the male reproductive system. *Midwifery* is the study of pregnancy, childbirth, and the postpartum period or the time following childbirth. *Obstetrics* encompasses midwifery as well as medical practices such as surgical procedures. Andrologists are urologists who focus on male fertility and sexuality. Urologists provide male healthcare because they specialize in both male reproductive and urinary systems.

ANATOMY

Basic anatomy of the reproductive system includes:
- Gonads—**gonads** are the primary reproductive organs; they include the testes in males and the ovaries in females.
- Gametes—**gametes** are sex cells; they include the spermatozoa in males and the oocytes in females.
- Ducts—the spermatic ducts in males and the fallopian tubes in females.
- Male accessory organs and glands—the penis, prostate and bulbourethral glands, and seminal vesicles.
- Female accessory organs and glands—these are the uterus, Bartholin glands, and the breasts.

PHYSIOLOGY

Important functions of the reproductive system are:
- Produces offspring—This involves sexual reproduction, which allows new individuals of a species to be produced and genetic material to be passed from one generation to the next. It also includes nourishment of the unborn and newborn by the female body.
- Hormone production and secretion—Hormones play a critical role in the reproductive process, in physical differentiation, and in maintenance of male and female characteristics.

MALE REPRODUCTIVE SYSTEM

The male reproductive system consists of gametes called sperm, gonads called testes, and a duct system called the

TABLE 25.1 Word Meanings

WORD	MEANING
bulbourethral glands	*L.* swollen root
cervix	*L.* neck
chromosome	*Gr.* color; body
corpus albicans	*L.* body; white
corpus luteum	*L.* body; yellow
Cowper gland	William Cowper, English surgeon, 1666–1709
cremaster	*Gr.* hanging
ejaculation	*L.* to hurl or throw out
embryo	*Gr.* in, to grow
epididymis	*Gr.* upon; pair
estrogen	*Gr.* sexuality; to produce
fallopian tubes	Gabriele Fallopio, Italian anatomist (1523–1562)
fertilization	*L.* fruitful
fetus	*L.* fruitful
gametes	*Gr.* to marry
gene	*Gr.* to produce
glans	*Gr.* acorn
gonads	*Gr.* seed
inheritance	*L.* within; to inherit
interstitial cells of Leydig	Franz von Leydig, German anatomist (1821–1908)
labia	*L.* lips
lactation	*L.* milk; process
mammary	*L.* breast
menstrual	*Gr.* monthly; *L.* moon
mons pubis	*L.* mountain; grown-up or hair
morula	*L.* mulberry or blackberry
oocyte	*Gr.* egg; cell
ovum	*L.* egg
placenta	*L.* cake
progesterone	*M.* produce; pregnancy
prostate	*Gr.* standing before
rugae	*L.* ridge
scrotum	*L.* a bag
semen	*L.* seed
seminiferous	*L.* seed; to bear
seminal vesicles	*L.* seed; bladder
spermatozoon	*Gr.* seed; life
testis	*L.* to bear witness
uterus	*L.* womb
vagina	*L.* sheath
vas deferens	*L.* to lead; to carry away
vulva	*L.* a covering
zygote	*Gr.* yoke

Gr., Greek; L., Latin.

spermatic duct that transports semen and sperm out of the body. External genitalia such as the scrotum and the penis facilitate this process. Male accessory glands secrete seminal fluid to nourish sperm (Fig. 25.1).

Sperm, Seminal Fluid, and Semen

Sperm, or *spermatozoa*, are sex cells that carry genetic information from the male who produced them. Sperm can

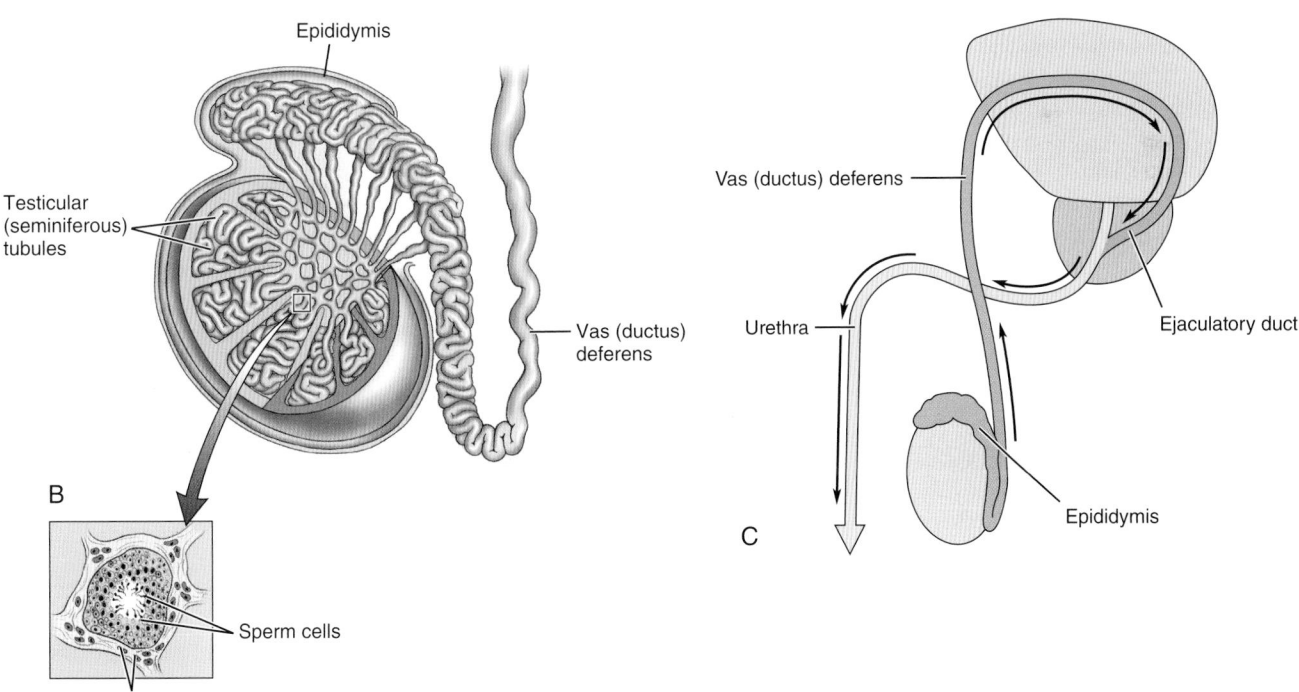

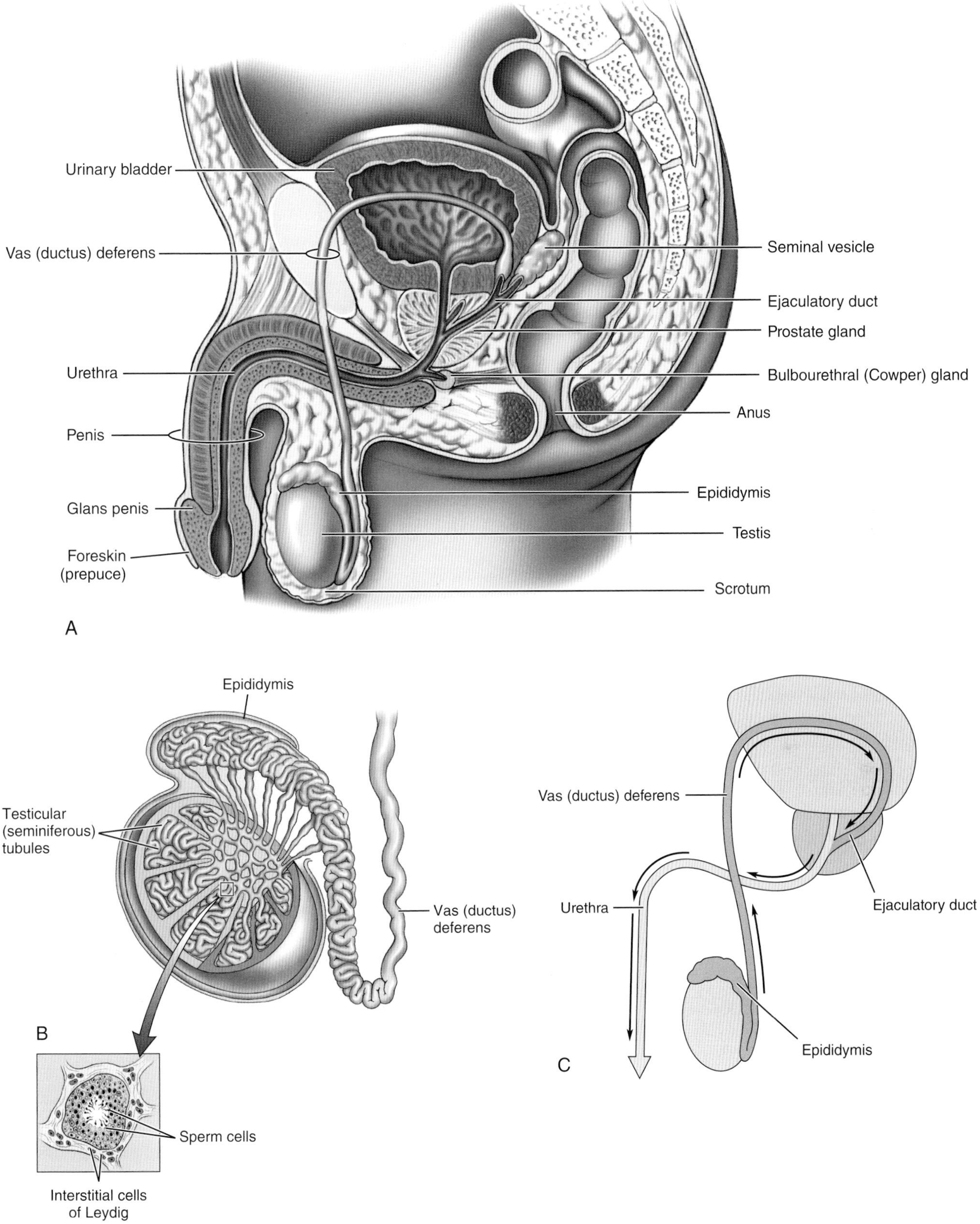

FIG. 25.1 (A) Male reproductive system (*lateral view*). (B) The testes, testicular tubules, and interstitial cells of Leydig (*cross-section view*). (C) The pathway for sperm. (Modified from Kirov, E. [2022]. *Herlihy's the human body in health and illness* [1st ANZ ed.]. Sydney, Australia: Elsevier.)

migrate or swim, and this property plays a key role in successful fertilization. Sperm cell production, or *spermatogenesis*, begins during puberty and continues throughout life. Sperm is produced in the testes. **Seminal fluid** is the milky white alkaline substance produced by the prostate and other male accessory glands. Seminal fluid is the transport medium and source of nutrients for sperm. **Semen** is a mixture of sperm and seminal fluid.

Testes

Testes, or *testicles*, are paired oval glands in the male scrotum at the base of the penis. The testes perform two functions: the production of sperm and hormones. Scattered between testicular (seminiferous) tubules are **interstitial cells of Leydig**. These cells secrete androgens. The principal androgen is testosterone. Testosterone stimulates sperm production and is responsible for the development and maintenance of male secondary sex characteristics throughout life. These characteristics include widening of the shoulders and narrowing of the hips; appearance of facial, axillary, pubic, and chest hair; and the enlargement of the larynx, which contributes to deepening of the male voice. Testosterone also stimulates the blood cell production, bone and muscle growth during and after puberty, and enhances libido or the desire for sexual activity. Follicle-stimulating hormone (FSH) and luteinizing hormone (LH) from the anterior pituitary stimulate the sperm and testosterone production.

Spermatic Duct

The **spermatic duct** transports semen out of the body during ejaculation. Sperm exits the testicles and enters the **epididymis**, a tightly coiled comma-shaped tube. Sperm remains in the epididymis for 2 to 3 months while they mature and become able to swim.

Next, sperm enter the **vas (ductus) deferens**, which joins the **ejaculatory duct**, a short tube that connects to the urethra about midway in the prostate gland. The **urethra** is a tube below the bladder that transports both semen and urine in males. A portion of the vas (ductus) deferens is removed or sealed during a sterilization procedure called a *vasectomy*. Once it is cut or sealed, sperm cannot get into the semen and out of the male body.

Male Accessory Glands

Male accessory glands secrete seminal fluid and include the prostate, the bulbourethral glands, and seminal vesicles. The **prostate** is a donut-shaped gland that lies inferior to the urinary bladder and surrounds the urethra. The prostate also prevents the flow of urine during ejaculation. **Bulbourethral (Cowper) glands** are pea-sized glands present on either side of the prostate. **Seminal vesicles** are at the base of the bladder.

Male External Genitalia

Male external genitalia include the penis and scrotum. The *penis* is composed of erectile tissues and contains the urethra. The end of the penis (*glans penis*) is covered with a loose flap of skin called the foreskin or prepuce. This foreskin is sometimes removed during a procedure called *circumcision.*

The *scrotum* is a divided pouch containing the testes. The scrotal sac is made of thin, loose, wrinkled skin hanging down behind the penis. The scrotum has a protective function, which includes maintaining the optimal temperature in the testes for sperm production. This temperature is slightly cooler than normal body temperature (approximately $\geq 4°$ F). Cremaster muscles in the wall of the scrotum contract and relax to help regulate temperature by moving the testes closer to or away from the body.

FEMALE REPRODUCTIVE SYSTEM

The female reproductive system consists of gametes called oocytes, gonads called ovaries, and a duct system called the fallopian tubes which transport oocytes to the uterus. The vagina and external genitalia help sperm enter the female body. Female breasts produce and secrete milk to feed any young resulting from sexual reproduction (Fig. 25.2).

Oocytes

Oocytes are sex cells that carry genetic information from the female who produced them. Oocytes, or *eggs*, are stored in fluid-filled sacs called ovarian (Graafian) follicles. When females are born, the ovaries contain all the oocytes they will ever have; their maturation does not occur until puberty. Beginning at puberty, FSH stimulates one oocyte to mature each month (sometimes more than one oocyte).

Ovaries

Ovaries are paired almond-shaped glands that produce oocytes and hormones; they are in the abdominopelvic cavity and connected to the lateral surface of the uterus by ligaments (Fig. 25.3). The ovaries secrete estrogen, which is responsible for regulating the menstrual cycle and for the development of female sex organs and secondary sex characteristics occurring during puberty, then maintains these characteristics throughout life. These characteristics include distribution of adipose tissue in the breasts, hips, and abdomen; a wide pelvis; and pubic and axillary hair. Progesterone maintains the uterine lining for implantation and pregnancy. Other ovarian hormones are relaxin and inhibin. Relaxin facilitates sexual reproduction and childbirth. Inhibin suppresses the release of FSH by the anterior pituitary after ovulation.

Fallopian Tubes

Fallopian (uterine) tubes are the paired passageways that extend laterally from the uterus toward the ovaries. The funnel-shaped end of the fallopian tube nearest the ovary is called the *infundibulum* that has fingerlike projections called *fimbriae*, to help the newly released oocyte enter the fallopian tube. The fallopian tube does not attach directly to the ovary. The lining of the fallopian tubes contains cilia, hair-like projections that sweep the ovum to the uterus. The fallopian tubes are the primary site of fertilization between an ovum

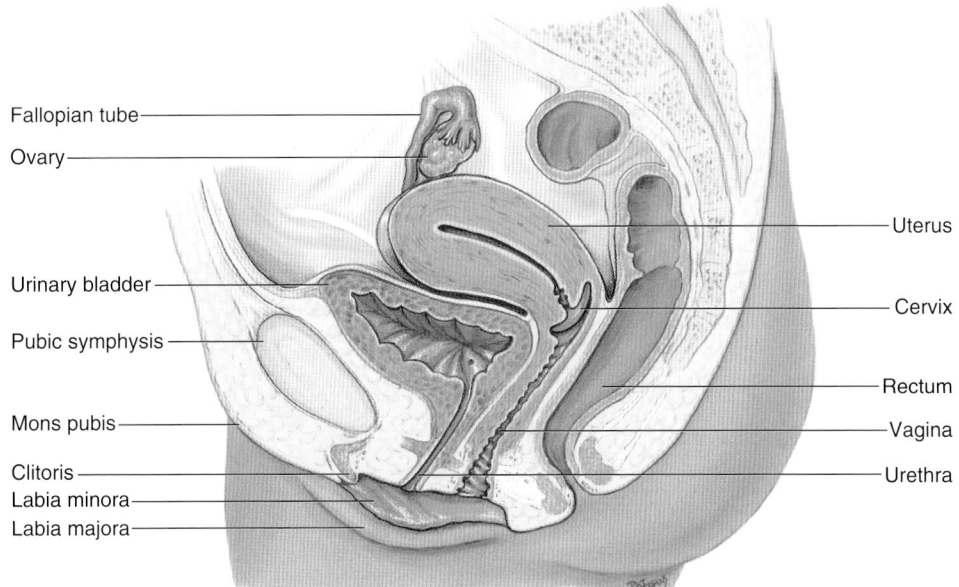

FIG. 25.2 Female reproductive system (*lateral view*). (From Applegate, E. [2011]. *The anatomy and physiology learning system* [4th ed.]. St. Louis, MO: Saunders.)

and the sperm. Fallopian tubes may be cut and sealed in a sterilization procedure called a *tubal ligation*, preventing the ovum from becoming fertilized by sperm after sexual intercourse.

Uterus and Vagina

The **uterus** is a hollow pear-shaped organ between the urinary bladder and the rectum. The uterus receives the fertilized ovum and allows the embryo to develop into a fetus during pregnancy or discharges its lining and the ovum if fertilization and implantation do not occur (see Fig. 25.3). The uterus has several regions—the *body,* or hollow cavity; the *fundus,* or uppermost region; and the *cervix,* or lower opening into the vagina. The **cervix** acts like a sphincter, allowing for the passage of semen, menstrual fluid, and a fetus during childbirth. The uterus contains several important ligaments, which are also discussed in Chapter 11 under Pregnancy Massage.

- **Round Ligament**. Arises from the anteroinferior surface of the uterus, passes through the groin region, enters the labia majora, and terminates at the mons pubis. The round ligament is composed of muscular as well as connective tissue, even though it is called a ligament, and may correspond to the cremaster muscle in males.
- **Broad Ligament**. Wide double-layered section of peritoneum that extends laterally from the uterus, surrounds the ovaries and fallopian tubes, and connects to the walls and floor of the pelvis.
- **Ovarian Ligament**. Lies within the broad ligament and attaches the ovaries to the lateral uterus.

The uterine wall consists of three layers.

- **Endometrium**. Inner lining that is shed during menstruation.

- **Myometrium**. Middle and thickest layer; composed of smooth muscle. During labor and childbirth, contractions of the myometrium widen or dilate the cervix to approximately 10 cm in diameter and contracts to push the fetus and the placenta out of the body.
- **Perimetrium**. Outer layer and essentially a part of the peritoneum, a serous membrane surrounding most abdominopelvic organs.

The **vagina** is the canal extending from the cervix to outside the body. The vagina, or *birth canal,* contains rugae, transverse folds allowing expansion during sexual intercourse and childbirth. Mucous-secreting Bartholin glands are on the sides of the vaginal opening; these glands are homologous to bulbourethral glands in males. Between the vaginal opening and the anus is the perineum, which can be torn or cut during childbirth; the latter is called an *episiotomy.*

Female External Genitalia

Female external genitalia, or *vulva,* include the labia majora and minora, the clitoris, and the mons pubis. The vulva facilitates the sperm's entry into the female body and provides sexual pleasure. The *mons pubis* is a mound of fatty tissue over the pubic symphysis, which becomes covered with hair after puberty. The *labia majora* are two folds of skin extending from the mons pubis and are homologous to the male scrotum. Like the mons pubis, the labia majora contain fat and are covered with hair after puberty. The *labia minora* are two folds of skin inside the labia majora and contain oil glands. The *clitoris* is a small cylindrical structure at the anterior junction of the labia minora. A small layer of foreskin covers the clitoris. The clitoris contains nerves and erectile tissue and, when stimulated manually, can enlarge

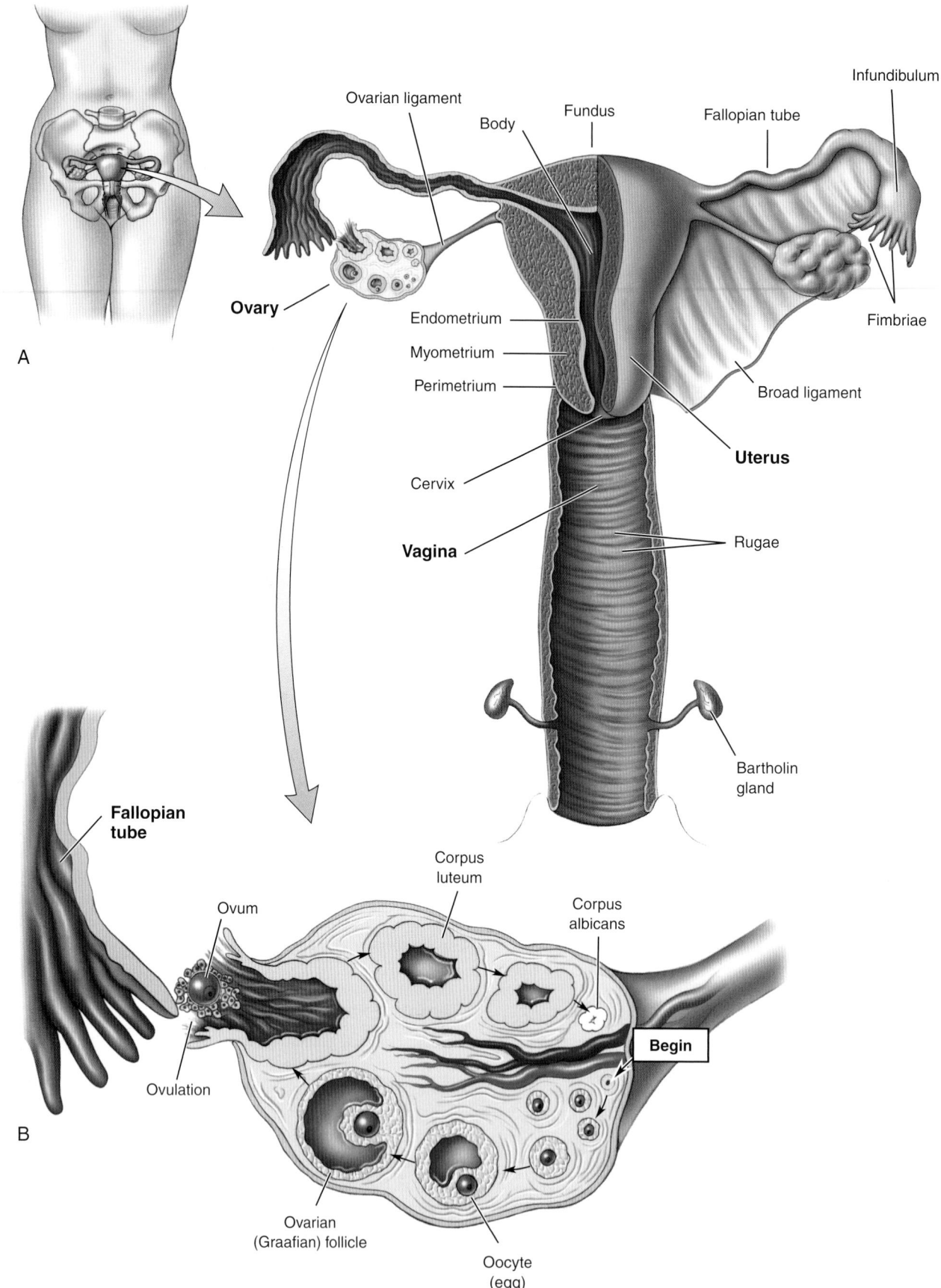

FIG. 25.3 (A) Female reproductive system with uterine layers and ligaments identified (*anterior and cross-section views*). (B) Maturation of the ovarian follicle, ovulation, and formation of the corpus luteum and corpus albicans. (Modified from Kirov, E. [2022]. *Herlihy's the human body in health and illness* [1st ANZ ed.]. Sydney, Australia: Elsevier.)

and produce sexual pleasure. The clitoris is homologous to the male penis.

Female Breasts

Breasts are two soft, protruding organs that cover the pectoralis major muscle in the upper chest wall. The outer portion of the breast is mostly adipose tissue. Each breast contains mammary glands, which consist of 15 to 20 lobules arranged in a circle. Each lobe is capable of producing milk, which passes through a system of ducts leading to an opening at the centrally located nipple. The pigmented area around the nipple is called the *areola* (Fig. 25.4). Lactation, or milk production by the breasts, is discussed later in the chapter.

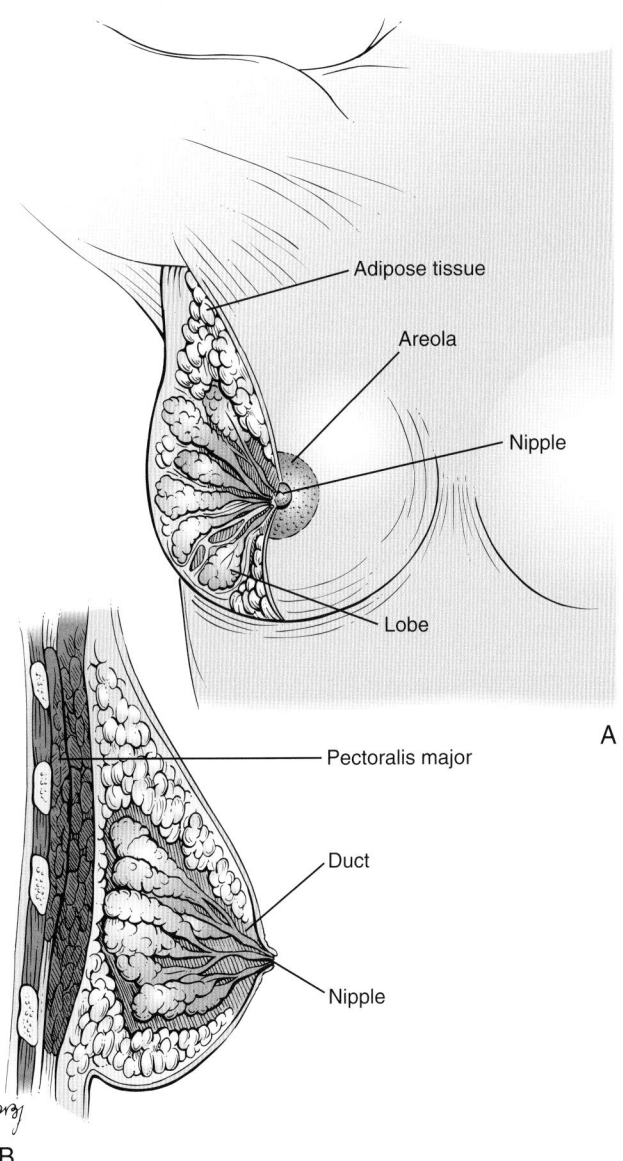

FIG. 25.4 Female breast and mammary glands. (A) Anterior view. (B) Lateral view. (From Swartz, M. H. [2010]. *Textbook of physical diagnosis: History and examination* [6th ed.]. Philadelphia, PA: Saunders.)

A loving person lives in a loving world. A hostile person lives in a hostile world: everyone you meet is your mirror.

Ken Keyes, Jr.

Menstrual Cycle

The **menstrual cycle** is a series of hormonal events that prepare the endometrium for the possibility of pregnancy. These cycles begin at **menarche**, or first menstruation, occur about every 28 days, and end at **menopause** about 40 years later, when menstruation stops. In the United States, the average age of menarche is 12, and the average age of menopause is 51. The menstrual cycle is also called the *reproductive* or *fertility cycle* (Fig. 25.5). The menstrual cycle has three phases.

Follicular Phase (Day 1 to 13)

The follicular phase begins with menstruation. **Menstruation** is the periodic discharge of the endometrium from a nonpregnant uterus through the vagina. Menstruation is caused by a sudden drop in estrogen and progesterone levels, which, in turn, cause constriction of uterine arteries and death of the endometrium. As a result, the lining detaches. The discharge, called **menses** or *menstrual fluid,* contains between 50 and 150 mL of blood, tissue fluid, mucus, and endometrial cells. Menstruation lasts approximately 5 days but varies between 2 and 7 days. FSH and LH begin to mature a new oocyte during this phase. After menstruation, estrogen levels slowly rise and the endometrium begins to proliferate again.

Ovulation (Day 14)

Ovulation occurs with a surge in LH levels, which stimulates the release of a mature oocyte from its follicle. The released oocyte (now called an **ovum**) enters the fallopian tube (see Fig. 25.3). If the ovum is fertilized by sperm, it travels to the uterus and implants in its lining. If the ovum is not fertilized, it is removed during menstruation.

Luteal Phase (Day 15 to 28)

The luteal phase occurs when the collapsed follicle forms into a hormone-secreting structure called the **corpus luteum**. The corpus luteum secretes estrogens and progesterone, which maintain the uterine lining for possible implantation of the fertilized ovum. Progesterone also slightly elevates body temperature, creating an incubating effect. Other ovarian hormones involved in this phase are relaxin and inhibin. Relaxin relaxes the uterus to facilitate implantation. Inhibin inhibits the secretion of FSH and LH. If the ovum is fertilized, hormones secreted by the corpus luteum will continue until the placenta develops and takes over this task. If the ovum is not fertilized, the corpus luteum degenerates after 10 days and becomes the *corpus albicans*, which is primarily scar tissue (see Fig. 25.3). Hormone levels then drop, leading to menstruation, removing the unfertilized ovum.

Love slays what we have been that we may be what we were not.

Saint Augustine

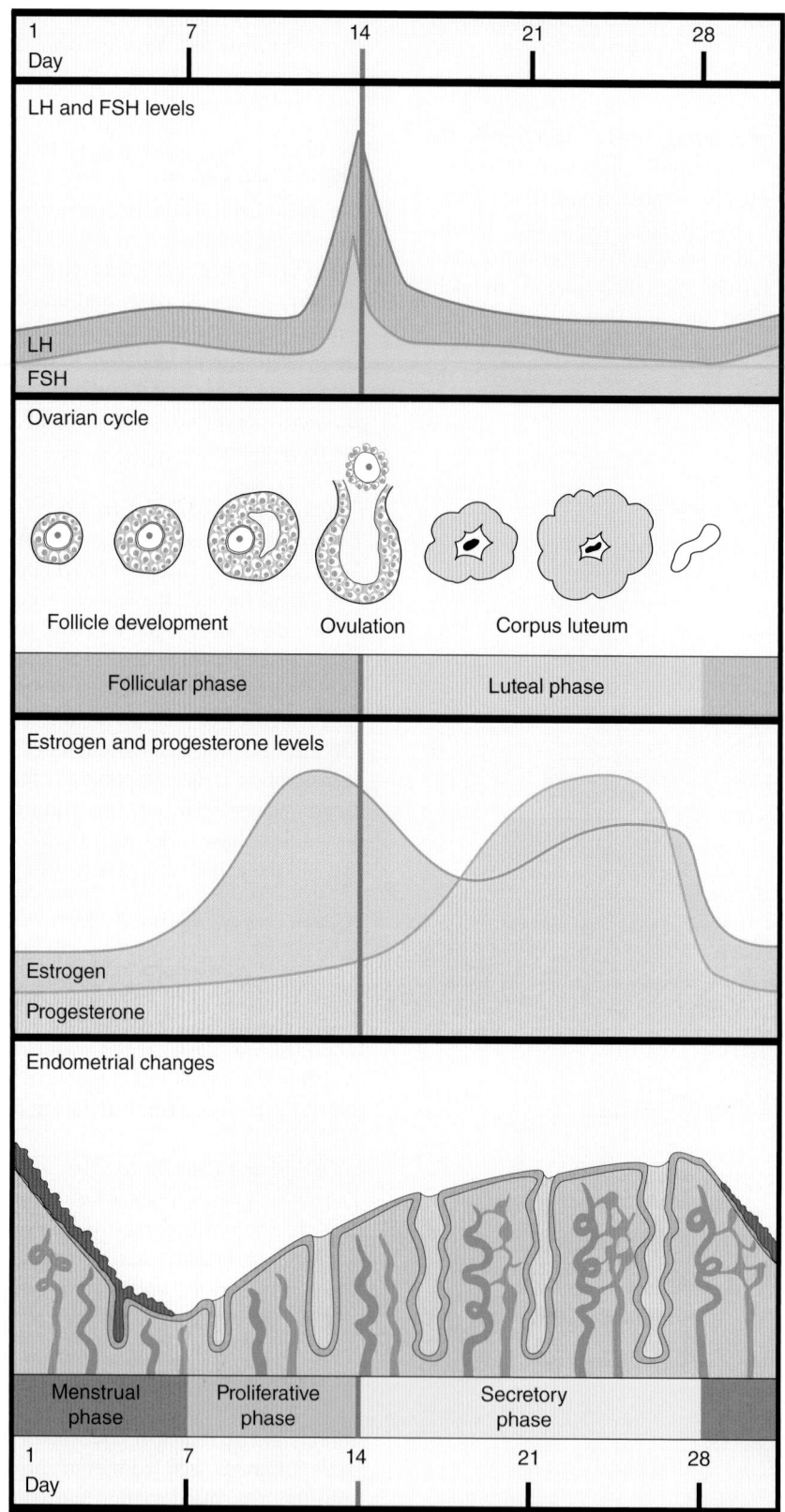

FIG. 25.5 The menstrual cycle. Hormonal changes, and changes in the ovaries and endometrial lining. (From Applegate, E. [2011]. *The anatomy and physiology learning system* [4th ed.]. St. Louis, MO: Saunders.)

SEXUAL INTERCOURSE AND FERTILIZATION

Sexual intercourse is the process of inserting and thrusting a usually erect male penis into a female's vagina, and often ends in orgasm and ejaculation of sperm. In males, sexual arousal causes penile arteries to dilate, causing large quantities of blood to enter penile sinuses, resulting in erection. Bulbourethral glands secrete mucus through the male urethra.

During ejaculation, impulses from the spinal cord stimulate muscles at the base of the penis to contract, which deposits semen outside the body. A sphincter at the base of the urinary bladder closes, preventing acidic urine from mixing with alkaline semen in the urethra—this closure also prevents semen from entering the bladder. The alkalinity of seminal fluid neutralizes the acidic environment of the vagina. Semen liquefies approximately 15 minutes after it is released. If intercourse occurs during ovulation, this liquefaction allows sperm to swim up a mucus thread, leading to an ovum in the fallopian tubes, where most fertilization occurs. This process is aided by vaginal and uterine contractions.

Female arousal is often dependent on both psychologic and tactile responses. Manual stimulation of the clitoris results in its erection and widespread sexual arousal. The cervical lining and Bartholin glands produce a lubricating fluid. Orgasm occurs as genital stimulation reaches maximal intensity and is accompanied by increased heart and respiration rates.

Fertilization is the penetration of the ovum by sperm, resulting in a *zygote.* Fertilization typically occurs approximately 24 hours after ovulation. The number of chromosomes in each ovum and each spermatozoon is one half of all other body cells. X and Y are designations for sex chromosomes. The most common configurations are XX and XY (other configurations may exist in intersex persons). XX means the offspring is female; XY means the offspring is male. The ovum contains one X (female) chromosome. Sperm contains either an X (female) or a Y (male) chromosome, so the male determines the sex of the offspring. When the sperm fertilizes the ovum or egg, the resulting offspring usually contains the same number of chromosomes as the parent cells. Therefore the zygote contains genetic information from each parent.

Approximately 36 hours after fertilization, the zygote undergoes division to form two cells; cells divide again to form four cells, then eight, then sixteen, and so forth. Although the number of cells increases, the size of the zygote does not. Finally, a solid mass of tiny cells, called a *morula,* is formed 3 to 4 days after fertilization. The solid mass eventually becomes a hollow fluid-filled ball of cells called *blastocyst.* During this process, the blastocyst continues to travel through the fallopian tube and enters the uterus about day 7 after fertilization, where it implants in the uterine wall (Fig. 25.6). The result of this process is pregnancy.

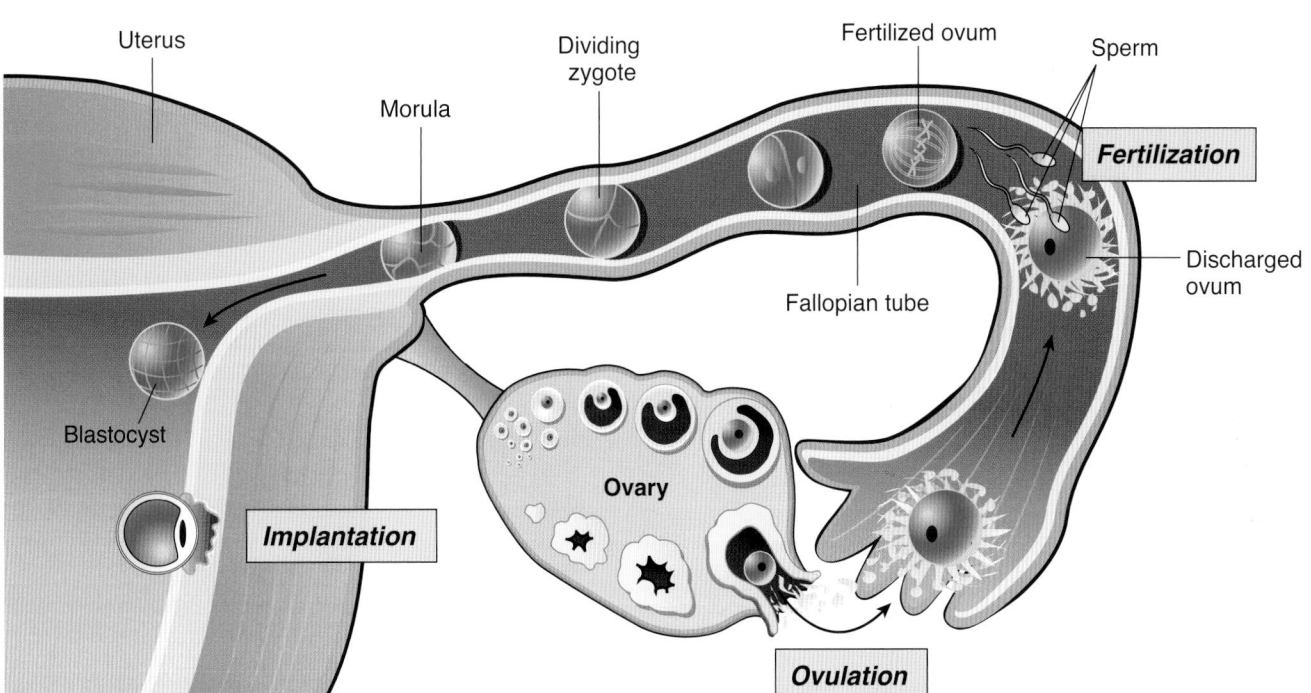

FIG. 25.6 Ovulation, fertilization, and implantation. At ovulation, an ovum is released from the ovary and travels through the fallopian tube where it might be fertilized by a sperm. The fertilized ovum becomes a zygote. After a few days of cell division, the zygote becomes a morula, then a blastocyst, and then the blastocyst implants into the uterine wall.

PREGNANCY, CHILDBIRTH, AND LACTATION

The next sections discuss pregnancy and childbirth. Pregnancy massage and infant massage are discussed in Chapter 11.

Pregnancy

Pregnancy is a sequence of events beginning with fertilization and implantation, continuing with embryonic development and fetal growth, and ending in childbirth. The pregnancy period is also called *gestation*. Normal gestation is approximately 10 lunar months (40 weeks, 9 calendar months, or 266 days) and is divided into trimesters (Fig. 25.7).

First Trimester (First 14 Weeks)

This is considered the *time of the embryo* because most embryonic development occurs in the first trimester and the pregnant female experiences few structural changes. By day 14, a connecting stalk forms, which later develops into the umbilical cord. By day 16, the inner cell mass of the blastocyst differentiates into three primary tissue layers. From superficial to deep, these layers are ectoderm, mesoderm, and endoderm (see Fig. 18.6). These layers will develop into tissues, organs, and glands. The embryo secretes human chorionic gonadotropin (HCG), stimulating the continual production of estrogens and progesterone, which help the uterine lining maintain the pregnancy. Pregnancy tests detect the presence of HCG in the female's urine or blood and are used to confirm pregnancy.

After week 8, the embryo is called a *fetus*. The fetus is contained within a fluid-filled amniotic cavity and is joined to the placenta by the umbilical cord. The **placenta** is a flattened organ in the pregnant uterus nourishing the developing fetus by exchanging nutrients and wastes between the fetus's and mother's blood (see Fig. 25.8). The placenta serves as a spongelike filter system because only small molecules (e.g., glucose, oxygen, amino acids) are allowed to enter the fetus's bloodstream. Maternal blood cells are too large to pass through the placenta. However, many drugs, alcohol, viruses, and other potentially harmful substances can pass through. The placenta also secretes estrogens, progesterone, HCG, placental lactogens, and relaxin.

Second Trimester (Week 15 to 28)

The female begins to "show," and should feel the baby move by the end of the second trimester (see Fig. 25.8). The baby grows to approximately 11 inches in length and weighs about 1.5 pounds.

Third Trimester (Week 29 to childbirth)

The baby grows to about 20 inches in length and between 5 and 9 pounds in weight (see Fig. 25.8). The female may experience occasional, preparatory contractions in which the uterus hardens and then returns to normal. Colostrum, the early form of breast milk, may leak from the breasts.

Childbirth

Childbirth is the process of delivering the baby, placenta, membranes, and umbilical cord to the outside world. Childbirth is also called *parturition* or *labor and delivery*. This process begins after the baby reaches a gestational age of approximately 40 weeks. Some births are by cesarean section (C-section), which is the surgical removal of the fetus and the placenta through the abdominal wall (Fig. 11.6). There have been quite a few scientific investigations on the effects of massage after C-section surgery; the results of these investigations are found on Evolve. There are three stages of childbirth.

- **First Stage: Dilation of the Cervix.** This stage is often called *labor* and begins with the onset of uterine contractions and continues until the cervix has dilated to approximately 10 cm (4 inches). Rupture of the amniotic sac often occurs during this stage.
- **Second Stage: Expulsion of the Fetus.** Time frame is from complete cervical dilation until birth of the fetus. The uterus contracts to push the fetus down the vagina and out of the body.
- **Third Stage: Expulsion of the Placenta.** Uterine contractions continue to push the placenta out of the body. These contractions also constrict blood vessels torn during childbirth to prevent hemorrhage.

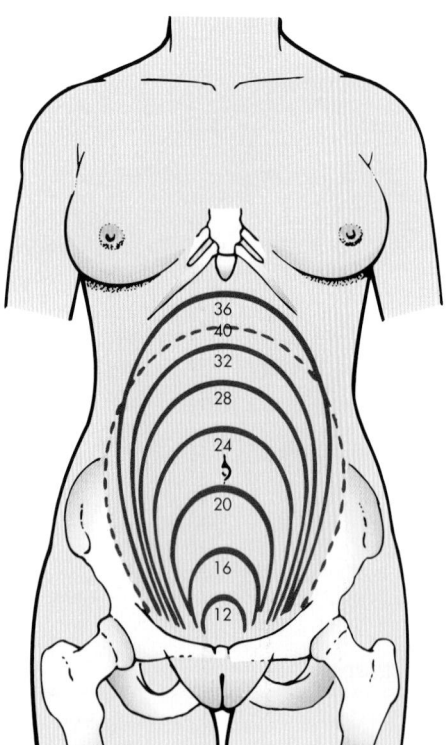

FIG. 25.7 Uterine growth by number of weeks during pregnancy (*anterior view*).

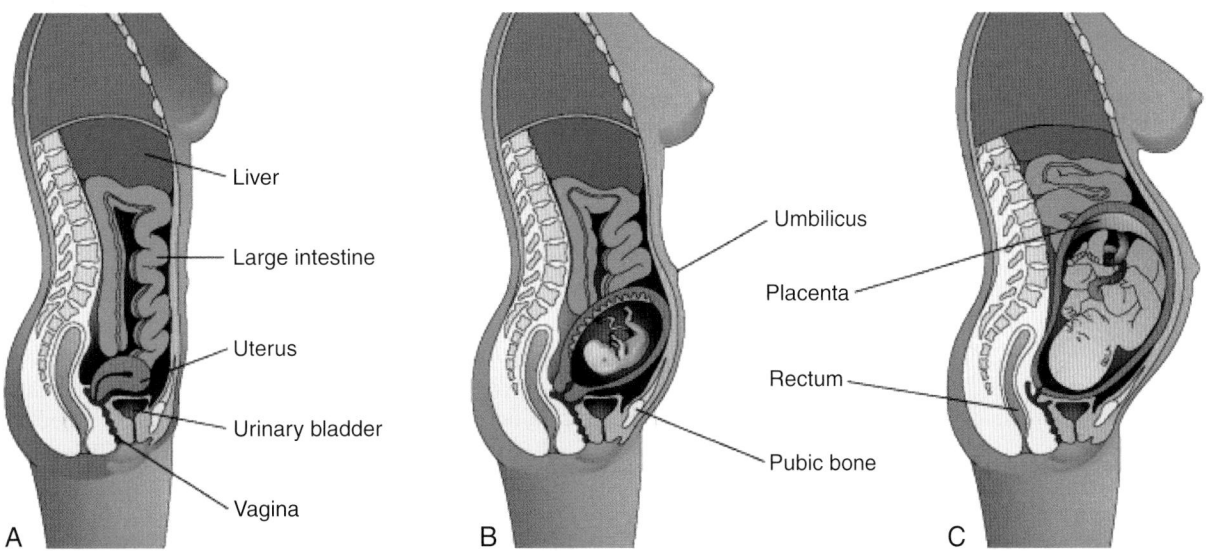

FIG. 25.8 Maternal changes during pregnancy. (A) Nonpregnant female. (B) Pregnant female at 20 weeks of gestation (second trimester). (C) Pregnant female at 30 weeks of gestation (third trimester). (Modified from Moore, K. L., & Persaud, T. V. N. [2008]. *The developing human: Clinically oriented embryology* [8th ed.]. Philadelphia: Saunders.)

Lactation

Lactation is the production and secretion of milk by the mammary glands within the breasts after childbirth, which can lead to breastfeeding. Lactation is facilitated by two pituitary hormones: prolactin and oxytocin. Prolactin assists milk production and oxytocin assists milk secretion, or expression. During late pregnancy and the first few days after childbirth, the glands secrete *colostrum* (first milk). True breast milk appears approximately day 4 postpartum. Breast milk contains antibodies that protect the newborn from diseases during the first few months of life.

REPRODUCTIVE PATHOLOGIES, CONDITIONS, AND DISORDERS

Featured next are common pathologies, conditions, and disorders of the female reproductive system listed alphabetically. Each item includes a brief description and their massage-related modifications. A more extensive list and related research is found in the current edition of *Mosby's Pathology for Massage Professionals* (2022).

Endometriosis

Endometriosis is the presence of functional endometrial tissue outside the uterus. The most common sites of endometrial tissue are the fallopian tubes and the ovaries, but it has been found throughout the body. Ectopic endometrial-like tissue responds to the hormone fluctuations of the menstrual cycle; it proliferates or thickens, degenerates or breaks down, and bleeds. Because there is no exit point for this blood (and blood is irritating to tissues when it is present where it does not belong), local inflammation and pain develop. This displaced tissue can lead to cyst formation, which can develop into scar tissue and adhesions. Scar tissue and adhesions related to endometriosis are a frequent cause of female infertility as they interfere with the transportation of the ovum or sperm within the fallopian tubes. Estimates indicate 10% to 15% of reproductive-age females may have endometriosis.

Massage and Endometriosis
See the entry for menstrual cramps.

Menopause

Menopause occurs when menstrual cycles and ovarian functions cease. Menopause is diagnosed when 12 months have passed since the last menstrual cycle. The time leading up to menopause is called *perimenopause*. Perimenopause usually begins in the fourth decade of life, when the person begins to notice changes in the menstrual cycle. In some females, cycles are less frequent, whereas others state their cycles are more frequent. The amount of discharge varies from lighter-than-normal to heavier-than-normal flow. This phase of irregular cycles may last 4 to 5 years or longer. The time after menopause is called *postmenopause*. Menopause occurs approximately 2 years sooner for smokers than for nonsmokers. Low to moderate alcohol consumption is related to later onset of menopause. When factoring life expectancy, females spend approximately one-third of their lives in postmenopause. Menopause can be induced with surgical removal of the ovaries or with certain medical treatments, such as radiation therapy and chemotherapy.

Massage and Menopause

Massage may reduce menopausal symptoms. Because 75% of females experience heat intolerance and hot flashes, avoid or limit the use of blankets, hot packs, hot immersion baths, or table warmers. Instead, use thinner, cooler fabrics to drape the client. The practitioner may uncover the client's arms and feet or use a cool washcloth over the forehead or across the base of the neck to help the client feel more comfortable. An oscillating fan may be used to circulate the air in a stuffy massage room.

Menstruation

Menstruation is part of the menstrual cycle and was discussed in a prior section of this chapter.

Massage and Menstruation

The client may elect to leave on undergarments because of the use of menstrual products such as pads or tampons. Keep disposable menstrual products in your office for client use. If the client has menstrual cramps, massage may reduce symptoms (see next entry).

Menstrual Cramps (Dysmenorrhea)

Menstrual cramps refer to severe cramping and pain in the abdominopelvic region that occur just before or during menses. Menstrual cramps are one of the most common gynecologic disorders, occurring occasionally in almost all menstruating females. In approximately 10% of females, menstrual cramps are severe enough to interrupt normal activities. The two main types of menstrual cramps are primary and secondary. Primary results from factors inherent to the menstrual process; therefore it is not regarded as a pathologic condition. These types of cramps tend to lessen with age. Secondary is related to pelvic pathology, such as endometriosis or pelvic inflammatory disease.

Massage and Menstrual Cramps

Massage, including abdominal massage, may reduce symptoms of menstrual cramps. While the client is supine, heat applied on the lower abdomen may decrease pain intensity. Coexisting conditions (endometriosis, pelvic inflammatory disease) should be factored into the treatment plan. A client experiencing severe menstrual cramps may not feel up to receiving a massage.

Ovarian Cysts and Polycystic Ovarian Syndrome

Ovarian cysts are fluid-filled sacs within the ovary or on its surface. Most ovarian cysts are related to the menstrual cycle, and are common during the reproductive years. The two types of ovarian cysts are follicular cysts and corpus luteum cysts. Follicles that do not rupture during ovulation may develop enlarged fluid-filled sacs called *follicular cysts*. Ruptured follicles (now called the corpus luteum) may be unable to degenerate into the corpus albicans. When this occurs, the corpus luteum may develop enlarged fluid-filled sacs called *corpus luteum cysts*. Most follicular and corpus

luteum cysts present little or no pain and reduce in size over several consecutive menstrual cycles. On rare occasions these cysts enlarge further and rupture or become cancerous. Ovarian involvement is typically unilateral.

Polycystic ovary syndrome (PCOS) is a condition of elevated hormone levels that produce irregular menstrual cycles and cause the ovaries to enlarge bilaterally and become studded with multiple cysts. Polycystic ovaries are two to five times larger than normal ovaries. The prevalence of PCOS is estimated to be between 5% and 10%, affecting 5 to 6 million females. Obesity is present in most cases. Complications of PCOS include infertility, type 2 diabetes, Cushing syndrome, high blood pressure, sleep apnea, nonalcoholic fatty liver disease, lipid and cholesterol disorders, and endometrial cancer. People with PCOS are also at higher risk for depression and anxiety.

Massage and Ovarian Cysts/PCOS

If the client has either ovarian cysts or PCOS, modify the massage according to the presenting signs and symptoms. For example, avoid the lower abdomen if applied pressure causes pain. Coexisting conditions (type 2 diabetes, Cushing syndrome, sleep apnea) should also be factored into the treatment plan.

Premenstrual Syndrome

Premenstrual syndrome (PMS) is a group of signs and symptoms that occur during the luteal phase of the menstrual cycle (last 2 weeks) and are relieved by its onset. More than 200 physical, emotional, and behavioral symptoms have been attributed to PMS, some of which may interfere with normal activities. The incidence of PMS increases with age and usually begins between the ages of 25 and 35. PMS affects approximately 75% of females. Several factors may cause or contribute to PMS including fluctuations in estrogens, progesterone, or serotonin; nutritional deficiencies; stress; and emotional disturbances.

Massage and Premenstrual Syndrome

Massage may reduce PMS symptoms. Position the client for comfort while prone to address breast tenderness. You may offer the client a rolled-up towel or cylindrical pillow to be placed under, above, or between the breasts, depending on what is most comfortable. Some positions may require a face rest frame adjusted above the level of the table. Several manufacturers now offer massage tables fitted with breast recesses that allow a client to lie prone more comfortably or offer specially designed bolstering systems that lie on top of the table. You may also use a side-lying position. Be prepared to take a comfort break or stop before the scheduled time if the client begins to cry during the massage.

E-RESOURCES

http://evolve.elsevier.com/Salvo/MassageTherapy

- Chapter challenge
- Flash cards

ABRAHAM MASLOW

Childhood can be tough for some people. From difficult family relationships to being the victim of social injustices and bullying at school, these painful experiences shape us and our future selves. In the case of Abraham Maslow, he learned very early in his life about the value and importance of safety, love, and acceptance.

Maslow never quite fit into the molds he found himself in. Nonetheless, his theory of the Hierarchy of Needs sensationalized the world of psychology in the mid-20th century—so much so we still see it pop up in conversations regularly today. In his words, "the purpose of education—and of all social institutions—is the development of full humaneness. If you keep this in mind, all else follows." He did not get perfect grades, nor did he have a sterling reputation, but he always held true to his ideal, synergistic humanity.

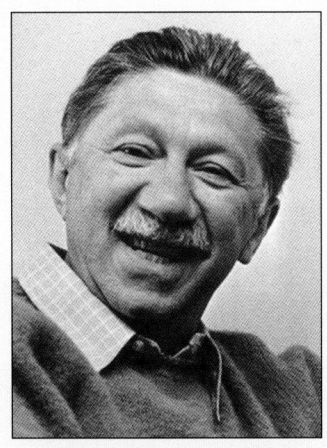

Courtesy Corbis, Inc. © Bettman

Maslow was born in Brooklyn, New York, on April 1, 1908. His parents were struggling Jewish folks who had recently fled from Kiev (what is now Ukraine but was then part of the Russian Empire) to avoid czarist persecution. Being the oldest of seven children, he often expressed feelings of isolation and coldness from both his parents and peers. By some accounts, he was even called "emotionally disturbed" by a psychologist as a child. He was subject to frequent anti-Semitism, which instilled an early passion for social justice and world peace. Maslow attended one of the most highly regarded high schools in Brooklyn at the time, participating in many academic clubs despite being chronically antisocial.

In 1926, Maslow began attending law school at the City College of New York. Dissatisfied with the program, he transferred to Cornell University. Uninspired by Cornell, he eventually dropped out and found his way to the University of Wisconsin. In 1931, he graduated with a master's degree in psychology and continued his research at Columbia University. At the age of 59, Maslow suffered the first of several heart attacks and on June 8, 1970, he died of a massive heart attack while jogging.

Much of Maslow's early studies were in the field of experimental-behaviorism, studying primate dominance and sexuality. This background gave him a strong lean toward positivist mindsets, meaning he was reliant on solid, empirical evidence and believed society operated on similar "laws" to those of physics and biology. Later in life, he would state most positivists were naïve in their failings to admit science was "relative to time, place, and local culture." Even today, some scientists argue his research was never quite tangible enough to qualify as science. He believed his research was far more meticulous than some other psychologists'. He was cut by the double-edged sword of his own theory: according to critics, his own time, place, and local culture provided as much bias as it did discovery.

In his Hierarchy of Needs model of psychology, Maslow developed a comprehensive ordered list of needs or attributes:

- **Level 1: Physiologic-Based Needs**. Food, safety, shelter, sex, and other survival needs.
- **Level 2: Security-Based Needs**. Safety of self, family, resources, and stability.
- **Level 3: Need for Love and Belonging**. Wellness and health in the social life, and the ability to "share" self with others.
- **Level 4: Need for Self-Esteem**. Comfort and pride in accomplishments, one's self, and surroundings.
- **Level 5: Need for Intellectual Stimulation**. Cognitive, new ideas, and philosophic fulfillment.
- **Level 6: Need for Esthetics**. Beautiful surroundings, self, and community.
- **Level 7: Need for Self-actualization**. Fulfillment of potential.

Maslow believed no one could successfully strive toward the higher few levels without first securing and mastering the first four, and he was the first to admit very few people ever made it to the top. Generally, he observed people did not intrinsically strive for the next "level" until the preceding one(s) had been fulfilled. His pyramid was representative of his consistent focus on studying the healthy human in order to heal the sick. His underlying ideology was humanistic, insisting all humans are worthy and capable of development and psychological health.

Maslow is important in the study of massage because he believed mental and physical health was intertwined and a more practical, accessible approach should be taken when tackling overall health. His theories, though frequently disputed, hold important truths: massage, touch, and basic contact are essential to human wellbeing and even may open doors for people to strive for things they thought they never would. People can be more than what society expects and are never exactly as simple as we would like them to be.

One can choose to go back toward safety or forward toward growth. Growth must be chosen again and again; fear must be overcome again and again.

REFERENCES

Salvo, S. G. (2022). *Mosby's pathology for massage professionals* (5th ed.). St Louis: Mosby.

BIBLIOGRAPHY

Abrahams, P. H., Spratt, J. D., Loukas, M., & van Schoor, A. N. (2003). *Abrahams' and McMinn's clinical atlas of human anatomy* (8th ed.). St Louis: Elsevier.

Applegate, E. (2010). *The anatomy and physiology learning system* (4th ed.). Philadelphia: Saunders.

Como, D. (Ed.). (2016). *Mosby's dictionary of medicine, nursing, and health professions* (10th ed.). St Louis: Elsevier.

Frazier, M. S., & Drzymkowski, J. W. (2015). *Essentials of human diseases and conditions* (6th ed.). St Louis: Elsevier.

Haubrich, W. S. (2003). *Medical meanings: A glossary of word origins* (2nd ed.). New York: American College of Physicians.

Herlihy, B. (2017). *The human body in health and illness* (6th ed.). St Louis: Saunders.

Hubert, R. J., & VanMeter, K. C. (2018). *Gould's pathophysiology for the health professions* (6th ed.). Philadelphia, PA: Saunders.

Huether, S. E., McCance, K. L., & Brashers, V. L. (2019). *Understanding pathophysiology* (7th ed.). St Louis: Mosby.

Kalat, J. W. (2013). *Biological psychology* (11th ed.). Belmont, CA: Cengage Learning.

Kapit, W., & Elson, L. M. (2013). *The anatomy coloring book* (4th ed.). New York: Benjamin Cummings.

Kumar, V., Abbas, A. K., & Aster, J. C. (2015). *Robbins & Cotran pathologic basis of disease* (9th ed.). St Louis: Mosby.

Marieb, E. N., Keller, S. M. (2018). *Essentials of human anatomy and physiology* (12th ed.). New York: Benjamin Cummings.

McCance, K. L., & Huether, S. E. (2019). *Pathophysiology: The biological basis for disease in adults and children* (8th ed.). St Louis: Mosby.

Myers, T. W. (2014). *Anatomy trains: Myofascial meridians for manual and movement therapists* (3rd ed.). Churchill Livingstone: Elsevier.

Netter, F. H. (2018). *Atlas of human anatomy* (7th ed.). St Louis: Mosby.

Patton, K. T. (2019). *Anatomy and physiology* (10th ed.). St Louis: Elsevier.

Patton, K. T., Thibodeau, G. A., & Douglas, M. M. (2012). *Essentials of anatomy and physiology* (4th ed.). New York: Pearson.

Porter, R. S. (2011). *The Merck manual of diagnosis and therapy* (19th ed.). Whitehouse Station, NJ: Merck Sharp and Dohme Corp.

Taber, C. W. (2021). *Taber's cyclopedic medical dictionary* (24th ed.). Philadelphia: FA Davis.

REVIEW AND APPLY YOUR KNOWLEDGE

MATCHING ONE: CONCEPT REVIEW

Place the letter of the answer next to the number of the term or phrase that best describes it.

A. Ovulation
B. Epididymis
C. Breasts
D. Prostate
E. Scrotum
F. Semen
G. Penis
H. Sexual reproduction
I. Sperm
J. Testes
K. Urethra
L. Menstruation

_____ 1. Pouch containing the testes; supports sperm production by regulating their temperature.

_____ 2. Process by which male sex cells and female sex cells unite, which may produce offspring.

_____ 3. Two soft, protruding organs in the upper chest wall that contain mammary glands.

_____ 4. Composed of erectile tissues and contains the urethra.

_____ 5. Paired glands within the scrotum that produce sperm and hormones.

_____ 6. Tightly coiled comma-shaped tube where sperm matures.

_____ 7. Sex cells that carry genetic information from the male who produced them.

_____ 8. Periodic discharge of the endometrial lining from the nonpregnant uterus.

_____ 9. Tube below the bladder that transports both semen and urine in males.

_____ 10. Phase of the menstrual cycle when the ovum is released from the ovarian follicle.

_____ 11. Gland that lies beneath the urinary bladder and secretes seminal fluid to nourish sperm.

_____ 12. Mixture of sperm and seminal fluid.

MATCHING TWO: CONCEPT REVIEW

Place the letter of the answer next to the number of the term or phrase that best describes it.

A. Lactation
B. Fallopian tubes
C. Follicular phase
D. Luteal phase
E. Menstrual cycle
F. Pregnancy
G. Oocytes
H. Ovaries
I. Ovum
J. Placenta
K. Uterus
L. Vagina

_____ 1. Mature oocyte that has been released during ovulation.

_____ 2. Canal extending from the cervix to outside of the body.

_____ 3. Paired almond-shaped glands that produce oocytes and hormones.

_____ 4. Flattened organ in the pregnant uterus that nourishes the developing fetus.

_____ 5. Series of hormonal events that begin at menarche, occurs approximately every 28 days, and ends at menopause.

_____ 6. Sex cells that carry genetic information from the female who produced them.

_____ 7. Hollow pear-shaped organ that receives the fertilized ovum and from which menses flows if pregnancy does not occur.

_____ 8. Secretion and ejection of milk by the mammary glands within the breasts.

_____ 9. Phase of the menstrual cycle that begins after ovulation and ends with menstruation.

_____ 10. Paired passageways that extend laterally from the uterus toward the ovaries.

_____ 11. Sequence of events that includes implantation, embryonic development, fetal growth, and ends in childbirth.

_____ 12. Phase of the menstrual cycle that begins with menstruation and last until approximately day thirteen.

MULTIPLE CHOICE: TEST YOUR KNOWLEDGE

Place the letter of the answer next to the number of the term or phrase that best describes it.

_____ 1. Testes and ovaries are examples of:
   A. gonads.
   B. gametes.
   C. ducts.
   D. accessory organs.

_____ 2. What do the interstitial cells of Leydig secrete?
   A. Relaxin
   B. Prolactin
   C. Estrogen
   D. Testosterone

_____ 3. A vasectomy procedure removes or seals a portion of the:
   A. prostate.
   B. urethra.
   C. vas deferens.
   D. penis.

_____ 4. Muscles in the wall of the scrotum that move the testes are called _____ muscles.
   A. prepuce
   B. cremaster
   C. fundus
   D. detrusor

_____ 5. Which hormone helps maintain the uterine lining for pregnancy?
   A. Relaxin
   B. Prolactin
   C. Inhibin
   D. Progesterone

_____ 6. The fingerlike projections that help the oocyte enter the fallopian tube are called:
   A. rugae.
   B. fimbriae.
   C. cilia.
   D. follicles.

_____ 7. Which ligament arises from the anteroinferior surface of the uterus, passes through the groin region, enters the labia majora, and terminates at the mons pubis?
   A. Round
   B. Broad
   C. Ovarian
   D. Flat

_____ 8. The uterine wall layer that contracts during labor is the:
   A. endometrium.
   B. myometrium.
   C. mesoderm.
   D. endoderm.

_____ 9. The average age of menarche, or first menstruation, is:
   A. 8
   B. 10
   C. 12
   D. 14

_____ 10. Fertilization results in a _____ that contains genetic information from each parent.
   A. zygote
   B. corpus
   C. oocyte
   D. menses

_____ 11. Normal gestation is approximately _____ weeks.
   A. 25
   B. 30
   C. 35
   D. 40

_____ 12. The condition involving pain in the abdominopelvic region just before or after menses.
   A. Menopause
   B. Lactation
   C. Dysmenorrhea
   D. Infertility

CRITICAL THINKING

Massage and Infertility

What role do you think massage plays in a couple struggling with infertility?

Answers can include but are not limited to:

Massage does not play a direct role in helping couples struggling with infertility. However, indirect effects include helping with stress management, increasing oxytocin release to support bonding, and supporting body awareness. These may all help decrease anxiety surrounding infertility issues.

PROFESSIONAL PRACTICE

A Personal Matter

Melinda is a healthy 24-year-old athlete. She initially used massage for lower back pain. Paul, her massage practitioner, was able to relieve Melinda's symptoms, allowing her to get back to her normal activities, and she has continued to see him for maintenance and general relaxation. Today, Melinda says she feels tired, nauseated, and is having trouble keeping her mind focused. She said she thought she might have a yeast infection and would see her doctor tomorrow if the symptoms did not go away. Paul suspects she might be pregnant. How should he proceed with this session? Would suggesting the possibility of pregnancy violate Melinda's privacy? Would discussing pregnancy with Melinda constitute an action outside of Paul's scope of practice? If he decides to discuss his concern with Melinda, how can he approach this sensitive issue?

DISCUSSION

The Linen Police

Your client walked out of the massage room and told you as he was getting redressed, he noticed a herpes sore on his private parts. If he did not wear undergarments during the massage, what would you do and why? If available, post your reflections on an internet-based discussion board monitored by your instructor.

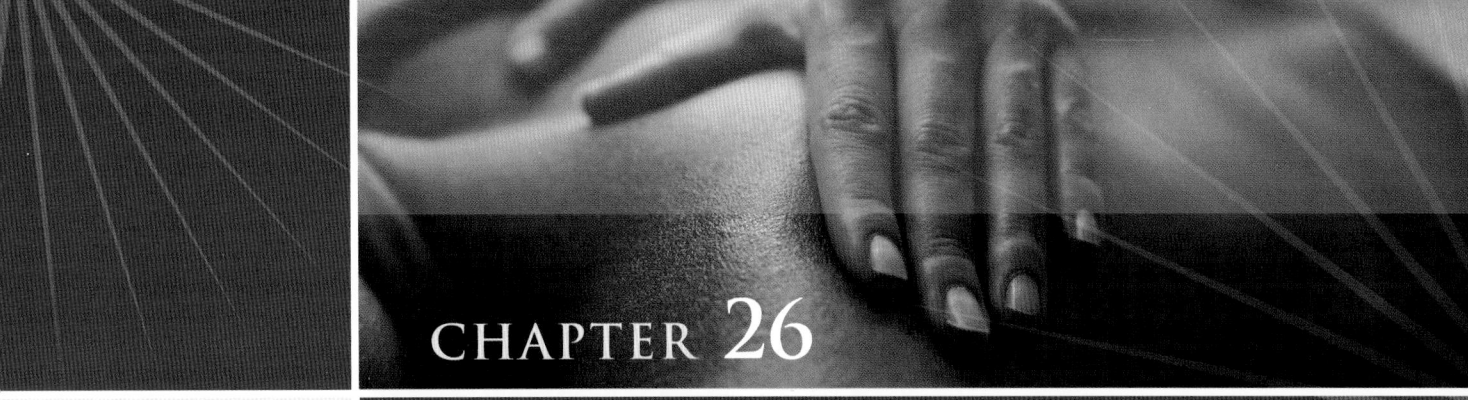

CHAPTER 26

Cardiovascular System, Pathologies, and Disorders

Be a lamp, a lifeboat, or a ladder.

—Rumi

LEARNING OBJECTIVES

After completing this chapter, the student should be able to:

1. List basic anatomy and physiology of the cardiovascular system and describe characteristics of blood.
2. Define the heart, its layers, chambers, valves, sounds, blood flow, heart rate, and heart rhythm.
3. Discuss blood vessels and paths of blood circulation.
4. Describe cardiovascular pathologies and disorders and state their massage modifications.

INTRODUCTION

Most of the body's cells are embedded in tissues and are stationary. They cannot move around to obtain oxygen and nutrients, or remove carbon dioxide, heat, and other wastes they produce. Instead, these stationary cells are served by interacting with fluids that include blood, lymph, and interstitial fluid. Blood is the fluid of the cardiovascular system, and it moves through a series of vessels and is pumped by a muscular organ called the heart. The cardiovascular system plays a major role in maintaining homeostasis, and the life of the individual is threatened if the heart loses its pumping efficiency for even a few minutes. *Cardiology* is the study of the cardiovascular system. Use Table 26.1 to help you understand terms of the cardiovascular system. Lymph and interstitial fluid are discussed in Chapter 27.

TABLE 26.1 Word Meanings

WORD	MEANING
aorta	*Gr.* a strap; to suspend
atrium	*L.* corridor
bicuspid	*L.* two; pointed
brady	*Gr.* slow
capillary	*L.* hairlike
cardio, cardia	*Gr.* heart
chordae tendineae	*Gr.* cordlike; *L.* tendon
coagulation	*L.* to curdle
coronary	*L.* shaped like a crown or circle
diastole	*Gr.* to expand
erythrocyte	*Gr.* red; cell
fibrinogen	*L.* fiber; *Gr.* to produce
hemoglobin	*Gr.* blood; *L.* globe
hemorrhage	*Gr.* blood; to burst forth
hemostasis	*Gr.* blood; stopping
intima	*L.* innermost
ischemia	*Gr.* to hold back blood
leukocytes	*Gr.* white; cell
lumen	*L.* light
mitral	*L.* headdress
plasma	*Gr.* a thing formed
platelet	*Fr.* flat
Purkinje fibers	Purkyne, Czech anatomist (1787–1869)
saphenous	*Gr.* the hidden
semilunar	*L.* half; moon
sphygmomanometer	*Gr.* pulse; thin; measure
systole	*Gr.* contraction
tachy	*Gr.* rapid, fast, or swift
thrombocyte	*Gr.* clot; cell
tricuspid	*Gr.* three; *L.* pointed
tunica	*L.* a tunic
vascular	*L.* a vessel or duct
vasoconstriction	*L.* vessel; a binder
vasodilation	*L.* vessel; to widen
vena cava	*L.* vein; cavity
ventricle	*L.* little belly

Fr., French; *Gr.,* Greek; *L.,* Latin.

ANATOMY

The basic anatomy of the cardiovascular system is:
- Blood
- Blood vessels—arteries, veins, and capillaries
- Heart

PHYSIOLOGY

Important functions of the cardiovascular system are:
- Transportation—Substances transported by the cardiovascular system include respiratory gases such as oxygen and carbon dioxide, nutrients from the digestive tract, waste, heat, and products, such as enzymes and hormones. The cardiovascular and lymphatic systems are regarded as "pick-up and delivery" because of their function of transportation.
- Protection—The body is protected by disease-fighting white blood cells (WBCs). These cells also assist in the removal of pathogens or foreign agents.
- Combating blood loss and hemorrhage—This is accomplished by several mechanisms that reduce blood loss from broken vessels.

BLOOD

Blood is the red fluid circulating through the heart and its vessels, and transporting products to and from body cells. The red color of blood varies from bright scarlet to dull maroon, depending on its oxygen content—the brighter the red, the more oxygen. Blood is thicker, more viscous, and more adhesive than water. Blood's pH is slightly alkaline, and it is slightly warmer than normal body temperature at approximately 100°F. Blood makes up approximately 8% of total body weight, and blood volume is approximately 5 L (6 quarts/12 pints) in an average-sized adult (Fig. 26.1). A unit of blood is approximately 0.5 L in volume, or just under a pint. This means a unit of blood donated to a blood center represents about 10% of total blood volume in an averaged-sized adult.

Blood drawn directly from the body is called *whole blood* and is a mixture of approximately 55% liquid plasma and 45% blood cells (see Fig. 26.1). Blood cell production, called *hematopoiesis,* occurs in red bone marrow, and blood itself is liquid connective tissue. Blood cells include erythrocytes, leukocytes, and thrombocytes. Blood flows in a circle. At rest, a single blood cell makes a round trip through the cardiovascular system every 60 seconds.

Blood Plasma

Blood plasma is a straw-colored liquid in which blood cells are suspended. Blood plasma is mostly water (90% to 95%). The remainder of plasma is solutes, mostly plasma proteins, such as albumin, globulins, and fibrinogen. In addition to plasma proteins, plasma contains other solutes, such as electrolytes (sodium, potassium, calcium ions), dissolved gases (oxygen, carbon dioxide), nutrients (vitamins, minerals,

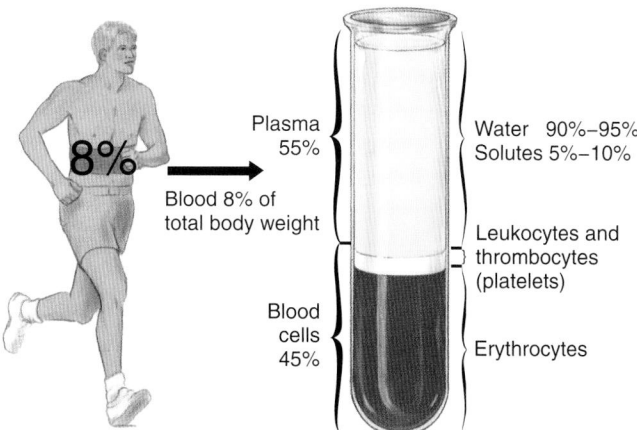

FIG. 26.1 Composition of blood. (From Applegate, E. [2011]. *The anatomy and physiology learning system* [4th ed.]. St. Louis, MO: Saunders.)

lipids, glucose, amino acids), hormones, and metabolic wastes. Nonprotein solutes make up only about 1% of the total volume of blood plasma.

Erythrocytes

Erythrocytes, or red blood cells (RBCs), transport oxygen and carbon dioxide to and from body cells. RBCs can perform this function because they contain **hemoglobin**, an iron-based protein that binds with oxygen and carbon dioxide, so it can be transported in blood. Hemoglobin also gives blood its characteristic red color. RBCs are the most numerous of all blood cells. They are shaped like biconcave discs with raised edges and a flattened middle (Fig. 26.2). This shape gives RBCs a greater surface area for gas exchange and helps them pass through narrow vessels called capillaries. RBCs lose their nucleus and other organelles as they emerge from bone marrow and enter the bloodstream, presumably so there is more room for hemoglobin. Because of this, RBCs cannot reproduce or carry out extensive metabolic activities. The lifespan of an RBC is 105 to 120 days, at which time it begins to fragment and is recycled or eliminated by the spleen and liver.

Blood Types

The surfaces of RBCs contain surface markers called *antigens* and are used to identify blood types. The two blood antigens are antigen A and antigen B. From this, we can group blood into four types:

- **Type A.** Contains antigen A.
- **Type B.** Contains antigen B.
- **Type AB.** Contains both antigen A and antigen B.
- **Type O.** Does not contain any antigens.

Blood plasma contains the antibody against the antigen not present. Categorizing blood according to types helps prevent reactions when someone gets a blood transfusion (Table 26.2). For example, the native antibody does not recognize the foreign antibody as familiar and attacks it. For example, if someone with type A blood is given type B blood, the type A antibody attacks foreign blood cells with

the type B antibody. During the attack, blood clots form, blocking off blood supply to vital organs, which may lead to death. Persons with type AB blood are called **universal recipients** because their plasma does not contain antigens. Persons with type O blood are called **universal donors** because their plasma contains both A and B antibodies, so it is compatible with all blood types (Fig. 26.3). Persons with type O blood can donate their blood to almost anyone. Blood is further classified as being either Rh positive (meaning it has Rh factor) or Rh negative (without Rh factor).

Leukocytes

Leukocytes, or white blood cells (WBCs), are the body's mobile army by destroying or deactivating pathogens and foreign agents. When needed, WBCs multiply quickly. The lifespan of a WBC ranges from a few hours to a few days to several years. WBCs have specific functions. For example, some WBCs combat irritants by producing histamine, a compound released in allergic and inflammatory reactions, and other WBCs produce antibodies, which help combat infection. There are several types of WBCs (see Fig. 26.2):

- **Granular Leukocytes (Granulocytes).** These contain abundant granules within the cytoplasm. They are *neutrophils, eosinophils,* and *basophils.*
- **Agranular Leukocytes.** While granules are not totally lacking in their cytoplasm, they are far fewer compared with granular leukocytes. They are *monocytes* and *lymphocytes.*

    LEARNING TIP: To help you remember all types of WBCs, use the phrase **N**ever **L**et **M**onkeys **E**at **B**ananas—for **N**eutrophils, **L**ymphocytes, **M**onocytes, **E**osinophils, and **B**asophils.

Thrombocytes

Thrombocytes, or platelets, are irregularly shaped blood cell fragments, have no nucleus, and are small compared with other blood cells (see Fig. 26.2). The lifespan of a platelet is between 7 and 10 days. Thrombocytes are involved in

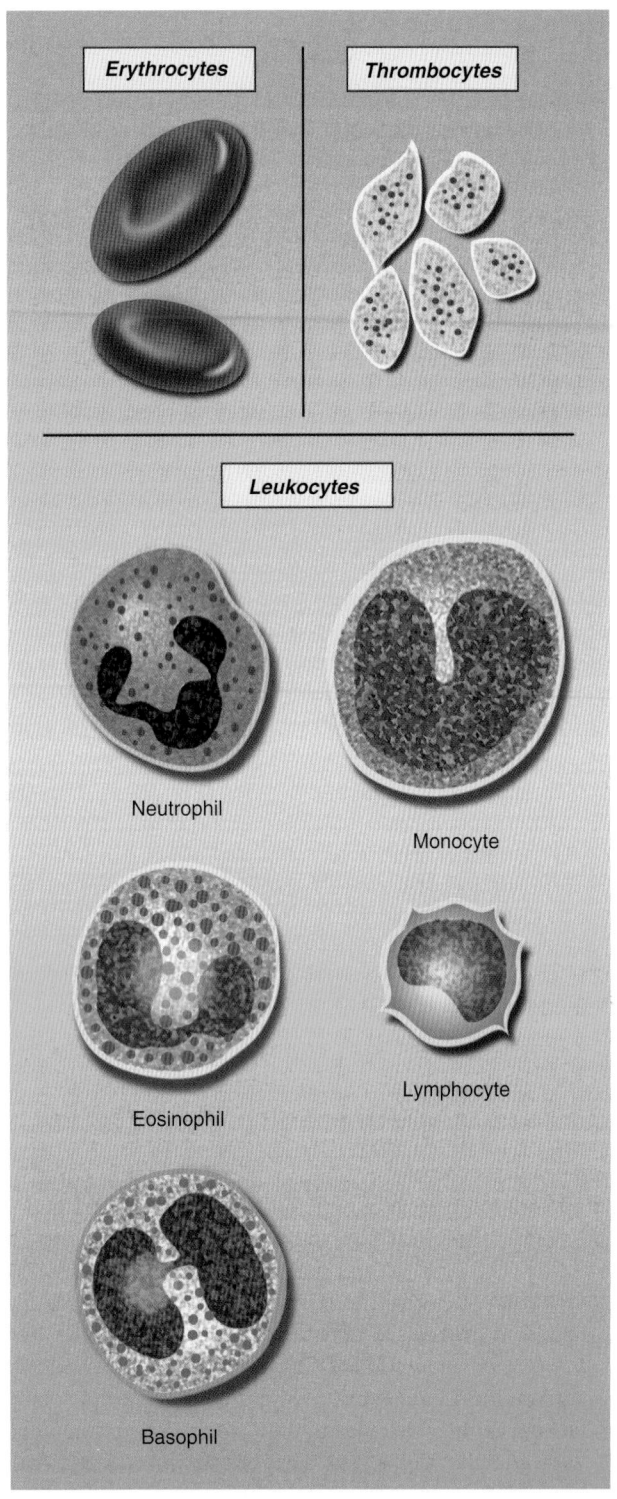

FIG. 26.2 Types of blood cells which include erythrocytes, thrombocytes, and leukocytes. Granular leukocytes (granulocytes) are neutrophils, eosinophils, and basophils. Agranular leukocytes are monocytes and lymphocytes.

hemostasis, mechanisms that stop bleeding. Thrombocytes also contain adhesive proteins that allow them to stick to the fibrin mesh at an injury site, which helps hemostasis. Wound healing, as described in Chapter 14, can only begin when bleeding from an injury has stopped.

Hemostasis

Hemostasis is a process that stops bleeding and helps keep blood within the damaged vessel. This is the first stage of tissue repair and wound healing. Hemostasis involves stages of vascular spasm or vasoconstriction, the formation of a platelet plug, and then a blood clot. When a blood vessel wall is broken, muscles in the vessel wall contract to reduce blood loss. Next, nearby platelets are activated and become sticky, which causes them to clump together to form a platelet plug over the break. Their jagged shape helps them adhere to rough or torn surfaces to seal the break in the wall. Fibrinogen within plasma changes into fibrin, which forms a mesh; this mesh traps blood cells as they float by the wound site (Fig. 26.4). The fibrin mesh tightens and shrinks it into a platelet plug, which acts like a cork to keep blood in the vessel. The platelet plug is not stable enough to stay in place without help. The next step, called coagulation, involves activation of blood clotting factors, which strengths fibrin and changes the plug into a stable clot. When the damaged vessel is repaired, the clot dissolves.

HEART

The **heart** is a hollow, muscular organ about the size of a clenched fist. It is located in the mediastinum region, which is behind the sternum and between the lungs. Pumping blood is the heart's main function. The heart is surrounded by a double-layered sac called the *pericardium* that has an outer parietal layer and an inner visceral layer. Between these layers is a pericardial space lined with a serous membrane that secretes serous fluid. This fluid helps reduce friction as the heart beats (Fig. 26.5).

Heart Layers

The heart has three layers. The *epicardium*, or outer layer, which contains fatty connective tissue and blood vessels called *coronary vessels*. The *myocardium*, or middle layer, contains cardiac muscle and makes up the bulk of the heart wall. Contraction of the myocardium forces blood from the heart chambers mentioned next. The *endocardium*, or inner layer, is continuous with the endothelium lining the heart chambers and blood vessels, as well as the valves of the heart.

> *Hippocrates had no means of recognizing the heart as a pump, because there was no such item in his world, and no such word in his vocabulary.*
> ~ **Guido Majno, MD**

Heart Chambers

The heart is divided into four chambers. The superior chambers are called atria (sing. atrium) and separated by an interatrial septum. The inferior chambers are called ventricles and are separated by an interventricular septum. The chamber walls contain special muscles to increase the power of contraction without significantly increasing the size of the

TABLE 26.2 ABO Blood Types

BLOOD TYPE	ANTIGEN (RBC MEMBRANE)	ANTIBODY (PLASMA)	PEOPLE WITH THIS BLOOD TYPE	
			CAN RECEIVE BLOOD FROM	CAN DONATE BLOOD TO
A	A antigen	Anti-B antibodies	A, O	A, AB
B	B antigen	Anti-A antibodies	B, O	B, AB
AB[a]	A antigen B antigen	No antibodies	A, B, AB, O	AB
O[b]	No antigen	Both anti-A and anti-B antibodies	O	O, A, B, AB

[a]Type AB blood characterizes the universal recipient.
[b]Type O blood characterizes the universal donor.

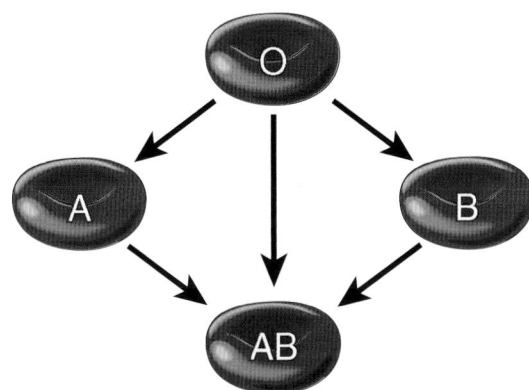

FIG. 26.3 Blood types: universal donor type O and universal recipient type AB.

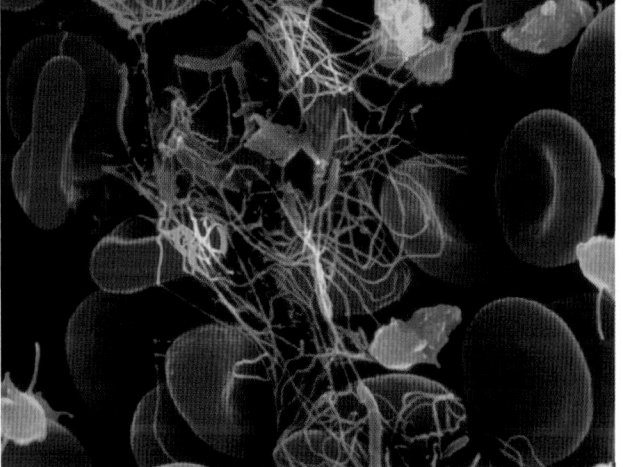

FIG. 26.4 Blood clot formation: Fibrinogen in plasma changes into fibrin, which forms a mesh. This mesh traps blood cells as they float by. Clotting factors then become activated, which strengths fibrin and changes the plug into a stable clot. (Copyright Dennis Kunkel Microscopy Inc.)

heart. Atrial walls contain *pectinate muscles*. Ventricular walls contain *trabeculae carneae*.

- **Right Atrium**. Receives oxygen-depleted blood from the superior and inferior vena and pumps it to the right ventricle.
- **Right Ventricle**. Receives blood from the right ventricle and pumps it to the pulmonary trunk, which divides into the right and left pulmonary arteries leading to their respective lungs.

- **Left Atrium**. Receives oxygen-rich blood from the right and left pulmonary veins and pumps it to the left ventricle.
- **Left Ventricle**. Receives blood from the left atrium and pumps it to vessels leading to every part of the body.

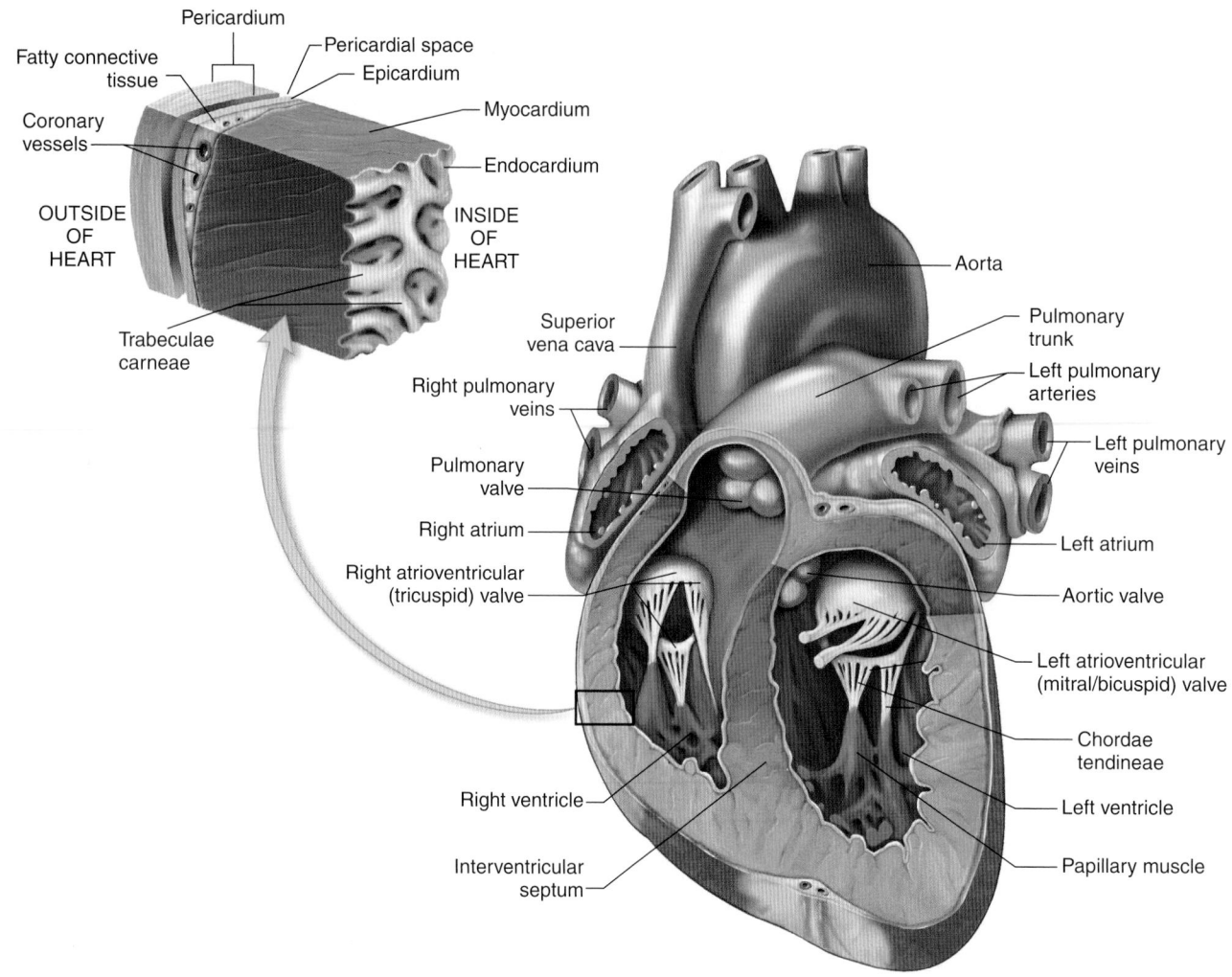

FIG. 26.5 The heart with major chambers, valves, and vessels *(right image)*; the heart sac and heart wall *(left image)*. (From Patton, K., & Thibodeau, G. [2014]. *The human body in health and disease* [6th ed.]. St. Louis, MO: Mosby.)

Even though the heart is a single organ, it is helpful to think of the heart as a double pump. The right atria and the right ventricle are the first pump. They carry oxygen-depleted blood to your lungs, where it releases carbon dioxide, picks up oxygen, and delivers oxygen-rich blood back to your heart. The left atria and the left ventricle are the second pump. They carry oxygen-rich blood to body tissues.

Heart Valves and Heart Sounds

Blood passes through a valve before leaving each chamber of the heart. The valves open and close to help prevent backward flow of blood, and keep it on a unidirectional course. The valves are actually pointed flaps or *cusps*. Most heart valves have three flaps, except the bicuspid or mitral valve, which has two. Closure of the heart valves produces the "lubb-dubb" sounds characteristic of the heartbeat.

- **Atrioventricular (AV) Valves**. Between the atria and the ventricles. Each AV valve is named for its location, number of cusps, or shape. The "lubb" is the low-pitched sound generated by blood turbulence from closure of both AV valves.
  - **Tricuspid Valve (Right AV Valve)**. Between the right atrium and the right ventricle.
  - **Bicuspid/Mitral Valve (Left AV Valve)**. Between the left atrium and the left ventricle. The bicuspid valve is also called the mitral valve because it is shaped like a miter or bishop's hat.
- **Semilunar (SL) Valves**. Between the ventricles and large blood vessels, such as the pulmonary trunk and the aorta. Each SL valve is named for the vessel it leads to. The "dubb" is the second higher-pitched sound caused by blood turbulence from closure of both the SL valves.
  - **Pulmonary Valve (Right SL Valve)**. Between the right ventricle and the pulmonary trunk.
  - **Aortic Valve (Left SL Valve)**. Between the left ventricle and the aorta.

The tricuspid and bicuspid/mitral valves are held in place by tendonlike cords called *chordae tendineae* that are attached to the heart wall by *papillary muscles*. Chordae tendineae keep the valve flaps from opening backward, or prolapsing, when the ventricles contract. This ensures blood moves forward through the heart instead of surging back into the atria. *LEARNING TIP:* To help you remember the right AV valve is the tricuspid valve, **R** has triple or **three** lines (two straight and one curved line). To help you remember the left AV valve is the bicuspid valve, **L** has double or **two** lines (two straight lines).

Cardiac Cycle and Blood Flow Through the Heart

Cardiac cycle is the sequence of events from the beginning of one heartbeat to the beginning of the next heartbeat. During the cardiac cycle, blood moves into and out of the heart in three well-coordinated and timed stages (Fig. 26.6). Blood is ejected from both atria and both ventricles at the same time (Fig. 26.7).

- **Stage 1**. Oxygen-depleted blood enters the right atrium from the superior and inferior vena cavae. The right atrium contracts and pushes blood through the tricuspid valve into the right ventricle.
- **Stage 2**. The right ventricle contracts and pushes blood through the pulmonary valve into the pulmonary trunk and pulmonary arteries and into the lungs. The pulmonary arteries are the only arteries that transport oxygen-depleted blood. Once blood is reoxygenated, the pulmonary veins transport blood from the lungs to the left atrium. The pulmonary veins are the only veins that transport oxygen-rich blood.
- **Stage 3**. Blood moves from the left atrium through the mitral valve and enters the left ventricle. The left ventricle contracts and blood moves through the aortic valve into the aorta and then to body cells.

Heart Rate and Heart Rhythm

Heart rate is the number of heart beats per minute. It varies from person to person—normal resting heart rate

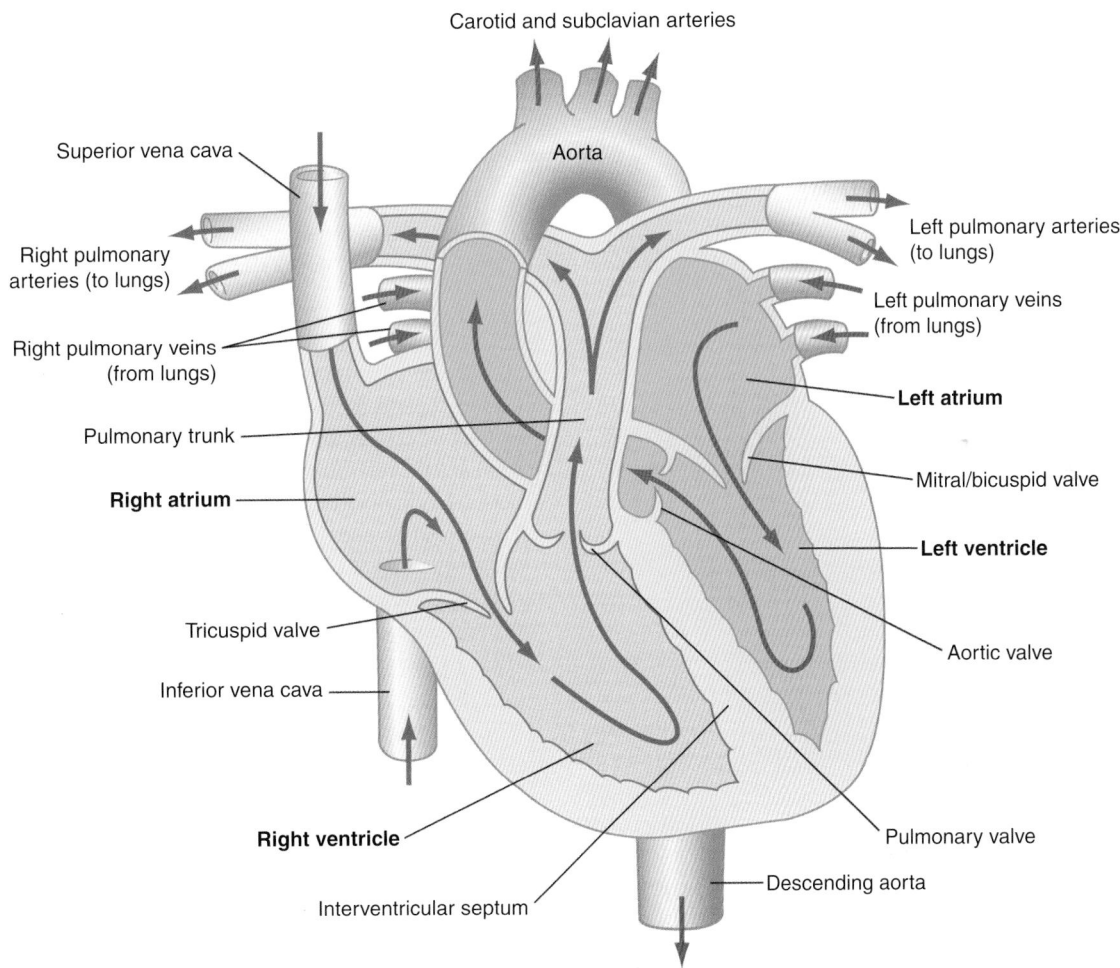

FIG. 26.6 Cardiac cycle (*cross-section view*) Oxygen-depleted blood *(blue)* enters the right atrium from the superior and inferior vena cavae. Blood moves through the tricuspid valve into the right ventricle. The right ventricle contracts and moves blood through the pulmonary valve into the pulmonary trunk, the pulmonary arteries, and into the lungs. Reoxygenated blood *(red)* is transported from the lungs to the left atrium by the pulmonary veins. Blood moves from the left atrium through the mitral valve and enters the left ventricle. The left ventricle contracts to push blood through the aortic valve into the aorta.

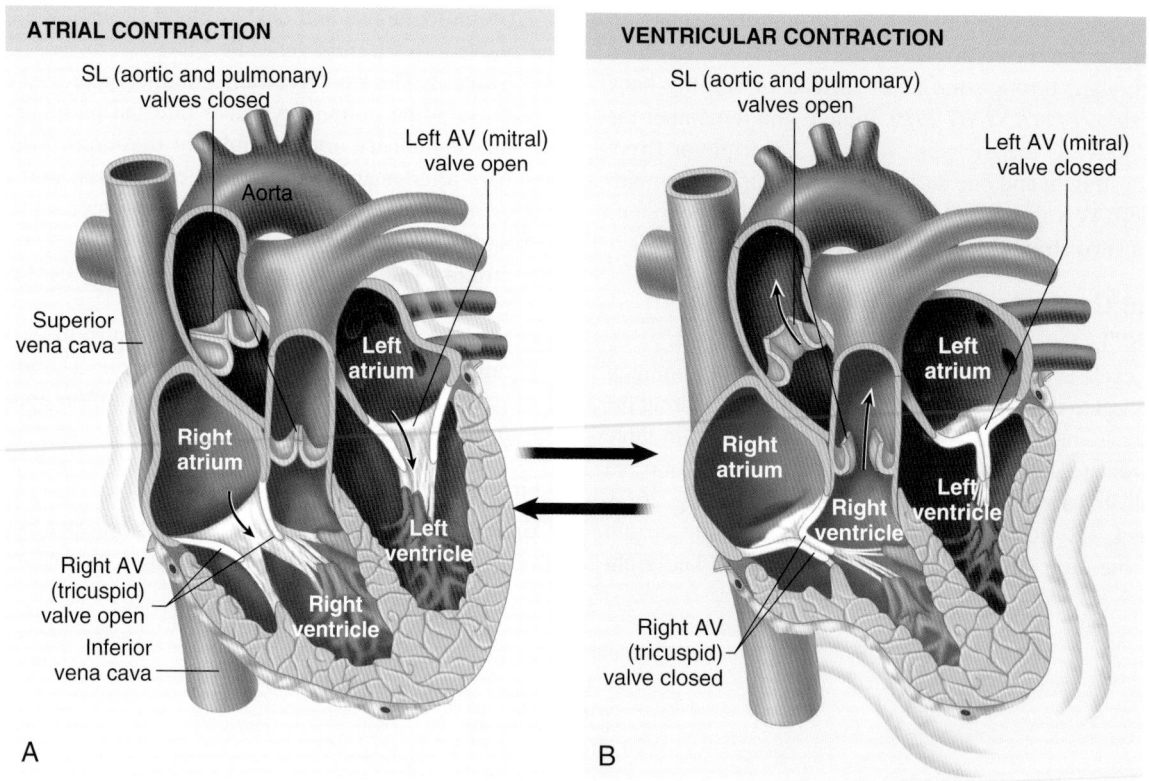

ATRIAL CONTRACTION	VENTRICULAR CONTRACTION

FIG. 26.7 Atrial and ventricular contractions during the cardiac cycle. (A) Both atria contract at the same time to eject blood while ventricles relax to fill with blood. (B) Both ventricles contract at the same time to eject blood while atria relax to fill with blood. (From Patton, K., & Thibodeau, G. [2014]. *The human body in health and disease* [6th ed.]. St. Louis, MO: Mosby.)

for adults is between 60 and 100 beats/min. Heart rate is also called *pulse rate*. Lower heart rate at rest implies a more efficient heart function and better cardiovascular fitness. For example, an athlete might have a normal resting heart rate of 40 beats per minute.

Heart rhythm is the pattern or regularity of electrical impulses that causes the heart to contract. These electrical impulses can be seen as electrical activity in an electrocardiogram (ECG). Heart rate and heart rhythm are coordinated by a group of cells in the heart wall called the heart's conduction system. This system generates and distributes nerve impulses throughout the myocardium in the heart's chambers, which causes them to contract. Main parts of the system are the sinoatrial (SA) node, the AV node, the bundle of His, and Purkinje fibers (Fig. 26.8). The SA node is in the superior surface of the right atrium, and the AV node is in the posterior surface. The bundle of His and the left and right bundle branches are in the interventricular septum, and the Purkinje fibers are in the walls of the right and left ventricles.

The SA node generates the nerve impulse and causes muscles in the atria to contract. The SA node is also called the *pacemaker* because it sets the pace of heart rate and heart rhythm. The nerve impulse then travels to the AV node through the bundle of His, down the bundle branches, and through the Purkinje fibers, which causes muscles in the ventricles to contract.

Heart Rate Variability

Heart rate variability (HRV) is the variation in time intervals between heartbeats. HRV is controlled by the autonomic nervous system, which regulates the stress response (sympathetic division) and the relaxation response (parasympathetic division). If a person has high HRV, it means their ANS is able to switch gears between stress and relaxation quickly, showing more resilience and adaptability. A person with low HRV is not adapting well and may stay in sympathetic arousal or the stress response longer than necessary. Research has shown a relationship between low HRV and conditions such as cardiovascular disease.

Heart Arrhythmia

A **heart arrhythmia** is an irregular heartbeat. Heart arrhythmias occur when the conduction system mentioned previously does not function properly and causes the heart to beat too fast or too slowly. Terms for abnormal heart rates are **tachycardia** (heartbeats ≥100 per minute) and **bradycardia** (heartbeats ≤60 per minute). Fibrillation is a type of arrhythmia in which faulty electrical signals cause the heart to beat fast and in an uncoordinated manner—the heart quivers instead of contracting forcefully and efficiently. **Atrial fibrillation (A-fib)** is irregular contractions of the atria. **Ventricular fibrillation (V-fib)** is irregular contractions of the ventricles. Fibrillations require medical treatment.

A man is only as old as his arteries.

~ **Pierre Cabanis, French physician**

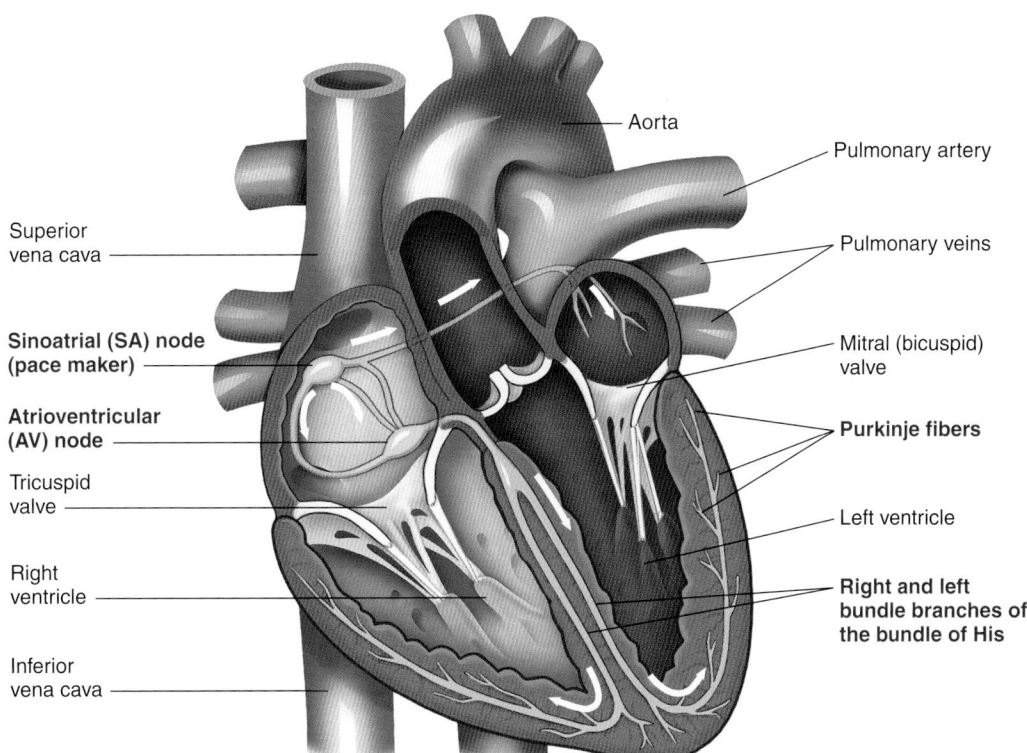

Aorta

Pulmonary artery

Pulmonary veins

Superior
vena cava

Mitral (bicuspid)
valve

**Sinoatrial (SA) node
(pace maker)**

Purkinje fibers

**Atrioventricular
(AV) node**

Tricuspid
valve

Left ventricle

**Right and left
bundle branches of
the bundle of His**

Right
ventricle

Inferior
vena cava

FIG. 26.8 Heart's conduction system (*white arrows denote path of conduction*). The impulse begins in the sinoatrial (SA) node, then travels to the atrioventricular (AV) node (causing the atria to contract), the bundle of His, the bundles branch and into Purkinje fibers (causing the ventricles to contract). (From Patton, K., & Thibodeau, G. [2014]. *The human body in health and disease* [6th ed.]. St. Louis, MO: Mosby.)

BLOOD VESSELS

Blood vessels are a closed network of tubes connected to the heart that transport blood (Fig. 26.9). These vessels are the blood's highway system and are comparable to hollow streets. There are three main types of blood vessels: arteries, veins, and capillaries. Arteries are vessels transporting blood away from the heart; veins are vessels returning blood toward the heart. Capillaries are vessels where blood exchanges gases, nutrients, and wastes with cells of the body. ***LEARNING TIP:*** To help you remember the direction blood is flowing in arteries and veins, blood in **A**rteries moves **A**way from the heart while blood in ve**IN**s moves **IN**to the heart.

Both arteries and veins have the same three distinct tissue layers, called tunics. The *tunica interna* is the innermost layer and is the endothelium. The middle layer, or *tunica media,* contains circularly arranged smooth muscle and elastic fibers. The outer layer, or *tunica externa,* is mostly connective tissue and collagen fibers (Fig. 26.10). *Lumen* is spaces within blood vessels. *Vasomotor* refers to actions of blood vessels to change their diameter. These actions are regulated by the medulla oblongata. There are two main types of action:

- **Vasodilation**. The lumen enlarges or widens. Smooth muscles in the walls of arteries or large veins relax, which leads to an increase in local blood flow (**hyperemia**) and a decrease in blood pressure.
- **Vasoconstriction**. The lumen becomes smaller or narrows. Smooth muscles in the walls of arteries or large veins contract, which leads to a decrease in local blood flow (**ischemia**) and an increase in blood pressure.

Most arteries and veins are named after structures they lie over or organs they serve. For example, the femoral artery and vein lie over the femur, and the renal artery and vein serve the kidneys. Names of many arteries and veins change as they enter and pass through regions of the body. For example, the axillary artery and vein become the brachial artery and vein as they move from the armpit to the arm. Arteries and veins are found on both sides of the body and are identified as right and left, such as the right and left subclavian artery and vein. Major arteries and veins are featured in their respective sections later in the chapter.

Arteries

Arteries are vessels transporting blood away from the heart. Blood within most arteries is oxygen-rich; the exceptions are the pulmonary arteries transporting oxygen-depleted blood from the heart to the lungs. Arterial lumen is narrower and arterial walls are thicker compared with their associated veins. These characteristics are important to keep blood

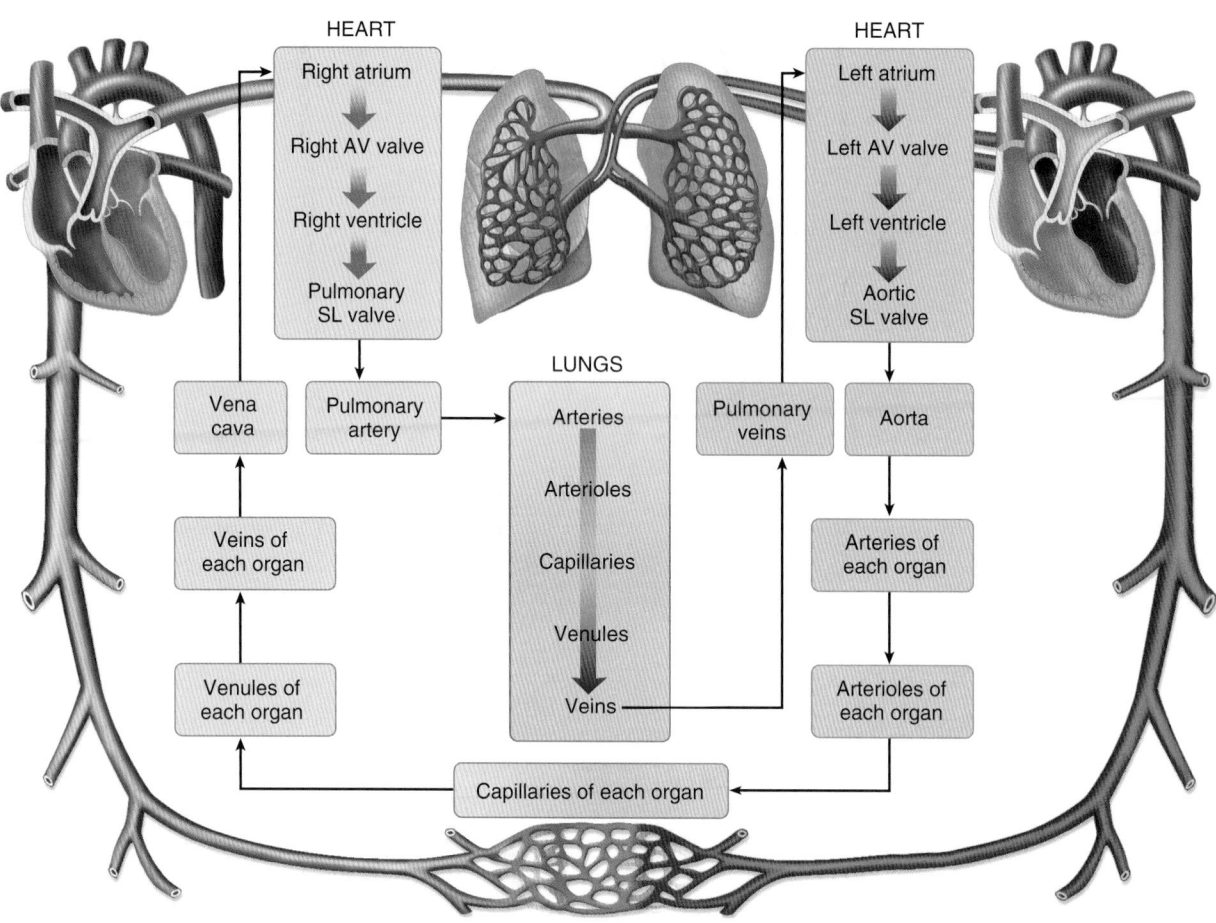

FIG. 26.9 Path of blood through the body using arteries, arterioles, capillaries, venules, and veins. (From Patton, K., & Thibodeau, G. [2014]. *The human body in health and disease* [6th ed.]. St. Louis, MO: Mosby.)

moving and withstand the force of blood pressure. Arteries branch off into smaller and thinner vessels called *arterioles*.

As the heart beats and ejects blood, the arterial walls expand and recoil. This arterial expansion is called a **pulse** and can be felt in arteries near the surface of the body. Common pulse points are named for their artery and are listed next (Fig. 26.11):

- **Temporal Pulse.** Front of the ear.
- **Facial Pulse.** On the mandible or jawbone in line with the corners of the mouth.
- **Carotid Pulse.** Sides of the neck.
- **Brachial Pulse.** Front of the elbow.
- **Radial Pulse.** In the wrist below the thumb.
- **Femoral Pulse.** Inner thigh between the pubic symphysis and anterior superior iliac spine.
- **Popliteal Pulse.** Behind the knee.
- **Posterior Tibial Pulse.** Between the medial ankle bone and the Achilles tendon.
- **Dorsalis Pedis Pulse.** Top of the foot lateral to extensor hallucis longus.

Blood Pressure

Blood pressure is the amount of force exerted by blood on vessel walls as the left ventricle of the heart contracts and relaxes. There are two ventricular phases: systole and diastole.

- **Systole (Systolic Pressure).** Pressure within arteries increases as the left ventricle contracts and ejects blood.
- **Diastole (Diastolic Pressure).** Pressure within arteries decreases as the left ventricle relaxes and fills with blood.

Blood pressure is usually measured in the brachial artery using a blood pressure cuff or *sphygmomanometer*. Blood pressure readings are expressed as two numbers: a higher number over a lower number as seen in a fraction. The higher number represents systolic pressure; the lower number represents diastolic pressure. A blood pressure reading of 120/80 mm Hg or less is considered within normal range. Blood pressure depends on many factors, such as efficiency of the heart muscle itself, blood volume, blood viscosity, age and health of the individual, and elasticity of arterial walls.

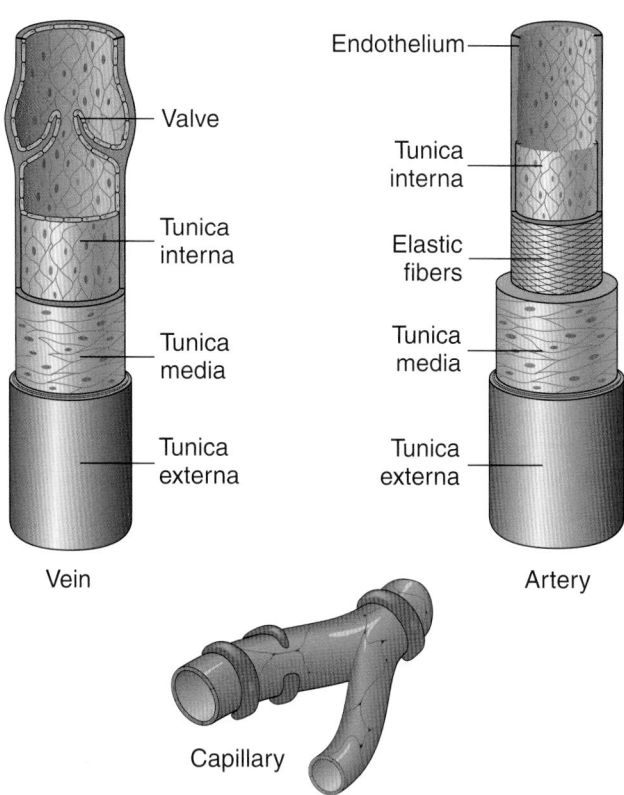

FIG. 26.10 Blood vessel walls with their respective tunics. The tunica interna is the innermost or endothelium. The tunica media contains circularly arranged smooth muscle and a layer of elastic fibers. The tunica externa is mostly connective tissue with collagen fibers.

Hypertension, or high blood pressure, is suspected when blood pressure readings reach or exceed 140/90. Hypertension is associated with cardiovascular disease.

Capillaries

Capillaries are the functional unit of the cardiovascular system because this is where gas exchange occurs between blood and body cells (see Fig. 26.10). To accomplish this, capillaries have thin, permeable walls. In addition, movement of blood within capillaries is slow and intermittent, which maximizes the exchange of gases. Blood flow to capillary beds is referred to as *microcirculation*. Exchange of gases at the capillary level is called *internal respiration* and is also discussed in Chapter 28.

Veins

Veins return blood to the heart. Blood within most veins is oxygen-depleted—the exceptions are the pulmonary veins transporting oxygen-rich blood from the lungs to the heart. Venous walls are thinner and collapse more easily compared with arteries. The walls also contain valves which prevent backflow of blood. Venous lumens are wider and provide less resistance to blood flow (see Fig. 26.10). Veins begin as small *venules* branching from capillaries (see Fig. 26.10). They gradually become larger in diameter until they reach the heart. Most blood in the body is within veins.

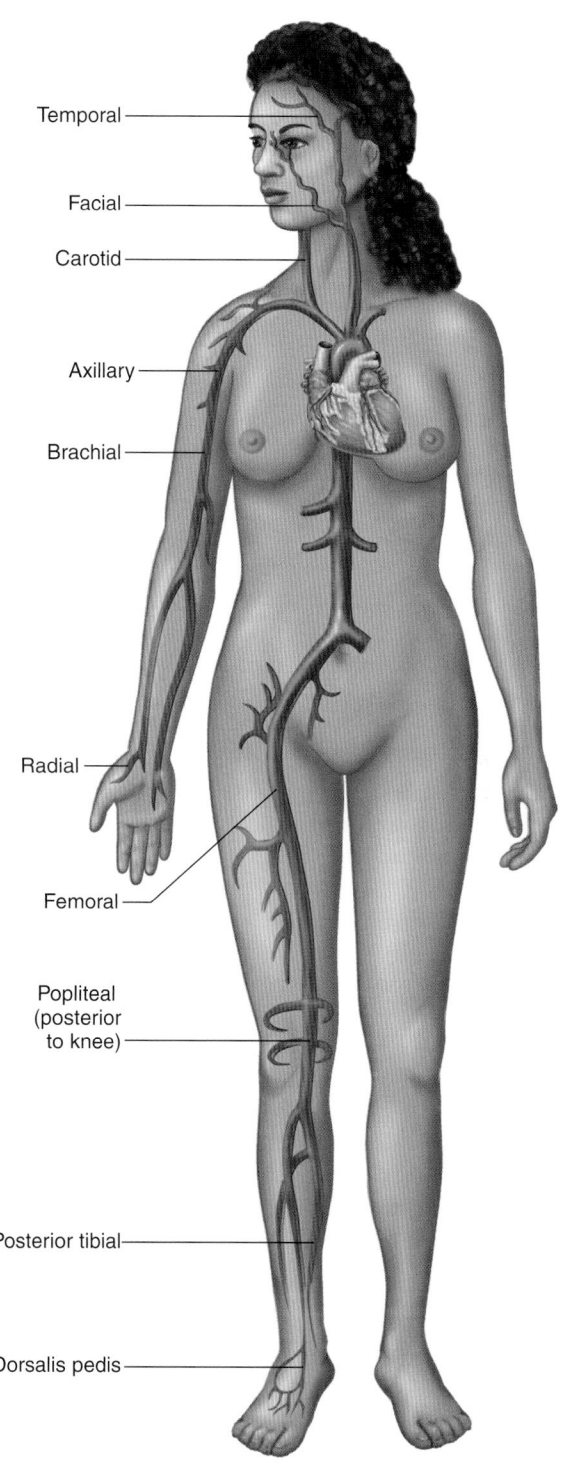

FIG. 26.11 Pulse points over major arteries *(anterior view)*. (From Patton, K., & Thibodeau, G. [2014]. *The human body in health and disease* [6th ed.]. St. Louis, MO: Mosby.)

Venous Return

Venous return is the rate blood flows back to the heart. Having good venous return is important because good cardiac output depends on good cardiac input. Veins do not have the heart pump to help push blood through its vessels as do arteries. Several mechanisms promote venous return. Gravity helps blood return to the heart. However, venous blood in the lower extremities must fight against gravity. This is why elevating the feet above the level of the heart promotes venous return. Venous valves help keep blood flowing in one direction—toward the heart. Another mechanism that assists venous return is the *skeletal muscle pump*, the squeeze-and-release action against venous walls that occurs when skeletal muscles contract and relax (Fig. 26.12). Lastly, the *respiratory pump* promotes venous return through pressure changes that occur during breathing. Inhalation causes a pressure decrease in the thoracic cavity and an increase in the abdominal cavity, creating an upward "sucking" effect, and pushing blood toward the heart.

Changes in muscle tone inside venous walls are called *venomotor tone*—this activity can affect blood flow and blood pressure. Lack of venomotor tone contributes to a sudden drop in blood pressure and resultant dizziness when sitting or standing upright from a recumbent position, a phenomenon called **postural (orthostatic) hypotension**.

PATHS OF BLOOD CIRCULATION

The heart pumps blood through blood vessels to the lungs to obtain oxygen and release carbon dioxide, and pumps blood to body cells to release oxygen and nutrients and to obtain carbon dioxide and other wastes. The heart performs these tasks proficiently because there are two separate circulatory paths, or circuits, with the heart as the common pump. These are the pulmonary circuit and a systemic circuit (Fig. 26.13).

Pulmonary Circuit

The **pulmonary circuit** delivers oxygen-depleted blood to the lungs, so it can be replenished with oxygen and eliminates carbon dioxide. Blood moves from the right ventricle through the pulmonary arteries to capillaries of the lungs and then returns blood through the pulmonary veins to the left atrium. Once blood returns to the heart, it enters the systemic circuit. As mentioned previously, pulmonary arteries transport blood away from the heart, and pulmonary veins transport blood back to the heart, but the oxygen content of blood is reversed in pulmonary arteries and veins—that is, pulmonary arteries transport oxygen-depleted blood, and pulmonary veins transport oxygen-rich blood.

Systemic Circuit

The **systemic circuit** delivers oxygen and nutrients to most of the body's organs and tissues and transports carbon dioxide and other wastes for elimination by various mechanisms, including respiration, urination, and perspiration. Blood moves from the left atrium to the left ventricle, then through the aorta into arteries and capillaries. From here, oxygen-depleted blood moves from capillaries to veins and returns blood to the heart to enter the pulmonary circuit at the right

atrium via the superior and inferior vena cavae. Some systemic organs and tissues, such as the liver and spleen, have a rich blood supply, whereas others are relatively avascular, such as cartilage.

Venous Portal Systems

Venous portal systems are found within the systemic circuit and consist of two capillary beds connected through a system of veins. Examples of venous portal systems are the *hepatic portal system* system in the gastrointestinal (GI) tract and the *hypophyseal portal system* between the hypothalamus and the pituitary within the brain (see Chapters 29 and 24, respectively). The hepatic portal system transports blood from parts of the GI tract to the liver via the hepatic portal vein, so absorbed substances can be processed before continuing to the heart. Not all sections of the GI tract are part of the hepatic portal system. The hepatic veins drain into the inferior vena cava (Fig. 26.14).

Major Systemic Arteries

All systemic arteries branch from one major artery, the *aorta,* which is the largest artery in terms of diameter. The first part of the aorta is the *ascending aorta,* then there is the *aortic arch* and then the *descending aorta.* The descending aorta, called the thoracic aorta, is above the diaphragm and the abdominal aorta below the diaphragm. The *carotid arteries* supply the brain, face, and neck. The *subclavian arteries* supply the upper regions of the body and the *external iliac arteries* supply the lower regions of the body. Additional major systemic arteries are featured in Fig. 26.15.

Major Systemic Veins

Veins begin at the capillary level and grow larger until they reach the superior vena cava or the inferior vena cava. The vena cavae are the largest veins in terms of diameter, and both drain into the right atrium. The *superior vena cava* drains blood from the upper half of the body. The *inferior vena cava* drains blood from the lower half of the body. The *great saphenous vein* is the longest vein in the body. The *jugular vein* drains the brain, face, and neck. The *subclavian veins* drain the upper regions of the body and the *common iliac veins* drain the lower regions of the body. Additional major systemic veins are featured in Fig. 26.16.

Wise men learn much from fools. Wise guys don't.
~ **Michel de Montaigne**

CARDIOVASCULAR PATHOLOGIES AND DISORDERS

Featured next are common pathologies and disorders of the cardiovascular system listed alphabetically. Each item includes a brief description and its massage-related modifications. A more extensive list and related research is found

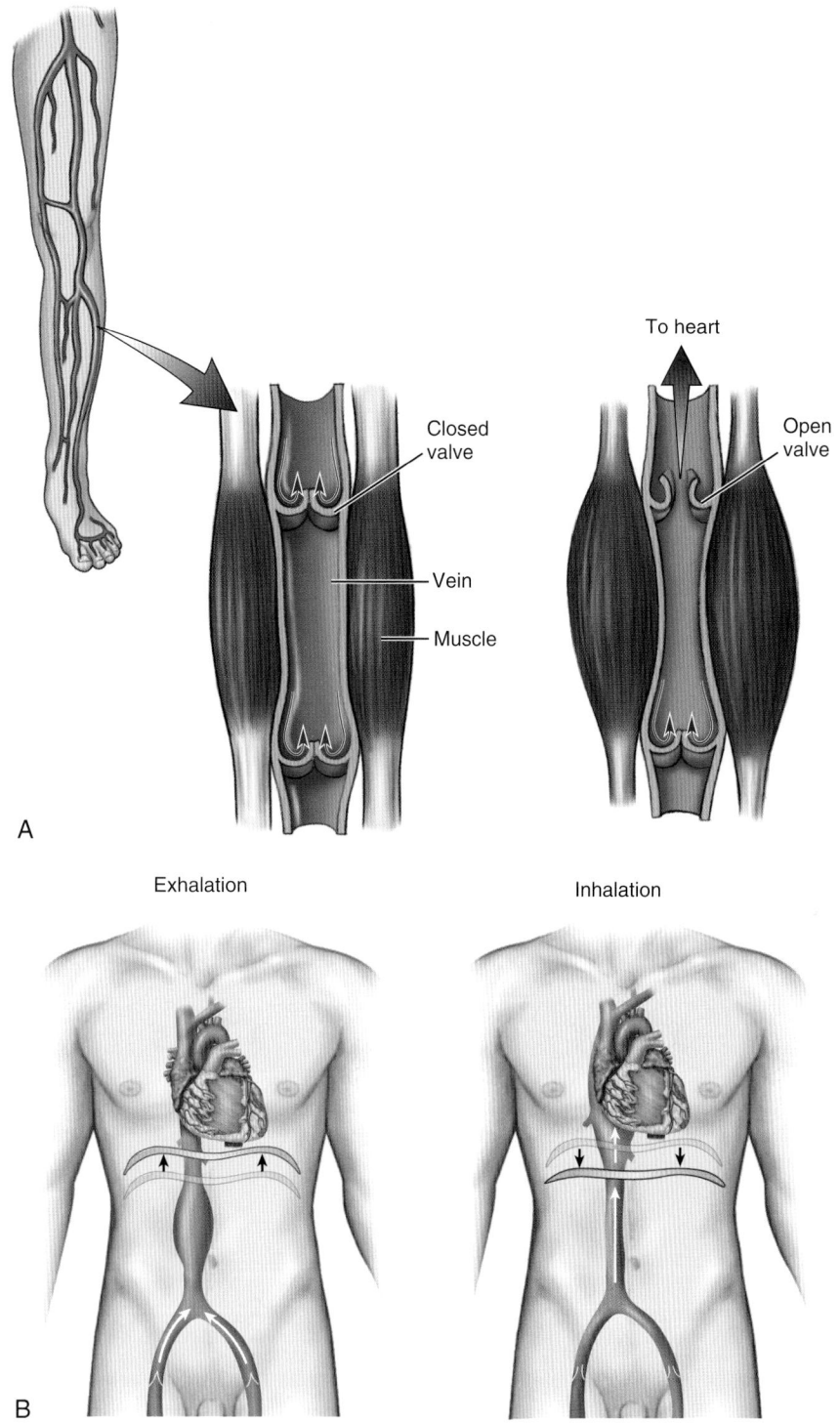

FIG. 26.12 Mechanisms that promote venous return. (A) Skeletal muscle pump. The squeeze-release action of skeletal muscle contraction against venous walls promotes venous return. Valves keep blood moving toward the heart. (B) Respiratory pump. During inhalation, pressure decreases in the thoracic cavity and increases in the abdominal cavity, creating an upward "sucking" effect that pushes blood toward the heart. (A, from Herlihy, B. [2011]. *The human body in health and illness* [4th ed.]. St. Louis, MO: Saunders. B, From Patton, K. T., & Thibodeau, G. A. [2010]. *Anatomy & physiology* [7th ed.]. St. Louis, MO: Mosby.)

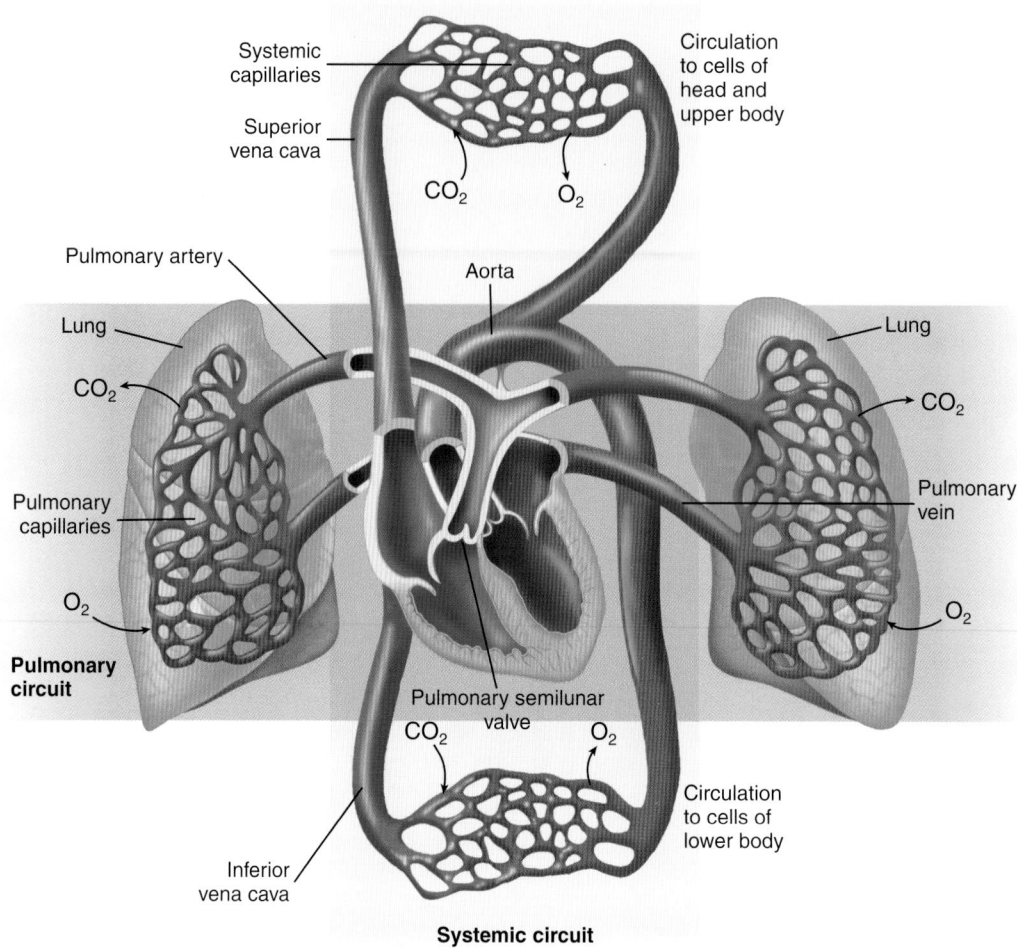

FIG. 26.13 Pulmonary and systemic circuits. The pulmonary circuit replenishes the blood's oxygen supply and eliminates carbon dioxide. The systemic circuit transports oxygen to body cells and transports carbon dioxide for their elimination. (From Patton, K., & Thibodeau, G. [2014]. *The human body in health and disease* [6th ed.]. St. Louis, MO: Mosby.)

in the current edition of *Mosby's Pathology for Massage Professionals* (2022).

Anemia

Anemia is reduced RBC count or reduced capacity of hemoglobin to carry oxygen to body cells. Anemia is a common blood disorder affecting approximately 3.5 million people in the United States. Many types of anemia have been identified. Most cases of anemia are classified by their causative factor (iron-deficiency, folate-deficiency, vitamin-deficiency anemia). Anemia can be temporary or long term and range from mild to severe. Another term for anemia is *erythrocytopenia*. The following are select anemias:

- **Iron-deficiency Anemia.** This is the most common type of anemia, and is associated with a low iron count, which interferes with hemoglobin production. This type of

anemia affects approximately 20% of all females, 50% of pregnant females, and 3% of males.
- **Folate-deficiency and Pernicious Anemias.** These are caused by folate (folic acid) and B-12 deficiencies, two of the B vitamins.
- **Anemia of Chronic Disease.** This can occur in people with chronic diseases such as autoimmune disease, kidney disease, or cancer.
- **Sickle Cell Disease.** This is characterized by RBC malformation; RBCs are shaped like a sickle instead of a disc. Sickle cells have shorter life spans (20 days instead of 120 days), and they may cause blood clots and block blood flow to the heart, brain, or other organs. Sickle cell disease is also called sickle cell anemia.
- **Aplastic Anemia.** This results from bone marrow failure, leading to a decrease in RBCs, and often reduces WBC and platelet counts as well.

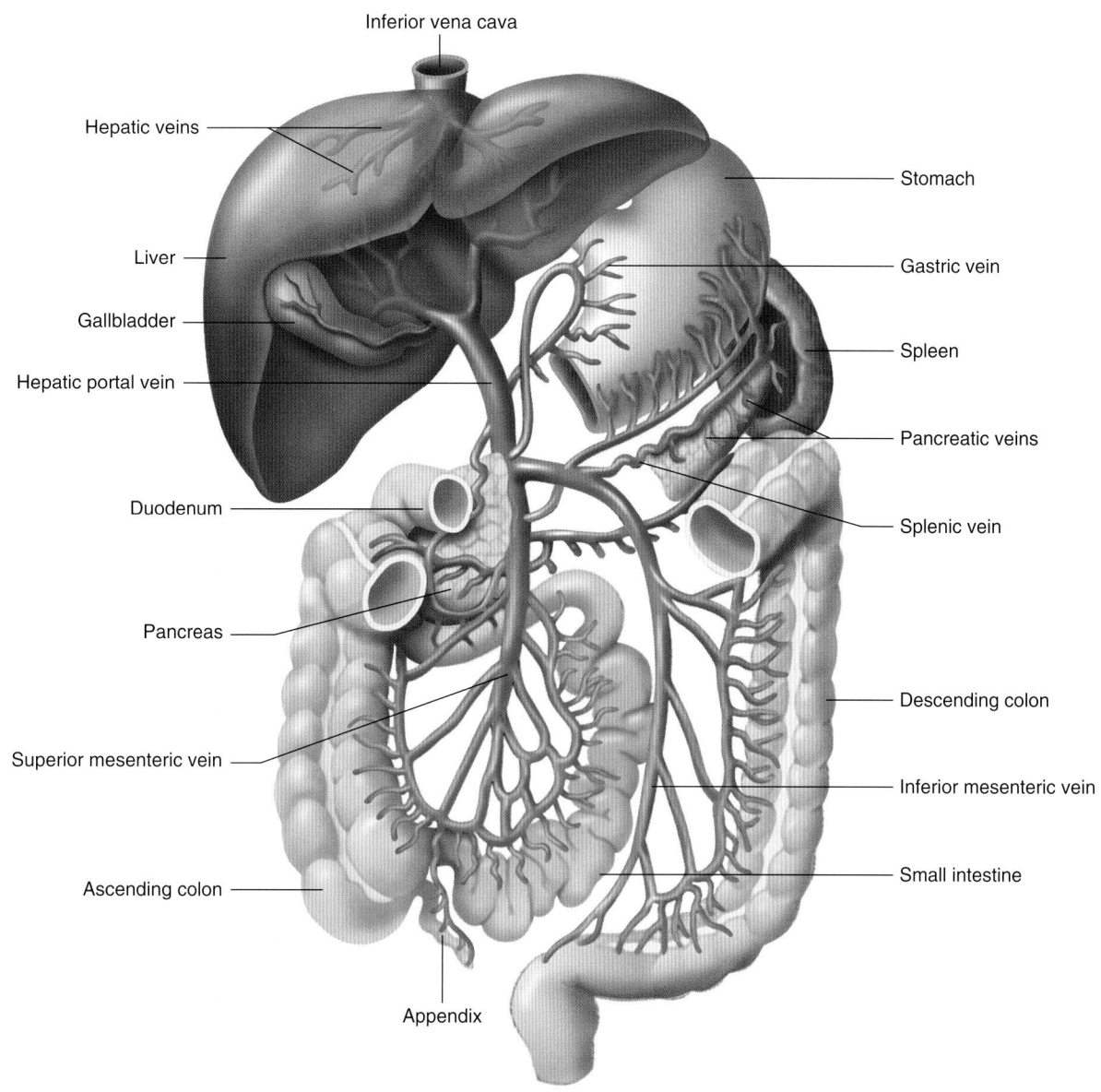

FIG. 26.14 Hepatic portal system. Blood from parts of the gastrointestinal tract travel to the liver so absorbed substances can be processed before continuing to the heart. The spleen, gallbladder, and pancreas also participate in the portal system. The hepatic veins drain into the inferior vena cava. (From Patton, K., & Thibodeau, G. [2014]. *The human body in health and disease* [6th ed.]. St. Louis, MO: Mosby.)

Massage and Anemia

The practitioner needs to modify the massage according to presenting signs and symptoms.

If the client has cold intolerance, provide comfort measures such as a blanket, an electric table warmer, raising the room temperature, or a combination of these. If the client has difficulty breathing, consider using body positions that help the client breathe more easily. Elevate the supine client's upper body and head while resting the knees on a bolster. Elevate the side-lying client's head and place a pillow between the knees; the back should be kept straight. The seated client's feet are flat on the floor with elbows resting on the knees (Cleveland Clinic, 2018). Because the client

may have orthostatic hypotension, ask the client to arise from the massage table in three stages: (1) sit up on the table for 1 minute; (2) sit on the side of the table with legs dangling for 1 minute; and (3) stand with care, holding onto the edge of the table or another nonmovable object for 1 minute. Coexisting medical conditions (autoimmune disease, kidney disease, cancer) should be factored into the treatment plan.

Angina Pectoris

Angina pectoris, or angina, is chest pain or discomfort caused by a temporary reduction of blood flow to the heart; the heart is not receiving enough blood. This pain or discomfort is also called an *angina attack.*

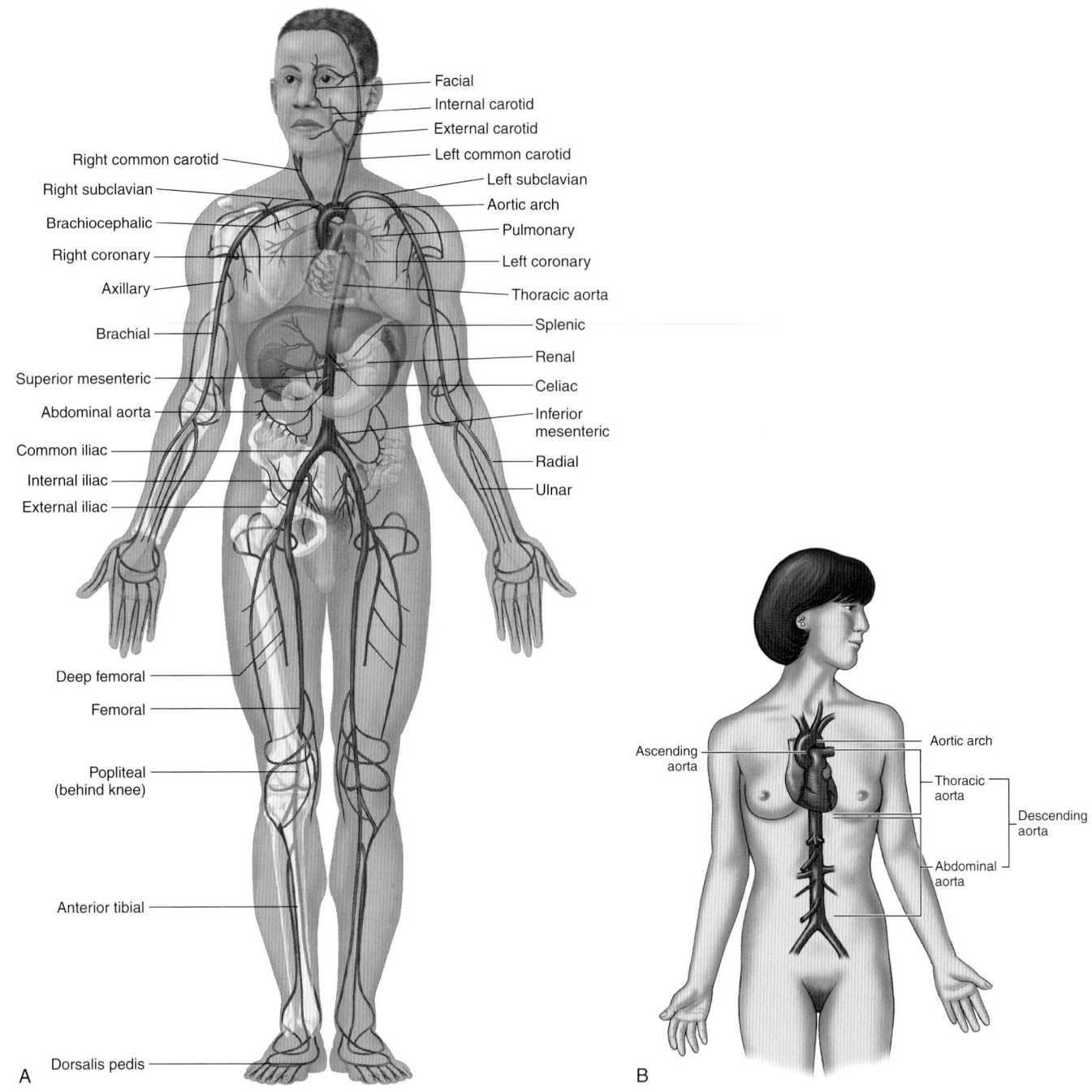

FIG. 26.15 (A) Major arteries (*anterior view*). (B) Branches of the aorta (*anterior view*). (A, From Patton, K., & Thibodeau, G. [2014]. *The human body in health and disease* [6th ed.]. St. Louis, MO: Mosby. B, From Herlihy, B. [2011]. *The human body in health and illness* [4th ed.]. St. Louis, MO: Saunders.)

Approximately 6.8 million people have angina, and approximately 400,000 new cases of angina are reported annually in the United States. Angina is the most common sign of coronary artery disease (CAD). Angina is also called ischemic chest pain.

Massage and Angina Pectoris

Massage may help reduce symptoms by promoting relaxation. Ask clients if they have medications with them (e.g.,

nitroglycerin) in case of an angina attack. Clients with a history of angina attacks may have medications with them, usually nitroglycerin, in the form of oral spray, sublingual powder, or sublingual tablets. These medications help dilate blood vessels, and restore blood flow to the heart, and work quickly to stop an angina attack that has already started. Because exposure to cold can bring on an attack, the practitioner needs to keep the client warm by using a blanket, an electric table warmer, raising the room temperature, or a combination of these measures. If prone

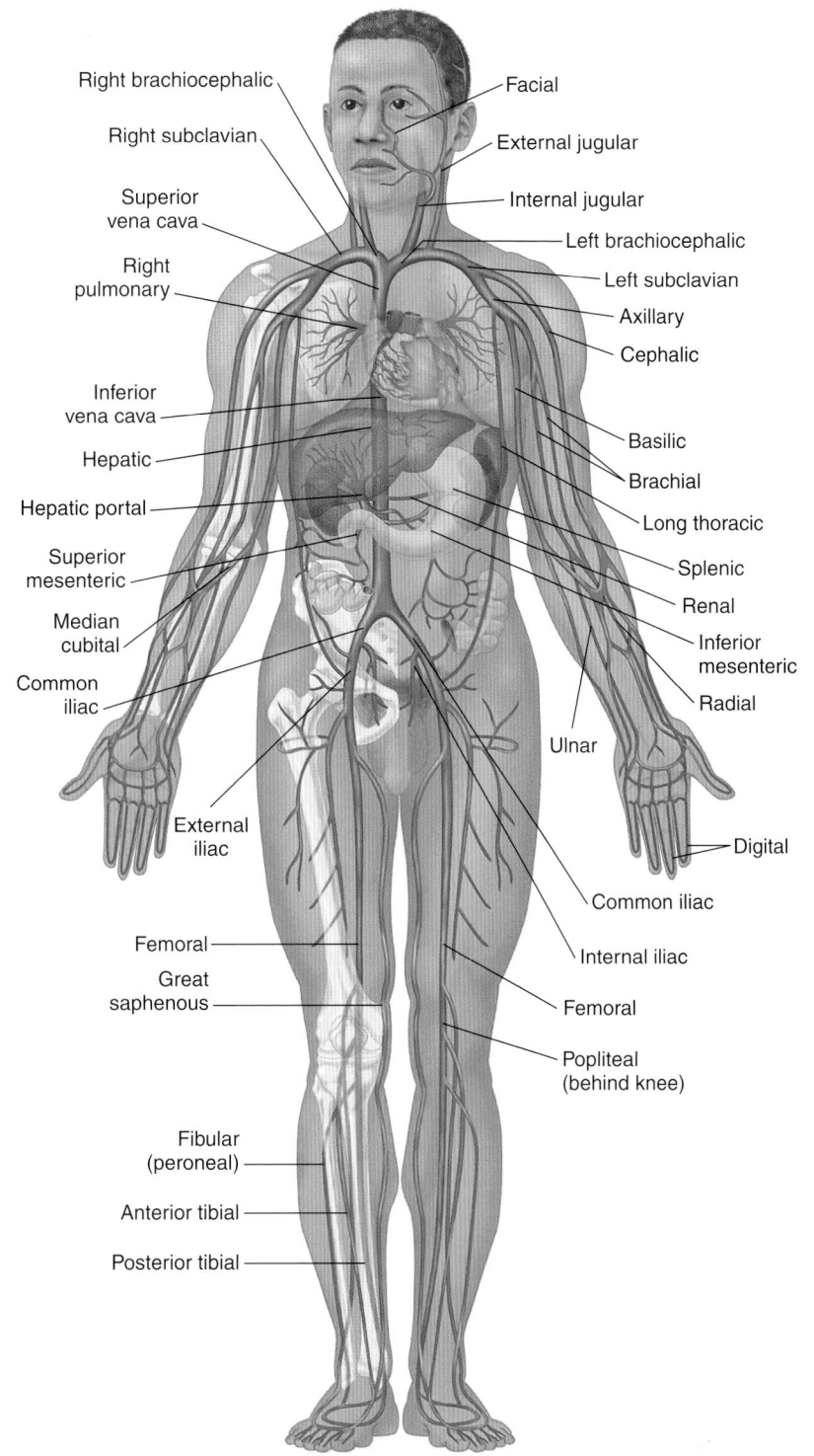

FIG. 26.16 Major veins (*anterior view*). (From Patton, K., & Thibodeau, G. [2014]. *The human body in health and disease* [6th ed.]. St. Louis, MO: Mosby.)

to dizziness related to OH, ask the client to arise from the massage table in three stages: (1) sit up on the table for 1 minute; (2) sit on the side of the table with legs dangling for 1 minute; (3) stand with care, holding onto the edge of the table or another nonmovable object for 1 minute.

The following protocol can be used if the client has an angina attack.
- Help the client to an upright position.
- Assist in the administration of medication (usually nitroglycerin). This step may require use of disposable gloves.

- Ask the client to remain seated during and after medication administration.

Nitroglycerin medication usually relieves symptoms 1 to 5 minutes after administration. The client may be instructed by a healthcare provider to take a second or third dose, if pain is not relieved within 5 minutes of taking a dose. If chest pain remains after a total of three doses, call 911 as chest pain may be related to a heart attack. Because of the risk of sudden cardiac arrest, do not allow the client to drive themselves to the emergency room.

Atherosclerosis

Atherosclerosis is the presence of atherosclerotic plaque within arteries. Plaque can increase blood pressure and clot formation. Plaque also causes partial or total obstruction of blood flow through arteries in the heart, brain, trunk, pelvis, or lower extremities. This can give rise to various diseases, including:

- **Atherosclerosis of the Coronary Arteries.** This can cause angina pectoris, CAD, congestive heart failure (CHF), and MIs.
- **Atherosclerosis of Cerebral Arteries.** This can lead to transient ischemia attacks and cerebrovascular events such as stroke.
- **Atherosclerosis of the Abdominal Aorta.** This can cause an abdominal aortic aneurysm.
- **Atherosclerosis of the Arteries of the Extremities.** This can cause peripheral artery disease.

Years are required for complications of atherosclerosis to become clinically evident; diabetes, hypertension, and smoking accelerate the process. *Arteriosclerosis* is the process of plaque accumulation within arterial walls causing them to become thick and rigid. In contrast, healthy arteries are thinner, flexible, and elastic. These two terms, atherosclerosis and arteriosclerosis, are often used interchangeably.

Massage and Atherosclerosis

Because atherosclerosis is related to other diseases, read applicable recommendations for specific diseases such as angina pectoris, CAD, CHF, TIA, and stroke (see Chapter 23).

Congestive Heart Failure

Congestive heart failure (CHF) is a chronic progressive heart condition affecting its ability to pump enough blood to meet the body's needs. Also known as heart failure, CHF is not a single disease, but rather a syndrome or complication associated with other diseases. The term "congestive" describes what happens when the left or right sides of the heart begin to fail; blood and other fluids back up into, or congest, organs such as the lungs, liver, as well as abdomen and lower extremities. CHF affects approximately 5.7 million people in the United States. Some heart conditions related to CHF may require a pacemaker or an implantable cardioverter defibrillator.

Massage and Congestive Heart Failure

Note the client's current signs and symptoms, such as shortness of breath and dizziness; modify the massage accordingly. For example, if the client is experiencing shortness of breath, consider using body positions that help the client breathe more easily. Elevate the supine client's upper body and head while resting their knees on a bolster. Elevate the side-lying client's head and place a pillow between the knees; the back should be kept straight. The seated client's feet are flat on the floor with elbows resting on the knees. Avoid or limit time spent in the prone position. If prone to dizziness related to OH, ask the client to arise from the massage table in three stages: (1) sit up on the table for 1 minute; (2) sit on the side of the table with legs dangling for 1 minute; (3) stand with care, holding onto the edge of the table or another nonmovable object for 1 minute.

If the client is frail, massage techniques should be applied slowly using light pressure. An example of light pressure is 3 on a 10-point pressure scale. If the client believes signs and symptoms have worsened, a referral should be made to a healthcare provider for medical evaluation.

If the client has a pacemaker or an ICD, avoid massage over or near the device (i.e., local contraindication). Consider placing a small pillow or cushion under the device while the client is lying prone if needed for comfort. Avoid passive shoulder movements on the side where the device is located for 6 to 8 weeks following surgery.

Coronary Artery Disease

Coronary artery disease (CAD) is the presence of atherosclerotic plaque within coronary arteries; these arteries supply the myocardium of the heart. Narrowed arteries reduce blood flow and create ischemia, sometimes leading to MI. CAD is the most common type of heart disease, causing over 370,000 deaths annually. CAD is also called *ischemic heart disease*, *coronary heart disease*, and *atherosclerotic heart disease*.

Massage and Coronary Artery Disease

No massage modifications are needed for clients with CAD.

Deep Vein Thrombosis, Thrombophlebitis, and Venous Thromboembolism

Deep vein thrombosis (DVT) is a thrombus or blood clot within a deep vein, usually in the legs (from knee to ankle). **Thrombophlebitis** occurs when the thrombus causes inflammation within a vein. Thrombi are composed of blood cells enmeshed in a fibrin network adhered to a vessel wall. An *embolus* is a mass floating through the intravascular space carried by blood. Emboli originating from a thrombus are called *thromboemboli*. Other types of emboli are bubbles of air, pieces of fat or bone marrow, tumor cells, and atherosclerotic plaque. Emboli can be classified by the vessel that carries them (venous or arterial). When an embolus lodges in and occludes a blood vessel, it is called *embolism*.

The most life-threatening acute complication of DVT is *pulmonary embolism* (PE), a partially or completely occluded artery in the lungs. Over time, PE causes the heart to work harder, which may lead to heart failure. The exact number of people affected by DVT/PE is unknown, but it is estimated as many as 900,000 people could be affected each year in the United States. **Venous thromboembolism** (VTE) is a collective term for DVT and PE. VTE and DVT are often used interchangeably.

Risk factors include personal or family history of DVT or PE, active cancer or cancer treatment, oral contraceptives, hormone replacement therapy, pregnancy or having given birth within the previous 6 weeks, immobility (e.g., bedrest, being chairbound, extended flights, or car travel), recent surgery or major injury, central venous catheters, inherited blood disorders, and obesity. People who smoke, people older than 60 years of age, and people previously diagnosed with COVID-19 are also at greater risk for DVT.

Massage and Deep Vein Thrombosis/Venous Thromboembolism

If the client has been diagnosed with DVT or VTE, prevent PE by avoiding massage to the affected lower extremity (thigh and leg). Leg massage has been linked to previous VTE incidents (Behera et al., 2018; Crump & Paluska, 2010; Jabr, 2007; Lim et al., 2009).

If the client is not diagnosed with DVT or VTE, identify clients at risk for DVT and look for signs and symptoms of DVT among clients identified as "at risk." Signs and symptoms of DVT include unilateral leg swelling, heat, redness or noticeable discoloration, pain, and tenderness. If present, avoid massage to the affected lower extremity (thigh and leg). Massage has been found safe with precautions taken, such as screening for DVT and avoiding the affected limb (Ng et al., 2018).

Hypertensive Heart Disease (Hypertension)

Hypertensive heart disease is heart disease caused by sustained high blood pressure or hypertension. Hypertensive heart disease can lead to other heart disorders, including CAD, heart failure, MI (heart attack), and other conditions. Approximately 75 million American adults (32%) have high blood pressure, or one in every three adults. Hypertensive heart disease is the leading cause of death from high blood pressure. Hypertension is often called the "silent killer" because it typically has no symptoms and is often undiagnosed until after significant damage to the heart and arteries—20% of Americans who have hypertension do not know they have it, which puts them at risk for not only hypertensive heart disease, but also diseases of the kidneys, eyes, and brain. Hypertension is suspected when systolic pressure exceeds 140 mm Hg, or diastolic pressure exceeds 90 mm Hg.

Massage and Hypertensive Heart Disease (Hypertension)

Massage is indicated for clients with hypertensive heart disease. Clients taking antihypertensive medications may be prone to orthostatic hypotension. If so, ask the client to arise from the massage table in three stages: (1) sit up on the table for 1 minute; (2) sit on the side of the table with legs dangling for 1 minute; (3) stand with care, holding onto the edge of the table or another nonmovable object for 1 minute.

Myocardial Infarction (Heart Attack)

A **myocardial infarction** (MI) occurs when blood flow to the heart is suddenly disrupted from a blocked or occluded vessel. Every year, approximately 735,000 Americans have a heart attack. Of these, 525,000 are a first-ever heart attack, and 210,000 occur in people who have had a heart attack previously. Sudden death occurs in approximately 25% of cases, usually from arrhythmias. CHF develops in many MI survivors because the heart does not pump blood as well as it did before the MI.

MIs can lead to **cardiac arrest**, sudden cessation of heartbeat, affecting blood flow to the brain and other vital organs. Other conditions that can disrupt heart rhythm and cause cardiac arrest are coronary heart disease, CHF, cardiomyopathy, and ventricular fibrillation (v-fib), a type of arrhythmia. Use of certain recreational drugs can cause sudden cardiac arrest, even in otherwise healthy people. Cardiac arrest can cause death if not treated within minutes.

Massage and Myocardial Infarction/Heart Attack

Heart attacks are medical emergencies requiring immediate intervention as they can progress to cardiac arrest. See Chapter 9 for first aid measures for cardiac arrest.

If the client has had an MI, ask when it occurred and how well recovery is proceeding. If the MI is recent and the client is frail, use slowly applied light pressure. An example of light pressure is 3 on a 10-point pressure scale. If the client is further along in the recovery or has completely recovered, massage is indicated. Clients should have their necessary medications (e.g., nitroglycerin) with them when they come for treatment. Coexisting medical conditions, such as CHF, should be factored into the treatment plan.

Peripheral Arterial Disease

Peripheral arterial disease (PAD) is the presence of atherosclerotic plaque within arteries outside the heart. Affected arteries can restrict blood flow and promote the formation of blood clots. PAD is a common disorder affecting approximately 8.5 million people in the United States, including 12% to 20% of individuals older than 60 years. PAD can occur in any blood vessel, but it is more common in the legs. Various metabolic disorders (e.g., diabetes, hypertension), high cholesterol, obesity, sedentary lifestyle, and cigarette smoking contribute to the disease. PAD is also called *peripheral arterial disease, peripheral vascular disease*, and *atherosclerosis of the extremities.*

Massage and Peripheral Arterial Disease

Look for signs and symptoms of DVT because of possible blood clots. These include unilateral leg swelling, heat, redness or noticeable discoloration, pain, and tenderness. If present, avoid massage to the affected lower extremity. If not present, massage can be applied with pressure adjusted according to the client's preferences.

Phlebitis

Phlebitis is inflammation of the veins without thrombus or blood clot formation. There are two forms of phlebitis. The most common form, *superficial phlebitis*, is inflammation of veins near the skin's surface. *Deep phlebitis* is inflammation of deep veins, usually in the leg. Deep phlebitis is a more serious condition because it can progress to DVT (see prior entry).

Massage and Phlebitis

Look for signs and symptoms of DVT because of possible blood clots. These include unilateral leg swelling, heat, redness or noticeable discoloration, pain, and tenderness. If present, avoid massage to the affected lower extremity.

Raynaud Disease

Raynaud disease is periodic episodes of vasospasms, usually in the fingers and toes. It also can affect the tip of the nose, parts of the ears, parts of the cheeks, and the tongue. During an attack, small and medium-sized arteries contract, which causes temporary ischemia. In light skin, a change in skin color (blue to purple) may be present. In dark skin, skin may appear paler. As vasospasms subside, blood flow is reestablished. An attack can be triggered by cold temperatures or emotional stress. Raynaud disease is more common in females than males. The condition is primary if it occurs without an underlying cause. Secondary Raynaud is caused by another disease, disorder, condition, or substance; secondary Raynaud is also called *Raynaud syndrome* or *Raynaud phenomenon.*

Massage and Raynaud Disease

To help prevent an attack, ensure the client is warm by using a blanket, an electric table warmer, raising the room temperature, or a combination of these. All forms of cryotherapy, including ice packs, are contraindicated as cold can trigger an attack. If the client experiences an attack during massage, apply superficial warming friction over the affected area. Warm towels can also be used. If hands or feet are involved during the attack, these can be submerged in warm water if available.

Varicose Veins

Varicose veins are enlarged veins caused by defective valves. The condition can affect superficial or deep veins; superficial veins lack the muscle support of deep veins and are therefore more susceptible to varicose veins. These are usually in the legs but are also found in other parts of the body, such as the esophagus (esophageal varices) and the rectum (hemorrhoids). Varicose veins are common, affecting approximately 40 million people in the United States. Spider veins are smaller varicose veins resembling a spider's web. Varicose veins are also called *varicosities*.

Massage and Varicose Veins

Avoid the affected area if pressure causes pain. Clients with varicosities may benefit from massage, especially techniques applied with light pressure. An example of light pressure is 3 on a 10-point pressure. Place the affected area on cushions to raise it above the level of the heart during the massage. Elevation may facilitate dependent drainage, which uses gravity to stimulate movement of fluids from a higher to a lower area.

E-RESOURCES

http://evolve.elsevier.com/Salvo/MassageTherapy

- Chapter challenge
- Flash cards

JACK MEAGHER

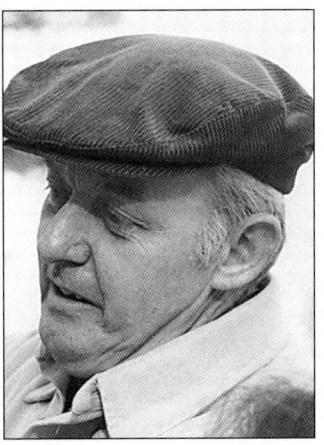

Many massage students first choose this career after receiving a professional massage. Other students choose massage as an initial introduction to the healthcare field because they plan to enter nursing, physical therapy, or medicine. Whatever your goals and motivations, it is important to receive a wide variety of massages by different practitioners and representing different styles. Doing so can give you a feel for the sort of massage you want to pursue further. The experience might just change your life. It certainly did for Jack Meagher, the father of sports massage.

Meagher's initial massage education consisted of a Swedish massage course. He was hoping to eventually study physical therapy, and it seemed like a good idea. He was an avid baseball player and saw how physical therapy could help athletes recover from injury. Shortly thereafter, he enlisted as a US Army medic and served for 4 years.

While overseas in Epernay, France, Meagher received a massage from a German prisoner of war. This massage, though, was different from any he had experienced before. Rather than relaxing him, it made him move more freely. It even improved his performance on the baseball field.

After he was discharged from the Army, Meagher went on to play baseball professionally, pitching for the Boston Braves. It was a dream come true but short-lived; a shoulder injury from the war landed him in physical therapy, unable to continue his athletic career. Remembering his experience in France, Meagher went searching for a similar massage. He finally found another German massage practitioner, an instructor at the Viennese Massage School in Connecticut. This practitioner was able to relieve Meagher's pain to such a degree he was able to play semipro baseball back in his hometown of Gloucester, Massachusetts.

Over the next 15 years, Meagher did a lot of work giving massages, thinking about them, and putting those reflections into action. The result was sports massage. Just like the defined techniques he learned in Swedish massage, Meagher categorized the various techniques he used, including direct pressure, friction, compression, and percussion. He worked in a YMCA on professional athletes and other people who were devoted to a life of exercise.

Taking his experiment one step further, Meagher tried the techniques he regularly used on human athletes on racehorses. It was a resounding success. The horses he worked on won two gold medals and one silver medal at the 1976 Olympics. Soon, people were clamoring for Meagher's expertise. He was interviewed extensively and asked to write a book. The American Massage Therapy Association invited him to speak at a conference.

The resulting book was *Sports Massage: A Complete Program for Increasing Performance and Endurance in Fifteen Popular Sports,* which has become a classic sports massage text. It introduces specific techniques and breaks them down step-by-step for the student. It also contains Meagher's warm sense of humor and humility.

Meagher attributed his success not to any innate talent but rather to ordinary hard work and a strong desire to help others. He said, "One time a chief of orthopedics told me I had a real gift, and I had to disagree. Gifts come easily. What I do is not a gift. I work hard. I developed my instincts through my failures and my successes." This was his philosophy whether on the ball field, on the field of battle, or standing at the massage table, and whatever his failures might have been, his legacy is absolutely a resounding success.

REFERENCES

Behera, C., Devassy, S., Mridha, A. R., Chauhan, M., & Gupta, S. K. (2018). Leg massage by mother resulting in fatal pulmonary thrombo-embolism. *The Medico-Legal Journal, 86*(3), 146–150.

Cleveland Clinic. (2018). *Positions to reduce shortness of breath*. Retrieved from https://my.clevelandclinic.org/health/articles/9446-positions-to-reduce-shortness-of-breath.

Crump, C., Paluska, S.A. (2010). Venous thromboembolism following vigorous deep tissue massage. *The Physician Sportsmedicine, 38*(4), 136–139.

Jabr, F. (2007). Massive pulmonary emboli after legs massage. *American Journal of Physical Medicine & Rehabilitation, 86*(8), 691.

Lim, D., Jayanthi, H., Money-Kyrle, A., & Ramrakha, P. (2009). Massaging the outcome: an unusual presentation of pulmonary embolism. *BMJ Case Reports*, bcr0120091505.

Ng, A.H., Francis, G.J., Sumler, S.S., Liu, D., & Bruera, E. (2018). The efficacy and safety of massage therapy for cancer inpatients with venous thromboembolism. Journal of Integrative Oncology, 7(1), 203.

Salvo, S.G. (2022). Mosby's *pathology for massage professionals* (5th ed.). St Louis: Mosby.

BIBLIOGRAPHY

Abrahams, P. H., Spratt, J. D., Loukas, M., & van Schoor, A. N. (2003). *Abrahams' and McMinn's clinical atlas of human anatomy* (8th ed.). St Louis: Elsevier.

Applegate, E. (2010). *The anatomy and physiology learning system* (4th ed.). Philadelphia: Saunders.

Como, D. (Ed.). (2016). *Mosby's dictionary of medicine, nursing, and health professions* (10th ed.). St Louis: Elsevier.

Frazier, M. S., & Drzymkowski, J. W. (2015). *Essentials of human diseases and conditions* (6th ed.). St Louis: Elsevier.

Hubert, R. J., & VanMeter, K. C. (2018). *Gould's pathophysiology for the health professions* (6th ed.). Philadelphia: Saunders.

Haubrich, W. S. (2003). *Medical meanings: A glossary of word origins* (2nd ed.). New York: American College of Physicians.

Herlihy, B. (2017). *The human body in health and illness* (6th ed.). St Louis: Saunders.

Huether, S. E., McCance, K. L., Brashers, V. L. (2019). *Understanding pathophysiology* (7th ed.). St Louis: Mosby.

Kalat, J. W. (2013). *Biological psychology* (11th ed.). Belmont, Calif: Cengage Learning.

Kapit, W., & Elson, L. M. (2013). *The anatomy coloring book* (4th ed.). New York: Benjamin Cummings.

Kumar, V., Abbas, A. K., & Aster, J. C. (2015). *Robbins & Cotran pathologic basis of disease* (9th ed.). St Louis: Mosby.

Marieb, E. N., & Keller, S. M. (2018). *Essentials of human anatomy and physiology* (12th ed.). New York: Benjamin Cummings.

McCance, K. L., & Huether, S. E. (2019). *Pathophysiology: the biological basis for disease in adults and children* (8th ed.). St Louis: Mosby.

Myers, T. W. (2014). *Anatomy trains: Myofascial meridians for manual and movement therapists* (3rd ed.). Churchill Livingstone: Elsevier.

Netter, F. H. (2018). *Atlas of human anatomy* (7th ed.). St Louis: Mosby.

Patton, K. T (2019). *Anatomy and physiology* (10th ed.). St Louis: Elsevier.

Patton, K. T., Thibodeau, G.A., & Douglas, M. M. (2012). *Essentials of anatomy and physiology* (4th ed.). New York: Pearson.

Porter, R. S., (2011). *The Merck manual of diagnosis and therapy* (19th ed.). Whitehouse Station, NJ: Merck Sharp and Dohme Corp.

Taber, C. W. (2021). *Taber's cyclopedic medical dictionary* (24th ed.). Philadelphia: FA Davis.

REVIEW AND APPLY YOUR KNOWLEDGE

 MATCHING ONE: CONCEPT REVIEW
Place the letter of the answer next to the number of the term or phrase that best describes it.

A. Atria
B. Blood
C. Erythrocyte
D. Hemoglobin
E. Leukocyte
F. Mitral
G. Myocardium
H. Plasma
I. Thrombocyte
J. Type AB
K. Type O
L. Ventricles

_____ 1. Universal blood donor and this type is compatible with all blood types.
_____ 2. Heart layer containing cardiac muscle.
_____ 3. Blood cell that helps reduce blood loss from damaged vessel walls.
_____ 4. Blood cell that transports oxygen and carbon dioxide to and from body cells.
_____ 5. Fluid circulating through the heart and its vessels that transports nutrients to and wastes from cells.
_____ 6. Universal blood recipient and this type has blood that does not contain antigens.
_____ 7. Superior chambers of the heart.
_____ 8. Left atrioventricular heart valve.
_____ 9. Iron-based protein in red blood cells that gives blood its characteristic red color.
_____ 10. Straw-colored liquid in which blood cells are suspended.
_____ 11. Inferior chambers of the heart.
_____ 12. Blood cell that are part of the body's defense mechanisms.

MATCHING TWO: CONCEPT REVIEW
Place the letter of the answer next to the number of the term or phrase that best describes it.

A. Aorta
B. Cardiac cycle
C. Vena cavae
D. Blood pressure
E. Lumen
F. Pulmonary circuit
G. Systemic circuit
H. Sinoatrial node
I. Skeletal muscle pump
J. Capillaries
K. Hyperemia
L. Tachycardia

_____ 1. Path of blood that replenishes oxygen and eliminates carbon dioxide.
_____ 2. Path of blood that transports oxygen to body cells and transports carbon dioxide for their elimination.
_____ 3. Generates the nerve impulse in the heart that causes the muscles in the atria to contract.
_____ 4. Heartbeats over 100 per minute.
_____ 5. Functional units of the cardiovascular system and where gas exchange occurs between blood and body cells.
_____ 6. Squeeze-and-release action against venous walls that occurs as skeletal muscles contract and relax.
_____ 7. Amount of force exerted by blood on vessel walls as the left ventricle of the heart contracts and relaxes.
_____ 8. Largest veins in diameter.
_____ 9. Largest artery in diameter.
_____ 10. Increased local blood flow.
_____ 11. Space within blood vessels.
_____ 12. Sequence of events from the beginning of one heartbeat to the beginning of the next heartbeat.

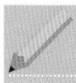

MULTIPLE CHOICE: TEST YOUR KNOWLEDGE

Place the letter of the answer next to the number of the term or phrase that best describes it.

_____ 1. The cardiovascular and lymphatic systems are regarded as _____ because of their function of transportation.
A. fight or flight
B. rest and digest
C. pick-up and delivery
D. stand and deliver

_____ 2. Which are red blood cells?
A. Erythrocytes
B. Leukocytes
C. Thrombocytes
D. Monocytes

_____ 3. What percentage of whole blood is liquid plasma?
A. 40%
B. 45%
C. 50%
D. 55%

_____ 4. Which is an electrolyte found in blood plasma?
A. Potassium
B. Oxygen
C. Glucose
D. Thrombus

_____ 5. What is the term for the process that stops bleeding and helps keep blood within damaged vessels?
A. Hematopoiesis
B. Hemoglobin
C. Hemostasis
D. Hemorrhage

_____ 6. The double-layered sac surrounding the heart is the:
A. pericardium
B. epicardium.
C. myocardium.
D. endocardium.

_____ 7. Which valve is between the left atrium and left ventricle?
A. Tricuspid
B. Bicuspid
C. Pulmonary
D. Aortic

_____ 8. The term that means irregular heart rate is:
A. anorexia.
B. sarcopenia.
C. arrhythmia.
D. ataxia.

_____ 9. Heart rate of less than 60 beats per minute is called:
A. tachycardia.
B. bradycardia.
C. atrial fibrillation.
D. ventricular fibrillation.

_____ 10. The normal range for a blood pressure reading is at or less than:
A. 140/90 mm Hg.
B. 90/140 mm Hg.
C. 120/80 mm Hg.
D. 80/140 mm Hg.

_____ 11. The blood vessels that supply blood to the brain, face, and neck are the:
A. subclavian arteries.
B. carotid arteries.
C. saphenous veins.
D. jugular veins.

_____ 12. What is the most common type of anemia?
A. Aplastic
B. Pernicious
C. Folate-deficiency
D. Iron-deficiency

CRITICAL THINKING

Watch That Blood Pressure

Your next client has indicated on his health history form he has hypertension. What is the best massage approach for this client?

Answers can include, but are not limited to:

You need to find out if the client's hypertension is being managed through diet, exercise, and medications. If it is, then the massage can proceed without modifications.

If the client's hypertension is not being managed successfully, then there are massage considerations to take into account. There is a chance certain massage techniques, such as trigger-point work or deep friction, can cause discomfort that may cause the client's heart rate to spike. Another area of concern is hypertension that is also called the "silent killer" because it can cause damage to body organs and structures without symptoms. It may be necessary to postpone massage until the client's blood pressure is under control, or it may be necessary to obtain clearance for massage from the client's healthcare provider. On the other hand, slow gentle techniques can be very relaxing for the client, and not cause a shift in blood pressure.

PROFESSIONAL PRACTICE

Congestive Heart Failure

Andre is a 55-year-old man who survived a heart attack a little over a year ago. About 4 months back, he was released by his cardiologist and began receiving weekly massages. Over his left pectoralis major muscle, he had a pacemaker inserted 3 months ago. Andre swims three times a week and is currently taking medications. When Andre arrives for his appointment today, he looks a little tired and pale. During the intake, he states he is fatigued, and you both decide a 30-minute massage is best.

As you pull back the sheet to place a bolster beneath his knees, you notice swelling around his ankles. You press your thumb into the skin, and as you pull your hand back to examine the area, your thumbprint remains for about 10 seconds. What modifications, if any, are needed?

DISCUSSION

Cardiac Medications and Massage

Heart disease and other cardiovascular disorders are the most prevalent diseases in industrialized countries. Without question, you will encounter clients with all manner of pathologies of the blood, heart, and blood vessels. Most of the clients will take medications to manage these conditions. Use the internet to locate two commonly used medications. List several side effects that might affect your massage treatment and indicate how you might modify your treatment. If available, post this information on an Internet-based discussion board monitored by your instructor.

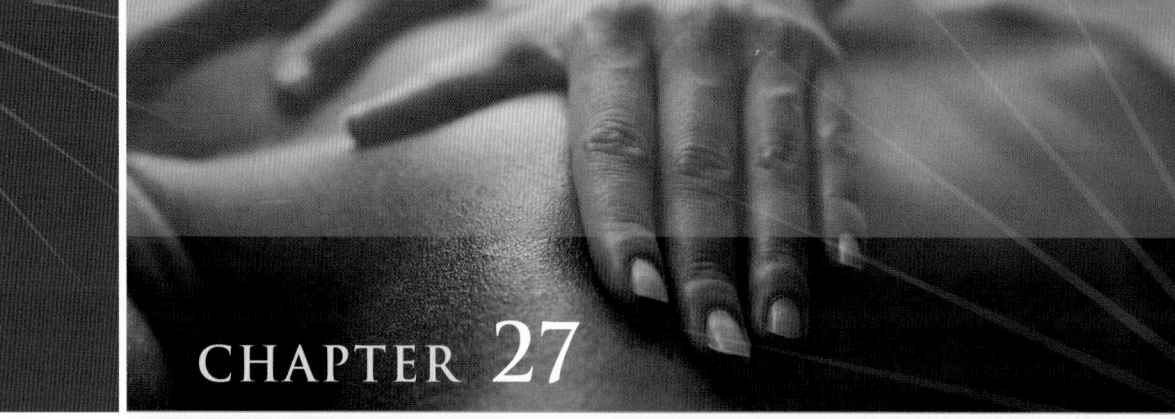

CHAPTER **27**

If you can't explain it simply, you don't understand it well enough.

—Albert Einstein

Lymphatic System, Pathologies, and Conditions

LEARNING OBJECTIVES

After completing this chapter, the student should be able to:

1. List anatomic structures; describe the physiologic processes of the lymphatic system; and discuss lymph, lymphatics, lymph movement, and lymphatic organs.
2. Discuss the body's resistance to disease, including nonspecific and specific mechanisms, immune dysfunctions, and diseases.
3. Describe lymphatic pathologies and conditions while stating their massage modifications.

http://evolve.elsevier.com/Salvo/MassageTherapy

INTRODUCTION

The lymphatic system is composed of lymph, lymphatics, lymph nodes, tissues, and organs. Each day, approximately 20 L of blood plasma flows through the arteries. However, only about 17 L are returned to the heart through the veins. The remaining 3 L leak through the capillary wall and into the surrounding tissues. The lymphatic system collects this excess tissue fluid and returns it to the bloodstream. The lymphatic system also moves select nutrients from the digestive tract, helps maintain fluid balance, and has disease-fighting functions. This chapter explores the lymphatic system and the body's defense responses. Use Table 27.1 to help you understand terms of the lymphatic system. *Immunology* is the study of the immune response.

ANATOMY

The basic anatomy of the lymphatic system includes:
- Lymph
- Lymphatics—the capillaries, vessels, trunks, and ducts
- Lymphatic structures—lymph nodes, bone marrow, thymus, and the spleen
- Lymphatic or lymphoid-related tissues—found in the gastrointestinal (GI) and the respiratory tract mucosae
- Lymphocyte—type of white blood cell

PHYSIOLOGY

Important functions of the lymphatic system are:
- Removes excess interstitial fluid—The lymphatic system collects accumulated interstitial fluid within tissue spaces and delivers this fluid into the bloodstream. This process helps prevent edema and maintains blood volume and blood pressure.
- Transports fats and fat-soluble vitamins—Specialized lymphatic vessels called *lacteals* in the small intestine absorb fats and fat-soluble vitamins from the GI tract and deliver them to the bloodstream.
- Protects the body through defense mechanisms—The lymphatic system helps defend the body against

disease-producing agents using barriers and specialized cells called lymphocytes.

LYMPH, LYMPHATICS, AND LYMPHATIC MOVEMENT

This section discusses lymph, lymphatics, and lymph movement through the body.

Lymph

One of the major ways the body maintains homeostasis is by the movement of fluid from the blood plasma to the interstitial spaces, to the lymphatic vessels, and then back to the blood plasma. **Lymph**, or *lymphatic fluid,* is the nearly colorless watery fluid in the lymphatic system. Lymph is made from interstitial fluid or fluid found between cells and tissues. When interstitial fluid enters lymphatic capillaries, it is called lymph. After lymph is filtered by lymph nodes, it is returned to the blood, becoming plasma once again. Therefore plasma, interstitial fluid, and lymph are basically the same fluid but called different names depending on where it is located. The composition of lymph continually changes as blood and surrounding cells continually exchange substances with the interstitial fluid.

Lymphatics

Lymphatics are all the lymphatic capillaries, vessels, trunks, and ducts along the lymphatic chain (Fig. 27.1). Lymph flows through lymphatics and enters the cardiovascular system at the right and left subclavian veins. With exception of the central nervous system, every organ of the body has a rich supply of lymphatics.

Lymph capillaries begin in the spaces between the tissues as close-ended sacs. Lymph capillaries are slightly larger in diameter compared with blood capillaries. The walls of lymph capillaries overlap to form a flapped one-way valve (Fig. 27.2). Attached to lymph capillaries are *anchoring fibers*, which secure the capillary to surrounding tissues. When tissues expand because of excess interstitial fluid, anchoring fibers become stretched, causing the flap to pull apart and open. This action allows surrounding interstitial fluid to enter the lymph capillary. When pressure inside the lymph capillary is greater compared with the surrounding tissues, the flap closes, preventing lymph from moving back into the interstitial spaces. **Lacteals** are lymphatic capillaries in fingerlike projections of the small intestines. Lacteals absorb dietary fats and fat-soluble vitamins (see Fig. 29.5).

Lymph capillaries merge with **lymphatic vessels**. These vessels contain internal valves that open in only one direction; this causes lymph in the capillary to move toward the center of the body (Fig. 27.3). There are more valves in lymph vessels compared with veins. Lymphatic vessels merge with larger structures called **lymphatic trunks**, which drain larger regions of the body. From here, lymph moves into one of two lymphatic ducts: right lymphatic duct and the thoracic duct. The distribution of lymphatics is like a tree with its progression

TABLE 27.1 Word Meanings	
WORD	**MEANING**
capillary	*L.* hairlike
cytotoxic	*Gr.* cell; poison
edema	*Gr.* swelling
immune	*L.* safe
macrophage	*Gr.* large; to eat
node	*L.* knot
phagocytosis	*Gr.* to eat; cell; condition
thymus	*Gr.* mind
vaccine	*L.* safe

Gr., Greek; *L.,* Latin

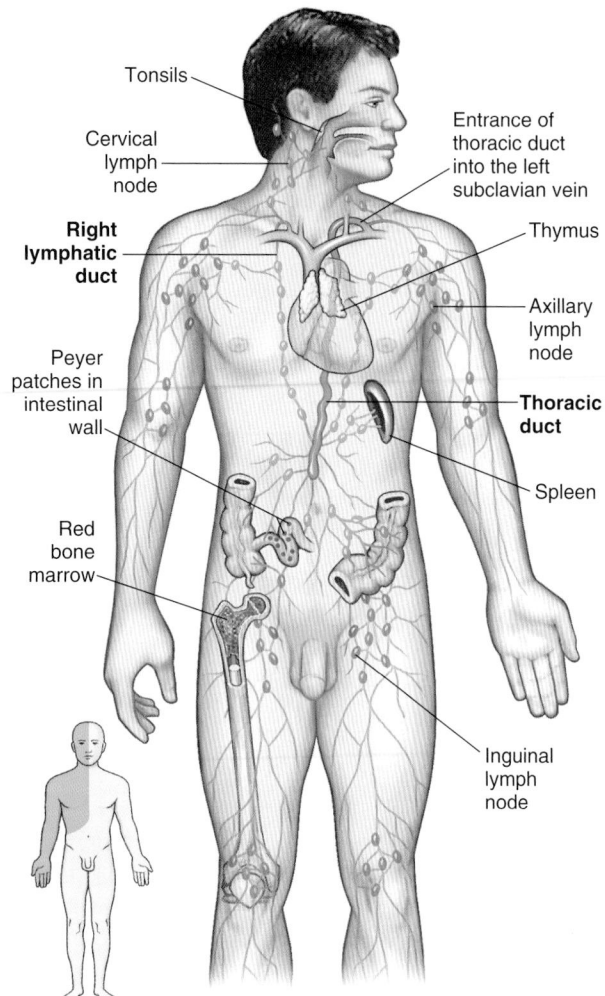

FIG. 27.1 The lymphatic system *(anterior view)*. Inset figure: green shading indicates areas drained by the right lymphatic duct. Blue shading indicates areas drained by the thoracic duct. (Modified from Patton, K., & Thibodeau, G. [2014]. *The human body in health and disease* [6th ed.]. St. Louis, MO: Mosby.)

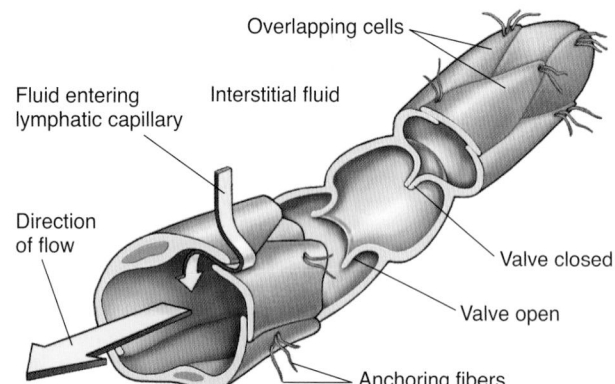

FIG. 27.2 A lymph capillary. Walls of lymph capillaries overlap to form a flap. Attached to lymph capillaries are anchoring fibers, which secures the lymph capillary wall to surrounding tissues. Valves help lymph move in one direction. (From Patton, K. T., & Thibodeau, G. A. [2010]. *Anatomy & physiology* [7th ed.]. St. Louis, MO: Mosby.)

from smaller twigs to bigger branches to finally larger trunks (see Fig. 27.1).

- **Right Lymphatic Duct**. This drains lymph from the right side of the head and neck, the right upper extremity, and the right half of the upper trunk and delivers it to the right subclavian vein.
- **Thoracic Duct**. This drains lymph from the rest of the body and delivers it to the left subclavian vein.

Movement of Lymph

Lymphokinesis is the movement of lymph through the body. The movement of lymph is different from the movement of blood in several ways. Lymph does not move in a circle. Instead, lymph flows in one direction toward two collecting ducts, entering the cardiovascular system at the right and left subclavian veins. The movement of lymph is slow and irregular compared with the movement of blood. Anything interfering with the flow of lymph, such as an obstruction, may cause fluids to accumulate, resulting in swelling.

Lymph does not have a centralized muscular pump such as the heart to help move it along its path. Lymph moves by the:

- Milking action of skeletal muscles;
- Pressure differences between the thoracic and abdominal cavities created by movements of the diaphragm and chest during breathing;
- Contraction and relaxation of smooth muscles within lymphatic walls;
- Presence of valves to help prevent backflow;
- Compressive forces such as massage, clothing, bandages, and hydrostatic pressure from water.

LYMPHOCYTES AND LYMPHATIC ORGANS

All blood cells, red blood cells or RBCs (erythrocytes), white blood cells or WBCs (leukocytes), and platelets (thrombocytes), are produced in red bone marrow. Twenty-five percent of WBCs are **lymphocytes**, cells vital to immune responses. Two types of lymphocytes are B-cells and T-cells.

- **B Lymphocytes (B-Cells)**. These cells remain in red bone marrow to complete their maturation. Once B-cells mature, they enter the bloodstream where they help the body defend itself against intruders.
- **T Lymphocytes (T-Cells)**. Some immature lymphocytes leave red bone marrow and travel to the thymus to complete their maturation. Once T-cells mature, they enter the bloodstream and travel to lymphatic organs where they facilitate defense mechanisms. The thymus produces thymosin and thymopoietin, hormones which stimulate the maturation of lymphocytes and their differentiation.

LEARNING TIP: To help you remember the difference between B-cells and T-cells, recall where they mature. **B**-cells mature in **bone marrow**. **T**-cells mature in the **thymus**.

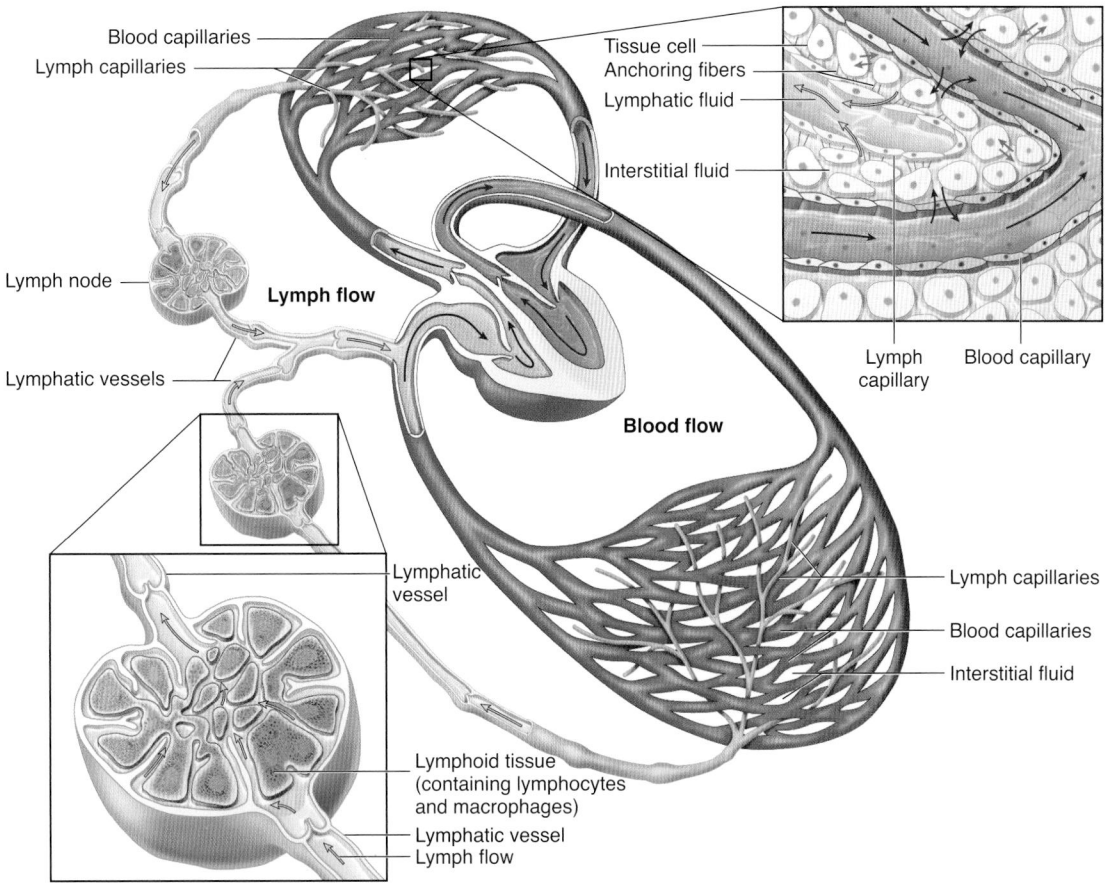

FIG. 27.3 The lymphatic system and how fluid enters the lymphatic system through a lymph capillary *(right image)* and how lymph flows through a node *(left image)*. (Modified from Patton, K., & Thibodeau, G. [2014]. *The human body in health and disease* [6th ed.]. St. Louis, MO: Mosby.)

Lymphatic organs are characterized by the presence of lymphocytes. Types of lymphatic organs are primary and secondary.

Primary Lymphatic Organs

Primary lymphatic organs are involved with the production and maturation of lymphocytes. Primary lymphatic organs are red bone marrow and the thymus (Fig. 27.4).

- **Red Bone Marrow.** This is in the spongy bone of the skeletal system.
- **Thymus.** This is behind the sternum in the chest area.

Secondary Lymphatic Organs and Structures

Secondary lymphatic organs and structures are populated by B-cells and T-cells. Secondary lymphatic organs include lymph nodes, mucosa-associated lymphoid tissue (MALT), and the spleen.

Lymph Nodes

Lymph nodes are bean-shaped structures found along the lymphatic chain (see Fig. 27.3). Lymph nodes filter lymph. In fact, lymph nodes are the only structures that filter lymph. As lymph moves through the node, pathogens, cancer cells, damaged cells, and cellular debris are destroyed or deactivated by

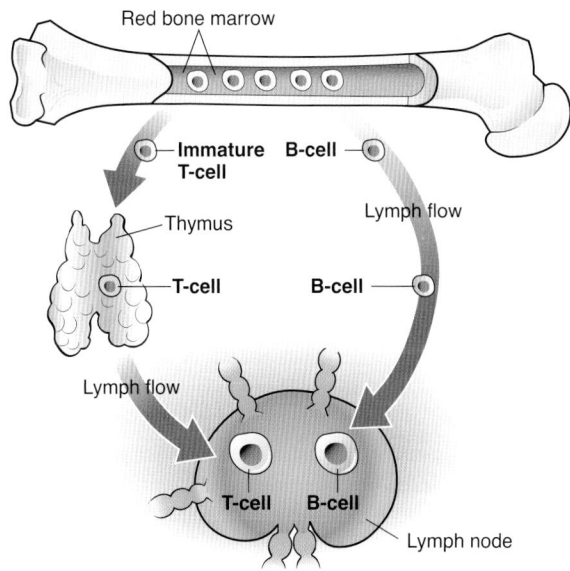

FIG. 27.4 B- and T-cells are formed in red bone marrow. Mature B-cells migrate to secondary lymphatic structures such as lymph nodes. T-cells complete their maturation in the thymus, and they also migrate to secondary lymphatic structures. (Adapted from McCance, K., & Huether, S. [2002]. *Pathophysiology* [4th ed.]. St. Louis, MO: Mosby. Patton, K. T., & Thibodeau, G. A. [2010]. *Anatomy & physiology* [7th ed.]. St. Louis, MO: Mosby.)

lymphocytes and macrophages present in the node. Lymph nodes may enlarge during infection. Several body regions contain clusters of superficial lymph nodes.

- **Cervical Lymph Nodes**. These are in the neck region.
- **Axillary Lymph Nodes**. These are in the armpit region.
- **Inguinal Lymph Nodes**. These are in the groin region.

Mucosa-Associated Lymph Tissues

MALTs are a collective term to describe small groups of lymphatic tissue along the respiratory and GI tracts. MALTs help protect the body from swallowed or inhaled pathogens and invaders.

- **Tonsils**. These are in the oral cavity and pharynx.
- **Peyer Patches**. These are in the small intestines and are also called *intestinal tonsils*.
- **Vermiform Appendix**. This is attached to the cecum, which is the first region of the large intestine.

Spleen

The **spleen** is the largest lymphatic organ and is in the upper left quadrant of the abdomen. Although much larger, the spleen resembles a lymph node and filters blood much like a lymph node filters lymph. Lymphocytes in the spleen react to pathogens in the blood and attempt to destroy or deactivate them. Macrophages engulf debris, damaged cells, and other microorganisms. The spleen releases stored lymphocytes when needed to assist in defense mechanisms. The spleen stores blood and can release small amounts into the bloodstream during blood loss. The spleen also destroys old, worn-out RBCs and is called the "graveyard of RBCs."

For peace of mind, resign as general manager of the universe.

—Larry Eisenberg

RESISTANCE TO DISEASE

Disease resistance is the body's ability to destroy or deactivate pathogens and foreign agents through defense mechanisms. In contrast, **disease susceptibility** is the lack of disease resistance and increased risk of acquiring disease. Two main defense mechanisms are nonspecific and specific. Immune dysfunctions and diseases can occur when immune responses are not working properly.

Nonspecific Defense Mechanisms

Nonspecific defense mechanisms target all pathogens and foreign agents. These defense mechanisms include barriers, cellular responses, and inflammation.

Barriers: Physical and Chemical

Physical and chemical barriers are the first line of defense. Intact unbroken skin and mucosa provide a physical barrier against many pathogens. Skin glands secrete sweat and sebum, which create a chemical barrier or hostile environment against many pathogens. Respiratory mucosae contain cilia,

which help move particles to be swallowed or pushed away by sneezing. Sticky mucus in the nose and mouth trap microorganisms, allowing them to be swallowed and destroyed by digestive enzymes and acids. Cerumen, or earwax, and hair in the ears and nose provide a physical barrier to foreign agents. Saliva, tears, and nasal secretions contain lysozyme, an enzyme with antibacterial properties. Vaginal secretions help maintain an acidic environment, which is inhospitable for many pathogens. Also, tears running over the eyes and urine flowing down the urethra flush microorganisms away from openings to these vulnerable areas.

Cellular Responses

Cellular responses are the body's second line of defense and are activated when microorganisms penetrate the body's first line of barrier defenses. Cellular responses include reactions from immune cells, nonimmune cells, and plasma proteins. Some WBCs destroy microorganisms through phagocytosis. The primary phagocytic cells are neutrophils and macrophages.

Some cells release cytokines, small proteins that control the immunologic and inflammatory responses of other cells. Some cytokines accelerate these responses and others slow down or reverse them, especially when they are out of control. Other cytokines recruit phagocytic cells to increase their numbers. Examples of cytokines are interleukins and interferons, the latter of which fight viral infections.

Cellular responses also include antigens found in blood plasma, called complementary proteins. These "complement" the ability of other cells to destroy pathogens and combat infection. Some antigens mark pathogens by coating them so antibodies can locate and destroy them later. Other antigens bore holes into pathogens such as bacteria, so their cell contents leak out, causing them to perish.

Inflammation

Inflammation is a protective response to tissue damage resulting from a variety of causes, including infection and trauma. The purpose of inflammation is to eliminate pathogens and foreign agents, remove damaged tissue, and prepare the area for repair. Inflammation can be classified by its extent as local or systemic, or by its duration as acute or chronic.

- **Local (Acute) Inflammation**. This type of inflammation is confined to a specific area. Characteristics of local inflammation are swelling, heat, a loss of function, redness, and pain. *LEARNING TIP:* To help you remember these, use the acronym **S-H-A-R-P** for **S**welling, **H**eat, **A** loss of function, **R**edness, and **P**ain. Acute inflammation is usually of short duration, lasting approximately 72 hours (3 days) after initial onset, but can last up to 5 days. Cytokines facilitate inflammation by promoting vasodilation, capillary permeability, and clotting mechanisms. Heat and redness occur during vasodilation as blood flows into the area. Swelling occurs as plasma moves into interstitial spaces. Swelling also causes pain from increased pressure. Loss of function may be associated with these events. Phagocytic cells destroy pathogens and foreign agents. Products of phagocytosis and other wastes combine with plasma to form *exudates,* substances accumulating and contributing to localized pain and swelling.

- **Subacute Inflammation**. Subacute inflammation can occur after acute inflammation. It is characterized by swelling and pain but lacks heat and redness. Subacute inflammation usually begins on day 4 and may last 2 to 6 weeks.

- **Systemic Inflammation**. This is widespread inflammation that may be associated with infection. Chemical mediators called *pyrogens* cause the hypothalamus to increase body temperature, causing fever. Fever also increases metabolism, facilitating inflammatory reactions. Systemic inflammation can range from 2 days to 2 weeks, depending on the cause. **Fever** is measured body temperature of 100.4°F (38°C) or higher. Fever is also called pyrexia. Normal body temperature ranges from 98°F to 100°F (36.5°C to 37.5°C).

- **Chronic Inflammation**. Chronic inflammation lasts longer than 2 weeks and may follow an unsuccessful acute inflammatory reaction. For example, if acute inflammation associated with a puncture wound later develops into a bacterial infection, this would be classified as chronic if it persists longer than 2 weeks. Chronic inflammation can occur as a distinct process without previous acute inflammation and is seen in cases of autoimmune diseases such as rheumatoid arthritis, respiratory diseases such as asthma, cardiovascular diseases such as atherosclerosis, and digestive diseases such as Crohn disease. Chronic inflammation is also found in some cancers such as lung and colorectal cancers.

If you listen long enough, the patient will tell you how to correct the problem.

—**William Osler**

Specific Defense Mechanisms

Specific defense mechanisms are the body's ability to develop immunity against specific pathogens and uses B lymphocytes (B-cells) and T lymphocytes (T-cells). **Immunity** is the body's ability to recognize and respond to pathogens and foreign agents. Once the body is exposed to a particular pathogen or foreign agent, it "remembers" and launches a quicker attack the next time the pathogen or foreign agent enters the body. This specific resistance, or immunity, is the third line of defense. Immunity can be acquired naturally from simple exposure or artificially by introducing substances into the body by vaccines.

T-Cells

T-cells attack pathogens or foreign agents directly by attaching themselves to their surfaces, often with the help of cytokines. This is called *cell-mediated immunity*. There are two main types of T-cells: helper T-cells and natural killer T-cells.

- **Helper T-cells**. These stimulate B-cells to make antibodies and increase the production of natural killer cells.

- **Natural Killer T-cells**. These cells kill abnormal cells such as tumor cells and cells that have already been infected by pathogens such as viruses.

Some T-cells are identified by the abbreviation CD, which means "cluster of differentiation." Examples are CD4 and CD8 cells. CD4 cells protect the body by activating other immune cells, including CD8 cells. CD8 cells, or *cytotoxic cells*, seek out and kill foreign cells such as cancer cells. CD4 and CD8 cell blood levels are often used to monitor the progression of HIV infection, discussed in the section "HIV Infection and AIDS."

B-Cells

B-cells do not directly attack invaders. They provide surveillance and produce proteins called *antibodies* that are specific to each pathogen or foreign agent. When antibodies encounter an invader, they mark it for destruction which will be carried out by other cells. This is called *antibody-mediated immunity*.

Immune Dysfunctions and Diseases

Dysfunctions of immunity can occur in several ways and include immunodeficiencies, hypersensitivities, and autoimmune diseases.

- **Immunodeficiencies**. These are failures of the immune response to protect the body from pathogens, causing increased risk of infections. Some immunodeficiencies are present at birth, but most arise later in life, such as AIDS discussed in the next section. Diabetes, advanced age, and chronic stress can also suppress immune responses and increase the risk of infections.

- **Hypersensitivities**. These are allergic reactions in which the body responds to harmless agents called *allergens* as if they were harmful. Allergies are discussed in the next section as well.

- **Autoimmune Diseases**. These occur from an inappropriate or excessive immune response. The body mistakenly attacks and destroys healthy tissue. Examples of autoimmune diseases are rheumatoid arthritis (involving synovial lining of joints), multiple sclerosis (involving myelin sheaths around neurons), and diabetes mellitus type 1 (involving pancreatic insulin-producing cells). These diseases are discussed in their respective chapters.

LYMPHATIC PATHOLOGIES AND CONDITIONS

Featured next are common pathologies and conditions of the lymphatic system alphabetically. Each item includes a brief description and their massage-related modifications. A more extensive list and related research is found in the current edition of *Mosby's Pathology for Massage Professionals* (2022).

Allergies

Allergies occur when the body's immune system overreacts to substances in the environment that are harmless to most people. Substances that cause allergic reactions are called allergens. There are several types of allergies such as *hay fever* (i.e., allergic rhinitis [see Chapter 28]), *sinusitis* and *asthma* (many cases are caused by allergens), *pet allergies*, *insect sting allergies*, *latex allergies*, *food allergies*, *drug allergies*, as well as *contact dermatitis* and *eczema* (i.e., allergic dermatitis and atopic dermatitis [see Chapter 22]).

The term *allergy* originally meant both aspects of the immune response—immunity, which is beneficial, and hypersensitivity, which is harmful. Now the term is used to indicate harmful immune responses and immunity to indicate its beneficial ones. Approximately 50 million people in the United States have allergies.

Allergies are classified as a hypersensitivity. The most harmful, but least common allergic reaction is anaphylaxis. *Anaphylaxis* is an acute allergic reaction that may include a swollen throat, chest tightness, shortness of breath, hives and, in severe cases, shock. If anaphylactic shock is not treated immediately, it can be fatal. Symptoms can occur within minutes of allergen exposure, but it can take up to an hour or longer. Anaphylaxis is more common in food allergies, insect stings, and drug allergies.

Massage and Allergies

Before the massage begins, ascertain environmental and product allergens; avoid contact between the client and the allergen if possible.

If the client is allergic to laundry detergents, eliminate contact with linens washed in the detergent identified. If clients are allergic to latex or wool, they may have an allergic reaction to products containing shea butter or lanolin, respectively. Latex allergies in particular have been linked to allergic reactions to shea butter caused by cross-reactivity (Grier, 2012). In these situations, avoid massage lubricants containing these ingredients and use a hypoallergenic lubricant. Avoid latex gloves on clients who have latex allergies.

If clients mention they have an epinephrine autoinjector such as an EpiPen with them, ask where it is in case it is needed. In addition, careful observation throughout treatment is recommended, noting possible allergic reactions such as skin reactions and changes in respiration. If signs and symptoms of anaphylaxis occur, call 911 immediately. Next, take steps to help keep the client safe and to prevent shock. Help your client lie down and elevate the feet approximately 12 inches. Loosen tight clothing. Cover the client with a blanket. Do not give the client anything to drink. If the client is not breathing or does not have a pulse, they may be in cardiac arrest, and you need to begin cardiopulmonary resuscitation (CPR).

Human Immunodeficiency Viral Infection

Human immunodeficiency viral infection is caused by HIV, a virus that destroys a type of T-cell called CD4. CD4 cells fight infection. The acronym "HIV" can refer to the virus or the infection. Over time, HIV can destroy so many CD4 cells that there is an increased risk of opportunistic infections (OI) and diseases, including cancer. *Opportunistic infections* (OI) are infections that are more common or more severe because of a weakened immune system. HIV can be transmitted through certain body fluids. A person is considered HIV-positive when blood tests positive for HIV antibodies, even if no symptoms are present. The three stages of HIV infection are:

- **Stage 1: Acute HIV Infection**. The first stage generally develops 2 to 4 weeks after initial infection. During this time, some people have flu-like symptoms, which last a few weeks. HIV multiplies rapidly and spreads throughout the body, and there is a slight drop in T-cell count. But most people are unaware they are infected at this stage, and the risk of HIV transmission to others is high.
- **Stage 2: Chronic HIV Infection**. In this stage, HIV is still active but reproduces at low levels, and many people do not have HIV-related symptoms. This is the longest stage, often described as the dormancy stage or clinical latency stage. People can still transmit HIV to others during this phase, but those taking antiretroviral therapy (ART) as prescribed and keep an undetectable viral load have little to no risk of transmitting HIV to their HIV-negative sexual partners. *Viral load* is a test measuring the amount of a virus in the blood. High viral loads are linked to disease progression and increased likelihood of opportunistic infections. For people taking ART as prescribed, this stage may last several decades. In people who are not taking ART, this period can last a decade or longer, but may progress to stage 3 as the viral load increases and T-cell levels decrease.
- **Stage 3: AIDS**. AIDS is the final and most severe phase of HIV infection. People with HIV are diagnosed with AIDS when they have a CD4 count of less than 200 cells/mm^3 (normal range is between 600 and 1000) or they develop opportunistic infections or diseases such as candida (fungal infection that causes thrush), pneumocystis carinii pneumonia or PCP (a lung infection), and certain cancers, including Kaposi sarcoma.

Massage and HIV Infection With AIDS

Determine if the client is robust or frail by applying Fried frailty criteria (2001), which include:
1. Slow walking speed
2. Muscle weakness evidenced by weak handgrip and sarcopenia
3. Self-reported exhaustion

4. Low level of physical activity
5. Underweight or unintentional weight loss

If clients have three or more of Fried's criteria, they are likely frail, which necessitates slowly applied light pressure. An example of light pressure is 3 on a 10-point pressure scale. Sessions may be shorter, with the client removing little if any clothing, and repositioning the client as little as possible. In general, individuals who are in the early stages of HIV infection are often robust, and individuals in later states of infection may be frail.

For all clients, inquire about areas to be avoided, including lesions, enlarged lymph nodes, and sites of most recent blood work. Ask about any secondary diseases (e.g., candida), which should be factored into the treatment plan. If the massage is given in the healthcare setting such as a hospital, follow all facilities guidelines when in direct contact with patients. Also, avoid forceful passive range of motion if the client has been inactive for prolonged periods because of possible reduced bone density.

Because the immune responses of these clients are deficient, they are more susceptible to infections. The practitioner is a greater health hazard to the HIV-infected client than the HIV-infected client is to the practitioner. If the practitioner has an infection such as a cold, they should reschedule the massage for the client's benefit.

Lymphedema and Edema

Both lymphedema and edema are swelling, but they have different causes. **Lymphedema** is swelling caused by removed or damaged lymphatic structures. Lymphedema usually affects a single limb, such as an arm or leg, and can be temporary or develop into a chronic condition. Infections are common complications of chronic lymphedema, especially if left untreated. These complications include *cellulitis* (bacterial infection of the skin and underlying tissues) and *lymphangitis* (bacterial infection of the lymph vessels). A small cut or wound in the affected limb can be an entry point for infection.

Edema is swelling caused by fluids moving from blood vessels into the interstitial spaces but, unlike lymphedema, the lymphatic system is intact and undamaged. Edema can occur anywhere in the body, but most cases are in the upper or lower extremities.

Lymphedema and edema can be pitting or nonpitting. *Pitting edema* leaves an indention or pit in the skin after firm digital pressure is applied for 2 to 3 seconds and removed. Most edema is nonpitting.

Lymphedema usually occurs from surgery or radiation therapy—lymphatic structures are removed or damaged during the process. Cancer cells or parasites can also enter lymph nodes, damaging them or blocking the flow of lymph. Edema is caused by a fluid imbalance as fluids move from the blood in blood vessels into interstitial spaces. Edema can occur from diet (salty foods or beverages), inactivity, recent injury, medication use (corticosteroids, nonsteroidal antiinflammatories, antihypertensives, hormone replacement

therapy [estrogens, insulin]), advanced pregnancy, or be a sign of underlying conditions such as liver, kidney, or cardiovascular disease.

Massage and Lymphedema

If you are not trained in lymphatic massage, avoid the area where lymph nodes have been surgically removed or damaged, and the area distal to this site (Ogawa, 2012). For example, if lymph nodes were removed or damaged in the left axillary region, do not massage the left arm, left forearm, or left hand. Massage pressure may exacerbate lymphedema.

Manual lymphatic drainage (MLD) techniques are beyond the scope of this book. The American Cancer Society (2016) recommends MLD as part of complex decongestive therapy for lymphedema resulting from cancer treatments.

Look for signs and symptoms of cellulitis, which include redness, warmth, and tenderness in the swollen area. If signs and symptoms of cellulitis are present, refer the client to a healthcare provider for medical evaluation. If left untreated, cellulitis may spread rapidly and become life-threatening.

Massage and Edema

For localized edema, place the affected area on cushions to raise it above the level of the heart. Elevation may facilitate *dependent drainage*, which uses gravity to stimulate movement of fluids from a higher area to a lower area. Light pressure effleurage and stretching of the skin may open lymph capillary valves, allowing interstitial fluid to enter. The recommended pressure to move lymph is approximately 5 g of pressure or about the weight of a nickel (Shepard, n.d.). Massage proximal to the affected area first, then proceed distally (e.g., massage the thigh, then the leg, then the ankle, and the foot last). In the upper extremities, lymph moves toward the armpit, and in the lower extremities, lymph moves toward the groin. All forms of thermotherapy (local heat applications and hot immersion baths such as spa tubs, steam baths, and saunas) are contraindicated because they can increase swelling.

Myalgic Encephalomyelitis/Chronic Fatigue Syndrome

Myalgic encephalomyelitis or **chronic fatigue syndrome** (ME/CFS) is a disorder characterized by extreme fatigue that is not relieved by rest and may worsen with physical or mental activity. Females are diagnosed more frequently than males and the age of diagnosis is between the ages of 30 and 50 years. ME/CFS is also called *systemic exertion intolerance disease* (SEID).

The cause of ME/CFS is unknown, but it appears to be linked to an overactive immune response. Other contributing factors are emotional stress, anemia, and a history of allergies or viral infections, including COVID-19 and Epstein-Barr virus, and hormonal imbalances.

Massage and Myalgic Encephalomyelitis/Chronic Fatigue Syndrome

Gentle to moderate pressure is recommended to avoid fatigue after treatment (Espejo et al., 2018). For returning clients, ask how they responded to the previous massage, making appropriate treatment modifications that may include changes in technique pressure and speed or changes in session duration. Because the client may have orthostatic hypotension, or dizziness from a drop in blood pressure when moving to an upright position, ask the client to arise from the massage table in three stages: (1) sit up on the table for 1 minute; (2) sit on the side of the table with legs dangling for 1 minute; and (3) stand with care, holding on to the edge of the table or other nonmovable object for 1 minute.

Systemic Lupus Erythematosus

Systemic lupus erythematosus (SLE or lupus) is a chronic autoimmune, inflammatory disease affecting the body's connective tissues. SLE commonly affects skin, joints, brain, kidneys, lungs, and other organs. Blood and blood vessels are often involved, leading to Raynaud disease, and reduced levels of red blood cells, white blood cells, and platelets (anemia, neutropenia, and thrombocytopenia, respectively). Lupus is the most common autoimmune disease, with periods of remission and exacerbation, which is typical with most autoimmune diseases. SLE may appear suddenly or take years to develop. SLE is also called *disseminated lupus erythematosus*.

Massage and Lupus

Massage is contraindicated during periods of exacerbation, or fever. During periods of remission, a gentle massage is indicated (Lupus Foundation of America [LFA], 2013). Use emollient lubricants to combat dry skin and avoid products containing alcohol. For returning clients, ask how they responded to the previous massage, making appropriate treatment modifications that may include changes in technique pressure and speed or changes in session duration. Coexisting medical conditions (Raynaud disease) should be factored into the treatment plan.

E-RESOURCES

http://evolve.elsevier.com/Salvo/MassageTherapy

- Chapter challenge
- Flash cards

EMIL VODDER

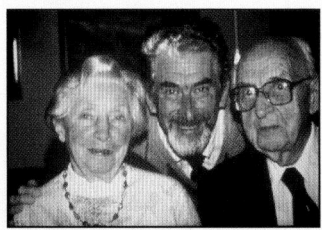

© Georg Thieme Verlag, Stuttgart

Sometimes, if you want to learn something nobody's talking about, you must search for answers in unusual places. For Emil Vodder, it was etchings of the lymphatic system created painstakingly by anatomists hundreds of years before he was born. This information had once been cutting edge but was uninteresting and pedestrian by the time Vodder developed his fascination with the movement of lymph. Today, lymphatic therapy has become an exciting area of study again, thanks to Vodder's creative quest for knowledge.

Vodder was born in 1896 in Copenhagen, Denmark. His education was initially focused on art, art history, and languages, but he then went on to study medicine at the University of Copenhagen. Midway through his program he became ill with malaria, and the university chose not to readmit him when he recovered, although he did receive a PhD from the University of Bruxelles in 1928.

Emil married a naturopathic doctor, Estrid, in 1925, and in 1929 the couple moved to France. They observed many of the patients who came to them with sinusitis and chronic colds had swollen lymph nodes. Might lymph be an essential part of immunity? Was it possible, by treating lymph nodes directly, one could improve immune function and help the body return to homeostasis? It was questions such as these that drove Vodder deeper into the study of human lymphatics.

Vodder read the papers and studied the drawings made when the lymphatic system was first being discovered and mapped. He came to believe lymph came from the loose connective tissue of the body: These tissues were present everywhere in the body, much as lymph was. As such, lymphatic congestion in one part of the body would negatively affect the entire body, and relieving it would result in a similarly universal positive effect.

At the time, direct treatment of the lymph nodes was rarely done, and often warned against. There was a concern that such treatment would cause toxins to spread throughout the body (a myth still circulated by misinformed massage practitioners today). The Vodders persisted in their research and gradually developed the gentle lymphatic drainage protocols still used today.

In 1936, Vodder had the opportunity to present his findings at a congress in Paris. They were not well received. In addition to flying in the face of conventional understanding about the lymphatic system, Vodder's credentials were called into question, as he was neither a medical doctor nor a physical therapist, or even a massage practitioner. Still the Vodders persisted, presenting here and there as the opportunities arose.

With the outbreak of World War II, the Vodders returned home to Copenhagen. Although their public presentations were curtailed by the war, this gave them more time to practice and refine their techniques. By the end of the war, Vodder started to receive invitations to teach, although his lack of credibility as a researcher still prevented his theories from being widely adopted.

This began to change in the 1960s, when Dr. Johannes Asdonk took an interest in Vodder's work. Using the statistical results from more than 2000 case studies, Asdonk developed a list of therapeutic applications, contraindications, and cautions for Vodder's method of lymphatic therapy. Together, Emil and Enid Vodder, Dr. Asdonk, and Gunther Wittlinger founded The Association of Dr. Vodder's Manual Lymphatic Drainage in 1967.

It was in 1976 that Vodder's methods finally received the final boost in credibility they had been waiting for. H. Mislin, a Swiss professor, published his research, titled "Active Contractility of the Lymphangion and Coordination of Lymphagion Chains." His findings about the nature of lymphangions, the functional units of lymphatic vessels, fully supported Vodder's theories, leading to their wider acceptance.

In 1985, Vodder was awarded the Rohrbach Medal by the German Massage and Physical Therapy Association. He died 1 year later, just days before his 80th birthday. Enid lived to be 99. The techniques they developed, once so controversial, are now used by professionals ranging from massage practitioners to speech pathologists to medical doctors. We no longer have to dig through centuries-old texts to learn about the impact the lymphatic system has on health and well-being, thanks to the commitment and thirst for knowledge of Emil Vodder.

REFERENCES

American Cancer Society. (2016). *For people with lymphedema*. Retrieved from https://www.cancer.org/treatment/treatments-and-side-effects/physical-side-effects/lymphedema/for-people-with-lymphedema.html.

Espejo, J. A., García-Escudero, M., & Oltra, E. (2018). Unraveling the molecular determinants of manual therapy: An approach to integrative therapeutics for the treatment of fibromyalgia and chronic fatigue syndrome/myalgic encephalomyelitis. *International Journal of Molecular Sciences, 19*(9), 2673.

Fried, L. P., Tangen, C. M., Walston, J., Newman, A. B., Hirsch, C., Gottdiener, J., et al. (2001). Frailty in older adults: Evidence for a phenotype. *The Journal of Gerontology Series: A Biological Sciences and Medical Sciences, 56*(3), 146–156.

Grier, T. (2012). *Is there cross-reactivity between shea butter and natural rubber latex?* American Latex Allergy Association, The Alert Newsletter. Retrieved from http://www.latexallergyresources.org/sites/default/files/newsletter-attachments/The%20ALERT%20Dec%202012.pdf.

Lupus Foundation of America. (2013). *Is massage therapy safe with cutaneous lupus?* Retrieved from https://www.lupus.org/resources/is-massage-therapy-safe-with-cutaneous-lupus.

Ogawa, Y. (2012). Recent advances in medical treatment for lymphedema. *Annals of Vascular Diseases, 5*(2), 139–144.

Salvo, S. G. (2022). *Mosby's pathology for massage professionals* (5th ed.). St Louis: Mosby.

Shepard, J. (n.d.). *What is lymph drainage therapy: What does it offer?* Retrieved from https://chiklyinstitute.com/sites/default/files/articles/What%20is%20Lymph%20Drainage%20Therapy%3B%20What%20Does%20it%20OfferJane%20Shepard%2C%20M.Ed_.%2C%20L.L.C.C%2C%20New%20Visions%20Magazine%2C%202001.pdf.

BIBLIOGRAPHY

Abrahams, P. H., Spratt, J. D., Loukas, M., & van Schoor, A. N. (2003). *Abrahams' and McMinn's clinical atlas of human anatomy* (8th ed.). St Louis: Elsevier.

Applegate, E. (2010). *The anatomy and physiology learning system* (4th ed.). Philadelphia: Saunders.

Como, D. (Ed.), (2016). *Mosby's dictionary of medicine, nursing, and health professions* (10th ed.). St Louis: Elsevier.

Frazier, M. S., & Drzymkowski, J. W. (2015). *Essentials of human diseases and conditions* (6th ed.). St Louis: Elsevier.

Haubrich, W. S. (2003). *Medical meanings: A glossary of word origins* (2nd ed.). New York: American College of Physicians.

Herlihy, B. (2017). *The human body in health and illness* (6th ed.). St Louis: Saunders.

Hubert, R. J., & VanMeter, K. C. (2018). *Gould's pathophysiology for the health professions* (6th ed.). Philadelphia: Saunders.

Huether, S. E., McCance, K. L., & Brashers, V. L. (2019). *Understanding pathophysiology* (7th ed.). St Louis: Mosby.

Kalat, J. W. (2013). *Biological psychology* (11th ed.). Belmont, CA: Cengage Learning.

Kapit, W., & Elson, L. M. (2013). *The anatomy coloring book* (4th ed.). New York: Benjamin Cummings.

Kumar, V., Abbas, A. K., & Aster, J. C. (2015). *Robbins & Cotran pathologic basis of disease* (9th ed.). St Louis: Mosby.

Marieb, E. N., & Keller, S. M. (2018). *Essentials of human anatomy and physiology* (12th ed.). New York: Benjamin Cummings.

McCance, K. L., & Huether, S. E. (2019). *Pathophysiology: The biological basis for disease in adults and children* (8th ed.). St Louis: Mosby.

Myers, T. W. (2014). *Anatomy trains: Myofascial meridians for manual and movement therapists* (3rd ed.). Churchill Livingstone: Elsevier.

Netter, F. H. (2018). *Atlas of human anatomy* (7th ed.). St Louis: Mosby.

Patton, K. T. (2019). *Anatomy and physiology* (10th ed.). St Louis: Elsevier.

Patton, K. T., Thibodeau, G. A., & Douglas, M. M. (2012). *Essentials of anatomy and physiology* (4th ed.). New York: Pearson.

Porter, R. S., (2011). *The Merck manual of diagnosis and therapy* (19th ed). Whitehouse Station, NJ: Merck Sharp and Dohme Corp.

Taber, C. W. (2021). *Taber's cyclopedic medical dictionary* (24th ed.). Philadelphia: FA Davis.

REVIEW AND APPLY YOUR KNOWLEDGE

MATCHING ONE: CONCEPT REVIEW

Place the letter of the answer next to the number of the term or phrase that best describes it.

A. Inguinal
B. Lymph
C. Lymph nodes
D. Lymphatics
E. Lymphokinesis
F. Peyer patches
G. Right lymphatic duct
H. Spleen
I. Thoracic duct
J. Thymus
K. Tonsils
L. Vermiform appendix

_____ 1. Term for superficial lymph nodes in the groin.
_____ 2. Duct that drains lymph from the right side of the head and neck, the right upper extremity, and the right half of the upper trunk.
_____ 3. Lymphatic tissue in portions of the small intestine.
_____ 4. Lymphatic tissue in the oral cavity and pharynx.
_____ 5. Only structure along the lymphatic chain that filters lymph.
_____ 6. Movement of lymph through the body.
_____ 7. Lymphatic tissue attached to the cecum of the large intestine.
_____ 8. Fluid in the lymphatic system.
_____ 9. Duct that delivers collected lymph to the left subclavian vein.
_____ 10. Largest lymphatic organ that releases stored lymphocytes when needed.
_____ 11. Collective term for all lymphatic capillaries, vessels, trunks, and ducts along the lymphatic chain.
_____ 12. Site of T-cell maturation.

MATCHING TWO: CONCEPT REVIEW

Place the letter of the answer next to the number of the term or phrase that best describes it.

A. Immunodeficiency
B. B-cells
C. Bone marrow and thymus
D. Disease resistance
E. Immunity
F. Inflammation
G. Lymphocyte
H. Lacteal
I. Nonspecific
J. Lymph nodes, MALTs, and spleen
K. Specific
L. T-cells

_____ 1. Lymphocytes responsible for cell-mediated immunity and includes CD4 and CD8 cells.
_____ 2. Type of defense mechanism that includes barriers, cellular responses, and inflammation.
_____ 3. Failure of immune responses to protect the body from pathogens, causing increased risk to infections.
_____ 4. Type of cell that comprises approximately 25% of the total WBC count.
_____ 5. The body's ability to counteract the effects of pathogens and foreign agents through defense mechanisms.
_____ 6. Lymphatic capillary in the small intestine that absorbs dietary fats and fat-soluble vitamins.
_____ 7. Type of defense mechanism that provides immunity and involves lymphocytes.
_____ 8. Secondary lymphatic organs and structures that are populated by lymphocytes, but do not produce them.
_____ 9. Primary lymphatic organs that produce and mature lymphocytes.
_____ 10. The body's ability to destroy or deactivate pathogens and foreign agents.
_____ 11. Protective response to tissue damage from a variety of causes and creates an environment that maximizes tissue repair.
_____ 12. Lymphocytes responsible for antibody-mediated immunity because they produce antibodies.

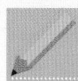

MULTIPLE CHOICE: TEST YOUR KNOWLEDGE

Place the letter of the answer next to the number of the term or phrase that best describes it.

_____ 1. Which cells are vital to immune responses?
A. Osteocytes
B. Lymphocytes
C. Erythrocyte
D. Oocytes

_____ 2. The colorless watery fluid that circulates through the body is called _____ when it is between cells and tissues.
A. lymph
B. blood plasma
C. interstitial fluid
D. synovial fluid

_____ 3. Which gland is behind the sternum in the chest area?
A. Pineal
B. Thyroid
C. Parathyroids
D. Thymus

_____ 4. Axillary lymph nodes are found in the ____ region.
A. neck
B. armpit
C. groin
D. knee

_____ 5. The spleen is in the _____ abdominal quadrant.
A. upper left
B. lower left
C. upper right
D. lower right

_____ 6. What organ is known as the "graveyard of red blood cells"?
A. Thymus
B. Spleen
C. Gallbladder
D. Pancreas

_____ 7. The lack of disease resistance and increased risk of acquiring disease is called:
A. immunity.
B. inflammation.
C. disease compliance.
D. disease susceptibility.

_____ 8. Which of the following occurs from an inappropriate or excessive immune response and the body mistakenly attacks and destroys healthy tissue?
A. Deficiency disease
B. Autoimmune disease
C. Metabolic disease
D. Degenerative disease

_____ 9. B-cells produce proteins called _____, which are specific to each pathogen or foreign agent.
A. cytotoxic cells
B. helper cells
C. antibodies
D. pyrogens

_____ 10. Another term for allergic reactions is:
A. immunodeficiency.
B. hypersensitivity.
C. autoimmunity.
D. antibody.

_____ 11. What is the term for an infection that is more common or more severe because of a weakened immune system?
A. Opportunistic
B. Cytotoxic
C. Anaphylactic
D. Lymphatic

_____ 12. Most harmful, but least common allergic reactions is called:
A. inflammation.
B. immunity.
C. phagocytosis.
D. anaphylaxis.

CRITICAL THINKING

Just What Type of Swelling Is This?

Esther is 46 years old and has arrived at Trevor's office for a massage. She has noticed her left ankle has been swollen lately. It is slightly swollen in the mornings, then gradually gets worse throughout the day. A friend of Esther's said Trevor had been able to relieve her swollen ankles with massage, so Esther thought she would give it a try. Trevor does an initial assessment of Esther's swollen ankle and notices a slight rash just proximal to it. He asks Esther if the area is tender, and she says it is more itchy than tender, but she does feel some discomfort. How should Trevor proceed?

Answers can include but are not limited to:

It is possible that Esther's swollen ankle is because of lymphedema, and the slight rash is cellulitis. For lymphedema, massage practitioners must screen the client for cellulitis. Cellulitis, a localized bacterial infection of the skin and underlying tissues, is a common complication of lymphedema. It is characterized by localized swelling, redness, warmth, abscess formation, and tender skin. The area of redness tends to expand over time, and red lines or streaks may appear proximal to the infection site or run along lymphatics. Systemic symptoms such as fever or malaise may develop. If the massage practitioner notices signs and symptoms of cellulitis in the affected limb, massage should not be done, and the client should be urged to seek medical attention immediately. If left untreated, cellulitis may spread rapidly and become life-threatening.

It is also possible that the rash is unrelated to Esther's swollen ankle, and she does not have lymphedema. In cases of edema rather than lymphedema, the massage practitioner should place the affected area on cushions to raise it above the level of the heart. Elevation may help promote dependent drainage or drainage from a higher area to a lower area under the influence of gravity. Light perpendicular and parallel pressure and stretching of the skin may open lymph capillaries, allowing interstitial fluid to enter the lymph capillaries. The massage practitioner should be sure that pressure is gradually moving in the direction of lymphatic flow. In the upper extremities, lymph moves toward the armpit and, in the lower extremities, toward the groin. Consider any coexisting medical conditions (cancer, congestive heart failure, cirrhosis, kidney disease) in the treatment plan. In addition, using heat and all forms of thermotherapy is contraindicated because it can increase swelling.

However, it is out of Trevor's scope of practice to determine whether Esther has lymphedema and cellulitis. The most appropriate course of action for Trevor is to refer Esther to her healthcare provider.

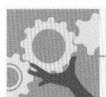

PROFESSIONAL PRACTICE
Lupus

Judy is a client referred to you by a local lupus support group. She was diagnosed with systemic lupus erythematosus when she was in her late 20. This was about 5 years ago. Because Judy is quite familiar with the disease, she calls you to make an appointment when her condition is in remission. She requests an appointment right away, because it is impossible to predict how long the remission state will last. You can see her today at 4 PM. Judy arrives with a big smile. She walked a mile this morning and swam a few laps after lunch, so she has good vitality. You inquire about any skin rashes; she shows you a reddish, slightly raised rash over her cheeks and across her nose. Judy also brushes her fingertips between her left and right clavicles and says there is a rash there. What are some treatment guidelines appropriate for Judy today?

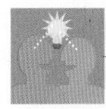

DISCUSSION
Indication or Contraindication?

During a massage session, you notice lymph nodes in your client's neck and armpits are swollen. Should you continue the massage as usual, alter the routine, or discontinue the massage entirely? What guides your decision? If available, post your reflections on an internet-based discussion board monitored by your instructor.

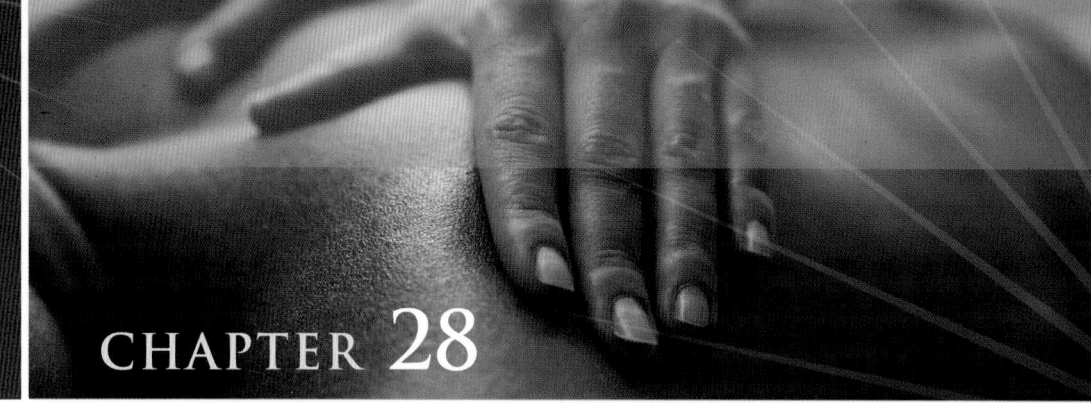

CHAPTER 28

Respiratory System, Pathologies, Conditions, and Disorders

When you own your breath, nobody can steal your peace.

— Author Unknown

LEARNING OBJECTIVES

After completing this chapter, the student should be able to:

1. List anatomic structures and the physiologic process of the respiratory system and describe specific structures of the upper and lower respiratory tracts.
2. Discuss breathing, respiration, and reflexes that affect breathing.
3. Name types of pathologies, conditions, and disorders of the respiratory system, giving massage modifications for each.

http://evolve.elsevier.com/Salvo/MassageTherapy

INTRODUCTION

Breathing has long been the inspiration of poets and philosophers. Books are filled with respiratory references, such as his dying breath, her breath rose and fell, his breath quickened, and he breathed life into them. Breathing is synonymous with life itself and is the most easily observed vital signs. Slow deep breathing can activate the parasympathetic nervous system, facilitating relaxation. Through the processes of respiration, we inhale air, extract oxygen from it, and exhale air filled with carbon dioxide and other wastes. Every cell needs oxygen, and the respiratory and cardiovascular systems work together to accomplish this via the bloodstream. Failure of either system has similar effects on the body—disruption of homeostasis and rapid cell death from oxygen deprivation and waste accumulation. Use Table 28.1 to help you understand terms of the respiratory system.

The respiratory tract moves air between the nose and the lungs and is divided into the upper and lower respiratory tracts. Accessory structures include the ribcage, the diaphragm, and other respiratory muscles (Fig. 28.1). *Phlegm* is mucus secreted by the respiratory tract, whereas *sputum* is phlegm mixed with saliva from the digestive tract. *Pulmonology* is the study of the respiratory system.

ANATOMY

The basic anatomy of the respiration system is:
- Nasal cavity
- Pharynx
- Larynx
- Trachea
- Bronchi
- Alveoli
- Lungs

TABLE 28.1 Word Meanings

WORD	MEANING
alveoli	*L.* little hollow
bronchus	*Gr.* windpipe
cilia	*L.* hairlike
conchae	*Gr.* shell
eustachian	Bartolomeo Eustachio, Italian anatomist (1524–1574)
glottis	*Gr.* mouthpiece of a pipe
meatus	*L.* passage
olfaction	*L.* to smell
pleura	*Gr.* rib; side
pneumo, pneum	*Gr.* air; lungs
pulmo	*L.* lung
ventilation	*L.* to air
volitional	*L.* will

Gr., Greek; *L.,* Latin.

PHYSIOLOGY

Important functions of the respiratory system are:
- Exchange of gases—Exchange of oxygen and carbon dioxide gases is the main function of the respiratory system.
- Olfaction—**Olfaction** is the sense of smell. Scent molecules enter the nose as we inhale. These molecules are forced against the olfactory nerves in the nasal cavity. Impulses travel from the olfactory nerves to the temporal lobe in the brain, which interprets the information (see Fig. 23.21).
- Sound production—Sound is produced by air moving over the vocal cords, causing them to vibrate. This action, combined with movements of the lips, facial muscles, and tongue, helps form words that produce speech. Nonspeech sounds such as gasping, sighing, moaning, laughing, and crying are also produced by the respiratory system; these sounds are essential for emotional expression.
- Maintains homeostasis—The respiratory system helps maintain homeostasis by supplying the body with oxygen and eliminating carbon dioxide and other gaseous wastes. Breathing also helps regulate blood pH by eliminating carbon dioxide.

UPPER RESPIRATORY TRACT

The upper respiratory tract includes the nasal cavity, the pharynx, and the larynx.

Nasal Cavity

The **nasal cavity** is the hollow space in the skull separated into right and left halves by a septum. The *anterior nares,* or nostrils, are the entrance into the nasal cavity, and the *posterior nares* are the nasal entrance into the pharynx. The walls of the nasal cavity contain ridged projections called *conchae* and grooved passageways called *meatuses.* A meatus lies beneath each of the conchae (Fig. 28.2).

Air enters the nasal cavities by inhalation. Air is warmed as it passes over superficial blood vessels, is moistened by mucus-producing *goblet cells,* and cleansed by passing over nasal hairs, which trap airborne particles. These particles become stuck in the mucus and are transported to the pharynx, where they are swallowed or expelled through coughing or sneezing. Hair-like projections of the mucosae called *cilia* help with these processes. The nasal cavity is often referred to as the "air-conditioning chambers" because of these functions. Because the nasal mucosa contains numerous superficial blood vessels, nosebleeds, or *epistaxis,* can occur from pressure or irritation on these vessels. Although they are dramatic, nosebleeds are seldom serious.

Paranasal Sinuses

Paranasal sinuses, or *sinuses,* are air-filled spaces lined with mucosa that open into the nasal cavities. Sinuses lighten the

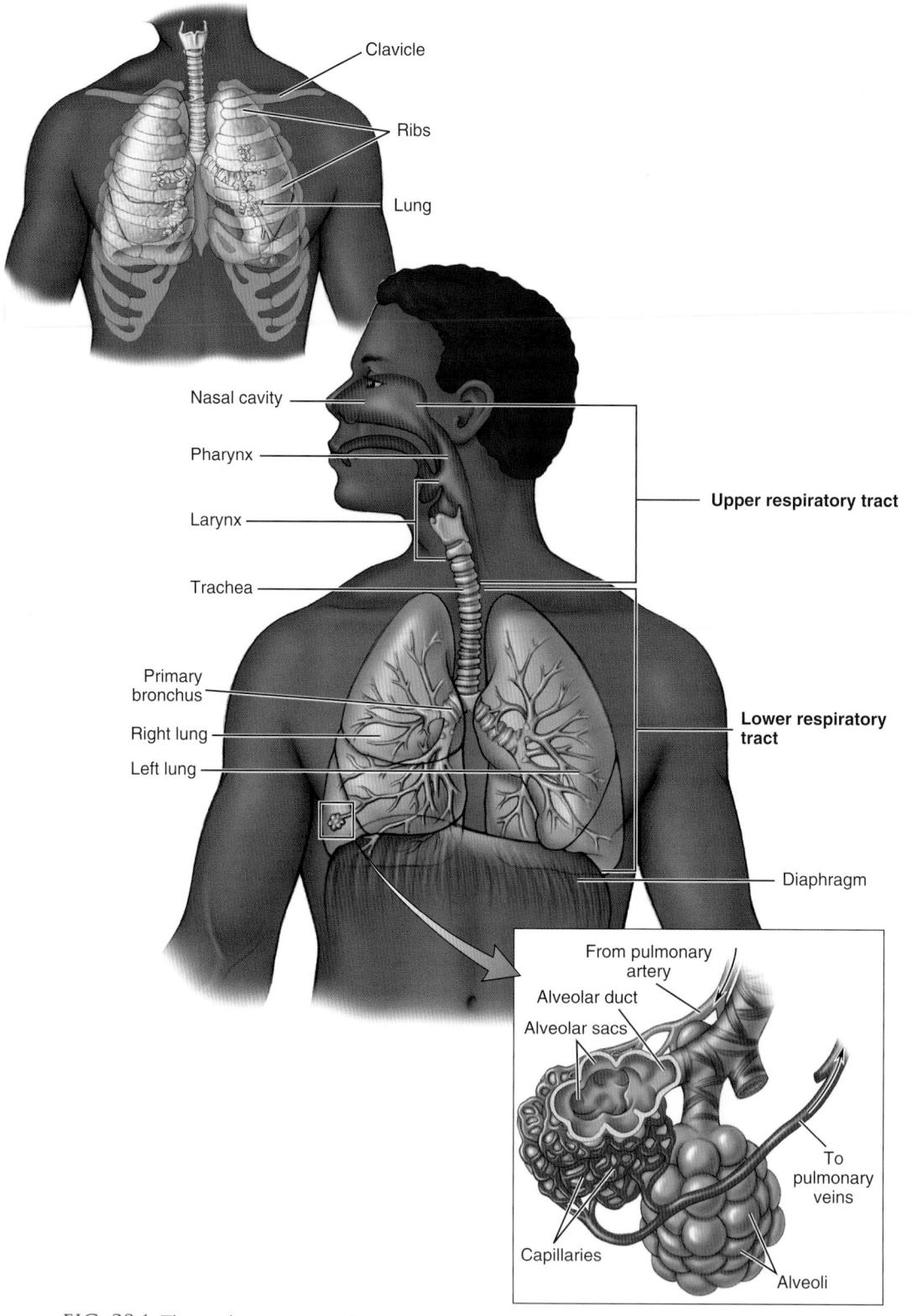

FIG. 28.1 The respiratory system. Upper and lower respiratory tracts, anterolateral view *(middle image)*, location of the lungs within the thorax *(superior image)*, and blood circulation to and from the alveoli *(inferior image)*. (From Herlihy, B. [2010]. *The human body in health and illness* [4th ed.]. St. Louis, MO: Saunders.)

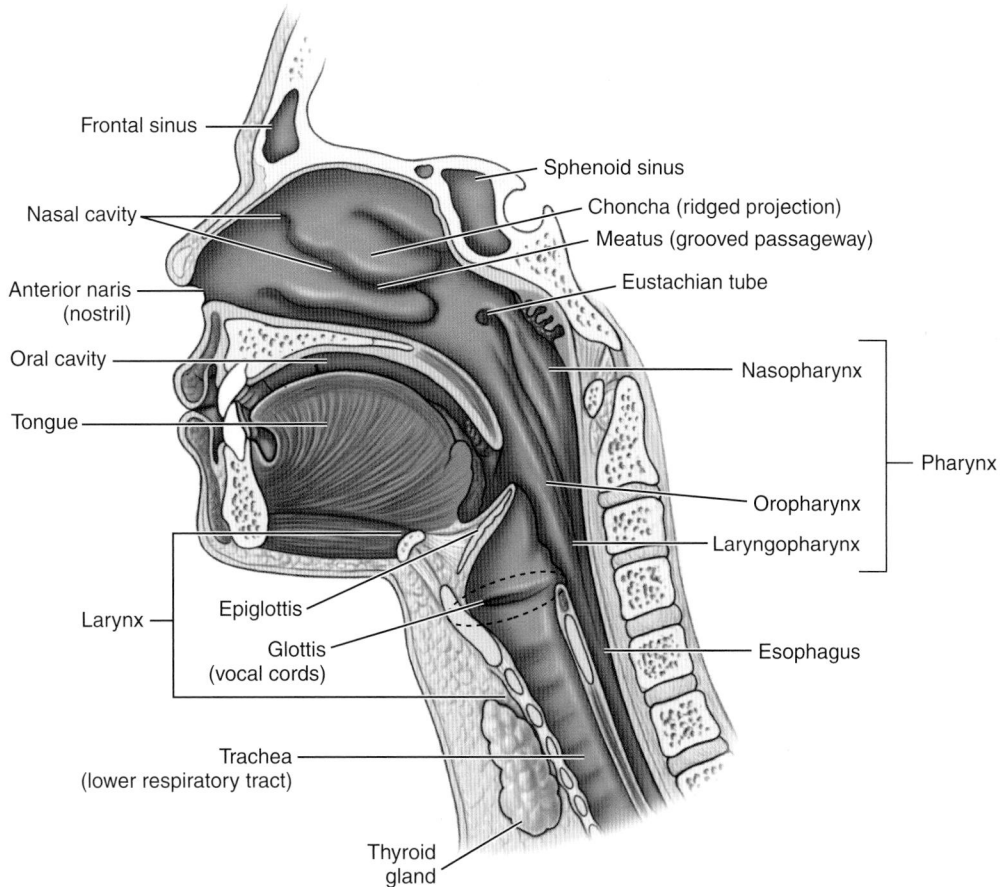

FIG. 28.2 Upper respiratory tract *(lateral view)*. (From Herlihy, B. [2010]. *The human body in health and illness* [4th ed.]. St. Louis, MO: Saunders.)

skull, act as resonance chambers for sound, and are named for the bones where they are located (Fig. 28.3).

- **Frontal Sinuses.** These are superior to the eyebrows.
- **Sphenoid Sinuses.** These are posterior to the eyes.
- **Ethmoid Sinuses.** These are between the nasal cavities and the eyes, and are essentially a collection of small air cells opening into the nasal cavities.
- **Maxillary Sinuses.** These are the largest and are inferior to the cheeks and superior to the teeth.

Pharynx

The **pharynx,** or throat, is the muscular tube extending from the nasal cavity to the larynx (see Fig. 28.2). The pharynx is approximately 5 inches in length and contains three regions: the nasopharynx, oropharynx, and laryngopharynx.

- **Nasopharynx**. This is the superior region and connects the nasal cavity with the pharynx. The Eustachian tubes open into the nasopharynx. Because of this close proximity, respiratory or sinus infections can easily spread to the middle ear and vice versa.
- **Oropharynx**. This is the visible part of the pharynx, when looking at the posterior oral cavity of an open mouth; this is where the tonsils are located.
- **Laryngopharynx**. This is the inferior region and is a passageway for both respiratory and digestive systems.

Larynx

The **larynx,** or voice box, connects the pharynx to the trachea (see Fig. 21.22). The larynx contains several structures.

- **Thyroid Cartilage.** This structure grows larger and more prominent in males during puberty. The thyroid cartilage is sometimes called the Adam's apple.
- **Glottis.** This contains the vocal cords, or vocal folds. Air passing over the vocal cords causes them to vibrate and produce sound. A narrower glottis produces higher-pitched sounds, and a wider glottis produces lower-pitched sounds.
- **Epiglottis.** This forms a flap over the glottis during swallowing, which helps food and liquids enter the esophagus (see Fig. 28.2). The epiglottis is referred to as the "guardian of the airways."

All things share the same breath.

—Chief Sealth, Duwamish tribe (1885)

THE LOWER RESPIRATORY TRACT

The lower respiratory tract includes the trachea, divisions of the bronchi, the alveoli, and the lungs.

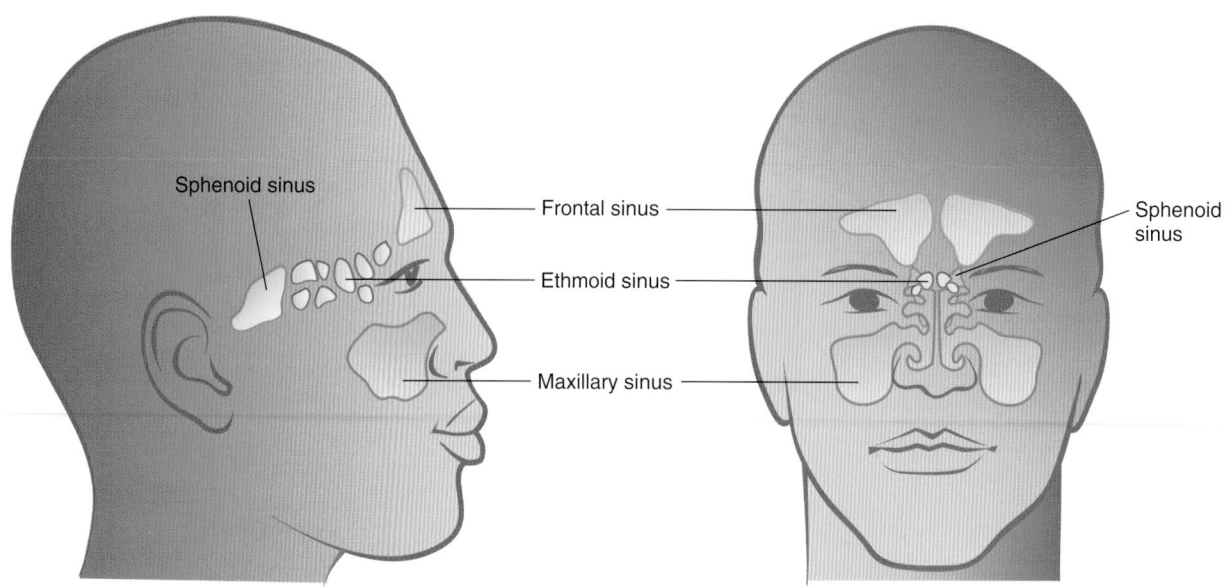

FIG. 28.3 The paranasal sinuses, lateral view *(left image)* and anterior view *(right image)*.

Trachea

The **trachea,** or windpipe, is anterior to the esophagus and connects the larynx to the bronchi. The trachea is approximately 9 inches in length and consists of 16 to 21 C-shaped cartilaginous rings at regular intervals. These rings serve several functions—they allow the esophagus to expand into the trachea as food is swallowed and keep the tracheal wall from collapsing as pressure changes during breathing. The trachea bifurcates at its base into right and left bronchi. The point of bifurcation is a cartilaginous ridge called the *carina.* This structure is highly sensitive to foreign objects and, when stimulated, causes violent reflexive coughing.

Bronchi

The right and left primary **bronchi** lead from the trachea to the right and left lung, respectively (primary means "first"). The right bronchus is wider and has a steeper downward angle compared with the left. Because of this characteristic, inhaled objects lodge on the right side more often. As each bronchus enters the lungs, they branch and become narrower, similar to a tree trunk with its branches and twigs—the bronchi are referred to as the *bronchial tree* (Fig. 28.4). Smaller branches of the bronchi are called **bronchioles.** At this level of the bronchi, the amount of cartilage in their walls decreases, and the amount of smooth muscle increases. These structural changes allow bronchioles to change their diameter to either increase or decrease air flow in response to signals from the autonomic nervous system or factors such air temperature, air pressure, or airborne irritants.

Alveoli

Alveoli are air sacs and the site of gas exchange in the lungs. Alveoli are attached to the bronchioles by a duct. The arrangement of an alveolar duct, along with the associated air sacs, resembles a cluster of grapes. Each alveolus contains a single layer of epithelium surrounded by numerous capillaries, each with their own single layer of endothelium. A basement membrane lies between them. These three structures, the alveolar epithelium, the basement membrane, and the capillary endothelium, are collectively referred to as the *respiratory membrane* (Fig. 28.5). Gas exchange occurs across the respiratory membrane, between the air in the alveoli and the blood in the capillaries. Each lung contains approximately 300 million alveoli, providing an immense gas-exchange surface area of approximately 1000 square feet (ft^2), or the size of a handball court.

Alveoli are coated with a fluid containing surfactants. *Surfactants* assist gas exchange by stabilizing the alveoli and reducing surface tension. Alveoli are similar to balloons. When they deflate, their walls collapse inward and, without surfactants, they stick together, making reinflation difficult. Lungs are one of the last organs to develop in utero. Infants born prematurely (28 weeks' gestation or earlier) may not have produced enough surfactants for their alveoli to function properly. Current medical advances enable healthcare providers to administer synthetic surfactants to improve survival rates among infants born prematurely.

Lungs

Lungs are the main organs of respiration. They extend from the clavicles to the diaphragm and lie against the interior ribcage (see Fig. 28.1). The inferior surface of the lungs is broad and concave to match the shape of the superior surface of the diaphragm. The spongy, elastic lungs fill most of the thoracic cavity, and each lung is separated into lobes. The right lung has three lobes; the left lung has two lobes. A depression called the *cardiac notch* is in the left lung to accommodate the heart.

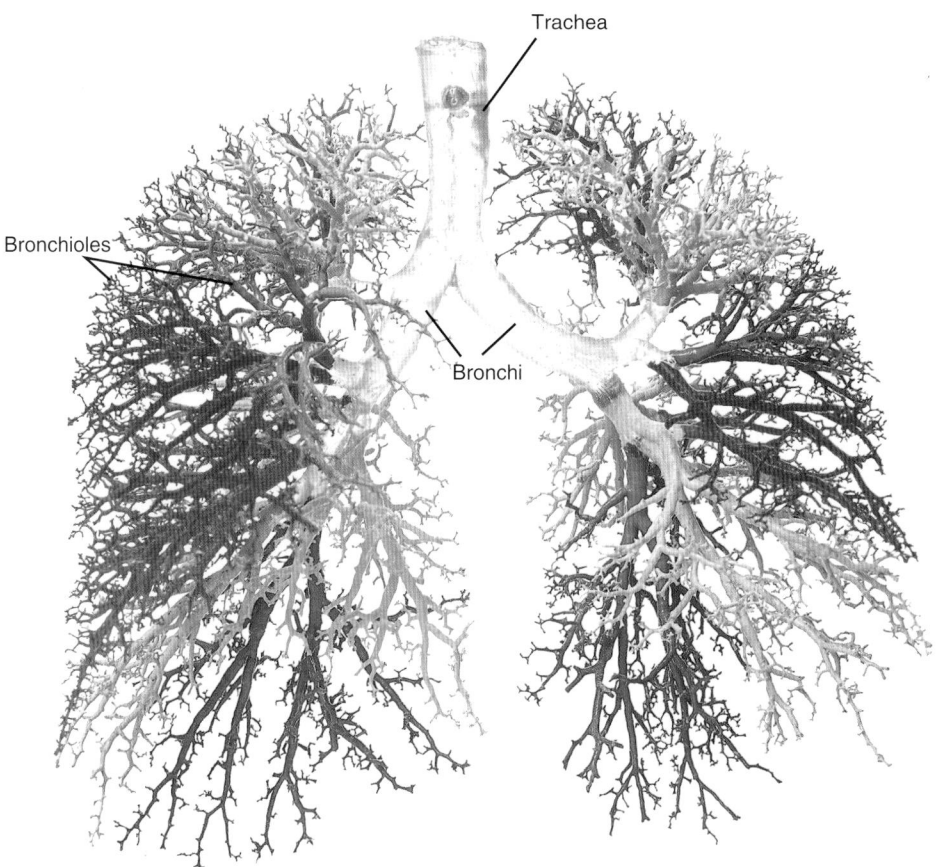

FIG. 28.4 Lower respiratory tract *(anterior view)*. As each bronchus enters the lungs, they branch and become narrower, similar to a tree trunk and its branches; this is sometimes referred to as the bronchial tree. (From Abrahams, P., Boon, J., Spratt, J., & Hutchings, R. [2008]. *McMinn's clinical atlas of human anatomy* [6th ed.]. Philadelphia, PA: Mosby.)

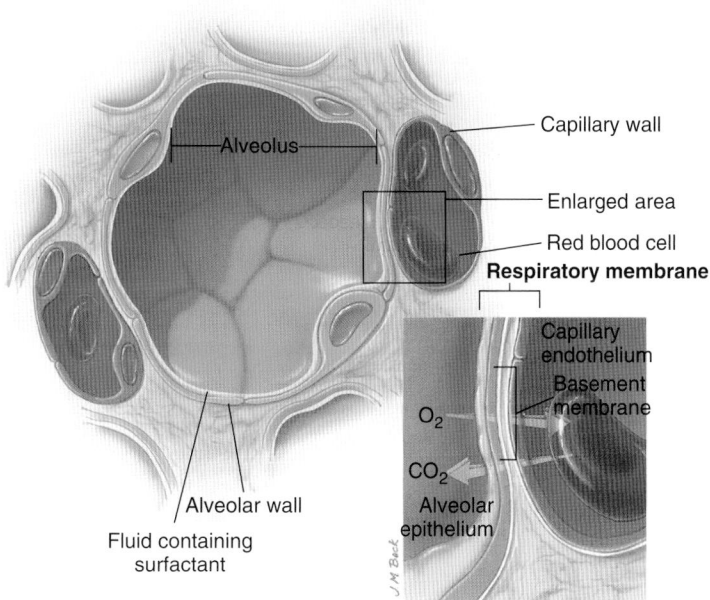

FIG. 28.5 Respiratory membrane includes the alveolar epithelium, the basement membrane, and the capillary endothelium *(cross-section view)*. This is where gas exchange occurs. (From Christensen, B. L. [2010]. *Adult health nursing* [6th ed.]. St. Louis, MO: Mosby.)

The exterior surfaces of the lungs are lined by a visceral and a parietal pleural membrane. The visceral pleura is attached to the lungs, and the parietal pleura is attached to the mediastinum and internal chest wall. Between these two membranes is a lubricating serous fluid, which reduces friction between these membranes as the lungs move during breathing. In review, air moves in the respiratory system by the following pathway:

Nose → Nasal cavity → Pharynx → Larynx →
Trachea → Bronchi → Bronchioles → Alveoli → Lungs

Diaphragm

The **diaphragm** is a broad muscle extending across the inferior ribcage and separates the thoracic cavity from the abdominopelvic cavity. The diaphragm is also called the *respiratory diaphragm*. The diaphragm attaches to several bony structures (L1 to L3, ribs 6 to 12, xiphoid process) and to the central tendon on its inferior surface. The diaphragm is the main muscle of respiration because when it contracts during inhalation, the volume of the thoracic cavity increases, which forces air into the lungs to fill the void.

The diaphragm contains three openings: the caval opening, the esophageal hiatus, and the aortic hiatus. The *caval opening* passes through the central tendon and contains the inferior vena cava and the phrenic nerve. The *esophageal hiatus* contains the esophagus. The *aortic hiatus* contains the aorta and the thoracic duct. Several accessory respiratory muscles facilitate breathing by changing the size of the thoracic cavity (i.e., external intercostals, internal intercostals, serratus posterior superior, serratus posterior inferior, pectoralis minor, scalenes, sternocleidomastoid, and the abdominals). Discussions of these muscles are in Chapter 21.

BREATHING

Breathing, or the *respiratory cycle*, is the process used to move air into and out of the lungs. At rest, adults breathe approximately 12 to 16 times a minute; children may breathe up to twice as fast as adults. The medulla oblongata in the brainstem contains the respiratory center, which regulates breathing. Nerve impulses from the medulla oblongata travel down the phrenic nerve to the diaphragm, causing the diaphragm to contract.

Several factors can temporarily change breathing patterns. Volitional, or voluntary, breathing allows individuals to hold their breath while swimming under water or take deep breaths to project their voice during public speaking, singing, or playing a musical instrument. How long individuals can hold their breath is largely determined by elevated levels of carbon dioxide in the bloodstream. Breathing can increase as body temperature rises (e.g., fever, exercise) and decrease as body temperature lowers (e.g., hypothermia, jumping into cool water). Emotions can change breathing patterns. Fear, grief, and shock reduce the number of breaths per minute, whereas excitement, anger, and sexual arousal increase it. A change in breathing patterns are needed to express emotions, such as when we laugh or cry. Reflexes such as sneezes, coughs, hiccups, and yawns also changes breathing patterns (discussed in a later section). Medical terms used to describe abnormal breathing patterns are listed in Box 28.1. Breathing consists of two phases: *inhalation* and *exhalation.*

Inhalation

Inhalation, or *inspiration*, is the process of moving air into the lungs. As the diaphragm contracts and moves inferiorly or descends, the external intercostal muscles contract and elevate the ribcage (Fig. 28.6). This action enlarges the thoracic cavity and causes the pressure in the lungs to be slightly lower than the atmospheric pressure. As a result, air moves from an area of high pressure (the atmosphere) to an area of low pressure (the lungs). Forced inhalation is aided by contraction of accessory muscles mentioned previously (i.e., external intercostals, internal intercostals, serratus posterior superior, serratus posterior inferior, pectoralis minor, scalenes, sternocleidomastoid, and the abdominals). The ease with which the thorax and lungs are able to stretch during inhalation is called **compliance**.

Exhalation

Exhalation, or *expiration*, is the process of moving air out of the lungs. The diaphragm relaxes and moves superiorly or ascends, which decreases the size of the ribcage (see Fig. 28.6B). This action causes pressure in the lungs to be slightly higher compared with atmospheric pressure. As a result, air moves from an area of high pressure (the lungs) to an area of low pressure (the atmosphere). The tendency of the thorax and lungs to return to their preinhalation size is called **elastic recoil**. Normal, quiet exhalation is a passive process because muscles relax and tissues recoil. However, exhalation, similar to inhalation, can also be forced. Forced exhalation is an active process, using contractions of the internal intercostal, serratus posterior inferior, and abdominal muscles.

How people treat you is their karma; how you react is yours.

—**Wayne Dyer**

BOX 28.1

Terms Used to Describe Abnormal Breathing Patterns

Apnea: Absence of normal, spontaneous breathing
Bradypnea: Slow breathing
Dyspnea: Labored or difficult breathing
Hyperpnea: Fast breathing
Orthopnea: Labored or difficult breathing when lying down flat
Tachypnea: Rapid but shallow breathing

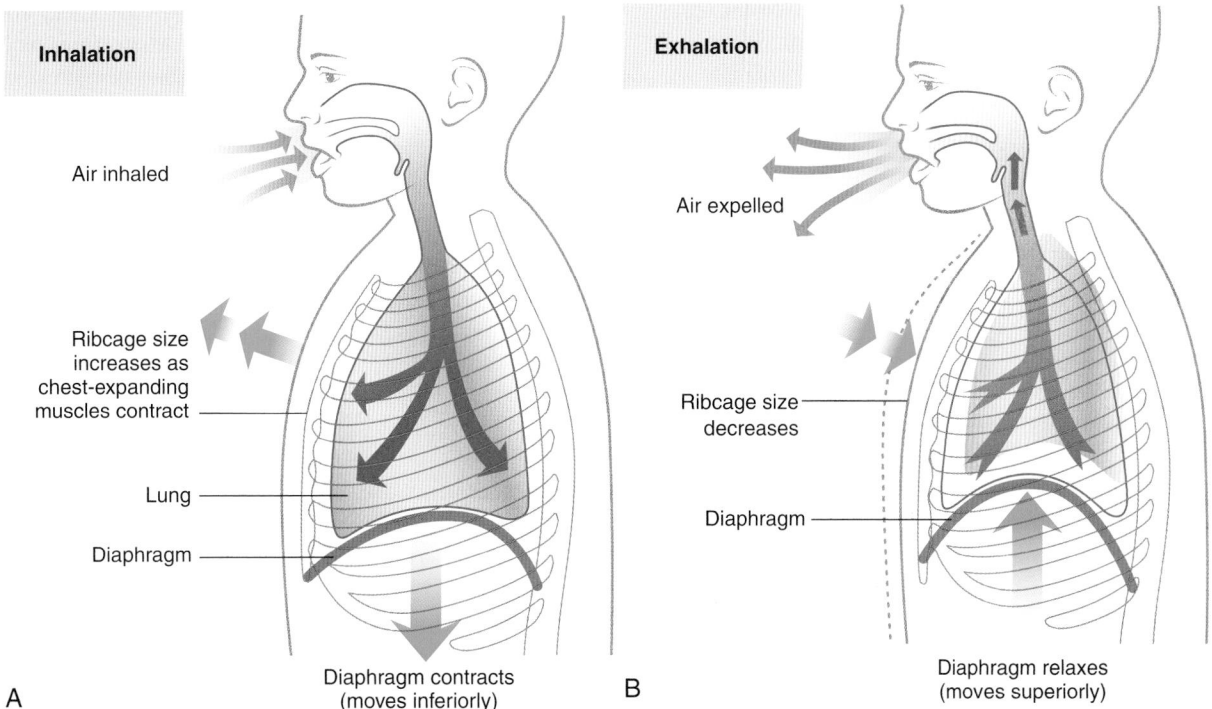

FIG. 28.6 Phases of breathing *(lateral view)*. (A) Inhalation. (B) Exhalation.

RESPIRATION

Respiration is the process of supplying body cells with oxygen and expelling carbon dioxide. For respiration to occur, oxygen must be continually extracted from the air and transported to body cells while removing carbon dioxide from these same cells. Exchange of gases occurs by *diffusion*, or the tendency of molecules to move from an area of high concentration to an area of low concentration. Both the respiratory and cardiovascular systems participate in the respiratory process. Two main types of respiration are: *external respiration* and *internal respiration.*

External (Pulmonary) Respiration

External respiration is gas exchange between the air in the alveoli and blood in capillaries. Deoxygenated blood within pulmonary arteries is transported from the heart to the alveoli. Oxygen diffuses from the air in the lungs, crosses the respiratory membrane, and moves into the bloodstream (see Fig. 28.5). Oxygen attaches to hemoglobin in red blood cells. At the same time, carbon dioxide moves in the opposite direction and is released during exhalation. Oxygenated blood within the pulmonary vein is transported from the alveoli back to the heart.

Internal (Tissue) Respiration

Internal respiration is gas exchange between blood in the capillaries and cells within tissues. Oxygen must be released first so carbon dioxide can attach to hemoglobin. Oxygen crosses the capillary wall and enters the cells. Carbon dioxide diffuses from cells, crosses the capillary wall, and enters the bloodstream. Most of the carbon dioxide diffuses in blood plasma to form carbonic acid, and some of the carbon dioxide attaches to hemoglobin. Just like in external respiration, oxygen and carbon dioxide are moving in opposite directions. Carbon dioxide is transported to the lungs to be expelled during exhalation.

REFLEXES THAT BREATHING PATTERNS

Reflexes that temporarily change breathing patterns are sneezing, coughing, hiccupping, and yawning.

Sneeze

Sneezing is the forceful expulsion of air through the nose and mouth to clear the *upper respiratory tract.* The sneeze reflex can occur by irritation from airborne particles such as dust or pollen, by sudden exposure to bright light, or by a sudden change in temperature, such as when exposed to a breeze of cold air.

Cough

Coughing is the sudden expulsion of air through the nose and mouth to clear the *lower respiratory tract* of irritants or particles. Coughing occurs after a brief inhalation. Productive coughing moves phlegm from the lower respiratory tract.

Hiccup

Hiccups, or *hiccoughs*, are spasmodic closures of the vocal cords after forceful contraction of respiratory muscles to assist the removal of air from the stomach (Howes, 2012). Hiccups may repeat several times per minute. Their sound occurs when inhaled air hits the closed vocal cords.

Yawn

A **yawn** is a very deep inhalation initiated by opening the mouth wide. The yawn reflex is triggered by the need to increase the oxygen content and decrease carbon dioxide in the blood, to reduce ear pressure, to stimulate arousal from drowsiness or boredom, and to socially empathize with fellow yawners as a well-known contagious effect (Gupta & Mittal, 2013), but the precise cause is unknown.

RESPIRATORY PATHOLOGIES, CONDITIONS, AND DISORDERS

Featured next are common pathologies, disorders, and conditions of the respiratory system, listed alphabetically. Each item includes a brief description and its massage-related modifications. A more extensive list and related research is found in the current edition of *Mosby's Pathology for Massage Professionals* (2022).

Asthma

Asthma is a chronic condition causing respiratory mucosa inflammation and bronchospasms that narrow the airway and lead to breathing difficulties called an *asthma attack*. More than 25 million Americans have asthma. This is 7.7% of adults and 8.4% of children. Asthma has been increasing since the early 1980s in all age, sex, and racial groups. Asthma is the leading chronic condition in children and one of the leading reasons for school absenteeism. Risk factors for asthma include having a first-degree relative (parent or sibling) with asthma; having allergic conditions such as hay fever or eczema; cigarette smoking or exposure to secondhand smoke; and exposure to occupational chemicals such as those used in farming, hairdressing, and manufacturing.

Massage and Asthma

During the intake, inquire about allergens to which the client is sensitive and eliminate them from the massage area. Ask about medications such as inhalers used during asthma attacks. If the client has an inhaler, put it in a location that is easy to access in case it is needed during the session. Long-term use of inhaled corticosteroids in the management of moderate to severe asthma is associated with decreased bone density and an increased risk of fractures. This risk is particularly high in postmenopausal females not on hormone replacement therapy. In these cases, reduce pressure over areas of known bone loss and avoid forceful passive range of motion. Avoid aromatherapy and essential oils, as these may trigger an asthma attack (Balekian & Long, 2015). These substances include scented soaps and deodorants used by the practitioner. The exception is inhaled lavender essential oil, which may suppress allergic airway inflammation and swelling (Ueno-Iio et al., 2014).

Consider using body positions to help the client breathe more easily (Cleveland Clinic, 2018). Elevate the supine client's upper body and head while resting the knees on a bolster. Elevate the side-lying client's head and place a pillow between the knees. The seated client's feet are flat on the floor with their elbows resting on their knees. Avoid or limit time spent in the prone position.

Consider teaching parents or caregivers how to massage the child with asthma, making massage more accessible to the child and giving parents/caregivers another way to care for and nurture the child. Limit techniques taught to gliding and kneading and convey the same precautions licensed practitioners follow, such as avoiding skin lesions.

Bronchitis

Bronchitis is inflammation of the bronchial mucosa with resultant swelling and overproduction of mucus. The two types of bronchitis are acute and chronic. Acute bronchitis, also called a *chest cold*, is common. Chronic bronchitis, a more serious condition, is usually caused by cigarette smoking. Chronic bronchitis is defined as a productive cough that lasts at least 3 months, with frequent episodes occurring for at least 2 consecutive years. Approximately 8.6 million Americans have chronic bronchitis.

Massage and Bronchitis

Massage is contraindicated if the client has acute bronchitis accompanied by a fever. The client can receive a massage after being fever-free for 24 hours without the use of fever-reducing drugs such as ibuprofen or acetaminophen (Centers for Disease Control and Prevention [CDC], 2018).

If the client has chronic bronchitis, ask about medications such as an inhaler used to improve breathing. If the client has an inhaler, put it in a location that is easy to access in case it is needed during the session. Consider using body positions to help the client breathe more easily. Elevate the supine client's upper body and head while resting the knees on a bolster. Elevate the side-lying client's head and place a pillow between the knees. The seated client's feet are flat on the floor with their elbows resting on their knees. Avoid or limit time spent in the prone position.

Common Cold

A **common cold** is a viral infection of the upper respiratory tract, usually confined to the nose and throat, although the larynx can be involved. There are millions of cases that occur each year in the United States. Adults have an average of two to three colds per year, while children have even more. Common colds are highly contagious during the onset of symptoms and then become less contagious. Other diseases can occur with a common cold, such as infections of the middle ears, sinuses, or lungs. The common cold is also called a *head cold*, *infectious rhinitis*, or an *upper respiratory tract infection*. The common cold is caused by one of more than 200 viruses that gain access through the nose or mouth. The virus can spread through airborne droplets or by contact with contaminated objects such as doorknobs, computer keyboards, and shopping cart handles, then touching the nose or mouth.

Massage and Common Cold

Massage is postponed until the client is no longer ill, usually 5 days from the onset of signs and symptoms.

Emphysema

Emphysema is a chronic obstructive pulmonary disease (COPD) that causes permanent enlargement of lower airways accompanied by destruction of alveolar walls. The damage is irreversible. Enlarged alveoli do not efficiently remove trapped air, which limits the space for fresh, oxygen-rich incoming air. Approximately 3.4 million Americans have emphysema. The major cause of emphysema is long-term cigarette smoking. Other causes include long-term exposure to airborne irritants such as air pollutants, chemical fumes, and dust.

Massage and Emphysema

Ask about medications such as inhalers used to improve breathing. If the client has an inhaler, put it in a location that is easy to access in case it is needed during the session. Consider using body positions to help the client breathe more easily. Elevate the supine client's upper body and head while resting the knees on a bolster. Elevate the side-lying client's head and place a pillow between the knees. The seated client's feet are flat on the floor with their elbows resting on their knees. If massage is part of palliative care or if the client is frail, use slowly applied light pressure. An example of light pressure is 3 on a 10-point pressure scale.

Hay Fever

Hay fever is a general term used to describe hypersensitivity of the nasal mucosa to allergens, usually plant pollen. Among adults, there are about 19.9 million new diagnoses of hay fever per year. Among children, new cases numbered approximately 5.6 million. Hay fever is also called *allergic rhinitis*. Allergens causing hay fever can be seasonal or environmental; the latter is present all year-round. Seasonal allergens include tree pollen (more common in spring), grass pollen (more common in late spring and summer), and weed pollen (more common in autumn). Allergens present year-round are dust mites, pet dander, cockroaches and their excrement, molds, and fungi.

Massage and Hay Fever

During the intake, inquire about seasonal/environmental allergens and eliminate them from the massage area. If clients mention they have severe allergic reactions such as respiratory distress, ask if they are carrying an epinephrine autoinjector, such as an EpiPen, with them and where it is in case it is needed.

Massage can help reduce facial pain related to nasal congestion. Apply pressure along the upper and lower edges of the cheekbones. This may help relieve pain over the maxillary sinuses. Next, apply along the upper and lower edges of the eyebrows. This may relieve pain over the frontal sinuses.

Pressure on each point is held for 10 seconds. Pressure should be firm but gentle. Request client feedback about levels of pressure and modify techniques according to comments (American Family Physician [AFA], 2004; Starkey, 2016).

Influenza

Influenza is an acute, highly contagious viral infection of the upper respiratory tract, but it can extend into the lower respiratory tract. The various forms of influenza, or "flu," such as Hong Kong or Beijing, are named after the areas where they were first recognized. Influenza is caused by different strains of viruses or influenza viruses—designated A, B, and C—transmitted by infected droplets or contact with contaminated objects (e.g., doorknobs, telephones, computer keyboards, shopping cart handles) and then touching the nose or mouth. Influenza can spread quickly because the incubation period is 1 to 3 days. Flu symptoms usually last 5 to 7 days.

Massage and Influenza

To prevent the spread of infection, massage is postponed until the client has been fever-free for 24 hours without the use of fever-reducing drugs such as ibuprofen or acetaminophen. This time frame is usually 5 to 7 days after the onset of symptoms.

Obstructive Sleep Apnea

Obstructive sleep apnea (OSA) is a sleep disorder characterized by temporary absence of normal breathing (or apnea) caused by a blocked upper airway. An estimated 22 million Americans have sleep apnea. When left untreated, OSA can lead to high blood pressure, chronic heart failure, atrial fibrillation, stroke, and other cardiovascular problems. OSA is associated with type 2 diabetes mellitus and is a factor contributing to numerous traffic accidents and accidents involving heavy machinery, owing to persistent tiredness experienced by many people before diagnosis and treatment. As carbon dioxide levels build up in the blood from improper breathing during sleep, the brain senses blood chemistry changes and rouses the person to breathe normally. People with sleep apnea may wake up as many as 20 to 30 times per hour, and they may be unaware of frequently waking.

Massage and Obstructive Sleep Apnea

Consider using body positions to help the client breathe more easily. Elevate the supine client's upper body and head while resting the knees on a bolster. Elevate the side-lying client's head and place a pillow between the knees. The seated client's feet are flat on the floor with their elbows resting on their knees. If clients fall asleep during massage and experience an apneic episode, they may wake suddenly while snorting or gasping. This is more likely to occur while clients are lying supine.

Pneumonia

Pneumonia is an infection or inflammation of the lungs. This disease is often preceded by common colds or influenza.

Severity ranges from mild to life threatening. Approximately 1 million people in the United States seek care in a hospital for pneumonia, and approximately 50,000 people die from the disease annually. Pneumonia is the most common infectious cause of death in the United States, affecting primarily older adults, infants, and immunocompromised individuals. Pneumonia is also called pneumonitis. Many types of pneumonia have been identified. Some types are named for their anatomic location, such as bronchial, lobar, or interstitial pneumonia; for their causative agent, such as bacterial or viral; or for the way in which it was acquired, such as community-acquired or aspiration pneumonia. Double pneumonia is pneumonia in both lungs. Walking pneumonia, a type of pneumonia, is associated with mild symptoms, and infected people are often unaware they are ill.

Massage and Pneumonia

Massage is contraindicated until the client has recovered completely. If a healthcare provider recommends postural drainage and percussion techniques, the following procedure can be used.

Place the client in each of the nine body positions featured in Fig. 28.7. Each position will help access lobes of the lungs during the application of percussion while taking advantage of gravity to help drain mucus from each lobe into larger airways so it can be expelled more readily through coughing.

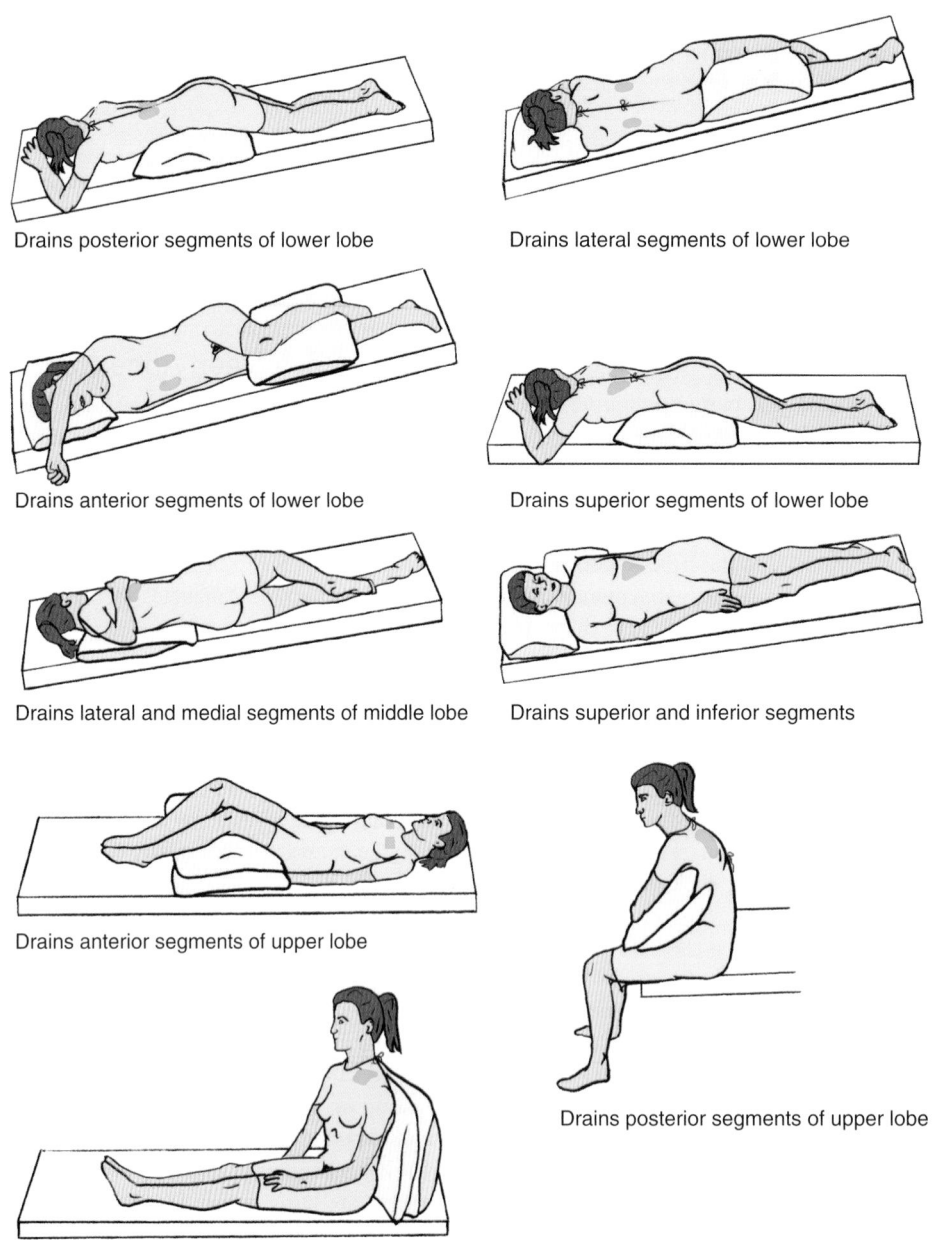

Drains posterior segments of lower lobe

Drains lateral segments of lower lobe

Drains anterior segments of lower lobe

Drains superior segments of lower lobe

Drains lateral and medial segments of middle lobe

Drains superior and inferior segments

Drains anterior segments of upper lobe

Drains posterior segments of upper lobe

Drains segments of upper lobe

FIG. 28.7 Body positions for postural drainage and percussion techniques. (From deWitt, S. [2009]. *Fundamental concepts and skills for nursing* [3rd ed.]. St. Louis: Saunders).

Apply percussion using cupped hands (cupping tapotement) over highlighted areas during exhalations for a few minutes. Next, apply vibration over the same area during five exhalations. Encourage the client to cough to help get the mucus out of the lungs. Do not percuss over bare skin, and do not percuss over the spine, sternum, or floating ribs. The movements should not illicit pain. If the client experiences pain, soften and adjust your hands. Do not perform this technique after eating (wait 1½ to 2 hours), if the client is nauseated, has experiences increased breathlessness, is wheezing, has blood in the sputum, or recent rib or spinal injury. If the client experiences symptoms of heartburn when the head is lower than the stomach, omit the position.

Sinusitis

Sinusitis, or *sinus infection*, is an acute or chronic inflammation of the mucosa lining in the paranasal sinuses. Most cases of sinusitis are acute and resolve within 4 weeks or less. When sinusitis is recurrent or lasts longer than 12 weeks, the condition is considered chronic. Causes of sinusitis are complications of an upper respiratory tract infection, which might be viral or bacterial in origin. Other causes are allergens, mold, and airborne fungi; these are called *allergic sinusitis*. Sinusitis can also be caused by a change in the atmosphere, as happens during air travel or underwater diving, sudden extreme changes in temperature, nasal polyps, or a structural defect such as a deviated septum.

Massage and Sinusitis

Massage is contraindicated during acute episodes when the client is experiencing fever. The client may receive massage after being fever-free for 24 hours without the use of fever-reducing drugs such as ibuprofen or acetaminophen.

For chronic sinusitis as well as fever-free acute cases, consider using body positions to help the client breathe more easily. Elevate the supine client's upper body and head while resting the knees on a bolster. Elevate the side-lying client's head and place a pillow between their knees. The seated client's feet are flat on the floor with their elbows resting on their knees (Cleveland Clinic, 2018). Avoid the prone position or limit time spent in this position.

Massage can help reduce facial pain related to nasal congestion. Apply pressure along the upper and lower edges of the cheekbones. This may help relieve pain over the maxillary sinuses. Next, apply pressure along the upper and lower edges of the eyebrows. This may relieve pain over the frontal sinuses. Pressure on each point is held for 10 seconds. Pressure should be firm but gentle. Request client feedback about levels of pressure and modify techniques according to comments (AFA, 2004; Starkey, 2016).

E-RESOURCES

http://evolve.elsevier.com/Salvo/MassageTherapy

- Chapter challenge
- Flash cards

ROBERT TISSERAND

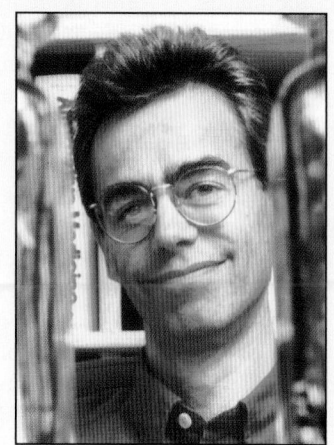

The sense of smell is intimately connected to our emotions and memories. Just one whiff of lily of the valley can remind you of snuggling up to your grandmother as a child, whereas the unmistakable antiseptic scent of a hospital room may take you back to the day you had your appendix removed. A revolting smell elicits disgust more quickly than an ugly sight or sound, and a pleasant scent encourages people to close their eyes and enjoy the moment.

Author and aromatherapist Robert Tisserand was born in London in 1948. Tisserand got his first "taste" of aromatherapy when he drank an entire bottle of perfume at age 2. Like many toddlers, he figured if it smelled "good enough to eat," it must be so. He still remembers the perfume, purchased at a Paris flea market before he was born, was called Creme de Zofali. Obviously, he survived. The bottle did not.

Tisserand's formal introduction to the study of aromatherapy occurred in 1967, when he and his mother attended a lecture on the subject given by Dr. Jean Valnet. Tisserand's mother purchased a copy of the speaker's book and had it signed by the author. A few years later, Tisserand decided to pursue training in massage with a focus on aromatherapy. In 1974, he started the Aromatic Oil Company in his home, bottling and hand-labeling each batch in his bedroom. The money was not great ("Basically, I starved for 20 years," he confesses), but he was following his passion and helping others in the process.

Today, Tisserand teaches aromatherapy around the world. His current business, Tisserand Aromatherapy Products, helps professional aromatherapists, massage practitioners, and enthusiastic amateurs learn about and get a hold of exactly the essential oil products they need. Tisserand's books include *The Art of Aromatherapy, Aromatherapy to Heal and Tend the Body, Aromatherapy for Everyone,* and *Essential Oil Safety.* His product line, greatly expanded since those early days of struggling to fill orders from his home, now includes essential oils, bath and beauty products, perfumes, and massage oils.

Clearly, the world is catching on that essential oils can be used to promote both psychologic and physiologic wellness. And to Robert Tisserand, widespread awareness is the sweet smell of success.

REFERENCES

American Family Physician. (2004). *Sinus infections.* Retrieved from https://www.aafp.org/afp/2004/1101/p1711.html.

Balekian, D., & Long, A. (2015). *American academy of allergy asthma and immunology: Essential oil diffusers and asthma.* Retrieved from https://www.aaaai.org/ask-the-expert/oil-diffusers-asthma.

Centers for Disease Control and Prevention. (2018). *Guidance for school administrators to help reduce the spread of infection.* Retrieved from https://www.cdc.gov/flu/school/guidance.htm.

Cleveland Clinic. (2018). *Positions to reduce shortness of breath.* Retrieved from https://my.clevelandclinic.org/health/articles/9446-positions-to-reduce-shortness-of-breath.

Gupta, A., & Mittal, S. (2013). Yawning and its physiological significance. *International Journal of Applied and Basic Medical Research, 3*(1), 11–15.

Howes, D. (2012). Hiccups: A new explanation for the mysterious reflex. *Bioessays, 34*(6), 451–453.

Salvo, S. G. (2022). *Mosby's Pathology for Massage Professionals* (5th ed.). St Louis: Mosby.

Starkey, J. (2016). *Cleveland clinic: Acupressure for allergy and sinus relief.* Retrieved from https://health.clevelandclinic.org/try-2-easy-acupressure-exercises-allergy-relief-video/.

Ueno-Iio, T., Shibakura, M., Yokota, K., Aoe, M., Hyoda, T., Shinohata, R., et al. (2014). Lavender essential oil inhalation suppresses allergic airway inflammation and mucous cell hyperplasia in a murine model of asthma. *Life Sciences, 108*(2), 109–115.

BIBLIOGRAPHY

Abrahams, P. H., Spratt, J. D., Loukas, M., & van Schoor, A. N. (2003). *Abrahams' and McMinn's clinical atlas of human anatomy* (8th ed.). St Louis: Elsevier.

Applegate, E. (2010). *The anatomy and physiology learning system* (4th ed.). Philadelphia: Saunders.

Como, D. (Ed.). (2016). *Mosby's dictionary of medicine, nursing, and health professions* (10th ed.). St Louis: Elsevier.

Frazier, M. S., & Drzymkowski, J. W. (2015). *Essentials of human diseases and conditions* (6th ed.). St Louis: Elsevier.

Hubert, R. J., & VanMeter, K. C. (2018). *Gould's pathophysiology for the health professions* (6th ed.). Philadelphia: Saunders.

Haubrich, W. S. (2003). *Medical meanings: A glossary of word origins* (2nd ed.). New York: American College of Physicians.

Herlihy, B. (2017). *The human body in health and illness* (6th ed.). St Louis: Saunders.

Huether, S. E., McCance, K. L., & Brashers, V. L. (2019). *Understanding pathophysiology* (7th ed.). St Louis: Mosby.

Kalat, J. W. (2013). *Biological psychology* (11th ed.). Belmont, CA: Cengage Learning.

Kapit, W., & Elson, L. M. (2013). *The anatomy coloring book* (4th ed.). New York: Benjamin Cummings.

Kumar, V., Abbas, A. K., & Aster, J. C. (2015). *Robbins & Cotran pathologic basis of disease* (9th ed.). St Louis: Mosby.

Marieb, E. N., & Keller, S. M. (2018). *Essentials of human anatomy and physiology* (12th ed.). New York: Benjamin Cummings.

McCance, K. L., & Huether, S. E. (2019). *Pathophysiology: The biological basis for disease in adults and children* (8th ed.). St Louis: Mosby.

Myers, T. W. (2014). *Anatomy trains: Myofascial meridians for manual and movement therapists* (3rd ed.). Churchill Livingstone: Elsevier.

Netter, F. H. (2018). *Atlas of human anatomy* (7th ed.). St Louis: Mosby.

Patton, K. T (2019). *Anatomy and physiology* (10th ed.). St Louis: Elsevier.

Patton, K. T., Thibodeau, G. A., & Douglas, M. M. (2012). *Essentials of anatomy and physiology* (4th ed.). New York: Pearson.

Porter, R. S. (2011). *The Merck manual of diagnosis and therapy* (19th ed). Whitehouse Station, NJ: Merck Sharp and Dohme Corp.

Taber, C. W. (2021). *Taber's cyclopedic medical dictionary* (24nd ed.). Philadelphia: FA Davis.

REVIEW AND APPLY YOUR KNOWLEDGE

MATCHING ONE: CONCEPT REVIEW

Place the letter of the answer next to the number of the term or phrase that best describes it.

A. Alveoli
B. Breathing
C. Bronchi
D. Diaphragm
E. Epistaxis
F. Larynx
G. Lungs
H. Nasal cavity
I. Pharynx
J. Respiratory membrane
K. Sinuses
L. Trachea

_____ 1. Hollow space in the skull separated into left and right halves by a septum.

_____ 2. Main muscle of respiration; between the thoracic and abdominopelvic cavities.

_____ 3. Main organs of respiration and extend from the clavicles to the diaphragm.

_____ 4. Located anterior to the esophagus and connects the larynx to the bronchi; also called the windpipe.

_____ 5. Muscular tube extending from the nasal cavity to the larynx; also called the throat.

_____ 6. Process of moving air into and out of the lungs.

_____ 7. Medical term for nosebleed.

_____ 8. Collective term for the alveolar epithelium, basement membrane, and capillary endothelium.

_____ 9. Respiratory passageways leading from the trachea to each lung.

_____ 10. Where gas exchange occurs in the lungs.

_____ 11. Connects the pharynx to the trachea; also called the voice box.

_____ 12. Air-filled cavities that lighten the skull and act as resonance chambers for sound.

MATCHING TWO: CONCEPT REVIEW

Place the letter of the answer next to the number of the term or phrase that best describes it.

A. Bronchioles
B. Compliance
C. Elastic recoil
D. Exhalation
E. External respiration
F. Inhalation
G. Internal respiration
H. Medulla oblongata
I. Olfaction
J. Pectoralis minor
K. Respiration
L. Surfactants

_____ 1. Accessory muscle of respiration and can help change the size of the thoracic cavity.

_____ 2. Process of moving air out of the lungs.

_____ 3. Sense of smell mediated by the temporal lobe in the brain.

_____ 4. Substances assisting in gas exchange by stabilizing the alveoli and reducing surface tension.

_____ 5. Area in the brainstem containing the respiratory center.

_____ 6. Process of moving air into the lungs.

_____ 7. Process used to supply body cells with oxygen and to expel carbon dioxide.

_____ 8. Tendency of the thorax and lungs to return to their preinhalation size.

_____ 9. Gas exchange between blood in the capillaries and body cells within tissues.

_____ 10. Gas exchange between air in the alveoli and blood in the capillaries.

_____ 11. Small branches of the bronchi.

_____ 12. Ease with which the thorax and lungs are able to stretch during inhalation.

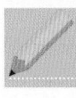

MULTIPLE CHOICE: TEST YOUR KNOWLEDGE

Place the letter of the answer next to the number of the term or phrase that best describes it.

_____ 1. Which is a function of the respiratory system?
   A. Heat production
   B. Mineral storage
   C. Sound production
   D. Vitamin D synthesis

_____ 2. The grooved passageways in the nasal cavity are the:
   A. anterior nares
   B. posterior nares
   C. conchae
   D. meatuses

_____ 3. The largest of the paranasal sinuses are the:
   A. frontal sinuses
   B. sphenoid sinuses
   C. ethmoid sinuses
   D. maxillary sinuses

_____ 4. Which area of the larynx contains the vocal cords/folds?
   A. Thyroid cartilage
   B. Glottis
   C. Adam's apple
   D. Epiglottis

_____ 5. The "guardian of the airways" is the:
   A. cilia
   B. glottis
   C. epiglottis
   D. hyoid

_____ 6. Because of its width and steep angle, inhaled objects tend to lodge in the:
   A. right bronchus
   B. left bronchus
   C. bronchioles
   D. alveoli

_____ 7. The left lung as ____ lobes and the right lung has ____ lobes.
   A. 3/3
   B. 2/2
   C. 2/3
   D. 3/2

_____ 8. At rest, adults breathe approximately _____ times a minute.
   A. 8 to 12
   B. 12 to 16
   C. 16 to 20
   D. 20 to 25

_____ 9. Exchange of gases during respiration occurs by:
   A. diffusion
   B. filtration
   C. osmosis
   D. photosynthesis

_____ 10. Spasmodic closure of the vocal cords after contraction of respiratory muscles is a:
   A. sneeze
   B. cough
   C. hiccup
   D. yawn

_____ 11. Which is the medical term for a chest cold?
   A. Bronchitis
   B. Rhinitis
   C. Emphysema
   D. Pneumonia

_____ 12. Which condition should a massage practitioner postpone the massage?
   A. Asthma
   B. Sinusitis
   C. Emphysema
   D. Influenza

CRITICAL THINKING

To Percuss or Not to Percuss

A client has recently recovered from pneumonia. She is no longer contagious but is having some difficulty clearing her lungs from residual congestion. She wants to know if there is anything you can do to help her. What treatment and legal considerations do you need to keep in mind?

Answers to this question can cover, but are not limited to:

Percussion on the client's back, and possibly performed lightly on the client's upper chest, can be helpful in breaking up congestion so the client can cough it up and eliminate it. Treatment considerations include whether the massage practitioner is qualified and proficient in percussion; the client's vitality (is she healthy enough to receive percussion); whether her doctor thinks the percussion would be helpful; whether the doctor gives permission for the massage practitioner to perform the percussion; and for the massage practitioner to be prepared for the mucus the client will be releasing by having tissues available or perhaps a towel, and tissues and towels need to be handled as contaminated by hazardous waste. Legal considerations include whether percussion for chest clearing is within the massage practitioner's legal scope of practice for the municipality in which the massage practitioner is working; whether a prescription from the client's doctor is needed for the percussion; and whether the percussion can be performed in the massage practitioner's office, or if it needs to be in a medical setting.

PROFESSIONAL PRACTICE

Gesundheit

On Monday morning, Wanda does not feel like her usual self as she heads to her massage office. She decides her sluggishness and stuffy nose are caused by the dusting she had done over the weekend when cleaning her condo. During her third massage of the day, Wanda suddenly feels worse. Her stuffy nose has turned into sniffles, and she begins to feel flushed. All at once, her nose starts running, not just a slight drip that could be sniffed away, but steady streams of mucus.

What should Wanda do now? Do you think she is contagious? If so, what are her obligations to herself and to her clients? Should Wanda excuse herself from the room and blow her nose, take some medication, and finish the massage? Should Wanda end the massage before the appointment is over? If so, should she charge the client for the incomplete session? How should Wanda handle her other clients for this day?

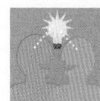

DISCUSSION
Treatment Plans and Respiratory Conditions

If your client discloses a respiratory condition such as asthma or chronic obstructive pulmonary disease (COPD), what types of assessment questions might you ask during the intake? What treatment modifications would be appropriate and why? If available, post your reflections on an internet-based discussion board monitored by your instructor.

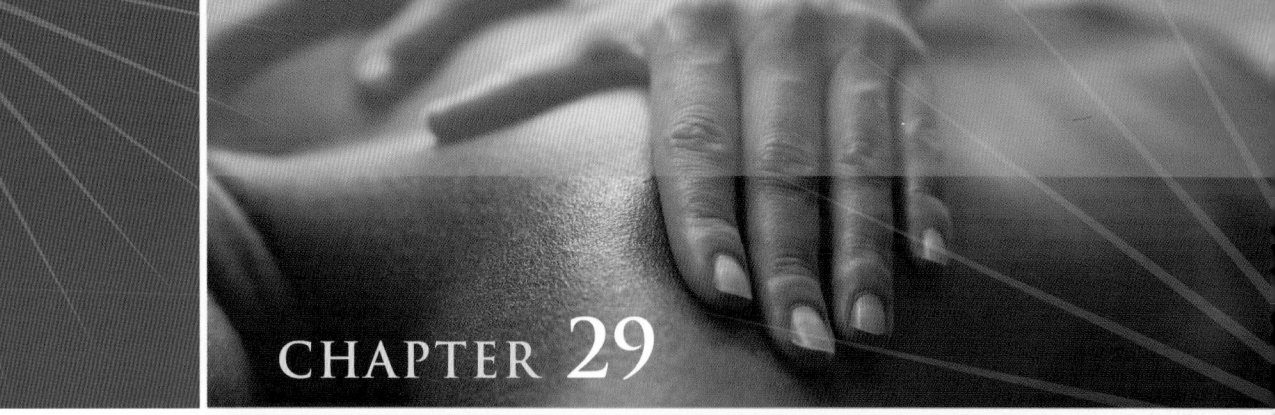

CHAPTER 29

Digestive System, Pathologies, Dysfunctions, and Disorders

Be careful about reading health books. You may die of a misprint.

—Mark Twain

LEARNING OBJECTIVES

After completing this chapter, the student should be able to:

1. List anatomic structures and physiologic processes related to the digestive system, and discuss layers of the gastrointestinal (GI) tract and peritoneum.
2. Discuss parts of the GI tract from the oral cavity to the large intestine, and their secretions.
3. Identify accessory organs and glands and their secretions.
4. Describe GI pathologies, dysfunctions, and disorders, and state their massage modifications.

http://evolve.elsevier.com/Salvo/MassageTherapy

INTRODUCTION

People consume more than 40 tons of food in an average lifetime. The digestive system takes this food and processes it into molecules more easily absorbed into the bloodstream and used by body cells. Essentially, the process of digestion is a *disassembly line* beginning in the mouth and ending at the anus, with major organs of digestion in the abdominopelvic cavity. Digestive functions are initiated by the parasympathetic division of the nervous system (see Chapter 23). Because digestion requires energy, it occurs primarily during periods of low activity; hence a nickname of the parasympathetic division is "rest and digest." Fortunately, digestion produces more energy than it uses, which is one of the purposes of eating food. Use Table 29.1 to help you understand terms of the digestive system. *Gastroenterology* is the study of the digestive system.

ANATOMY

The basic anatomy of the digestive system is:
- Oral cavity
- Pharynx
- Esophagus
- Stomach
- Small intestine
- Large intestine
- Accessory structures—these include the pancreas, liver, and gallbladder

TABLE 29.1 Word Meanings

WORD	MEANING
Amylase	*Gr.* starch; enzyme
Bolus	*Gr.* a lump
Cecum	*L.* blindness
Chyme	*Gr.* juice
Deglutition	*L.* to swallow
Duodenum	*L.* 12 fingers (refers to its length)
Haustra	*L.* to draw, drink
Hepato	*Gr.* liver
Jejunum	*L.* empty
Mastication	*L.* to chew
Omentum	*L.* a covering or apron
Peristaltic	*Gr.* contracting around
Plicae circulares	*L.* a fold or little ring
Pylorus	*Gr.* gatekeeper
Rectum	*L.* straight
Rugae	*L.* a crease or fold
Sacchar	*Gr.* sugar
Sigmoid	*Gr.* letter *sigma*, meaning S-shaped
Sphincter	*Gr.* a binder
Taenia coli	*L.* band of the colon
Tonsils	*L.* almond
Vermiform appendix	*L.* wormlike appendix
Villi	*L.* tuft of hair

Gr., Greek; *L.,* Latin.

PHYSIOLOGY

Important functions of the digestive system are:
- **Ingestion**—The process of taking materials into the mouth by eating and drinking
- **Digestion**—The process of breaking materials down into molecules that can be used by the body. It includes both mechanical and chemical digestion. Mechanical digestion includes chewing food with the teeth, churning it in the stomach, and localized mixing actions within the oral cavity and in the digestive tube. Chemical digestion is the chemical alteration of food facilitated by the effects of acids, bases, and enzymes. An **enzyme** is a substance acting as a catalyst in chemical reactions.
- **Secretion**—Cells in the gastrointestinal (GI) tract secrete mucus, chemicals, and enzymes. Secretions are supplied by salivary glands, the stomach, the liver and gallbladder, the pancreas, and the intestines.
- **Absorption**—The process of molecules moving from the GI tract into blood or lymph vessels and then into body cells
- **Defecation**—The process of eliminating indigestible or unabsorbed materials from the body

GASTROINTESTINAL TRACT

The **gastrointestinal tract** is a long muscular tube from the mouth extending through the body, and ending at the anus (Fig. 29.1). This open tube is known as the *alimentary canal* or *digestive tube*. The GI tract contains various cells, organs, and glands secreting substances into its internal hollow space or lumen. *Goblet cells* are the mucus-producing cells in the GI tract. These cells are found in greater numbers in the large intestine and distal small intestine (i.e., ileum) compared with the rest of the GI tract. The GI tract includes various organs and glands, such as the salivary glands, pancreas, liver, and gallbladder.

Layers of the Gastrointestinal Tract

The GI tract has four layers: the mucosa, submucosa, muscle layer, and serosa.
- **Mucosa Layer**—The innermost layer that is composed of mucus membranes
- **Submucosa Layer**—Lies next to the mucosa and contains loose connective tissue along with blood and lymph vessels, nerves, and some glands
- **Muscle Layer**—Composed of circular and longitudinal smooth muscle (see Fig 29.5A)
- **Serosa Layer**—The outermost layer that is attached to the peritoneum (discussed next)

Peritoneum

The **peritoneum** is a large, flat, folded serous membrane within the abdominopelvic cavity (Fig. 29.2). The peritoneum serves as an anchor for digestive organs, blood and lymph vessels, and nerves. Although it is one continuous membrane, the peritoneum contains two layers—a parietal

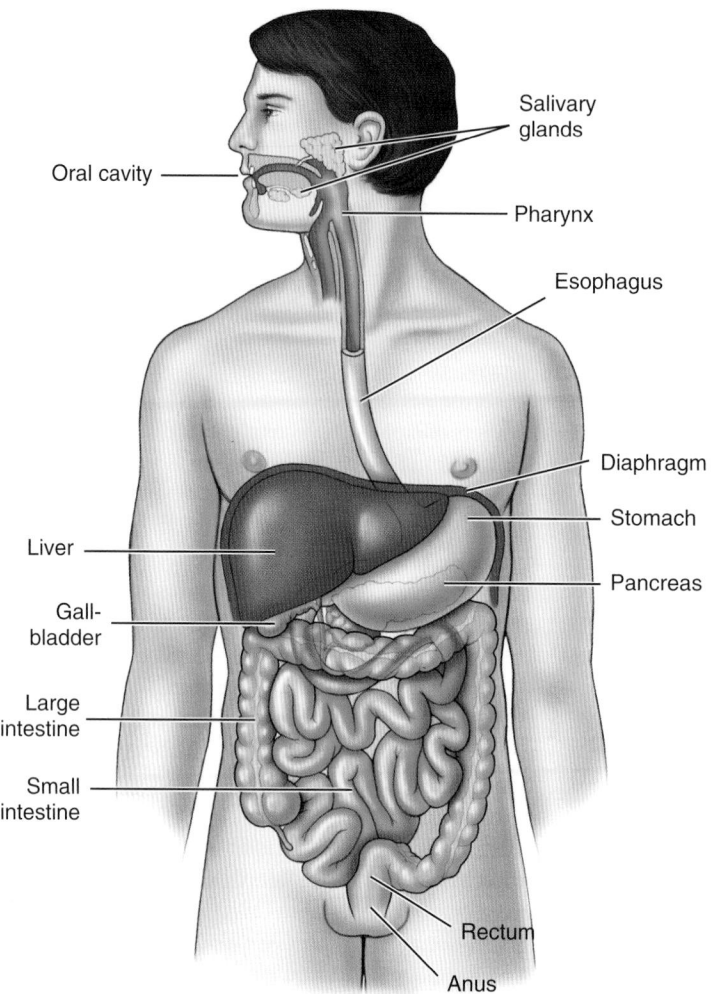

FIG. 29.1 The gastrointestinal tract (*anterior view*). Parts of the GI tract including accessory digestive organs and glands. (From Herlihy, B. [2011]. *The human body in health and illness* [4th ed.]. St. Louis, MO: Saunders.)

and visceral layer. The visceral peritoneum covers the external surfaces of most abdominal organs, including the GI tract. These layers secrete serous fluid, which lubricates the viscera and allows structures to slide over each other.

The intestines are suspended from the posterior portion of the parietal peritoneum called the *mesenteries*. Subsections of the mesenteries are named for their respective attachments (e.g., mesogastrium for the stomach, mesocolon for the large intestines). The omentums are similar to mesenteries but suspended from the anterior portion of the parietal peritoneum, and contain prominent patches of fat. The *greater omentum* extends from the stomach and duodenum to the transverse colon and resembles an apron. The *lesser omentum* extends from the stomach and the duodenum to the liver (see Fig. 29.2.). Some organs in the abdominopelvic cavity are not encased in peritoneum. The kidneys, pancreas, and small portions of the intestines lie in the retroperitoneal space.

ORAL CAVITY

The **oral cavity** or mouth is the first portion of the GI tract and contains the teeth and tongue and openings for the salivary glands. Here, food is chewed or *masticated*; this action is aided by the teeth and tongue. Teeth are enamel-coated structures used to bite and chew to help break up large pieces of food into smaller ones. Adults usually have 32 secondary, or permanent, teeth. Children have about 20 primary, or deciduous, teeth usually shed between 6 and 12 years of age. Teeth are classified according to shape and function: incisors, cuspids (canines), bicuspids (premolars), and multicuspids (molars). The third molars are also called wisdom teeth because they erupt when a person is old enough to be "wise" (usually between the ages of 17 and 25).

As food is chewed, the tongue mixes it with saliva to form a **bolus**, which is a small round mass of food. Once formed, the tongue directs the bolus toward the back of the throat.

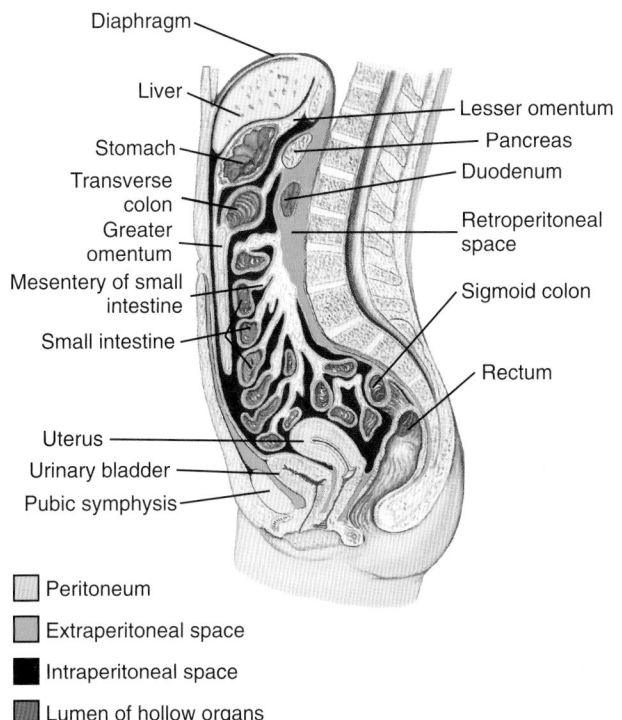

FIG. 29.2 Peritoneum of a female (*lateral cross-section view*). Note some organs and portions of the intestines lie behind the peritoneum (From Thibodeau, G. A. & Patton, K. T. [2007]. *Anatomy & physiology* [6th ed.]. St. Louis, MO: Mosby.)

With the exception of a few substances (e.g., medications, such as nitroglycerin, administered *sublingually* or beneath the tongue), no absorption takes place in the oral cavity.

Secretions

The salivary glands in the oral cavity are responsible for the production and secretion of *saliva*, a watery liquid whose moisturizing effects preserve oral hygiene and allows taste, speech, and mastication. Saliva also helps form the bolus, and lubricates it so it is easier to swallow. *Sputum* is saliva mixed with phlegm—the latter is mucus secreted by the respiratory mucosa. Saliva contains digestive enzymes, such as salivary amylase and lingual lipase.

- **Salivary Amylase (Ptyalin)**—Initiates carbohydrate digestion
- **Lingual Lipase**—Initiates fat digestion by breaking down lipids into glycerol and fatty acids

There are several salivary glands. The *submandibular glands* are below the mandible. The *sublingual glands* are below the tongue. The *parotid glands* are below and in front of each ear. These glands drain their secretions into the mouth through the parotid duct, which is located superficial to the masseter muscle. The enzymatic breakdown of carbohydrates and lipids in the oral cavity is why we taste food. There is no enzyme in the oral cavity that breaks down protein; high-protein food, such as tofu or eggs, have little to no flavor.

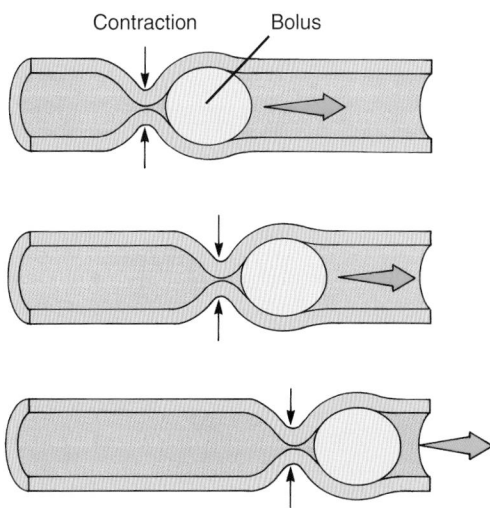

FIG. 29.3 Peristalsis. Smooth muscle contractions begin behind the bolus to move it further into the gastrointestinal tract. (From Thibodeau, G. A. & Patton, K. T. [2007]. *Anatomy & physiology* [6th ed.]. St. Louis, MO: Mosby.)

PHARYNX

The **pharynx**, or throat, is approximately 5 inches in length and contains three regions: the nasopharynx, oropharynx, and laryngopharynx. The *nasopharynx* is the superior region and connects the nasal cavity to the pharynx. The *oropharynx* contains the tonsils and is visible when looking at the posterior oral cavity of an open mouth. The *laryngopharynx* is the inferior region, and is a passageway for both the digestive and respiratory systems.

The pharynx is involved with swallowing or *deglutition*. During swallowing, the bolus and liquids are transported from the oral cavity through the pharynx and toward the esophagus via **peristalsis**, the mixing and propulsive movements in the GI tract (Fig. 29.3). Propulsion contractions begin behind the bolus and these contractions occur in the smooth muscle layer of the GI tract.

Secretions

The lining of the pharynx secretes only mucus.

ESOPHAGUS

The **esophagus** aids in transporting food and liquids from the pharynx to the stomach. It is behind the trachea, and pierces the diaphragm at the esophageal hiatus. The *lower esophageal sphincter* (LES) is between the base of the esophagus and the stomach. A **sphincter** is a ring-shaped muscle that relaxes or tightens to open or close an opening in the body. As food is pushed toward the stomach, the LES relaxes and opens, permitting food to enter the stomach. The LES is also called the *cardiac sphincter* or the *gastroesophageal sphincter.*

Secretions

The lining of the esophagus secretes only mucus.

STOMACH

The **stomach** is a J-shaped saclike organ between the esophagus and the small intestine. It is essentially an enlargement of the GI tract, and serves as an expandable food storage tank. When empty, the stomach is approximately the size of a large sausage. When full, it can expand, and hold up to 1 gallon of food and liquid.

The stomach has three main regions. The superior dome-shaped region is the *fundus,* the central region is the body, and the narrow inferior region is the *pylorus.* The stomach also contains a *greater curvature* on its lateral aspect and *lesser curvature* on its medial aspect. The stomach's lining contains folds called *rugae* enabling it to enlarge as food is ingested. Rugae are typical of expanding structures, such as the stomach, gallbladder, urinary bladder, and vagina. The stomach is bound at both ends by the LES between the esophagus and the stomach, and by the *pyloric sphincter* between the stomach and the small intestines.

The stomach churns and mixes the food with gastric juice, which is a blend of enzymes and acids, until it becomes a semiliquid substance called **chyme.** Chyme then passes through the pyloric sphincter (Fig. 29.4). The process of

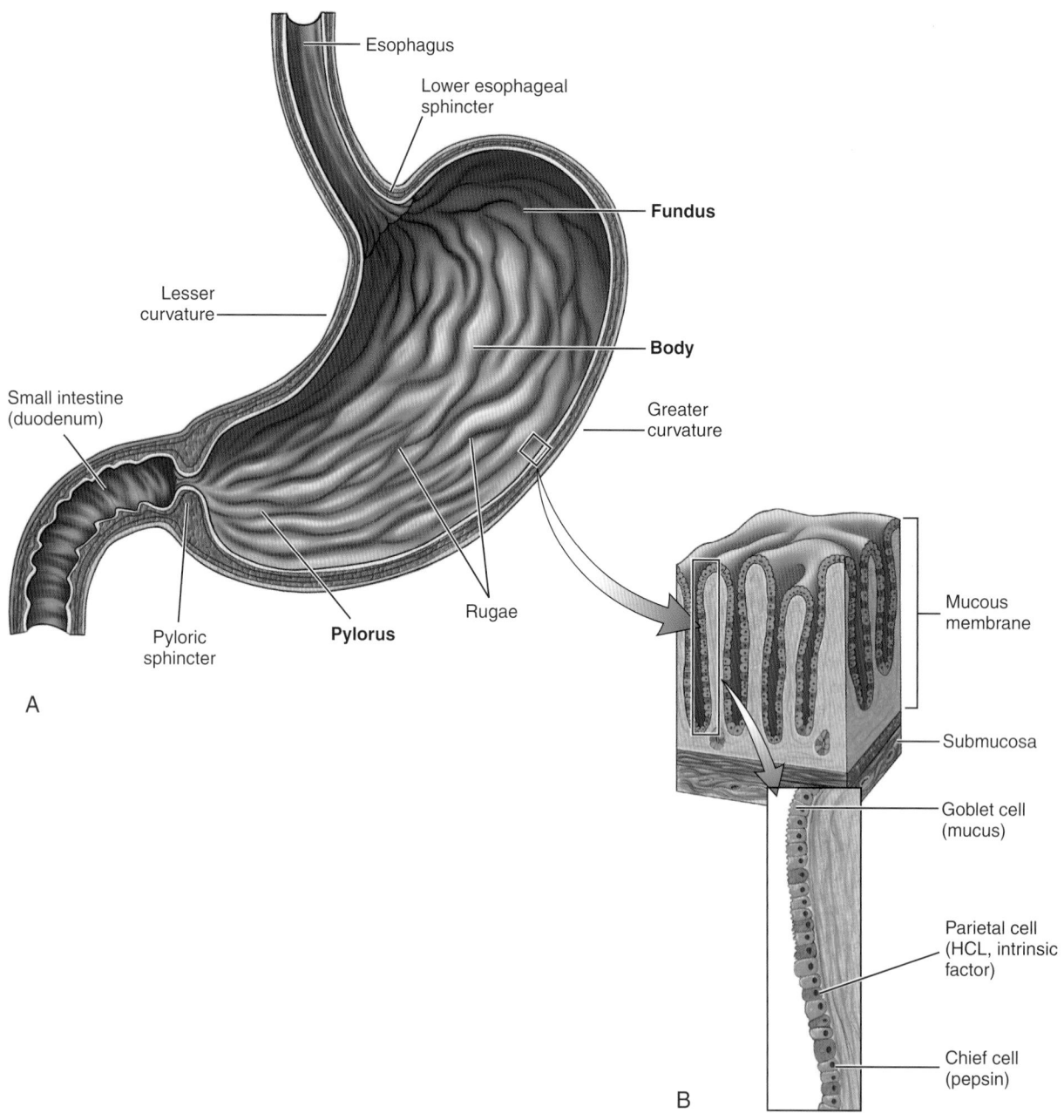

FIG. 29.4 The stomach. (A) Structures of the stomach (*cross-section view*). (B) Stomach lining (*microscopic view*). *HCL,* Hydrochloric acid. (From Herlihy, B. [2011]. *The human body in health and illness* [4th ed.]. St. Louis, MO: Saunders.)

TABLE 29.2 Enzymes and Substances Affecting Digestion

NAME AND SUBSTANCE	LOCATION PRODUCED	ACTION(S)
Bile	Liver	Physically breaks apart large fat globules into smaller ones
Carboxypeptidase	Pancreas	Breaks down proteins
Chymosin/rennin	Stomach	Aids in milk curdling
Chymotrypsin	Pancreas	Breaks down proteins
Enterokinase	Small intestine	Promotes protein and carbohydrate digestion
Enteropeptidase	Small intestine	Converts inactive trypsinogen to active trypsin
Hydrochloric acid	Stomach (parietal cells)	Breaks down protein, kills many bacterial pathogens, and converts inactive pepsinogen to active pepsin
Intrinsic factor	Stomach (parietal cells)	Promotes absorption of vitamin B_{12}
Lactase	Small intestine	Promotes protein and carbohydrate digestion
Lingual lipase	Oral cavity	Breaks lipids down into glycerol and fatty acids
Maltase	Small intestine	Promotes protein and carbohydrate digestion
Pancreatic amylase	Pancreas	Breaks down carbohydrates and converts polysaccharides into disaccharides
Pancreatic lipase	Pancreas	Converts fats into fatty acids
Pepsin	Stomach (chief cells)	Protein digestion
Peptidase	Small intestine	Promotes protein and carbohydrate digestion
Salivary amylase/ptyalin	Salivary glands	Breaks down carbohydrates
Sucrase	Small intestine	Promotes protein and carbohydrate digestion
Trypsin	Pancreas	Protein digestion

moving chyme into the small intestine may take up to 4 hours—food with higher fat content will stay in the stomach longer. Because of the slow release, the body is able to maintain energy needs with only two or three meals a day instead of requiring a steady supply of food, like grazing animals and birds. The only substances absorbed by the stomach are water, some minerals, alcohol, and some medications.

Secretions

The stomach lining contains gastric glands secreting several substances important to the digestive processes. Secretions of all gastric glands are collectively referred to as *gastric juices.*

- **Pepsin**—Gastric enzyme that facilitates protein digestion. Pepsin is secreted by *chief cells* as inactive pepsinogen and, upon mixing with the hydrochloric acid, becomes active pepsin.
- **Hydrochloric Acid**—Breaks apart proteins so they are more easily digested, activates gastric enzymes, and kills pathogenic bacteria. Hydrochloric acid is secreted by *parietal cells.* Hydrochloric acid also converts pepsinogen into its active form of pepsin, which facilitates protein digestion.
- **Intrinsic Factor**—Binds to vitamin B_{12}, and temporarily protects it from deactivation by gastric juice until it reaches the small intestine, where B12 is absorbed. Intrinsic factor is secreted by *parietal cells*
- **Gastrin**—Hormone secreted by endocrine cells that promotes digestion by stimulating gastric glands to secrete their products (Table 29.2)

SMALL INTESTINE

The **small intestine** or small bowel is a coiled tube between the stomach and the large intestine. The small intestine is called small because of its smaller diameter compared with the larger diameter of the large intestine. However, the small intestine is longer than the large intestine; it occupies most of the abdominopelvic cavity (approximately 20 feet [6 meters] in length). The main function of the small intestine is chemical digestion and the absorption of digested food. The small intestine has three sections:

- **Duodenum**—First and shortest portion of the small intestine and approximately 10 to 12 inches in length; it contains ducts from the liver, gallbladder, and pancreas
- **Jejunum**—Middle section, approximately 7 to 8 feet long
- **Ileum**—Last and longest section at approximately 12 feet; contains groups of lymphatic tissue called *Peyer patches*

Walls of the small intestine contain circular folds called *plicae circulares* housing numerous fingerlike projections called *villi.* Each villus contains a blood capillary and a lymphatic capillary called a *lacteal* (Fig. 29.5). The blood capillaries absorb nutrients, transporting them to the liver via the hepatic portal system; the liver processes these nutrients before they are distributed throughout the body. The lacteals absorb fat, transporting it to the lymphatic system, where it enters the bloodstream and is distributed throughout the body. The surfaces of villi contain projections called *microvilli,* giving the small intestine a velvety appearance called brush border. Peristalsis in the small intestine is distinct, and not only contracts to propel its contents forward but also contracts locally to mix and move nutrient-rich materials back and forth, which increases the timeframe for absorption. Approximately 90% of absorption occurs in the length of the small intestine (Fig. 29.6). The *pyloric sphincter* is the beginning of the small intestine, and the *ileocecal sphincter* is the end,

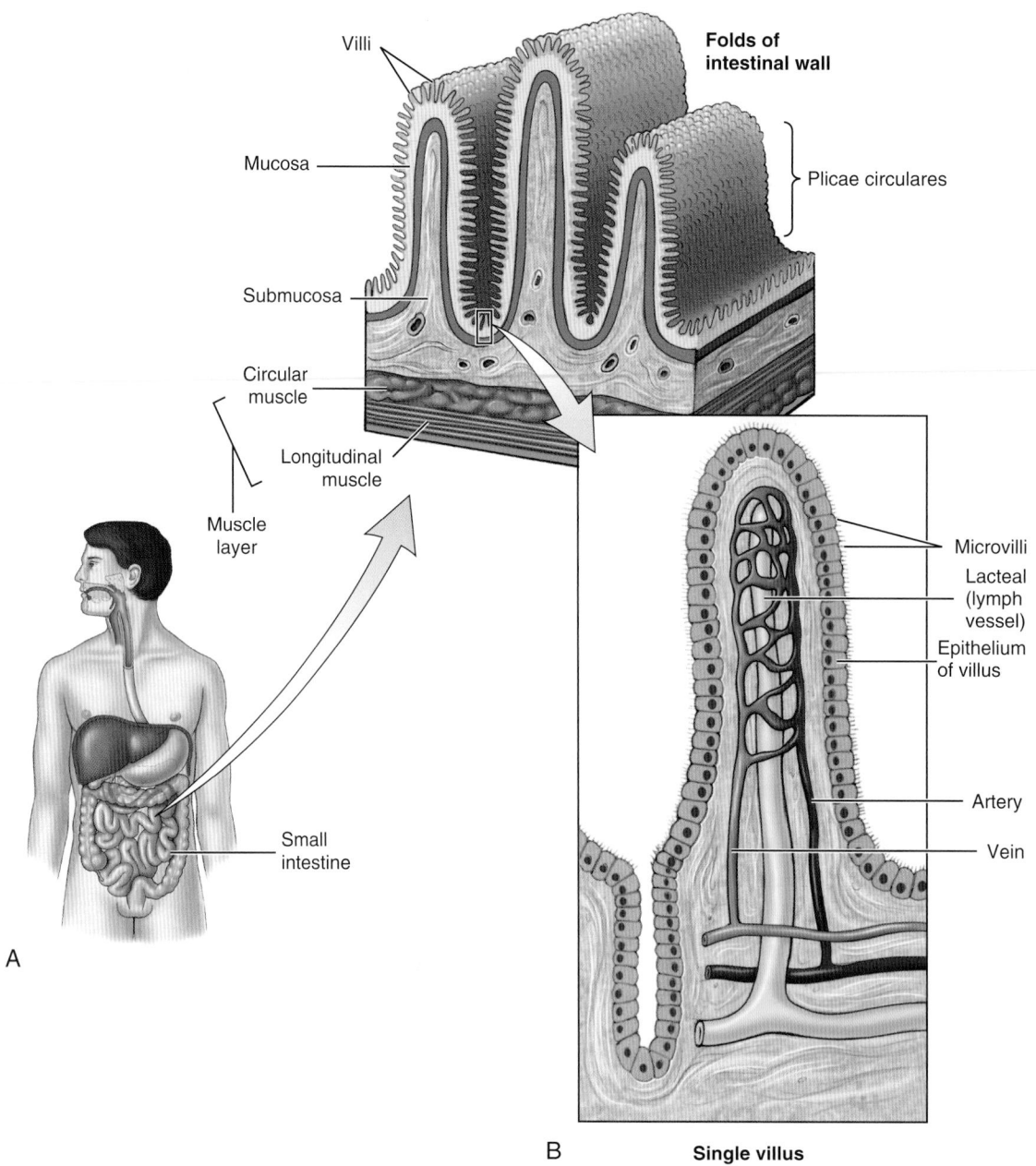

FIG. 29.5 Small intestinal wall. (A) Plicae circulares, villi, and several layers of the gastrointestinal tract (*cross-section view*). (B) Single villus showing microvilli, blood vessels, and a lacteal (*microscopic view*). (From Herlihy, B. [2011]. *The human body in health and illness* [4th ed.]. St. Louis, MO: Saunders.)

between the ileum and the cecum or first section of the large intestine.

Secretions

The lining of the small intestine secretes several substances promoting digestion and absorption. Secretions by all intestinal glands are called *intestinal juice.*

- **Peptidase**—Splits proteins into small peptides and amino acids
- **Enteropeptidase (Enterokinase)**—Converts trypsinogen into its active form of trypsin (a pancreatic enzyme), which facilitates protein digestion

- **Maltase**—Breaks down maltose (malt sugar) into glucose (simple sugar)
- **Sucrase**—Breaks down sucrose (cane or table sugar), fructose (sugar in honey, many fruits, and some vegetables), and glucose (simple sugar)
- **Lactase**—Breaks down lactose (sugar in dairy products) into glucose and galactose (simple sugars). *Lactose intolerance* is the inability to digest lactose due to a lactase deficiency, which manifests as bloating, abdominal pain, and diarrhea. A large portion of Middle-Easterns and Asians lack this enzyme. This enzyme also decreases with age. Lactose intolerance is common in these populations.

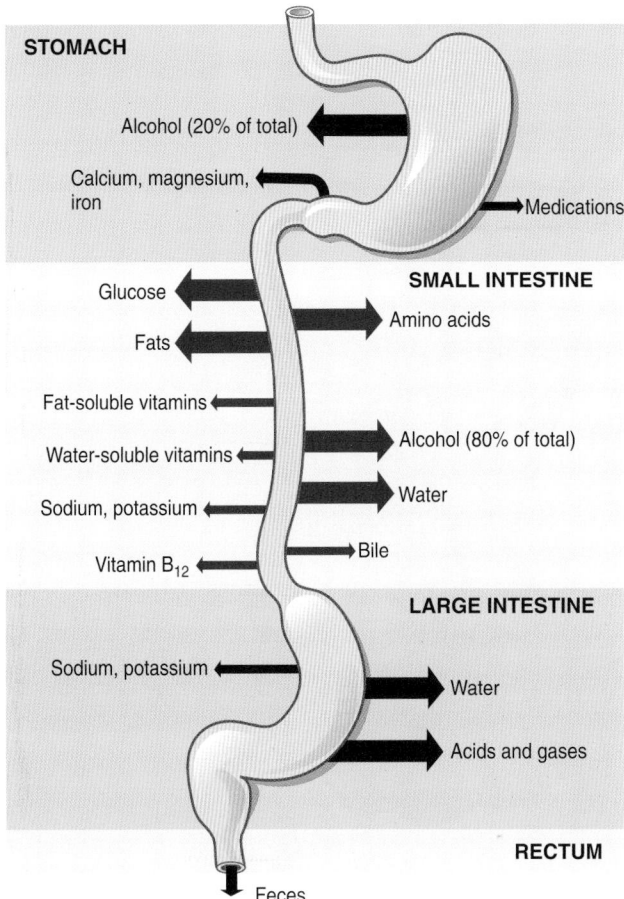

FIG. 29.6 Absorption in the gastrointestinal tract with most occurring in the length of the small intestine.

- **Cholecystokinin**—Intestinal hormones that stimulate the secretion of bile and pancreatic enzymes; slows down the discharge of gastric contents into the small intestines
- **Secretin**—Intestinal hormone that stimulates the pancreas to secrete an alkaline liquid neutralizing acidic chyme, and making it more alkaline, which facilitates enzymatic digestion (see Table 29.1)

LARGE INTESTINE

The **large intestine**, large bowel, or colon is the tube beyond the small intestine. The large intestine is called large because of its diameter compared with the small intestine, and it is actually shorter—approximately 5 to 6 feet. The *ileocecal sphincter* is the beginning of the large intestine and the *external anal sphincter* is the end. Functions of the large intestine are absorption of water and electrolytes, production of vitamins, such as K and some B vitamins, formation and elimination of *feces* or stools. The sections of the large intestine are featured next (Fig. 29.7):

- **Cecum**—Blind pouch in the lower right quadrant of the abdomen; the vermiform appendix, which contains lymphatic tissue, is suspended from the inferior surface of the cecum (see Chapter 27)

- **Ascending Colon**—Section that ascends upward to the liver
  - **Hepatic Flexure (Right Colic Flexure)**—Bend between the ascending colon and the transverse colon found inferior to the liver
- **Transverse Colon**—Horizontal section from the liver at the right to the spleen at the left
  - **Splenic Flexure (Left Colic Flexure)**—Bend between the transverse colon and the descending colon found inferior to the spleen
- **Descending Colon**—Section that descends downward from the spleen
  - **Sigmoid Flexure**—Bend between the descending colon and the sigmoid colon found at the top of the iliac crest
- **Sigmoid Colon**—S-shaped section from the middle of the abdomen to the rectum
- **Rectum**—Contains overlapping circular folds when empty, and expands to become straight as it fills with feces
  - **Anus**—Section of the rectum where feces exits the body. It contains two sphincters. The *internal anal sphincter* has involuntary smooth muscle. As feces fills the rectum and presses against the internal anal sphincter, the urge to defecate occurs. The *external anal sphincter* is voluntary muscle, which stays contracted until defecation, when feces is eliminated from the body.

Two distinguishing features of the colon are taeniae coli and haustra. *Taeniae coli* are thick, longitudinal bands resembling a thread-gathering fabric. *Haustra* are pouches formed by taenia coli, giving the colon a segmented appearance. Contents of the large intestine are moved by intermittent peristaltic waves pushing the contents of one haustrum to the next in a patterned sequence. Water is continually absorbed through the intestinal wall, changing its contents from a semiliquid to a semisolid mass before defecation.

Secretions

The lining of the large intestine secretes only mucus.

The body tells the story. It is, in fact, a living autobiography.

—Elaine Mayland

ACCESSORY ORGANS AND GLANDS

The accessory organs of digestion are the liver, gallbladder, and pancreas (Fig. 29.8). They produce and secrete substances aiding in the chemical digestion of food while in the small intestine.

LIVER

The **liver** is inferior to the diaphragm in the upper right quadrant of the abdomen. The liver is the largest organ within the body, weighing between 3 and 4 pounds. It has two main lobes, a larger one and a smaller one, separated by

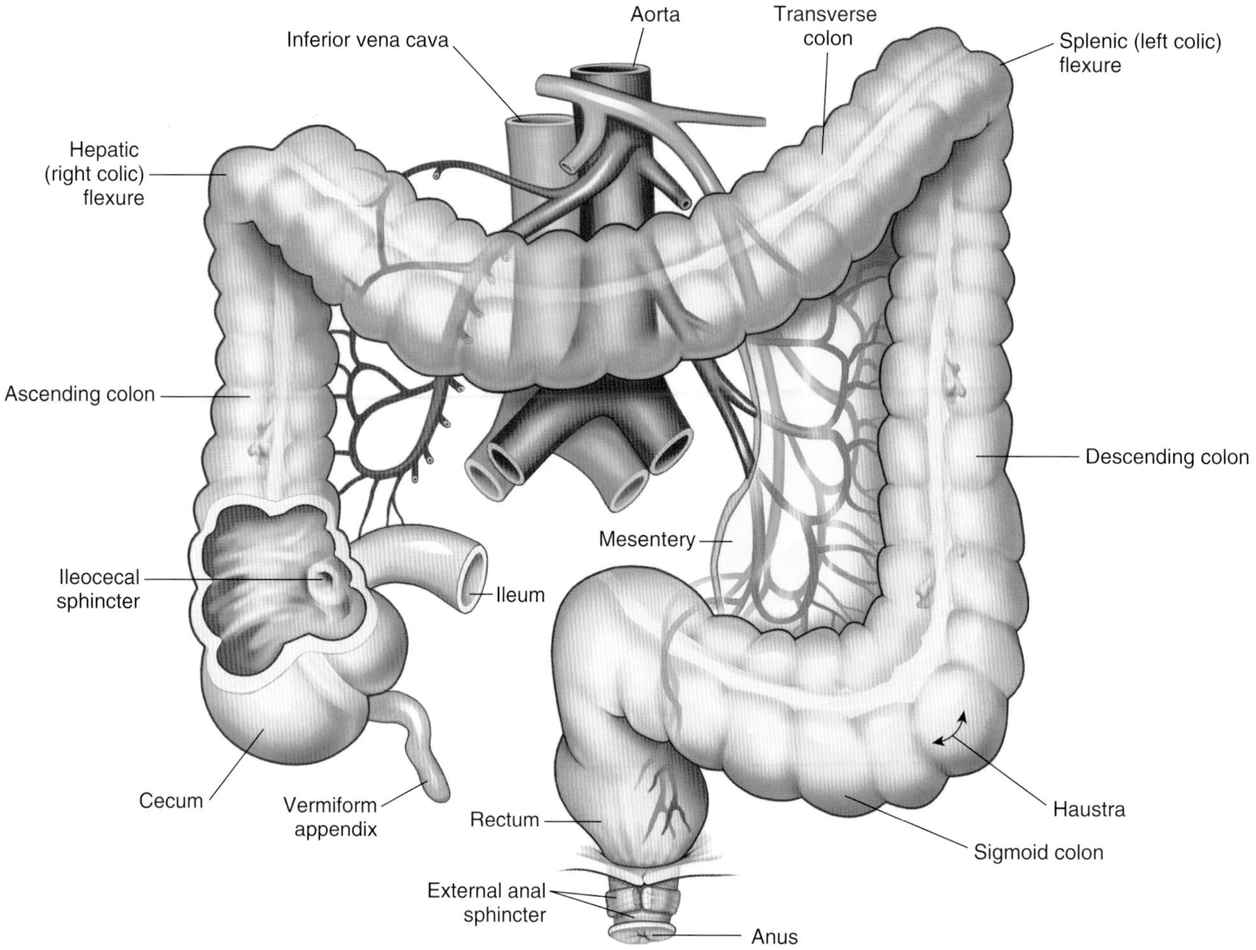

FIG. 29.7 Large intestine with sections and flexures identified (*anterior view*); the mesentery, part of the peritoneum, lies behind the intestines and digestive organs. (From Thibodeau, G. A. & Patton, K. T. [2007]. *Anatomy & physiology* [6th ed.]. St. Louis, MO: Mosby.)

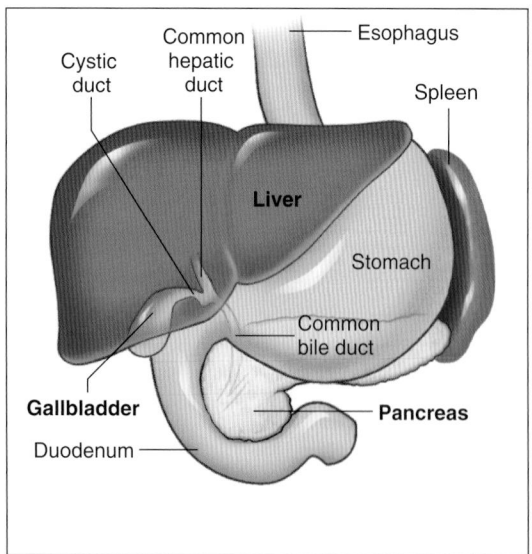

FIG. 29.8 Accessory digestive organs, which include the liver, gallbladder, and pancreas (*anterior view*). (Modified from Patton, K. T. [2013]. *Anatomy & physiology* [8th ed.]. St. Louis, MO: Mosby.)

a ligament. The functions of the liver include (1) metabolizing proteins, carbohydrates, and fats; (2) producing plasma proteins; (3) storing nutrients including glycogen (stored glucose), minerals, such as iron and copper, fat-soluble vitamins, and B_{12}; (4) detoxifying certain harmful chemicals; (5) excreting substances, such as bilirubin, cholesterol, and drugs; (6) producing bile; and (7) providing defense through phagocytosis by Kupffer cells. Hepatic means liver.

The liver has a unique arrangement of blood vessels called the *hepatic portal system*, which carries blood from the capillaries of the GI tract, the spleen, gallbladder, and pancreas to the liver (see Fig. 26.14).

Secretions

The main secretion serving a digestive function is bile.

- **Bile**—Greenish-yellow liquid emulsifying fat, which means separating large globules into small droplets. This allows pancreatic lipase, a fat-digesting enzyme, to work more efficiently. The result is increased absorption of fatty acids and fat-soluble vitamins A, D, E, and K.

GALLBLADDER

The **gallbladder** is a hollow pear-shaped sac on the inferior surface of the liver. The gallbladder stores and concentrates bile produced by the liver. The lining of the gallbladder contains *rugae* similar to the lining of the stomach. Rugae enable the gallbladder to expand as it fills with bile.

The **biliary tract**, or *biliary system*, refers to the liver, gallbladder, and bile ducts that store bile and release it into the small intestine. Bile is released by the liver and enters the common hepatic duct. The common hepatic duct joins the cystic duct from the gallbladder to form the common bile duct. The common bile duct terminates at the duodenum. During a meal, bile is secreted into the duodenum to help break down the fats. Some of the bile is stored in the gallbladder. When needed, the gallbladder contracts and releases stored bile into the duodenum. The common bile duct is later joined by the pancreatic duct before entering the duodenum at the major duodenal papilla.

Secretions

The gallbladder does not produce the bile it stores or secretes.

PANCREAS

The **pancreas** is a pinkish-gray gland approximately 6 to 9 inches in length that lies posterior to the stomach. The pancreatic duct runs the length of the pancreas, joins the common bile duct, and enters the duodenum at the major duodenal papilla. The pancreatic duct carries digestive enzymes from the pancreas to the duodenum (Fig. 29.9).

Secretions

The pancreas secretes enzymes breaking down all categories of digestible food. The pancreas also secretes substances rich in bicarbonate, which neutralizes the highly acidic chyme released from the stomach into the duodenum.

- **Trypsin**—Facilitates protein digestion; trypsin is secreted as inactive trysinogen and, upon mixing with the hydrochloric acid, becomes active trypsin
- **Chymotrypsin**—Facilitates protein digestion; chymotrypsin is secreted as inactive chymotrypsinogen and, upon mixing with trypsin, becomes active chymotrypsin
- **Pancreatic Amylase**—Facilitates carbohydrate digestion
- **Pancreatic Lipase**—Facilitates fat digestion

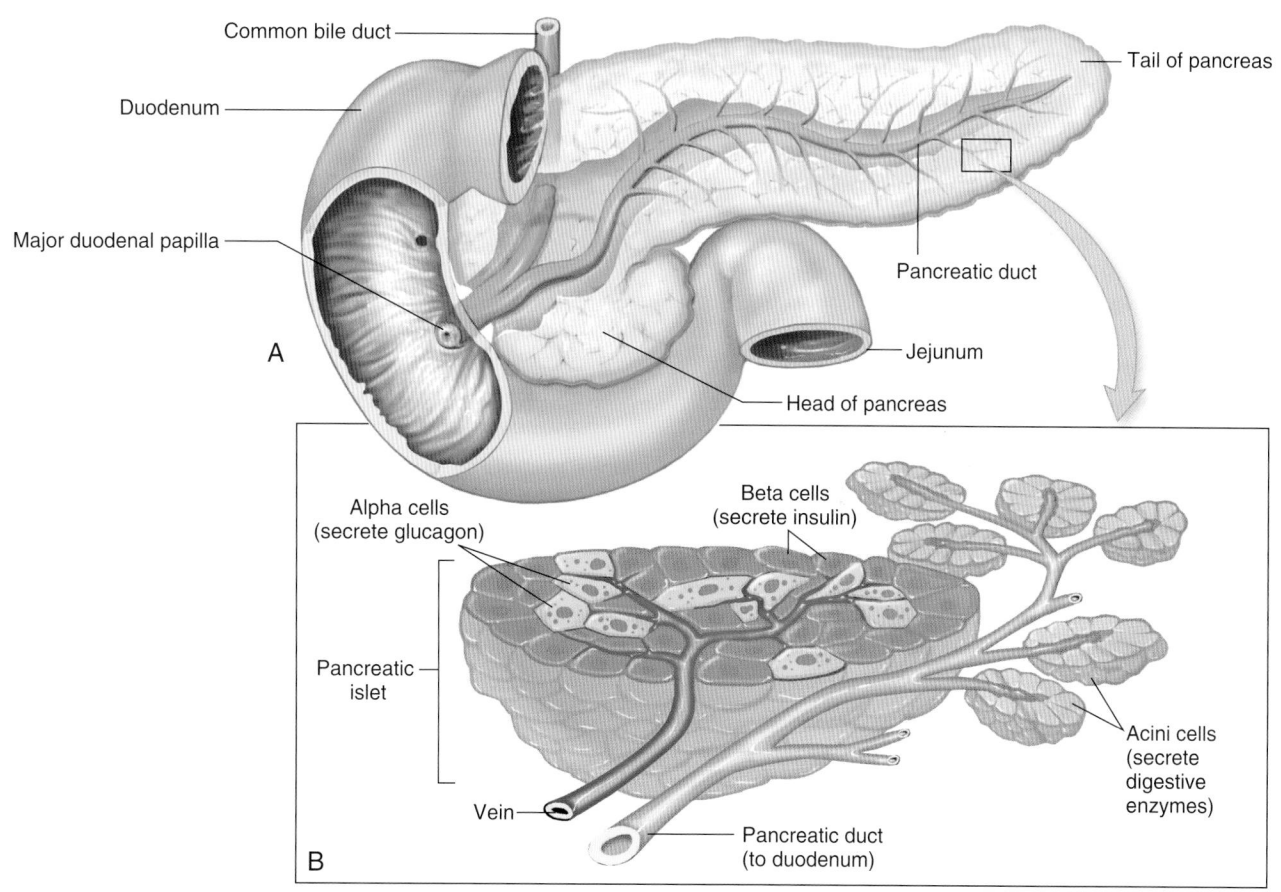

FIG. 29.9 Pancreas. (A) Locations of the pancreas, pancreatic and common bile ducts, and the major duodenal papilla (*anterior view*). (B) Enzyme-producing Acini cells and their relationship to the hormone-producing alpha and beta cells (*microscopic view*). (Modified from Patton, K. T. [2013]. *Anatomy & physiology* [8th ed.]. St. Louis, MO: Mosby.)

- **Somatostatin**—Inhibits secretion of pancreatic hormones including glucagon and insulin
- **Pancreatic Polypeptides**—Inhibits the activity of other pancreatic secretions, gallbladder contraction, intestinal motility, and satiety or feelings of fullness after consuming food

GASTROINTESTINAL PATHOLOGIES, DYSFUNCTIONS, AND DISORDERS

Featured next are common pathologies, dysfunctions, and disorders of the digestive system, listed alphabetically. Each item includes a brief description and its massage-related modifications. A more extensive list and related research is found in the current edition of *Mosby's Pathology for Massage Professionals*.

Cirrhosis

Cirrhosis is a progressive disease in which liver cells degenerate and are replaced by fibrotic scar tissue, giving it a yellow-orange color and cobbled appearance (called a "hobnail liver"). Cirrhosis is twice as common in males as females. The affected person bruises easily because the liver stops producing proteins that help blood clot. Small, red, spidery marks on the skin that itch may appear on the skin. Cirrhosis is usually the result of viral hepatitis (usually hepatitis B or C virus [HBV or HCV]), nonalcoholic fatty liver disease, or alcoholic hepatitis. In some cases, cirrhosis is idiopathic.

Massage and Cirrhosis

If the client is uncomfortable lying prone due to abdominal swelling, use a different position, such as side-lying or seated, to massage the back. Inform the client of the possibility of bruising from the massage. However, if the client is frail, use slowly applied light pressure. An example of light pressure is 3 on a 10-point pressure scale. Avoid skin rashes.

Constipation

Constipation is infrequent or difficult passing of stools, usually described as having fewer than three bowel movements a week. Normal bowel habits range from two to three evacuations daily to three a week, and depend on various factors, including diet and activity. Constipation is common among all ages and populations in the United States. Constipation is regarded as harmless, but it can indicate an underlying disease. Constipation may be considered chronic if it lasts for 3 months. Common causes of constipation are insufficient intake of fluid or dietary fiber, lack of physical activity, irritable bowel syndrome (IBS), diverticulitis, diabetes, advanced pregnancy, and advancing age. Other causes are consistent suppression of the defecation reflex because of pain, such as from anal fissure or hemorrhoids, or inconvenience, such as no access to a toilet. Medication side

effects may reduce bowel motility and lead to constipation, particularly with narcotic pain relievers. Some neurologic conditions, such as multiple sclerosis, Parkinson disease, and spinal cord injury, contribute to constipation.

Massage and Constipation

Abdominal massage is an effective intervention for constipation. The following massage procedure can help relieve constipation symptoms. Modify or discontinue any massage movements that cause pain. Coexisting conditions (e.g., multiple sclerosis, Parkinson disease) should be factored into the treatment plan. The client should be in the supine position with the knees resting on a bolster, which helps relax the abdominal muscles. This procedure has six steps, and uses medium pressure and vibrational movements that follow the colon route.

1. With the finger pads of one or both hands, apply effleurage over the descending colon starting from the left lower ribs to the left pelvis. Repeat this movement 10 to 15 times.
2. With the palms of one or both hands, apply effleurage over the transverse colon starting from the right lower ribs before moving to the left lower ribs and include the area to the navel. Repeat this movement 10 to 15 times.
3. With the finger pads of one or both hands, apply effleurage over the ascending colon starting from the right pelvis to the right lower ribs. Repeat this movement 10 to 15 times.
4. With the finger pads of one or both hands, apply small circular effleurage in a clockwise direction over all three sections of the colon. Begin at the left pelvis, moving backwards up the descending colon, across the transverse colon, and down the ascending colon. Repeat the movement series 10 to 15 times.
5. With the finger pads of one or both hands, apply effleurage over all three sections of the colon starting from the right pelvis to the right lower ribs, to the left lower ribs, to the left pelvis. The shape is an upside-down "U," and movements will be applied in a clockwise direction. Repeat this movement 10 to 15 times.
6. With the finger pads of one or both hands, apply vibration over the abdomen for 30 seconds to conclude the massage.

This procedure can be taught to clients for self-application or taught to client caregivers. This massage should be done daily at home for the best results. Remind clients to follow any treatments recommended by other members of their healthcare team.

Crohn Disease

Crohn disease (CD) is an inflammatory bowel disease causing long-term inflammation and ulcer formation. CD most commonly affects the end of the small intestine or ileum, but any part of the GI tract can be affected, including the large intestine, stomach, esophagus, or even the mouth. Typically, normal segments are separated by diseased segments called *skip lesions.* CD can occur at any age, but it is most common between the ages of 15 and 30. The cause of CD is unknown, but it is thought to be an autoimmune disease. Approximately one-third of people with CD also have other autoimmune conditions. Individuals with Crohn disease are at a higher risk for reduced bone density and osteoporosis; the risk increases if the person takes corticosteroids for disease management.

Massage and Crohn Disease

Avoid massaging the abdomen if pressure causes pain or discomfort. Position the client for comfort. Because periods of exacerbation may be linked to stress, relaxing massage is indicated using techniques of even pressure and slower speed. Rhythmic effleurage (gliding) may enhance the relaxation effect. Some clients develop osteoporosis as a disease complication. In these cases, reduce bone stress by decreasing the amount of applied massage pressure over areas of known bone loss and avoid forceful passive range of motion (PROM).

Diarrhea

Diarrhea is frequent passing of unformed, loose, watery stools. Diarrhea can be acute, and last a few days, or chronic, and last a few weeks, depending on the cause. Diarrhea is also considered a protective response, especially acute cases, in an attempt to remove harmful ingested substances. Most acute cases of diarrhea are caused by infection from viruses (especially noroviruses), parasites, and bacteria (especially *Escherichia coli*). Possible causes of chronic diarrhea include digestive disorders, such as CD, ulcerative colitis, celiac disease, and irritable bowel syndrome. Other causes include stress, diet, medication side effects (particularly antibiotics and hypoglycemics), and sweeteners, such as fructose, and artificial sweeteners, such as Sorbitol and Mannitol.

Massage and Diarrhea

Ask the client about what caused the diarrhea. For acute gastritis, massage is postponed until the client has been fever-free for 24 hours without the use of fever-reducing drugs, such as ibuprofen or acetaminophen (Centers for Disease Control and Prevention [CDC], 2021).

For chronic cases, avoid the abdomen if pressure causes uneasiness or discomfort, and suggest the client use the toilet before massage as a comfort measure. Be prepared for a toilet break during the session. Offer drinking water before and after the massage because chronic diarrhea can cause dehydration.

Diverticulosis and Diverticulitis

Diverticulosis is the presence of small herniations called diverticula in the colon, usually the sigmoid colon. Once they form, they are permanent. Diverticula range from 1/10 of an inch to a full inch in diameter. Complications, such as rectal bleeding and diverticulitis, affect about 20% of people

with diverticulosis. **Diverticulitis** is inflammation or infection of diverticula. Fecal matter plugs the diverticula and predisposes the area to infection with colonic bacteria. A perforation can develop in an infected diverticula, leading to peritonitis, a serious complication.

Massage and Diverticulosis/Diverticulitis

For clients with diverticulosis, avoid the abdomen during the massage if pressure causes the client discomfort. For clients with diverticulitis, massage is postponed until the condition has resolved.

Gallstones

Gallstones are masses of solid material or stones called calculi that form in the gallbladder or bile duct. Gallstones can be tiny (the size of a grain of sand) or may be as large as a golf ball. Some people develop a single gallstone, whereas others develop many gallstones at the same time. Gallstones may remain undetected or become lodged in the common bile duct. Risk factors include obesity, middle age, being female, and having Native American ancestry. They are also seen in females who are pregnant or use oral contraceptives. Losing weight too rapidly or eating a very low-calorie diet also can cause gallstones. Gallstones recur in approximately 50% of people within 5 years if nonsurgical treatment is used.

Massage and Gallstones

Clients can receive massage if they currently have gallstones or have had gallstones previously. However, massage is postponed if the client exhibits signs and symptoms of gallstone obstruction, such as nausea, vomiting, and intermittent or steady pain in the upper right quadrant, often radiating to the right shoulder. A referral to the client's primary care provider is then indicated.

Gastroesophageal Reflux Disease

Gastroesophageal reflux disease (GERD) is periodic regurgitation of gastric contents into the esophagus. GERD is most often caused by one of two scenarios: Relaxation of the LES or increased intraabdominal pressure. Either scenario allows stomach acids to enter the lower esophagus. Situations that increase intraabdominal pressure are overeating and obesity, pregnancy-related weight gain, frequent vomiting, and lifting heavy objects. Medications that weaken the LES include sedatives, calcium channel blockers for high blood pressure, birth control pills, antihistamines, and several other asthma medications. Some cases of GERD are idiopathic.

Massage and Gastroesophageal Reflux Disease

The client should wait 3 hours after consuming a meal before lying down for a massage. Discuss this with your client and consider scheduling the massage appointment accordingly. If this is not possible, elevate the upper body in a semireclining position while lying supine to reduce symptoms (Mayo Clinic, 2018). When side lying, position the client on their left side with the head elevated with a pillow, as this position makes it easier for acids to flow from the LES into the stomach because of gravity.

Hepatitis

Hepatitis is inflammation of the liver. Most cases of hepatitis are caused by viruses, and named after the first five letters of the alphabet (A, B, C, D, and E). Hepatitis A (HAV), hepatitis B (HBV), and hepatitis C (HCV) are the most common forms of viral hepatitis. Hepatitis can either be acute (lasting less than 6 months) or chronic (lasting more than 6 months). Although most people recover from hepatitis, it is considered a serious health risk because it can destroy liver cells, weaken the body's immune response, and cause liver cancer or liver failure. As the disease progresses, the liver stops producing proteins that help blood clot, causing easy bruising.

- **Hepatitis A**—Most cases are mild, with recovery within 2 months and no lasting liver damage. Infection recovery provides lifelong immunity. However, some HAV infections are severe and life threatening. In 2017, a widespread outbreak occurred among people who used intravenous drugs and were experiencing homelessness. Vaccines are available to reduce the risk of HAV infection.
- **Hepatitis B**—Most cases are mild, with recovery within 6 months. The person may be asymptomatic; the virus can still be transmitted during this time. Some cases cause chronic, lifelong infection. The earlier in life HBV is contracted, the more likely it is to become chronic. Vaccines are available to reduce the risk of HBV infection.
- **Hepatitis C**—Most cases of HCV are chronic. HCV is one of the most common causes of liver disease in the United States and the number one reason for liver transplant. The person may be asymptomatic, but the virus can still be transmitted during this time. No vaccine is yet available to reduce the risk of HCV infection.

Types of nonviral hepatitis include alcoholic hepatitis caused by drinking too much alcohol and autoimmune hepatitis caused by the body attacking healthy liver cells.

Massage and Hepatitis

The appropriateness of massage is determined by the client's symptoms. Massage is contraindicated if clients have fever until they have been fever-free for 24 hours without the use of fever-reducing drugs, such as ibuprofen or acetaminophen. If the client is uncomfortable lying prone due to abdominal swelling, use a different position, such as sidelying or seated, to massage the back. If the client is nauseated, consider using a semireclining (semi or standard Fowler) or upright (high Fowler) position while the client is supine to reduce the severity of nausea. In addition, avoid techniques that cause the client to rock or shake because excessive body motion may worsen nausea. Consider having a disposable emesis bag in the massage room in case it

is needed. Inform the client of the possibility of bruising from the massage.

Irritable Bowel Syndrome

Irritable bowel syndrome (IBS) is characterized by abnormal muscular contractions of the colon. It occurs more often in females than males, and generally begins before the age of 35. Unlike UC and CD, IBS does not cause inflammation, or permanently damage the intestines. Endometriosis may accompany IBS, which complicates diagnosis of either condition. IBS is also called irritable bowel disease or spastic colon.

Massage and Irritable Bowel Syndrome

Avoid the abdomen if pressure causes pain or discomfort. Because many cases of IBS are related to stress, a relaxing massage is indicated, which includes techniques using even pressure and slower speed. If the client is nauseated, use a semireclining (semi or standard Fowler) or upright (high Fowler) position while the client is supine to reduce the severity of nausea. In addition, avoid techniques that cause the client to rock or shake because excessive body motion may worsen nausea. Consider having a disposable emesis bag in the massage room in case it is needed.

Peptic Ulcer Disease

Peptic ulcer disease (PUD) is ulcerations or open sores in parts of the GI tract exposed to acidic gastric juice. The word "peptic" refers to the enzyme pepsin, which breaks down proteins. Ulcers can be found in the lower esophagus (esophageal ulcers), stomach (gastric or stomach ulcers), or duodenum (duodenal ulcers). All peptic ulcers have the same appearance: a sharply punched-out round hole, which can extend into deep mucosal layers. Normally, a thick layer of mucus protects the stomach lining from the effect of gastric juice. But many things can reduce this protective layer, allowing for ulcers to occur. Peptic ulcers of all types have a tendency to recur.

Massage and Peptic Ulcer Disease

Ask the client about symptoms, such as abdominal discomfort and heartburn. If the client has heartburn, they should wait 3 hours after consuming a meal before lying down for a massage. Discuss this with your client and consider scheduling the massage appointment accordingly. If this is not possible, elevate the upper body in a semireclining position while lying supine to reduce heartburn symptoms (Mayo Clinic, 2018). When side lying, position the client on their left side with their head elevated with a pillow, as this position makes it easier for acids to flow from the LES into the stomach because of gravity. If the client has abdominal discomfort, avoid the abdomen.

Ulcerative Colitis

Ulcerative colitis (UC) is an inflammatory bowel disease causing long-term inflammation and ulcer formation in the colon. UC usually begins in the rectum and then spreads proximally. How much of the colon is affected varies from person to person. UC is characterized by alternating periods of exacerbation or flare-ups and remission. Periods of exacerbation are often precipitated by emotional stress and can last from weeks to years. Individuals with ulcerative colitis are at a higher risk for reduced bone density and osteoporosis; the risk increases if the person takes corticosteroids for disease management.

Massage and Ulcerative Colitis

Massage is postponed until the client has been fever-free for 24 hours without the use of fever-reducing drugs, such as ibuprofen or acetaminophen. Avoid massaging the abdomen if pressure causes pain or discomfort. Because periods of exacerbation may be linked to stress, relaxing massage is indicated using techniques of even pressure and slower speed. Rhythmic effleurage (gliding) may enhance the relaxation effect. Some clients develop osteoporosis as a disease complication. In these cases, reduce bone stress by decreasing the amount of applied massage pressure over areas of known bone loss, and avoid forceful PROM.

In dwelling, live close to the ground. In thinking, keep it simple. In conflict, be fair and generous. In governing, don't control. In work, do what you enjoy. In family life, be completely present.

—Tao Te Ching

E-RESOURCES

http://evolve.elsevier.com/Salvo/MassageTherapy

* Chapter challenge
* Flash cards

JOHN BARNES

Sometimes we do things that work and only later understand why. Discovering this "why" is one of the great pleasures of massage school and continuing education. It is also key to becoming better at our work because it enables us to make educated choices rather than relying on blind luck. John Barnes successfully treated people for years as a physical therapist and massage practitioner, but it was only after he began learning more about fascia in the body that the work that has spread his name across the globe took shape.

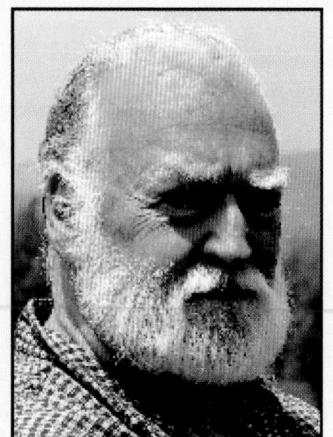

Born in 1939 and raised in Philadelphia, Barnes knew since high school he wanted to be a physical therapist. Lifting weights in the gym, he loaded the barbell with too much weight and found he was unable to rise from his deep squat. Stuck, he attempted to roll backward but landed on his tailbone with 300 pounds on his shoulders. He brushed off the injury at first, thinking it minor, but his condition worsened with multiple reinjuries. Surgery reduced but did not eliminate his pain.

Of this experience Barnes would later say to Robert Calvert, "I don't really mean this should happen, but in a way, every physician or practitioner should be severely injured, and not just hurt for a week or two or a month but a couple years. It's a whole different story when you are a prisoner in your own body. I felt broken, and I was broken. It was a horrible, horrible experience."

Barnes graduated from the University of Pennsylvania as a physical therapist in 1960 and began his practice. His style was slow, rhythmic, and focused, and he was able to help many patients with their pain. But it was learning about fascia that truly illuminated the process for him. Fascia, the thin, iridescent connective tissue surrounding and permeating various structures of the body, proved to be the missing connection between treatment and result. Further study and practice resulted in the development of the John F. Barnes myofascial approach to massage.

Barnes began teaching others his approach in the mid-1970s and continues to teach it today. His method is systematic yet holistic, and he encourages his students to give up the compulsion to fix everything: Massage practitioners cannot fix anything; they can only offer the body and mind tools to change themselves.

To massage students and new graduates, Barnes advocates for advanced continuing education. Reading about a technique or taking an introductory class is a nice start but insufficient and can lead to bad habits and dangerous mishandling of the technique. He also recommends learning many different forms of massage and bodywork. That way, no matter the needs of your client, you always have a skill that may be able to help.

Barnes's advice for new massage practitioners is to continue learning advanced methods after graduation. Simply reading about a bodywork concept or a basic introduction to a modality is insufficient to practice it successfully, and, in some cases, may lead to bad habits or faulty techniques. Barnes suggests learning as many forms of bodywork as possible to adapt to the wide range of client needs.

Barnes has written two books and many articles, and continues to teach his method all over the world. *Massage Magazine* named him one of the most influential people in the profession in the last century. He is the president of The Sanctuary, the Myofascial Release Treatment Center in Malvern, Pennsylvania, and Therapy on the Rocks in Sedona, Arizona.

Given the choice between treatment that seems to work and treatment that does not, choose the one that works. But do not give up on trying to understand what makes things work, even if it leads you down some uncomfortable roads. Follow the example of John Barnes and never stop learning. Never stop asking why.

REFERENCES

Centers for Disease Control and Prevention. (2021). *Guidance for school administrators to help reduce the spread of infection.* Retrieved from https://www.cdc.gov/flu/school/guidance.htm. Accessed June 21, 2022.

Mayo Clinic. (2018). *Heartburn.* Retrieved from https://www.mayoclinic.org/diseases-conditions/heartburn/diagnosis-treatment/drc-20373229.

Salvo, S. G. (2022). *Mosby's Pathology for Massage Professionals* (5th ed.). St Louis: Mosby.

BIBLIOGRAPHY

Abrahams, P. H., Spratt, J. D., Loukas, M., & van Schoor, A. N. (2003). *Abrahams' and McMinn's clinical atlas of human anatomy* (8th ed.). St Louis: Elsevier.

Applegate, E. (2010). *The anatomy and physiology learning system* (4th ed.). Philadelphia: Saunders.

Como, D. (Ed.), (2016). *Mosby's dictionary of medicine, nursing, and health professions* (10th ed.). St Louis: Elsevier.

Frazier, M. S., & Drzymkowski, J. W. (2015). *Essentials of human diseases and conditions* (6th ed.). St Louis: Elsevier.

Hubert, R. J., & VanMeter, K. C. (2018). *Gould's pathophysiology for the health professions* (6th ed.). Philadelphia: Saunders.

Haubrich, W. S. (2003). *Medical meanings: A glossary of word origins* (2nd ed.). New York: American College of Physicians.

Herlihy, B. (2017). *The human body in health and illness* (6th ed.). St Louis: Saunders.

Huether, S. E., McCance, K. L., & Brashers, V. L. (2019). *Understanding pathophysiology* (7th ed.). St Louis: Mosby.

Kalat, J. W. (2013). *Biological psychology* (11th ed.). Belmont: Cengage Learning.

Kapit, W., & Elson, L. M. (2013). *The anatomy coloring book* (4th ed.). New York: Benjamin Cummings.

Kumar, V., Abbas, A. K., & Aster, J. C. (2015). *Robbins & Cotran pathologic basis of disease* (9th ed.). St Louis: Mosby.

Marieb, E. N., & Keller, S. M. (2018). *Essentials of human anatomy and physiology* (12th ed.). New York: Benjamin Cummings.

McCance, K. L., & Huether, S. E. (2019). *Pathophysiology: The biological basis for disease in adults and children* (8th ed.). St Louis: Mosby.

Myers, T. W. (2014). *Anatomy trains: Myofascial meridians for manual and movement therapists* (3rd ed.). Churchill Livingstone: Elsevier.

Netter, F. H. (2018). *Atlas of human anatomy* (7th ed.). St Louis: Mosby.

Patton, K. T (2019). *Anatomy and physiology* (10th ed.). St Louis: Elsevier.

Patton, K. T., Thibodeau, G. A., & Douglas, M. M. (2012). *Essentials of anatomy and physiology* (4th ed.). New York: Pearson.

Porter, R. S., (2011). *The Merck manual of diagnosis and therapy* (19th ed). Whitehouse Station, NJ: Merck Sharp and Dohme Corp.

Taber, C. W. (2021). *Taber's cyclopedic medical dictionary* (24th ed.). Philadelphia: FA Davis.

REVIEW AND APPLY YOUR KNOWLEDGE

 **MATCHING ONE: CONCEPT REVIEW**

Place the letter of the answer next to the number of the term or phrase that best describes it.

A. Absorption
B. Bolus
C. Defecation
D. Digestion
E. Enzyme
F. Esophagus
G. Gastrointestinal tract
H. Ingestion
I. Mucosa
J. Peristalsis
K. Saliva
L. Sphincter

_____   1. Substance that acts as a catalyst in chemical reactions.
_____   2. Long muscular tube that begins in the mouth and ends at the anus.
_____   3. Innermost layer of the GI tract.
_____   4. Small round mass of food.
_____   5. Watery liquid whose moisturizing effects preserve oral hygiene and allows taste, speech, and mastication.
_____   6. Process of taking materials into the mouth by eating and drinking.
_____   7. Tube behind the trachea that aids in the transport of food and liquids from the pharynx to the stomach.
_____   8. Process of eliminating indigestible or unabsorbed materials from the body.
_____   9. Mixing or propulsive movements caused by smooth muscle contraction in the GI tract.
_____ 10. Process of breaking materials down into molecules that can be used by the body.
_____ 11. A ring-shaped muscle that relaxes or tightens to open or close an opening in the body.
_____ 12. Process by which molecules move from the GI tract into blood or lymph vessels and then into body cells.

MATCHING TWO: CONCEPT REVIEW

Place the letter of the answer next to the number of the term or phrase that best describes it.

A. Bile
B. Duodenum
C. Gallbladder
D. Lipase
E. Amylase
F. Liver
G. Pancreas
H. Peritoneum
I. Pyloric
J. Rugae
K. Small intestine
L. Villi

_____   1. Pinkish-gray gland that lies posterior to the stomach.
_____   2. Hollow pear-shaped sac that stores and concentrates bile.
_____   3. First and shortest portion of the small intestines and contains ducts from the liver, gallbladder, and pancreas.
_____   4. Fingerlike projections that house blood and lymph capillaries.
_____   5. Enzyme that promotes carbohydrate digestion.
_____   6. Sphincter between the stomach and small intestine.
_____   7. Enzyme that promotes fat digestion.
_____   8. Coiled tube between the stomach and large intestine and where most absorption occurs.
_____   9. Large serous membrane within the abdominopelvic cavity and serves as an anchor for digestive organs, blood and lymph vessels, and nerves.
_____ 10. Folds that permit expansion found in the stomach and gallbladder.
_____ 11. Organ that produces bile and is the largest organ within the body.
_____ 12. Digestive fat emulsifier that separates large fat globules into smaller droplets.

MULTIPLE CHOICE: TEST YOUR KNOWLEDGE

Place the letter of the answer next to the number of the term or phrase that best describes it.

_____ 1. Which function of the digestive system involves producing mucus, chemicals, and enzymes?
   A. Ingestion
   B. Digestion
   C. Secretion
   D. Absorption

_____ 2. Which is the outermost layer of the GI tract?
   A. Mucosa
   B. Submucosa
   C. Muscle
   D. Serosa

_____ 3. Saliva mixed with phlegm is called:
   A. Pepsin
   B. Sputum
   C. Chyme
   D. Bile

_____ 4. Which of the following is a passageway for both digestive and respiratory systems?
   A. Pharynx
   B. Larynx
   C. Esophagus
   D. Mesentery

_____ 5. The cecum is in the _____ quadrant.
   A. Upper right
   B. Upper left
   C. Lower left
   D. Lower right

_____ 6. Which stomach secretion aids in B12 absorption?
   A. Pepsin
   B. Hydrochloric acid
   C. Intrinsic factor
   D. Gastrin

_____ 7. Which sphincter begins the large intestine?
   A. Cardiac
   B. Pyloric
   C. Ileocecal
   D. Anal

_____ 8. Which is the correct order of the large intestine?
   A. Ascending, descending, transverse, sigmoid
   B. Ascending, transverse, descending, sigmoid
   C. Descending, ascending, transverse, sigmoid
   D. Descending, transverse, ascending, sigmoid

_____ 9. The liver is in the _____ quadrant.
   A. Upper left
   B. Lower left
   C. Upper right
   D. Lower right

_____ 10. The liver, gallbladder and ducts that make and store bile, and release it into the small intestine are collectively called the:
   A. Gastrointestinal tract
   B. Biliary tract
   C. Hepatic portal
   D. Digestive portal

_____ 11. Which degenerative pathology creates the appearance of a "hobnail liver"?
   A. Cirrhosis
   B. Crohn
   C. Hepatitis A
   D. Hepatitis C

_____ 12. Which pathology would cause the practitioner to postpone massage until the condition is resolved?
   A. Irritable bowel syndrome
   B. Peptic ulcer disease
   C. Diverticulosis
   D. Diverticulitis

CRITICAL THINKING

Orange Means Warning

You notice your next client has skin with an orange tint. There is nothing on the health history form to indicate what this could be from. What are possible reasons for the client's appearance? What questions would you ask during the pretreatment interview to design the best treatment plan for the client?

Answers can include but are not limited to:

An orange tint to the client's skin can be from something simple, such as a spray-on tan or ingestion of foods high in carotene. It can also be from more serious conditions, such as jaundice, which is an indicator of possible hepatitis infection or cirrhosis of the liver.

Pretreatment interview questions can include asking the client if they are aware of the orange tint of their skin and if the cause is known. (Sometimes people who ingest foods high in carotene are unaware their skin has changed color.) The questions should be asked in a professional and nonjudgmental manner.

If the client is hesitant to answer questions, it may be because of a more serious condition, such as hepatitis or cirrhosis of the liver. Clients are not always comfortable revealing information about themselves, and sometimes think they will not be able to receive massage if they do. It is important to explain that the treatment will be designed according to the client's needs, and adapted according to their health.

PROFESSIONAL PRACTICE

Oh No, Not Now

Sandy arrives at your office at 4:45 for her 5 a.m. massage appointment. She is 29 years old and has just found out she is pregnant. After she fills out the intake form, she heads for the toilet, and does not return for about 10 minutes. During the interview, Sandy says she has diarrhea and some cramping today, adding, "But that's normal with IBS, you know." Because of her pregnancy, her doctor has taken her off her medications. What is an appropriate treatment plan for Sandy?

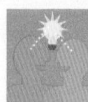

DISCUSSION

Lifestyle Diseases

Americans are among the most obese individuals in the world. Many causes have been cited, including advertising, industrial farming practices, chronic stress, artificial sweeteners, sedentary lifestyle, genetically modified foods, and a culture accustomed to modern conveniences. What do you think may be contributing to this epidemic? Where do you feel the responsibility lies? With the individual? Parents? Advertising? What impact does obesity have on healthcare costs? Can this problem be solved? If so, what do you propose? Are other countries discouraging obesity? How? If available, post your reflections on an internet-based discussion board monitored by your instructor.

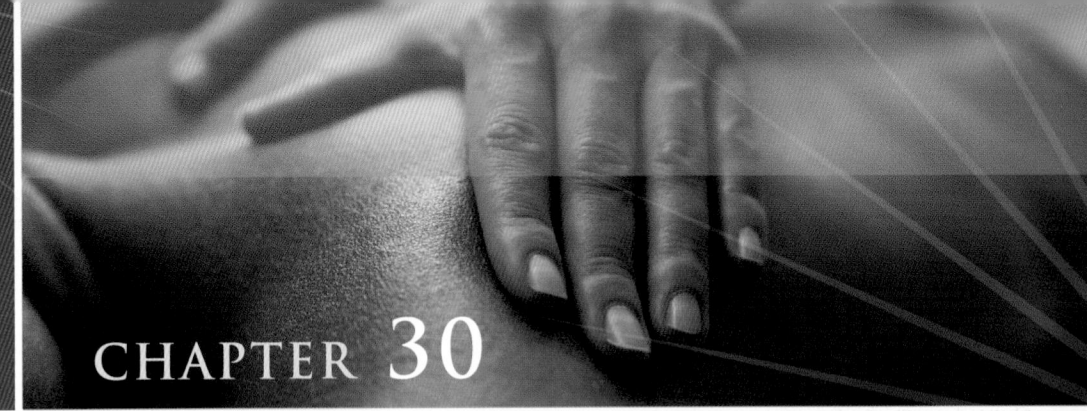

CHAPTER 30

Urinary System, Pathologies, and Disorders

One doesn't discover new lands without consenting to lose sight of the shore for a very long time.
—Andre Gide

LEARNING OBJECTIVES

After completing this chapter, the student should be able to:

1. List anatomic structures and physiologic processes of the urinary system and describe the kidneys and nephrons.
2. Discuss ureters, urinary bladder, urethra, urine formation, urine, urination, body fluids, and fluid balance.
3. Name types of urinary pathologies and disorders, giving massage modifications for each one.

INTRODUCTION

The human body is a complex machine, and when cells metabolize nutrients, they produce wastes such as ammonia and urea. These wastes can be harmful in large amounts, so they must be excreted from the body for homeostasis to be maintained. Excretion of wastes is an important and complex task, and no single body system can handle it alone. Several body systems contribute to waste excretion, including the respiratory, integumentary, and digestive systems, as well as the urinary system.

In general, the kidneys filter wastes from the blood and reabsorb many filtered nutrients back into the blood. Wastes filtered by the kidneys exit the body in the form of urine. Urine travels through the ureters into the urinary bladder, where it is stored until released through the urethra out of the body. Use Table 30.1 to help you understand terms of the urinary system. *Urology* is the study of the urinary system, and *nephrology* is the study of kidney function.

ANATOMY

The basic anatomy of the urinary system is:
- Kidneys
- Ureters
- Urethra
- Urinary bladder

PHYSIOLOGY

Important functions of the urinary system are:
- Eliminates wastes—Waste products produced by metabolism and foreign substances such as drug metabolites are eliminated.
- Regulates chemical composition of blood—As wastes are filtered from blood, substances such as glucose, sodium, vitamins, and minerals are reabsorbed back into blood to adjust its chemical composition.
- Regulates blood pH—The kidneys possess cells that monitor the acid–base balance of the blood and assist with pH regulation by eliminating and reabsorbing acids and ions.
- Regulates blood volume and fluid balance—The kidneys adjust blood volume by conserving or eliminating water and electrolytes. In this way, both blood volume and body fluids stay balanced to maintain homeostasis.
- Regulates blood pressure—The kidneys continuously monitor and regulate blood pressure by secreting the hormone renin. This hormone is discussed in Chapter 24. Blood pressure regulation is complex and involves the cardiovascular and nervous systems.
- Regulates red blood cell production through secretion of the hormone erythropoietin. This hormone is discussed in Chapter 24.
- Maintains homeostasis—Because the kidneys remove waste products, regulate the blood's chemical composition and blood volume, and maintain electrolyte balance and blood pressure, they are considered the most homeostatic organs of the body. Malfunction of the kidneys cause dangerous changes in blood composition, which may lead to death.

KIDNEYS

The **kidneys** are the principal organs of the urinary system. They process blood and form urine to be excreted. The kidneys are located bilaterally at the spinal level of T11 and L3 (Fig. 30.1). Kidneys are reddish-brown in color and lima bean–shaped (convex laterally and concave medially), and each kidney is approximately the size of a bar of bath soap. Both kidneys are behind the peritoneum, or *retroperitoneal,* and lie against the posterior wall of the abdominal cavity. The kidneys are surrounded by a fibrous capsule and are embedded in adipose tissue, which serve as a barrier against both trauma and the spread of infection. Because of the presence of the liver, the right kidney is slightly lower than the left. On top of each kidney is an adrenal gland (see Fig. 24.5).

Each kidney has two main regions (see Fig. 30.1). The outer region is the **renal cortex** and the inner region is the **renal medulla**. Two distinct kidney structures are the renal pyramids and renal columns. *Renal pyramids* are numerous tubules organizing themselves into a dozen or so triangular wedges. *Renal columns* are cortical tissue between the renal pyramids. The *hilus* is the medial indentation where the renal arteries, veins, and ureters enter and exit.

In the average person, the kidneys filter about 180 L of blood and produce about 1 L of urine per day. Each kidney is a separate organ functioning independently of the other. If one kidney is removed, the other will increase its filtering capacity up to 80% of the capacity of two normal kidneys.

TABLE 30.1 Word Meanings

WORD	MEANING
Antidiuretic	*Gr.* against or opposed; urine flow
Bowman capsule	Bowman, English physician (1816–1892)
Calyx	*Gr.* Cup
Cortex	*L.* bark or rind
Diuretic	*Gr.* urine flow
Glomerulus	*L.* little ball
Juxtapose	*L.* close by, adjacent, side by side
Loop of Henle	Henle, German anatomist (1809–1885)
Macula densa	*L.* spot; thick
Medulla	*L.* middle
Nephro, nephra	*Gr.* Kidney
Pelvis	*L.* basin
Peritubular	*Gr.* around, about; as a tube
Renal	*L.* kidney
Retroperitoneal	*L.* backward; the peritoneum

Gr., Greek; *L.,* Latin.

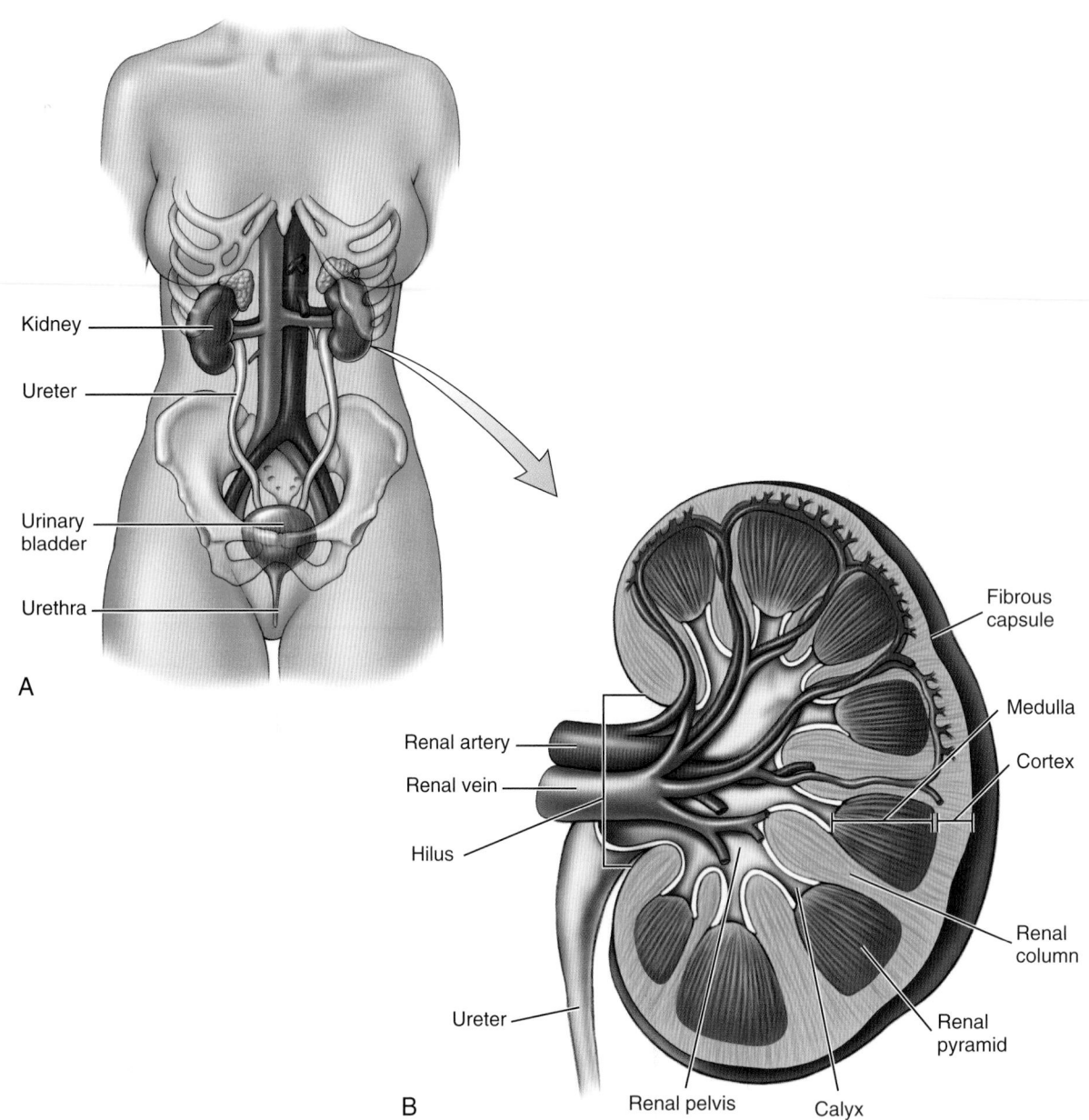

FIG. 30.1 The urinary system. (A) General urinary structures (*anterior view*). (B) Kidney and neighboring structures (*cross-section view*). (From Herlihy, B. [2011]. *The human body in health and illness* [4th ed.]. St. Louis, MO: Saunders.)

Nephrons

Nephrons are specialized tube-shaped structures in the kidneys that filter blood, reabsorb nutrients, and form urine. There are approximately 1 million nephrons in each kidney, and 85% of the nephron is in the renal cortex; the remainder lies in the renal medulla. The number of nephrons does not increase after birth, and once they are damaged, they are not replaced.

Each nephron has a glomerulus, a Bowman capsule, and a renal tubule (Fig. 30.2). The combined glomerulus and Bowman capsule are called the *renal corpuscle*.

Glomerulus and Peritubular Capillaries

Two main blood vessel networks are the *glomerulus* and the *peritubular capillaries*. Blood flows to the kidney through the renal artery, which arises from the abdominal aorta. After entering the kidney at the hilus, the renal artery branches into smaller arteries called arterioles. Afferent arteriole brings blood to the glomerulus. The **glomerulus** is a small cluster of capillaries at the beginning of the nephron. Efferent arteriole drains blood from the glomerulus.

The efferent arteriole branches out and becomes the **peritubular capillaries**, a network of capillaries surrounding

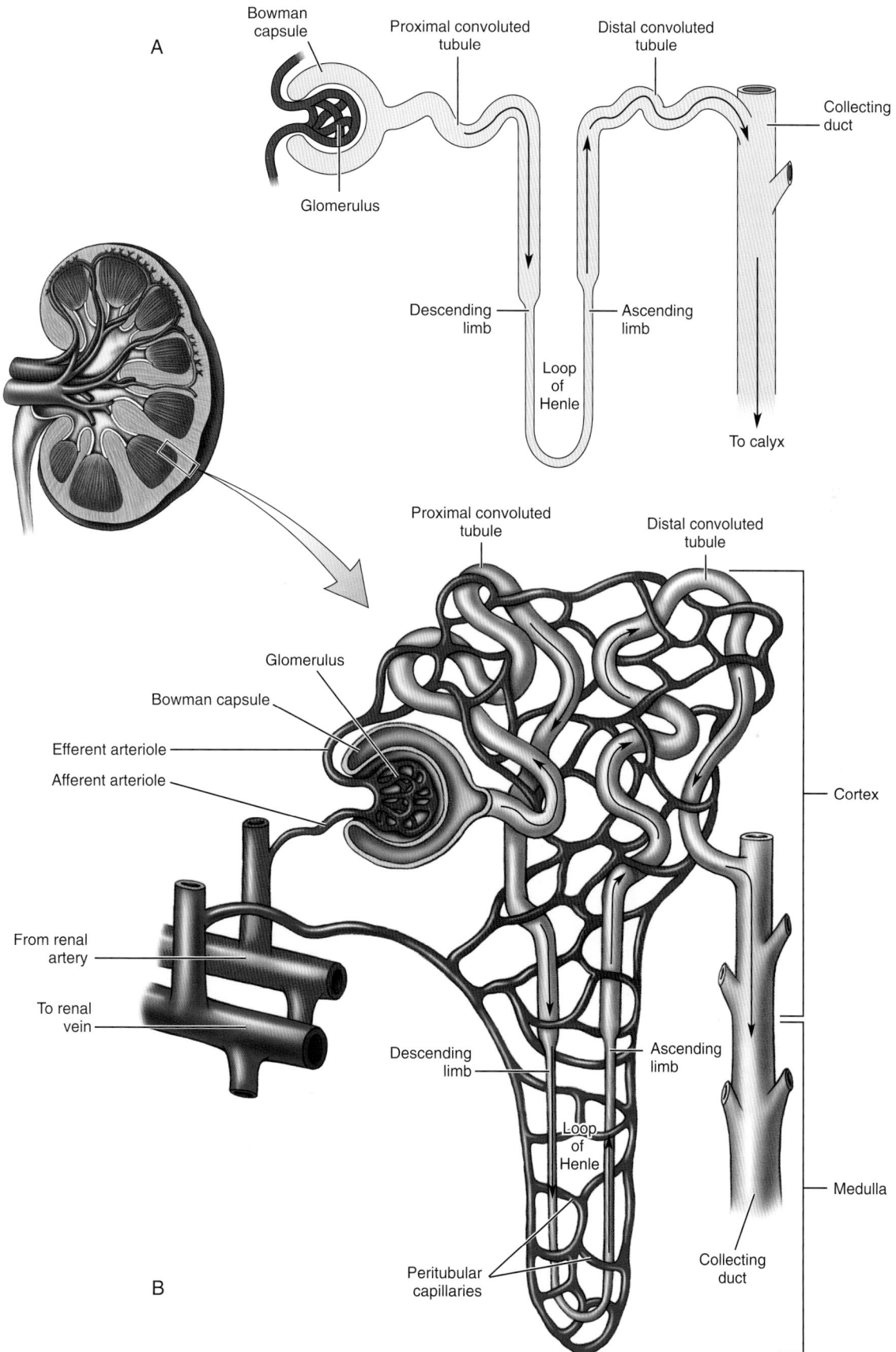

FIG. 30.2 Nephron. (A) The nephron contains a glomerulus, a Bowman capsule, and a renal tubule, which joins a collecting duct. (B) The renal blood vessels, which include the glomerulus, the peritubular capillaries, the afferent and efferent arterioles, and the renal artery and vein. (From Herlihy, B. [2011]. *The human body in health and illness* [4th ed.]. St. Louis, MO: Saunders.)

the nephron's renal tubules, which are discussed next. The placement of an arteriole between two capillary beds (i.e., glomeruli and peritubular capillaries) is unique and found only in the kidneys. The peritubular capillaries later join the renal vein, which empties into the inferior vena cava (see Fig. 30.2B). To review, the sequence of blood vessels in the kidneys is as follows:

Abdominal aorta → Renal artery → Afferent arteriole → Glomerulus → Efferent arteriole → Peritubular capillaries → Renal vein → Inferior vena cava

Bowman Capsule, Renal Tubule, Collecting Ducts, Calyxes, and Renal Pelvis

The kidney's tubular structures are discussed next. The **Bowman capsule** is the double-walled, hollow, cup-shaped section of the nephron surrounding the glomerulus. The **renal tubule** attaches the Bowman capsule and contains several structures—the *proximal convoluted tubule*, the *loop of Henle* (or nephron loop), and the *distal convoluted tubule.* The loop of Henle, which extends into the renal medulla,

possesses a descending limb, a hairpin turn, and an ascending limb. Distal convoluted tubules of several nephrons join a *collecting duct*, which is where the renal tubule ends.

Several collecting ducts merge to form a larger cavity called a *calyx,* a cuplike structure at the base of a renal pyramid. The narrower beginning of the cavity is called a minor calyx, which widens to become a major calyx. Several major calyxes (also spelled calyces) combine to form a reservoir called the *renal pelvis*—the upper region of the ureter.

Juxtaglomerular Apparatus

The **juxtaglomerular apparatus** is between the afferent arteriole and the renal tubule. This structure monitors blood pressure and filtrate concentration levels and, when needed, helps increase blood pressure to promote glomerular filtration. This juxtaglomerular apparatus contains the juxtaglomerular cells and the macula densa (Fig. 30.3).

- **Juxtaglomerular Cells**. These are mechanoreceptors within the afferent arteriole that monitor blood pressure. The kidneys are involved in blood pressure regulation

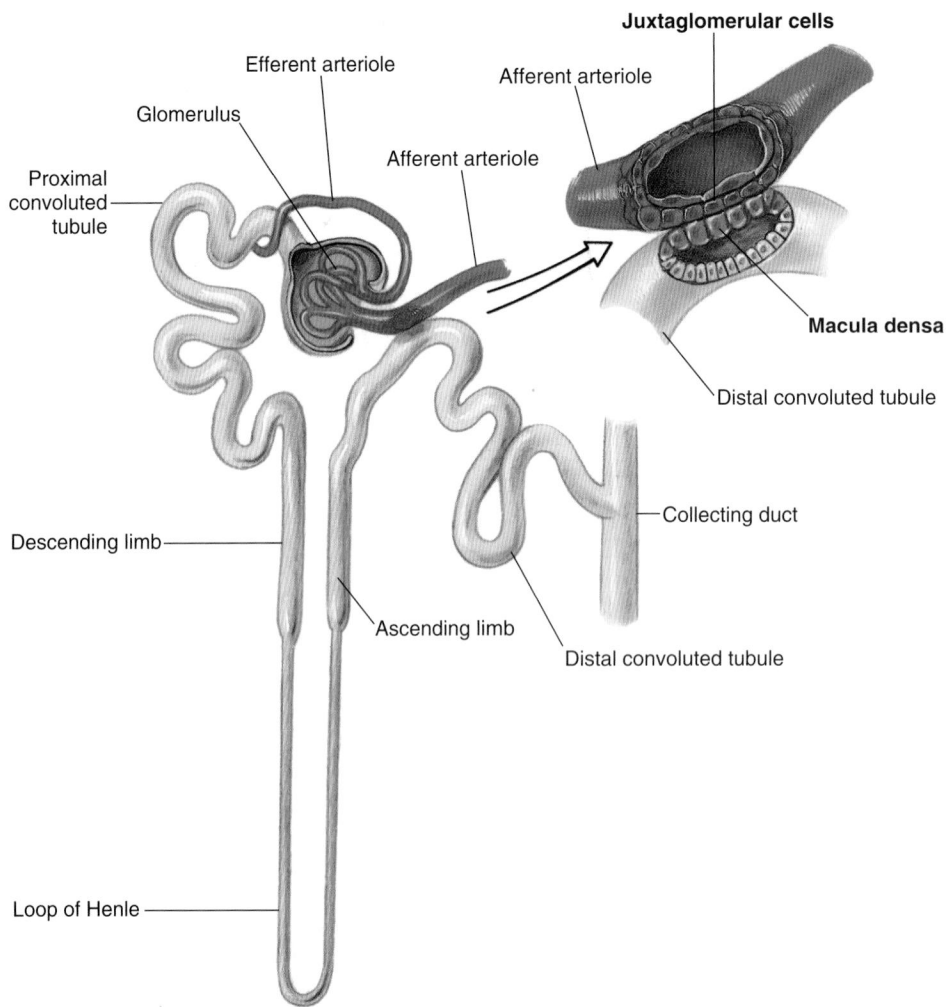

FIG. 30.3 Juxtaglomerular apparatus. Positional relationship of the juxtaglomerular apparatus within the afferent arteriole (mechanoreceptor monitoring blood pressure) and the macula densa within the distal convoluted tubule (chemoreceptor monitoring sodium chloride concentration levels). (From Applegate, E. [2011]. *The anatomy and physiology learning system* [4th ed.]. St. Louis, MO: Saunders.)

because this is the force used to push substances from the blood across the filtration membrane located between the glomerulus and the Bowman capsule. When blood pressure drops, the filtration rate decreases. The juxtaglomerular cells release renin to raise blood pressure. Other ways to stimulate the release of renin are activation of the sympathetic nervous system and the macula densa. Juxtaglomerular cells are also called *granular cells*.

- **Macula Densa**. These are chemoreceptors within the distal convoluted tubule and monitor sodium chloride concentration levels. When concentration levels are low, filtration rate decreases. The macula densa releases prostaglandins, which stimulates juxtaglomerular cells to release renin, which raises blood pressure.

URETERS

The **ureters** are two slender narrow tubes extending from the renal pelvis to the urinary bladder. Urine flow is facilitated by gravity and peristalsis, or smooth muscle contraction, within ureteral walls. As the bladder fills, the distal ends of the ureters contract, preventing backflow of urine into the ureters and the kidneys. The following diagram represents how fluids flow in the renal tubules to the ureters:

Bowman capsule → Proximal convoluted tubule → Loop of Henle → Distal convoluted tubule → Collecting duct → Minor calyx → Major calyx → Renal pelvis → Ureter

URINARY BLADDER

The **urinary bladder** is an expandable sac that temporarily stores urine. The empty bladder is in the abdominopelvic region of the body behind the pubic symphysis (Fig. 30.4). In females, the bladder is positioned anterior to the vagina and posterior to the uterus (see Fig. 25.2). In males, the bladder is superior to the prostate (see Fig. 25.1).

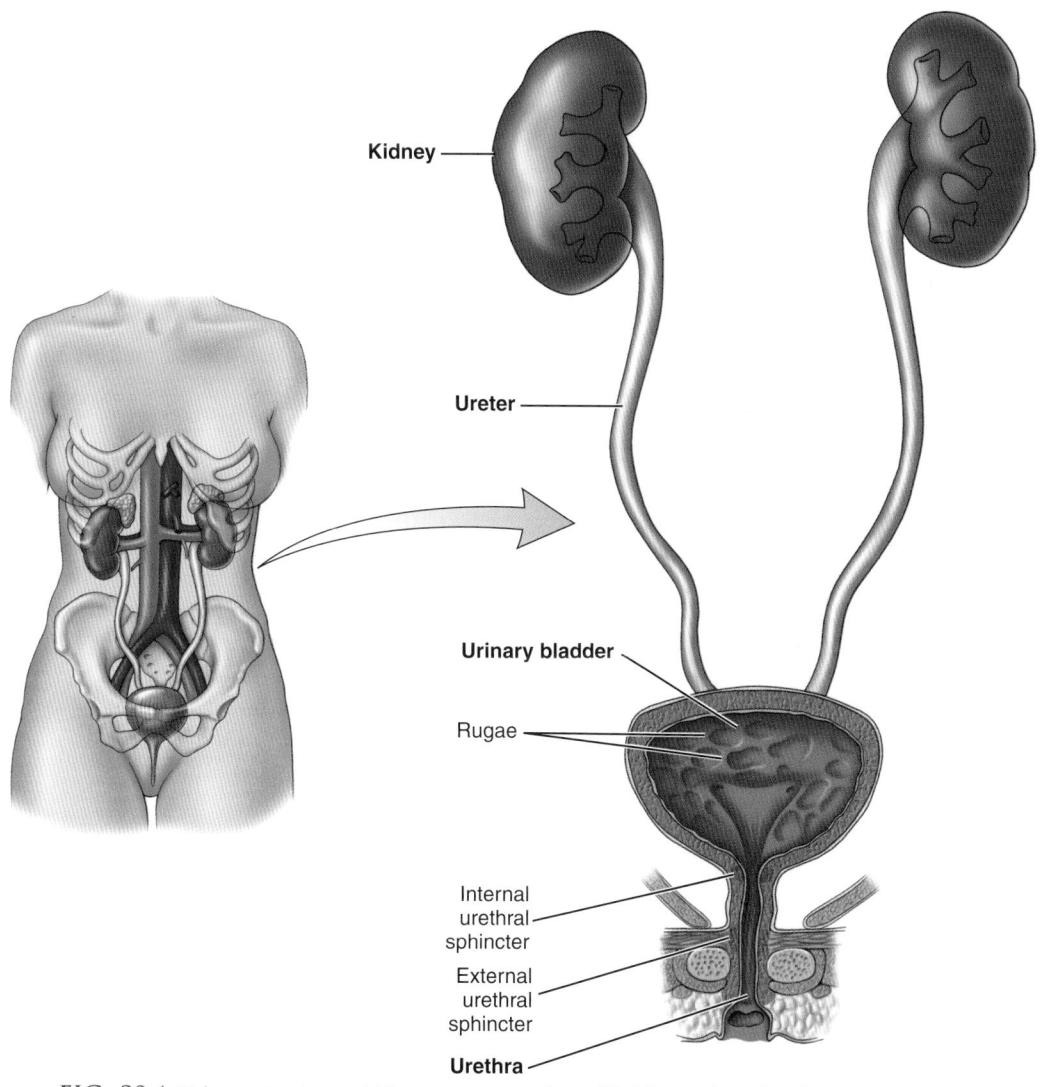

FIG. 30.4 Urinary structures: kidneys, ureters, urinary bladder, and urethra (*anterior and cross-section views*). (From Herlihy, B. [2011]. *The human body in health and illness* [4th ed.]. St. Louis, MO: Saunders.)

The interior lining of the bladder contains *transitional epithelium* and folds called *rugae*, both of which help the bladder expand as it fills with urine. Rugae are typical of expanding structures such as the stomach, gallbladder, and vagina. The urge to urinate usually begins when it has accumulated approximately 200 mL of urine. The bladder contains the *detrusor muscle*, which contracts to help the bladder release urine into the urethra.

URETHRA

The **urethra** is a narrow tube below the urinary bladder and transports urine out of the body. In males, the urethra extends through the prostate and penis; both urine and semen travel down the male urethra. In females, the path of the urethra is between the vaginal opening and the clitoris; it functions only to pass urine. The female urethra is relatively short (approximately 1.5 inches) compared with the male urethra (approximately 4 inches). The shorter length in females means less opportunity to flush out pathogens such as bacteria. This and the female urinary orifice being close to the anal opening are some reasons why females tend to have a higher incidence of urinary tract infections (UTIs) compared with males.

URINE FORMATION

The formation of urine is complex and occurs during several phases: glomerular filtration, tubular reabsorption, and tubular secretion. The end result is urine. These processes are discussed next.

Glomerular Filtration

The first phase of urine formation is **glomerular filtration**, the transfer of water and wastes from the blood into the nephron. Between the glomerulus and the Bowman capsule is a filtration membrane. This membrane contains numerous pores that act like a sieve or strainer. As blood enters the nephron and is forced against the filtration membrane, small molecules such as sodium, potassium, chloride, glucose, uric acid, creatinine, and water pass easily. Blood cells and large proteins do not pass in normally functioning kidneys. Fluid in the renal tubule is called *filtrate*. Approximately 45 gallons (180 L) of filtrate are produced in a 24-hour day. Glomerular filtration is also called *renal ultrafiltration*.

As discussed in Chapter 18, filtration is the movement of water and molecules across a cell membrane because of pressure. Blood pressure is the force used to push blood against the filtration membrane. Filtration occurs when the pressure on the glomerular side of the filtration membrane is higher than the pressure on the tubular side of the membrane.

Tubular Reabsorption

The next phase is **tubular reabsorption** or the reabsorption of molecules, ions, and water from the filtrate into peritubular blood—these substances are necessary to maintain body homeostasis. Approximately 99% of the substance initially filtered is reabsorbed. Substances reabsorbed include glucose; amino acids; and varying amounts of vitamins, minerals (electrolytes), and water, depending on the body's needs. Although tubular reabsorption happens through the entire length of the renal tubule, most reabsorption occurs in the proximal convoluted tubule. Blood cells and glucose are not normally found in urine.

Tubular Secretion

The final phase or urine formation is **tubular secretion**, the transfer of hydrogen ions, creatinine, drugs, and urea from the peritubular blood back into the renal tubule. The kidneys have one more opportunity to adjust the chemical composition of filtrate before they are secreted from the kidneys. When tubular secretions reach the collecting duct, it is called *urine*.

All feelings, both positive and unpleasant, come out of the same faucet. To turn down the faucet on pain is to slow the flow of pleasant feelings as well.
—**Gay and Kathlyn Hendricks**

URINE AND URINATION

Urine is liquid excrement made in the kidneys and released through the urethra. Urine is 95% water and 5% dissolved wastes (e.g., urea, creatinine, uric acid, sodium chloride, potassium, sulfates, phosphates, drug residue). The color of urine is caused by a yellow-tinted substance called *urochrome*, which is formed by the breakdown of hemoglobin by the liver. The average adult produces 1 L of urine per day.

Urination is the expelling of urine from the urinary bladder. Urination is also called *voiding* or *micturition*. The internal and external urethral sphincters regulate and control the release of urine from the urinary bladder.

The *internal urethral sphincter* is between the bladder and the proximal end of the urethra; this sphincter is made of smooth muscle and is involuntary. As the bladder fills with urine and compresses against the internal urethral sphincter, the urge to urinate occurs.

The *external urethral sphincter* is at the distal end of the urethra in females and inferior to the prostate in males; this sphincter is made up of skeletal muscle and is under voluntary control. During urination, the external urethral sphincter relaxes, the bladder's detrusor muscle contracts, and urine is forced from the urinary bladder, through the urethra, and out of the body.

Neuromuscular, physical, and chemical factors can affect urine production and excretion. Nerves and muscles of the urinary system and pelvic floor work together to hold and release urine. Movements used to cough, sneeze, laugh, or participate in physical activity can put pressure on your bladder and cause urine to leak. Carrying extra weight in the body's midsection (e.g., obesity, advanced pregnancy) can put pressure on the bladder and pelvic floor and cause urine leakage. Some caffeinated and alcoholic beverages have a mild diuretic effect. Alcohol inhibits the secretion of antidiuretic hormone (ADH). A **diuretic** is a substance promoting urine production and excretion.

BODY FLUIDS AND FLUID BALANCE

Body fluids can be found in two main compartments—outside the cells or *extracellular fluids* and inside the cells or *intracellular fluids*. **Extracellular fluids** include blood plasma, interstitial fluid, lymph, and transcellular fluids, the latter of which helps transport substances to and from cells. Approximately 34% of body fluids are extracellular. **Intracellular fluids** facilitate chemical reactions within cells. Approximately 66% of body fluids are intracellular (Fig. 30.5).

The input of water must closely equal the output of water to maintain fluid balance and homeostasis. Hormones are essential to these processes. *Antidiuretic hormone* (ADH) secreted by the posterior pituitary stimulates the kidneys to reabsorb more water, which decreases urine output and concentrates urine. *Aldosterone* secreted by the

adrenal cortex causes the kidneys to reabsorb sodium and excrete potassium. Because of these effects, aldosterone is called the *salt-retaining hormone.* In addition, specialized cells in the atrial walls of the heart produce *atrial natriuretic hormone* (ANH), which increases urine production and decreases blood volume and blood pressure. ANH is an antagonist to ADH and aldosterone.

Fluid imbalance can also occur when there is inadequate fluid intake, inadequate ADH production, diseases such as diabetes mellitus, cirrhosis, and hypertensive heart disease, or conditions such as lymph blockage. Examples of fluid imbalance are dehydration and edema.

Dehydration

Dehydration is excess loss of body fluids. This can occur when water is unavailable or with certain conditions, such as severe diarrhea or vomiting and excessive sweating. Severe dehydration occurs when water loss exceeds 5% to 10% of total body weight. A 20% loss of water is often fatal. Common causes of water loss are infection, fever, and severe burns.

If you suspect your client is dehydrated, check their skin turgor. **Skin turgor** is the degree of elasticity of the skin. Turgor is assessed by pinching the skin and then observing how quickly it flattens. In an individual who is well

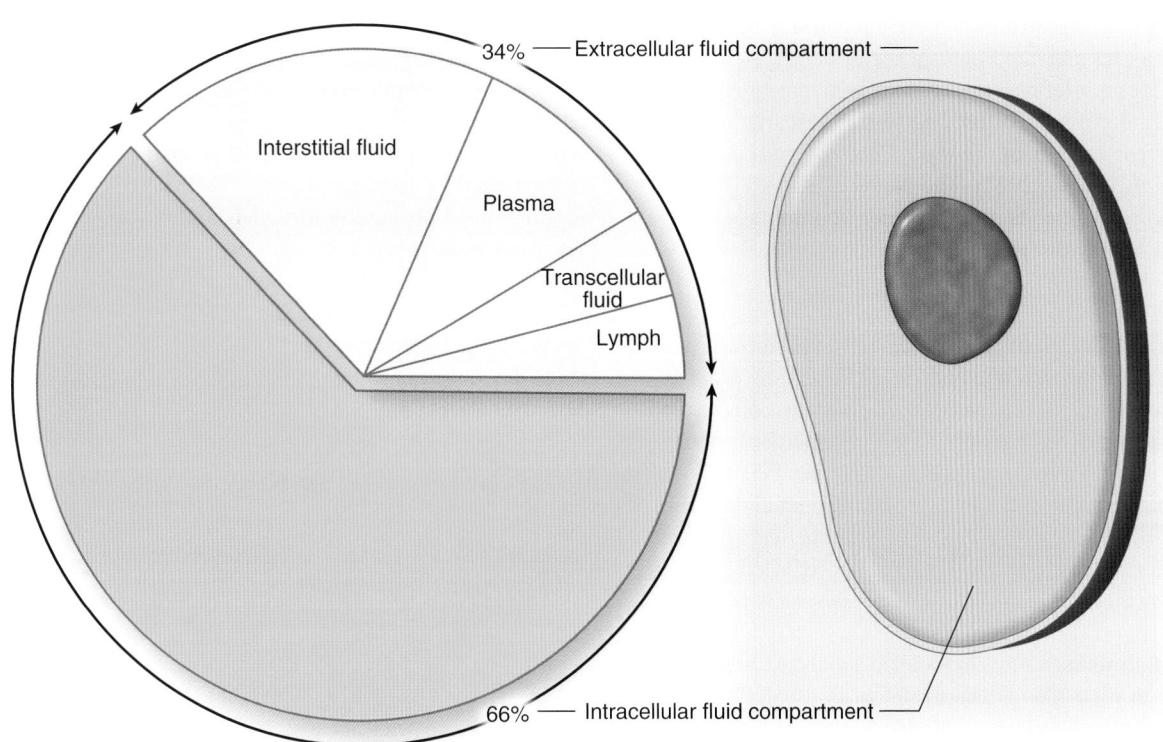

FIG. 30.5 Distribution of extracellular and intracellular fluids within the body. (From Patton, K. & Thibodeau, G. [2014]. *The human body in health and disease* [6th ed.]. St. Louis, MO: Mosby.)

hydrated, pinched skin flattens quickly. In individuals who may be dehydrated, skin will flatten more slowly, giving it a tented appearance. Common places to assess skin turgor are over the back of the hand, lower arm, and abdomen. Keep in mind that elderly people have decreased skin elasticity, so wrinkled, loose skin on the back of the hand should not be mistaken for dehydration.

Edema and Lymphedema

Edema is swelling caused by fluids moving from blood vessels into the interstitial spaces when the lymphatic system is intact and undamaged. Edema can occur anywhere in the body, but most cases are found in the upper or lower extremities. Extreme generalized edema may occur with serious medical conditions such as preeclampsia and liver, kidney, or heart failure.

Lymphedema is swelling caused by removed or damaged lymphatic structures. Lymphedema usually affects a single limb, such as an arm or leg, and can be temporary after surgery or develop into a chronic condition.

Lymphedema and edema can be pitting or nonpitting. Pitting edema leaves an indention or pit in the skin after firm digital pressure is applied for 2 to 3 seconds and removed. Most edema is nonpitting. See Chapter 27 for more information on edema and includes discussions of lymphedema.

URINARY PATHOLOGIES AND DISORDERS

Listed next in alphabetical order are a few of the more common pathologies and conditions of the urinary system. Each entry includes a brief description and basic massage modifications. A more extensive list and related research is found in the current edition of *Mosby's Pathology for Massage Professionals* (Salvo, 2022). The National Kidney Foundation (2013) recommends avoiding deep abdominal massage in cases of kidney disease.

Dialysis

Dialysis is a method of filtering wastes from the blood through a semipermeable membrane and dialysis solution when the kidneys are not functioning properly. Dialysis also can be used to remove drugs or poisons during medical emergencies. Over 700,000 Americans have kidney failure and need dialysis or a kidney transplant to survive (National Kidney Foundation [NKF], 2014). More than 500,000 of these patients received dialysis. Renal dialysis is also called renal replacement therapy. Two methods of dialysis are hemodialysis and peritoneal dialysis.

- **Hemodialysis** uses a machine called a dialyzer, or artificial kidney, to filter blood. The treatment is usually provided in a hospital or dialysis center. An access site is used to remove unfiltered blood and return filtered blood. Types of access sites are an arteriovenous (AV) fistula or graft usually in the forearm or a central venous catheter in the neck or groin region. During the process, waste products from the blood cross over a semipermeable membrane into the dialysis solution. The filtered blood is returned to the body. Anticoagulants such as heparin are administered to prevent the blood from clotting during the procedure. The entire process takes approximately 3 to 4 hours to complete and is usually performed three times a week.

- **Peritoneal dialysis** uses the peritoneum (located in the abdomen) as the semipermeable membrane; the treatment is usually administered at home. Compared with hemodialysis, peritoneal dialysis requires more time and is done daily. Peritoneal dialysis can be administered while the person is asleep, depending on the type of dialysis prescribed. A flexible catheter is implanted through the abdomen and into the peritoneal cavity and serves as the entry and exit site for the dialysis solution. The process of filling and draining the peritoneum is called an exchange and takes approximately 30 to 40 minutes.

Massage and Dialysis

Massage can be given, with massage modifications made according to the type of dialysis the client is receiving. In cases of hemodialysis, avoid the arm with the fistula (NKF, 2014). In cases of peritoneal dialysis, avoid the site containing the dialysis catheter, which is usually in the abdomen (NKF, 2014). Infection at the access site is a concern; the massage practitioner is advised to observe the area, monitoring it for signs and symptoms of local infection (swelling, heat, redness, pain), with referral made to the client's healthcare provider when noted.

Clients with an abdominal catheter can receive a massage with a few positional modifications. To reduce pressure on the catheter while the client is prone, place a pillow across the abdomen above the catheter and another pillow below the catheter. A soft crescent-shaped face rest cushion can be used as catheter support. If these prone positional modifications are uncomfortable for the client, use a side-lying position.

It is important to discuss the timing of massage sessions. Each client will experience dialysis differently. Depending on client preference, you may provide massage on the same day or at the same time as dialysis, or you may wait a few days or even a week or more. Some clients may feel progressively worse as waste products build up between dialysis treatments, and other clients may feel tired before or immediately after a dialysis treatment.

Because of the possibility of orthostatic hypotension, ask the client to arise from the massage table in three stages: (1) sit up on the table for 1 minute; (2) sit on the side of the table with legs dangling for 1 minute; and (3) stand with care, holding onto the edge of the table or other nonmovable object for 1 minute. Offer drinking water before and after the session because of increased thirst.

Kidney Failure

Kidney failure, or renal failure, is loss of kidney function. Two types are acute and chronic; most cases are chronic.

Acute renal failure (ARF) is the sudden and usually temporary loss of kidney function. Most people who experience ARF are critically ill, already hospitalized, and often in intensive care; treatment is usually expedient. Chronic kidney failure, called chronic renal failure (CRF), has a gradual onset, is usually irreversible, and often goes undetected until kidney function has decreased to less than 25% of normal. Months to years may be required to reach end-stage renal failure. More than 661,000 Americans have kidney failure. Several important terms are used in the discussion of kidney failure. *Kidney insufficiency*, or renal insufficiency, occurs when kidney function has diminished by 75%, and only 25% of function remains. *End-stage kidney disease*, or end-stage renal disease (ESRD), occurs when only 10% or less of kidney function remains. Diabetes mellitus and hypertension are the two most common causes of CRF and ESRD, accounting for approximately two-thirds of cases.

Massage and Chronic Kidney Failure

Massage is contraindicated for cases of ARF, as immediate medical attention is needed. Massage is postponed until the condition resolves. For cases of CRF, and if the client is frail, use slowly applied light pressure. An example of light pressure is 3 on a 10-point pressure scale. Because the client may have orthostatic hypotension, ask the client to arise from the massage table in three stages: (1) sit up on the table for 1 minute; (2) sit on the side of the table with legs dangling for 1 minute; (3) stand with care, holding onto the edge of the table or other non-movable object for 1 minute.

Kidney Stones

Kidney stones are small, hard masses that form inside the kidney. Kidney stones are made of minerals and salts and come in various shapes and sizes; most are found in the renal pelvis. The greatest risk for stone formation is in the second and fourth decades of life. In the United States, the lifetime incidence of kidney stones is nearly 11% in males and 6% in females. Once an individual has formed a stone, the likelihood of recurrence is 50% or greater. Several factors influence a person's tendency to form kidney stones. These factors include genetics; low water intake; and a diet high in calcium, vitamin D, protein, or oxalate, which is a compound found in some fruits and vegetables and in caffeinated beverages. Gout and hyperparathyroidism are illnesses that increase a person's likelihood of developing kidney stones. The tendency to form kidney stones is also seen in people undergoing chemotherapy or gastric bypass surgery and in chronically immobilized people.

Massage and Kidney Stones

Massage is postponed during the acute phase. Massage can begin once the stone has passed or has been addressed by medical procedures and the client has recovered. In addition, if a client has a history of kidney stones but none currently, there are no special massage considerations. Consult with the client before massage to devise a treatment plan, as you would for any other client. Encourage the client to increase fluid intake.

Urinary Incontinence

Urinary incontinence (UI) is a general term for loss of bladder control and involuntary leakage of urine. Approximately 25 million Americans have some form of UI; 75% to 80% of these cases are females. There are several types of UI: stress incontinence; urge incontinence; mixed incontinence; and overflow incontinence.

- **Stress Incontinence.** This is urine leakage from increased intraabdominal pressure alone or in combination with weak pelvic floor muscles. Stress incontinence is the most common type of UI.
- **Urge Incontinence.** This is frequent, sudden, strong urges to urinate with little or no chance to postpone urination, and is the second most common type of UI. Urge incontinence is also called overactive bladder.
- **Mixed Incontinence.** This is a combination of both stress incontinence and urge incontinence.
- **Overflow Incontinence.** This is the inability to completely empty the bladder during urination, causing retained urine to leak or dribble out slowly.

Massage and Urinary Incontinence

Avoid the abdominopelvic region if pressure causes pain or discomfort. Suggest the client void before the massage begins as a comfort measure. Be prepared for a toilet break during the session.

Urinary Tract Infections (Urethritis and Cystitis)

Urinary tract infection (UTI) is an infection and inflammation of one or more structures of the urinary tract. UTIs are common, affecting females more than males. A female's urethra is shorter than a male's, allowing bacteria quicker access to the urethra and bladder. Also, a female's urethral opening is near the main source of bacteria, which is at the anus; bacteria can be transported from the anus to the female urethra from improper toilet habits (i.e., wiping from back to front rather than from front to back). Most UTIs involve lower urinary tract structures. Urethritis is infection or inflammation of the urethra. Cystitis is infection or inflammation of the urinary bladder. Escherichia coli bacterium is the most common cause of bacterial UTIs. UTIs can also occur as a reaction to chemotherapeutic drugs, radiation, or irritation from instrumentation such as catheters, or chemicals such as those used in feminine hygiene sprays, or contraceptives such as spermicidal products, but these cases are rare. Urethritis is usually caused by a sexually transmitted disease or infection.

Massage and Urinary Tract Infections

Massage is contraindicated if the client is experiencing fever. Once clients have been fever-free for 24 hours without the use of fever-reducing drugs such as ibuprofen or acetaminophen, they may receive massage (Centers for Disease Control and Prevention [CDC], 2018). Suggest the client void before the massage begins as a comfort measure. Be prepared for a toilet break during the session.

E-RESOURCES

http://evolve.elsevier.com/Salvo/MassageTherapy
- Chapter challenge
- Flash cards

DIANNE POLSENO

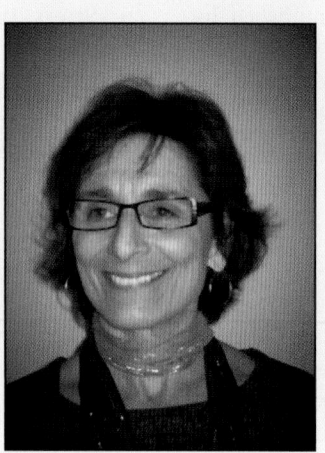

"We touch people!" There are many professions making this claim, but none can mean it on so many levels as massage. This sentiment echoed passionately and often through the hallways at Bancroft School of Massage Therapy in Worcester, Massachusetts, for well over a decade.

Dianne Polseno was born in 1951 into a loving family living in a Providence, Rhode Island, suburb. When Polseno was a child, her family bought and moved to a 20-acre orchard in rural Rhode Island, the place she considered home, wherever she lived, for the rest of her life. Complete with apple cider and a bakery full of goods made from the fruits of the land, the orchard provided the quintessential New England experience.

On finishing high school, Polseno went to work at a top-notch bank in Providence. She worked her way from teller to assistant bank manager before leaving Rhode Island for Florida. It was there she went to nursing school and became a Licensed Practical Nurse. Ultimately, New England called her back, and she worked at a few prestigious hospitals in Rhode Island before making the decision to study massage.

When she announced this to her family in the late 1980s, they were mortified. As they pictured brothels disguised as "massage parlors," Polseno insisted, "You have no idea, this is the up-and-coming thing." She could see where massage was going, how it could be integrated into healthcare, and she wanted to be a part of it.

Upon graduating from Bancroft School of Massage Therapy in 1990, Polseno started her private practice, which she maintained until the end of her life. Only 1 year after graduation, she combined her nursing knowledge with her newfound massage skills and began teaching at her alma mater.

With her ferocious love of anatomy paving the way, Polseno brought massage students to the cadaver lab at the University of Rhode Island for an unparalleled learning experience. Her teaching was not limited to massage practitioners, however. She taught pelvic floor anatomy to medical residents and Introduction to Massage to physical therapy students, even bringing massage students into the class to assist and build rapport between the professions. Polseno's passion was not limited to anatomy. She provided guidance to practitioners worldwide with her "Ethically Speaking" column in the AMTA's Massage Therapy Journal and served as chair of the AMTA National Ethics Subcommittee. She also taught ethics continuing education across the United States, was a regular presenter and devoted supporter of the AMTA New England Regional Conference.

In 2006, Polseno received the AMTA Jerome Perlinski Teacher of the Year Award. That same year she became the education director at Cortiva Institute in Boston. She was quickly promoted to vice president, then president of the campus, and she left her mark on the school in many ways. As a member of the Cortiva Curriculum Committee, she was open-minded, fair, and rational. She welcomed the input of less-seasoned practitioners and educators, and mentored scores of those who also wished to elevate massage education.

Polseno was devoted to the success of her students, and she had high expectations for both individual practitioners and the profession as a whole. She empowered practitioners and educators to speak up and gave them a voice.

Polseno was diagnosed with esophageal cancer in September 2011, and chronicled her journey through treatment with her characteristic humor, hope, and pragmatism. She passed away in May 2012, and in true form, gifted her body to Brown University for anatomic study.

"We touch people!" It's a mantra many massage practitioners repeat when sharing their enthusiasm for the profession. But none can say it as truly as Dianne Polseno, the memory of whose knowledge, courage, and passion continues to touch her students and colleagues around the world.

REFERENCES

Centers for Disease Control and Prevention. (2018). *Guidance for school administrators to help reduce the spread of infection.* https://www.cdc.gov/flu/school/guidance.htm.

National Kidney Foundation. (2014). *Ask the doctor: Can a person on dialysis receive massage?* https://www.kidney.org/blog/ask-doctor/i-have-person-who-dialysis-3-times-week-requesting-massage-therapy-we-are-taught-it.

National Kidney Foundation. (2013). *Is massage therapy safe for someone with kidney disease?* https://www.kidney.org/blog/ask-doctor/massage-therapy-safe-someone-kidney-disease-specifically-multicystic-dysplastic.

Salvo, S. G. (2022). *Mosby's pathology for massage professionals* (5th ed.). St Louis: Mosby.

BIBLIOGRAPHY

Abrahams, P. H., Spratt, J. D., Loukas, M., & van Schoor, A. N. (2003). *Abrahams' and McMinn's clinical atlas of human anatomy* (8th ed.). St Louis: Elsevier.

Applegate, E. (2010). *The anatomy and physiology learning system* (4th ed.). Philadelphia: Saunders.

Como, D. (Ed.). (2016). *Mosby's dictionary of medicine, nursing, and health professions* (10th ed.). St Louis: Elsevier.

Frazier, M. S., & Drzymkowski, J. W. (2015). *Essentials of human diseases and conditions* (6th ed.). St Louis: Elsevier.

Hubert, R. J., & VanMeter, K. C. (2018). *Gould's pathophysiology for the health professions* (6th ed.). Philadelphia: Saunders.

Haubrich, W. S. (2003). *Medical meanings: A glossary of word origins* (2nd ed.). New York: American College of Physicians.

Herlihy, B. (2017). *The human body in health and illness* (6th ed.). St Louis: Saunders.

Huether, S. E., McCance, K. L., & Brashers, V. L. (2019). *Understanding pathophysiology* (7th ed.). St Louis: Mosby.

Kalat, J. W. (2013). *Biological psychology* (11th ed.). Belmont: Cengage Learning.

Kapit, W., & Elson, L. M. (2013). *The anatomy coloring book* (4th ed.). New York: Benjamin Cummings.

Kumar, V., Abbas, A. K., & Aster, J. C. (2015). *Robbins & Cotran pathologic basis of disease* (9th ed.). St Louis: Mosby.

Marieb, E. N., & Keller, S. M. (2018). *Essentials of human anatomy and physiology* (12th ed.). New York: Benjamin Cummings.

McCance, K. L., & Huether, S. E. (2019). *Pathophysiology: The biological basis for disease in adults and children* (8th ed.). St Louis: Mosby.

Myers, T. W. (2014). *Anatomy trains: Myofascial meridians for manual and movement therapists* (3rd ed.). Churchill Livingstone: Elsevier.

Netter, F. H. (2018). *Atlas of human anatomy* (7th ed.). St Louis: Mosby.

Patton, K. T (2019). *Anatomy and physiology* (10th ed.). St Louis: Elsevier.

Patton, K. T., Thibodeau, G. A., & Douglas, M. M. (2012). *Essentials of anatomy and physiology* (4th ed.). New York: Pearson.

Porter, R. S., (2011). *The Merck manual of diagnosis and therapy* (19th ed). Whitehouse Station, NJ: Merck Sharp and Dohme Corp.

Taber, C. W. (2021). *Taber's cyclopedic medical dictionary* (24th ed.). Philadelphia: FA Davis.

REVIEW AND APPLY YOUR KNOWLEDGE

MATCHING ONE: CONCEPT REVIEW

Place the letter of the answer next to the number of the term or phrase that best describes it.

A. Renal cortex
B. Glomerular filtration
C. Hilus
D. Juxtaglomerular cells
E. Kidneys
F. Loop of Henle
G. Macula densa
H. Renal medulla
I. Nephrons
J. Detrusor
K. Renal tubule
L. Retroperitoneal

_____   1. Term meaning behind the peritoneum and describes the location of the kidneys.
_____   2. Structures in the kidneys that filter blood, reabsorb nutrients, and form urine.
_____   3. Outer region of the kidneys.
_____   4. Structure within the nephron that begins at the Bowman capsule and ends at the collecting duct.
_____   5. Muscle that helps the urinary bladder release urine into the urethra.
_____   6. Lima bean-shaped organs located bilaterally that process blood and form urine to be excreted.
_____   7. Chemoreceptors within the distal convoluted tubule that monitor sodium chloride concentration levels.
_____   8. Inner region of the kidneys.
_____   9. Mechanoreceptors within the afferent arteriole that monitor blood pressure.
_____ 10. Medial indentation of the kidneys where renal arteries, veins, and ureters enter and exit.
_____ 11. The transfer of water and wastes from the blood into the nephron and the first phase of urine formation.
_____ 12. Part of the renal tubule that contains a descending limb, a hairpin turn, and an ascending limb.

MATCHING TWO: CONCEPT REVIEW

Place the letter of the answer next to the number of the term or phrase that best describes it.

A. Kidneys
B. Tubular secretion
C. Diuretic
D. Edema
E. Turgor
F. Glomerulus
G. Peritubular
H. Ureter
I. Urethra
J. Urinary bladder
K. Micturition
L. Urine

_____   1. Swelling caused by fluids moving from blood vessels into the interstitial spaces.
_____   2. Tube extending from the renal pelvis of the kidneys to the urinary bladder.
_____   3. Expelling urine from the urinary bladder.
_____   4. Expandable sac that temporarily stores urine.
_____   5. Most homeostatic organs of the body.
_____   6. Substance that promotes urine production and excretion.
_____   7. Tube below the urinary bladder that transports urine out of the body.
_____   8. Liquid excrement which is made in the kidneys and released through the urethra.
_____   9. The elasticity of the skin.
_____ 10. The transfer of hydrogen ions, creatinine, drugs, and urea from the peritubular blood back into the renal tubule and the final phase of urine formation.
_____ 11. Network of capillaries surrounding the nephron's renal tubules.
_____ 12. Small cluster of capillaries at the beginning of the nephron.

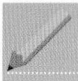

MULTIPLE CHOICE: TEST YOUR KNOWLEDGE

Place the letter of the answer next to the number of the term or phrase that best describes it.

_____ 1. Which is a function of the urinary system?
   A. Regulates hormone production
   B. Regulates blood volume
   C. Regulates body temperature
   D. Regulates blood oxidation

_____ 2. Which organs of the urinary system are located beneath the adrenal glands?
   A. Kidneys
   B. Ureters
   C. Parathyroids
   D. Testes

_____ 3. Cortical tissue between the renal pyramids is the:
   A. Hilus
   B. Medulla
   C. Cortex
   D. Columns

_____ 4. Each kidney contains approximately 1 million _____ .
   A. Sarcomeres
   B. Melanocytes
   C. Nephrons
   D. Lymph nodes

_____ 5. Which of the following is synonymous with infection or inflammation of the urinary bladder?
   A. Cystitis
   B. Urethritis
   C. Meningitis
   D. Phlebitis

_____ 6. What structure monitors blood pressure and filtrate concentration levels, and can increase blood pressure when needed to promote glomerular filtration?
   A. Ureters
   B. Urethra
   C. Bowman capsule
   D. Juxtaglomerular apparatus

_____ 7. The folds in the urinary bladder are called:
   A. Calyx
   B. Glomeruli
   C. Meatus
   D. Rugae

_____ 8. What are the components of the renal corpuscle?
   A. Renal cortex and renal medulla
   B. Renal pyramids and renal columns
   C. Juxtaglomerular cells and macula densa
   D. Bowman capsule and glomerulus

_____ 9. The hormone secreted by the posterior pituitary that stimulates the kidneys to reabsorb more water is:
   A. Antidiuretic Hormone
   B. Aldosterone Hormone
   C. Salt-Retaining Hormone
   D. Atrial natriuretic hormone

_____ 10. Excessive loss of body fluids is:
   A. Dehydration
   B. Micturition
   C. Renal Failure
   D. Incontinence

_____ 11. Hemodialysis patients usually receive dialysis ___ times per week:
   A. 1
   B. 3
   C. 5
   D. 7

_____ 12. Which is the appropriate massage modification for an acute phase of kidney stones?
   A. Lighter pressure
   B. Side-lying position
   C. Semireclining position
   D. Postponing the massage

CRITICAL THINKING

Do Cranberries Really Work?

Melissa is 21 years old and is Donna's next client. During the pretreatment interview, Melissa confides she has had several UTIs in the past 2 years. She is currently symptom free but is worried about getting another infection. She asks Donna if cranberries really do prevent UTIs and if there is anything else she can do to prevent them. What is Donna's most appropriate response?

Answers can include but are not limited to:

It is likely giving dietary advice is outside of Donna's scope of practice. However, she can recommend Melissa drink plenty of water and void frequently rather than "holding it." She should recommend Melissa consult with her healthcare provider about other ways to prevent UTIs. Donna can also recommend Melissa do an online search for credible sources about cranberries and the prevention of UTIs. In addition, a referral to a registered dietician may be helpful for Melissa.

PROFESSIONAL PRACTICE

Time Out for Tom

Tom is a 26-year-old man with a history of recurrent kidney stones. He is currently in college and is working two jobs to help support his wife and newborn daughter. When Tom arrives at your office, he asks to use the toilet. During Tom's intake, he complains of lower back pain, which he would like you to focus on. He also states he has gained a few pounds this week. You complete the intake and begin to escort him to the massage room. He asks to use the toilet once more. He returns from the toilet, but this time you notice his face is a little flushed. Do you proceed with the massage? What are appropriate modifications you might implement for him? If not, why?

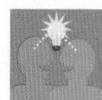

DISCUSSION

Tapotement Over the Kidneys?

Many massage practitioners feel tapotement/percussion should be avoided over the kidney area of the lower back. Do you feel this is valid? Why or why not? If available, post your reflections on an internet-based discussion board monitored by your instructor.

GLOSSARY

Abdominopelvic cavity Cavity that contains abdominal cavity and the pelvic cavity.

Abduction Movement of a joint so that a body part moves away from the midline of the body.

Absolute contraindications Conditions which make receiving a massage absolutely inadvisable; these situations include presence of a contagious disease that can be transmitted to others or when client has a condition that could become more severe with application of massage.

Abstract Presented at the beginning of a paper, and provides a brief overview of the entire study.

Abuse Any action by a person in a position of trust or power that causes harm to another person.

Accounting Process of measuring, processing, and communicating financial and nonfinancial information.

Acetylcholine (ACH) Principal neurotransmitter involved in muscle contraction.

Acne Bacterial infection of skin containing hair follicles and sebaceous glands that become clogged, producing lesions called comedones (e.g., whiteheads and blackheads or pimples).

Active assisted movements Client actively performs joint mobilization or stretch while the practitioner assists and "guides movement" in same direction client is moving.

Active process Cell process that requires a cell to expend energy to help move molecules across its membrane.

Active range of motion Movement produced by voluntary muscular contraction; the person themselves moves the limb or body part.

Active resisted movements Client actively performs joint mobilization or stretch while the practitioner provides resistance to client's movement.

Active transport See *Active process.*

Acute disease Disease which occurs suddenly, persists for a brief period of time (less than 3 months), then resolves or, in some cases, causes death.

Acute inflammation An immediate response to tissue damage characterized by localized swelling, heat, redness, pain, and a loss of function.

Acute pain Pain that lasts less than 30 days and is usually related to injuries, disease, or invasive procedures such as surgery.

Adduction Movement of a joint so that a body part moves toward the midline of the body.

Adenosine triphosphate (ATP) Main sources of energy for muscle contraction.

Adhesion Bands of scar tissue that bind together two or more previously separated structures.

Adhesive capsulitis Chronic inflammation and thickening of the shoulder joint capsule, causing pain and limited range of motion.

Adipose tissue Connective tissue type that is predominately fat and serves as storage for surplus food, insulation to conserve body heat, as well as support and protection for certain structures such as heart, kidneys, and some joints.

Adrenal cortex Outer region of the adrenal gland.

Adrenal medulla Inner region of the adrenal gland.

Adrenals Endocrine gland located superior to each kidney and divided into two regions called the cortex and medulla.

Adverse events (massage) Rare but serious massage-related injuries, and often require medical treatment and can cause varying degrees of temporary or permanent disability; also called adverse effects.

Advertising Use of persuasive messages to influence consumer buying habits, usually by paid announcements.

Afferent (sensory) neuron Neuron that transmits information toward the central nervous system (CNS); also called receptors.

Agonists See *Prime movers.*

Airborne precautions Methods to reduce or prevent transmission of pathogens transmitted by the airborne route.

Allergies Body's immune response to substances in the environment called allergens that are otherwise harmless.

All-or-none law (muscle) Law that states when an individual muscle fiber receives a stimulus to contract, it will contract to its fullest ability or will not contract at all.

All-or-none response (neuron) Principle that states that once nerve impulse begins, it will be conducted at maximum capacity without fluctuations in membrane potential and without any decrease in magnitude.

Allostasis The process of achieving homeostasis through physiologic and behavioral changes.

Alveoli Gas exchange structures of respiratory tract; attached to alveolar ducts.

Alzheimer disease Progressive neurodegenerative disease; produces a typical profile of mental deterioration and affects processes of thinking, memory, and communicating.

Americans with Disabilities Act (ADA) Law that prohibits discrimination of individuals with disabilities and guarantees that these individuals have the same opportunities as nondisabled individuals.

Amphiarthrotic joints Joints that are slightly movable, such as joints between the ribs and their cartilage, joints between vertebrae, and the joints between the two pubic bones.

Anatomic position Standard posture in which body stands upright and faces forward, arms at sides, palms face forward with thumbs to side; feet-hip distance apart with toes pointing forward.

Anatomy The study of the structures of the human body and their positional relationships to one another.

Anecdote A description of a personal experience.

Anemia Reduction in quantity of either RBCs or hemoglobin, which impairs blood's ability to carry oxygen to cells.

Angina pectoris Chest pain from temporary reduced blood flow to heart.

Antagonists Muscles that relax and lengthen while prime movers and their synergists contract to produce movement.

Anterior Located on front side of a structure. Also known as *ventral*.

Aortic valve Left semilunar valve located between the aorta and the left ventricle.

Aponeurosis Broad, flat tendon that attaches muscle to bone, muscle to other muscle, or muscle to superficial fascia beneath the skin.

Appendicular skeleton Bones of shoulder and pelvic girdles, and bones of upper and lower extremities; 126 named bones in appendicular skeleton.

Arachnoid mater Middle meningeal layer, composed of loosely arranged collagen fibers which gives it a weblike appearance.

Archer stance Foot stance used when the target area(s) of the applied technique is toward one side of the practitioner's body.

Areolar tissue Most widely distributed connective tissue and functions like elastic glue; connects structures to each other and permits movement between them.

Aromatherapy Use of fragrant essential oils by inhalation or by blending with products such as massage lubricant for topical application.

Arrector pili Muscles attached to hair follicles that contract to pull hair upright.

Arteries Vessels that move blood away from the heart; blood within arteries is oxygenated (except pulmonary arteries).

Articular cartilage Covers the articulating surfaces of bones.

Asian bodywork therapy Use of pressure and/or soft tissue manipulation to treat the body, mind, and spirit, including the electromagnetic or energetic fields in and surrounding the body.

Assessment A systematic process of gathering information in order to make informed decisions about treatment.

Assets Valuable economic resources to which an individual or business has a legal claim.

Asthma Bronchospasms that cause breathing difficulties in susceptible people.

Atherosclerosis Presence of atherosclerotic plaque within arteries can restrict blood flow and promote blood clot formation.

Athlete Someone who possesses a natural or acquired ability needed to participate in a sport.

Athlete's foot Fungal infection of foot, most often sole and between toes.

Atrioventricular valves Heart valves located between the atria and the ventricles.

Attention-deficit/hyperactivity disorder (ADHD) Neurologic disorder; affected person displays behavior associated with inattentiveness, hyperactivity, impulsivity, or combination of these.

Authenticity The ability to be oneself while in a professional role.

Autism spectrum disorder (ASD) Syndrome present in early childhood characterized by difficulty communicating and forming relationships.

Autogenic inhibition reflex Involuntary reduction of motor activity caused by high levels of tension from either prolonged stretching or excessive contraction.

Autoimmune disease Disease marked by an inappropriate or excessive immune response; body mistakenly attacks and destroys healthy tissue.

Autonomic nervous system (ANS) Part of peripheral nervous system (PNS); regulates the involuntary activities of organs, glands, and smooth muscles, with the exception of breathing, which is both voluntary and involuntary.

Autonomy Respecting the rights of competent individuals to make their own decisions.

Axial skeleton Bones located along the body's central axis; 80 named bones in axial skeleton.

Axon Part of neuron that transmits impulses away from the cell body.

Bacteria Single-cell organisms; can be spherical, spiral, or rod-shaped; may appear singly or in chains.

Baker cyst Accumulation of synovial fluid behind knee.

Balance sheet An overview of a business's assets, liabilities, and shareholder equities on a specific date.

Ball-and-socket joints Joints with one bone containing a ball-shaped head that fits into a rounded socket-shaped surface of another bone; these joints offer the greatest range of motion and permit all movement in all planes, including flexion, extension, abduction, adduction, circumduction, and rotation.

Bartering The nonmonetary exchange of goods or services; there is no exchange of cash.

Base of support All points of contact on which an object rests.

Bell palsy Sudden unilateral facial paralysis in areas supplied by cranial nerve 7 or facial nerve. Causes weakness or paralysis of muscles on one side of face, and may be transient, lasting only a few months, or permanent, and can recur.

Belly (muscle) Wide central portion of muscle that contains contractile units or sarcomeres, which produce movement.

Bending Compressive and tension forces combined, usually by pushing and pulling tissues in a C shape.

Beneficence Actions that benefit the well-being of others.

Biarticular muscles Muscles that cross two joints.

Bias (research) Researcher's preference for an outcome.

Biaxial joints Joints that provide movement around two perpendicular axes and in two perpendicular planes. Types include saddle, condyloid/ellipsoidal.

Bicuspid valve See *Mitral valve*.

Biliary tract (system) Refers to the liver, gallbladder, and bile ducts that make and store bile, and release it into the small intestine.

Blog Discussion or informational website often written using diary-style entries called *posts*.

Blood Liquid connective tissue that transports respiratory gases, nutrients, and waste products.

Blood plasma Straw-colored liquid in which blood cells are suspended.

Blood pressure Amount of force exerted by blood on vessel walls; usually expressed as a fraction.

Blood vessels Closed network of tubes connected to heart that help transport blood and include arteries, veins, and capillaries.

Blood-brain barrier (BBB) Tightly packed group of cells in the lining of blood vessels that supply the central nervous system and allow the passage of some molecules such as oxygen and glucose, but prevent the passage of some harmful molecules, like viruses, drugs, and even blood itself.

Board certification The examination of a person's professional qualifications by a group of peers, often in a specialty of practice, and granting the person a title if qualifications are met.

Body cavity A hollow space or compartment that can house organs and other structures.

Body diagram Outline of a body on which a client is asked to indicate where pain is experienced.

Body mechanics Use of one's body that is safe, energy-conserving, and reduces physical stress and strain.

Body shampoo Gentle scrubbing of a client's skin using a cloth or brush dipped in warm, soapy water.

Body wrap The application of products to a client's body, which is then wrapped in large wet or dry sheets and blankets.

Boils Infected hair follicles that manifest as a painful pus-filled mass or abscess.

Bolsters Pillows and other cushioned devices used to support certain client positions.

Bolus Small round mass of food.

Bone remodeling The process of bone destruction by osteoclasts and bone formation by osteoblasts.

Bones Hard connective tissues making up the skeletal system.

Bony markings Areas on bone where muscles, tendons, and ligaments attach and where nerve and blood vessels pass.

Bookkeeping Recording financial transactions.

Bowman capsule Hollow cup-shaped mouth of nephron that contains glomerulus.

Brain Organ located in the skull; it interprets sensory information and governs intellectual activity and is also seat of consciousness, memories, and emotions.

Brainstem Stalklike region of the brain and connects the cerebrum to the spinal cord; contains midbrain, pons, and medulla oblongata.

Brainwaves Rhythmic patterns of cerebral electrical activity that can be displayed using an electroencephalogram (EEG).

Breastfeeding Feeding a child with milk from lactating breasts; also called nursing.

Breasts Two soft protruding organs in the upper chest wall of the female body that contain mammary glands.

Breathing Process of taking in air and expelling it from the lungs; consists of two phases: inhalation and exhalation.

Bronchi Two passageways leading from the trachea to each lung.

Bronchioles Small branches of bronchi that lead to alveolar ducts and eventually to alveoli.

Bronchitis Inflammation of the bronchial mucosa with resultant swelling and mucus hypersecretion.

Bruise Skin discoloration caused by blood leaking from broken capillaries and collecting in interstitial spaces. Also called contusion.

Bulbourethral glands Pea-sized pair of glands located on either side of the prostate that secretes seminal fluid.

Bulging disc Tear within the annular fibrosus of an intervertebral disc; less severe than herniated disc because nucleus pulposus remains contained within the annular wall.

Burn Tissue damage from heat (including fire, hot liquid, steam, and hot objects including metal or glass), extreme cold, radiation (including sunlight exposure, tanning beds, and radiation therapy), chemicals (strong acids, drain openers, toilet bowl cleaners, and paint thinner), electricity, or friction; four degrees of burns have been identified, depending on depth of injury.

Burnout State of emotional exhaustion, depersonalization, and diminished sense of personal accomplishment resulting from chronic workplace stress not successfully managed.

Bursae Flattened, saclike structures located between ligaments and bones within joints; contain synovial fluid; bursae provide cushion that prevents muscle tendons from rubbing against bones during contraction.

Bursitis Inflammation of a bursa.

Business coach An individual who has business experience and oversees, assists, and guides a novice business person in developing, starting, or growing a business.

Business partnerships A business owned by two or more entities.

Business plan A document that describes a business's organization, services and products, marketing strategy, management style, financial projections, future plans, and strategies for achieving them.

Calorie Units of energy received from nutrients.

Cancer Growth of abnormal cells possessing uncontrolled cell division, lack programmed cell death, and can accumulate into masses or tumors; can spread or metastasize, and invade other tissues of the body.

Capillaries Functional unit of the cardiovascular system where gas exchange occurs between blood and body cells; possess thin, permeable walls.

Cardiac arrest Sudden cessation of heartbeat, affecting blood flow to the brain and other vital organs.

Cardiac cycle Cycle of events from the beginning of one heartbeat to the beginning of the next; contains two ventricular phases: diastole and systole.

Cardiac muscle Muscle tissue type located in heart wall; helps heart contract repeatedly to pump blood.

Cardiorespiratory exercises Activities involving prolonged body movements to increase heart and respiration rates to improve stamina, lose or maintain weight, and reduce the risk of heart disease, lung cancer, type 2 diabetes, and stroke; levels range from low, moderate, and high intensity.

Career longevity Length of time spent in service or employment within a field.

Carpal tunnel syndrome (CTS) Median nerve compression within the carpal tunnel, causing numbness, tingling, and other symptoms in the affected hand.

Cartilage Strong protective tissue capable of withstanding repeated stress; has tough, rubbery matrix and is found chiefly in thorax, joints, and certain rigid structures (trachea, nose, ears).

Cartilaginous joints Joints united by cartilage.

Case report Study describing a single case the intervention used, and the treatment outcome.

Case series Collection of case reports in which the same intervention was used or participants had the same condition.

Cash flow statement A statement that reports movement of money into and out of a business.

Cautionary sites See *Endangerment site.*

Cell Smallest structural and functional unit existing as a self-sustaining entity; cells are building blocks of human body.

Cell body Part of neuron that contains nucleus and other organelles.

Cell membrane The membrane that separates intracellular fluid from extracellular fluid; membrane is semipermeable and allows some materials to pass freely and blocks passage of others.

Cellular level Biologic level that encompasses cells and provides functions vital for life (e.g., muscle and nerve cells).

Center of gravity The exact center of an object's mass.

Central nervous system Part of nervous system that occupies a central or medial position in body and includes brain, spinal cord, meninges, and cerebrospinal fluid (CSF).

Central neuropathy Type of neuropathy originating in the central nervous system.

Central sensitization Increased responsiveness and reduced pain threshold in the central nervous system.

Centrioles Paired, tubular structures that assist cell division by organizing chromosomes.

Centripetal Toward the center.

Cerebellum Cauliflower-shaped structure located posterior and inferior to cerebrum and is responsible for balance, posture, coordination, equilibrium, and muscle tone.

Cerebrospinal fluid Clear, colorless fluid surrounding the central nervous system and is found within the subarachnoid space.

Cerebrum Largest and most superior portion of brain where sensations are consciously perceived, where skeletal muscle motor movements are initiated, and where emotional and intellectual processes occur.

Ceruminous glands Specialized sudoriferous glands that produce cerumen or earwax; these glands are found in the ear canal.

Cervix Lower, narrow portion of uterus that opens into the vagina.

Cesarean childbirth Surgical removal of a fetus, placenta, membranes, and umbilical cord through an incision in the abdominal wall; also called a C-section.

Chain of infection Model used to explain transmission of infectious diseases.

Chemical level Biologic level that encompasses chemical elements or biochemistry of the body.

Chemoreceptors Receptors that detect chemical stimuli or changes in chemical concentrations of fluids; they are located in nose, on tongue, and within some arterial walls.

Childbirth The process of delivering a fetus, placenta, membranes, and umbilical cord to the outside world.

Choking Trachea is blocked and affected person cannot breathe.

Chondromalacia patellae Softening and degeneration of articular cartilage on the posterior patella.

Chronic diseases Diseases that have an insidious onset, gradual increase in signs and symptoms and last for a long time (perhaps for life).

Chronic fatigue syndrome (CFS) Disorder characterized by extreme fatigue without any identifiable cause or underlying condition. Also called myalgic encephalomyelitis (ME).

Chronic inflammation Inflammation that lasts longer than 2 weeks and may follow unsuccessful acute inflammation.

Chronic pain Pain that persists past the normal healing time and reflects the state of the person's nervous system rather than the condition of the tissues.

Chyme Mixture of churned food and gastric juice.

Circular muscle fibers Muscle fibers with a rounded fiber arrangement.

Circumduction Conical movement in which distal end of a structure moves in a circle and proximal end remains relatively fixed; circumduction is actually a combination of several movements, including flexion, extension, adduction, and abduction.

Cirrhosis Progressive liver disease in which liver cells degenerate and are replaced by fibrotic scar tissue.

Class 1 levers Levers where fulcrum is positioned between the load and the pull like a seesaw or pair of scissors.

Class 2 levers Levers where the pull is at one end, the load is in the middle, and the fulcrum is at the opposite end like a wheelbarrow.

Class 3 levers Levers where the load is at one end, the pull is in the middle, and the fulcrum is at the opposite end like a shovel.

Cleaning Removal of adherent visible soil, blood, and other substances, usually with soap (i.e., detergent), water, and friction. Cleaning may involve the use of heat (warm to hot water).

Client positioning Positions that ensure comfort through proper body alignment, allowing a client to receive a massage in ways that promote stability and enhance the practitioner's body mechanics.

Client preferences A collection of goals, expectations, predispositions, social and cultural values, and religious or spiritual beliefs creating partiality for certain decisions and their outcomes.

Clinical massage Massage used to help rehabilitate injuries, manage diagnosed medical conditions and their treatments or complications, and manage issues related to surgery. Can also refer to the practice settings where massage services are provided.

Clinical significance Practical importance of statistical significance to professional practice.

Close-ended questions Precise questions and require affirmative, denial, or specific answers such as "yes," "no," or "the right shoulder."

Code of ethics A code that represents a set of standards of ethical conduct for members of a profession.

Cohort A group of individuals who share a common characteristic.

Cold gel packs Strong vinyl pouches filled with gel composed of silica or a mixture of saline and gelatin used to transfer cold.

Cold plunge A brief submersion in a pool or tub of cold water.

Cold sores Recurrent viral infections affecting skin and mucous membranes caused by herpes simplex.

Colon See *Large intestine.*

Commercial general liability (CGL) insurance A type of liability insurance that helps protect businesses from bearing the full cost of defending against claims for damages.

Common cold Viral infection of upper respiratory tract, usually confined to nose and throat, although larynx can be involved as well.

Communication Act of exchanging information by encoding and decoding verbal and nonverbal messages within a defined cultural, physiological, relational, and perceptual context.

Compact bone The hard outer shell of bone and constitutes approximately 80% of the total adult bone mass.

Compassion fatigue Emotional strain from working with those who are suffering from the consequences of traumatic events.

Compensatory patterns Conscious or unconscious movements used to correct imbalances and reduce discomfort.

Complications Conditions that arise as a disease progresses.

Compression (technique) Nongliding technique of pressure application.

Concentric contractions Muscles that shorten while generating force.

Conceptual definitions Definitions that clarify what is measured and the population or condition/pathology under investigation.

Conduction Transfer of heat between objects or substances that are in direct contact with each other.

Condyloid joints Possess an oval-shaped surface or condyle of one bone that fits into a depression or socket of another bone.

Confidentiality The obligation of professionals or professional organizations to safeguard entrusted information.

Conflict of interest Any financial or other interest which conflicts with the service of the individual because it (1) could significantly impair the individual's objectivity or (2) could create an unfair competitive advantage for any person or organization.

Confounding variables Type of extraneous variable related to the independent variable but may affect the dependent variable.

Congenital disorders Disorders present at birth. May be caused by genetic abnormalities, by a maternal diet deficient in nutrients, or by habits of the mother while the fetus is in utero, such as use of recreational drugs, alcohol, or tobacco.

Congestive heart failure (CHF) Inability of heart to pump blood to meet body's demands.

Connective tissue Tissue that connects, supports, transports, and defends; it connects tissues to each other (e.g., muscles to muscles, muscles to bones, bones to bones); it forms a supporting mesh framework for organs and glands, and for the body as a whole, and helps transport nutrients and wastes, as well as providing defensive functions such as blood clotting and immune responses.

Connective tissue membranes Membrane composed solely of connective tissues such as synovial and meningeal membranes.

Constipation Infrequent or difficult passing of stools.

Contact dermatitis Inflammation of the skin that develops at the site of contact with the causative agent.

Contact precautions Procedures used to reduce or prevent transmission of pathogens that spread by direct or indirect contact.

Contact transmission The most common method of disease transmission involving some form of touch, either by direct or indirect contact.

Continuing education (CE) Education to ensure ongoing competence relevant to professional practice after leaving a system of formal education such as a college, university, or trade/vocational school.

Continuous conduction Nerve impulse conducted along unmyelinated axons.

Contract Written agreements that outline expectations, duties, and responsibilities in business relationships, and can be legally binding and enforceable by law.

Contraindication A condition which could be aggravated by the application of massage.

Contralateral Related to opposite sides of body.

Contrast method Combining cold and heat in the same treatment.

Control group Population sample that does not receive an intervention under investigation, or receives comparison or alternative treatment.

Convection Transfer of heat by circulating currents of water or air between a warmer object or substance and a cooler object or substance.

Convergent muscle fibers Muscle fibers that join at one end with fibers spreading out like a fan at other end.

Conversion Transfer of heat using a nonthermal form of energy (e.g., mechanical, electrical, chemical) and converts it to heat in the body.

Core stability The ability to control the position and motion of the trunk, which allows for optimum production and transfer of force.

Coronal plane See *Frontal plane.*

Coronary artery disease (CAD) Presence of atherosclerotic plaque within coronary arteries.

Corporation Legal business entity who is granted a charter by the state in which they operate.

Coughing Sudden expulsion of air to clear lower respiratory passageways of irritants or foreign materials.

Countertransference Practitioner transfers past feelings, conflicts, and attitudes onto the client.

Cowper glands See *Bulbourethral glands.*

Cranial nerves Cranial nerves emerge from the inferior surface of the brain and are named by Roman numerals, for the areas they supply, or the type of signal they carry.

Cranial cavity Cavity within the skull that contains brain.

Cranial reflex Reflexes mediated by cranial nerves and include blinking, changes in pupil diameter, salivation, gagging, and sneezing.

Crepitus Joint sounds, sometimes described as creaking, cracking, grating, crunching, or popping.

Crohn disease (CD) Type of inflammatory bowel disease causing long-term inflammation and ulcer formation; may affect any part of gastrointestinal tract with small intestine being most common.

Cross bridging (muscle) The cycle that begins with excitation by a motor neuron, which causes thick filaments to cross and bridge the gap between them and then pulls the thin filaments toward the center of the sarcomere.

Crossed extensor reflex Reflexive activation of muscles in the contralateral limb to compensate for loss of support when the opposite limb withdraws from a painful stimulus during the withdrawal reflex.

Cryokinetics Combining cold applications with joint mobilizations.

Cryostretch Combining cold applications before stretching.

Cryotherapy Therapeutic application of cold.

Cultural competency A set of behaviors, attitudes, and policies enabling professionals to interact effectively with others in cross-cultural situations.

Culture An accumulated pattern of values, beliefs, and behaviors shared by an identifiable group of people with a common history and verbal/nonverbal symbol system.

Cupping therapy Involves placing glass, plastic, or silicone cups on the skin to create suction and lift tissue.

Current procedural terminology (CPT) List of codes used to report medical services and procedures administered to patients.

Curriculum vitae In-depth overview of an individual's education, experience, and accomplishments and are organized in reverse chronologic order.

Cutaneous membranes Tissue layer that covers external body surfaces and includes the skin.

Cyanosis Blue or purple-tinted skin from low oxygen levels in blood or decreased blood flow.

Cytoplasm Intracellular gel-like fluid within cells.

Cytoskeleton Network of microfilaments and microtubules within cells; network serves as scaffolding material to provide an internal structure to cell.

Data Recorded factual information used to validate research results.

de Quervain tenosynovitis Inflammation of tendinous sheath located on radial side of wrist.

Decubitus ulcers Localized injuries to the skin from sustained pressure.

Deep Relative to or situated within the body.

Deep fascia Fascia that extends from superficial fascia and surrounds deeper structures.

Deep tissue massage The use of deep pressure to reduce tension; some define this as the application of massage techniques that reaches a client pain threshold by applying more pressure.

Deep vein thrombosis (DVT) Inflammation of a vein with blood clot formation, which restricts blood flow.

Deficiency disease Disease caused by lack of an essential nutrient in individual's diet or by inability to digest and absorb a particular nutrient properly; this deficiency typically interferes with body's growth, development, and metabolism.

Degenerative disease Disease that involves tissue breakdown caused by overuse or those that occur naturally as a result of the aging process.

Dehydration Excess loss of body fluids.

Delayed-onset muscle soreness Pain or discomfort in skeletal muscles following unaccustomed or strenuous physical activity; also called *post-exercise muscle soreness.*

Delegation Assignment of a task or task completion from one person to another person.

Delimitations Things the researcher can control (choice of variables, population studied).

Dendrites Short and narrow extensions of neuron that transmit impulses to the cell body.

Dendritic (Langerhans) cells Epidermal cells that stimulate immunologic responses when skin is injured or invaded by pathogens; this response is aided by helper T cells.

Dense irregular tissue Similar to *Dense regular tissue*, but fibers are stronger, thicker, and arranged irregularly; found in areas where tension is exerted from multiple directions.

Dense regular tissues Connects muscle to bone (tendons, aponeurosis) and bone to bone (ligaments). Protein fibers are arranged in parallel rows and are slightly wavy, which gives them elasticity and tensile strength and the ability to resist pulling forces in one or two directions.

Dependent variable The condition expected to change because of the independent variable.

Depression Movement at a joint in an inferior or downward direction; essentially it is lowering or dropping a body part.

Dermatomes Areas of skin supplied by a specific sensory spinal nerve root.

Dermis Thicker inner region of skin; contains blood vessels, sensory nerve receptors, hair follicles, muscles, skin glands, and connective tissue.

Descriptive study A study which describes a phenomenon or characteristic of a population (e.g., demographics, educational levels, socioeconomic factors).

Diabetes mellitus Group of disorders characterized by chronic elevated blood glucose levels and disturbances in protein, fat, and carbohydrate metabolism.

Diabetes mellitus type 1 Type of diabetes in which pancreatic beta-cells are damaged or destroyed, creating a lack of insulin.

Diabetes mellitus type 2 Type of diabetes in which cells are resistant to insulin produced by pancreatic beta-cells; also called insulin resistance.

Diagnosis The process of identifying a particular disease and includes evaluation of signs and symptoms, medical and surgical histories, physical examination, laboratory tests, and other procedures.

Dialysis Method of filtering wastes from blood through a semipermeable membrane and dialysis solution when kidneys are not functioning properly; can also be used to remove drugs or poisons during medical emergencies.

Diaphragm Main muscle of respiration located between thoracic and abdominal cavities.

Diaphragm line In reflexology, the horizontal line located below the ball of the foot. These lines are used to delineate treatment areas containing reflex points.

Diaphysis The cylindrical shaft of long bones, usually narrower than the epiphyses.

Diarrhea Frequent passing of unformed, loose, watery stools.

Diarthrotic joints Freely movable joints such as knees, wrists, hips, and shoulders.

Diastole (diastolic pressure) Pressure within arteries as the left ventricle relaxes and fills with blood.

Diencephalon Structure located in the brain and contains thalamus, hypothalamus, pituitary gland, and pineal gland.

Diffusion Movement of molecules from an area of high concentration to an area of low concentration to equalize concentrations; during diffusion, molecules simply spread out or diffuse in a given space or across a cell membrane.

Digital citizenship Responsible and ethical use of technology by anyone who uses computers, the Internet, and digital devices.

Direct contact Disease transmission that occurs from physical contact between an infected person and a noninfected person; this includes touching, kissing, or sexual acts.

Disability An impairment or condition that makes it more difficult to participate in one or more major life activity.

Disability insurance A form of insurance that provides income protection if a person is unable to work because of disease or injury.

Disclosure Sharing information such as thoughts, feelings, and personal history.

Discrimination The unjust or prejudicial treatment of others based on a perceived difference, such as a person's race, nationality, age, marital status, gender, gender identity, sexual orientation, religion, disability, cognitive reasoning, level of physical fitness, political affiliations, socioeconomic factors, pregnancy status, employment status, veteran's status, immigration status, or history.

Disease A condition of abnormal function involving anatomic structures or body systems.

Disease outbreak Disease occurrence in excess of what is normally expected within a community, geographic area, or season; may last for a few days, weeks, or several years.

Disease resistance Body's ability to destroy or deactivate pathogens and foreign agents through defense mechanisms.

Disease susceptibility The lack of disease resistance and increased risk of acquiring disease.

Disinfection Use of chemicals to destroy pathogens and may include heat. Disinfection kills most bacterial spores.

Dislocation Temporary displacement of bones within a joint, with complete loss of contact between articulating surfaces.

Disorders Disruptions of normal body function and may not involve structural change.

Distal Located farther from the point of reference, usually away from the trunk of the body.

Distress Stress perceived as negative and beyond our capacity to cope with the situation.

Diverticulitis Inflammation or infection of diverticula when fecal matter plugs and predisposes the area to infection with colonic bacteria.

Diverticulosis Presence of small herniations in the colon, usually in the sigmoid colon.

Document release form Form that must be signed and dated by a client before a company or individual can legally share client information with other parties.

Documentation Process of collecting, confirming, and recording information.

Dorsal cavity Cavity located on backside or posterior aspect of body; divided into cranial and spinal cavities.

Dorsiflexion Movement of the ankle as the foot moves superiorly—toes are moving toward the shin or tibia.

Double crush syndrome (DCS) Compression of a single peripheral nerve at multiple sites.

Downward (inferior) rotation Scapular movement that occurs as glenoid cavity rotates to orient inferiorly.

Draping Utilization of linens or similar fabrics to cover the client's body, the massage table, and table accessories.

Droplet precautions Methods to reduce or prevent transmission of pathogens transmitted by respiratory droplets generated by speaking, coughing, or sneezing.

Dual relationships Situations when two or more different relationships exist; there are several types of dual relationships, such as social, professional, business, communal, and sexual.

Ductus deferens See *Vas deferens.*

Dura mater Outermost meningeal layer that lies against the central nervous system; thick and dense and creates partitions within the brain.

Eccentric contractions Muscles that lengthen while generating force.

Ectoderm Embryonic outermost layer that gives rise to structures of the nervous system, including special senses and epidermis of the skin.

Eczema Noncontagious inflammatory skin condition commonly found on the hands, scalp, face, nape of neck, creases of elbow and knees, and ankles and feet.

Edema Swelling, typically occurring in the legs, ankles, and feet, and caused by an imbalance in the distribution of body fluids but, unlike in lymphedema, lymphatic vessels are still intact.

Efferent (motor) neuron Neuron that transmits impulses away from the central nervous system toward muscles or glands; also called effectors.

Effleurage The application of gliding movements that follow the contours of the body.

Ejaculatory duct Short tube that passes through the prostate to join the urethra.

Elastic cartilage Cartilage type that is soft and pliable; this flexible cartilage gives shape to external nose and ears and is found in internal structures, such as larynx (voice box).

Elastic connective tissue Found in the walls of blood vessels and bronchi and recoil after being stretched by blood or air during breathing.

Elastic therapeutic tape Thin, stretchy, elastic tape applied to the skin.

Elevation Movement at a joint in a superior or upward direction; essentially it is raising or lifting a body part.

Ellipsoidal joints Joints that contain an oval-shaped surface that fits into a concave surface allowing bone to travel back and forth (flexion and extension) and side to side (abduction and adduction).

Emergency preparedness Process of providing first and immediate responses during health or medical emergency situations to minimize loss of life.

Emotional boundaries The capacity to be aware of, to control, and to express one's emotions.

Emotional wellness Involves the capacity to be aware of, to control, and to express one's emotions, and to handle interpersonal relationships judiciously and empathetically.

Empathy The desire to understand what another person is experiencing without mistaking it for your own experience.

Emphysema Permanent enlargement of lower airways accompanied by destruction of alveolar walls, affecting its elasticity.

End-feel Quality of resistance felt by the practitioner at the end of passive range of motion.

Endangerment site Areas containing structures vulnerable to injury from applied pressure because they are not well protected by bones and muscles; also called cautionary sites or areas of caution.

Endemic disease A disease which occurs regularly in particular regions or populations.

Endochondral ossification Bone development from cartilage.

Endocrine glands Glands that secrete products called hormones directly into the bloodstream; they do not use ducts and are also called ductless glands.

Endocytosis Process of moving substances inside cells.

Endoderm Embryonic innermost layer that forms the lining of the body's cavities, passages, and covering for most internal organs.

Endometriosis Presence of functional endometrial tissue outside uterus.

Endoneurium Inner layer of connective tissue layer that surrounds the axons of neurons.

Endoplasmic reticulum (ER) Network of curved sacs arranged in parallel rows found near center of a cell; types are rough or smooth; rough ER is spotted with ribosomes and resembles sandpaper; smooth ER does not contain ribosomes and has a smooth appearance.

Enzyme Substances that aid in digestion by acting as catalysts in chemical reactions.

Epicondylitis Inflammation of a tendon where it attaches to a bone, often an epicondyle. Types are lateral epicondylitis, or tennis elbow, and medial epicondylitis, or golfer's elbow.

Epidemics Disease outbreaks affecting many individuals at about the same time and often spread to one or more communities.

Epidermis Thin, outer region of skin composed of epithelial tissue.

Epididymis Tightly coiled comma-shaped tube that lies behind and on top of each testicle.

Epineurium Dense outermost layer which surrounds groups of fascicles within a peripheral nerve.

Epiphyseal line Line of ossified bone indicating where previous bone growth occurred at the epiphyseal plate in long bones.

Epiphyseal plate Hyaline cartilage found near the ends of growing bone, allowing them to increase in length.

Epiphyses Ends of a long bone.

Epithelial membranes Layer of epithelial cells with an underlying supportive layer of connective tissue; subclassifications of epithelial membranes are cutaneous, mucous, and serous.

Epithelial tissue Tissue that lines or covers external and internal body structures, lines open body cavities such as digestive, respiratory, urinary, and reproductive tracts, as well as closed body cavities such as heart and abdomen.

Equity An individual's or business's net worth.

Ergonomics Adapting the work to the worker.

Erythrocytes Red blood cells that transport oxygen and carbon dioxide to and from body cells.

Esophagus Muscular tube that connects the pharynx to the stomach.

Essential oils Concentrated essences of plants and possess characteristic fragrances of plants.

Ethics Moral principles that govern behavior.

Ethnocentrism The evaluation of other cultures according to preconceptions originating in the standards and customs of one's own culture.

Etiology Causes or origins of disease.

Eustress Stress perceived as positive and within our ability to meet the demands of the situation; it helps keep us focused on a goal, improves performance, and improves our sense of personal satisfaction.

Evaporation Transfer or loss of heat when a liquid changes into a gas or a vapor.

Eversion Elevation of the lateral edge of the foot so it turns outward or away from the midline of the body.

Evidence Information that supports an idea or conclusion.

Evidence-informed A problem-solving approach used when making treatment decisions that integrates relevant evidence, the client's preferences and values, and the practitioner's professional expertise to achieve desired patient/client goals.

Exacerbations Periods of time when signs and symptoms of disease worsen or become more severe; also called *flare-ups* or *relapses*.

Exclusion criteria Characteristics that disqualify participants from inclusion in an experiment.

Excursion (massage) The distance a massage technique travels over the body.

Excursion (movement) Side-to-side movements of the jaw or mandible.

Exhalation Process of expelling air from the lungs.

Exocrine glands Glands that produce and secrete their products into ducts that open to body cavities, center of a hollow organ, or on surface of body; examples are sudoriferous glands, sebaceous glands, and ceruminous glands.

Exocytosis Process of moving substances outside a cell.

Expert opinion Opinions from people who have acquired vast amounts of information and offer experienced views on specified topics.

Expertise A combination of formal education, knowledge accumulation, previous treatment decisions, and past outcomes.

Expiration See *Exhalation.*

Exploratory questions Questions used to gain deeper understanding of the client's health and preferences.

Extension Straightening a joint so that the angle of a joint increases.

External respiration Gas exchange between air in the alveoli and blood in the capillaries.

Exteroceptors Receptors located on or near the surface of the body, such as in skin and mucosa, and receive stimuli from the external environment.

Extracellular fluids Fluids located outside of body cells such as plasma, interstitial fluid, lymph, and transcellular fluids.

Extraneous variables Variables not under investigation but may influence the outcome or the relationship between the dependent and the independent variables.

Fallopian (uterine) tubes Paired tubes extending laterally from the uterus and used as a passageway for ova to travel from the ovaries to the uterus.

Fascia Sheets of connective tissue enveloping the body beneath the skin and enclosing muscle and nerve cells, and compartmentalizing muscle into muscle groups, and provides for their attachments to bone and other structures.

Fast twitch Muscles that contract more quickly, for shorter periods of time, and fatigue faster compared with slow twitch muscle.

Fat pads Structures that protect articular cartilages and act as packing material to fill spaces that occur as the joint cavity changes shape during movement.

Fertility cycle See *Menstrual cycle.*

Fertilization Penetration of an ovum by sperm, resulting in a zygote.

Fibroblasts Precursor cells that produce the protein fibers found in connective tissues and also contribute to wound healing and tissue repair.

Fibrocartilage Cartilage type that is strong and durable; fibrocartilage discs serve as shock absorbers and are found between vertebrae (intervertebral discs) and in the knee (meniscus).

Fibromyalgia syndrome A chronic condition characterized by widespread pain and joint stiffness, restless sleep, and chronic fatigue.

Fibrous connective tissue Connective tissue type that supports structures, attaches them to each other, fills in spaces between structures, and helps keep them in their proper places.

Fibrous joints Joints that are joined by dense fibrous connective tissue and do not have a joint capsule.

Fidelity Professionals should be loyal and dedicated to their clients, keep their promises, and honor commitments.

Filtration Movement of water and molecules across a cell membrane due to pressure.

Financial boundaries Encompasses money and includes fee schedules, payment arrangements and procedures, and policies of nonpayment.

Financial statements Written records that convey financial information and financial performance of individuals, businesses, and corporations.

Fixators Muscles that act like specialized synergists to stabilize joints or help maintain posture so prime movers can exert their action; fixators are also called stabilizers.

Flat bones Bones that possess a broad flat surface; flat bones found in chest, upper back, ribcage, pelvis, and skull.

Flexibility exercises Activities that lengthen and stretch muscles to improve range of motion and balance;

includes static stretching, dynamic movement, and ballistic stretching/movement.

Flexion Bending a joint so that the angle of a joint decreases.

Floatation therapy Activity wherein the client floats in a foot or less of warm salt water within a dark, soundproof tank.

Fomite A contaminated object or material.

Food labels Panels on packaged foods that contain information about its nutritional value and are required by the Food and Drug Administration.

Foot stances Positions of the practitioner's feet used to provide a base of support while applying massage.

Force The push or pull upon an object resulting from one object's interaction with another.

Fracture Any crack or break in a bone.

Friction Massage technique which involves rubbing one body surface against another while maintaining constant and equal pressure in all directions.

Frontal lobe Brain region that regulates executive functions such as judgment, problem-solving, planning, concentration, self-awareness, cognition, intelligence, as well as personality. Also contains Broca's area, critical for speech production.

Frontal plane Plane that bisects the body side to side and divides it into front (anterior) and back (posterior) sections.

Functional reversibility Occurs when muscles reverse their relationship between attachment sites and muscle origins move toward their insertions.

Fungi Include molds, yeast, and dermatophytes; only a few varieties are pathogenic.

Gait The pattern of movement used while walking or running.

Gait cycle A repetitive movement pattern which begins when one foot contacts the ground and ends when the same foot contacts the ground again, which begins the next cycle.

Gait disorders Altered gait patterns caused by deformities, amputations, muscle weakness or contracture, pain, or loss of motor control.

Gallbladder Hollow pear-shaped sac that lies on inferior surface of the liver.

Gallstones Masses of solid material or stones (calculi) that form in gallbladder or bile duct.

Ganglion cyst Fluid-filled pouch that forms on tendons or joints, usually the wrists or hands.

Gastroesophageal reflux disease (GERD) Periodic regurgitation of gastric contents into the esophagus.

Gastrointestinal tract Long open muscular tube from the mouth, extending through the body, and ending at the anus.

Gate control theory of pain Theory that states that the spinal cord acts like a neurologic gate and controls whether or not pain signals enter the brain, which results in the experience of pain.

General partnerships An agreement between two or more individuals who conduct the business for profit and each partner contributes money, property, labor, or skill, and share the business's profits and losses.

Genetic disease Disease caused by abnormalities in the genetic code; genetic diseases can pass from one generation to next, which means they are inherited; some result from mutation (either natural or induced).

Geriatric massage Modification of basic massage techniques and body positions to meet needs of older and aging adults; takes into account physical, psychological, and socioeconomic factors.

Gestational diabetes mellitus (GDM) Diabetes that develops during pregnancy in females who did not already have diabetes.

Gift cards Vouchers given as a "gift" to pay for services and/or products. Also called gift certificates.

Gliding joints Joints that allow interaction of relatively flat surfaces of articulating bone; gliding joints allow limited movement along all axes.

Glomerular filtration The first step in the process of filtering blood and manufacturing urine.

Glomeruli Cluster of capillaries at the beginning of the nephron in the kidneys; plural form of glomerulus.

Goiter Enlargement of the thyroid gland.

Golgi body Series of separate horizontal membranous sacs that are stacked on top of each other found in cells. Golgi bodies synthesize proteins and lipids, then pack and store them.

Golgi complex See *Golgi body*.

Golgi tendon organs Tension-sensitive receptors located at musculotendinous junctions; if tension is too great, motor nerves are inhibited and muscle contraction is prevented.

Gout A type of arthritis caused by the accumulation of uric acid crystals in joints.

Graves Disease Overproduction of thyroid hormones called hyperthyroidism, causing a generalized increase in the body's metabolism.

Gravity The force that pulls objects toward the center of the earth.

Gross income The total amount of income earned over a period of time by an individual/household or a company.

Hair Keratinized filaments arising from pouchlike hair follicles in the dermis.

Hair follicle receptor See *Hair root plexus*.

Hair root plexus Receptors that detect hair movement and may alert us to slight breezes or intrusive insects; they wrap around hair follicles and resemble a net or web.

Hand hygiene General term for cleaning or disinfecting the hands by handwashing or by alcohol-based hand rubs.

Hashimoto disease An underactive thyroid gland leading to a thyroid hormone deficiency.

Hay fever Hypersensitivity of nasal mucosa to allergens (usually plant pollen).

Health insurance Insurance that covers part or all of the medical expenses for diseases, conditions, and injuries.

Health Insurance Portability and Accountability Act of 1996 (HIPAA) Created by the Department of Health and

Human Services to protect client rights and targets the storage, transmission, and dissemination of personal health information, which includes information that is written, spoken, recorded, or electronically stored that pertains to the past, present, or future care of clients.

Health literacy Capacity of an individual to obtain, communicate, and understand health information and services when making decisions.

Healthcare-associated infections Infections acquired while a person is receiving healthcare for another condition.

Healthy Eating Plate Developed by the Harvard School of Public Health to help consumers make food choices and plan portions at meal times.

Hearing impairment Decreased capacity to hear; may occur in one or both ears.

Heart Hollow, muscular organ located in the mediastinum region, which is behind the sternum and between the lungs.

Heart arrhythmia Irregular heartbeat; occurs when the conduction system does not function properly and causes the heart to beat too fast or too slow.

Heart attack Sudden disruption of blood flow to the heart caused by a blocked or occluded blood vessel; also called myocardial infarction.

Heart rate Number of cardiac cycles that occur in 1 minute.

Heart rate variability (HRV) Variation in time intervals between heartbeats; controlled by the autonomic nervous system.

Heart rhythm Pattern or regularity of electrical impulses that causes the heart to contract.

Heartburn Burning sensation in the chest or epigastrium behind the sternum.

Hemoglobin An iron-based protein that binds with oxygen and carbon dioxide so they can be transported in blood.

Hemostasis Process that stops bleeding and helps keep blood within the damaged vessel.

Hepatitis Inflammation of the liver usually caused by viruses.

Herniated disc Protrusion of the nucleus pulposus through a tear in the annulus fibrosus within the intervertebral disc.

Hiccups Intermittent involuntary contractions of the diaphragm followed by a spasmodic closure of the vocal cords.

Hierarchy of evidence System used to rank the strength of research according to its possibility of bias; there are several levels within the hierarchy; lower level studies tend to have weaker evidence and more bias, while higher level studies have stronger evidence and less bias.

High-risk pregnancy Pregnancy that is more likely to experience complications, including disease and death to the mother, the developing fetus, or both.

Hinge joints Joints that possess a convex surface that fits into the concave surface of another bone; movements allowed by hinge joints are flexion and extension.

Homeostasis The constant and stable internal environment within a narrow range despite changes that occur in the external environment.

Homolateral See *Ipsilateral*.

Horizontal abduction Movement which occurs as the shoulder or hip moves the extremity away from the midline in the transverse/horizontal plane.

Horizontal adduction Movement which occurs as the shoulder or hip moves the extremity toward the midline in the transverse/horizontal plane.

Horizontal plane See *Transverse plane.*

Hormonal regulation Release of hormones from one gland regulating the release of hormones from another gland.

Hormones Chemical messengers that regulate physiologic activity of other cells and influence growth, metabolism, digestion, reproduction, and mood.

Horse stance Foot stance used when the target area(s) of the applied technique is directly in front of the practitioner's body. Feet are symmetric and pointing in the same direction, usually beneath the massage table.

Hospice care Type of medical care that provides palliative services to patients and their families who are facing a life-limiting illness.

Hospital-based massage therapy Massage services provided in hospital or medical settings.

Host susceptibility How vulnerable an individual is to developing infection after exposure to pathogens.

Hot packs Heated packs that range from electrical plug-in heating pads, chemical heating pads, to packs warmed in a microwave or cabinet, to packs filled with hot water.

Hot stone massage A treatment where smooth, flat heated stones are placed on the skin or used as hand-held massage tools; sometimes cold stones are also used.

Human immunodeficiency viral infection (HIV) Caused by the HIV, a virus that destroys a type of T-cell called CD4, which fight infection; can refer to the virus or the infection, the final stage of which is AIDS.

Human trafficking Form of modern-day slavery in which traffickers use force, fraud, or coercion to obtain some type of labor or commercial sex acts.

Hyaline cartilage Cartilage type that is elastic, rubbery, smooth and is composed of cells in a translucent, pearly blue matrix; covers articulating surfaces of bones, connects ribs to the sternum, and is found as supportive tissues in the nose, ears, trachea, and smaller respiratory tubes.

Hydrostatic pressure Pressure exerted by fluids on an immersed object; according to Pascal's law, a fluid exerts equal pressure at a given depth, and this pressure will increase as depth increases.

Hydrotherapy Use of water in any of its forms for health promotion or treatment of various diseases and conditions.

Hyperemesis gravidarum Severe and uncontrollable nausea and vomiting during pregnancy.

Hyperemia Skin reddening from vasodilation and increased local blood flow.

Hyperextension Overextending a joint beyond its normally straightened position, as in moving the head back to look upward.

Hyperkyphosis (Kyphosis) Exaggeration of the normal kyphotic (posterior) curvature in the thoracic spine.

Hyperlordosis (Lordosis) Exaggeration of the normal lordotic (anterior) curvature in the lumbar spine.

Hypersensitivities Overly sensitive immune reactions to substances that are usually harmless; include allergies.

Hypertension Elevated blood pressure, usually suspected when blood pressure readings reach or exceed 140/90. Also called hypertensive heart disease.

Hypoglycemia Abnormally low blood glucose levels, usually below 70 mg/dL.

Hypothalamus Brain structure located in the diencephalon of the brain that regulates the autonomic nervous system as well as controls behavioral patterns and 24-hour cycle called circadian rhythm.

Hypothesis Presumed outcome of an experiment and what is expected to happen given a certain set of circumstances.

Ice massage Combining ice application with friction massage.

Ice packs Plastic bags filled with ice or icy water.

Idiopathic A disease that does not have a known cause.

Illness The feeling of ill health a person identifies themselves, often based on self-report.

Immunity Body's ability to recognize and respond to pathogens and foreign agents.

Immunodeficiency Failure of the immune response to protect the body from pathogens.

Impetigo Highly infectious bacterial skin infection seen primarily in children and occurs mainly around the mouth, nose, hands, and in skin folds such as the axillae.

Impingement syndrome Occurs when the supraspinatus tendon and the subacromial bursa become compressed between the narrow space beneath the acromion process and the humeral head, and leads to pain and dysfunction during shoulder adduction. Also known as *shoulder impingement syndrome*.

Incidence The number of new cases of a given condition within a population per unit of time, usually a calendar year.

Inclusion criteria Characteristics that participants must possess to be included in an experiment.

Income tax Taxes owed on personal and business income and on unearned income such as dividends and rental property.

Incubation period Time interval between initial exposure to pathogens and the first appearance of disease signs and symptoms.

Independent contractors Individuals who have specialized skills, training, or license that allows them to work without supervision.

Independent variable Focus of an experiment or intervention under investigation.

Indirect contact Disease transmission from contaminated fomites or objects and infected droplets.

Infant massage Modifications of massage techniques and body positions to meet the needs of the child and the child's family (newly born to age 3).

Infectious disease Disease caused by pathogens, such as bacteria, fungi, viruses, protozoa, prions, and pathogenic animals.

Inferior Situated below or toward the tail end.

Inflammation Protective response to tissue damage resulting from a variety of causes, including infection and trauma.

Influenza Acute, highly contagious viral infection of the upper respiratory tract, but it can extend into the lower respiratory tract.

Informed consent Permission given by a client to receive treatment after they have been informed of all relevant facts related to treatment.

Inhalation Process of taking air into the lungs.

Insertion (muscle) Tendinous attachment on the bone that is movable during contraction; insertions are usually lateral or distal compared with origins.

Inspiration See *Inhalation.*

Instrument-assisted soft tissue mobilization (IASTM) Handheld, round-edged tools used to scrape the skin in multiple directions.

Insurance Agreement by a company or governmental agency to provide compensation for specified losses, damages, illness, or death in return for payments called premiums given to the insurance provider.

Intellectual boundaries Encompass beliefs, thoughts, and ideas as well as safeguarding self-esteem.

Intellectual wellness The continuous acquisition, development, and creative application of critical thinking in the quest for a more satisfying existence.

Intercultural communication Communication between people of different cultures and ethnicities.

Intercultural communication competency The degree to which you can effectively adapt verbal and nonverbal messages to the appropriate cultural context.

Internal respiration Gas exchange between blood in capillaries and body cells and tissues.

International Classification of Disease (ICD) Comprehensive database used in healthcare and research to classify and monitor incidence and prevalence rates of diseases, disorders, and injuries.

Interneurons (association neurons) Neurons that lie between sensory and motor neurons and participate in integrative functions.

Interoceptors (visceroceptors) Receptors located internally and respond to stimuli such as heartbeat, breathing, hunger, satiety, thirst, and the urge to defecate or urinate.

Interstitial cells of Leydig Endocrine cells scattered between testicular tubules.

Interstitial fluid Fluid found in extracellular spaces between tissues; this fluid is primarily water and contains substances, such as salts, sugars, fatty acids, amino acids, hormones, and neurotransmitters; interstitial fluid bathes cells and provides a transport medium for nutrients, gases, and wastes.

Intracellular fluids Fluids located within body cells and facilitates chemical reactions.

Intramembranous ossification Bone development from membranes such as those found in the flat bones of the skull.

Introception Awareness of thoughts, feelings, and sensations related to the internal environment, through mindfulness; includes the perception of physical sensations such as heartbeat, respiration, and satiety or fullness from eating.

Inversion Elevation of the medial edge of foot so it turns inward or toward the midline of the body.

Ipsilateral Related to same side of body.

Irregular bones Odd-shaped bones that do not fit well in other categories; these types of bones are found in the skull and the spine.

Irritable bowel syndrome (IBS) Common disorder characterized by abnormal muscular contractions of the colon.

Ischemia Decreased local blood flow.

Islets of Langerhans See *Pancreatic islets*.

Isometric contractions Muscles whose lengths remain the same as they generate force; movement does not occur.

Isotonic contractions Muscles generating force, which causes muscle length to change; can become shorter or longer depending on desired action.

Joint capsule Double-layered joint structure; outer layer of the capsule is fibrous and surrounds the joint like a sleeve, and the inner layer of the capsule is lined with synovial membrane that secretes synovial fluid. Also called an *articular capsule*.

Joint cavity Space between the two layers of a joint capsule.

Joint play Small involuntary joint movements that are independent of muscle contraction, due to joint capsule laxity, and are limited to approximately 1/8 inch in any plane and occur along the contours of the joint surfaces.

Joints Where bones come together or join; joints allow body to move in response to muscle or outside forces.

Justice Acting on the basis of fairness, equality, and non-discrimination.

Juvenile rheumatoid arthritis (JRA) Rheumatoid arthritis that develops in children and adolescents. Clinical manifestations unique to JRA include large joints are most affected, fusion or ankylosing of cervical spine is common if the disease progresses, joint pain is less severe, and subcutaneous nodules are absent.

Juxtaglomerular apparatus Structure located between the afferent arteriole and the renal tubule; contains juxtaglomerular cells located in afferent arteriole and macula densa located in distal convoluted tubule.

Juxtaglomerular cells Cells in the afferent arteriole that act as mechanoreceptors and monitor blood pressure.

Keratin Substance that waterproofs the skin.

Keratinocytes Cells that produce keratin, a tough fibrous protein that protects skin; keratinocytes secrete a lipid substance that forms a waterproof barrier between cells.

Kidney (renal) failure Loss of kidney function.

Kidney stones Small, hard masses composed of minerals and salts that form inside the kidney.

Kidneys Two reddish-brown lima bean-shaped organs located bilaterally at or about spinal level T11 to L3.

Kinesiology Study of human motion.

Krause (bulboid) corpuscles Receptors that detect deep pressure, cold or reduced temperatures, low-frequency vibration, and textural sensations.

Kyphosis See *Hyperkyphosis*.

Labrum A ring of fibrocartilage around the edge of the articular cartilage to increase the surface area of the articular surface of the joint.

Lactation The production and secretion of milk by mammary glands after childbirth, which can lead to breast-feeding.

Lacteals Lymphatic capillaries located in fingerlike projections of the small intestine called villi.

Landmarks (foot reflexology) Four horizontal lines that traverse the bottom or plantar surface of each foot.

Langerhans cells See *Dendritic cells*.

Large intestine Last section of gastrointestinal tract.

Larynx Tube that connects the pharynx to the trachea.

Lateral Oriented farther away from the midline of the body.

Lateral recumbent See *Side-lying position*.

Lateral rotation (external rotation) Refers to the outward rotation of joints in the appendicular skeleton, such as the shoulder, hip, and knee (the knee can be rotated slightly when flexed), and occurs in the transverse/horizontal plane.

Left lateral recumbent Client side-lying position when lying on left.

Leukocytes The body's mobile army and serves as part of the body's defense mechanism by destroying or deactivating pathogens and foreign agents.

Liabilities Debts or obligations an individual or business owes to another individual or business and are payable in money, goods, or services.

Lice Wingless parasites that live their entire life cycle on a single human host and depend on its blood for survival; three forms of human lice are head lice, body lice, and pubic lice (crabs).

License Official permission granted to an individual by a legal authority to do, to use, or to own something; this term also refers to the document issued to the licensee.

Ligaments Connective tissue that unites articulating bones, which strengthens the joint.

Limbic system Areas of the brain that regulate behavioral and emotional responses, especially those needed for survival, and include the hypothalamus, thalamus, amygdala, hippocampus, and the olfactory bulbs.

Limitations Things the researcher cannot control (participant compliance, dropout rate).

Limited liability companies A company that is a blend of partnerships and corporations.

Limited partnerships A business partnership which limits the personal liability of partners according to the amount that partner invested into the company.

Line of gravity Vertical line that extends through the center of an object to its base of support.

Literature review A study, or survey, of existing scholarly work with the aim of discussing all published information about a specific topic or research question.

Liver Largest organ in body and is located beneath right side of diaphragm in right upper quadrant of the abdomen.

Local contraindication Condition which makes receiving massage to a local area of the body inadvisable.

Local disease Disease affecting only one area of the body.

Local inflammation See *Acute inflammation*.

Location boundaries Encompasses where professional activities are conducted, and include an office, clinic, spa or wellness center, client residence, or institutional care facility.

Long bones Bones longer than they are wide and found in arm, forearm, thigh, and leg.

Longitudinal study A study which looks at the effect of a condition(s) over an extended period of time (e.g., low carb diets and weight loss).

Lordosis See *Hyperlordosis*.

Lungs Main organs of respiration and extend from just above the clavicles to the diaphragm.

Lyme disease Recurrent form of arthritis that affects not only joints but also skin, heart, and nervous system; large joints, such as the knee and hip, are most commonly involved.

Lymph Nearly colorless watery fluid that circulates through lymphatic vessels.

Lymph capillaries Small lymphatic vessels found in the spaces between the tissues.

Lymph nodes Bean-shaped structures located at intervals along the lymphatic chain that filter lymph.

Lymphatic fluid See *Lymph*.

Lymphatic trunks Larger lymphatic vessels along the lymphatic chain; these trunks converge to form one of two regionally draining lymphatic ducts.

Lymphatic vessels Vessels containing internal valves that open in only one direction, causing lymph to flow toward the center of the body, and are what lymph capillaries merge into.

Lymphatics All lymphatic capillaries, vessels, trunks, and ducts along the lymphatic chain.

Lymphedema Swelling caused by abnormal accumulation of fluids within interstitial spaces because lymphatics or nodes are malformed, damaged, or have been surgically removed.

Lymphocytes Type of white blood cells; types are B lymphocytes (B cells) and T lymphocytes (T cells) and are vital to immune responses.

Lymphokinesis Movement of lymph through the body.

Lysosomes Membranous organelles that have broken off from Golgi bodies, break down unneeded proteins, and engulf and destroy pathogens with enzymes.

Macula densa Cells located in the distal convoluted tubule that act as chemoreceptors and monitor concentration of the filtrate.

Malpractice insurance See *Professional liability insurance*.

Mammary glands See *Breasts*.

Mandatory reporting Legislative mandate that applies to individuals who have regular contact with vulnerable populations to file a report with protection services when abuse or neglect is observed or suspected.

Manual lymphatic drainage (MLD) Gentle superficial skin stretching applied along lymphatic pathways to promote lymph flow and reduce or prevent swelling.

Marketing Activities used to create, communicate, deliver, and exchange products and services that have value for consumers, clients, and the society at large.

Massage (Massage Therapy) Method of manipulating soft tissue using compression and decompression/traction for clinical, therapeutic, and palliative purposes or for wellness and self-care purposes.

Massage Practitioner Trained individual who practices massage.

Maternity massage See *Pregnancy massage*.

Mechanoreceptors Type of proprioceptors that detects mechanical stimuli such as pressure and sound, and are found in skin, blood vessels, ears, muscles, joints, and fascia; includes muscle spindles and Golgi tendon organs.

Medial Oriented toward or near the midline of the body.

Medial rotation (internal rotation) Refers to the inward rotation of joints in the appendicular skeleton, such as the shoulder, hip, and knee (the knee can be rotated slightly when flexed), and occurs in the transverse/horizontal plane.

Medulla oblongata Most inferior portion of brainstem, and transmits sensory and motor impulses between parts of the brain and the spinal cord; contains the respiratory, cardiovascular, and vasomotor centers, and regulates autonomic functions such as blood pressure, gastric secretions, sweating, sneezing, swallowing, and vomiting.

Medullary cavity Hollow space within the diaphysis filled with red and yellow bone marrow.

Meissner (tactile) corpuscles Receptors that detect light pressure, textural sensations, and low-frequency vibration.

Melanin Substance that darkens the skin.

Melanocytes Cells that produce melanin or pigment, which contribute to skin color; melanin also serves as a semi-protective shield from the damaging effects of sunlight.

Membranes Thin, soft, pliable sheets of tissue that cover the body, line body cavities, and cover organs within body cavities. They protect internal and external surfaces and anchor structures to each other; most membranes secrete lubricating fluids.

Menarche First menstruation.

Meningeal membranes (Meninges) Connective tissue coverings that surrounding the brain and spinal cord.

Menisci Crescent-shaped fibrocartilaginous pads located in select joints such as knees and jaw; menisci help joints to move smoothly and serve as a shock absorber.

Menopause Period of life when menstrual cycles end and ovarian functions cease.

Menses Menstrual fluid discharged during menstruation containing blood, tissue fluid, mucus, and endometrial cells.

Menstrual cramps Severe cramping and pain in the abdominopelvic region occurring just before or during menses.

Menstrual cycle Series of hormonal events that begin at menarche during puberty, occur approximately every 28 days, and ends at menopause.

Menstruation Periodic discharge of endometrial lining from a nonpregnant uterus through the vagina, and lasts approximately 5 days.

Mentor An experienced and trusted advisor who provides counsel, guidance, support, and encouragement.

Merkel (tactile) discs Receptors that detect light pressure as well as subtle changes in surface topography such as depressions and elevations or contours, and low-frequency vibrations; have small receptive fields and can make subtle tactile distinctions and adapt slowly.

Mesoderm Embryonic middle layer that develops into muscles and connective tissues.

Meta-analysis Type of systematic review that uses statistics to determine the strength of evidence.

Metabolic disease Occurs when the metabolism fails, causing the body to have too much or too little of an essential substance, such as hormones.

Metabolism Biochemical processes that occur within a living organism to maintain life.

Methicillin-resistant *Staphylococcus aureus* (MRSA) infection Caused by staph bacteria resistant to antibiotics commonly used to treat ordinary staph infections; commonly occur in healthcare settings.

Micturition See *Urination*.

Midbrain Brainstem structure that conducts nerve impulses from the cerebrum to the pons and from the spinal cord to the thalamus.

Midsagittal plane Plane that runs through the midline of the body, dividing it into equal right and left halves.

Migraine headaches Severe and recurrent headaches often accompanied by symptoms such as visual disturbances and nausea.

Mindfulness Heightened self-awareness and focused attention given to present moments characterized by curiosity, openness, acceptance, and engagement.

Miscarriage Noninduced embryonic or fetal death or passage of conception products before 20 weeks of gestation; occurs in approximately 20% to 30% of all pregnancies.

Mission statement Single statement of a business's purpose.

Mitochondria Oval organelles found in cells and involved in cellular respiration; provides most of the cell's ATP, which is the cell's energy or power molecule.

Mitral valve Left atrioventricular valve located between the left atrium and the right ventricle.

Mobility impairment Decreased capacity to move or use one or more of the extremities, or a lack of strength needed to walk, grasp objects, or lift objects.

Mobilizations Movements passively applied to a joint without a manual thrust at the end of available motion.

Mode of transmission Transfer of pathogens by contact (direct and indirect), through vehicles, such as food or water, or by vectors, such as insects or animals to spread pathogens between two or more hosts.

Morbidity Departure from a state of physiologic or psychologic well-being.

Morbidity rate Number of persons who are diseased, ill, injured, or disabled within a population or region.

Morning sickness Nausea with or without vomiting during pregnancy; affects 75% of pregnancies and can occur any time of day or night.

Mortality Condition of being dead.

Mortality rate Number of deaths within a population or region.

Motor end plate Folded sections of the sarcolemma or covering of a muscle fiber.

Motor neuron Neuron responsible for sending impulses to stimulate muscle contraction or glandular secretion.

Motor unit Single motor neuron and all muscle fibers to which it attaches.

Mucosa-associated lymph tissue Collective term to describe small groups of lymphatic tissue positioned strategically along respiratory and digestive tracts; includes tonsils, Peyer patches, and vermiform appendix.

Mucous membranes Tissue layer that lines open body cavities; examples are linings of digestive, respiratory, and urogenital tracts; mucous membranes secrete mucus.

Multiarticular muscles Muscles that cross three or more joints.

Multiaxial joints Permit movement around three axes and in three planes.

Multiple sclerosis (MS) Progressive degeneration and demyelination of nerves in the brain, spinal cord, and cranial nerves (especially the optic nerve).

Muscle Groups of fasciculi that are surrounded by a layer of connective tissue called *epimysium* and anchored to bones by tendons.

Muscle contraction The generation of tension in muscle fibers through cross-bridging, or connection, between actin and myosin filaments.

Muscle energy techniques Uses energy produced by muscle contraction to improve musculoskeletal function and reduce pain.

Muscle fatigue The decline in muscle's ability to generate force.

Muscle fibers Muscle cells and they are as long as the length of the entire muscle.

Muscle spindles Stretch-sensitive receptors that monitor changes in muscle length and cause reflexive contraction.

Muscle tissue Tissue type that possesses properties of excitability or ability to respond to a stimulus; when stimulated, muscle tissue has the ability to contract or shorten; when relaxed, muscle can extend or stretch and lengthen, and is quite elastic and returns to its original shape after movement; types are smooth, skeletal, and cardiac.

Muscle tone Continuous and partial muscle contraction even while muscles are at rest; also called *tonus*.

Myelin White fatty substance that insulates axons and prevents impulse "leakage" to adjacent neurons.

Myocardial infarction Sudden disruption of blood flow to the heart muscle or myocardium caused by an occluded blood vessel or hemorrhage from a broken blood vessel; see also *heart attack*.

Myofascial pain syndrome A chronic pain disorder characterized by the presence of myofascial trigger points and muscular pain; points can produce both pain and referred pain when pressed.

Myofascial release (MFR) Low-load, long-duration skin stretching.

Myofibrils Slender strands within muscle fibers that contain sarcomeres.

Myofilament Fine filaments within sarcomeres, namely thin filaments and thick filaments.

Myoglobin Red respiratory pigment in muscle cells similar to hemoglobin in red blood cells.

Myotomes Groups of skeletal muscles supplied by specific motor spinal nerve root.

Nails Compact keratinized cells that form thin, hard plates found on distal surfaces of fingers and toes.

Nasal cavity Hollow space in the skull separated by a septum into left and right halves.

Neck/shoulder line In reflexology, the horizontal line located between the base of the toes and the ball of the foot. These lines are used to delineate treatment areas containing reflex points.

Negative feedback regulation Response to stimulus that moves something in opposite or negative direction.

Neglect Failure by a caregiver to provide necessary food, shelter, healthcare, or supervision to the person for whom they are caring.

Nephrons Specialized tube-shaped filtering units in kidneys.

Nerve impulse Electrical signal that conveys information along a neuron.

Nerve plexus Network of nerves, formed by some ventral rami from the spinal cord.

Nerve tracts Bundles of nerve fibers in the central nervous system.

Nerves Bundles of nerve fibers located in the peripheral nervous system.

Nervous tissue Tissue type that possesses characteristics of excitability and conductibility; located in the brain, spinal cord, and within nerves.

Net income The amount an individual/household or a company makes after deducting allowable expenses and taxes.

Neural regulation Release of hormones by nerve impulses.

Neurilemma Outer layer of a myelin sheath.

Neuroglia Connective tissue that supports, nourishes, protects, and insulates neurons. Types in the central nervous system are astrocytes, ependymocytes, microglia, and oligodendrocytes, and in the peripheral nervous system are Schwann cells and satellite cells.

Neuromatrix theory of pain Theory that pain is a multidimensional experience produced by a person's "neurosignature" or unique pattern of nerve impulses within a widely distributed network in the brain called the body-self neuromatrix.

Neuromotor exercises Activities that incorporate resistance and flexibility with slow, focused movements and/or sustained body postures.

Neuromuscular junction Point where a motor neuron excites the sarcolemma of a muscle and initiates contraction.

Neurons Impulse-conducting cells of the nervous system, and possess properties of excitability or irritability, conductivity, and secretion.

Neuropathic (neurogenic) pain Pain originating from nonnociceptive nerve activation; also called *neuropathy*.

Neuroplasticity The brain's ability to form and reorganize synaptic connections, especially in response to learning or experience.

Neurotransmitters Classes of chemical messengers involved in synaptic transmission and stored in synaptic vesicles of presynaptic neurons.

Nociception The encoding of a painful event.

Nociceptive pain Pain originating from nociceptors.

Nociceptors Receptors that detect actual or potential tissue damage, are sensitive to pain, and serve a protective function by sending signals of a possible threat.

Nodes of Ranvier Unmyelinated spaces between myelinated sheaths, which increases the speed of the nerve impulses.

Nonmalfeasance Actions that "do no harm" and avoid harm.

Nonspecific defense mechanisms Targets all pathogens and foreign agents and include barriers, cellular responses, and inflammation.

Nonspecific pain Pain without an inflammatory, structural, or disease-related cause, commonly experienced in the lower back, neck, shoulders, hips, and knee; most pain is nonspecific.

Nucleus Cell structure that contains clusters of proteins, deoxyribonucleic acid (DNA), and ribonucleic acid (RNA), which helps form chromosomes or our genetic code, and directs most metabolic activities, including growth and reproduction.

Numeric rating scale (NRS) A line of numbers between 0 and 10 with 0 representing *no pain* and 10 representing *worst pain possible*.

Nutrients Substances necessary for life and can be grouped into two categories (macronutrients and micronutrients) and six subcategories (proteins, carbohydrates, fats, vitamins, minerals, and water).

Nutrition Ingesting food and drink to help our bodies function properly, to support tissue growth and repair, and to supply the energy needed to perform daily activities.

Objective information Information that is measurable and verifiable.

Observational study A study that simply observes a phenomenon (e.g., how many people use massage).

Obstructive sleep apnea (OSA) Sleep disorder characterized by temporary absence of normal breathing caused by a blocked upper airway.

Occipital lobe Brain region which contains the centers for visual perception including distance, depth, color, form, motion, and facial recognition.

Occupational wellness The ability to achieve balance between work and leisure time, to manage workplace stress, and to build relationships with colleagues.

Olfaction The sense of smell.

Oocytes (eggs) Sex cells that carry genetic information from the female who produced them; oocytes mature within ovarian follicles and one (sometimes more) is released during ovulation.

Open-ended questions Questions that offer little restriction when answering.

Operational definitions Definitions that describe how dependent variables were measured.

Opposition Movement in which the thumb comes into contact with any finger on the same hand.

Oral cavity First portion of the gastrointestinal tract; contains teeth, tongue, and openings for salivary glands.

Organ system level Biologic level that encompasses groups of related organs with complementary functions arranged into systems performing physiologic processes, such as respiration and digestion.

Organelles Structures within cells, and can function in reproduction, material storage, or metabolizing nutrients.

Organism level Biologic level that represents a living entity; each organism is composed of several organ systems that promote life; examples of organisms are *Homo sapiens*, fish, frogs, butterflies.

Origin (muscle) Tendinous attachment on the bone that is stable and less movable during contraction; origins are usually medial or proximal compared with insertions.

Orthopedic assessments Used to determine the presence or absence of musculoskeletal or neurologic conditions; also called *special tests*.

Osgood–Schlatter disease Patellar tendinitis in immature bone at the tibial tuberosity where the quadriceps attach.

Osmoreceptors Receptors that detect changes in electrolyte concentrations in blood plasma and are located in the hypothalamus.

Osmosis Movement of water across a cell membrane from an area of low concentration to high concentration to equalize fluid concentration on both sides of the membrane.

Ossification Process of bone tissue development by osteoblasts that begins during fetal development and continues throughout adulthood. Also called *osteogenesis*.

Osteoarthritis Age-related arthritis characterized by inflammation of the joint capsule and progressive joint damage leading to loss of articular cartilage.

Osteoblasts Bone-forming cells that fill small cavities left by osteoclasts.

Osteoclasts Bone-destroying cells that help dissolve bone and its minerals, especially calcium and phosphate.

Osteocytes Mature bone cell.

Osteoporosis Loss of normal bone density and increased bone porosity.

Ovarian cysts Fluid-filled cystic sacs within the ovary.

Ovaries Paired almond-shaped glands located in the abdominopelvic cavity of the female body, and secrete the hormones progesterone and estrogen responsible for regulating the menstrual cycle and for female secondary sex characteristics that occur during puberty.

Ovum Mature oocyte that has ovulated.

Pacini (lamellar) corpuscles Receptors that detect deeper pressure, vibration, and stretch, and receive proprioceptive information about joint position.

Pain Unpleasant sensory and emotional experiences associated with, or resembling, actual or potential tissue damage.

Pain management Process of providing care that alleviates or reduces pain to a level of comfort acceptable to a patient.

Pain perception The subjective reporting of a painful experience.

Pain threshold The *minimum* intensity of a stimulus perceived as painful.

Pain tolerance The *maximum* intensity of a pain-producing stimulus an individual is willing to accept in any given situation.

Palliative Noncurative measures used to improve a patient's quality of life.

Pallor Pale or ashen skin.

Pancreas Pinkish-gray gland that lies behind the stomach.

Pancreatic islets Specialized cells located on the pancreas that provide endocrine functions.

Pandemics Epidemics that spread across many regions, often worldwide.

Paraffin bath The dipping of a limb into a heated mixture of paraffin wax and mineral oil.

Parallel muscle fibers Muscle fibers arranged along the long axis of a bone; usually tapered at both ends or are spindle-shaped.

Paranasal sinuses Air-filled cavities lined with mucosa that open into the nasal cavity; sinuses lighten the skull and act as resonance chambers for sound.

Parasympathetic division Division of the autonomic nervous system that dominates during restful and calm situations to help the body conserve and restore energy; also called the craniosacral division.

Parathyroids Endocrine gland located in the throat on posterolateral surface.

Paresthesia Abnormal sensations, such as burning, itching, numbness, tingling or pricking, often called "pins and needles," which may or may not include the sensation of pain.

Parietal lobe Cerebral lobe that possesses centers for taste and touch.

Parkinson disease Progressive neurodegenerative disease characterized by tremors, rigidity, slowness of movements, and postural instability.

Passive process Cell process that does not require energy or activity of the cell membrane.

Passive range of motion Movement produced by external forces without voluntary muscle contraction.

Patellofemoral pain syndrome Pain and stiffness in front or around the kneecap.

Pathogen Biologic agent capable of causing infectious diseases.

Pathogenic animals Live on or within the host and depend on it for nourishment and replication; parasitic diseases are called infestations.

Pathology The study of disease.

Patient The recipient of medical/healthcare services; includes inpatient (a person admitted to a hospital to receive services and who stays overnight) and outpatient (a person not admitted to a hospital).

Peer review Evaluation of scientific, academic, or profession work by group of experts in the same or similar field.

Pelvic line (reflexology) In reflexology, the horizontal line located above the heel. These lines are used to delineate treatment areas containing reflex points.

Pennate muscle fibers Muscle fibers arranged with a central tendon and muscle fibers emerging diagonally, giving them a featherlike appearance; types are unipennate, bipennate, and multipennate.

Peptic ulcer disease (PUD) Ulcerations of gastrointestinal mucosa exposed to acidic gastric juice.

Perineurium Middle connective tissue layer that surrounds bundles of neurons; provides vascularization.

Periosteum Dense, fibrous sheath surrounding the diaphysis and is noticeably absent on the epiphyses; periosteum is the bone's life support system, containing blood and lymphatic vessels, nerves, and osteoblasts for growth and fracture healing.

Peripheral See *Superficial.*

Peripheral arterial disease Presence of atherosclerotic plaque within arteries outside the heart.

Peripheral nervous system Part of nervous system composed of cranial nerves emerging from the brain and spinal nerves emerging from the spinal cord.

Peripheral neuropathy Type of neuropathy originating in the peripheral nervous system.

Peripheral sensitization Increased responsiveness and reduced pain threshold in the peripheral nervous system.

Peristalsis Movements of mixing and propulsion in the gastrointestinal tract.

Peritoneum Large, flat, folded serous membrane that envelops the abdominal cavity.

Peritubular capillaries A network of capillaries surrounding the renal tubules.

Personal protective equipment Clothing and other items worn to protect the wearer's body from infection or injury.

Petrissage Massage technique involving compression, lifting or decompression, and then releasing soft tissues such as skin and muscle.

Petty cash A small amount of cash a business keeps on hand to pay for minor expenses.

Peyer patches Lymphatic tissue located in the small intestines; also called intestinal tonsils.

Phagocytosis Cell process that uses a piece of cell membrane to wrap large molecules, then pulls them inside the cell; once inside, it is digested by lysosomes.

Pharynx Muscular tube that extends from the nasal cavity to the larynx; functions as a passageway for both digestive and respiratory systems.

Phasic muscles Muscles that provide movement.

Phlebitis Inflammation of veins without thrombus or blood clot formation.

Photoreceptors Receptors that detect light stimuli; located in the retina of the eye.

Physical activity Movement produced by skeletal muscles and requires energy expenditure.

Physical boundaries The circumstances under which practitioners physically touch clients; this includes the who, when, where, how, and under what circumstances of professional touch.

Physical rehabilitation The restoration of an individual to a normal or near-normal function after a disabling disease or injury.

Physical wellness Promotes proper care of our bodies for optimal health and functioning.

Physiology The study of how the body and its individual parts function in normal body processes.

Pia mater The innermost meningeal layer attached to the surface of the central nervous system; thin and contains a rich supply of blood vessels, as well as helps circulate cerebrospinal fluid.

Pineal gland Endocrine gland located in diencephalon of brain; helps maintain the body's circadian rhythm.

Pinocytosis Cell process that uses a piece of cell membrane to wrap a liquid molecule and then pulls it inside cell; once inside, it is digested by lysosomes.

Piriformis syndrome Compression of the sciatic nerve caused by a hypertonic piriformis muscle; can be a cause of sciatica.

Pituitary gland Endocrine gland located in the diencephalon of brain; helps regulate energy, mood, reproduction, growth, and metabolism.

Pivot joints Joints that possess a ringed or notched surface of one bone that fits into a projection of another bone; movement limited to rotation.

Placenta Flattened organ located in the pregnant uterus that nourishes a developing fetus by exchanging nutrients and wastes with the mother; also secretes hormones required to maintain pregnancy.

Placenta previa Condition wherein the placenta partially or completely covers the cervix.

Planes Transparent flat surfaces that divides the body into three dimensions of up/down, left/right, and front/back; planes lie at right angles to each other and provide references for height, depth, and width. Three cardinal planes are sagittal, frontal, and transverse.

Plantar fasciitis Chronic inflammation of the plantar fascia; this thick band of fascia is located on plantar surface of foot, inserts on calcaneus and fans towards the toes.

Plantar flexion Movement of ankle so the foot moves inferiorly—toes are pointing downward.

Pneumonia Infection or inflammation of the lungs.

Polycystic ovary syndrome (PCOS) Bilateral enlargement of the ovaries as they become studded with multiple cysts.

Pons Brainstem structure that connects the cerebellum and the cerebrum with the spinal cord.

Portal of entry The route pathogens use to enter a new host after transmission has occurred.

Portal of exit The pathway pathogens use to leave a reservoir.

Positional release therapy (PRT) The placement of a target muscle into a shortened, comfortable position; also called *strain-counterstrain (SCS)*, *passive positioning*, or *orthobionomy*.

Posterior Located on back of a structure. Also known as *dorsal*.

Postpartum The time frame after childbirth and lasts for approximately 6 weeks.

Postural assessment An observational evaluation of a client's relaxed, barefoot, standing posture and is used to determine postural abnormalities that may cause or contribute to a client's complaint.

Postural (orthostatic) hypotension A sudden drop in blood pressure and resultant dizziness when sitting or standing upright from a lying down position.

Postural muscles Skeletal muscles that maintain body posture.

Posture Positions of the body, such as standing and sitting, over a base of support, and are maintained by a skeletal framework and muscle tone.

Power differential An imbalance of power in the professional relationship, with clients in the vulnerable position.

Preceptor An experienced individual within a healthcare facility who is paired with a newly hired individual during the orientation period.

Preeclampsia Persistent high blood pressure with protein in urine that develops after 20 weeks of gestation and returns to normal after childbirth.

Prefix Letters in front of a root word to elaborate, qualify, or change the meaning of the word.

Pregnancy Sequence of events that begins with fertilization and implantation, continuing with embryonic development and fetal growth, and ending in childbirth. Process of gestation takes approximately 40 weeks and is divided into trimesters.

Pregnancy massage Modification of techniques and body positions to meet the needs of clients as they undergo changes during pregnancy and the postpartum period; pregnancy massage is also called prenatal massage.

Premenstrual syndrome Group of signs and symptoms that occur during the luteal phase of the menstrual cycle and are relieved by its onset.

Prenatal massage See *Pregnancy massage.*

Prescription Authorization and instruction from a medical practitioner for drugs, procedures (e.g., physical or massage therapy), or devices (e.g., hearing aids, eyeglasses).

Pressure Application of gliding or nongliding force, and varies from light to moderate/medium to deep.

Preterm labor Regular uterine contractions that result in changes in cervical size or length after week 20 gestation and before week 37.

Prevalence Number of all existing cases (new and old) of a given condition within a population per unit of time.

Prime movers Muscles causing specific or desired movement; movements produced by prime movers describe muscles action.

Prions Proteinaceous infectious particles that can affect the central nervous system; these infections are currently untreatable and fatal.

Prodromal period The period where the host begins to experience signs and symptoms of disease from the activation of the immune response.

Professional boundaries Spaces between the practitioner's power and the client's vulnerability.

Professional liability insurance A form of insurance that helps protect a service-provider from bearing the full cost of a legal defense and helps pay for damages awarded by the courts if the provider was found negligent; also called *malpractice insurance* and *errors and omission insurance.*

Professional license A license which restricts the practice of an occupation to those who hold a license.

Professional profile Written summary of professional skills, strengths, and key experiences.

Professionalism Adherence to a set of values and obligations, formally agreed-upon codes of conduct, and reasonable expectations of clients, colleagues, and co-workers; key values of professionalism include acting in client's best interest and putting that interest before your own, maintaining standards expected of other members of profession, and staying current with changes and discoveries in field.

Profit and loss statement (P&L) A statement which reports an individual's or business's financial performance during a particular period of time.

Prognosis A prediction of how a disease will progress and chances of recovery based on the person's condition and the usual course of the disease.

Pronation Medial rotation of the forearm so that the palm is facing downward or backward.

Prone position Client position when the body is lying face down on the abdomen.

Proposal Plans or suggestions put forward for consideration and discussion in business relationships.

Proprioception Self-awareness of body movements and body position.

Proprioceptive neuromuscular facilitation (PNF) Or *PNF stretching*; a group of techniques developed by physical therapists Kabat and Knott in the late 1940s to increase motor function and activities of daily living among individuals who have mobility impairments.

Proprioceptors Specialized interoceptors found in muscles, joints, fascia, and ears that detect body movements, body position in space, and muscle stretch.

Prospective study A study which looks at outcomes during a period of time in relation to suspected risk or protective factors (e.g., vaccines).

Prostate Gland that lies beneath bladder, surrounds the urethra, and secretes seminal fluid.

Protozoa Simplest form of animal life and causes protozoal diseases.

Protraction Movement at a joint in an anterior or forward direction.

Protrusion See *Protraction*.

Proximal Located nearer to the point of reference, usually toward the trunk.

Psoriasis Noncontagious chronic inflammatory skin condition in which the proliferation rate of epidermal cells is greatly accelerated; instead of skin renewing every month, it occurs every few days; because old skin cells do not slough off quickly, they build up in thick patches.

Publicity Free media exposure.

Pulmonary circuit Movement of blood from the right ventricle, through pulmonary arteries, to lung capillaries and returns from the lungs through pulmonary veins to the left atrium to replenish oxygen and to eliminate gaseous wastes.

Pulmonary valve Right semilunar valve located between the pulmonary trunk and the right ventricle.

Pulse Expansion of the arterial walls as the heart beats and can be felt in arteries that lie near the surface of the body.

Qualitative research Type of research that is used to explore ideas; subjective and narrative-based.

Quality of life Perception people have regarding their position in life in the context of their culture and their value systems, and the degree to which a person is able to participate in and enjoy life events.

Quantitative research Type of research that is used to establish generalizable facts about a topic; focuses on testing theories and hypotheses and is largely objective. Emphasizes objective measurements and statistic, mathematic, or numeric data analysis.

Radial deviation Hand movement away from the midline of the body in the anatomic position.

Radiation Transfer of heat through heat rays.

Radiculopathy Type of neuropathy originating in the spinal nerve roots; if originating in the cervical region, it is called *cervical radiculopathy*; if originating in the lumbar region, it is called *lumbar radiculopathy*.

Rami One of two spinal nerve extensions emerging from the sides of the spinal cord. Dorsal rami innervate skin and muscles of the posterior surfaces of the head, neck, and trunk. Ventral rami innervate the extremities and the anterolateral trunk.

Randomized controlled trial Study design that randomly assigns participants to an experimental/treatment group or a control group. By randomly assigning participants, confounding factors are randomized which significantly reduce bias, placebo effect, and individual participant results.

Range of motion The amount of motion that occurs when one segment of the body moves in relationship to another segment of the body.

Rapport Emotional bond people experience when concerns, feelings, and ideas are mutually expressed.

Rate The number of times or speed at which a technique is repeated.

Raynaud disease Periodic episodes of vasospasms in the fingers and toes.

Receptive field Areas of the body where a single receptor can detect stimuli.

Reciprocal inhibition Neurologic principle which states while a muscle spindle is reflexively contracting a stretched muscle, motor activity is inhibited in its antagonist or opposing muscle, so contraction can occur.

Recruitment Process of motor unit activation based on need.

Recumbent position A position where clients lie down, and usually involves positioning equipment, such as bolsters, for client comfort.

Red bone marrow Primary lymphatic structure and involved with the production and maturation of lymphocytes.

Referral Act of recommending a product or service to help clients achieve treatment goals.

Reflective questions Questions confirming that the client's response was received and understood, also allowing the opportunity for the client to clarify information if the practitioner misunderstood the meaning of the client's message.

Reflex Rapid, often protective, involuntary response to a stimulus.

Reflex arc Neural pathway used to produce a reflex.

Reflex points (reflexology) Points that correspond to body structures, including organs and glands.

Reflexology Application of pressure to specific points on the feet or hands; these points are believed to correspond with certain areas of the body.

Relaxin A hormone that alters the properties of connective tissues by activating collagenase, an enzyme that breaks down collagen and reduces its strength; also works synergistically with progesterone to maintain pregnancy by relaxing the uterus, and helps relax and dilate the cervix, as well as pelvic ligaments, to assist in childbirth.

Reliability Consistency of a study and indicates that if an experiment or test were repeated by the same or different investigators, the results would be the same.

Remissions Periods of time when signs and symptoms of disease disappear or diminish significantly.

Renal tubule Hollow tube between the renal corpuscle and the collecting duct; divided into three main regions: proximal convoluted tubule, loop of Henle, and distal convoluted tubule.

Renin Increases blood pressure, leading to the restoration of pressure in the kidneys needed to filter blood.

Reposition Returning the thumb to its anatomic position next to the index finger.

Reproductive cycle See *Menstrual cycle.*

Research Systematic inquiry using prescribed methods to validate or refine existing knowledge or to develop new knowledge.

Research literacy Cognitive and social understanding of the purpose, process, and value of research.

Reservoir The person, animal, or environment where pathogens live and reproduce, or depend on for survival.

Resistance exercises Activities involving contracting skeletal muscles against resistance.

Respect Ability to accept another person's beliefs despite your own personal feelings, and the choice to treat them with value and consideration.

Respiration Process used to supply body cells with oxygen and to dispose of carbon dioxide.

Respiratory hygiene Methods used to reduce or prevent transmission of pathogens spread by droplet or airborne transmission.

Rest Behaviors used to promote health and well-being by temporarily discontinuing a previous stressful or demanding activity; both a process (to rest) and a condition (being in rest).

Results (research) Outcome of study; written carefully and applies only to what was found after data analysis.

Resume Brief summary of an individual's education, experience, and accomplishments related to a particular skill set.

Reticular tissue Connective tissue type that provides supportive framework for bone, bone marrow, lymph nodes, and organs such as liver and spleen; functions as part of body's defense system; reticular fibers trap harmful substances as they travel in blood and lymph.

Retinaculum A band of connective tissue surrounding tendons to help keep them in place and stabilize them; retinacula are found primarily around elbows, knees, ankles, and wrists.

Retraction Movement at a joint in a posterior or backward direction.

Retrospective study A study which looks back in time and examines exposures to suspected risk or protective factors in relation to an outcome (e.g., lung cancer).

Reuptake Reabsorption of released neurotransmitters by the presynaptic neuron.

Rheumatoid arthritis Arthritis caused by an autoimmune response in which the body attacks, inflames, and destroys synovial joint membranes; over time, joint inflammation spreads through the joint capsule, to articular cartilages and surrounding ligaments, then to underlying bone.

Rhythm The pattern or regularity of applied massage techniques.

Ribosomes Small granules of ribonucleic acid found in cells.

Right lymphatic duct Lymphatic duct that drains lymph from the right arm, right side of head, and right half of the thorax into the right subclavian vein.

Ringworm Fungal infection of the skin transmitted by direct contact with infected skin, infected domestic animals, such as cats and dogs, or with fomites.

Risk factors Factors that increase or decrease the chances of getting a particular disease.

Root The main or most basic part of a word; also called the stem.

Rosacea Progressive, inflammatory skin condition causing facial redness.

Rotation Movement that occurs when a bone pivots or rotates around its own central axis.

Rotator cuff tear Occurs when one or more rotator cuff muscles are partially or completely torn from its attachment on the humerus; more common in the dominant arm.

Ruffini (bulbous) corpuscles Receptors in the dermis that detect deeper pressure, continuous touch, stretching of skin, and warmth.

Saddle joints Joints that possess a concave surface of one bone that fits into a convex surface of another; positional relationship resembles a rider in a saddle; movements allowed are flexion, extension, abduction, adduction, opposition, reposition, and circumduction, but not rotation.

Sagittal plane Plane that bisects the body from front to back and divides it into right and left sections.

Saltatory conduction Nerve impulse conducted along myelinated axons.

Sample (research) A subset of a population used to represent the entire population as a whole.

Sanitation Removal of impurities and harmful agents to promote health and safety, and usually refers to the environment (e.g., soil, water). Sanitation does not indicate a specific level of cleanliness.

Sarcolemma Covering of muscle fiber; equivalent to a cell membrane in a typical cell.

Sarcomeres Basic unit of muscle contraction.

Sarcoplasm Cellular fluid within muscle fibers; equivalent of cytoplasm in typical cells.

Sarcoplasmic reticulum System of interconnected hollow tubes surrounding myofibrils, stores and releases calcium, and plays a role in muscle contraction.

Sauna bath Dry heat bath received in a wood-lined room or cabinet.

Scabies infestation Skin infestation caused by burrowing parasitic mites.

Scar Mark left on damaged skin or other tissues after it is healed; damage may result from trauma, burns, surgery, or disease. Types are hypertrophic, keloid, and contracture.

Sciatica Inflammation or irritation of the sciatic nerve.

Scleroderma Chronic disease characterized by hardening and tightening of the skin and connective tissues, caused by overproduction and accumulation of collagen and leads to fibrosis accompanied by inflammation.

Scoliosis Lateral curvature in the normally straight vertical line of the spine, usually in the thoracic region.

Scope of practice Professional activities that can be performed legally by members of a licensed profession and the context these activities can be applied.

Seated massage Massage performed on a seated, clothed individual usually in an open, public space.

Seated position Client position where the client is seated usually with the torso erect, knees bent, with glutes supported.

Sebaceous glands Skin glands connected to hair follicles by small ducts that produce sebum; also called oil glands.

Seborrheic dermatitis Chronic inflammatory condition of the sebaceous glands marked by an increase in the amount of and changes in the quality of their secretions.

Seizure Episodes of uncontrolled and excessive electrical activity in the brain resulting in a sudden change of behavior and level of consciousness; include focal (partial) and generalized seizures.

Seizure disorders Characterized by episodes of uncontrolled and excessive electrical activity in brain called a seizure.

Self-care Learned, proactive, deliberate, purposeful, and continuous activities to reduce stress, avoid burnout, prevent illness and injury, and live a more balanced life.

Self-disclosure Revealing our own thoughts, feelings, and personal history.

Self-employment taxes Taxes levied on small business owners who derive income directly from consumers as opposed to individuals who are employees.

Semen Mixture of sperm and seminal fluid produced by male accessory glands.

Semilunar valves Heart valves located between the ventricles and the aorta or pulmonary trunk.

Seminal fluid Milky white alkaline substance produced by the prostate and other male accessory glands; transport medium and source of nutrients for sperm.

Seminal vesicles Structures located at the base of bladder that secrete seminal fluid.

Semireclining position The client is half lying down and half sitting up instead of completely reclining.

Senescence Period of life from old age to death.

Sensitization Condition of a lower pain threshold, which results in pain hypersensitivity.

Sensory adaptation Gradual decrease in receptor responsiveness to a constant or prolonged stimulus.

Serous membranes Tissue layer that lines closed body cavities; examples of serous membranes are the pericardium which surrounds heart, the pleura which surrounds lungs, and the peritoneum, which surrounds organs in the abdominopelvic cavity; serous membranes secrete serous fluid.

Sesamoid bones Small, round bones embedded in tendons and ligaments; sesamoid bones are found in the hands, feet, and in the throat (hyoid); largest sesamoid bone is located in the knee.

Sexual harassment Sexual or sexually suggestive unwanted behavior perceived as offensive, threatening, or embarrassing.

Sexual intercourse Process of inserting and thrusting the erect male penis into a female's vagina, often ending in orgasm and ejaculation of sperm.

Sexual misconduct Range of sexual behaviors, consensual and nonconsensual, between someone in an authoritative role and someone in a subordinate role.

Sexual reproduction Process by which male sex cells and female sex cells unite and combine genetic material to create a new organism.

Shearing Sliding force, usually by compressing and gliding two surfaces against each other in the same or opposite directions.

Shin splints Term used to describe pain along the medial tibia.

Shingles Acute, localized viral infection of the skin; essentially reactivation of the varicella zoster or chickenpox virus.

Shirodhara Ayurvedic treatment where the client lies on a table with the upper portion of the head over the table's edge, and a steady stream of warm oil pours over the client's forehead into a vessel below.

Short bones Bones that are generally small and cube-shaped and contain multiple articulating surfaces; short bones are located in the wrists, feet, and ankles.

Side effect (massage) A nonharmful and unintended but predictable effect that occurs after a massage session.

Side-lying position Position where the client is lying on their side, usually with the hips and knees flexed.

Signs Objective evidence that can be measured and observed by others.

Sinusitis Acute or chronic inflammation of the mucosal lining of paranasal sinuses.

Skeletal muscle Muscle tissue attached to bones and can produce movement at joints.

Skin turgor Degree of elasticity of the skin; assessed by pinching the skin and observing how quickly it flattens.

Sleep Recurring state of relaxation characterized by an altered state of consciousness, inhibited sensory activity, muscular inhibition, and reduced interactions.

Slow twitch Muscles that contract more slowly, for longer periods of time, and are fatigue-resistant compared with fast twitch muscles.

Small intestine Coiled tube located between the stomach and the large intestine.

Smooth muscle Muscle tissue type located in walls of hollow organs, such as the stomach, bladder, and uterus and within tubes, such as the intestines and blood vessels.

Sneezing Forceful expulsion of air through the nose and mouth to clear upper respiratory passageways.

Social media Websites where members of virtual communities can interact with other individuals.

Social wellness The positive interaction with others involving the use of good communication skills, developing and maintaining meaningful relationships, valuing diversity and treating others with respect, and creating a social support system that includes family, friends, teachers, classmates, and others.

Sodium-potassium pump Mechanism that actively transports sodium out and potassium into the neuron at unequal rates.

Soft tissue injuries Trauma to muscles, tendons, and ligaments.

Sole proprietorship Single-owner business.

Somatic nervous system Part of the peripheral nervous system that transmites sensory input, such as vision, hearing, taste, smell, and touch, and the voluntary function of skeletal muscles, with the exception of cranial and spinal reflexes, which are involuntary.

Spa A place where water treatments and other services are administered to encourage relaxation and rejuvenation of mind and body.

Special populations Groups of individuals who are disadvantaged, vulnerable, and/or at risk for harm. Can include physical limitation (severe illness, impairment, disability) or life stage (pregnancy, minor, elderly); can also arise from situations that can restrict some rights and privileges (institutionalized persons such as prisoners and mentally incompetent).

Specific defense mechanisms Body's ability to develop immunity against specific pathogens and uses B and T lymphocytes (B- and T-cells).

Specific pain Pain that has a specific cause, such as tissue damage, deformity, disease, or a condition such as disc herniation.

Specificity theory of pain Theory that states pain is a specific sensation transmitted by specific receptors.

Sperm Sex cells that carry genetic information from the male that produced them.

Spermatic duct Passageway used to transport semen from the epididymis and out of the body during ejaculation.

Sphincter Ring-shaped muscle that relaxes or tightens to open or close a passage or opening in the body.

Spinal cavity Cavity within vertebrae of the spinal column and contains the spinal cord.

Spinal cord Cylindrical bundle of nerve fibers extending from the brainstem.

Spinal nerves Emerge from the left and right sides of the spinal cord and are numbered by their location along the spine.

Spinal reflex Reflexes mediated by spinal nerves and includes stretch reflexes, autogenic inhibition reflexes, withdrawal reflexes, and crossed extensor reflexes, and can be influenced or modified by the brain to either exaggerate or suppress the reflex.

Spiral muscle fibers Muscle fibers that twist between their points of attachment.

Spiritual wellness Searching for meaning and purpose of human existence with or without religious affiliation.

Spleen Largest lymphatic organ and lies within the upper left quadrant of the abdomen; filters blood much in the same way a lymph node filters lymph.

Spondylosis Osteoarthritis of spine, affecting the intervertebral discs and facet joints.

Spondylolisthesis Anterior displaced vertebra, usually L4 or L5; types are isthmic (spondylolytic) and degenerative.

Spondylolysis A type of isthmic spondylolisthesis caused by a fracture in a thin portion of the lamina called the pars interarticularis.

Spongy bone Thin latticework beams within bone, giving it a spongy appearance; lighter and less dense than *compact bone*. Also called *cancellous bone*.

Sports massage The application of massage techniques to address the needs of athletes in competitive and recreational settings.

Sprain An injury caused by an overstretched or torn ligament.

Stabalizers See *Fixators*.

Standard of care The degree and level of care given by similarly trained and qualified individuals who are in the same or similar line of work or in the same or similar work setting.

Standard precautions Minimum infection control practices to prevent occupational transmission of disease.

Standards of practice A document which includes guidance for business practices, prevention of sexual misconduct, and ethical principles such as confidentiality.

Startup cost Expenses incurred before a business opens.

Statistical significance Indicates there was a relationship between variables and it was caused by something other than chance.

Statistical insignificance Indicates there was no relationship between variables or small differences can be accounted for by chance.

Steam baths A vapor bath taken in a ceramic-tiled room, cabinet, or canopy; temperatures range between 105°F and 120°F.

Sterilization Destruction of all microorganisms, pathogenic and nonpathogenic, and can be achieved through heat, chemicals, irradiation, high pressure, and other means.

Stomach J-shaped saclike organ located between the esophagus and the small intestine; bound at both ends by sphincters and serves as an expandable food storage tank.

Strain Occurs when muscles or tendons become overstretched or torn; the most commonly injured areas are the hands, thighs (hamstrings), and lower back.

Strain-counterstrain (SCS) See *Positional release therapy.*

Stress Response of the body to any demand placed on it which triggers sympathetic arousal or the stress response; stress can include environmental, societal, situational, or chemical factors, all of which require a response from the body.

Stretch marks Indented lines or bands from overstretched skin; most commonly located on breasts, hips, thighs, buttocks, and the abdomen.

Stretches reflexes Reflexive muscle contractions caused by sudden passive stretch.

Stretching Passively positioning muscle attachments as far apart as possible to elongate the muscle in the direction opposite of its action.

Stroke Sudden disruption of cerebral blood flow from an occluded or ruptured blood vessel leading to irreversible brain damage or, in some cases, death.

Subacute inflammation The period after acute inflammation and is characterized by swelling and pain, but lacks heat and redness.

Subacute pain Pain that may follow acute pain; occurs when inflammation subsides, but the person still experiences pain and impaired function.

Subluxation Partial loss of contact between two articulating surfaces in a joint.

Subjective information Information obtained from the client or client's family and friends; based on opinions, attitudes, and beliefs.

Sudoriferous glands Skin glands that produce sweat or perspiration; also called sweat glands.

Suffix Letters at the end of a root word to change the meaning of the word or denotes a type of word, such as an adjective or a noun.

Superficial Relative to the outside or external surface of a structure.

Superficial fascia Fascia located on the body's periphery just beneath the skin.

Superior Situated above or toward the head end.

Supination Lateral rotation of the forearm so that the palm is facing upward or forward.

Supine hypotensive syndrome Drop in blood pressure caused by compression of the pregnant uterus against major abdominal blood vessels.

Supine position Client position when the body is lying face up on the back.

Swiss shower Warm water sprayed over a client standing or sitting in a shower stall.

Sympathetic division Division of the autonomic nervous system that dominates during dangerous or stressful situations and helps the body produce the energy needed for physical exertion; also called thoracolumbar division.

Sympathy The commingling of your own feelings and the feelings of others without differentiation.

Symptoms Subjective evidence perceived only by the individual experiencing them.

Synapse Junction between two neurons or between a neuron and a muscle or gland, where nerve impulses are transmitted.

Synaptic bulbs Budlike structures located on the ends of axons that contain synaptic vesicles filled with neurotransmitters.

Synaptic cleft See *Synaptic gap.*

Synaptic gap Small space between the synaptic bulb on the presynaptic neuron and the cell membrane on the postsynaptic cell membrane of a neuron, muscle or gland.

Synaptic transmission Process of transmitting signals from one neuron to another neuron, muscle, or gland.

Synarthrotic joints Joints that have extremely limited movement; synarthrotic joints are common in the axial skeleton and include joints between cranial bones and joints that hold teeth into their sockets.

Synergists Muscles that facilitate movement caused by prime movers by performing the same movement at the same time.

Synovial fluid Viscous-lubricating, shock-absorbing, and joint-nourishing fluid that fills joint cavities and is secreted by synovial membranes.

Synovial joints Joints that contain a fluid-filled cavity between articulating bones.

Synovial membrane Tissue layer that lines joint cavities or spaces between bones and joints; synovial membranes secrete a thick clear liquid called synovial fluid.

Synovial sheaths Elongated bursae that surround long tendons located in the forearms, legs, wrists, ankles, hands, and feet; these tubular structures are lined with synovial membranes to increase their gliding capacity.

Systematic review Critical analysis of many studies from different researchers to assess what is known about a specific research question; statistical analysis of these studies, or meta-analysis, is often used to produce the results of the review.

Systemic circuit Blood moving from the left atrium to the left ventricle through arteries into capillaries and through veins and to the right atrium to transport nutrients, hormones, and oxygen; carries wastes from cells for their elimination.

Systemic disease A disease distributed throughout the body rather than isolated to one area.

Systemic inflammation Widespread inflammation, and usually associated with an infection.

Systemic lupus erythematosus (SLE or Lupus) Chronic autoimmune, inflammatory disease affecting the body's connective tissues.

Systole (systolic pressure) Pressure within arteries as the left ventricle contracts and ejects blood.

T tubules Indentations that extend transversely across the sarcoplasmic reticulum at right angles; this allows impulses to travel deep into the cell during muscle contraction.

Tactical athletes People in service professions who have physical fitness and performance requirements associated with their job.

Tapotement Massage technique that consists of repetitive striking movements.

Target cells Cells that possess receptor(s) for hormones or other signaling molecules.

Target market A group of consumers that are more likely to want or need products or services.

Tax deduction Expenses that reduce taxable income and usually result from expenses incurred to produce the income.

Taxes Sums of money paid on income, property, and sales of goods and services, which are then given to a government agency to carry out its functions, such as expenditures on war, law enforcement, protection of property, public transportation, and the operation of government itself.

Temporal lobe Brain region which controls hearing, taste, smell, and contains the Wernicke's area, which is critical to speech comprehension; also helps to form memories and integrates them with sensations of taste, sound, sight, and touch.

Temporomandibular disorders Generalized term to describe disorders affecting the jaw, its musculature, or both.

Tendinitis Inflammation of the tendon(s); can occur in any tendon, but the most commonly involved areas are wrists, elbows, shoulders, knees, and heels.

Tendinosis Degeneration of a tendon; often mislabeled as tendinitis, but inflammation is not present in tendinosis.

Tendon Dense band of connective tissue that attach muscles to bones.

Tendon sheaths See *Synovial sheaths.*

Tenosynovitis Inflammation that involves the synovial sheath surrounding the tendon.

Tension Elongating or lengthening force, usually by pulling an object in opposite directions.

Tension headaches Pain or discomfort in the head, scalp, or neck from muscle tension.

Testes Paired oval glands in the male scrotum.

Testicles See *Testes.*

Thalamus Largest portion of the diencephalon; relays sensory information (except olfaction) to appropriate parts of the cerebrum.

Thalassotherapy The external use of seawater specifically in hydrotherapy.

Therapeutic Curative measures used to treat diseases, disorders, or injuries.

Therapeutic relationship Relationship between a practitioner and a client that allows practitioners to apply their professional knowledge and expertise to help clients achieve their treatment goals.

Thermogenesis The mechanism by which skeletal muscles produce heat and are important for maintaining body temperature. When the body is chilled, skeletal muscles contract rapidly (i.e., shivering) to produce additional heat.

Thermoreceptor Receptors that detect changes in environmental temperature; located beneath the skin and mucosae.

Thermoregulation Constant maintenance of internal body temperature independent of the external environmental temperature.

Thermotherapy Therapeutic application of heat.

Thick filaments Myofilament within sarcomeres shaped like golf clubs with shafts of the club bundled together and myosin heads sticking out from the bundle.

Thin filaments Attached to Z lines at the ends of the sarcomere and extend partway toward the sarcomere's center; thin filaments are made of three proteins: actin, tropomyosin, and troponin.

Thoracic cavity Cavity that contains the pleural cavities, which surround the lungs and mediastinum, which is the space between the lungs.

Thoracic duct Lymphatic duct that drains lymph from all parts of body not drained by the right lymphatic duct and delivers it to the left subclavian vein.

Thoracic outlet syndrome (TOS) Disorder caused by brachial nerve compression alone or with compression of the subclavian artery and vein.

Thrombocytes Blood cell fragments that release substances to activate blood clotting and to form platelet plugs.

Thrombophlebitis Occurs when the thrombus causes inflammation within a vein.

Thymus Primary lymphatic structure and involved with the production and maturation of lymphocytes.

Thyroid Endocrine gland located in the throat below the larynx, and around the front and sides of the trachea.

Time boundaries Encompasses when appointments are scheduled, and the duration of time spent on professional activities.

Tips Discretionary (optional or extra) payments given to service providers by the customer. Also called *gratuities.*

Tissue level Biologic level that encompasses groups of cells, all of which possess similar structure and perform specific functions.

Tissues Groups of similar cells that act together to perform specific functions; tissues organize themselves into organs; there are four tissue types: epithelial, connective, muscular, and nervous.

Tonsils Lymphatic tissue located in the oral cavity and pharynx.

Torsion Twisting or rotational force, usually by compressing and moving tissues in the same or opposite directions.

Torticollis Group of disorders involving spasms of the sternocleidomastoid muscle.

Touch Ability to perceive objects or forces through physical contact.

Trachea Tube that connects the larynx to the bronchi; located anterior to the esophagus.

Tracking The ability to notice and respond to changes that a client experiences during a massage session.

Transference Client *transfer* of past feelings, conflicts, and attitudes into present relationships, situations, and circumstances.

Transmission-based precautions Practices used in addition to standard precautions and are only applied to patients/clients who are infected or colonized with pathogens that can be transmitted by droplet or airborne transmission or by contact with skin or contaminated surfaces.

Transverse plane Plane that bisects the body and divides it into top (superior) and bottom (inferior) sections.

Transverse tubules See *T tubules.*

Traumatic disorders Injuries to the body often from violence or accidents.

Treatment group Population sample that receives an intervention under investigation.

Treatment planning Documented process by which the practitioner or healthcare team plans an appropriate treatment or course of treatment for a client.

Tricuspid valve Right atrioventricular valve located between the right atrium and the right ventricle.

Trigeminal neuralgia Excruciating episodic pain in areas supplied by the trigeminal nerve (CN V).

Trigger point therapy The use of pressure over trigger points.

Trigger points Hyperirritable tender spots in taut palpable bands within skeletal muscle and its associated fascia.

Trust Confidence in and reliance upon others, whether individuals or organizations, to act in accordance with accepted social, ethical, or legal norms.

Tubular reabsorption Second step of the kidney's filtration process as filtered molecules are reabsorbed from the renal tubule into the peritubular blood.

Tubular secretion Third and final step of the kidney's filtration process as certain molecules move from peritubular blood into the renal tubule.

Type 1 muscles Muscle fibers that contain large amounts of myoglobin and mitochondria; also called red muscle.

Type 2 muscles Muscle fibers that have fewer myoglobin, mitochondria, and blood capillaries compared to type 1 fibers; also called white muscle.

Ulcerative colitis (UC) Inflammatory bowel disease causing long-term inflammation and ulcer formation of the large intestine.

Ulnar deviation Hand movement toward the midline of the body in anatomic position.

Uniarticular muscles Muscles that cross only one joint.

Uniaxial joints Joints that provide movement around only one axis and in only one plane.

Universal donors Persons with type O blood.

Universal recipients Persons with type AB blood.

Upward (inferior) rotation Scapular movement that occurs as the glenoid cavity rotates to orient superiorly.

Ureters Two slender, hollow tubes that extend from the renal pelvis of the kidneys to the urinary bladder.

Urethra Narrow tube located below the bladder that transports urine (females) or urine and semen (males).

Urinary bladder Expandable sac that stores urine located in the pelvis.

Urinary incontinence (UI) Loss of bladder control and involuntary leakage of urine.

Urinary tract infection General term for infection and inflammation of one or more structures of the urinary tract.

Urination Release of urine from the urinary bladder.

Urine Liquid excrement made in the kidneys and released through the urethra; 95% water and 5% dissolved waste.

Uterus Hollow pear-shaped organ that receives the fertilized ovum and allows the embryo to grow and develop into a fetus during pregnancy, and from which menses flows during menstrual cycle.

Vagina Canal that extends from the cervix to the outside of the body.

Vaginal childbirth Childbirth that occurs when the fetus, placenta, membranes, and umbilical cord are delivered out of the mother's vagina.

Value-added services Services offered to consumers for little or no cost.

Validity Accuracy of a study, and indicates the experiment measured what it was supposed to measure.

Variable Anything that can vary or change in an experiment and is measurable.

Varicose veins Enlarged veins caused by incompetent vascular valves.

Vas deferens Tube that connects the epididymis to the ejaculatory duct.

Vasoconstriction Narrowing of a lumen, usually a blood vessel.

Vasodilation Enlargement or widening of a lumen, usually a blood vessel.

Vector transmission Disease transmission through a vector (usually an animal or insect) to spread pathogens between two or more hosts; most vector-borne diseases are transmitted by bites, stings, or infestation of tissues.

Vehicle transmission Disease transmission through a common vehicle or source, such as food, water, air and in some cases, blood distributed by a transfusion service; vehicle transmission can be classified as foodborne, waterborne, or airborne.

Veins Vessels that return blood to the heart; blood within arteries is deoxygenated (except pulmonary veins).

Venous portal systems Found within the systemic circuit and consist of two capillary beds connected through a system of veins.

Venous return Rate at which blood flows back to the heart.

Ventral cavity Cavity located on the front side of the body; the ventral cavity is divided into the thoracic and abdominopelvic cavities.

Veracity The obligation to tell the truth.

Verbal descriptor scale (VDS) A series of descriptive phrases such as *mild, moderate, severe*, and *worst* to indicate the client's current pain level.

Vermiform appendix Lymphatic tissue attached to the cecum, the first region of the large intestine.

Vibration Massage technique that uses shaking or trembling motions.

Vichy shower Warm water sprayed over a client lying on a shallow table.

Virus Nonliving entities that depend on a host cell for growth and replication.

Visceral muscle See *Smooth muscle*.

Visceroreceptors See *Interoceptors*.

Visual analog scale (VAS) A straight horizontal or vertical line with the endpoints defining extreme limits such as *no pain* and *worst pain possible*.

Visual impairment Decreased capacity to see, and cannot be corrected by usual means, such as glasses or contact lenses.

Voiding See *Urination*.

Waistline (reflexology) In reflexology, the horizontal line located at the base of the fifth metatarsal. These lines are used to delineate treatment areas containing reflex points.

Wart Small, rough, raised, viral-induced skin growth; the causative virus is the human papillomavirus.

Websites Places on the Internet where one or more pages of information are located.

Well being The experience of health and includes feelings of comfort, safety, contentment, happiness, high life satisfaction, sense of meaning or purpose, and the ability to manage stress.

Wellness Activities, choices, and lifestyles oriented toward optimal health and well-being to live more fully within a community.

Wellness massage Self-care to reduce stress, promote relaxation, improve function, and decrease pain and muscle soreness unrelated to diagnosed medical conditions.

Whiplash-associated disorder A collective term describing neck injuries caused by rapid forceful back-and-forth movements of the cervical spine, similar to cracking a whip.

Whirlpool bath A bath in a tub containing heated water that is continuously circulated.

Withdrawal reflex Sudden withdrawal of an extremity from a painful stimulus.

Wolff law The phenomena by which bone in a healthy person will adapt to the loads under which it is placed. If loading on a bone increases, the bone can remodel to become stronger. However, if loading on a bone decreases, the bone will become less dense and weaker.

Wong-Baker FACES Scale (WBS) A series of faces ranging from a happy face at 0 which represents *no hurt* to a sad crying face at 10 which represents *hurts worst*.

Workers compensation A type of insurance that provides income to employees who are unable to work because of a job-related injury.

Yawn Very deep inhalation initiated by opening the mouth wide.

Zoning The dividing of geographic areas into zones so a city or municipality can restrict the number of and types of buildings within the zone, as well as how these buildings are used.

BIOGRAPHY INDEX

Page numbers followed by "*f*" indicate figures, "*t*" indicate tables, and "*b*"indicate boxes.

A

A bands, 441
Abdomen
    access to, 127–128, 130*f*
    in endangerment sites, 140
Abdominal aorta, 704*f*
Abdominal area, in foot reflexology, 280
Abdominal massage, 96–97
Abdominal quadrants, 403*f*, 406
Abdominal regions, 403*f*, 406
Abdominals, 583, 582*f*
Abducens nerve, 636, 637*f*
Abduction, 422, 424*f*, 516
Abductor digiti minimi, 524*f*, 531*f*, 546
Abductor pollicis brevis, 524*f*, 533*f*, 545
Abductor pollicis longus, 472*f*, 524*f*, 533*f*, 545
Abnormal end-feel (pathologic), 290
ABO blood types, 693*t*
Abortion, spontaneous, 228
Absence seizures, 194
Absolute contraindications, 143, 203
Absorption, epithelial tissue for, 395
Abstract, 82
Abuse, 18
Accessory glands, male, 676
Accessory nerve, 637, 637*f*
Accounting, 375–376
Acetabulofemoral joint, 477, 479
Acetabulum, 476*f*, 477
Acetylcholine (ACh), 440, 443, 627, 628*t*
Achilles tendon, 494*f*
Acini cells, 753*f*
Acne, 613
Acquired immunodeficiency syndrome (AIDS), 720
Acromial region, 406
Acromioclavicular (AC) joint, 465
Acromion, 465–466*t*, 466*f*
Actin, 440–441, 440*f*
Active assisted range of motion (AAROM), 161
Active range of motion (AROM), 161, 289
Active resisted range of motion (ARROM), 161
Active trigger points, 307
Acupoints, 333–347
Acute disease, definition of, 182
Acute inflammation, 302, 718–719
    protocols during, 302
Acute pain, 288
Adam's apple, 731
Adduction, 422, 424*f*
Adductor brevis, 535*f*, 546*f*, 570
Adductor hiatus, 545*f*, 569
Adductor longus, 494*f*, 535*f*, 545*f*
Adductor magnus, 494*f*, 535*f*, 545*f*, 567–569
Adductors, 544*f*, 566
Adductor stretch, 170, 172*f*
Adductor tubercle, 478–479*t*, 478*f*
Adenohypophysis, 661
Adenosine triphosphate (ATP), for muscle contraction, 444, 445*f*
Adhesions, 617
Adhesive capsulitis, 427

Adipocytes, endocrine cells in, 666
Adipose tissue, 395*t*, 396*f*, 397
Adjustable frames, face rest, 45
Adolescent massage, 236–237
Adrenal cortex, 663
Adrenal glands, 663–664, 663*f*
    hormones from, 663–664
    mnemonics for, 658
Adrenal medulla, 663
Adrenocorticotropic hormone, 660*t*, 662
Adson test, 295, 295*f*
Advanced beginners, 82
Adverse events, 139–140
Advertising, 370
Aerobic glycolysis, 446
Afferent arteriole, 766–767
Afferent neurons, 627–629
Age-related macular degeneration, 241
Age spots, 608
Aging, 237–247
    in elderly, 237–247
    massage and, 99
Agonists, 449
Agranular, 691
Ah shi, 348
AIDS, 720
Airborne precautions, 187
Airborne transmission, 185
Air sacs, attachment of, 732
Albinism, 609
Alcohol-based hand rubs, 187
Aldosterone, 660*t*, 664
Allen, Tina, 250*b*
Allergies, 720
Alliance for Massage Therapy Education (AFMTE), 8
All-or-none response, 445, 630
Ally (straight ally), 22
Alpha cells, 664
Alpha wave, 634, 635*f*
Alternate-hand compression, 155
Alternate hand effleurage, 144–145, 146*f*, 147*f*
Alternate hand pétrissage, 150, 150*f*
Alternative treatment, 78
Alveoli, 730*f*, 732
Alzheimer disease (AD), 238, 630, 647
American Association of Masseurs and Masseuses (AAMM), 7
American Massage Therapy Association (AMTA), 7
Americans with Disabilities (ADA) Act, 227
Amma, 2
Amphiarthrotic joints, 419
Anaerobic glycolysis, 446
Anatomical neck (of humerus), 467*f*, 467*t*
Anatomic position, 400, 401*f*
Anatomic snuffbox, 543
Anatomy, 384
Anchoring fibers, 715
Anconeus, 514*f*, 520*f*, 529
Andrology, 674
Anecdote, 79